W9-COL-822

# THE PRACTICE OF GERIATRICS

EVAN CALKINS, M.D.

Professor of Medicine and Clinical Professor of Family Medicine,
Head, Division of Geriatrics / Gerontology,
State University of New York at Buffalo School of Medicine
Chief, Section of Gerontology,
Buffalo Veterans Administration Medical Center,
Buffalo, New York

PAUL J. DAVIS, M.D.

Co-editor
Professor and Vice Chairman, Department of Medicine and
Head, Endocrinology Division, Department of Medicine,
State University of New York at Buffalo School of Medicine
Chief, Medical Service, Veterans Administration Medical Center,
Buffalo, New York

AMASA B. FORD, M.D.

Co-editor
Professor of Epidemiology and Biostatistics,
Associate Dean for Geriatric Medicine, and
Director, Office of Geriatric Medicine,
Case Western Reserve University, School of Medicine,
Cleveland, Ohio
Chairman, Geriatric Medicine and Gerontology
Advisory Committee, Ohio Board of Regents

W. B. SAUNDERS COMPANY

Philadelphia London Toronto Mexico City Rio de Janeiro Sydney Tokyo Hong Kong

**W. B. SAUNDERS COMPANY**
Harcourt Brace Jovanovich, Inc.

The Curtis Center
Independence Square West
Philadelphia, PA 19106

**Library of Congress Cataloging in Publication Data**

Main entry under title:

The Practice of geriatrics.

1. Geriatrics. I. Calkins, Evan. II. Davis, Paul J. III. Ford, Amasa B., 1922– . [DNLM: 1. Geriatrics. WT 100 P8957]

RC952.P64 1986 618.97 83-25520

ISBN 0-7216-2329-8

*Editor:* Bill Lamsback
*Designer:* Bill Donnelly
*Production Manager:* Bill Preston
*Manuscript Editor:* Ann Binder
*Illustration Coordinator:* Walt Verbitski
*Indexer:* Dorothy Stade

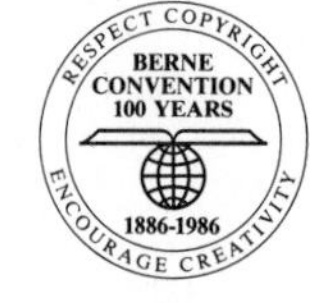


The Practice of Geriatrics ISBN 0-7216-2329-8



Last digit is the print number: 9 8 7 6 5 4 3

# Contributors

**Sonia Ancoli-Israel, Ph.D.**
Assistant Adjunct Professor, Department of Psychiatry, University of California, San Diego School of Medicine, San Diego, California; Assistant Director, Sleep Disorders Clinic, San Diego Veterans Administration Medical Center, San Diego, California
*Sleep and Aging*

**Robert G. Anderson, M.D., F.A.C.S.**
Associate Professor of Otolaryngology, Department of Otolaryngology; University of Texas Southwestern Medical School, Dallas, Texas; Attending, Children's Medical Center, Dallas, Texas; Teaching Consultant, John Peter Smith Hospital, Fort Worth, Texas; Associate Attending, Parkland Memorial Hospital and Baylor University Medical Center, Dallas, Texas; Active Attending, Dallas Veterans Administration Hospital, Dallas, Texas
*Otologic Disorders*

**William Applegate, M.D., M.P.H.**
Associate Professor of Medicine and Community Medicine and Chief, Division of Geriatric Medicine, University of Tennessee, Memphis
*Sexuality and the Elderly*

**David Baylink, M.D.**
Professor of Medicine, Loma Linda University School of Medicine, Loma Linda, California; Chief, Mineral Metabolism, Jerry Pettis Veterans Administration Hospital, Loma Linda, California
*Osteoporosis*

**J. Andrew Billings, M.D.**
Assistant Clinical Professor of Medicine, Harvard Medical School, Boston, Massachusetts; Assistant Physician, Massachusetts General Hospital, Boston, Massachusetts
*Home Care*

**Jeffrey Blumberg, Ph.D.**
Associate Professor, School of Nutrition, Tufts University, Boston, Massachusetts; Acting Associate Director, U.S.D.A. Human Nutrition Research Center on Aging at Tufts University, Boston, Massachussets
*Drug Nutrient Interrelationships*

**Robert N. Butler, M.D.**
Brookdale Professor of Geriatrics and Adult Development and Chairman, Gerald and May Ellen Ritter Department of Geriatrics and Adult Development, Mount Sinai School of Medicine, New York, New York; Formerly Director, National Institute on Aging, National Institutes of Health, Bethesda, Maryland; Mount Sinai Hospital, New York, New York
*Principles of Care in the Nursing Home*

**Bertram N. Buxton, M.D.**
Professor and Chief, Division of Gynecology, University of Tennessee Center for Health Sciences, Memphis, Tennessee; Active Staff, Regional Medical Center and William F. Bowld Hospital, Memphis, Tennessee; Consulting Staff, Baptist Memorial Hospital, St. Joseph's Hospital, Le Bonheur Children's Medical Center, and Veterans Hospital, Memphis, Tennessee
*Gynecologic Problems*

**Evan Calkins, M.D.**
Professor of Medicine, Clinical Professor of Family Medicine and Head, Division of Geriatrics/Gerontology, Department of Medicine, State University of New York at Buffalo School of Medicine, Buffalo, New York; Director, Western New York Geriatric Education Center, Buffalo, New York; Head, Gerontology Section, Buffalo Veterans Administration Medical Center, Buffalo, New York; Attending Physician, Erie County Medical Center, Buffalo General Hospital, Presbyterian Homes of Western New York, and Rosa Coplon Jewish Home, Buffalo, New York
*Aging and Disease; Confusion (Delirium); Falls; Musculoskeletal Diseases in the Elderly; Protein-Calorie Malnutritional Therapy*

**Paul Carbone, M.D.**
Professor and Chairman, Department of Human Oncology, University of Wisconsin Medical School, Madison, Wisconsin; Director, University of Wisconsin Clinical Cancer Center, Madison, Wisconsin

**Christine K. Cassel, M.D.**
Associate Professor of Medicine, University of Chicago Pritzker School of Medicine, Chicago, Illinois; Chief, Section of General Internal Medicine, University of Chicago Hospitals and Clinics, and Director, Center on Aging, University of Chicago, Chicago, Illinois
*Ethical Dilemmas in the Clinical Care of the Elderly*

**Hanimi R. Challa, M.D.**
Clinical Instructor, State University of New York, Buffalo, New York, and Clinical Assistant Professor, Hahnemann University, Philadelphia, Pennsylvania; Staff Member, Private Practice, Seven Rivers Community Hospital, Crystal River, Florida, and Citrus Memorial Hospital, Inverness, Florida
*Musculoskeletal Diseases in the Elderly*

**Donna Cohen, Ph.D.**
Associate Professor, Department of Psychiatry, Montefiore Medical Center and Albert Einstein College of Medicine, New York, New York; Division Head, United Division of Aging and Geriatric Psychiatry, Montefiore Medical Center and Albert Einstein College of Medicine, New York, New York
*Depression; Dementing Disorders; Paranoia*

**Harvey Jay Cohen, M.D.**
Professor of Medicine, Chief Geriatrics Division, and Director, Center for the Study of Aging and Human Development Duke University School of Medicine, Durham, North Carolina; Director, Geriatrics Research Education and Clinical Center, Veterans Administration Medical Center, Durham, North Carolina
*Hematologic Problems*

**Jeffrey Crawford, M.D.**
Assistant Professor of Medicine, Duke University Medical Center, Durham, North Carolina; Hematologist-Oncologist, Veterans Administration Medical Center, Durham, North Carolina
*Hematologic Problems*

**John J. Cunningham, M.D.**
Associate Professor of Family Medicine and Associate Chairman, Department of Family Medicine, Brown University, Providence, Rhode Island; Physician and Associate Chairman, Department of Family Medicine, Memorial Hospital, Pawtucket, Rhode Island
*Social Factors and Family Supports*

**Barry J. Cusack, M.D.**
Assistant Professor of Medicine, Division of Gerontology and Geriatric Medicine, University of Washington, Seattle, Washington; Director, Clinical Geriatrics, Veterans Administration Medical Center, Boise, Idaho; Associate Medical Director, Veterans Nursing Home Care Unit, Boise, Idaho
*Clinical Pharmacology: Special Considerations in the Elderly*

**Faith B. Davis, M.D.**
Associate Professor of Medicine, State University of New York at Buffalo School of Medicine, Buffalo, New York; Endocrinologist, Erie County Medical Center, Buffalo, New York
*Endocrine Diseases*

**Paul J. Davis, M.D.**
Professor and Vice-Chairman, Department of Medicine and Head, Endocrinology Division, State University of New York at Buffalo School of Medicine, Buffalo, New York; Chief, Medical Service, Buffalo Veterans Administration Medical Center, Buffalo, New York
*Endocrine Diseases*

**Ananias C. Diokno, M.D.**
Clinical Professor, Section of Urology, Department of Surgery, The University of Michigan, Ann Arbor, Michigan; Chief, Department of Urology, William Beaumont Hospital, Royal Oak, Michigan; Program Project Director NIH-NIA Grant on "Medical, Epidemiologic, and Social Aspects of Urinary Incontinence in the Elderly 1983–1988"
*Urinary Incontinence in the Elderly; Prostate Gland Disease*

**Gerald F. Dixon, M.D.**
Medical Director of Respiratory Services, Memorial Hospital of Union County, Marysville, Ohio
*Pulmonary Disease*

**Roy L. Donnerberg, M.D.**
Associate Professor of Medicine and Director of Clinical Geriatrics, Department of Medicine, College of Medicine, Ohio State University, Columbus, Ohio; Attending Staff, University Hospital, Columbus, Ohio; Courtesy Staff, Grant Hospital, Columbus, Ohio; Medical Director, Westminster Thurber Community Retirement Center and Nursing Home, Columbus, Ohio
*Pulmonary Disease*

**David Dube, M.D.**
Assistant Professor of Medicine, State University of New York at Buffalo, Buffalo, New York; Staff Physician, Erie County Medical Center and Veterans Administration Medical Center, Buffalo, New York; Associate Medical Director Amherst Presbyterian Home and Rosa Coplon Nursing Home, Buffalo, New York
*Aging and Disease; Protein-Calorie Malnutrition Therapy*

**Carl Eisdorfer, Ph.D., M.D.**
Professor and Chairman, Department of Psychiatry, University of Miami School of Medicine, Miami, Florida
*Depression; Dementing Disorders; Paranoia*

**Amasa B. Ford, M.D.**
Professor of Epidemiology and Biostatistics, Associate Dean for Geriatric Medicine, and Director, Office of Geriatric Medicine, Case Western Reserve University School of Medicine, Cleveland, Ohio; Board of Eliza Bryant Center, Cleveland, Ohio; Medical Director, Benjamin Rose Hospital, Cleveland, Ohio; Associate Physician, University Hospitals of Cleveland, Cleveland, Ohio; Chairman, Geriatric Medicine and Gerontology, Advisory Committee, Board of Regents, and NIA Geriatrics Review Committee
*The Aged and Their Physicians*

**Barbara A. Gilchrest, M.D.**
Professor and Chairman, Department of Dermatology, Boston University School of Medicine, Boston, Massachusetts; Chief, Cutaneous Gerontology Laboratory, U.S.D.A. Human Nutrition Research Center on Aging, Tufts University, Boston, Massachusetts; Chief of Dermatology, University and Boston City Hospitals, Boston, Massachusetts
*Skin Diseases in the Elderly*

**Carl V. Granger, M.D.**
Professor of Rehabilitation Medicine, State University of New York at Buffalo, Buffalo, New York; Head, Rehabilitation Medicine, Buffalo General Hospital, Buffalo, New York
*Rehabilitation for the Elderly*

**Charles J. Gudas, D.P.M.**
Clinical Professor of Surgery, University of Chicago Medical Center, Chicago, Illinois; Surgeon, University of Chicago Medical Center, Ravenswood Hospital, Hinsdale Surgical Center, and Norwood Nursing Home and Care Facilities, Chicago, Illinois
*Common Foot Problems in the Elderly*

**John Hedley-Whyte, M.D., F.A.C.P.**
David S. Sheridan Professor of Anaesthesia and Respiratory Therapy, Harvard University, Boston, Massachusetts; Anaesthetist-in-Chief, Beth Israel Hospital, Boston, Massachusetts
*Anesthesiology*

**Shirley B. Hesslein, M.A., M.L.S.**
Librarian Emeritus, State University of New York at Buffalo, Buffalo, New York; Library Resource Specialist, Western New York Geriatric Education Center, Buffalo, New York
*Patient Information in Geriatrics*

**John Jennings, M.D.**
Assistant Professor of Medicine, Loma Linda University School of Medicine, Loma Linda, California; Staff Physician, Jerry Pettis Veterans Administration Hospital, Loma Linda, California
*Osteoporosis*

**Paul Katz, M.D.**
Assistant Professor, Division of Geriatrics/Gerontology, Department of Medicine, and Geriatric Fellowship Coordinator, State University of New York at Buffalo, Buffalo, New York; Medical Director, Rosa Coplon Nursing Home, Buffalo, New York; Assistant Medical Director, Amherst Presbyterian Nursing Home and Nursing Home Care Unit, Veterans Administration Medical Center, Buffalo, New York
*Aging and Disease; Protein-Calorie Malnutritional Therapy*

**Carol R. Kollarits, M.D.**
Clinical Associate Professor Medical College of Ohio, Toledo, Ohio; Medical Director, Eye Institute of Northwestern Ohio, Toledo, Ohio; Attending, Medical College of Ohio Hospital, Toledo, Ohio, St. Luke's Hospital, Maumee, Ohio, and Flower Memorial Hospital, Sylvania, Ohio
*The Aging Eye*

**Daniel F. Kripke, M.D.**
Professor of Psychiatry, University of California, San Diego School of Medicine, San Diego, California; Staff Psychiatrist and Director, Sleep Disorders Clinic, San Diego Veterans Administration Medical Center, San Diego, California; Affiliated with UCSD Teaching Nursing Home, San Diego, California
*Sleep and Aging*

**Jacqueline Levitt, M.D.**
Assistant Professor of Medicine, State University of New York at Buffalo, Buffalo, New York; Associate Head, Division of Geriatrics, Buffalo Veterans Administration Medical Center, Buffalo, New York; Attending Physician, Rosa Coplon Jewish Home and Amherst Presbyterian Home, Buffalo, New York
*Patient Information in Geriatrics*

**Robert J. MacGregor, M.D., M.B.B.S., B.Sc., F.R.A.C.S., F.A.C.S.**
Formerly Assistant Professor of Surgery, University of Michigan, Ann Arbor, Michigan; Visiting Urologist, Albury Base Hospital, Albury Mercy Hospital, Wodonga District Hospital, Albury Private Hospital, Deinliquin District Hospital, and Yarrawonga District Hospital, Albury, Australia
*Prostate Gland Disease*

**Mark J. Magenheim, M.D., M.P.H., F.A.C.P.M., C.C.F.P.**
Graduate School Faculty, University of South Florida, Tampa, Florida; Director, Sarasota County Health Department, Florida Department of Health and Rehabilitative Services, Sarasota, Florida; Attending Physician, Memorial Hospital of Sarasota and Doctors Hospital of Sarasota, Sarasota, Florida
*Screening the Elderly*

**Maury Massler, D.D.S., M.S., D.Sc.**
Professor Emeritus, Tufts University, School of Dental Medicine, Boston, Massachusetts
*Oral Aspects of Aging*

**Fletcher H. McDowell, M.D.**
Professor of Neurology, Cornell Medical School, New York, New York; Director, Burta Rehabilitation Center, New York, New York; Attending Neurologist, the New York Hospital, New York, New York; Consulting Staff in Neurology, Memorial Sloan Kettering Hospital, New York, New York
*Neurologic Diseases—Stroke and Other Cerebrovascular Conditions; Other Neurologic Diseases of the Elderly*

**Jack H. Medalie, M.D., M.P.H.**
The Dorothy Jones Weatherhead Professor and Chairman, Department of Family Medicine, Case Western Reserve University School of Medicine, Cleveland, Ohio; Attending Physician, University Hospitals and Cuyahoga County Hospital, Cleveland, Ohio
*An Approach to Common Problems in the Elderly; Confusion (Delirium)*

**William L. Meyerhoff, M.D., Ph.D.**
Professor and Chairman, Department of Otorhinolaryngology, University of Texas Health Science Center at Dallas, Dallas, Texas; Attending Physican, St. Paul Hospital, Parkland Memorial Hospital, Dallas, Texas
*Otologic Disorders*

**Arthur J. Moss, M.D.**
Clinical Professor of Medicine, University of Rochester School of Medicine and Dentistry, Rochester, New York; Attending Physician, Strong Memorial Hospital, Rochester, New York; Director, Heart Research Follow-Up Program, University of Rochester, Medical Center, Rochester, New York; Editorial Board, American Geriatrics Society
*Cardiac Disease in the Elderly*

**Rudolph M. Navari, M.D., Ph.D.**
Simon-Williamson Clinic, P.A., Birmingham, Alabama; Hillhaven Convalescent Center, Birmingham, Alabama
*Hypothermia*

**Theodore Papademetriou, M.D.**
Clinical Professor of Orthopaedic Surgery, State University of New York at Buffalo, Buffalo, New York; Attending, Orthopaedic Surgeon, Erie County Medical Center and Buffalo General Hospital, Buffalo, New York
*Musculoskeletal Diseases in the Elderly*

**H. Reddy Pasem, M.D.**
Former Fellow, State University of New York at Buffalo Veterans Administration Medical Center, Buffalo, New York; Staff Physician, Central State Hospital, Petersburg, Virginia
*Confusion (Delirium)*

**W. Bradford Patterson, M.D.**
Visiting Professor of Surgery, Harvard Medical School, Boston, Massachusetts; Chief, Division of Cancer Control, Dana-Farber Cancer Institute, Boston, Massachusetts; Surgeon, New England Deaconess Hospital, and Consultant in Surgery, Brigham and Women's Hospital, Boston, Massachusetts
*Malignant Diseases*

**C. Carl Pegels, M.S., Ph.D.**
Professor and Chairman, Department of Management Science and Systems, School of Management, State University of New York at Buffalo, Buffalo, New York; Consultant to Millard Fillmore Hospital Corporation, Buffalo, New York; Board Member, Western New York Health Planning Corporation, Buffalo, New York
*Issues in Paying for Health Care of the Aged*

**John B. Redford, M.D.**
Professor and Chairman, Department of Rehabilitation Medicine, University of Kansas, Kansas City, Kansas; Attending, University of Kansas Medical Center, Kansas City, Kansas, Veterans Administration Medical Center, Truman Medical Center, and Swope Ridge Rehabilitation Center for Long-Term Care, Kansas City, Missouri
*Assistive Devices for the Elderly*

**John W. Rowe, M.D.**
Associate Professor of Medicine and Director, Division on Aging, Harvard Medical School, Boston, Massachusetts; Chief, Division of Gerontology, Joint Department of Medicine, Beth Israel and Brigham and Women's Hospitals, Boston, Massachusetts; Director, Geriatric Research Education Clinical Center (GRECC), West Roxbury/Brockton Veterans Administration Medical Center, Boston, Massachusetts
*Renal and Lower Urinary Tract Diseases in the Elderly*

**Fred Rubin, M.D.**
Instructor in Medicine, Harvard Medical School, Boston, Massachussets; Assistant Physician, Massachusetts General Hospital, Boston, Massachusetts
*Home Care*

**Robert M. Russell, M.D.**
Associate Professor of Medicine, Tufts University School of Medicine and Adjunct Associate Professor of Nutrition, Tufts University School of Medicine, Boston, Massachusetts; Staff Physician, Department of Medicine, Section of Gastroenterology, New England Medical Center, Boston, Massachusetts; Director of Human Studies, Acting Director (HNRC), Human Nutrition Research Center on Aging, Boston, Massachusetts
*Nutritional Assessment*

**George Ryan, Jr., M.D., M.P.H**
Professor of Ob/Gyn and Community Medicine, University of Tennessee College of Medicine, Memphis; Active Staff, City of Memphis Hospital, Baptist Memorial Hospital, and St. Joseph Hospital, Memphis, Tennessee; Courtesy Staff, Methodist Hospital, Memphis, Tennessee
*Gynecologic Problems*

**Nadine R. Sahyoun, M.S., R.D.**
Research Dietition, U.S.D.A. Human Nutrition Research Center on Aging at Tufts University, Boston, Massachusetts
*Nutritional Assessment*

**Jay S. Schinfeld, M.D.**
Chief, Reproductive Endocrinology, Infertility, and Menopause and Associate Professor, Obstetrics and Gynecology, University of Tennessee College of Medicine,

Memphis, Tennessee; Junior Staff, Baptist Memorial Hospital, Memphis, Tennessee; Active Staff, William F. Bowld Hospital and Regional Medical Center at Memphis, Memphis, Tennessee; Consultant, St. Jude's Children's Hospital, Le Bonheur Children's Hospital, and Methodist Hospitals of Memphis, Memphis, Tennessee
*Gynecologic Problems*

**Madeline H. Schmitt, Ph.D., R.N.**
Associate Professor of Medical-Surgical Nursing and of Sociology, School of Nursing, University of Rochester, Rochester, New York
*The Team Approach in the Elderly*

**Thomas W. Sheehy, M.D.**
Professor of Medicine, School of Medicine, and Acting Director, Center for Aging, University of Alabama in Birmingham, Birmingham, Alabama; Chief of Medicine, Birmingham Veterans Administration Medical Center, Birmingham, Alabama
*Hypothermia*

**Manuel Sklar, M.D., F.A.C.P.**
Associate Professor of Medicine, Wayne State University School of Medicine, Detroit, Michigan; Chief, Section of Gastroenterology, Sinai Hospital of Detroit, Detroit, Michigan
*Gastrointestinal Diseases*

**Ian M. Smith, M.D., F.R.C.P. (G), F.A.C.P., F.R.C. Path.**
Professor of Internal Medicine and Family Practice, University of Iowa Hospitals and Clinics, Iowa City, Iowa; Attending, Veterans Administration Hospital, Iowa City, Iowa; Medical Director, Oak Noll Retirement Home, Iowa City, Iowa; Recipient, NIA Geriatric Medicine Academic Award
*Host Resistance Impairment and Protection Against Infection; Prevalence, Diagnosis, and Treatment of Infectious Diseases*

**Donald L. Spence, Ph.D.**
Professor of Gerontology, University of Rhode Island, and Adjunct Associate Professor of Community Health, Brown University Program in Medicine, Providence, Rhode Island; Visiting and Consulting Staff, Rhode Island Medical Center General Hospital, Providence, Rhode Island; Faculty Participant, New England Long-Term Care Gerontology Center, Brown University, Providence, Rhode Island
*Social Factors and Family Supports*

**Jonathan M. Stein, M.D.**
Clinical Assistant Professor of Anesthesiology, Boston University School of Medicine, Boston, Massachusetts; Visiting Staff in Anesthesiology, Framingham Union Hospital, Framingham, Massachusetts
*Anesthesiology*

**John D. Stoeckle, M.D.**
Professor of Medicine, Harvard Medical School, Boston, Massachusetts; Physician, Massachusetts General Hospital, Boston, Massachusetts
*Home Care*

**Robert C. Tarazi, M.D.**
Late Head, Clinical Science Department and Vice Chairman, Research Division, Cleveland Clinic, Cleveland, Ohio
*Hypertension in the Elderly*

**Robert E. Vestal, M.D.**
Associate Professor of Medicine, Division of Gerontology and Geriatric Medicine, University of Washington, Seattle, Washington; Associate Chief of Staff for Research and Development and Chief, Clinical Pharmacology and Gerontology, Veterans Administration Medical Center, Boise, Idaho; Associate Medical Director, Idaho State Veterans Nursing Home, Boise, Idaho
*Clinical Pharmacology: Special Considerations in the Elderly*

**Stanley Wallach, M.D.**
Chief, Medical Service, Veterans Administration Medical Center, Bay Pines, Florida; Professor of Medicine, University of South Florida College of Medicine, Tampa, Florida
*Paget's Disease of Bone*

**Thelma J. Wells, R.N., Ph.D.**
Associate Professor, University of Michigan School of Nursing, Ann Arbor, Michigan; Associate Research Scientist, Institute of Gerontology, Ann Arbor, Michigan
*Major Clinical Problems in Gerontologic Nursing*

**Rosalind Whinston-Perry, M.S.**
Research Assistant, Human Nutrition Research Center on Aging at Tufts University, Boston, Massachusetts
*Nutritional Assessment*

**Henry M. Wieman**
Clinical Assistant Professor, Medical Center of New York at Syracuse, Binghamton Clinical Campus, Binghamton, New York; Member, Medical Staff, United Health Services, Johnson City, New York
*Falls*

**T. Franklin Williams, M.D.**
Director, National Institute on Aging, National Institutes of Health, Bethesda, Maryland; Professor of Medicine, University of Rochester, Rochester, New York
*Comprehensive Assessment of Frail Elderly in Relation to Needs for Long-Term Care*

**Sheldon Winkler, B.A., D.D.S., F.A.C.D.**
Professor and Chairman, Department of Removable Prosthodontics, Temple University, School of Dentistry, Philadelphia, Pennsylvania; Consultant in Prosthodontics, Temple University Hospital, Philadelphia, Pennsylvania
*Oral Aspects of Aging*

**Rosemary Yancik, Ph.D.**
Assistant Director, Centers and Community Oncology, Division of Cancer Prevention and Control, National Cancer Institute, Bethesda, Maryland

# Contents

# *Introduction: The Challenge of Geriatrics*

The provision of good medical care to elderly persons provides a difficult and exciting challenge. It is now well known that the structure and physiology of cells and organs of persons of advanced age are as different from those of a person of mid-life as an adult is different from a young child. These changes affect all aspects of bodily function, including, particularly, the response to stress and to drugs. These biological changes have a major influence on the incidence and frequency of disease and on the clinical and laboratory manifestations, course, and management of specific disorders. Older persons who become ill seldom suffer from a single disease. Knowledge is beginning to accumulate concerning the effect that the presence of one disease has on the manifestations, course, and treatment of a second or third disorder. Similarly, the psychological and social aspects of aging play an important role in the health and happiness of elderly persons and in their ability to remain independent. The interrelationship between the biological and behavioral aspects of human existence, important at all ages, is particularly important for the elderly.

Unfortunately, in the development of American medicine to date, a full understanding of the implications of each of these age-related problems is possessed by only a limited number of specialists in a given field, be it cardiology or other "medical" or surgical specialties, the neurosciences, psychology, physiology, rehabilitation medicine, nursing, social work, sociology, or medical economics. However, because of the multiplicity of their problems, limited economic and physical resources, and the importance of a preventive approach to the medical problems of aging, older persons do not fare well in a pattern of care that is dependent on the individual efforts of a range of subspecialists. Some one individual or, in certain instances, a closely integrated team, needs to assume overall responsibility for the health care of an older person. To do this job in a responsible fashion, the primary care physician needs to possess an enormous range of knowledge, encompassing a wide variety of disciplines. Few physicians in this country have had sound preparation for this task.

This book has been designed to assist the primary care physician in fulfilling this role and in doing it well and enjoying it. It includes 48 chapters written by specialists who are well versed in their own discipline as it applies to the elderly. In most instances, these specialists serve as members of a well-organized geriatric program within their respective universities. Twenty-nine chapters relate to individual organ systems, 19 to broader issues of health care. In each instance, the authors have sought to present material that is authoritative, complete, stimulating, and clinically applicable. The book includes extensive bibliographies, and articles of special importance for background reading are annotated to guide the reader in further study. Clinical presentations are based, to a large extent, on reviews of published work, coordinated and prioritized in accordance with the author's clinical experience. An effort has been made to delineate therapeutic recommendations in a clear-cut and practical fashion.

Material that may prove useful in providing family and patient education has been assembled in the final chapter.

Although the clinical topics have been assigned to authors on the basis of a traditional organ-system format (authorities tend to specialize in organ systems rather than in patient complaints), many chapters have included a problem-oriented approach. The index has been developed on a problem-oriented basis; through use of the index the reader should have little difficulty in locating individual sections relevant to major symptom complexes that affect the elderly.

The book has not been designed for fireside reading. It is intended to be kept in the physician's or other health care provider's office for handy reference. Each chapter has been reviewed by four generalist reviewers prior to final acceptance. The reviewers included in each instance the senior editor, one of the associate editors, a young geriatrician, and a geriatric fellow, medical student, or other health professionals. The editors are indebted to the following for assistance in this regard: Dr. Hanami Reddi Challa (who reviewed each of the chapters in the book), and Drs. David Dube, Paul Katz, Margaret Mitchell, and Reddy Pasem (geriatric fellows). Many chapters were also reviewed by a specialist in the area in question. We wish to thank Drs. Donald Gregory, Gloria Heinemann, Gerald Logue, Basab Mookerjee, Kevin Pranikoff, Alan Saltzman, Robert Scheig, Monica Spaulding, and Bradley Truax of SUNY/Buffalo, Mr. William Reichman (medical student), Dr. Thelma Wells of the University of Michigan School of Nursing, and Dr. Alan Tisdale of the University of Vermont for these helpful reviews. The editors are greatly indebted to the authors for their patience with this reviewing process and their willingness to try to present their material in a fashion that will be understood by a generalist reader.

We are also indebted to the staff of W.B. Saunders Company for their encouragement and cooperation: Kay Dowgun, Priscilla Estes, Cynthia Fazzini, Evelyn Weiman, and Bill Preston. We also wish to thank Pat Baier, Joan Manley, Barbara Lannen, and Elizabeth Webb for assistance in typing correspondence and some of the manuscripts and Ms. Shirley Heslein for library assistance.

The book reflects, particularly, the efforts of faculty members from 32 different medical centers across the country, specialists in the fields of anesthesiology, business administration, dermatology, family medicine, internal medicine, neurology, orthopedic surgery, ophthalmology, psychiatry, and urologic surgery. Six of the authors are recipients of the Geriatric Medicine Academic Award of the National Institute on Aging. One author is a former Director and one the present Director of the National Institute on Aging. One author helped develop many of the questions pertaining to geriatric medicine that were included in a recent certifying examination of the American Board of Internal Medicine. The senior editor served as a member of the drafting committee for a document on geriatric medical education developed by the Association of American Medical Colleges. An effort has been made to include clinical material from these two sources (the Board examinations in Internal Medicine and the AAMC document) in the pages of this book. Thus, at the very least, we hope that this book will provide a vista into the broad, lively, and growing field of American geriatrics.

EVAN CALKINS, M.D.

Section I

# GENERAL ASPECTS

Chapter 1

## Aging and Disease

*Paul Katz*
*David Dube*
*Evan Calkins*

This volume is directed toward geriatric medicine. It does not attempt to serve alone as a text on the biology of aging. Readers who wish to learn more about the subject are referred to a number of excellent volumes and reviews, some of which are cited at the end of this chapter. It should be recognized, however, that effective clinical practice in elderly patients is based on a solid understanding of the biologic changes of aging and the way in which these changes influence the presentation, manifestations, course, and treatment of disease. In the past, considerable emphasis was placed on the need to differentiate the changes of "normal aging" from those of disease. Increasingly, however, studies of selected older people, carefully screened to exclude the presence of *any* disease, have failed to demonstrate many of the changes previously attributed to "normal aging." Because of the infrequency with which one encounters elderly persons who are devoid of *any* disease, the concept of "normal aging" is receiving less emphasis and is being replaced by a consideration of the changes to be expected in a representative sampling of elderly populations. This is the concept that prevails throughout most of this volume.

Individual chapters in this book include a review of these changes as they pertain to the organ system in question. Since aging affects the body as a whole, not merely its individual parts, this chapter will present a brief overview of age-related changes as they are understood at this time.

Aging is a lifelong process. It does not begin at any specific time, such as at age 60 or 70, but, instead, is a developmental process that starts at the very outset of life. Aging is accompanied by profound changes in the number, configuration, and composition of cells and by comparable changes in the intracellular matrix and extracellular fluid.[1] These changes follow one of two courses, as illustrated in Figure 1–1. In some instances, the individual starts life with a superabundance, such as in the number of cells in a given area of the skin[2] or in segments of the brain.[3] This superabundance is followed by a progressive decline (see line A, Fig. 1–1). In other instances,[4] the individual cells start out "small," achieve a maximum in early adult life, and then decline along a curve, depicted schematically in line B, Figure 1–1. In addition to pertaining to number or size, configuration, and composition of individual cells and organs, these developmental curves also describe certain physiologic processes, such as the progressive decline with age in renal function[5] and in myocardial response to exercise.[6]

Although one or the other of these two curves characterizes the developmental pattern of most bodily tissues and physiologic processes, it must be stressed that there is a marked degree of individual variation. This variation increases with

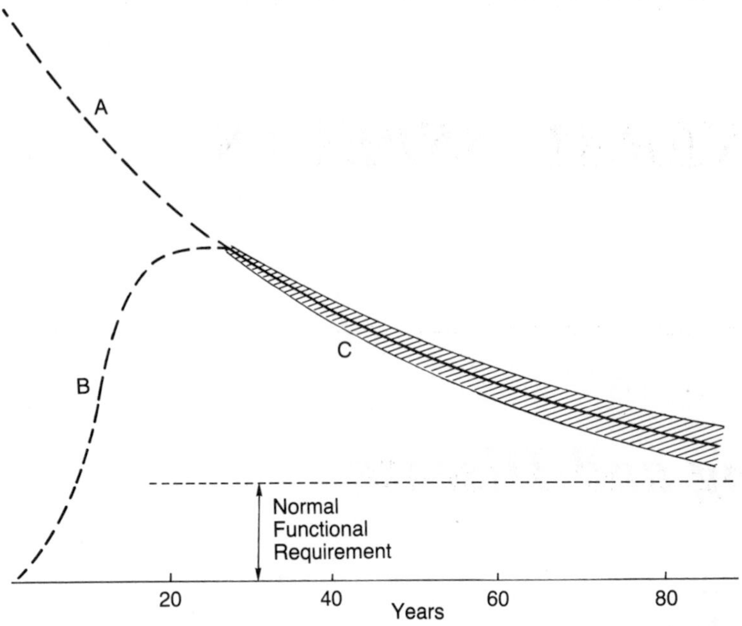


**Figure 1–1.** Normal development and aging.

age (see shaded area, Fig. 1–1). Thus, older people differ from each other to a greater extent than is true for the young or middle-aged.

Despite these changes, in the unstressed condition, the healthy individual's body continues to function well up to very advanced age. This is due to the fact that, at the outset of life, people are endowed with an ample reserve of physiologic capacity (see area between line C and the dotted horizontal line in the lower third of Fig. 1–1). As one proceeds through life, the functional capacity decreases, becoming progressively close to that necessary to sustain life functions (see dotted horizontal line, Fig. 1–1). However, the slope of this functional decline is not fixed and is potentially modifiable, certainly for the worse and probably for the better. Individual differences in environmental exposure, nutritional intake, and fitness are but a few of the parameters contributing to this plasticity of aging.[7]

As a corollary of the preceding, most people as they advance in age are not significantly limited in overall function. However, stresses, such as infection, trauma, and certain drugs may serve to highlight previously masked decrements, resulting in single and multiple organ failure and causing illness. This illness may further stress the dwindling social and psychologic as well as physiologic reserves.

## ROLE OF THE PHYSICIAN

Viewed in this light, the role of the physician interested in geriatric medicine is *first* to encourage his or her patient to establish a pattern of living early in life that will allow the downward slope in function to be as gradual as possible. Measures that will decrease the impact of disease, such as appropriate immunization, use of safety equipment, maintenance of physical fitness, good dietary habits, and achievement of a stable personality and an inquiring active mind, will go far in maintaining viability into old age. In addition, early identification of organ systems with minimal functional reserve and of marginal reserve in social and economic support systems will permit the physician to assist the individual in deferring or avoiding physiologic and psychosocial decompensation. An example of a way in which age-related decrements may be lessened or averted by appropriate intervention is the use of supplemental dietary calcium or estrogen in people with postmenopausal osteoporosis (see Chapter 39).

Although the clinician is often preoccupied with the biologic processes of aging, it is essential that he or she also recognize the psychosocial dynamics of growing older (see Chapter 5). Such an appreciation has important implications for therapy, which may involve psychologic intervention, family and patient counseling, and the team care approach to patient management (see Chapter 3).

## BIOLOGY OF AGING

In all likelihood, there is no "unitary" theory of aging. Aging probably depends on the interaction of multiple factors, including individual gene expression, mutation, accumulation of intracellular and extracellular toxins, and decline in immune function. Death appears to be an inherent property of normal life, both for cells in tissue culture[8] and for the body as a whole.[9]

**Changes in Body Composition.** With age, changes in body composition are evident in the well-known physiognomic changes of advanced age.[1] Lean body mass declines progressively with age, replaced in large part by an increase in fat stored primarily in the omentum and other central portions of the body. This accounts for the seemingly cachectic appearance of many elderly people despite adequate nutrition. Concomitantly, there is a decrease in body water. Changes in body composition have multiple ramifications, particularly in regard to drug distribution and elimination (see Chapter 12), organ reserve, muscle bulk, and overall strength.

**Contour Changes.** Contour changes of the face, pelvis, and chest reflect skeletal changes accompanying normal aging. The increase in chest anteroposterior diameter, often resulting in obscuration of heart sounds and displacement of the apical impulse, makes cardiac examination in the elderly much more difficult.[10] The decline in bone mass accompanying aging is often reflected in decrements in vertebral height and overall stature[11] (see Chapter 39). Gait and posture must accommodate to those changes. Changes in bone mass also lead to an increased susceptibility to fractures. Fractures in both the axial and appendicular skeleton contribute substantially to morbidity and mortality in the elderly. Changes in articular surface lead to the almost ubiquitous presence of osteoarthritis (see Chapter 36).

**External Environmental Forces.** The elderly are also at a disadvantage in relation to external environmental forces. The skin, the largest organ of the body, becomes less resistant to trauma and to toxins, secondary to a decrease in melanocyte number, vasculature, and subcutaneous fat (see Chapter 41).[12] Concomitant loss of sebaceous and sweat glands, increase in pain threshold, and decrease in sensory acuity predispose the elderly to an increased risk of trauma, infection, decubitus ulceration, and abnormalities of temperature regulation (see Chapter 28).

**Sensory Input.** Changes in sensory input include decrements in vision, hearing, taste, and smell.[13] Although cataracts account for much of the loss of visual acuity, decrease in accommodative ability and in the speed of dark adaptation also contribute to the overall decrement in vision (see Chapter 24). Hearing loss, which affects primarily the high-frequency tones, contributes much to the social isolation of the elderly (see Chapters 5 and 25). Indeed, it is not surprising that some elderly patients are labeled demented and incompetent largely as a consequence of this type of sensory deprivation. Decrements in taste and smell have important nutritional implications.

**Immune Function.** Age-related changes in immune function include decreased cell-mediated immunity, as evidenced by decreased hypersensitivity and rejection of tumors and allografts; decreased antibody response to foreign antigens; and increased incidence of autoantibodies and benign monoclonal gammopathy.[14] These changes result in increased incidence of infection among the elderly and may contribute to increased frequency of cancer and cardiovascular disease.

**Renal Function.** The kidney, like most organs, decreases in size with age. Related to this is a progressive decrease in the number of functional nephrons, which is accompanied by a decrease in the glomerular filtration rate[5] (see Chapter 31). A decreased glomerular filtration rate, which is often not reflected in an increased serum creatinine, must be considered in determining optimum doses of drugs eliminated by the renal route. Sclerosis of glomeruli and renal vasculature, basement membrane thickening, and decreased levels of renin and aldosterone all contribute to decreases in normal regulation of water and electrolytes and account, in large part, for the high incidence of perioperative renal failure secondary to hypoperfusion or drug nephrotoxicity (see Chapter 31). The decrease in bladder capacity and the presence of prostatic hypertrophy and alterations in pelvic support and vaginal mucosal integrity further compromise genitourinary function. Obstructive and infectious complications of the genitourinary tract and incontinence are among the most common and important concomitants of advanced age (see Chapters 33–35).

GI age-related changes in the alimentary tract are varied, although the significance of many such changes has not yet been delineated clearly.[15] Although the liver and pancreas atrophy with time, the effects on absorption and endocrine function are usually not clinically significant. However, the effects on drug metabolism may be important, even in the absence of chemical indices of liver dysfunction (see Chapter 46). Altered intestinal mobility contributes to functional bowel syndrome, constipation, esophageal spasm, and diverticular disease. Gastric atrophy, with decreased parietal cell mass, leads to a decline in the secretion of acid and of intrinsic factor. Older people may exhibit decreased absorption of iron, calcium, and vitamin $B_{12}$, even in the presence of adequate absorption of other nutrients. Changes in cholesterol secretion, mucus production, and gallbladder emptying predispose elderly people to an increased frequency of cholelithiasis and cholecystitis.

**Respiratory Function.** Respiratory function in the aged is marked by alterations in gas exchange secondary to a decline in both thoracic cage compliance and airway elasticity (see Chapter 30).[1,16] Although alveolar size increases, the overall surface area of alveolar capillary membranes decreases, contributing to ventilation perfusion mismatch. Such changes result in a redistribution of lung volumes in the elderly, with an increase in functional residual capacity and residual volume despite normal total lung capacity. Values for $PaO_2$ decline with age. Declines in respiratory muscle strength and mucociliary clearance predispose to pulmonary infection (see Chapter 45). Decreased responsiveness to hypoxia and hypercarbia, which is often aggravated by drugs, predisposes to breathing disorders and to increased risk of perioperative respiratory complications (see Chapter 47).

**Cardiovascular Function.** Cardiovascular changes associated with aging have recently become clarified (see Chapter 29).[6] Age-related decreases in arterial elasticity lead to increased peripheral resistance. The resulting increased impedance is thought to contribute to the myocardial hypertrophy and fibrosis commonly seen in the aged heart and may contribute to an increased risk of ischemia and hypertension in the elderly. Calcification and sclerosis of the fibrous cardiac skeleton and heart valves may adversely affect conduction pathways and valvular integrity. Despite such changes, myocardial performance at rest, when corrected for lean body mass, appears to be little affected. However, under stress, overall performance may be decreased, characterized by a decline in the response of heart rate and cardiac output.

**Hematology.** Despite a decrease in bone marrow cellularity by approximately one third, normal people of advanced age exhibit normal peripheral cell populations and, in most instances, normal hematologic response to stress[17] (see Chapter 43). Although the size, number, and metabolic activity of erythrocytes decrease slightly with age, such changes are of little practical significance. Coagulation remains intact within the geriatric patient.

**Nervous System.** Aging is accompanied by very significant changes in the nervous system (see Chapters 18, 21, and 22). These changes include decreased deep tendon reflexes and altered dorsal column function, which might otherwise be misinterpreted as pathologic.[18] Results of an examination of the mental status of an elderly patient must be interpreted in the context of the patient's altered sensory input, past personality, educational background, and current use of medication. Although elderly patients may exhibit certain changes in cognitive function, such as minor loss of recent memory, cognitive ability generally remains intact in the normal elderly, even in persons of very advanced age. Anatomic changes in the normal aging brain include atrophy of gray and white matter, ventricular dilatation, selective neuronal loss, and decreased dendritic arborization. There is also a decrease in nerve conduction velocity. It is becoming increasingly evident that normal aging is also accompanied by alterations in brain neurotransmitter systems, including a generalized decrease in cholinergic activity.

**Endocrine Changes.** Endocrine changes with age are varied (see Chapter 38).[19] Certain plasma hormone levels decrease with increasing age (e.g., estrogen) as a result of a depressed rate of secretion. Serum concentrations of most other hormones remain unchanged (e.g., thyroxin, cortisol), reflecting, in most instances, declines in rates of both secretion and degradation. The response of most endocrine glands to appropriate stimuli, such as stress, remains intact with age. A notable exception is the hyporesponsiveness of the renin angiotensin system to sodium restriction on upright posture in most elderly people. However, end-organ response to hormonal stimulation may be decreased in people of advanced age. Examples include decreased sensitivity of the renal tubules to antidiuretic hormone (ADH), and of the testes to gonadotropin or luteinizing hormone (LH). Impaired glucose tolerance with increasing age may also reflect a decrement in tissue sensitivity to insulin action as well as independent changes in body composition.

Responsiveness of the pituitary gland to perturbations of the steady state generally remains intact. Exceptions include a decrease in thyroid-stimulating hormone (TSH) output to thyrotropin-releasing hormone (TRH) administration in elderly males and a decrease in growth hormone levels under stress (e.g., hypoglycemia, dopaminergic stimulation).

## THERAPEUTIC IMPLICATIONS

It is to be hoped that the preceding outline will serve as a guide to a better understanding of geriatric medicine. As will become apparent throughout this book, rational treatment of the elderly relies heavily on a knowledge of the interaction of multiple systems. Successful treatment may depend less on the recognition of dysfunction in any one particular physiologic parameter than on an understanding of how such dysfunction relates to the "whole person." Functional status and adaptability often take precedence over the concept of disease and will frequently dictate the overall management of the elderly patient.[20]

## References


1. Rossman I: Anatomic and body composition changes with aging. *In* Finch CE, Hayflick L (eds.): Handbook of the Biology of Aging. New York, Van Nostrand Reinhold Co., 1977, pp. 189–221.
   *Morphologic and anthropometric changes of aging are delineated, as is the change in body composition.*
2. Andrew W, Behnke RH, Sato T: Changes with advancing age in the cell population of the human dermis. Gerontologia 10:1, 1965.
3. Brody H: Organization of the cerebral cortex III. A study of aging in the human cerebral cortex. J Comp Neurol 102:511, 1955.
4. Dagliotti Z: Anat Entw 76:716, 1931. Referred to on page 696. *In* Finch CE, Hayflick L (eds.): Handbook of the Biology of Aging. New York, Van Nostrand Reinhold Co., 1977.
5. Rowe J: Renal function and aging. *In* Reff ME, Schneider EL (eds.): Biological Markers of Aging. Washington DC, NIH Publication No. 82-2221, 1982, pp. 228–236.
   *A concise review of basic anatomic and functional changes of the kidney associated with aging.*
6. Lakatta EG: Determinants of cardiovascular performance modification due to aging. J Chronic Dis 36:15, 1983.
   *An excellent overview of age-related changes in the cardiovascular system, including increased blood pressure, cardiac hypertrophy, and decreased ventricular compliance and responsiveness to catecholamines. Pharmacologic intervention in cardiac disease is discussed in the context of aforementioned changes.*
7. Fries J: Aging, natural death, and the compression of morbidity. N Engl J Med 303:130, 1980.
   *This article highlights differences between life span and life expectancy and discusses the "rectangularization" of the survival curve. It introduces the "plasticity" theory of aging and the implications of this theory for health care for the aged and directions for future research.*
8. Hayflick L: Future directions in aging research. Proc Soc Exp Biol Med 165:206, 1980.
   *This article evaluates current trends and goals in biologic research. Theories of aging are discussed, as are the extension of human longevity and its social and biologic implications.*
9. Strehler BL: Implications of aging research for society. *In* Thorbecke GJ (ed.): Biology of Aging and Development. Bethesda, FASEB, New York and London, Plenum Press, 1975.
   *This article clearly illustrates the fact that despite extraordinary increases in the percentage of people reaching advanced age (80–100 years) over the past 20 or more centuries, there has been no increase in total duration of life. It also illustrates the fact that most of the improvement in life expectancy is attributable to improved housing, sanitation, antisepsis, immunization, nutrition, and health education. Relatively little change in total life expectancy can be attributed to recently developed biotechnical interventions, such as cancer chemotherapy, coronary care units, and organ transplantation. The key figure in this article is reproduced on page 5 of this book. The entire volume provides an excellent background in biomedical changes of aging. Chapter authors include Leonard Hayflick, T. Makinodan, Roy Walford, H.N. Munro, Richard Adelman, George Roth, Jay Roberts, and others.*
10. Caird FI, Judge TG: Chapters on physical examination. *In* Caird FI, Judge TG (eds.): Assessment of the Elderly Patient. Kent, England, Pitman Medical Publishing Co., 1976, pp. 22–86.
    *A practical guide to the interpretation of physical signs and symptoms in the geriatric population.*
11. Raisz LG: Osteoporosis. J Am Geriatr Soc 30:127, 1982.
    *A comprehensive review of normal bone physiology and the clinicopathologic changes characteristic of osteoporosis.*
12. Gilchrest BA: Age associated changes of the skin. J Am Geriatr Soc 30:139, 1982.
    *A concise outline of changes in skin physiology and morphology with aging. Well illustrated.*
13. Welford AT: Sensory, perceptual, and motor processes in older adults. *In* Birren JE, Sloan RB (eds.): Handbook of Mental Health and Aging. Englewood Cliffs, Prentice-Hall, 1980, pp. 192–213.
    *An outline of sensory and motor changes related to aging, with an emphasis on psychosocial ramifications.*
14. Siskind G, Weksler ME: The effect of aging on the immune response. *In* Eisdorfer C (ed.): Annual Review of Gerontology and Geriatrics. New York, Springer Publishing Co., 1982, pp. 3–26.
    *The relative state of immunodeficiency in the geriatric population is comprehensively reviewed, along with its attendant biologic implications.*
15. Schumaker DL, et al (eds.): Gastrointestinal physiology. *In* Masaro EJ (ed.): Handbook of Physiology in Aging. Boca Raton, CRC Press, 1981, pp. 231–285.
    *A compilation of annotated references for several basic physiologic parameters. Outline format facilitates review of data.*
16. Klocke RA: Influence of aging on the lung. *In* Finch CE, Hayflick L (eds.): Handbook of the Biology of Aging. New York, Van Nostrand Reinhold Co., 1977, pp. 432–444.
    *Morphologic changes of the aging lung are examined, with emphasis on overall pulmonary function.*
17. Freedman ML, Marcus OL: Anemia and the elderly: Is it physiology or pathology? Am J Med Sci 280:81, 1980.
    *A reduction in red cell count with age is unlikely to reflect normal physiologic change. Anemia in the elderly deserves a full medical work-up.*
18. Wolfson LI, Katzman R: The neurologic consultation at age 80. *In* Katzman R, Terry RD (eds.): The Neurology of Aging. Philadelphia, FA Davis Co., 1983, pp. 221–244.
    *This article describes normal age-related changes in the neurologic examination and describes commonly encountered clinical problems, including cognitive*

*loss, gait disturbance, falls, temperature dysregulation, and seizures.*

19. Gregerman RI, Bierman EL: Aging and hormones. *In* Williams RH (ed.): Textbook of Endocrinology. 6th ed. Philadelphia, WB Saunders Co., 1981, pp. 1193–1212.
*This article outlines the current state of knowledge in geriatric endocrinology and has extensive references.*
20. Cape R: Aging: Its Complex Management. Hagerstown, Cape R Medical Department, Harper and Rowe, 1978.
*This book provides an excellent perspective on the impact of biologic changes of aging on the normal elderly and on the diseases of aging and their management. Special emphasis is placed on confusion, falls, incontinence, homeostatic impairment, and the iatrogenic disorders.*

Chapter 2

# The Aged and Their Physicians

Amasa B. Ford

Physicians who care for adults know from their own experience and from popular and medical literature that the United States, lagging only slightly behind other industrialized nations, is in the midst of an unprecedented expansion, in both numbers and proportion, of the aged population. However, some details of this massive demographic change and its implications for the future of medical practice are not familiar to physicians. This chapter, therefore, will provide an overview of the elderly population in the United States, their health problems, and their geographic and social situations and will examine how physicians encounter them. Finally, looking ahead, we will consider the professional and personal qualities physicians of the future will need to become more competent and efficient providers of health care to the aged.

## THE MODERN AGED

Who are the aged of today, and what are their needs for medical care? The general outlines of demographic change are quite familiar.[1] Life expectation has increased at all ages (except for young male adults), although the maximum life span has probably not changed. Eleven per cent of the population are now aged 65 or over, up from 4 per cent in 1900. More significantly in terms of health services, the proportion of the "old-old" (those aged 75 and over) among the elderly has risen from 29 per cent in 1900 to 38 per cent in 1970 and is expected to reach 44 per cent by 2000. A striking and unexpected exaggeration of this trend has been caused by a recent decline in mortality among the very old, which has been greater than that for any other age groups.[2,3]

One is impressed not only by the sheer numbers of the old (especially the very old) but also by the large and increasing proportion of women in this group. The sex ratio of 77 men for every 100 women in the total aged group (over age 65) drops to 50 men per 100 women above age 85, and the disproportion is continuing to increase because the sex difference in expectation of life at birth, which was 2.0 years in 1900, had risen to 7.7 years by 1974.[1] Similarly, racial differences in mortality over the life span have, until now, resulted in proportionately fewer nonwhites among the aged than in the general population.[4]

Another striking characteristic of the aged is that most are relatively poor. For example, in a 1975 survey of a representative sample of people age 65 and over in the city of Cleveland, Ohio, a third reported incomes below the poverty level (then approximately $3,000), another third reported incomes at near-poverty levels ($3,000 to $5,000), and only a third had incomes of over $5,000.[5] Nationally, the median income of elderly women is only about half that of elderly men.[1] The complexity, cost, and fragmentary character of our health care financing system is a great and, at times insuperable, obstacle to obtaining prompt and appropriate care (see Chapter 16).

What is the state of health of these aged people, and what are their needs for health care and other services? It is important to bear in mind that a large majority of the elderly are living at home and consider themselves to be in good health and that even outside observers find a high proportion to be functioning well. Trained interviewers from the Cleveland survey, for example, found that 41 per cent of the elderly were unimpaired or only slightly impaired in general well-being, and only 7 per cent were rated as extremely impaired.[6] The continuing National Health Survey records that two thirds of the noninstitutionalized elderly describe their health as good or excellent compared with other people their age, whereas only 9 per cent consider their health to be poor.

Of course, certain subgroups of the elderly do not fare as well as the average. Nonwhite elderly report poor health twice as frequently as whites, and those with lower incomes and those who live in the South and in nonmetropolitan areas also say that they have poor health more frequently than the average elderly person. Men and women report about the same amount of poor health, but, in terms of a different criterion, namely, inability to carry out a major activity (such as a job or housework) because of health problems, men are very much more limited than women. The conditions that most frequently cause disability among the elderly are of two kinds: (1) those that are also the leading causes of death, such as heart disease, cancer, and cerebrovascular disease, and (2) chronic conditions that are generally nonfatal, such as dementia, arthritis, and orthopedic, visual, and hearing impairments.[1]

The survival of many more people into old age will inevitably result in more chronic conditions and disabilities that will call for treatment. Even though death due to some life-shortening conditions, notably the cardiovascular diseases, appears to have been postponed, it is unlikely that the onset of other kinds of morbidity has likewise been deferred. The whole task of caring for the elderly will certainly become greater and more complex in the years immediately ahead.

Risk factors for both morbidity and mortality in old age include advancing age itself and being male, black, and poor, or poorly educated.[4,7] There are also certain specific risk factors, such as hypertension for heart disease and stroke[8] and cigarette smoking for lung and other types of cancer. Improper nutrition may also increase the risk of cancer.[9] The genesis of some of the major health problems of old age, such as coronary disease and malignancy, probably lies as far back as malnutrition in childhood or occupational exposures during the working years.

If some of the trends visible in successive cohorts of the elderly persist, the elderly people whom medical students and young physicians of today will have to care for in the future will be significantly different from those now under our care. They will certainly be older, and more of them will be women. There will be more blacks among the elderly, since race-specific mortality differentials are decreasing. Fewer will be foreign-born (until Spanish-speaking immigrants take the place of the European immigrants of the early twentieth century), and most will be better educated because they grew up in the era of public education. Most significantly, when the large "baby-boom" generation reaches age 65 (about the year 2030), they will have substantially fewer children to look after them, and the wives and daughters who have so often cared for aging men in the past will be more likely to be employed or to be removed by divorce. The financial impact of these changes will also be great, raising costs, limiting access for the individual, and increasing the burden for society.

Both the physical location of the elderly and their place in the social network affect how they encounter physicians. The proportion of old people (65 years and over) is highest in nonmetropolitan counties (11.4 per cent), nearly as high in central city counties (10.8 per cent), and distinctly lower in the suburbs (noncentral city metropolitan counties without central cities [8.0 per cent]). Thus, the aged are often those who have been left behind by the two great immigration trends of our recent history: (1) the movement of young people away from farms and into the cities and (2) the subsequent movement of successful young families from inner cities into the suburbs.[10] Primary care physicians, on the other hand, have progressively left rural and inner city locations during these years, with the result that the elderly, who generate much of the demand for primary care, are more concentrated in the two areas where there are the fewest physicians to provide it. The fact that many older people frequently live in stagnant rural areas or deteriorating central cities also subjects them to housing and transportation problems, aggravated by economic recession, which in turn affect their health and restrict their access to care.

The fact that about one third of older people live alone suggests that they are socially isolated. For many widows, this may be true, but there are also a significant number of never-married persons, many of them men, who live alone by choice or by habit and who are relatively healthy and independent. The most disabled among the noninstitutionalized elderly are more likely to move in with children or other relatives.[11] This sequence points to the increasing importance of the vertically extended family. A high proportion of older people are now members of three- and four-generation families, and the man or woman who reaches retirement age today is often responsible for the care of surviving parents. Elderly people who have children may not live with them, but they generally live near them and see them often or keep in frequent telephone contact if the distance is great (see Chapter 6).[12]

## THE AGED AND THE HEALTH CARE SYSTEM

For the old person who becomes physically or mentally disabled, particularly if he or she has no close family, the nursing home offers a symbolic and often a real "last resort."[13] About 6 per cent of people aged 65 years and older live in institutions, mainly nursing homes, but this relatively low proportion may be misleading, since 20 to 27 per cent of those who reach the age of 65 are admitted to such an institution before they die.[14] Most families in the United States make sustained, often very taxing efforts to care for their older members at home, turning to the nursing home only when the combined economic, physical, and psychologic burden surpasses their capacities.[6] The myth that families commonly "dump" their relatives in nursing homes persists, even though facts refute it.[12] The nursing home, or some organized (and not inexpensive) equivalent, is an indispensable part of a humane system of care in a developed society in which increasing numbers of individuals are surviving into advanced old age, often with severe disability (see Chapter 10). In spite of the well-publicized costs and abuses of the nursing home system as it has evolved in this country, we need to develop more stable and equitable means of financing such services and of assuring their quality.[15]

The flow chart in Figure 2–1, which is based on estimates from a variety of sources, gives an idea of the dynamics of movement of the elderly population into and through the health care system. Some of the data presented may be unfamiliar and even surprising to the hospital- or office-based practitioner. The high proportion of older persons who die in hospitals and nursing homes may not be unexpected, but do the 18 per cent who die at home receive adequate terminal care? We know that 94 per cent of old people are not institutionalized, but how many physicians realize that 28 per cent of people discharged from nursing homes go to a residence in the community? How often are these discharges medically planned and followed up? At most of the nodal points in this system, the physician is likely to be the decision-maker or at least to be involved in making the decision. Whether and when to hospitalize, discharge, or transfer a patient to a nursing home or mental hospital or whether to return the patient home and plan and participate in home care are critical issues that affect the allocation of the physician's efforts, as well as the survival and quality of life of the patient.

Compared with the options available to the elderly in Great Britain and other countries, the system in the United States is relatively inflexible, with "placement" into the life-altering nursing home likely to be thrust hurriedly upon a patient and family still stunned by the impact of a stroke or a hip fracture. Economic pressures, sound medical and rehabilitation principles, and respect for the dignity of the aged person require that we provide a more flexible framework for their care in the future. Options to be considered include extensive development of home care, day care, respite care, and active rehabilitation paced to the prolonged recovery cycle that is characteristic of old age. Ideas that are relatively new to the United States, such as sheltered housing and "nursing homes without walls" are beginning to be experimented with.[16] The Veterans Administration, confronted with the imminent aging of the World War II cohort, is starting to develop a comprehensive, multilevel system.[17] Systems such as this will not evolve without active encouragement by physicians, and they will require more direct participation by physicians in nursing homes and in home care, as well as earlier, better informed, and more thoughtful planning for hospital discharges.

In spite of the fact that currently practicing physicians are active at critical junctures of the health care system and are providing more health care for old people, particularly since the introduction of Medicare and Medicaid,[18] most were never trained to practice geriatric medicine or to respond to the large social and demographic changes just described. A partial mismatch between clinical practice and the perceived needs of the elderly has therefore developed. Many old people believe that doctors have little time or patience for them. Indeed, an honest self-appraisal will result in the acknowledgment that often, in our preoccupation with specialization and the demands of practice, we have allowed barriers to develop between ourselves and our elderly patients.[19] Indifference and a pessimistic attribution of all problems to "old age" can set the stage for overlooking treatable causes of "senility," for failure to notice the "hidden patient" who is bearing the brunt of caring for the elderly person, or for contributing to the large pool of iatrogenic illness due to the prescription of multiple potent drugs. Many of us know very little about what goes on in nursing homes because we are unac-

## OLDER PERSONS AND THE HEALTH CARE SYSTEM (IN THOUSANDS)

POPULATION OF THE UNITED STATES
1975-- 229,195

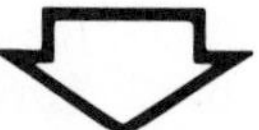

PERSONS 65 AND OVER
24,275 (10.6% OF TOTAL)

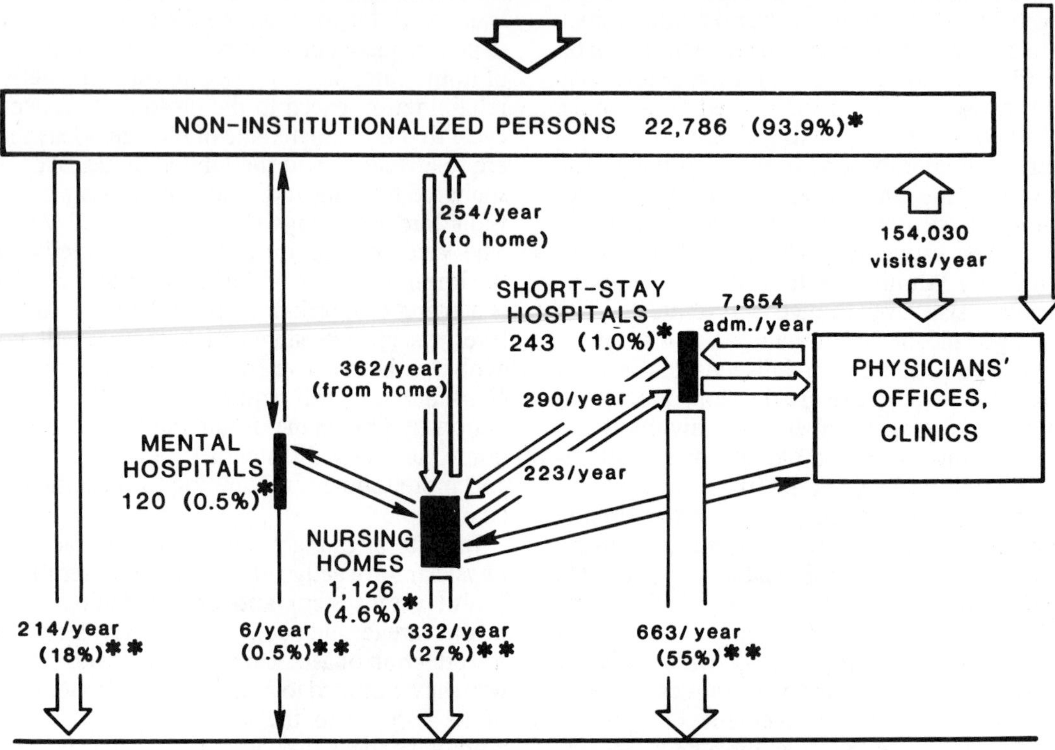


ALL DEATHS-- 1,217/YEAR

(AGE-SPECIFIC MORTALITY RATE 50.1 PER THOUSAND)

* -% OF OLDER PERSONS

** -% OF DEATHS

**Figure 2-1.** Location and flow of older persons in and through the health care system in the United States. Only major trends and locations are shown.

Data are estimates for 1975 to 1978, from the following sources: U.S. Department of Commerce, Bureau of the Census: Population Profile of the United States: 1980, Current Population Reports. Series P-20, No. 363, Washington, D.C., U.S. Government Printing Office, 1981. Kata BP, Zdeb MS, Therriault GD: Where people die. Public Health Rep 94:522-527, 1979. Kovar MG: Health of the elderly and use of health services. Public Health Rep 92:9-19, 1977. Ranofsky AL: Utilization of Short-Stay Hospitals: Annual Summary for the United States, 1975. Vital and Health Statistics, Series 13, No. 31, DHEW Publication No. (HRS) 77-1782, Washington, D.C., U.S. Government Printing Office, 1977. National Center for Health Statistics: Health, United States: 1978. DHEW Publication No. (PHS) 78-1232, Washington, D.C., U.S. Government Printing Office, 1978. Van Nostrand JF, Zappolo A, Hing E, et al: The National Nursing Home Survey: 1977 Summary for the United States. U.S. National Center for Health Statistics. Vital and Health Statistics, Series 13, No. 43, DHEW Publication No. (PHS) 79-1794, Washington, D.C., U.S. Government Printing Office, 1979. Kramer M: Psychiatric Services and the Changing Institutional Scene, 1950-1985. National Institutes of Mental Health, Series B, No. 12, Washington, D.C., U.S. Government Printing Office, 1977. National Center for Health Statistics: Vital Statistics of the United States: 1975. Vol II. Mortality, Part A. Washington D.C., U.S. Government Printing Office, 1979.

customed to visiting patients there, although there are nearly as many nursing home beds as there are hospital beds in the United States, and the nursing home is where one fifth to one quarter of old people die. A great deal of serious mental illness exists among the elderly in our communities that is not brought to medical attention.[20] The practice of preventive medicine and health promotion is just beginning to be advocated for the aged, in part because these activities have not been reimbursable,[21] and many physicians appear to be unaware of the rehabilitation needs of their patients.[22]

Remedies are required for these deficiencies. Many of these remedies are being actively incorporated into clinical practice. Inquiry into the patient's living arrangements and social resources is increasingly recognized as essential in the present economic climate (Chapter 5). The dangers of polypharmacy and the proper use of drugs in the elderly are being brought to physicians' attention by leading medical journals (Chapter 12).[3] The value of the house call is being rediscovered (Chapter 11), and physicians and medical schools are being called upon to pay more attention to nursing homes (Chapter 10).[24] Important details of the older person's personal life are beginning to receive overdue attention, such as sexual function (Chapter 27), sleep patterns (Chapter 23), dental problems (Chapter 40), and foot problems (Chapter 37). Especially, it is being shown that the physician's scope of understanding of a given patient's problems can be greatly enhanced when he shares information with a professional team (Chapter 3). Although some of the problems alluded to here will require long-term solutions involving public policy and structural social change, there is one further step that must be taken in which physicians are intimately involved, that is, better education in geriatric medicine for future practitioners.

## PHYSICIANS TO THE AGED

A great many physicians practicing today are self-taught geriatricians. Internists in particular have had considerable experience with the aged and have tended to be favorably oriented toward them.[25] According to one estimate, 80 to 85 per cent of the care provided to the elderly is furnished by primary care physicians (i.e., internists, family practitioners, or general practitioners),[26] but medical subspecialists, surgeons, gynecologists, and psychiatrists also have a significant number of the elderly among their patients. Lack of training in geriatrics, affecting most of the current generation of practitioners, and specific recommendations for dealing with this lack were clearly formulated in a 1978 report from the Institute of Medicine.[27] Extended and improved educational content in geriatrics is unmistakably required at all levels, from basic science courses in medical school through residency training and on into continuing medical education.[28] The American Geriatrics Society, the Veterans Administration, and others are developing and offering geriatrics fellowships.[29] Doubts about whether there exists a definable body of relevant knowledge have been resolved, and outlines of curricular content have been provided.[30,31] Several textbooks of geriatric medicine have been published, some of them designed specifically for medical students.[32,33] The issue of whether geriatrics will develop into an autonomous specialty or a certified subspecialty of medicine and family medicine is much debated and is at present unresolved.

Is geriatric medicine simply good medical practice applied to the health problems of the aged? Much evidence, some of it cited previously, indicates that we need more than an extension of what we are doing now. In addition to specialized knowledge, a future physician to the aged will need to develop what amounts to a new set of skills and attitudes.[19] A prime need is to revitalize an old tradition: the perspective of a generalist (see Chapter 6). The accumulated impairments and chronic conditions of the older patient must be seen comprehensively, with due attention to the psychologic and social setting in which they occur. Comprehensiveness does not imply lack of attention to details, but the key details may include variables and measurements that have not been part of traditional medical practice. The physician must have a good basic knowledge of internal medicine, especially as it applies to the aged, and must be aware of the special diseases that afflict the elderly, the atypical presentations of common diseases, the altered physiology of the aged body, and the special requirements of clinical pharmacology in treating the elderly. Expertness will be needed in synthesizing complex sets of information and in the use of functional scales and standardized definitions that permit effective communication of information among various professional workers (see Chapters 8 and 14).[34]

The ideal geriatrician of the future will also have a keen appreciation of the role of the family in resolving the patient's problem, an awareness of such critical factors as the role-reversal experienced by children who have to become parents to their own parents, and a working knowledge of the psychiatry of the aged and of the social, economic, and institutional aspects of old age and the care of the aged. The practitioner must be well endowed with patience, since convalescence is often slow, and the hope for improvement must not be prematurely abandoned. The importance of small gains is salient in geriatrics, since apparently minor improvements, such as relief from painful bunions, the achievement of urinary continence, or training in the use of a walker, may make the difference between staying at home and having to go to a nursing home. The patient must be involved as much as possible in major decisions, and this is easy for the physician to forget, especially when the patient is demented.

Skills that belong to the whole of medical practice assume particular importance with the elderly. These include teamwork with other professionals, continuity of care, and the consistent practice of preventive medicine. Priorities must be established; not every problem on the patient's list can or should be given a thorough diagnostic evaluation, but critical ones may require urgent attention. Unnecessary intervention, whether diagnostic or therapeutic, is often dangerous to a frail old person. Modern medical technology increasingly raises the question of whether to initiate and when to discontinue life-support measures. The physician's traditional function of providing symptomatic relief and comfort during a terminal illness is becoming a more complex task, involving decisions with troubling ethical implications (see Chapter 9). More than ever, wisdom, sound judgment, and compassion will be called for.

Rich rewards in personal satisfaction await the practitioner who approaches his or her elderly patients with respect for their personal dignity and who understands the critical importance of maintaining their independence. The exercise of true professionalism on behalf of the elderly can be one of the most difficult and gratifying accomplishments in the whole of clinical medicine.

## References


1. Kovar MG: Health of the elderly and use of health services. Public Health Rep 92:9, 1977.
   *A basic source of information. Data assembled by the National Center for Health Statistics.*
2. Rosenwaike I, Yaffe N, Sagi PC: The recent decline in mortality of the extreme aged: An analysis of statistical data. Am J Public Health 70:1074, 1980.
3. Fingerhut LA: Changes in Mortality Among the Elderly: United States, 1940–78. National Center for Health Statistics, (PHS) 82-1406, Washington, DC, U.S. Government Printing Office, 1982.
4. Palmore E: Predictors of longevity. *In* Haynes SG, Feinlieb M (eds.): Second Conference on Epidemiology of Aging. NIH Publication No. 80-969, Washington, DC, U.S. Government Printing Office, 1980, pp. 57–64.
5. U.S. General Accounting Office: Survey of Cleveland Elderly, 1975 (unpublished data).
6. U.S. General Accounting Office: Profiles of older people. Washington DC, U.S. Government Printing Office, 1981.
   *A summary report of the 1975–76 surveys of older persons in Cleveland. See also General Accounting Office reports HRD 77-70 (4/19/77), HRD 78-19 (12/30/77), and HRD 79-95 (9/20/79).*
7. Eisdorfer C: Some variables relating to longevity in humans. *In* Ostfeld AM, Gibson DC, Donnelly CP (eds.): Epidemiology of Aging. DHEW Publication No. (NIH) 75-711. Washington DC, U.S. Government Printing Office, 1972, pp. 97–107.
8. Kannel WB: Cardiovascular risk factors in the aged: The Framingham Study. *In* Hayne SG, Feinlieb M (eds.): Second Conference on Epidemiology of Aging. NIH Publication No. 80-969. Washington, DC, U.S. Government Printing Office, 1980, pp. 65–89.
9. Doll R, Peto R: The causes of cancer: Quantitative estimates of avoidable risks of cancer in the United States today. J Natl Cancer Inst 66:1191, 1981.
10. Ford AB: Urban Health in America. New York, Oxford University Press, 1976, p. 79.
11. Zyzanski SJ, Medalie JH, Ford AB, Grava I: Household composition and the well being of the elderly patient (manuscript in preparation).
12. Shanas E: Social myth as hypothesis: The case of the family relations of old people. Gerontologist 19:3, 1979.
13. Vicente L, Wiley JA, Carrington RA: The risk of institutionalization before death. Gerontologist 19:361, 1979.
14. Kastenbaum R, Candy S: The four percent fallacy. Aging Hum Dev 4:15, 1973.
15. Rango N: Nursing-home care in the United States: Prevailing conditions and policy implications. N Engl J Med 307:883, 1982.
16. Williams TF: Clinical and service aspects of geriatric teaching programs. *In* Somers AR, Fabian DR (eds.): The Geriatric Imperative. New York, Appleton-Century-Crofts, 1981, pp. 295–313.
    *The book in which this chapter occurs is an up-to-date collection of essays by experts in a variety of geriatric and gerontologic fields. A stimulating, wide-ranging survey, with an exceptionally diverse set of perspectives. See also reference 21.*
17. Calkins E: Role of Veterans Administration hospitals as bases for academic units in geriatric medicine—a historical perspective. *In* Steel K (ed.): Geriatric Education. Lexington, MA, Collamore Press, 1981, pp. 53–58.
18. Rogers DE, Blendon RJ, Moloney TW: Who needs Medicare? N Engl J Med 307:13, 1982.
19. Williams TF: The physician viewpoint. *In* Haug MR (ed.): Elderly Patients and Their Doctors. New York, Springer Publishing Co., 1981, pp. 42–46.
20. Blazer D: The epidemiology of mental illness in life. *In* Busse EW, Blazer D (eds.): Handbook of Geriatric Psychiatry. New York, Van Nostrand Reinhold Co., 1980, pp. 249–271.
21. Filner B, Williams TF: Health promotion for the elderly: Reducing functional dependency. *In* Somers AR, Fabian DR (eds.): The Geriatric Imperative. New York, Appleton-Century-Crofts, 1981, pp. 187–204.
22. Brogan DR: Rehabilitation service needs: Physicians'

perception and referrals. Arch Phys Med Rehabil 62:215, 1981.

23. Ouslander JG: Drug therapy in the elderly. Ann Intern Med 95:211, 1981.
24. Butler RN: The teaching nursing home. JAMA 245:731, 1981.
25. Ford AB, Liske RE, Ort RS, Denton JC: The Doctor's Perspective: Physicians View Their Patients and Practice. Cleveland, Press of Case Western Reserve University, 1967, pp. 130–133.
26. Kane RL, Solomon DH, Beck JC, et al: Geriatrics in the United States: Manpower projections and training considerations. Rand Report R-2543-HJK. Santa Monica, CA, The Rand Corporation, 1980.
27. Institute of Medicine: Aging and Medical Education. Washington, DC, National Academy of Sciences, 1978.
    *The landmark report of a committee, chaired by Paul B. Beeson, M.D., that stated the need for and gave impetus to the movement toward improved geriatric education.*
28. Steel K (ed.): Geriatric Education. Lexington, MA, Collamore Press, 1981.
29. Robbins AS, Vivell S, Kane R, et al: Geriatric Medicine: An Educational Resource Guide. Cambridge, MA, Ballinger, 1981.
30. Association of American Medical Colleges: Incorporating Geriatric Knowledge in Medical Education Programs. Washington, DC, AAMC, 1983.
31. Robbins AS, Fink A, Kosecoff J, et al: Studies in geriatric education: I. Developing educational objectives. J Am Geriatr Soc 30:281, 1982.
32. Brocklehurst JC, Hanley T: Geriatric Medicine for Students. London and New York, Churchill Livingstone, 1976.
33. Libow LS, Sherman FT (eds.): The Core of Geriatric Medicine: A Guide for Students and Practitioners. St. Louis, CV Mosby, 1981.
34. Kane RA, Kane RL: Assessing the Elderly: A Practical Guide to Measurement. Lexington, MA, Lexington Books, 1981.
    *A basic methodologic handbook that assembles and evaluates most of the scales and instruments currently in use.*

*Chapter 3*

# *The Team Approach in the Elderly*

*Madeline H. Schmitt*

## THE PROBLEM OF TEAM DELIVERY APPROACHES

Because of the scope and complexity of the problems that geriatric patients present, physicians have been encouraged to adopt new conceptual models for diagnosis and management.[1,2] These new models not only demand a broader awareness of the elderly patient and his or her needs but also implicate a host of strategies for care and a demand for resources not usually encompassed in a primary care practice in the United States. One of the strategies commonly proposed for dealing with the elderly person's broad and complex needs is the utilization of a multidisciplinary health care team.[1,3-6] Although definitions of a multidisciplinary team vary, some common elements of the definitions are identifiable. A multidisciplinary team is a small group whose members (1) share common goals, (2) possess the diversity of skills and professional orientations needed to achieve the goals, and (3) coordinate their efforts to provide services to a patient or group of patients through systematic communication.[7]

Although there is a strong commitment reflected in geriatric literature to the "team approach" in the provision of care to geriatric patients in the United States, a variety of problems prevent the easy development of teams in primary care settings. The dilemma of the sensitive primary care physician can probably best be understood by contrasting the situation of the physician in this country with that of the British general practitioner caring for the elderly patient. A practitioner in Great Britain has available "a geriatric consultant, the nurse, the physical therapist, the occupational therapist, and the health visitor who meet regularly to solve patient care problems arising in a defined area."[8] In addition, there are likely to be several varieties of institutional facilities, home care services, and other supports available as needed for individual patients.[8] The process of "attachment" of various health-care personnel to the general practitioner has been encouraged by legislation.[9] Examples of the range of problems of the elderly that concern such teams include basic health needs, such as dental, hearing, and eye care, nutrition, housing and home support services, preventive screening, hazards of multiple drug prescriptions, identification and management of psychiatric illness, and financial problems in maintaining health.[6,10]

One of the key differences between British primary health care and the American system is that of overall organization. Whereas the British system benefits from a centralized organization of primary care services and reimbursement for those services and coordinated utilization of local health care institutions, the American system has been labeled as "not organized,"[8] "disorganized," and "chaotic."[5] A major impediment to the rational organization of primary care services for the elderly is the third-party reimbursement mechanism.[8] Our present reimbursement patterns emphasize institutional, particularly acute, care.[3] Less than one per cent of Medicare and Medicaid budgets are used for home health services.[6] As a consequence, the availability of multidisciplinary personnel outside of institutions and the development of community resources vary enormously from one community to another.[11] This lack of coordinated effort of various disciplines and underdevelopment of community resources are serious problems for the delivery of comprehensive care to the elderly in the United States, since 95 per cent of our elderly population reside in the community at large at any given time. An estimated 10 per cent of these people are in need of long-term home support services.[12] In 1977, the Institute of Medicine of the National Academy of Sciences presented a proposed national plan for the elderly that emphasized the development of programs and services supportive of primary health care of the elderly person in the home setting; rational planning for the utilization of all resources, including institutional ones; and expansion of those institutional resources to include multiple levels of care appropriate to the individual elderly person's needs.[13]

Results of demonstration projects may suggest the effectiveness and potential cost benefits of multidisciplinary teams in meeting the health needs of the elderly in community settings. However, these are not sufficient to bring about lasting changes in health care delivery. A variety of mechanisms for recovering the costs of such services need to be explored. Incorporating such services into third-party reimbursement mechanisms is a difficult issue and requires awareness of the potential benefits by primary care physicians, consumers, and third-party agencies; organized community planning; and political action. Community-based demonstration programs and some services have been developed. A key dimension of these programs and services is that they are frequently organized as multidisciplinary teams.

## TYPES OF TEAM APPROACHES AVAILABLE IN COMMUNITY SETTINGS

### *Home Health Services*

Probably the oldest type of team resource available and familiar to the primary care physician is the community health nurse. These generalist nurses have provided home health care since 1886.[14] Studies in the 1970s demonstrated the impact of home nursing services on the health and well-being of the chronically ill and elderly. In one study,[15] the availability of visiting nurses led to physical and psychologic improvement in a cohort of patients with chronic illness who were not severely ill and disabled. For those who were more severely ill and disabled, the availability of the visiting nurse was associated with the greater use of an array of professional services, reflecting the nurse's "coordinator of care" role. In another study,[16] three combinations of visiting nurse and medical nurse practitioner services were delivered in three high-rise elderly housing units. Those residents involved in the most comprehensive nursing program reported greater increases in positive perceptions of their own health and learned to respond effectively to a dental health screening program, and there was an increase in the numbers of elderly who were under primary care.

Medicare and Medicaid certification requirements have promoted the availability of a more comprehensive array of services in Home Health Agencies. Such services now typically include nursing, physical therapy, visits by home health aides, and speech therapy, and, on a less frequent basis, others.[12,14] These services are coordinated through a team effort.[14] Availability of such services to patients depends on physician referral, and the maintenance of contact between the physician and the rest of the team by way of written and telephone communication is essential to successful delivery of services.

Comparative data utilizing statistics from countries where there is a greatly expanded home care service program and from communities in the United States with a comparable percentage of elderly suggest that the presence of greater amounts of home care services are associated with far less institutional care.[12] In addition, studies are beginning to demonstrate the sizeable cost reductions of such team-based home care strategies compared with institutional care.[12,17]

### *"Channeling" Services*

Channeling refers to organizational devices created in a community to link elderly people in need of services to the appropriate level of services.[17] At a minimum such services involve a comprehensive team evaluation of the needs of the individuals referred. The goal is to maintain people at the appropriate level of care. A pioneer project demonstrating the effectiveness of comprehensive team evaluation is described by Williams and associates.[12,18,19] Only 35 per cent of a group of 315 elderly persons originally headed for nursing homes were placed there, as a result of evaluation efforts. The comprehensive evaluation teams outperformed two other sources of evaluation for the same patients.

Freestanding nonprofit corporations have expanded the channeling concept by assuming responsibility for continued coordination of services as well as evaluation. Again, the principle is to provide the appropriate level and range of services, in the community if at all possible.

TRIAGE, organized to serve a seven-town area in central Connecticut, evaluates need; coordinates medical, mental health, and social services at the institutional, ambulatory, and home care levels; creates new services as needed; and streamlines the reimbursement process. The clinical staff consists of teams composed of a nurse-clinician, and a social worker.[17] Such channeling agencies have had the capability, missing in traditional community resources such as Home Health Agencies, to experiment with the expansion of services needed to maintain someone in a home setting.

### *Alternative Team-Delivered Primary Care Services*

For over 30 years some chronically ill and elderly patients have received their primary care through hospital-based outpatient programs organized around a team approach. In some instances this care was extended into the home.[20] A few early studies provided empirical support for the improvement of care as the result of a team effort.[20] Giorgi[5] provides a description of some of these model programs using the team approach for primary care in medical center settings, such as those existing at Cedar Sinai and Orange County Medical Center in California.

A newer approach has a community-based primary care team going to the patient's home, rather than the patient coming to the hospital for care (see Chapter 11). In an experimental program funded by the National Center for Health Services Research, a team composed of a physician, geriatric nurse practitioner, and social worker provided primary medical care in the home—including 24-hour phone consultations to 81 chronically and terminally ill elderly. Using a randomized control trial design, these patients were compared with a group receiving conventional care. Patients receiving team care had fewer acute hospital days and fewer nursing home days, and patients and family members were both more satisfied with care.[21]

### *Specialized Teams*

Some teams are being developed to respond to special needs of the elderly in the community. An example of a team of this type is the geriatric abuse intervention team. A model team composed of a physician, clinical psychologist, educator, social worker, nurse clinician, and clinical pharmacist is based in the Family Medicine Program at the University of Tennessee.[22] Since physicians often are unlikely to suspect abuse as an etiology,[22] such teams can serve both educational and clinical functions in a community.

## TYPES OF TEAM APPROACHES AVAILABLE IN INSTITUTIONAL SETTINGS

### *Acute Care Settings*

A variety of team approaches have been used to assist the elderly in both acute and long-term care institutions. In the acute care setting rehabilitation teams may provide comprehensive evaluation and treatment for stroke patients and plan for their continuing care needs.[23,24] Gresham[23] points out that standard medical practice has been to give stroke patients a trial period of several weeks in a hospital-based or freestanding medical rehabilitation unit. Currently, many pressures exist to change this practice, and a wider array of alternatives (e.g., skilled nursing facilities, home care, day care), suited to the patient's needs and potential, are being utilized. Comprehensive multidisciplinary team assessment is the key to matching services with patient needs. At least one study has demonstrated the comparative effectiveness of such team approaches for stroke patients.[24]

Unit-based geriatric consultation teams have been formed to help hospital staff to assess needs comprehensively.[25] Such an approach needs to be compared with both the usual care on hospital units and another approach increasingly employed. This is the geriatric evaluation unit. These units admit patients on a relatively short-term basis and provide comprehensive multidisciplinary assessment and treatment, with the goals of maximizing functional ability and minimizing institutional care. An example of the potential of such units is described within the Veterans Administration (VA) system.[26] Data on 74 patients indicated that placement location was improved over expectations for 48 per cent of the patients.

In an attempt to provide an opportunity for multidisciplinary education and simultaneously evaluate the effectiveness of the team approach to geriatric care in the VA institutional setting, in 1979 the VA initiated a system-wide program for interdisciplinary team training and geriatric team care.[27,28] Currently, twelve VA medical centers are sites for this Interdisciplinary Team Training in Geriatrics (ITTG) program.

Even within the specialized setting of a rehabilitation hospital where all patients receive multidisciplinary care, some differential effectiveness has been found by establishing a separate unit staffed with multidisciplinary team with expertise in geriatrics for patients over age 70. In comparing 50 patients treated on such a unit with 50 patients matched by sex, age, and diagnosis treated elsewhere in the hospital and who had similar levels of functioning on admission, significantly more patients on the unit were discharged to a home setting. More of these patients were independent in activities of daily living and ambulation, improved in mental orientation, and continent at discharge than those treated elsewhere in the hospital.[29]

### *Long-Term Care Settings*

There are few reports of the implementation of the team approach in long-term care settings. However, one reported use of physician, nurse, and dietitian teams to deliver care to diabetic patients living in the health-related section of a large chronic care facility. Compared with a randomized control group, over a year's time, patients cared for by the teams showed significantly more positive change and less negative change across a variety of health outcomes encompassing physiologic, physical, social, and emotional function than those cared for in the usual fashion.[30,31]

In England, where case conferences held by multidisciplinary teams in geriatric units are more common and have been studied, problems with the team approach have been identified.[32] Although the approach was observed to work well for those patients for whom the goal was cure or rehabilitation, it was not effective for the majority of long-term patients. In the latter instance, nurses carrying major responsibilities for care did not have the authority for it, and effective team functioning broke down as the physician retreated from problems not manageable by traditional treatment approaches.

In the United States, the absence of teams in long-term care institutions may reflect a similar problem. Nationally, statistics are cited suggesting that only 17 per cent of physicians participate in nursing home care.[33] Although the percentage of participating primary care physicians has been noted to be higher in some areas of the country,[34] nationally, primary care physicians are cited as spending an average of less than 1.5 hours per month in this type of care.[33] Since most of the problems present in long-term care are nursing problems, a proposed solution has been to strengthen the capabilities of nurses. The use of gerontologic nurse clinicians and nurse practitioners working in consultative relationships with physicians could reduce the use of costly acute care services.[33,35,36] In addition, since much of the care in long-term care institutions is provided by aides, any team approach should consider the complex relationship between patients, aides, and professional staff.[37]

## GENERAL CONSIDERATIONS IN WORKING WITH TEAMS

Reports of the use of multidisciplinary teams have shown this to be an effective approach that may be employed by a primary care physician in specific aspects of the comprehensive care of geriatric patients. Many more studies exploring their potential are needed. Such studies should examine a variety of unanswered evaluation and research questions about the nature of teams and their functioning, costs, and acceptability to patients.[38,39] Several classes of variables can affect the productivity of the team approach in specific situations. Bass[40] identifies these as (1) the biographic characteristics of members, (2) the knowledge and skills of the members, (3) the positions of members in the team, (4) the interaction processes, (5) the properties of the team, and (6) the conditions imposed on the team. All these can separately and interactively affect the task performance of individual members and the total team. Few studies to date have examined any of these variables systematically in health care settings. Specific team variables commonly perceived as creating problems for the team delivery of health care are a lack of clarity of roles, lack of clearly defined common goals, inability of some members to communicate their expertise, and disagreements over leadership and the distribution of authority.[14,41-43] Primary care physicians should be aware of these factors affecting productivity in team situations. A variety of techniques have been developed to improve the ability of health professionals to work effectively in teams.[43,44]

For teams to function effectively, each team member's capabilities and responsibilities in relation to specific patient care goals should be explicit. Regular communication should foster awareness and coordination of various team members' efforts and assessment of progress in reaching the goals. The process by which decisions are made and by whom for various aspects of care should be clear. Assignments of responsibility for care and decision-making should be consistent. Identification of someone as coordinator of the team's efforts who understands the mechanics of teamwork is important in maintaining the patient care efforts of the total group.

The relationship between the physician and an existing team, such as an assessment team, a rehabilitation team, or a geriatric abuse team, should be clarified. What services will the team provide? Who is the coordinator of the team's efforts? What regular communication may be expected about the patient? What does the team expect of the physician's involvement while the team's efforts are being carried out? Since the team approach to the care of the elderly in the United States has not been formally "attached" to the primary care physician, the activation of a team approach depends on the physician's knowledge, referral, active involvement, and follow-up. Unless the primary care physician abdicates responsibility, the ultimate authority for the patient's well-being remains with him or her in collaboration with the patient.

Finally, a central aspect of the success of any patient care effort is that it must be patient-centered. The implementation of any plan of care requires agreement on the patient's part that problems important to him or her have been identified and are being dealt with in acceptable ways. The team approach may present some special problems for the elderly individual. Several authors have pointed out that patients may have difficulty relating to multiple providers of health care services.[14,20] It is important, therefore, that the primary care physician orient the patient about what to expect from a team approach and help the patient to understand the benefits of such an approach.

## References


1. Katz S, Papsidero J, Halstead L: Team care and chronic illness: A framework for teaching comprehensive health care. *In* Clark DW, Williams TF (eds.): Teaching of Chronic Illness and Aging. Bethesda, MD, DHEW No. (NIH) 75-876, pp. 45–58.
   *This article offers several models for understanding the comprehensive health care needs of the chronically ill and aging. It also contains an extended discussion of the team approach to managing comprehensive care needs.*
2. Engel GL: The clinical application of the biopsychosocial model. *In* Haug MR (ed.): Elderly Patients and Their Doctors. New York, Springer Publishing Co., 1981, pp. 3–21.
   *Based on systems theory, the biopsychosocial model is presented as an alternative to the biomedical model. Through an extended clinical example, Engel demonstrates how this new model can "extend application of the scientific method" by expanding the range of variables relevant to accurate diagnosis and management.*
3. Somers AR: The geriatric imperative: A major challenge to the health professions. *In* Somers AR, Fabian DR (eds.): The Geriatric Imperative: An Introduction to Gerontology and Clinical Geriatrics. New York, Appleton-Century-Crofts, 1981, pp. 3–19.
4. Butler RN: The national institute on aging. *In* Spieler C (ed.): Care of the Aging. Report of a Macy Conference. New York, Josiah Macy Jr. Foundation, 1978, p. 9.
5. Giorgi EA: Utilizing the health team in the care of the aged. *In* Psychosocial Needs of the Aged: Selected Papers. Los Angeles, University of Southern California, Ethel Percy Andrus Gerontology Center, 1973, pp. 61–66.
6. Sherman FT: Clinical problems in geriatric medicine: A team approach. Allied Health and Behav Sci 2:1, 1979.
7. Kane RA: Interprofessional Teamwork. Syracuse, Syracuse University School of Social Work, Manpower Monograph Number Eight, 1975.
   *This is a widely cited comprehensive and critical review of teams: definition, rationale, dimensions of teams as small groups, descriptive data based on 229 "team" articles, and problems of evaluation of team modalities.*
8. Estes EH Jr: The team context. *In* Haug MR (ed.): Elderly Patients and Their Doctors. New York, Springer Publishing Co., 1981, pp. 132–136.
   *This brief, well-organized chapter examining environmental, organizational, and functional problems discouraging the formation of geriatric teams is part of a unique book on aspects of the relationship between elderly patients and their doctors.*
9. Reedy BLEC: The health team. *In* Fry J (ed.): Trends in General Practice. 2nd ed. London, Royal College of General Practitioners, 1979, pp. 111–141.
10. Shukla RB: The role of the primary care team in the care of the elderly. The Practitioner 225:791, 1981.
11. Ball RM: Rethinking national policy on health care for the elderly. *In* Somers AR, Fabian DR (eds.): The Geriatric Imperative: An Introduction to Gerontology and Clinical Geriatrics. New York, Appleton-Century-Crofts, 1981, pp. 21–38.
12. Williams TF: Clinical and service aspects of geriatric teaching programs. *In* Somers AR, Fabian DR (eds.): The Geriatric Imperative: An Introduction to Gerontology and Clinical Geriatrics. New York, Appleton-Century-Crofts, 1981, pp. 295–313.
    *This review of the role of a team approach in comprehensive assessment of the elderly examines the potential of this approach for maintaining elderly individuals in the community and describes a successful, pioneering project.*
13. The Elderly and Functional Dependence. Washington, DC, Institute of Medicine, National Academy of Sciences, 1977.
14. Pesznecker BL, Paquin R: Implementing interdisciplinary team practice in home care of geriatric clients. J Gerontol Nurs 8:504, 1982.
    *This well-written article describes how home health services are organized and delivered by a team process and examines a variety of problems encountered, including reimbursement issues, patient acceptance, and team procedures.*
15. Katz S, Ford AB, Downs TD, et al: Effects on Continued Care: A Study of Chronic Illness in the Home. Bethesda, MD, National Center for Health Services Research and Development, DHEW No. (HSM) 73-3010, 1972.

16. Sullivan JA, Armignacco F: Effectiveness of a comprehensive health program for the well-elderly by community health nurses. Nurs Res 28:70, 1979.
17. Quinn J, Segal J, Raisz H, Johnson C (eds.): Coordinating Community Services for the Elderly. New York, Springer Publishing Co., 1982.
*This full report is of an innovative program in a community setting that is one of several demonstration projects emphasizing a systems approach to coordinating services to the elderly. It includes a coordinated reimbursement mechanism.*
18. Williams TF, Hill JG, Fairbank MF, et al: Appropriate placement of the chronically ill and aged: A successful approach by evaluation. JAMA 226:1332, 1973.
19. Bentley DW, Williams ME, Williams TF: Assessment of the elderly for long term care. J Am Geriatr Soc 30:71, 1982.
20. Katz S, Halstead L, Wierenga M: A medical perspective of team care. *In* Sherwood S (ed.): Long-term Care: A Handbook for Researchers, Planners and Providers. New York, Spectrum Publications, 1975, pp. 213–252.
*This chapter includes useful sections on the history of team care and elements of team care. It reviews a number of studies focusing on the effectiveness of team care.*
21. Feins ML, Zaenglein N, Groth-Junker A: Interdisciplinary team functioning: Descriptive analysis of a home health care team. *In* Pisaneschi JI (ed.): Proceedings of the Fourth Annual Conference on Interdisciplinary Health Team Care. Lexington, University of Kentucky, 1982, pp. 113–129.
22. Clark CB: Geriatric abuse intervention team. *In* Bachman JE (ed.): Proceedings of the Third Annual Conference on Interdisciplinary Health Team Care. Kalamazoo, Western Michigan University Center for Human Services, 1982, pp. 13–19.
23. Gresham GE: Rehabilitation of the geriatric patient. Primary Care 9:239, 1982.
24. Pendarvis JF, Grinnell RM Jr: The use of a rehabilitation team for stroke patients. Soc Work Health Care 6:77, 1981.
25. Blumenfield S, Morris J, Sherman FT: The geriatric team in the acute care hospital: An educational and consultation modality. J Am Geriatr Soc 30:660, 1982.
26. Rubenstein LZ, Abrass IB, Kane RL: Improved care for patients on a new geriatric evaluation unit. J Am Geriatr Soc 29:531, 1981.
*This is an excellent data-based description of the potential impact of a multidisciplinary geriatric evaluation unit in an acute care setting.*
27. Campbell LJ: Approaches to staff and student interdisciplinary team training on a geriatric evaluation unit. *In* Bachman JE (ed.): Proceedings of the Third Annual Conference on Interdisciplinary Health Team Care. Kalamazoo, Western Michigan University Center for Human Services, 1982, pp. 81–85.
28. Mather JH, Waltraut FD: Veterans Administration's development of health professions education programs in geriatrics and gerontology. *In* Somers AR, Fabian DR (eds.): The Geriatric Imperative: An Introduction to Gerontology and Clinical Geriatrics. New York, Appleton-Century-Crofts, 1981, pp. 329–335.
29. Lefton E, Bonstelle S, Frengley JD: Success with an inpatient geriatric unit: A controlled study of outcome and follow-up. J Am Geriatr Soc 31:149, 1983.
30. Feiger SM, Schmitt MH: Collegiality in interdisciplinary health teams: Its measurement and its effects. Soc Sci Med 13A:217, 1979.
*This study is unusual in examining the impact of team versus usual care in a long-term care institution and, also, in examining the relative effectiveness of four similar multidisciplinary teams working with similar samples of chronically ill diabetics.*
31. Schmitt MH, Watson NM, Feiger SM, Williams TF: Conceptualizing and measuring outcomes of interdisciplinary team care for a group of long-term, chronically ill, institutionalized patients. *In* Bachman JE (ed.): Interdisciplinary Health Care: Proceedings of the Third Annual Conference on Interdisciplinary Team Health Care. Kalamazoo, Western Michigan University Center for Human Services, 1982, pp. 169–181.
32. Evers HK: Multidisciplinary teams in geriatric wards: Myth or reality? J Adv Nurs 6:205, 1981.
*This article reports the results of qualitative research in geriatric wards of several English hospitals. Using case examples, the author illustrates the difference between team rhetoric and effective team practice and speculates on the purposes that team rhetoric may serve.*
33. Mechanic D, Aiken LH: A cooperative agenda for medicine and nursing. N Engl J Med 307:747, 1982.
34. Callen K, Ingman SR, Lower DJ: Physicians' attitudes toward geriatric medical education. Gerontol Geriatr Educ 2:207, 1982.
35. Walsh J, Walsh E: Summary of the conference. *In* Spieler C (ed.): Care of the Aging. Report of a Macy Conference. New York, Josiah Macy Jr. Foundation, 1978, pp. 17–36.
36. Abdellah F: New nurse practitioners and care of the aging. *In* Spieler C (ed.): Care of the Aging. Report of a Macy Conference. New York, Josiah Macy Jr. Foundation, 1978, pp. 37–55.
37. Dawes PL: The nurses' aide and the team approach in the nursing home. J Geriatr Psychiatry 14:265, 1981.
*This article sensitively explores the stereotypes of the nursing home aide, conditions of employment, and anticipated reactions of aides to being included in a team approach to long-term care.*
38. Spitzer WO, Roberts RF: Twelve questions about teams in health services. J Community Health 6:1, 1980.
39. Ducanis AJ, Golin AK: The Interdisciplinary Health Care Team: A Handbook. Germantown, MD, Aspen Systems Corporation, 1979.
*This is presently the only comprehensive text on the multidisciplinary team approach to health care. It incorporates relevant research excellently and is written in a straight-forward manner.*
40. Bass BM: Team productivity and individual member competence. Small Group Behav 11:431, 1980.
*This is a lengthy article to be reserved for the serious reader interested in basic research on teams from a social science perspective.*
41. Bottom WD: Teaming up in geriatrics. Geriatrics 35:106, 1980.
42. Nagi SZ: Teamwork in health care in the U.S.: A sociological perspective. Milbank Mem Fund Q 53:75, 1975.
43. Lister L: Role training for interdisciplinary health teams. Heath Soc Work 7:19, 1982.
44. Rubin IM, Plovnick MS, Fry RE: Improving the Coordination of Care: A Program for Health Team Development. Cambridge, MA, Ballinger Publishing Co., 1975.
*This workbook was developed by social scientists at Massachusetts Institute of Technology, based on their experience training health care teams. It is designed for use by all team members, without the necessity of outside consultants or facilitators.*

## Chapter 4

# Major Clinical Problems in Gerontologic Nursing

*Thelma J. Wells*

The beginning of modern gerontologic nursing can be traced to 1864, when Agnes Jones, a Nightingale-trained nurse, provided radically improved care to the poor, ill, elderly at the Liverpool Infirmary.[1] Progress in the field has paralleled advances in general nursing and geriatric medicine. The following are some highlights, which may provide a useful perspective. The first nursing textbook that focused on the care of the elderly appeared in 1950.[2] Specialization in nursing is at the Master's degree level, and the first such program in gerontologic nursing began in 1966. The American Nurses' Association recognized nursing care of the elderly that same year with the formation of a Geriatric Nursing Practice Division, later renamed Gerontological Nursing Practice in 1976. The field of gerontologic nursing has rapidly expanded in the 1980s, with a proliferation of educational programs, textbooks, and research.[3] In many ways this specialty is coming of age. It is timely that it does so because the care problems are formidable, extensive, and complex. This chapter discusses the major clinical problems in gerontologic nursing: physical dependence, confusion, urinary incontinence, and pressure sores. A broad perspective will be explored with an emphasis on management. Although this chapter focuses on nursing, the problems discussed involve the whole interdisciplinary team. Modern, progressive geriatric care requires the expertise of many professionals and, thus, creates a challenge for communication and understanding across different disciplines (see Chapter 3).

## PHYSICAL DEPENDENCE

Physical dependence has been defined as reliance (on someone else) for support or aid. Blenkner[4] described it as the normal dependency of aging, which is a consequence of numerous physiologic losses, resulting in diminished strength, ability, and energy to perform required and desired activities. Traditional and useful measures of physical dependence focus on function and are described as activities of daily living (ADL): The ability of an individual to perform skills of personal hygiene, dressing, eating, toileting, and often ambulation.

Unpublished data from the 1978 National Health Interview Survey reveal that 1 to 4 per cent of noninstitutionalized individuals 65 years of age and older require help in the following activities: bathing (3 per cent), dressing (4 per cent), eating (1 per cent), and toileting (2 per cent).[5] When only those 85 years of age and older are considered, those requiring assistance increases as follows: bathing (11 per cent), dressing (18 per cent), eating (4 per cent), and toileting (7 per cent). The same source finds that 17 per cent of noninstitutionalized people 65 years of age and older report inability to carry out major activity; this figure increases to 31 per cent if only those 85 years and older are considered. Studies of institutions in which assistance of the elderly is required report the following data: 50 to 94 per cent need help in bathing; 72 to 76 per cent, dressing; 30 to 50 per cent, eating; 55 to 68 per cent, toileting; and 18 to 28 per cent, walking, with 54 to 69 per cent of patients chairfast or bedfast.[6-10] These figures support the statement by the Institute of Medicine that "functional dependency among the elderly is emerging as a critical challenge to our society."[11]*

The need for assistance is not surprising, con-

* The data are intercategory specific and do not distinguish individuals with multiple dependencies across categories.

sidering that 86 per cent of the noninstitutionalized elderly have at least one chronic disease, most commonly arthritis, heart disorders, hypertension, or diabetes.[12] The 1977 National Nursing Home Survey[9] reported the primary diagnosis of patients at last physical examination as follows: Forty per cent had diseases of the circulatory system; 20 per cent, mental disorders and senility without psychosis; 6 per cent, diabetes; 4 per cent, arthritis and rheumatism; 2 per cent, cancer, 2 per cent, hip fractures, and 2 per cent, Parkinson's disease. As expected, the primary reason for care in 78 per cent of patients was poor physical health. Apart from the pervasiveness of chronic disease, with its negative impact on mobility, common decremental changes in perception, notably vision and hearing, add to physical dependence.

## Management Considerations

### *Interdependence*

Progressive geriatric medicine advocates a rehabilitative approach to care, i.e., "management of loss of function with the dual objectives of regaining and maintaining the maximum ability to function and preventing or delaying additional decline."[11] Sometimes a rehabilitative approach yields only the targeted patient goal of independence, and the simplicity of this attitude can lead to conflict between and among patients and professionals. It may be more helpful to conceive of dependence and independence not as opposite ends of a continuum but as unstable behavioral states that fluctuate in a wide variety of circumstances, with "interdependence" best describing the dynamic action. Interdependence refutes an all-or-none philosophy and espouses negotiation and acceptance of the coexistence of dependence (needing another) and independence (self-reliance). It is a useful concept for geriatric medicine because it accommodates changing physical, social, and psychologic states and emphasizes the uniqueness of the individual. Nursing has traditionally used an interdependent mode with patients but has only recently begun to formulate its theoretic basis, developmental patterns, and related clinical problems.

### *Energy*

Energy is the currency of the aged; strength and endurance are its underpinning. As physical debility increases, more energy is necessary just to function, and the individual makes compensatory adjustment, choosing various forms of assistance in order to carry out a personalized selection of required and desired activities. Emphasis should be put on compensation mechanisms that fit the individual's personal preference and life-style. For example, an elderly individual may be able to walk but prefers to use a wheelchair in order to travel a greater distance in less time and have more energy remaining. Although the ability to walk should be maintained, the desire to be more mobile should be respected and a wheelchair provided to permit a wider range of social opportunities.

To determine the true "cost" of an activity, energy should be conceived of as an expenditure over a specific time period. Table 4-1 displays the energy cost per minute in calories and metabolic equivalents (METS) for activities of daily living and several light recreational activities.[13] METS are the customary measure of energy cost. One MET is the amount of oxygen required by a seated person at rest who is not using either his arms or legs, and it equals 3.5 to 4.0 ml of oxygen per kilogram of body weight per minute. Ideally an elderly person with physical dependence should have activities spaced, with rest periods throughout the day, and have flexible availability of assistance relevant to ability and desires. For example, a person may prefer the privacy of self-toileting and wish to use considerable energy in that activity but may receive assistance dressing. Another individual may do best if fed lunch, although able to feed himself or

**Table 4-1.** ENERGY COSTS OF ACTIVITIES OF DAILY LIVING AND OTHER SELECTED ACTIVITIES

| Activity | cal/min | METS* |
|---|---|---|
| Bathing | | |
| Hands and face | 2.5 | 2 |
| Showering | 4.2 | 3.5 |
| Dressing/Undressing | 2.3 | 2 |
| Eating | 1.4 | 1 |
| Toileting | | |
| Bedside commode | 3.6 | 3 |
| Bedpan | 4.7 | 4 |
| Walking | | |
| 2.5 mph | 3.6 | 3 |
| Wheelchair propulsion | 2.4 | 2 |
| Conversation | 1.4 | 1 |
| Sitting painting | 2.0 | 1.5 |
| Playing piano | 2.5 | 2 |

* MET = Metabolic equivalents. 1 MET is the amount of oxygen required by a seated person at rest, who is not using arms or legs (3.5-4.0 ml of oxygen per kilogram of body weight per minute).

herself, in order to use limited energy resources for recreational activities in the afternoon.

Unfortunately, institutional environments do not always consider the individuality of patients and either provide total assistance, thought to be more efficient, or stress self care in ADL to the exclusion of energy use for other endeavors. Professional perspectives can become distorted because of fixed institutional routines, little to no personal information about the patient, or a failure to consider overall functional ability of the patient. For example, patient placement or support discussions often revolve around whether or not the patient has attained a particular skill involved in dressing, often considered an important self-care activity. However, if this skill is not seen in the context of time and other functions, a false assessment occurs. Clearly there is a difference between a patient who can dress himself or herself in 30 minutes and one who takes 3 hours and is too tired afterward to eat lunch. Recall also the proverbial case in which great effort was put into teaching an elderly woman the institution's goal for independence in living, i.e., climbing stairs unassisted. The woman finally attained the skill at considerable cost to all other activity and was discharged to her single-level, elevator-serviced apartment unable to get into either her high, old-fashioned bed or her bathtub.

## *Discomfort and Pain*

Kenshalo,[14] reviewing the literature on sensitivity to pain as a function of age, noted variance in findings but concluded from animal studies that there is diminished perception of pain with advancing years. Geriatricians confirm that often the pain threshold appears to be raised in the elderly, with distressful conditions more easily tolerated among older rather than younger individuals.[15,16] Hodkinson[16] acknowledges that in part this can be due to greater stoicism with age and that memory impairment might impede the recall of pain. However, given these considerations, both he and Agate[15] discuss the great difficulty that most elderly people have in accurately describing pain, noting that it is rare to have a clear account correlated with specific activities. This difficulty is compounded among those elderly with cognitive impairment or multiple potentially painful conditions.

Part of the difficulty with understanding pain perception in the elderly may arise as a result of the clinician's own experience with acute rather than chronic pain. Acute pain is time-limited and arises directly from a known stimulus, e.g., a wound. Chronic pain has no time frame; it continually recurs or persists at various levels of intensity. The source of chronic pain is usually not specific or readily observable.[17] The multiple disease states affecting the elderly can account for numerous potential sources of chronic pain. In addition, immobility either as a result of physical dependence or restriction of behavior can cause painful conditions such as stiff or contracted joints, osteoporosis, and skin pressure areas.[18] Multiple foot problems, including toenail conditions, bunions, corns, plantar warts, and shortened Achilles tendons, may make walking painful even without musculoskeletal disease. Patients with hemiplegia or general weakness may develop shoulder subluxation, as a result of inappropriate assistance from well-meaning helpers. These and numerous other circumstances create continuing potential sources of painful conditions in older people.

Pain in the elderly can increase physical dependence, cause sleeplessness and fatigue, or be camouflaged as combativeness or noncooperation, withdrawal, or depression. It is probable that hypnotics, sedatives, and tranquilizers are often given for behavior that actually arises from pain. An assumption of some degree of underlying chronic pain in most elderly patients with physical dependence is helpful in the approach to management. A limited trial course of analgesics, taking into consideration underlying disease and present behavior, may yield an improvement in many areas of function and warrant regular use of such medication and, when appropriate, discontinuance of mood or consciousness-altering drugs.

## *Falls*

A common concern among elderly people is that of sustaining a fall. Community studies confirm that the incidence of falls does increase with age.[19,20] Several age-related physiologic changes may account for this finding, such as loss of perception, musculoskeletal dysfunction, and increased postural sway.[21–23] However, recurrent falls are symptomatic of a wide variety of possible underlying conditions, such as diabetes, myocardial or cerebral dysfunction, Parkinson's disease, and various neurologic disorders.[16,24] Thus, every fall should be followed by a careful history and physical examination.

Among the institutionalized elderly, the high percentage described as chairfast may be the consequence of staff concern for safety rather than recognition of actual loss of ambulatory ability. Retrospective studies of institutional incident reports reveal that fall rates of elderly patients vary from 12 to 24 per month, 422 per 1000 patients, and 42.7 per 10,000 patient days.[25-28] Interestingly, only a minor percentage of falls (1.6 to 3.2 per cent) resulted in fractures. However, the fear of injury to patients and the concern of possible litigation may act to significantly deter adequate efforts at mobility and promote excessive use of restraints. Ironically, standard safety measures do not necessarily prevent falls among the old. Walshe and Rosen[26] studied falls from bed and found that 51 per cent had occurred when both side rails were up and 13 per cent when a posey restraint was on the patient. Foerster[29] analyzed falls prospectively in a setting characterized by a vigorous ambulation program, e.g., periods for marching around the halls to music and a policy that limited the use of restraints. One hundred and fifty-eight elderly nursing home residents who were able to walk without staff assistance were followed, and 25 per cent fell a total of 105 times in the 10-week study period. Those who fell were 75 years of age and older and were likely to fall more than once. However, only 39 per cent of falls resulted in injury and all injuries were minor, e.g., "reddened area."

It seems reasonable to suspect that there might be fewer falls among the institutionalized if patients were not trying to struggle out of cloth restraints or barrier chairs and were encouraged to ambulate as possible in supervised situations. Patients with ambulatory ability who are apt to arise from bed at night should have beds that are close to the floor and without side rails. Clearly, use of consciousness-altering drugs should be as limited as possible. Restricting a patient's mobility through chemical or mechanical restraint is a serious infringement of human rights and is too seldom challenged in institutional settings. Its consequences may be more grave than the falls it aims to prevent, e.g., incontinence, pressure sores, and greater physical dependence.

## *Environment*

Filled with people, objects, and defined spaces, the environment itself may greatly affect patient outcome.

### People

Most nursing personnel in the long-term care environment are not registered nurses. The United States Special Committee on Aging[30] reported that only 7 per cent of nursing home staff were licensed at the level of registered nurse. The most common employees in such settings are nursing helpers (e.g., aides, orderlies) who have little to no education in nursing. They are necessary workers who perform useful assistance by doing a variety of tasks. Unfortunately, there is a tendency outside of nursing to endow these workers with abilities that they do not have. Unprepared and unsupervised helpers can easily retard or destroy rehabilitation goals of patients. Nursing care of the elderly should be planned, directed, and evaluated by a registered nurse who appropriately teaches and models quality care by demonstration of her clinical practice skills in direct patient care activities. Ideally, this registered nurse should have theoretic knowledge about aging and clinical experience with older patients.

### Objects

The objects surrounding a nurse ought to help her to provide care, but this is frequently not the case. Although it may appear impossible that anyone would expect another to do a complex job without adequate or sufficient tools, this is the unfortunate situation for many nurses caring for the physically dependent elderly. Nursing education has tended to foster a "make do," noncomplaining attitude and often does not directly teach about equipment and furniture. It is assumed that all nursing care environments are superbly equipped with well-functioning items, which the nurse intuitively knows how to use. In reality, many nursing care environments lack requisite basic equipment and furnishings.

Table 4–2 presents selected guidelines for the use of basic equipment and furniture in long-

**Table 4–2.** SELECTED GUIDELINES FOR EQUIPMENT AND FURNITURE FOR LONG-TERM CARE PATIENTS

| Item | Recommendation |
|---|---|
| Beds | Adjustable |
| Chairs | Height 14–21 in.* |
| | Average height 16 in.* |
| | Arms that come fully forward |
| | A variety of models |
| | A minimum of one easy chair per bed plus a dining or work area chair |
| Commodes | One for every two beds beyond 40 ft from a toilet |
| Overbed tables | One per bed |
| | Cantilever model |
| Bedside tables | One per bed |
| | Height 4–6 in. above top of mattress |

* Height based on patients wearing 1-in.-heel shoes.

term patient care. Fundamental design principles stress comfort and safety; for example, in a seated position one's feet should be flat on the floor with a 90- to 100-degree angle of knee flexion. Thus, lower leg or popliteal length determines the appropriate height of a seat. The depth of a seat is determined by upper leg length (knee to slightly beyond the greater trochanter), with hip flexion between 90- and 110-degrees. All dimensions of furniture are based on average body measures applicable to specific use. The most recent anthropometric data for the United States were compiled in 1962.[31] Relevant subset data for lower leg length rounded to the closest inch, plus one inch for heels of shoes, range from 11 to 19 in. for women (average 15 in.) and from 15 to 21 in. for men (average 17 in.).

**Beds.** The typical modern commercial bed is 18- to 19-in. high at mattress level, but many elderly people have considerably higher beds, reflecting older bed styles or box spring and multiple mattress use. Nonadjustable hospital beds vary in fixed height but are usually at least 23 in. Modern adjustable-height hospital beds often do not lower sufficiently for older individuals to sit with their feet flat on the floor. Thus, in general, the height of the bed is too great for safe and comfortable use by older people. Also, alternating pressure devices or other bed surface equipment can increase the functional height of the bed.

Beds for physically dependent individuals serve as work areas for care providers who find it best if bed height is at a table-surface level. Historically, patients with physical dependence seldom left their beds, and the tradition of fixed-height hospital beds was formed to facilitate the activities of nurses. In more recent times, an emphasis has been placed on patient self-care, with the result that beds are sometimes fixed low, at patient-comfort levels. In long-term care nursing environments, there is no substitute for or better item of equipment than an adjustable-height bed. Its height should range from a low height, based on elderly lower-leg length, to a high height, based on parallel alignment with hospital stretchers for patient transfer.

**Chairs.** Chairs and wheelchairs in long-term care nursing institutions are typically of one design; this would not be problematic if patients had a single, uniform functional ability. In practice, however, one notes chair-footstool use or dangling, edematous feet (seat too high); the use of extra pillows between the patient and the back of the chair or restraints to prevent forward sliding (seat too long); and the need for team efforts to extract a patient from a chair (seat too low and angled back). Chairs are often the underlying cause of falls, foot and leg circulatory problems, pressure sores, contractions, and various increased dependence needs.

In selecting a chair, the uses to which the chair will be put and the dimensions and needs of the user should be considered. Chairs in long-term care settings are used primarily for dining or other table work activity or for extended periods of relaxed sitting. Basic principles apply to both, but the following list of major design requirements was developed specifically for easy chairs[32]: Desirable chair features include sturdiness, durability, stability, back height that supports the head and shoulders, closed arm sides with padded arms that come fully forward, comfortable seat height, no cross rail behind the front legs, and fabric coated with polyvinyl chloride to ease cleaning. Unfortunately, there has not been either a comprehensive cataloguing or a comparative testing of chairs for the elderly in the United States. Thus, institutions have to develop their own sources and evaluation processes. By involving all staff, including cleaning personnel, in addition to patients, a selection of potentially suitable chairs can undergo user trial, after which a variety of preferred chairs will be selected for more frequent purchase.

Since it is seldom possible to anticipate all potential needs or the correct balance of suitable chairs matched to appropriate patients, a central chair pool can be developed to hold a small surplus of the standard chair mix as well as selected special chairs. Special chairs have less generalized use but serve specific therapeutic functions. Several will be discussed to illustrate the range of chairs available. A combination chair, often called a "geri" or geriatric chair, attempts to be multipurpose by providing a removable tray table surface, adjustable back and leg support, and staff-dependent mobility (leg casters). Such a chair is suitable for the very frail, dependent person who cannot walk. Assisted rise chairs are spring-loaded, hydraulic, or electric units that are adjusted for the individual patient's use. In these chairs, the activated cushion lifts forward to slide the patient to his or her feet; this is especially helpful for those with arthritis. A bean bag chair (loose polyvinyl chloride material filled with polystyrene beads) has been found to be very useful for either contracted or frail geropsychiatric patients. This chair is very low unless supported on a frame.[33]

**Commodes.** Commodes are toilet substitutes that can be fully mobile, with four wheels; partially mobile, with two rear wheels; or fixed, with no wheels. A mobile commode facilitates transport from patient to patient but engenders some safety hazard because braking mechanisms seldom secure it. Fixed commodes have fewer safety hazards but must be carried from patient to patient; they are best kept at a bedside. Lightweight models of commodes provide ease in maneuverability but are not suitable for large, immobile patients, for whom wooden commodes are safer. Variation in commode features include padded and nonpadded seat and arms, removable arms, and bucket/bedpan receptacle; some are designed to be stackable, to fold, or to convert to chairs or to be adjustable in height. It is suggested that in patient units without in-room toilets, one commode should be available for every two beds beyond 40 feet from communal toilets.[34] Even with in-room toilets, a supply of commodes is still needed for those patients who have severely limited mobility or the need for frequent, sudden nighttime voiding.

**Overbed Tables and Bedside Tables.** Although to many, overbed and bedside tables are standard unit furnishings, long-term nursing care wards have sometimes been denied these necessities or use discarded, frequently broken models rejected by other wards.

## SPACE

Space can be a barrier or facilitator to both patients and nurses. Too little space fosters dependence and immobility because it bars self-help equipment and requires that major communal service activities, such as food and supply transport, be given high priority rather than individual mobilizing functions. Too much space may isolate patients and result in large energy expenditure of patients and staff to meet simple needs. Minimum space requirements for long-term care or other health-providing facilities are set by a variety of local, state, and federal agencies. Unfortunately, the tendency has been to accept minimum standards as definitive, with little effort directed toward optimizing the environment. Table 4–3 provides recommendations for space utilization that stress increased space needs in problematic areas.

**Bed Areas.** Whether there should be single-bed rooms or multiple-bed rooms is frequently an issue. Desire for privacy and the establishment of one's visually bounded personal space often make single rooms most popular. For patients requiring frequent observation, it is useful for several single units to be situated in front of or close to the central nursing position. Couples or individuals seeking companionship usually prefer double rooms. Multibed units can also be useful for cognitively impaired individuals who can be more self-supporting in a group-guided setting. A common design error is underestimation of the amount of space needed for the equipment for the physically dependent. For example, walking frames, wheelchairs, specialized geriatric chairs, and commodes all require considerable space and cannot or will not be used in crowded areas because they demand constant path clearing and other manipulation of furnishings.

**Table 4–3.** SPACE UTILIZATION: RECOMMENDATIONS AND CONSIDERATIONS

| | |
|---|---|
| Bed areas | Consider needs for direct nurse observation and physical dependence aides |
| Toilet areas | Cubicle area: 6 ft. 7 in. by 4 ft. 11 in.<br>Location: in room or not more than 40 ft. from patient areas<br>Design: outward opening door and wall grab bars or other supportive aid |
| Bathing equipment | A selection of options (e.g., free-standing bath tub, shower, cabinet bath) |
| Storage areas | Additional space frequently needed, e.g., for clothing owned by patients (coats, dresses, etc.), high disposable product utilization, active mobility regimens with high wheelchair and walking frame use |
| Nurse functions | Teaching area for ward staff<br>Conference room for families |

**Toilet Areas.** In *Designing for the Disabled,* Goldsmith[35] states that the standard small toilet (5 ft 7 in. × 4 ft 7 in.) allows only lateral or oblique wheelchair transfer and does not provide adequate space for assistance by an attendant. He recommends a cubicle area of 6 ft 7 in. by 4 ft × 11 in., which permits lateral, frontal, or oblique wheelchair transfer plus adequate space for an attendant. This larger cubicle also provides the turning circle required by a person who uses a walking frame. Toilet doors that open outward allow more cubicle room for function. An ideal toilet door would have a weighted, gravity-assisted close mechanism because many people with walking aides and a sense of urgency cannot take time to turn and close toilet doors. Grab rails are essential, and other assistive structures are useful; several additional publications provide advice.[36,37] The standard toilet seat is 16 in. high, too low for many older individuals with arthritic hips who experience difficulty rising from the toilet. Plastic or metal toilet seat inserts are available that can raise seat height up to 20 in.

**Bathing Equipment.** Since each patient presents with a variety of dysfunctions and preferences, methods of bathing should be tailored to suit the individual. Few institutionalized elderly people require a bed bath and most appear to prefer the familiar tub bath. Bath tubs should be available for both patient-assisted transfer, using a bath board or seat, and dependent transfer, using hydraulic, crank, or electric assistive devices. Bath tubs used for those requiring bathing assistance must be at a comfortable work level for the nurse (bath rim 31 to 32 in.). Showers with a hand-held spray provide a helpful cleaning option, especially for chairfast incontinent patients. Care must be taken with drainage, i.e., the stall must be adequately angled to control water volume but not so sharply angled as to cause danger in use. If nursing assistance is needed for showering, staff members must be provided with suitable shoe coverings and protective clothing. Development in design of bathing equipment has yielded a variety of innovative products that offer considerable help in bathing the physically frail or dependent. Correctly using new devices in clinical practice requires careful consideration of patient needs and staff behaviors. In-service education on the use of a new product combined with a guided utilization framework is essential.

**Storage Areas.** Availability of ward level storage depends on overall facility storage space, supply turnover, and ward servicing. Traditionally, ward storage space is inadequate even with an ideal support environment. Various new equipment/product items and progressive rehabilitation programs incidently utilize considerable space.

**Nurse Functions.** In-service on-ward education programs are major needs in long-term care facilities. Basic teaching is not facilitated in noisy work areas. Nursing staff members require a quiet staff teaching area on every unit, with space for resource material and learning aids. Family members are important participants in long-term care. Communication needs are frequent and often not best done in corridors or at the bedside. A family conference room provides privacy and can also be used for quiet communication or teaching sessions with residents from multi-bed units.

**Table 4–4.** ADDITIONAL ENVIRONMENTAL FACTORS

| Item | Recommendations | Considerations |
|---|---|---|
| Lighting | Increase illumination | Self-management ideal<br>Keep toilets and corridors well lighted |
| | Avoid glare | Tinted glass<br>Flexible window shading<br>No gloss floors |
| Color | Careful use of blue, green, and purple | Use bright contrast, e.g., orange or yellow next to blue hued shades |
| | Use colored lines or symbols for location guides | Symbol size adequate and at wheelchair viewing level |
| Sound | Reduce work noise | Carpeting reduces sound but increases mobility friction |
| | Provide listening aids for TV and radio for the hard of hearing | Self-management ideal |
| | Avoid amplified, continuous background noise (music) | Self-management ideal |

## Additional Factors

Table 4–4 notes several additional environmental factors that must be considered. Fozard and associates[38] reviewed visual perception and communication in the aged and concluded that determining suitable levels of illumination for a variety of elderly people for a variety of activities was probably the single most difficult environmental design problem. In general, older people require more illumination than younger people, but there is individual variation. Providing standard lighting for total areas but individual control of lighting for specific tasks is the best arrangement. Thus, long-term care settings should have numerous adjustable individual lamps and dimmer/brightener wall switches.

Glare is not tolerated well by older people, and the typical multi-glass, highly glossed modern environment is perceptually dysfunctional. Tinted glass and flexible window shading allow for visual enjoyment with reduced glare. Highly polished floor surfaces reflect overhead light and create visual distortion for old people. No known health code requires highly buffed floors, and the practice should be stopped.

The lens of the eye yellows with age and in so doing tends to filter out the blue-green end of the color spectrum. As a result, discrimination of these colors is more difficult for older people.[38] Therefore, it is hazardous to carpet stairs used by older persons with blue-green surfaces because step boundaries may not be perceived. If such colors are used in decoration, it is best to offset them with brightly contrasting colors. Color can also be a helpful guide to locations, e.g., "follow the red line to the dining room."

Although long-term care environments should not be hushed and tranquil, excessive noise is tiring to patients and staff and distracts from activities that demand concentration. Carpeting reduces noise and looks nice but requires a good cleaning method and creates more friction for moving surfaces, making self-propelling a wheelchair require more energy and contributing to tripping among patients able to walk. Inexpensive listening devices can be provided for the hard of hearing who enjoy radio and television. Devices are available from the telephone company to aid those who are hard of hearing. Continuous public address systems or loud radio background music violates the individual's freedom to choose listening matter and serves to distract from communication.

## CONFUSION—THE NURSING PERSPECTIVE*

### *Negative Labeling*

An individual is thought to be confused when his or her behavior or speech seems to be inappropriate. We are usually surprised or puzzled if we perceive confusion in another individual and we quickly act to resolve the difficulty and realign our communication. However, this pattern is often not followed in communication with an older person; negative stereotyping may persuade the listener that what appears to be inappropriate is acceptable, being consistent with typical cognitive dysfunction in the old. The listener labels the older individual "confused" but does not evaluate the actual circumstance that appeared to be inappropriate. Yet the first principle when encountering seemingly inappropriate behavior or speech is to assume that the listener is confused until proved otherwise. It is critical that the listener relate his or her confusion to the interactant and seek the interactant's help in resolving the difficulty. Most often the listener has misunderstood because vocabulary, cultural variance, regional dialect, speech patterns, and complex ideas combine to make communication a difficult process. The older individual, like any individual, deserves the assumption that he or she is not cognitively impaired even though what he or she says puzzles the listener. To label someone "confused" is to discredit him or her at the most fundamental level.

In addition to negative stereotyping, loss of perception and various stressors also result in old people being labeled "confused." Both visual and auditory acuity have been found to correlate with mental status measures in the institutionalized old.[39,40] This is a logical finding in that sensory input is essential for time orientation. Illness, requiring a visit to strangers in a strange setting, or overall physical frailty, requiring a move to a place where assisted care is provided, acts as a significant stress to further distort communication. Thus, the elderly may misunderstand or misinterpret the environment. Such situations can be reduced by the following actions: (1) Maximize perceptual ability through the use of appropriate devices, such as eyeglasses and hearing aids; (2) keep these devices in working order, e.g., clean eyeglasses, fresh battery in hearing aid; (3) practice good communication techniques, e.g., face the individual when speaking, enunciate clearly; and (4) utilize patient self-pacing for communication input. Self-pacing is a communication process in which the listener is allowed sufficient time to comprehend a message and respond to it before additional messages are sent, and the rate of communication is controlled by the patient.[41] In the often hectic institutional atmosphere, communication is usually dominated by a hurried provider who overloads the patient with rapid, multiple questions or directions. A slower, patient-controlled process is frequently more efficient and more productive.

### *Definition and Prevalence of Confusion*

Stereotyping and perceptual distortion can lead to negative attitudes on the part of relatives and staff and to inaccurate labeling of the behavior of older people. These aspects aside, there is a condition described as confusion. Wolanin and Phillips recognize the difficulty in defining this term but provide a working definition of confusion as "a condition characterized by the client's disorientation to time and place, incongruous conceptual boundaries, paranormal awareness, and seemingly inappropriate verbal statements that indicate memory defects."[42] Various studies yield figures that highlight the frequency of confusion or mental dysfunction in the institutionalized old. The 1977 National Nursing Home Survey[9] found that 20 per cent of patients were diagnosed as having mental disorders and "senility." A prior nursing home survey described 54 per cent of patients as being disoriented and 41 per cent as having inappropriate behavior.[8] Previously noted British studies of long-term care found that nursing staff de-

* See also Chapter 20.

scribed between 18 and 46 per cent of patients as confused.

### *Management of Confusion*

Brocklehurst and Hanley[43] stress that mental confusion is not a diagnosis or disease entity but is a disturbance of cerebral function. Two types of confusion are typically distinguished: (1) acute, symptomatic, or reversible confusion, characterized by fairly rapid onset and often associated with an acute physical illness, an unstable or undetected chronic condition, or drug therapy, and (2) chronic brain failure or irreversible confusion, characterized by gradual onset and continuing progressive functional loss (see Chapter 20).[16] Obviously, the management of the chronically confused will be more difficult if a superimposed acute confusional state exists as well. Numerous physiologic disturbances can cause temporary cerebral dysfunction in the old; these commonly include infections, hypovolemia, electrolyte alterations, hypoglycemia, anemia, drug interactions, or adverse reactions to drugs. When the underlying disorder is detected and treatment begun, the confusion typically clears. It is critical that the nursing staff evaluate baseline mental function in older people and are alert to changes. Careful attention to adequate fluids and nutrition, with appropriate health monitoring and drug therapy overview, may prevent or more readily yield appropriate response to acute confusional states.

Depression is considered the most common affective disorder and its incidence rises with age (see Chapter 17). Its symptoms can mimic confusion, especially the chronic type.[44] It is a reasonable assumption that many elderly people confined to a nursing home are depressed and grieving over multiple losses. Such behavior can manifest as dysfunctional apathetic disinterest or as aggressive anger. Nurses must be careful observers to distinguish the sources of dysfunctional behavior in the old. Various nurse actions can prevent or alleviate emotional stress and, in conjunction with appropriate referral, reduce or manage depression in the elderly.

Chronic confusion is a consequence of progressive cerebral deterioration; combined with physical dependence, it creates the most demanding of all nursing care situations. Little study has been directed toward this complex care group. Until recently, nursing literature was surprisingly unhelpful in suggestions for management of chronic confusion. However, texts by Burnside[44] and by Wolanin and Phillips[42] offer considerable, helpful advice. Architectural interest has been directed toward designing environments more supportive of the confused elderly, and these environments hold promise to facilitate management.[45] Placement of chronically confused elderly in a nursing home has always engendered discussion about issues of segregation versus integration. Interestingly, a study by Wiltzius and associates[46] found that placing mentally incompetent patients with those who were mentally competent significantly reduced the mental and emotional status of the latter.

## URINARY INCONTINENCE—THE NURSING PERSPECTIVE*

### *Definition and Prevalence*

The International Continence Society defines incontinence as "a condition where involuntary loss of urine is a social or hygienic problem and is objectively demonstrable."[47] Recent studies indicate that the prevalence of urinary incontinence is about one in ten among community elderly and about one in two among the institutionalized elderly.[48]

Although this clinical problem is well known to those who nurse the elderly, very little has been done for its resolution or reduction. A sense of hopelessness often pervades those who care for the old. Convinced that all age changes are decremental and irreversible, they believe it is kinder to clean elderly wet patients rather than expect or strive for urinary continence by elderly patients. It is typical to find unquestioning acceptance of urinary incontinence, with a concomitant "change" routine, that is, a repetitive exchange of wet pads or diapers for dry. Ignorance is the common denominator of this unhelpful behavior. It should be noted that a chapter on urinary incontinence in the elderly did not appear in a nursing textbook until 1979.[49]

### *Management of Urinary Incontinence*

Various physiologic, psychosocial, and environmental factors can act as barriers to urine control in the elderly. Positive findings in one or more of these can cause a temporary inconti-

* See Chapter 33.

nence or worsen an underlying urologic disorder.

### Physiologic Factors

Urinary tract infections are a common finding in elderly living in the community and especially in the institutionalized old, often presenting without typical symptoms.[50-52] A clean-catch, midstream urine is used in the standard diagnostic test. Care should be taken with specimen collection. Skin cleansing with a material oversaturated with antiseptic or other cleaning agent can leave excess solution on the skin, which falls into the collecting container, altering the subsequent urine specimen. Damp cleaning materials, applied with a firm mechanical action (front to back), provide the most satisfactory cleansing approach. Patients receiving morning diuretics should provide urine specimens after the first morning void but before lunch. The nurse should assist the frail or mentally confused elderly, or do the necessary skin cleansing and hold the container. This can be an extremely difficult, if not impossible, task in uncooperative patients. Occasionally, in such cases, cleansing followed by use of a commode-held sterile container yields a fairly satisfactory specimen. However, catheterization is often the only reasonable means to obtain an appropriate urine sample, risks being outweighed by specimen need and improbability of patient cooperation. Because of the importance of this diagnostic test and the often great effort needed to obtain a satisfactory specimen, staff members must stress the requirement of immediate specimen refrigeration or laboratory analysis.

Fecal impaction or severe constipation can cause obstruction to urine outflow at the bladder neck, as firm stool exerts pressure across soft tissue. In such cases, examination of the abdomen will reveal a distended bladder, and the rectum will contain a large volume of firm stool. History usually includes dribbling urinary incontinence, infrequent bowel movements, and sometimes the presence of a watery, mucus-laden diarrhea. Once the wedge or volume of firm stool is removed, the bladder spontaneously empties.

The direct or side effect of numerous drugs has an impact on urinary control. It is essential that patients explain exactly how they take medications because error is not infrequent, e.g., diuretics may be taken more often than prescribed or at incorrect times. Patients may still be taking urologic drugs prescribed correctly for a short-term episode in the distant past. Drugs that act on the central nervous system, on cholinergic or adrenergic receptors, or directly on smooth muscle can affect urine control. Bissada and Finkbeiner[53] reviewed nonurologic drugs that affect the lower urinary tract and included the following that are frequently used in the elderly: levodopa (outlet obstruction), phenothiazines (difficulty voiding or retention), and tricyclic antidepressants (retention). Hypnotics, sedatives, and tranquilizers can cause incontinence because they alter conscious bladder inhibition and decrease attention to bladder cues. Many over-the-counter medications contain drugs that can affect urination; for example, phenylpropanolamine hydrochloride, a common ingredient in nasal and sinus preparations, can cause voiding difficulties or retention.

### Psychosocial Factors

The lack of personal assistance or positive attitudes in helpers may be the most frequent psychosocial cause of urinary incontinence in the elderly. The need for help in toileting, discussed earlier, in combination with urge symptomatology almost always results in incontinence. Assistance may not be available at the moment the urge is felt, delay time is short, and mobility may be slow even with help. Frequent failed attempts to get to the toilet or commode in time may create a sense of hopelessness for both the older person and the helpers. Subsequently, padding or a diaper is used, incontinence is accepted, and no serious toileting effort is attempted.

It seems reasonable that if urine control requires considerable conscious attention in the elderly, anything disrupting that attention, such as reaction to a significant irreplaceable loss, might result in urine control difficulty. Sutherland[54] also notes the following possible psychosocial etiologies: regression, dependency, rebellion, insecurity, attention-seeking, sensory deprivation, the vulnerability of the bladder for symptom selection, and disturbance of conditioned reflexes, i.e., paradoxical behavior with the individual emptying the bladder on the wrong stimulus.

Patients with chronic confusion, such as in Alzheimer's disease, eventually present with established urinary incontinence. Initially, such individuals may have difficulty anticipating bladder needs and prophylactically toileting. Later, there may be difficulty locating the toilet or in remembering how to correctly respond to bladder cues. In addition to cognitive impairment, urge incontinence (uninhibited neurogenic bladder) may be present, decreasing voiding delay time.[55]

Techniques of behavior modification and habit training have been tried with mixed response in the management of urinary incontinence in the elderly.[56] Behavior modification is an educative process, with social or material reinforcement of correct behavior; habit training is a process of discovering a patient's voiding pattern and establishing a regular toilet visit at the patient's usual voiding time. Small sample size, little replication, and significant methodologic problems have precluded adequate evaluation of these techniques thus far.

#### Environmental Factors

Environmental needs discussed in the section on physical dependence (Tables 4–2 to 4–4) are germane for urine control management. Recognizing bladder signals and responding appropriately in time requires energy and mobility, especially if the bladder relays its signals often or gives little warning before imperative emptying. Toilets that are close to patient areas, have ample cubicle space, and, if in communal areas, are clearly labeled are most helpful. Chairs from which patients can easily rise or that assist standing are required to promote self-toileting behaviors. Clothing should be such that it facilitates toilet use, e.g., skirts for women, overlap flies for men.

Toilet aids and alternatives provide a variety of flexible options. Since many older people have stiff or painful hips, the standard 16-in. toilet seat may be too low for comfort. Plastic or metal toilet seat inserts can be obtained from supply companies to raise toilet seat height to 20 in. Commodes allow for bedside voiding when even a short distance to the toilet is too far to travel. There are at least three significantly different designs of bed pans, with the shovel model particularly useful. Commonly called a "fracture pan," it requires minimal hip flexion for use and comes in both large and small sizes. There are both male and female urinals; the latter are less well known but are available with a wide or narrow mouth. Selection of a urinal for either sex requires special attention to urinal neck angle for ease of voiding without run back and handle design for use with potentially weak or arthritic hands.

#### Protective Garments and Devices for Management of Urinary Incontinence

In the past several years, great progress has been made in protective garments, pads, and devices for the management of urinary wetting in adults. Protective garments are designed as either diapers or pants. Numerous diaper products are available. These come in either disposable or washable forms and vary in size, closure, and urine containment capacity. Diapers are useful for contracted or bedfast patients and those with fecal incontinence. For the ambulatory, individual protective pants are usually the more suitable choice. These garments are all washable, with disposable pads, and vary by size, pant material, degree of pad absorbency, and color, model (male/female). Other optional design features include flushable pads and separation of skin from urine containment. Protective pads are also either washable[57] or disposable, with the latter more commonly found. Disposable pads, commonly thought to be similar, actually vary in a number of important features. There are a range of sizes available with the larger usually more suitable. Polypropylene backing material is preferred in pads because it is heat resistant and thus not likely to damage a clothes dryer if not separated from bed linen during washing. Pad backing may also be smooth or raised (embossed), with the latter more likely to stay in place over sheets. Pad-absorbent surfaces are of various compositions; the synthetic fiber (nonwoven) hydrophobic cover is most popular as it tends not to adhere to skin and passes urine through it to give a "dry to the touch" surface. The fill in pads differs by amount and composition; polymers ("gelling effect") usually provide greater absorbency and less squeeze back of urine.

Devices used in management of urinary continence consist of those that occlude and those that collect. Penile clamps are appropriate for some male patients but require mental competence and adequate hand function. Female occluding devices are not generally available in the United States. External urinary collecting devices have had the most use with males. Partially molded condoms attached with an elastic foam, Velcro adjustable strap are least likely to twist, split, detach, or impede penile blood flow. Female external devices have been unsuccessful in the past, but recent developments may be more useful. Internal catheter drainage is a suitable management technique for urologic disorders that are characterized by retention, for extensive pressure sores, or as a means to improve the quality of patient life when other management techniques prove unhelpful or undesirable.

## PRESSURE SORES

### *Definition, Prevalence, and Incidence*

Pressure sore is the more accepted term for what has been called bed sore or decubitus (from the Latin term "decumbere," to lie down). Characterized by an area of damaged tissue overlying a bony prominence, a pressure sore can be limited to an acute epidermal inflammatory response or may progress to an infectious necrotic stage, which can involve deep fascia and cause osteomyelitis or septic dislocated joints.[58] Information on the prevalence and incidence of pressure sores in the institutionalized elderly has been provided by several studies.[6,8,9,59–62] Prevalence, the number of patients with pressure sores on a specific survey day, ranges from 3 to 20 per cent. Incidence, the number of patients developing a pressure sore after admission, ranges from 6 to 24 per cent. The fact that prevalence is not greater is explained by the mortality associated with pressure sores in older people. This has been reported as 24 to 60 per cent[62,63] and 73 per cent for those who develop sores within the first 2 weeks of admission.

In studies that explore age as a variable in pressure sore development, the consistent finding is that both prevalence and incidence of pressure sores are higher among the elderly.[64–67] Apart from age, time since admission is a significant factor, with patients greatly at risk during the first month. The first week or two are the most critical.[6,59,62,66,67] A variety of disease states are associated with the development of pressure sores, but all are characterized by decreased mobility or difficulty with wound healing.

## *Etiology and Course*

The name of these sores highlights their primary cause, which is pressure. Kosiak[69] found that tissue showed cellular infiltration, extravasation, and hyaline degeneration after application of 60 mm Hg of pressure for 1 hour.[68] However, in a later study, he showed that increased pressure (70 to 240 mm Hg) sustained for 5 minutes, alternating with pressure relief for a similar time, created no or minimal tissue change when continued over 1 to 3 hours in both normal and paraplegic rats.[69] Pressure is significant when it exceeds capillary levels, usually considered to be 30 mm Hg at the arteriolar and 15 mm Hg at the venous end.[70] Lying on a firm mattress yields pressure levels of 77 mm Hg at the shoulder and 37 mm Hg at the sacrum, as soft tissue is compressed between the surface and bony prominence,[71] but typically these pressures are of short duration because the individual turns often or shifts his body weight. Indeed, Exton-Smith and Sherwin[72] found that the number of body movements made per night in elderly hospitalized patients was related to pressure sores; nine of ten individuals having 20 or fewer spontaneous body shifts developed a sore. It should be noted that restraints, either standard models applied too tightly or improvised gown/sheet versions, severely restrict body movement and in some cases may decrease circulation in the extremities.

Friction has been implicated in pressure sore development, e.g., when the head of a bed is raised, a patient typically slides toward the foot, and in the process, friction occurs between the skin and the bed surface. Dinsdale[73] studied pressure and friction in ulcer formation among paraplegic swine and concluded that friction increased susceptibility to ulceration because of additional epidermal mechanical trauma. Others have postulated that, in addition to the friction, a specific shearing force is created when a semirecumbent patient slides down in bed.[74,75] Such a force causes progressive relative tissue displacement, with excessive stretching of blood vessels and tissue fibers and multiple capillary thromboses.

Pressure sores can occur over any bony prominence but are most typically located on the hips, sacrum, heels, and ankles. Initial signs of a pressure sore are those of acute inflammation of soft tissue: an irregular area of redness, pain, heat, and swelling. If pressure continues, the overlying skin blisters, sloughs, and an area of necrosis is evident. Tissue damage extends into subcutaneous fat and is frequently accompanied by foul-smelling, infected drainage. The size and depth of the wound continue to increase, involving deep fascia and ultimately bone. This extensive tissue damage occurs because pressure is transmitted from the bone to the overlying skin in a cone shape, with the base over the bone and the cone tip at the surface.[76]

It is useful to classify the extent of a pressure sore in some descriptive manner. Most popular is to make the simple distinction between superficial and deep, superficial describing erythematous, blistered, or abrased tissue involving only the dermal layers and deep describing any sore extending below the dermis. However, Shea[59] distinguishes a four-grade classification system that offers greater specificity. Clinically, the grades appear as follows: Grade I is an irregular area of soft tissue swelling and induration; grade II, a shallow, full-thickness skin ulcer; grade III, a skin ulcer extending into subcutaneous fat, with foul drainage and a necrotic base; and grade IV, a deep ulcer with bone evident, profuse drainage, and necrosis.[58] The ulcers of grades I and II are reversible with appropriate treatment. Grade III and IV ulcers are life-threatening. Although a diagnosis of pressure sore is usually evident from examination and history, Reuler and Cooney[77] note several differential diagnoses: ischial-rectal abscess, vasculitis, mycotic infection, and a necrotic malignant lesion.

## *Management of Pressure Sores*

### Prevention

Prevention starts with recognizing those individuals at risk for pressure sore development. Norton and associates[6] developed a simple assessment tool, which has proved clinically useful (Fig. 4–1). Patients are described on four different levels within five major categories: physical condition, mental condition, activity, mobility, and incontinence. Overall scores can range from 5 to 20; the lower the score, the more dysfunctional the individual. It was found that patients scoring under 14 were at risk and those at 12 or less were likely to develop a pressure sore.

Once patients at risk are identified, preventive measures can be instituted; these are principally directed toward reducing the amount and/or duration of pressure. Pressure reduction can be facilitated through special support surface options, a variety of which are available, including foam, gel, and water. The latter can be a heavy and awkward aid, requiring special nursing techniques and monitoring. Pressure duration can be limited by frequent nurse turnings or by use of an alternating pressure mattress. If the latter is used, it must have a wide cell/tube area to lift off body weight adequately. Such a mattress should be inflated before the patient is placed on its surface, and at best, only a single, loose-fitting sheet should be used as covering. In no case does a piece of equipment replace the need for frequent nursing observation of skin areas. Indeed, nurse-assisted turning procedures can be an extremely effective technique to prevent pressure sores, but this technique must be done more often than is typical. The Conduct and Utilization of Research in Nursing (CURN), Project,[78] a DHEW Division of Nursing supported study to implement research in practice settings, has produced an instructional nursing guide that uses the pressure sore assessment chart and a nursing technique to produce small shifts of body weight between traditional 2-hourly turning times to prevent pressure sores in patients at risk. Friction can be significantly reduced by having patients lie on sheep skins; natural sheep skins have been found to be superior to simulated products.[79] Footboards that can be adjusted to a patient's position rather than fixed at the end of the bed or a firm pillow rolled in a sheet, fixed against the patient's feet and tied under the mattress, can serve as an excellent body-slide reducer and help prevent foot-drop.

There are a variety of nursing skin-care procedures aimed at preventing pressure sores. Some involve frequent washing of vulnerable skin. Although such a practice fosters careful observation, the washing away of skin oils and the frequent addition of a soap residue dries elderly skin unnecessarily and may cause itching. Another questionable skin technique uses alcohol or alcohol-based applications to "toughen" skin against possible tissue damage. Norton and colleagues[6] found that elderly patients for whom witch hazel (alcohol-based) was used as part of skin care were more likely to develop an early pressure sore, perhaps due to the astringent effects of alcohol on older skin. No topical application can prevent or delay skin damage from pressure. Good skin care for the elderly should consist of minimizing pressure, frequent observation, minimal soap washing, and applications to restore oil and retain skin moisture. Tradi-

Name ______________________ Date ______________

| | Physical Condition | Mental Condition | Activity | Mobility | Incontinence |
|---|---|---|---|---|---|
| | Good 4<br>Fair 3<br>Poor 2<br>Very bad 1 | Alert 4<br>Apathetic 3<br>Confused 2<br>Stupor 1 | Ambulant 4<br>Walks/help 3<br>Chair-bound 2<br>Bed 1 | Full 4<br>Slightly limited 3<br>Very limited 2<br>Immobile 1 | Continent 4<br>Occasional 3<br>Usually urine 2<br>Doubly 1 |
| Total* | | | | | |

* > 14 points = patient at risk; > 12 points = patient greatly at risk.

**Figure 4–1.** Pressure sore assessment chart. (From Norton D, McLaren R, Exton-Smith AN: An Investigation of Geriatric Nursing Problems in Hospital. London, National Corporation for Old People, 1962; reprinted by Churchill Livingstone, New York, 1976.)

tional skin massage techniques may create a shearing force and cause underlying skin damage. Massage is part of an ancient nurse belief system that holds that systematic rubbing of vulnerable skin will prevent pressure sores. It appears more likely that the turning and observation basic to any massage technique are the more essential factors.

Prevention considerations should also include hydration, nutrition, general mobility, and reduction of any behavior, such as incontinence, that may potentially damage skin. Environmental factors should be carefully checked to reduce falls (sudden excessive skin pressure) and limit heel damage, e.g., correct chair height and use of footboards. Heel sores are also less likely if patients wear shoes when standing up because the firm shoe both protects and better positions the foot.

### TREATMENT

A pressure sore is a wound and its management should be no more mystifying than any other wound: (1) Stop the cause of the trauma, i.e., relieve pressure, and (2) follow classic wound healing techniques, i.e., keep the wound clean, keep the wound moist, and ensure that blood supply to the area has adequate oxygen and nutrients.[80] Yet it is not uncommon to find no systematic management of pressure sores, typically in combination with an atmosphere of medical indifference. Poor nursing staff morale and lack of medical assistance foster unlikely and bizarre treatments. In reviewing the literature of topical treatment for pressure sores, Morgan[81] reported over 30 different applications in 11 major categories. She concluded that improvements were associated with control of infection, debridement of dead tissue, and absence of pressure rather than any one specific topical agent. Just as there is no magic in prevention, there is no magic in treatment.

Uncontrolled bacterial contamination of grade I and II ulcers (superficial), with continued pressure, leads to the frank tissue infection of grades III and IV (deep) sores. Thus, basic cleansing and antiseptic/bactericidal agents employed at an early stage in conjunction with relief of pressure and general health measures may allow for resolution of an ulcer. The infection of deeper ulcers is a serious problem, often associated with bacteremia and mortality, even with appropriate antibiotic therapy.[82] Despite the seriousness of this infection and the necessity of surgical debridement, management is typically by enzymatic debriding agents. Although chemical debridement may augment or facilitate deep ulcer cleaning, such agents are not as effective or efficient as surgical methods and may further impede resolution by blockage of drainage or by causing allergic reactions.[76] Surgical debridement is a technique that can be done at the bedside, and it can be taught to qualified nurses who work in collaboration with physicians. Once necrotic tissue has been surgically removed, cleaning may need to be continued using the mechanical debridement that occurs when wet saline dressings are allowed to dry so that removal pulls necrotic tissue away. Enzymatic agents or hypochlorite solutions may be useful at this stage but require saline rinsing after use, protection of good tissue, and careful observation for negative tissue reaction. Deep wounds must be inspected with a flashlight and probe to assess for tracts, sinuses, and tissue response.

Healing by secondary intention is possible in clean superficial ulcers, once pressure is relieved and general health status maintained. Deep clean wounds are best healed by surgical closure. Robson and Haggers[83] showed that delayed wound closures of deep pressure ulcers with bacterial estimates of $10^5$ or less per gm of tissue were highly successful. Surgical consultation should be obtained early in the course of a deep ulcer.

Treatment of pressure sores should include attention to systemic needs, with special attention to anemia, dehydration, protein depletion, and general metabolism. Blood transfusion or intravenous hyperalimentation may be essential components in the management of deep pressure sores. Supplemental ascorbic acid and zinc sulfate may facilitate healing, especially in patients with low intakes.[84,85]

## References


1. Wells TJ: Nursing committed to the elderly. *In* Reinhardt A, Quinn M (eds.): Current Practice in Gerontological Nursing. St. Louis, C.V. Mosby Co., 1979, pp. 187–196.
   *A review of the development and status of gerontologic nursing.*
2. Newton K: Geriatric Nursing. St. Louis, C.V. Mosby, 1950.
3. Wells TJ: What does committment to gerontological nursing really mean? J Gerontol Nurs 8: 434, 1982.
   *A review of progress and problems in gerontologic nursing.*
4. Blenkner M: The normal dependencies of aging. *In* Kalish R (ed.): The Dependence of Old People. Ann Arbor, Michigan, Institute of Gerontology, 1969, pp. 27–38.
5. U.S. Department of Health and Human Services: The Need for Long-term Care. A Chartbook of the Federal Council on the Aging. Washington, DC, National Center for Health Statistics (OHDS81-20704), 1981, p. 31.

*A collection of demographic, health status, health service, and informal support data about the elderly.*

6. Norton D, McLaren R, Exton-Smith AN: An Investigation of Geriatric Nursing Problems in Hospitals. London, National Corporation for Old People, 1962. Reprinted by Churchill Livingstone, New York, 1976.
*A classic inductive study of nursing problems arising from care of old people in a British geriatric hospital unit.*
7. Adams GF, Mcllwraith PL: Geriatric Nursing. A Study of the Work of Geriatric Ward Staff. London, Oxford University Press, 1963.
*A study using systematic activity sampling to describe nurses' work in a British 200-bed geriatric unit.*
8. U.S. Office of Nursing Home Affairs: Long-term Care Facility Improvement Study. Introductory Report. Bethesda, Md., U.S. Office of Nursing Home Affairs, July 1975.
*A survey of 288 nursing homes with skilled personnel, describing characteristics of facilities and patient data.*
9. U.S. Department of Health and Human Services: The National Nursing Home Survey: 1977 Summary for the United States. Hyattsville, Md., Office of Health Research, Statistics, and Technology, National Center for Health Statistics, July 1979.
*A survey of 1451 nursing homes, describing characteristics of facilities and providing patient data.*
10. Wells TJ: Problems in Geriatric Nursing Care. New York, Churchill Livingstone, 1980.
*An exploratory, descriptive study of geriatric nursing in a British geriatric hospital unit.*
11. Institute of Medicine: A Policy Statement. The Elderly and Functional Dependency. Washington, DC, National Academy of Sciences, June 1977, p. 1.
12. Soldo BJ: America's Elderly in the 1980s. Popul Bull 35:17, 1980.
*A presentation and discussion of demographic data about the elderly.*
13. Rusk HA: Rehabilitation Medicine. St. Louis, C.V. Mosby Co., 1977, p. 557.
14. Kenshalo DR: Age changes in touch, vibration, temperature, kinesthesis and pain sensitivity. *In* Birren J, Schaie K (eds.): Handbook of the Psychology of Aging. New York, Van Nostrand Reinhold Co., 1977, pp. 562–579.
15. Agate J: The Practice of Geriatrics. London, W. Heinemann Medical Book, 1970.
16. Hodkinson HM: Common Symptoms of Disease in the Elderly. Oxford, Blackwell Scientific Publications, 1976.
17. Fordyce W: Chronic pain. *In* Stolov W, Clowers M (eds.): Handbook of Severe Disability. Washington, DC, U.S. Government Printing Office, 1981, pp. 219–229.
18. Corcoron PJ: Disability consequences of bed rest. *In* Stolov W, Clowers M (eds.): Handbook of Severe Disability. Washington, DC, U.S. Government Printing Office, 1981, pp. 55–63.
19. Campbell AJ, Reinken J, Allan BC, Martinez GS: Falls in old age: A study of frequency and related clinical factors. Age Aging 10:264, 1981.
*An analysis of falls experienced by a stratified British population sample of 553 subjects who were 65 years and over.*
20. Prudham D, Evans JG: Factors associated with falls in the elderly: A community study. Age Aging 10:141, 1981.
*A survey of 2793 British individuals aged 65 and over living in communities, which provides data about falls in the preceding year.*
21. Sheldon JH: Falls in old age. *In* Agate J (ed.): Medicine in Old Age. London, Pitman Medical Publishing Co., 1966, pp. 199–207.
*A classic anecdotal paper on sway, drop attacks, and patterns of recovery from falls in old people.*
22. Hasselkus B, Shambes G: Aging and postural sway in women. J Gerontol 30:661, 1975.
23. Fernie GR, Gryfe CI, Holliday PJ, Llewellyn A: The relationship of postural sway in standing to the incidence of falls in geriatric subjects. Age Aging 11:11, 1982.
*A double-blind study to determine the relationship between the extent of postural sway and frequency of falling in subjects 63 to 99 years old.*
24. Sabin TD: Biologic aspects of falls and mobility limitations in the elderly. J Am Geriatr Soc 30:51, 1982.
*A review of gait disorders in the elderly.*
25. Feist RR: A survey of accidental falls in a small home for the aged. J Geront Nurs 4:15, 1978.
26. Walshe A, Rosen H: A study of patient falls from bed. J Nurs Admin 9:31, 1979.
27. Morris EV, Isaacs B: The prevention of falls in a geriatric hospital. Age Aging 9:181, 1980.
28. Berry J, Fisher R, Lang S: Detrimental incidents, including falls in an elderly institutional population. J Am Geriatr Soc 29:322, 1981.
*An analysis of 2177 untoward accidents in a Canadian geriatric hospital.*
29. Foerster J: A Study of Falls: The Elderly Nursing Home Resident. Unpublished Master's Thesis, University of Rochester, Rochester, New York, 1978.
30. Subcommittee on Long-term Care of the Special Committee on Aging, United States Senate: Nursing Home Care in the United States. Supporting Paper No. 4. Nurses in Nursing Homes: The Heavy Burden. Washington, DC, U.S. Government Printing Office, 1975, p. 360.
31. U.S. Department of Health, Education, and Welfare: Weight, Height, and Selected Body Dimensions of Adults. Washington, DC, June, 1965.
32. The Disabled User: RICA Comparative Test Report No. 6, Easy Chairs. London, The National Fund for Research into Crippling Diseases, July 1970.
33. Dench J, Heath P: Are you sitting comfortably? NT 70:922, 1974.
34. Scottish Home and Health Department: Geriatric Accommodation Report. Edinburgh, Scotland, 1970.
35. Goldsmith S: Designing for the Disabled. 3rd ed. London, RIBA Publications, 1976.
*A comprehensive and detailed guide to environmental design for wheelchair, walker, and other equipment of the disabled.*
36. Jordan JJ: Senior Center Design. Washington, DC, National Council on the Aging, 1978.
*A guide to community senior centers, with helpful checklists.*
37. Veterans Administration: Handbook for Design. Washington, DC, 1978.
*A design guide developed for the physically handicapped veteran, which includes useful ideas for the elderly.*
38. Fozard J, Wolf E, Bell B, et al: Visual perception and communication. *In* Birren J, Schaie KW (eds.): Handbook of the Psychology of Aging. New York, Von Nostrand Reinhold Co., 1977, pp. 497–534.
39. Snyder L, Pyrek J, Smith KC: Vision and mental function in the elderly. Gerontologist 16:491, 1976.
*An investigation of the relationship between vision and mental functioning in 295 elderly nursing home residents.*
40. Ohta RJ, Carlin MF, Harmon BM: Auditory acuity and performance on the mental status questionnaire in the elderly. J Am Geriatr Soc 29:476, 1981.

*An investigation of the relationship between hearing and mental function in 27 nursing home residents.*
41. Panicucci CL, Paul PB, Symonds JM, Tambellini JL: Expanded speech and self-pacing in communication with the aged. *In* ANA Clinical Sessions, New York, Appleton-Century-Crofts, 1968, pp. 95–101.
42. Wolanin M, Phillips L: Confusion. St. Louis, C.V. Mosby Co., 1981, p. 8.
*A comprehensive discussion of confusion as a clinical nursing problem. Contains helpful guides.*
43. Brocklehurst J, Hanley T: Geriatric Medicine for Students. New York, Churchill Livingstone, 1976.
44. Burnside I: Depression and grief in the aged person. *In* Burnside I (ed.): Nursing and the Aged. New York, Macmillan Co., 1981, pp. 122–136.
45. Liebowitz B, Lawton M, Waldman O: Evaluation: designing for confused elderly people. AIA Journal 68:59, 1979.
46. Wiltzius F, Gambert S, Duthie E: Importance of resident placement within a skilled nursing facility. J Am Geriatr Soc 29:418, 1981.
47. International Continence Society: First report on the standardization of terminology of lower urinary tract function. Br J Urol 48:39, 1976.
48. Wells T: Promoting urine control in older adults: Scope of the problem. Geriatr Nurs 1:236, 1980.
49. Specht J, Cordes A: Incontinence. *In* Carnevali D, Patrick M (eds.): Nursing Management for the Elderly. Philadelphia, J.B. Lippincott, 1979, pp. 387–398.
50. Walkey FA, Judge TG, Thompson J, Sarkari NB: Incidence of urinary infection in the elderly. Scott Med J 12:411, 1967.
51. Sourander LB, Kasanen A: A 5-year follow-up of bacteriuria in the aged. Gerontol Clin 14:247, 1972.
52. Brocklehurst JC, Bee P, Jones D, Palmer MK: Bacteriuria in geriatric hospital patients: Its correlates and management. Age Aging 6:240, 1977.
53. Bissada N, Finkbeiner A: Lower Urinary Tract Function and Dysfunction. New York, Appleton-Century-Crofts, 1978, pp. 127–134.
*A review of classic and more recent research contributions to the evaluation and treatment of lower urinary tract disorders.*
54. Sutherland SS: The psychology of incontinence. *In* Willington FL (ed.): Incontinence in the Elderly. New York, Academic Press, 1976, pp. 52–69.
55. Coni N, Devison W, Webster S: Lecture Notes on Geriatrics. Oxford, Blackwell Scientific Publications, 1977.
56. Wells TJ, Brink CA: Urinary continence: Assessment and management. *In* Burnside I (ed.): Nursing and the Aged. New York, McGraw Hill, 1981, pp. 519–548.
*A review of urinary incontinence as a clinical nursing problem. Contains assessment and intervention guides.*
57. Williams TF, Foerster JE, Proctor JK, et al: A new double-layered launderable bed sheet for patients with urinary incontinence. J Am Geriatr Soc 29:520, 1981.
58. Shea JD: Pressure sores: Classification and management. Clin Orthop Relat Res 112:89, 1975.
*A clinical discussion of pressure sore presentation and recommended treatment.*
59. Irvine RE, Memon AH, Shera AS: Norethandrolone and prevention of pressure-sores. Lancet 2:1333, 1961.
60. Rosin AJ, Boyd RV: Complications of illness in geriatric patients in hospitals. J Chronic Dis 19:307, 1966.
61. Gosnell DJ: An assessment tool to identify pressure sores. Nurs Res 22:55, 1973.
62. Welten JB: Pressure sores: Prevention and treatment. Gerontol Clin 15:234, 1973.
63. Vasile J, Chaitin H: Prognostic factors in decubitus ulcers of the aged. Geriatrics 27:126, 1972.
64. Hicks DJ: An Incidence Study of Pressure Sores Following Surgery. ANA Clinical Sessions 1970, Miami. New York, Appleton-Century-Crofts, 1971, pp. 49–54.
65. Gerson LW: The incidence of pressure sores in active treatment hospitals. Int J Nurs Stud 12:201, 1975.
66. Michocki RJ, Lamy PP: The problem of pressure sores in a nursing home population: Statistical data. J Am Geriatr Soc 24:323, 1976.
67. Manley MT: Incidence, contributory factors and cost of pressure sores. S Afr Med J 53:217, 1978.
68. Kosiak M: Etiology and pathology of ischemic ulcers. Arch Phys Med Rehabil 40:62, 1959.
*A classic paper reporting studies of ischemic ulcer formation in dogs.*
69. Kosiak M: Etiology of decubitus ulcers. Arch Phys Med Rehabil 42:19, 1961.
70. Ganong WF: Review of Medical Physiology. Los Altos, Calif., Lange Medical Publications, 1975.
71. Redfern SJ, Jeneid PA, Gillingham ME: Local pressures with ten types of patient-support systems. Lancet 2:277, 1973.
*An analysis of local tissue pressure on eight body sites produced by different support systems, including a water bed, foam mattress, and an alternating pressure mattress.*
72. Exton-Smith AN, Sherwin RW: The prevention of pressure sores: Significance of spontaneous bodily movements. Lancet 2:1124, 1961.
73. Dinsdale SM: Decubitus ulcers: Role of pressure and friction in causation. Arch Phys Med Rehabil 55:147, 1974.
74. Reichel SM: Shearing force as a factor in decubitus ulcers in paraplegics. JAMA 15:762, 1958.
75. Tepperman PS, De Zwirek CS, Chiarcossi AL, Jimenez J: Pressure sores: Prevention and step-up management. Postgrad Med 62:83, 1977.
76. Argis J, Spira M: Pressure ulcers: Prevention and treatment. Clinical Symposium. Vol. 31(5), 1979.
77. Reuler JB, Cooney TG: The pressure sore: Pathophysiology and principles of management. Ann Intern Med 94:661, 1981.
*A comprehensive discussion of the clinical settings, causative factors, complications, and principles of prevention and management of pressure sores.*
78. CURN Project: Preventing Decubitus Ulcers. New York, Grune & Stratton, 1981.
*One of a series of instructive guides developed out of a DHEW Division of Nursing grant to facilitate the implementation of research in practice.*
79. Denne WA: An objective assessment of the sheepskins used for decubitus sore prophylaxis. Rheum and Rehabil 18:23, 1979.
80. Winter GD: Some factors affecting skin and wound healing. *In* Kenedi R, Cowden J (eds.): Bedsore Biomechanics. Baltimore, University Park Press, 1976.
81. Morgan JE: Topical therapy of pressure ulcers. Surg Gynecol Obstet 141:945, 1975.
*A review of topical therapy of pressure sores in the English literature from 1900 to 1974.*
82. Galpin JE, Chow AW, Bayer AS, Guze LB: Sepsis associated with decubitus ulcers. Am J Med 61:346, 1976.
83. Robson MC, Heggers JP: Delayed wound closures based on bacterial counts. J Surg Oncol 2:379, 1970.
84. Taylor TV, Rimmer S, Day B, Butcher J, Dymock IW: Ascorbic acid supplementation in the treatment of pressure sores. Lancet 2:544, 1974.
85. Fulghum DD: Ascorbic acid revisited. Arch Dermatol 113:91, 1977.

## Chapter 5

# Social Factors and Family Supports

*Donald L. Spence*
*John J. Cunningham*

This chapter is about the involvement of community and family in the support of geriatric patients. It presents the physician with a challenge to view the geriatric patient in a way that is not necessarily consistent with traditional medical education and training. Multiple diagnoses combined with situational factors present the physician with problems that vary in relation to the individuality of the aging patient.

Sorting out the various dimensions of these problems is further complicated by the different traditions through which our understanding of aging has developed. Geriatrics, which focuses on disease, tends to equate aging with disease. Gerontology, on the other hand, looks for developmental changes associated with the aging process. The geriatric tradition tends to overlook the role of environmental and social factors in the disabilities manifested by the aged. The gerontologic tradition tends to discount the importance of medical intervention in the restoration and maintenance of the impaired older person.

There are three assumptions that govern the presentation of the material in this chapter. First, the geriatric patient must be approached from both traditions, developmental and pathologic. It is not enough just to deal with the disease or diseases presented by the patient. One must also be aware that social circumstances affect the way in which disease presents. The physician must become aware of and learn how to refer to social services.

Second, a rehabilitative approach is essential in the treatment of the geriatric patient. All too often, when it comes to treating geriatric patients, physicians have a pessimistic attitude. There is little or no recognition by physicians of therapies appropriate to an individual's age and situation. As a consequence, people who could regain or maintain a considerable degree of independence if rehabilitated, are relegated to custodial institutions.

Third, there has to be active communication between the physician, the geriatric patient and his family. A patient responds better to treatment if he understands his illness and can participate in his health care. This is especially true with geriatric patients. Without an accurate understanding of what the physician is trying to do, the patient and his family may work at cross purposes on the objectives of the prescribed medical regimen.

This chapter begins with a presentation of what is known about family and social supports for the elderly. It then looks at some problems in geriatric medicine and the practice of medicine in relation to geriatric patients and their families. Finally, gaps in the availability of services to support geriatric patients and their families are identified in such a way as to present the physician with some challenges to improve the system.

## SUPPORTS FOR THE ELDERLY

An understanding of social and family supports for the care of frail and chronically ill elderly people living in the community should help the physician to maximize the effectiveness of these supports in order to maintain older patients in their own homes. This is not meant to negate the appropriate use of institutional care but to begin to minimize its inappropriate use. There is no question that many who are institutionalized could remain in the community if there were adequate services available. Lawton[1] estimates that between 10 and 40 per cent of those in nursing homes receive unnecessarily high levels of health care, whereas Eggert and associates[2] have demonstrated that the source of payment and not the level of care required is primary in determining who is admitted to these homes. Since the physician generally legitimizes the decision to place a patient in an institution, his or her influence could be critical in altering the present situation. However, this cannot occur without some essential changes in the structure of social supports.

## *Family Supports for the Elderly at Home*

It has been estimated that between 60 and 85 per cent of all disabled or impaired older persons are helped by their families in a significant way.[3] Children are the primary providers, taking a secondary role only when a functional spouse is present.[4] At the same time, it can be shown that families represent a limited resource, which can be rapidly eroded without some type of supplemental social service, such as respite from what is often a taxing physical burden.[5] What is known about family interaction patterns, however, is not necessarily the information needed to assess the potential role of families in caring for members who require long-term care.[6] Recent studies are just now beginning to provide some data on this important topic.[7-10]

Most large survey studies are limited in the detail of the data they collect or else they focus on a specific area and fail to provide the breadth of understanding required in such a complex topic as family support systems. These studies help one to understand that most older people (84 per cent) live less than 1 hour away from one or more of their adult children[4,11] and that shared households occur infrequently, mostly among the poorest families or in response to functional dependence.[12] They show that patterns of interactive behavior occur daily for about one half and weekly for over three fourths of the older people interviewed.[4] Contrary to the assumption that a person's social network contracts with age, studies show no difference in the interactive patterns of those over and those under age 65. They show patterns of mutual aid and support,[12] with the nature of the exchange consistent with need and available resources.[13,14] In almost every study of the elderly and their families, emotional support is the most important service provided, whereas financial help is seen as relatively unimportant.[3] What these studies fail to show is the developmental dynamics associated with the patterns of mutual involvement during or in response to a crisis or functional decline.

As effective and responsive as the family structure might be, it is extremely frail and will require substantial bolstering if it is to assume a greater significance in providing for the long-term care needs of older people. The research in this area is growing, and although some consistent patterns of behavior are emerging, two cautions are worth noting. First, there is the potential bias of the subjects studied. For a variety of reasons, most subjects studied tend to be urban, of lower than average socioeconomic status, and over-representative of minorities. Second, there is the problem of forming generalizations about individual families on the basis of collective data. The uniqueness of an individual family may totally belie the statistical norms. With these cautions in mind, a descriptive understanding of the typical family process is still useful.

The tasks of care-giving can vary widely.[15] It is important to distinguish normal reciprocal relations within the family from those provided in response to long-term health care needs. Care-giving, under these circumstances, varies in accordance with the relationship of the care-giver to the elderly person. Spouses devote the most time to care-giving, with children next and other relatives providing somewhat less time. According to the Horowitz and Dobrof study,[7] the average amount of time spent care-giving was 22 hours per week. When the care-giving was provided in the home of a care-giver, the time spent was 40 or more hours a week.[16] The burden of care appears to fall on one member of the family, usually a female and in the following order: spouse, child, and other relative, depending on availability. The costs of care-giving are significant, with emotional exhaustion or stress being mentioned most frequently.[17,18] A restructuring of schedules and the loss of free time,[19,20] combined with the consequent stress on marital and family relations,[21] indicate the precarious nature of this form of long-term care. Care-giving is provided out of obligation or affection for the patient; care-giving as a means to avoid nursing home placement is mentioned in only 3 per cent of cases.[7] When one adds to the preceding the fact that family willingness to provide care erodes by almost 50 per cent after a second hospitalization (from 70 to 38 per cent), the role of complementary support by social provision becomes paramount.[5]

## *Social Supports for the Elderly at Home*

Any discussion of the way social services support families in the long-term care of the chronically impaired older person is speculative at best. Neither policy with respect to program development nor research objectives with respect to program evaluation is sufficiently uniform to allow appropriate comparisons.[22,23] Even in relation to Medicare coverage in nursing homes, the variation from state to state in reviewers' decisions to cover or not to cover patients is sufficiently great as to question the uniform applicability of Federal law.[24] Since agreement among reviewers varies directly with the skilled-nursing requirements of the patients, additional support is given to the notion that social factors rather than level of impairment are primary determinants of who is served.

The way that long-term care is currently paid for adds to the problem. Medicare offers only limited support for extended rehabilitative services following hospitalization for an acute illness. It specifically prohibits custodial and most long-term care services. Private insurance, including major medical, has also avoided any significant involvement. Less than a fraction of 1 per cent of home and nursing home expenditures were covered during 1980; most of these expenditures were for full-time private duty nursing following acute illness. Medicaid, which is limited to institutional, custodial care for the very poor or those who are willing to impoverish themselves, is essentially the only system of public support.[25]

With passage of the Pepper/Waxman Medicaid Community Care Act in 1981, it is now possible for states to apply for waivers to the Medicaid statutory requirements in order to cover a wide range of home and community-based services.[26] The law emphasizes the coordination and targeting of services to individuals who would otherwise be institutionalized. Given the consequences of the 1981 Omnibus Budget Reconciliation Act, which places limits on the Federal share of Medicaid, and the fear by state legislatures that an expansion of services would produce an add-on of eligible recipients, most states are moving cautiously. Although community-based services may delay institutionalization, evidence that they will prevent institutionalization is inconclusive.[26]

Current Federal research and demonstration projects are directed at more systemic reform (1) to extend the coverage to include the Medicare as well as the Medicaid population, (2) to effect the necessary linkages between the acute and chronic care systems, and (3) to provide limitations on total costs.

Five channeling demonstration projects have been designated as "complex" models. The project administrators have the authority to prescribe and directly pay for services based on client need, not income eligibility. The income eligibility requirements have limited these demonstration studies in two ways. First, although approximately one half of those in nursing homes supported by Medicaid were not initially "poor,"[27] by the time they became eligible for services, institutionalization had altered their potential for responding to community supports. Second, since those who are eligible for Medicaid are least likely to have an abundance of informal supports, there has been little experience in assisting families in care-giving. These demonstration projects are important because they represent a radical change in existing health policy.

Present policy directs patients to services. The channeling projects direct services to patients. Therefore, the channeling alternative is specific to individuals. Since it is known that there are at least one and one-half individuals in the community for every one in an institution, all equally impaired, services to support those in the community must exist. The ability to channel those services according to the specific needs of geriatric patients may provide an alternative to long-term institutional care.

A second alternative to long-term institutional care is being advocated by the American Hospital Association's Office on Aging and Long-Term Care. In response to results of a Health Care Financing Administration (HCFA)-supported demonstration project at Mount Zion Hospital and Medical Center in San Francisco, hospitals are being encouraged to develop appropriate in-home services and case management suited to the multiple, multifaceted, and chronic conditions of the elderly. Preliminary findings from the Mount Zion study show that a demonstration group was able to maintain levels of functioning, whereas controls who were subject to traditional extended care showed reduced activities of daily living, reduced social supports, and reduced environmental satisfaction. The superior results with the demonstration group were effected with a savings of over 5 per cent in part-A Medicare costs.[26] The Robert Wood Johnson Foundation, in conjunction with the American Hospital Association, is funding up to 10 not-for-profit, voluntary or public hospitals to provide "comprehensive and coordinated long-term medical care and social services to individuals within a defined, elderly population."

A third alternative to long-term institutional care is based on the capitation principle of the health maintenance organization, the social HMO. By putting the provider at risk, it encourages the most appropriate and lowest cost alternative for all health and social services. As a system, the social HMO delivers service on the basis of individual need rather than income. As of the beginning of 1982, three sites had been designated to try out this system: Brooklyn Metropolitan Jewish Geriatric Center, Kaiser Portland Health Plan, and the Ebenezer Society in Minneapolis. The project is supported by HCFA, with Brandeis University designing and developing the sites.[26]

It is important to understand that most older individuals have limited access to the programmatic resources supported under the various Federal programs. Medicare, with its limitations and deductibles, is generally available to older individuals, but Medicaid is limited to the poor (15.7 per cent in 1980) or those willing to impoverish themselves.

Programs supported under Title XX of the Social Security Act are also directed toward low-income people. The law requires that at least one half of the Federal dollars be used for welfare recipients while the other half is limited to those whose incomes do not exceed 115 per cent of a particular state's median income. Fees are required for individuals or families with incomes between 80 and 115 per cent of the state's median income. Title XX provides reimbursement for the costs incurred by states in providing social services to all low-income people. Because these services are administered under a social service grant, they vary from state to state, and it is difficult, if not impossible, to determine the number of elderly served as well as the types of services they have received.[26]

Older Americans Act programs, with the exception of the congregate and home-delivered nutrition services, provide very limited support for long-term care. For example, in 1980, less than 3 per cent of all older people were served by the home care service component of Title III.[26] Although Older Americans Act programs are aimed at improving the lives of all older Americans, their emphasis on those who have the greatest social or economic needs is quite evident. Of the 9 million older persons served in 1980, 54 per cent were designated low-income and 22 per cent minorities.[26]

## PRESENT CIRCUMSTANCES AND FUTURE PROJECTIONS

There are several characteristics of the older population and their families that may affect long-term care needs. Basically these characteristics are related to demographic processes, economic circumstances, and health status. A brief examination of these factors may help in understanding the dynamics and significance of geriatric long-term care.

The demographic circumstances of older people can be predicted with a great deal of accuracy. In 1980, those who will be 65 or older through the year 2045 are already living. The conditions that attended the different age cohorts are known and can be used to make some projections of number and circumstance. For example, those who will be old-old (75 years or over) in the year 2000 were born in 1925 or earlier, when the total fertility rate was well over three children per female of reproductive age. Those in the age range of 65 to 74 years (young-old) were born between 1920 and 1930, a period of declining fertility. The implications of this for the distribution of age among the older population are significant. Although the total older population will increase by 7.4 million between 1977 and 2000, an increase of 32 per cent, the number of young-old will increase by 25 per cent, whereas the number of old-old will increase by almost 60 per cent.[28]

The shifts in population combined with such factors as life expectancy by sex, age-specific mortality rates, the proportion of people ever married, marriage and divorce rates specific to age groups, and projected fertility rates can be used to forecast the future for the aged with respect to marital status and living arrangements,[28] family support systems,[29] and the dependency burden of the overall kin structure.[30] Clearly there are increasing numbers of unmarried older women who are living alone. The adult children of aging parents are fewer in proportion. With growing numbers of women in the workforce, there is a general reduction in the availability of family members to support the long-term care needs of the elderly. On the other hand, if some general assumptions are made with respect to the dependency needs of those under 18 and over 70, it can be shown that even with a "high fertility projection" to the year

2000, the total "dependency burden" on the middle generation will not differ significantly from what it was in 1950. With a "low fertility projection," the position of the middle generation will improve.[30] However, since increases in life expectancy will produce a family structure of four rather than three generations, with the adult children of the frail elderly themselves either into or fast approaching their own retirement, some careful thought must be given to the use of the family as an economic resource in support of dependent older individuals.

The primary economic concerns with respect to long-term care are the escalating costs. Between 1976 and 1981, nursing home costs to Medicaid increased by $12.8 billion, a 112 per cent increase.[31] The proportion of institutionalized elderly has remained relatively constant, with about 5 per cent over the age of 65. However, with the population aging and the largest increases occuring after age 80, when the probability of institutionalization increases to at least one in eight,[32] the nursing home industry will continue to grow. Even the successful development of alternatives, including the effective development of family involvement in the long-term care of the frail elderly, cannot totally offset this trend.

At least 20 per cent of nursing home residents are without family. Spouses of nursing home residents are already making significant payments and are therefore considered a poor source of additional support. In fact, it is estimated that less than 10 per cent of all nursing home residents have children with incomes that would permit them to make financial contributions to the care of their parents.[3] The primary contributions that families can make are in the form of aid provided through the informal support network and therefore affect those elderly living in the community.

The studies available and the questions that they leave unanswered about long-term care of the elderly are a clear indication that more research is needed and a caution to those who would generalize prematurely from a limited data base. Comparisons between the elderly in the Cleveland sample[9] and those in the Massachusetts sample[10] concerning their use of such services as personal care (basic activities of daily living), housekeeping, meal preparation, and transportation (instrumental activities of daily living) produce differences that leave a number of unanswered questions. By examining a modest but carefully conducted study of what it means for families to take care of their sick elders,[8] one is led to understand the diversity and flexibility of family care; the need for major policy shifts if social services are to support family care; and, most important in relation to practice, the need to understand family circumstances when prescribing for individual patients.

Clearly the health status of older people will improve. There are those who have gone so far as to suggest that most people will be well and vigorous until about age 85, after which there will be a short period of debility leading to death.[33] Others have suggested that life-style changes will reduce malignant disease, chronic obstructive lung disease, and arteriosclerotic disease, and suffering from hypertension will be reduced through extensions in the application of therapy. However, the increases in life expectancy accompanying these changes will increase the rates of bone and joint disease and senile dementia.[34] Even with some significant breakthroughs in medical research, it is probably overly optimistic to assume that people will stay healthy until age 85 and then die quickly. At the same time, a focus on the chronic health problems of the older population is changing the preferred measure of health status from one based on the presence of disease to one based on functional ability. Even among individuals 85 years of age and older, only a relatively small proportion have severe degrees of disability.[32] This information should improve the outcome expectations of physicians' practicing geriatric medicine.

## PATIENTS AND THEIR FAMILIES: PROBLEMS IN GERIATRIC PRACTICE

Thirty-five per cent of patients seen by internists and 25 per cent of those seen by family physicians are 65 years or older. The practice of geriatric medicine, therefore, should be integrated into already established medical service delivery systems rather than segregated as a specialty. People will specialize in geriatrics to fill academic needs and to serve as consultants in relation to specific problem areas. The segregationist approach ignores the necessary role that must be provided by most medical specialties in the care of older patients.

### *Issues in Geriatric Practice*

Older patients challenge physicians. They are not like other patients. Although age alone should not imply disease, the incidence of chronic disease increases dramatically with age. What is most important to recall is that pathologic conditions and disability are not synonymous. The world is alive with examples of political and scientific leaders who function at above normal levels in spite of the presence of serious medical problems, such as vascular, pulmonary, or endocrine disease. The other side of this coin is that many older people are classified as disabled because their physical status is inappropriately compared with that of younger people. If thought about appropriately in relation to the social and economic status of the elderly, the implications of so-called handicaps appear to be much less negative.[35]

## Stereotypes, Prejudices, and Social Breakdown

An objective in the care of older patients is to maximize the functional abilities of the elderly so that they maintain their independence. This does not mean that patients must do everything for themselves. A lack of physical stamina or the inability to perform personal care activities may justify the need for appropriate assistance. What should be avoided is the provision of service in such a way as to indicate to older patients that their inability to function is their fault. If patients blame themselves for their disability rather than believe that expectations are inappropriate, the consequence may be patient decline.

It is assumed that family, friends, or neighbors would be more inclined to put out the garbage, change the bed, and assist with bathing or with cutting toenails or even paying bills or shopping if they were made aware of how these activities help in the maintenance of their relative, friend, or neighbor. Historically, if there is not an appropriate understanding of the role of support activities, reinforcement of negative stereotypes about aging occurs. Since older patients share the same conceptions and prejudices about aging, the lack of appropriate expectations in the presence of impairment has led to what the gerontologic literature has called the "social breakdown hypothesis."[36]

Social breakdown is not really an hypothesis but an heuristic device. The term is being used because of its descriptiveness in relation to the way social relationships foster and support the stereotypic view of aging, particularly the notion of aging as ever-increasing pathologic condition. Without this social reinforcement, many of the traumas of aging would be responsive to treatment, with a proportionate improvement in the quality of life for the aged.

The consequences of social breakdown are as damaging to the family or other caretakers as they are to the patient. Because of the prejudices and negative stereotypes about aging generally held within our society, the family or caretaker usually believes that providing any assistance is tantamount to assuming responsibility for the total care of the geriatric patient. The physician has a major responsibility in helping the patient and his or her family define and accept appropriate expectations for the patient and understand the contribution that family assistance can provide. If there is no effective family, knowing the available service agencies and their philosophies of service delivery is necessary to ensure that their actions are not fostering social breakdown.

Social breakdown results from older people accepting as their own self-image the negative stereotypes of aging. Since some older people manage to resist this process, understanding both sides of the issue should help the physician to be more effective in his or her work with older patients. For example, better educated, affluent older people are more likely to be perceived as middle-aged rather than old. This generally means that they are active in the process of their health care, responding to the prescription of a medical regimen as a "good" patient should. They continue to perceive themselves as middle-aged rather than old. The physician perceives them as sharing his world view and reinforces their younger self image.

There are any number of reasons why patients fail to follow their medical regimen. Some are not sure what to do even as they leave the physician's office. Most patients do have their prescriptions filled, but Libow and Sherman[37] estimate that between 30 and 50 per cent of geriatric patients fail to take their medication as prescribed. This aspect of geriatric practice can be most frustrating to the medical practitioner. If repeated noncompliance leads to what the physician sees as unnecessary medical crises, a probable response is to place the patient in an environment where the medical regimen can be controlled, thus contributing to a loss of independence for the patient and inappropriate use of acute hospital or long-term institutional care.[38] This action says to the patient that he or she is no longer in control of his or her life. Working with families and the community to produce better support for ambulatory medical practices with geriatric patients is one of the major challenges faced today. This issue is discussed in the final section of this chapter.

### Finding the Appropriate Mode of Intervention

Reichel[39] suggests that intelligent treatment of geriatric patients involves the application of Seegal's principle of minimal interference. In fact, when it comes to family or social arrangements in support of the elderly, adherence to the philosophic advice of Archie Bunker, "if it ain't broke, don't fix it," is probably quite sound.

Traditional medical training prescribes intervention in the presence of disease. With geriatric patients, one had better be sure that intervention will improve things or at least not make matters worse. The extreme example, as it relates to patient care, is the prescription of drugs to treat drug-induced symptoms. Historically we have erred by giving up on the aged patient too soon, and ignoring the rehabilitative potential.[40] The opposite error can be just as damaging. We must allow the patient the dignity of his or her person. Institutional custodial care denies a person's independence. Intensive medical heroics do the same thing. Choosing the appropriate intervention should be decided *with* the patient if possible. If there is a supportive family, they must be involved. Developing effective communication with the patient or with the patient's family is what makes geriatric practice so challenging. It has little to do with age, as the following case study illustrates.

**Case Study.** Trudy is a 76-year-old divorced businesswoman and community leader. She has several children who are married and scattered about the country. She lives alone. She is a highly intelligent woman who was treated unprofessionally by the medical system when she was found to have a mass in her breast.

Shortly after the mass was detected, she was told to have the proper laboratory evaluation, but she did not receive the results for several days. Trudy then received a call from the physician's office asking her to come in and discuss "her problem." When the doctor appeared, his greeting was: "Pack your bags, I have a hospital bed for you." The significance of the physical and laboratory findings was not discussed with the patient, and, to make matters worse, it was recommended that she enter a hospital in another town and see a surgeon she did not know. The patient was angry and resentful at this approach to her problem. She believed that she was intelligent enough to discuss the pros and cons of the laboratory and clinical findings with her physician, but she was never offered the opportunity. She felt that she had not been allowed to express or discuss her feelings and opinions about the problem, the recommended surgery, and the recommended surgeon.

Trudy knew that she had a serious medical problem. She had a close friend who was a surgeon, so she called him. She has undergone surgery and is presently receiving chemotherapy.

Trudy had been dealt with in a manner that was unnecessarily unjust and unkind. There was no need for her to experience worry, frustration, and fear while awaiting information that was rightfully hers. The cavalier, condescending attitude that followed was thoughtless. This can happen to anyone at any age, but all too often age alone prompts the doctor or caretaker to make decisions for the elderly without properly discussing the problem with the patient.

In the course of treating a geriatric patient, the physician may only be able to obtain information about the patient's behavior prior to the acute episode from the patient's family. Even though the physician may feel comfortable making judgments about patients he has known and treated for the past 20 years, the family's feelings still must be considered. If, however, the patient is seen for the first time in the hospital under the circumstances of an acute episode, then the input of family or friends is essential. Decisions cannot be made on the basis of the patient's age. If the physician does not know the patient, then he or she must work with those who do or risk practicing in a manner governed by stereotypes and prejudices.

## *The Role of Patients and Their Families in the Practice of Medicine*

Families are naturally concerned about illness in the older family member. What is going to happen? Will he feel pain? Will he suffer? Will he be up all night? Will he scream or cry out? Will he be able to eat? Will he lose control of his bowels? Will he know what day it is? Will he go into a coma? Will I be able to manage alone? Can the family feed and bathe him and look after his bowels? Should we try to get him out of bed? He likes beer; can he have a drink? How long can this go on? Should I give up my job to stay home, or should I get a homemaker? Does Medicare cover homemakers? How about major medical insurance?

All physicians are asked questions of this sort by families. The answers are never simple. They must be tailored to the patient, the patient's problems, and the family.[41] Some families are happy to be kept informed and will leave all decision-making to the doctor. Frequently, however, some or all in a family will have very strong feelings and will insist on a particular course of action. It takes diplomacy, patience, and time to work with families in relation to the needs of the patient as well as in relation to the way family situations affect those needs. With national policy changes, families will be expected to assume a greater role and not to be so substantially relieved of caring tasks as in the past. As Morris[42] has stated, "Policy has changed from one that included government responsibility in response to group-identified needs in improving the quality of life for frail, chronically ill older people to one that sees government involvement as undesirable." Given this change, working with families of geriatric patients with varying functional abilities will become critical in geriatric practice.

### Family and Physician Involvement with Progressive Illness

One of the most difficult problems in all of medicine is Alzheimer's disease.[43] Early on, manifestations of the disorder are subtle. Both the patient and the caretaker know something is wrong, but they do not understand what it is, and often the physician is unable to explain what is going on. By the time diagnosis becomes clear, families are often distrustful and angry with the physician. Even with adequate explanation, anxiety and denial often make it difficult for family members to understand or accept the explanation. The characteristics of the disease, i.e., irritability, lack of initiative, impulsiveness, lability, and belligerent behavior, are not understood. Family members often feel responsible or guilty for a behavioral problem that really is part of the disease. Family members with unrealistic expectations are often angry and hostile toward the patient whom they regard as consciously choosing to have symptoms rather than being affected by an illness.

Looking after the patient day and night can easily isolate a spouse or a whole family, creating feelings of frustration, resentment, guilt, anxiety, despair, depression, or anger directed toward the patient, the doctor, other family members, or maybe toward one's self.

There is no scheduled time in the course of caring for the elderly when these feelings may emerge, but an alertness on the part of the physician to this possible development and a sharing of this concern with family members will do much to minimize such problems.

### The Decision to Institutionalize

The patient usually prefers to remain at home rather than be institutionalized. Knowing when the condition of the patient and the resources of the family have reached the critical point at which the balance of judgment shifts in favor of institutional care is always problematic, and there is no simple solution. By planning ahead with patients and their families, the physician can avoid some of the usual pitfalls.

The transfer or relocation of a patient is often one of the most traumatic events in the life of that person.[44] The move is usually abrupt; one day you are here, the next you are there. Usually "there" is completely unknown to the patient, who suddenly finds himself or herself in a new building, surrounded by unfamiliar faces, and, more often than not, living in a room with a total stranger. This can be devastating. This is the time for families to become involved. Getting to know the facility and the people working there and, above all, visiting the patient frequently during the early days in the nursing facility are important.

Once the patient is established in the place that will be his or her home, the physician should consider and discuss the plans for care of this patient with the family. The physician must determine whether the patient's condition and function are good enough to warrant health maintenance and prevention efforts, such as priodic laboratory screenings or x-ray studies, or whether the patient has progressed to a point at which any response by the physician to change in the patient's physical status should be minimal. Proper family preparation often makes it possible to avoid hospitalization of a vegetating, demented patient in whom an acute problem, such as bleeding or high fever, develops and to allow nature to take its course. It is very important to understand the patient's feelings and those of the family about resuscitation and heroic measures. Periodic meetings with the family are valuable in planning the course of action to be followed in the terminal illness of an Alzheimer's patient. During these meetings, it is valuable to assess the feelings of the family members toward the patient, toward the illness, and toward each other.

### Services That Help the Older Patient in the Community

Fortunately most older patients will not require a great deal of assistance in their later years. Even those without effective family ties can be helped to maintain their independence. Visiting nurse associations provide a wide range of health and social support services. Day programs can provide social supports and, in some cases, therapy to help patients to maintain fitness, or to rehabilitate patients so that they regain lost functions. Senior transportation services are available to take individuals to medical appointments, shopping, or other destinations. Nutritional services and Meals-on-Wheels are available in most communities. For patients with families, in addition to the preceding services, respite services are becoming available, including homemaker services as well as short-stay residential care. If all these services are available, what then are the problems with respect to effective alternatives to long-term institutional care?

First, with the exception of a few scattered demonstrations, there is often no program for the coordination of services. Issues of territoriality, program administration, and eligibility requirements, as well as the reduction of supports for social services as a policy perspective, make it highly unlikely that this maze will sort itself out in the immediate future. Second, similar to long-term care support in general, without public programs, the costs of community-based services are beyond the reach of all but the most affluent older patients. Forcing family support of these long-term care costs fails to consider the projected abilities of families to participate in their own future maintenance.

Older patients and their families could coordinate their own service needs. Since this is already happening in a significant way,[3] the development of a policy that would build on this resource rather than destroy it appears only logical.[8] Unfortunately, the concepts involved are sufficiently different as to require changes in the way aging and the aging process are viewed.

## A CHALLENGE TO PHYSICIANS

Physicians must take the lead in initiating developments that are necessary to improve care for geriatric patients. If the physician advocates the necessary changes, there is a chance that they will be realized. The principal objective is the integration of health services and social services into a system that will offer real alternatives to institutional care.

However, before anything else can be accomplished, the prejudice that the frailties of age preclude the active contribution of older people must be eliminated. The assumption that aging is an ever-increasing pathologic condition is built into the structure of our society. Even those who advocate for the aged do so in such a way as to perpetuate this stereotype.[45] The fact that vulnerability increases with age[46] does not mean that all people at an advanced age will become impaired.

Three things are needed: (1) the means of determining objectively the services needed by the patient, (2) a system for managing service delivery, and (3) public policies that encourage the necessary social and economic supports.

1. In the area of functional assessment, scales have been constructed in such a way as to direct the physician's attention toward objectives for therapeutic intervention.[47] These include scales of physical functioning,[48] cognitive functioning,[49] and activities of daily living[50] (see Chapters 8 and 14). These measure only physical or mental impairments in the patient. They do not measure or evaluate environmental supports or deficiencies. Disability, however, is the result of a patient's impairment plus environmental setting. Intervention on the part of the physician to change either the patient or his or her environment can contribute to the independence of the patient. Simple modifications in the environment can, for example, enable the wheelchair patient to achieve far greater independence. Good, simple techniques to screen for problem areas are also needed. An example might be a simple way to assess gait and posture to identify individuals who are likely to fall. Proper exercise therapies could be developed to counter this tendency.

2. Physicians must become knowledgeable concerning services and service agencies that provide geriatric care. The physician does not have to do it all. Just as pharmacists, social workers, nurses, nutritionists, psychologists, audiologists, and others are involved in care of the aging, so, in the area of social support, a wide range of services are available. Unfortunately, the quality and appropriateness of the care provided by different agencies also differ. Many agencies provide only a limited range of service and lack effective means for networking with complementary services. Turf issues create competitive attitudes and vested interests that do not necessarily serve the patient's needs. With the present system of support or lack of support for noninstitutional services, those that are *available* rather than those that are *needed* are the services often provided.

It is important to maximize the participation of the patient in his own health care. Even the services required by the geriatric patient should be managed, if possible, by the patient. If the physician working with the patient helps him understand his health problems and their relationship to his functional status, then there is every reason to encourage the patient to arrange for his own service needs. When there is a supportive family, the physician's responsibility is to help family members understand how they can back up the patient rather than assume responsibility for him. Working with the patient to help him maintain maximum functional capability should aid in countering the tendency toward social breakdown.

In the relatively few instances in which the patient is compromised in such a way as to require management, it is the physician's role to encourage the caretakers to maximize the patient's input so that whatever function that remains is preserved. This applies to nursing homes, home health agencies, or family members providing care in their own home. This approach is likely to ensure that the care being provided is the appropriate level of care for the functional needs of the patient in question.

3. Developing a new policy to support long-term health care and social services is probably our most pressing problem. If practicing physicians can make a difference in relation to those patients and families whom they currently serve, the supporting policy will follow. This may be optimistic, but functional criteria are the appropriate criteria to determine service delivery needs and maintaining function will reduce the need for institutional care.

## CONCLUSION

Our general understanding of the "at risk" older person must be altered. Professional and lay people alike must understand that much of what has been assumed in relation to the inevitable decline associated with old age is not true. Chronic health and age-related mental health problems *can* be managed. The disabilities of aging are predominantly the consequence of an impairment in interaction with the environment. Functional and social assessments as ways of identifying disabilities should allow us to combine health and social services in a new approach to long-term care of the elderly that is both beneficial to quality of life and economically feasible.

Eventually, understanding and knowledge of aging will take the place of the prejudices that currently dominate geriatric health care and social practices. The physician's involvement will be interesting and rewarding; he or she will perhaps practice in such a way as to follow the philosophy of the Harvard psychiatrist Avery Danto Weisman, who advocates "safe conduct." The physician conducts his patient and the caretakers through the maze of uncertain, perplexing, and distressing events.

## References


1. Lawton MP: Institutions and alternatives for older people. Health Soc Work 3:123, 1978.
2. Eggert GM, Bowlyou JE, Nichols CW: Gaining control of the long term care system: First returns from the ACCESS experiment. Gerontologist 20:356, 1980.
3. Callahan JJ Jr, Diamond LD, Giele JZ, Morris R: Responsibility of families for their severely disabled elders. Health Care Financing Review 1:29, 1980.
4. Shanas E: The family as a social support system in old age. Gerontologist 19:169, 1979.
5. Eggert GM, Granger CV, Morris R, Pendleton SF: Caring for the patient with long-term disability. Geriatrics 32:102, 1977.
6. Maddox GL: Families as context and resource in chronic illness. *In* Sherwood S (ed.): Long Term Care: A Handbook for Researchers, Planners and Providers New York, Behavioral Publishers, 1975.
7. Horowitz A, Dobrof R: The role of families in providing long-term care to the frail and chronically ill elderly living in the community. Final report submitted to the Health Care Financing Administration, Department of Health and Human Services. New York, Brookdale Center on Aging of Hunter College, May 1982.
8. Frankfather DL, Smith MJ, Caro FG: Family care of the elderly. Lexington, MA, D.C. Heath and Co., 1981.
9. Comptroller General of the United States: The Well-Being of Older People in Cleveland, Ohio (HCD 77-70). Washington, DC, U.S. General Accounting Office, 1977.
10. Branch LG, Jette AM: Elders' use of long-term care assistance. Gerontologist 23:51, 1983.
11. Cantor M: Life space and the social support system of the inner city elderly of New York. Gerontologist 15:23, 1975.
12. Schorr A: . . . thy father and thy mother . . . a second look at filial responsibility and family policy. Washington, DC, Department of Health and Human Services, Social Security Administration, no. 13-11953, July 1980.
13. Sussman MB, Burchinal L: Parental aid to married children: Implications for family functioning. Marriage and Family Living 24:320, 1962.
14. Sussman MB: Social and Economic Supports and Family Environments for the Elderly. Final report to Administration on Aging. Washington, DC, Department of Health and Human Services, 1979.
15. Danis BG: Stress in individuals caring for ill elderly relatives. Paper presented at the 31st Annual Gerontological Society of America Meeting, Dallas, Texas, 1978.
16. Newman S: Housing adjustments of older people: A report of findings from the second phase. Ann Arbor, Institute for Social Research, University of Michigan, 1976.
17. Cicirelli VG: Personal strains and negative feelings in adult children's relationship with elderly parents. Paper presented at the 33rd Annual Gerontological Society of America Meeting, San Diego, California, 1980.
18. Cantor M: Caring for the frail elderly: Impact on family, friends, and neighbors. Paper presented at the 33rd Annual Gerontological Society of America Meeting, San Diego, California, 1980.
19. Weiler P, Rathbone-McCuan E: Adult Day Care: Community Work with the Elderly. New York, Springer Publishing Co., 1978.
20. Archold PG: Impact of caring for an ill-elderly parent

on the middle-aged or elderly offspring caregiver. Paper presented at the 31st Annual Gerontological Society of America Meeting, Dallas, Texas, 1978.
21. Seelbach WC: Correlates of aged parents filial responsibility, expectations, and realizations. Fam Coord Sci 27:341, 1978.
22. Kane RL, Kane RA: Care of the aged: Old problems in need of new solutions. Science 200:913, 1978.
23. Streib GF: The frail elderly: Research dilemmas and research opportunities. Gerontologist 23:40, 1983.
24. Smitz HL, Feder J, Scanlon W: Medicare's nursing-home benefit: Variations in interpretation. N Engl J Med 307:855, 1982.
25. Somers A: Long-term care for the elderly and disabled: A new health priority. N Engl J Med 307:221, 1982.
26. Senate Special Committee on Aging: Volume I Developments in Aging: 1981. Washington, DC, U.S. Government Printing Office, 1982.
27. Comptroller General of the United States: Entering a nursing home: Costly implications for medicaid and the elderly. Report to the Congress. Washington, DC, 1979.
28. Glick PC: The future marital status and living arrangements of the elderly. Gerontologist 19:301, 1979.
29. Treas J: Family support systems for the aged: Some social and demographic considerations. Gerontologist 17:486, 1977.
30. Hammel EA, Wachter KW, McDaniel CK: The kin of the aged in A.D. 2000: The chickens come home to roost. *In* Kiesler SB, Morgan JN, Oppenheimer VK (eds.): Aging: Social Change. New York, Academic Press, 1981.
31. Pepper CD: The search for alternatives. Internist 23:6, 1982.
32. Neugarten BL: Older people: A profile. *In* Neugarten BL (ed.): Age or Need? Public Policies for Older People. Beverly Hills, Sage Publications, 1982.
33. Fries JF, Crape LM: Vitality and Aging. San Francisco, WH Freeman, 1981.
34. Cobb S, Fulton J: An epidemiologic gaze into the crystal ball of the elderly. *In* Kiesler SB, Morgan JN, Oppenheimer VK (eds.): Aging: Social Change. New York, Academic Press, 1981.
35. Comfort A: A Good Age. New York, Crown, 1976.
36. Kuypers J, Bengston V: Social breakdown and competence: A model of normal aging. Hum Dev 16:181, 1973.
37. Libow LS, Sherman FT: The Core of Geriatric Medicine: A Guide for Students and Practitioners. St. Louis, C.V. Mosby, 1981.
38. Butler RN: Why Survive? Being Old in America. New York, Harper and Row, 1975.
39. Reichel W: Family practice and the care of the elderly. Proceedings of Family Medicine Curriculum and Care of the Elderly. East Lansing, MI, Michigan State University, 1979.
40. MacMillan D: Features of the senile breakdown. Geriatrics 24:109, 1969.
41. Fortinsky R: Bibliography on health, age and the family. Mimeographed. Kingston, RI, Program in Gerontology, University of Rhode Island, 1981.
42. Morris R: Forward. *In* Frankfather DL, Smith MJ, Caro FG: Family Care of the Elderly. Lexington, MA, D.C. Heath and Co., 1981.
43. Aronson M, Lipkowitz R: Alzheimer's type: The family and the health care delivery system. J Geriatr Soc 29:568, 1981.
44. The Gerontologist. Relocation—interpretation and application: A symposium. [Eustis NN (coordinator)] 20:481, 1981.
45. Estes C: The Aging Enterprise. San Francisco, Jossey-Bass, 1979.
46. Department of Health, Education, and Welfare: A Staff Report: Public Policy and the Frail Elderly. Washington, DC: Federal Council on the Aging, Publication No. 79-20959, 1978.
47. Granger C, Albrecht G, Hamilton B: Outcome of comprehensive medical rehabilitation: Measurement by PULSES profile and Barthel index. Arch Phys Med Rehabil 60:145, 1979.
48. Mahoney F, Barthel D: Functional evaluation: The Barthel index. MD State Med J 14:61, 1965.
49. Pfeiffer E: Functional Assessment: The OARS Multidimensional Functional Assessment Questionnaire. Durham, NC, Duke University, 1975.
50. Katz S, Ford A, Moskowitz R, et al: Studies of illness in the aged: The index of ADL, a standardized measure of biological and psychosocial function. JAMA 185:914, 1963.

## Chapter 6

# An Approach to Common Problems in the Elderly

Jack H. Medalie

*"It is more important to know the patient who suffers from the disease, than to know the disease from which the patient suffers."*

ATTRIBUTED TO SIR WILLIAM OSLER

The title of this chapter implies that the elderly differ from other age groups in important respects and that these differences demand an approach by physicians that is geared to the specific needs of the aged. This approach is the result of a number of factors. The first of these is the attitude and behavior of the physician toward the elderly. This in turn depends on an understanding of the aging process, the diseases from which the elderly suffer, and the elderly themselves, as well as the imperative need for the physician to come to terms with his or her own aging. In addition, the physician should follow a biopsychosocial diagnostic process appropriate to the complaints or problems of the elderly, and do so in an environment that is suitable for interviewing and examining elderly patients (for example, longer appointments, different types of examining equipment and furniture).

It must also be emphasized that the diagnostic process is part of the management process because from the initial portion of the interview, the relationship between the patient and physician has begun. The physician is a vitally important therapeutic agent for all patients, but perhaps even more so for the elderly.

This chapter reviews some background material that contributes to an understanding of the elderly and provides a diagnostic approach to some of the common clinical syndromes with which the elderly present.

## SPECIAL FEATURES OF THE ELDERLY

### The Aging Process

The process of aging is a multifactorial one in which tissues, organs, and cells age at different rates, with much individual variation (see Chapter 1). The genetic programming specific to Homo sapiens, with their built-in metabolic clock, is influenced by a number of factors at the DNA-RNA-protein cellular-molecular level either directly or indirectly.[1-4] These vary from environmental hazards such as radiation, toxic chemicals, and viruses to stressful life events such as the bereavement period following the death of a spouse, to risk factors such as alcoholism and social isolation. Some of the effects of these factors can be modified through appropriate social support systems, but when they affect the body they do so by way of the neuroendocrine and/or immune system or directly at the molecular level in the cells. In Figure 6-1, an attempt has been made to portray this integrated model of the aging process.

### Results of Aging

The major results of the aging process are as follows:

1. A reduced physiologic reserve of many bodily functions, e.g., cardiac, respiratory, and renal.
2. An impaired homeostatic mechanism by which certain bodily activities are kept adjusted, e.g., fluid balance, temperature control, and blood pressure control.

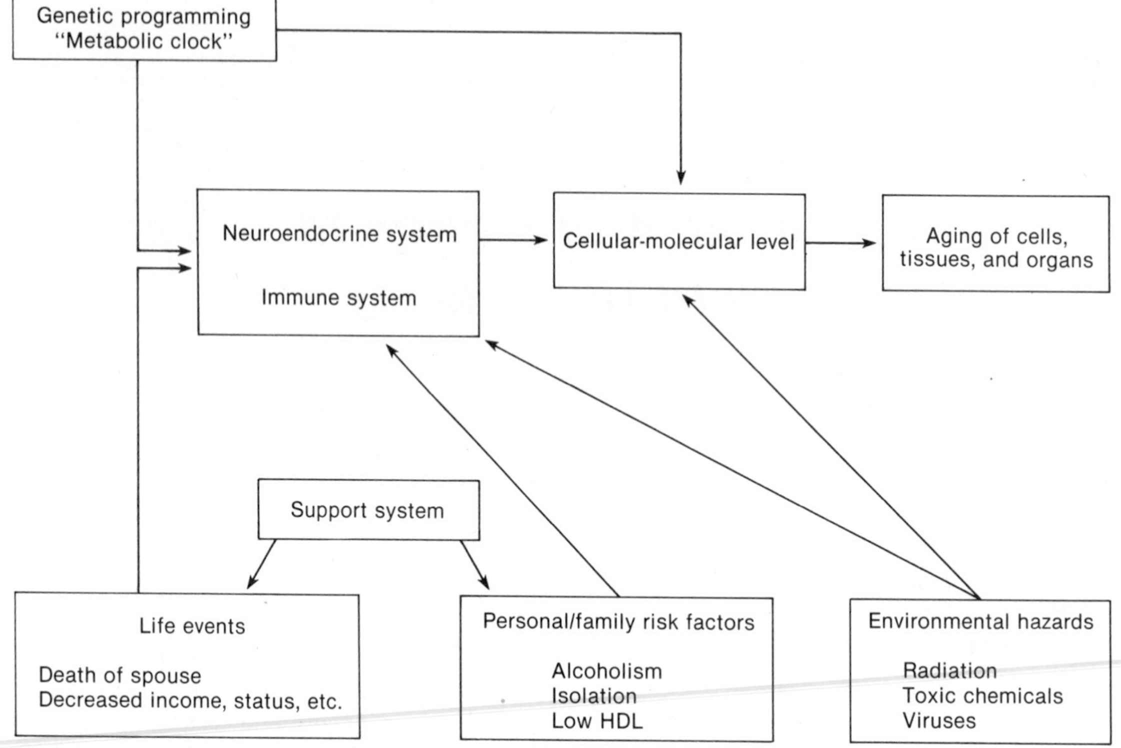


**Figure 1.** A proposed integrated model of the processes involved in aging.

3. Added to this (or perhaps part of the preceding) is the impaired immunologic system as well as a related, increased incidence of neoplastic and age-related autoimmune processes and diseases.

These results become slowly apparent over a long period of time, but sometimes moderate or severe unexpected stressors might precipitate symptoms and signs, or even failure of bodily functions due to this impairment of reserves and homeostatic mechanisms.

## *Individual and Family Development*

Experience during medical training frequently exposes graduates of American medical education to only one side of the geriatric picture—that is, the frail, confused, incontinent, dependent, very ill, disabled, elderly person who evokes in us ambivalent feelings of sadness and sympathy mixed with periods of disgust and rejection. It is only after we enter practice, outside of the tertiary care teaching centers, that we begin to appreciate that the vast majority of elderly can function independently and we realize that the last stage of the life cycle can be an active one of growth and satisfaction.

It is interesting to reflect on the large number of artists, intellectuals, and statesmen, such as Picasso, Freud, Wright, Toscanini, Rubinstein, Michelangelo, and Churchill, whose enthusiasm for their work and their achievements continued into the eighth and ninth decades of their lives. Similarly, in the past 10 years, as a result of new training methods and life-styles, elderly people are performing sporting activities and achieving results that were previously unthinkable.

The last stage of the life cycle is marked by the reality of bodily decline in strength and vitality, punctuated by marker events (not necessarily crises) such as illness; retirement; repeated loss of family members, friends, and colleagues; and often a diminution of personal recognition, authority, status, and control over one's own situation.[5] Sometimes this state is not ameliorated, and the person becomes lonely, isolated, disabled and mentally dysfunctional and dies in a manner that leaves the family feeling both guilty and relieved. On the other hand, the majority of the elderly do very well as a result of a combination of their own inner strength, the support of intimate associates (spouse, children, grandchildren), the use of community resources, and their participation in community activities. The married elderly with close family members do far better on almost all outcome measures compared with the widowed, divorced, or childless.[6] The last stage of the life cycle is a period of active adaptation in which the elderly person finds his or her place somewhere along Erikson's continuum that has "integrity" at one end and "despair" at the other.[7] It is to be hoped that the integrated person achieves the states of "personal wisdom" and "balanced relationships" with his or her family, for this allows death to be faced with equanimity.

Another misconception is that the elderly are often abandoned and that their families do not play an important role in their lives. As pointed out in Chapter 5, nothing is further from the truth. Approximately 80 per cent of the elderly have children and grandchildren and the overwhelming majority sustain frequent contact, reciprocal emotional ties, and mutual support with their offspring. If they do not live together or very close to each other, the elderly and their families often have a pattern called "intimacy at a distance," with ready availability of family members in a crisis situation.[8]

It is also important to remember that the response of the family system to the challenges of later life evolves from earlier family patterns. Relationship conflicts, as well as coping patterns of the family, are repeated throughout the life cycle but can often be modified even in the last stage of the cycle during a terminal crisis.

Duvall[9] defines "family development tasks" of the elderly (presumably middle-class) family to include the following areas: making satisfying living arrangements; adjusting to retirement income; establishing comfortable routines; safeguarding physical and mental health; maintaining love, sex, and marital relations; remaining in contact with other family members; keeping active and involved; and finding meaning in life. Although these tasks apply to most elderly, the lower socioeconomic groups often are so busy trying to survive on a daily basis that all other features are inconsequential.

Walsh[8] includes the following events or processes as development tasks: launching the last child from home, empty-nest transition, retirement (important distinction between forced or desired), residential change, menopause, adjustment to widowhood, remarriage (common occurrence), and grandparenthood.

The understanding of these developmental processes and tasks is most important in gaining a perspective of the elderly patient. Thus, the taking of a family history in the context of a family tree, or genogram, is often a key to the understanding of elderly patients.

## *Perceived Health and Life Problems*

There is increasing evidence that a person's perception of his or her own health and other problems significantly influences the person's own well-being and health status. A recent study by Mossey and Shapiro[10] of over 3000 elderly people showed that self-rating of health was significantly related to the mortality rate in the subsequent 7-year period. This self-rated health status declined with age and was positively associated with life satisfaction, income, and objective health status. Even when controlled for age, sex, and objective health status, the association between self-rated health and mortality remained significant. The mortality rate of the group reporting a poor self-rating was three times the rate of the group reporting an excellent rating. The implication of this and other studies is that, in interviewing elderly patients, we must ascertain how they perceive their own health and life situation. In this connection, it is interesting to note the results of a random sample of 1598 Cleveland residents aged 65 and over.[11] In their self-rating of health, 59.6 per cent declared that it was excellent (11.0 per cent) or good (48.6 per cent), whereas 34.2 per cent thought it was fair, and only 6.2 per cent rated their health as poor. In this same survey, 55.7 per cent indicated that they were highly satisfied with life and 73.3 per cent found life exciting!

The correlation between self-report, or rating, of health and evaluations from medical records, or a special examination, varies from marginal[12] to fairly great.[10] Linn and colleagues[12] looked at self-assessed health among Caucasians, Black, and Cuban elderly patients attending a university center outpatient clinic and found that self-rating of health was associated with the patients' level of functioning (daily activities), the way they reacted to an illness, and their overall health status. However, there has been no deliberate attempt to determine if enhancing a person's self-rating of health will contribute to improved health and survival.

## EVALUATION AND ASSESSMENT OF THE ELDERLY PATIENT

The complaints or presenting problems of the elderly patient are determined by multiple, interrelating factors associated with the patient, his or her intimate associates and cultural subgroup, and society. These factors are depicted in Figure 6–2, using a venn diagram based on epidemiologic principles. The innermost area (d) represents the patient's adjustment to the interacting factors and projects his or her outlook on life, as well as the pattern or type of presenting problems or complaints. It is clear from this concept that the traditional biomedical model used so successfully for acute medical emergencies is totally inappropriate for dealing with elderly patients in primary care. Engel[13] speaks about the need for a biopsychosocial model but does not appear to place sufficient emphasis on the cultural aspects, as do Kleinman and others.[14] In addition, prevention and rehabilitation emerge as important aspects of the care of the elderly, as does the need for continuity of care. The "family epidemiologic model," as well as comprehensive and holistic medicine models, attempts to incorporate these factors.[15]

An important aspect of primary care is the assessment of the new patient (see Chapter 8). Although the new patient often presents with serious complaints or, rarely, with a life-threatening situation, the physician generally has time

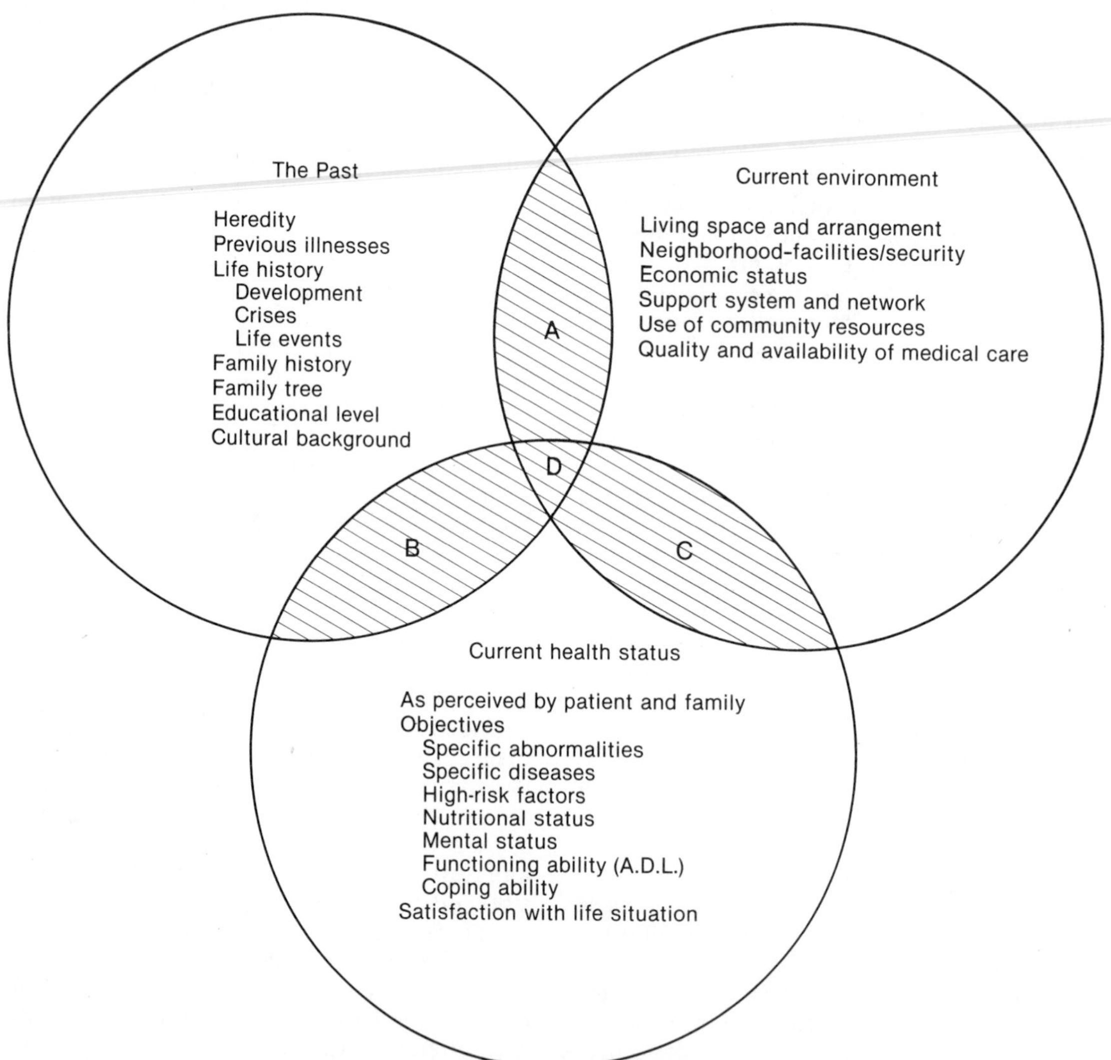


**Figure 2.** Factors determining the problems presented by the elderly: the information required for a comprehensive examination. *A*, Personal habits, attitudes, and behavior. *B*, Past medical care and utilization pattern. *C*, Participation in community activities. *D*, Resultant adjustment.

(i.e., a number of visits over a period of weeks) to make the assessment. The goals of the assessment include determining the patient's current health status and diagnosis; establishing a data base against which future developments and changes can be compared; establishing a good relationship with the patient and the patient's family; and, based on the preceding, determining the priorities for management and intervention in order to prevent or alleviate disease and improve the quality of the patient's life situation.

### *Determination of the Patient's Current Health Status and Diagnosis*

The major factors involved in the assessment of the patients are depicted in Figure 6–1; this assessment covers so much ground that no primary care practitioner has the time to complete it in one session. Depending on the type of practice, the information can be collected by a number of workers (physician, nurse, receptionist, laboratory technician) over a period of time.

Some aspects of the history and examination that are important in respect to the elderly have been emphasized by Steel,[16] Kerzner,[17] Cutler,[18] Nowlin and Busse,[19] Kennie,[20] and Schneiderman.[21] Important aspects of taking a history are as follows:

1. Sufficient time must be scheduled.
2. Patience is not only a virtue but also a necessity!
3. Empathy is essential. Nowlin and Busse believe that the good practitioner must have come to terms with his or her own aging (as well as dealing with aged patients), otherwise the physician-patient relationship, which is the key to the therapeutic relationship, will be deficient.
4. The patient's intelligence should not be underestimated.
5. It is always a good policy to ask one of the patient's intimate associates to accompany the patient and participate in the interview or be in the waiting room if parts of the history need to be validated.
6. If possible, the summaries of previous hospitalizations and other important medical data should be included in the patient's folder.
7. Many of the young elderly (up to 75 years) can review the medicinal drugs they are taking without difficulty but usually they will be easier to review accurately if the patient brings the medicine.
8. Make sure the patient can hear you. This may involve sitting close to the patient rather than having a table or couch between you.
9. Make sure the patient can understand you.
10. If the patient comes in with a third person, arrange seating so that all of you can see and hear each other without difficulty and without having to rotate the head or body unduly.

Points outlined below will make the examination more productive for the physician and more comfortable for the patient.

1. Whenever possible observe the patient undressing and later dressing himself. This is a valuable aid in assessing daily activities.
2. If you have an examination table that is narrow and uncomfortable, do as much of the examination as possible with the patient sitting in a chair. A wider examination table or one that can be pushed up against the wall often gives the elderly person a secure feeling. In the same context, make sure the elderly person can get onto the table without difficulty or support.
3. Make sure that the temperature of the room is comfortable.
4. Many elderly patients prefer rectal examinations in the left lateral position rather than supine or bending over. Ask them which position is preferred.
5. The question of what is normal for the elderly is often troublesome. Some changes with aging are well-known: kyphoscoliosis, brown spots on dorsum of hand, slight tremor, diminution in hearing and vision, barrel-shaped chest, and loss of abdominal and Achilles reflexes. Care must be taken not to accept these changes as due merely to aging without a careful examination to exclude treatable conditions, such as diminished hearing due to impacted wax, diminished vision due to cataracts, or constipation due to impacted feces.

The data base on each elderly patient should include all the relevant items from Figure 6–2 relating to the patient's past, current environment, and current health status. When the data base is established, future changes in functioning, laboratory results, and so forth can be evaluated better. In addition, intangible but vital ingredients of the physician-patient relationship should be in place. Mutual trust, understanding, and acceptance should be established, and this will lay the foundation for a future satisfying relationship between the physician and the patient as well as between the physician and the patient's closest associates (e.g., family, friends).

With these facts and information available, a comprehensive biopsychosocial evaluation can be made and a management plan adopted with the patient, the patient's family, or, when necessary, community agencies and institutions. A family conference centering on the problems of the aged member plays a very important role in reducing tension, anxiety, and guilt and improves the situation of many elderly patients and their families.

## COMPLAINTS, ILLNESSES, AND DISEASE

### *Distinguishing Between Complaints, Illnesses, and Disease*

It is important to differentiate between subjective complaints of patients and/or their families, i.e., "illness," which is the interpretation and understanding of symptoms of the patient, and "disease," which is the structural and functional changes in body organs and systems as diagnosed and classified by physicians.[14]

A clinical-problem list in the problem-oriented record system might contain diseases, illnesses, and complaints.

### *Categories of Presenting Complaints or Problems*

Presenting complaints can be classified as follows.

1. Associated with a disease process. Some examples are pain from pleurisy or arthritic joint and cough from bronchitis.
2. Associated with the aging process. These could include impaired visual acuity, diminished hearing ability, senile purpura, wax in ears, nocturnal leg cramps, decline in physical strength, and kyphosis.
3. A mixture of 1 and 2 or an interaction 1 on 2.
4. Loss of mobility or disability, e.g., a decreased ability to carry out the activities of daily living such as dressing or walking.
5. Reflection of, or association with, a breakdown or dysfunction of personal resources, family relationships, social support system, or environmental conditions.
6. Asymptomatic conditions found during periodic health examinations, e.g., high blood pressure, hyperglycemia, breast lump, enlarged lymph glands, and anemia.
7. Complaints related to cultural interpretation of symptoms (illness).

These presenting problems will vary depending on many factors, from cultural beliefs and behavior of the patient population to the type and quality of the medical care system available. The frequency of the different types of presenting problems will be discussed later.

### *Presentation of Symptoms*

The manner in which symptoms are presented varies but can be classified under the following headings.

1. Direct complaint. The patient complains about the major problem(s) that are worrying him or her.
2. Indirect complaint. The patient complains in medically acceptable terms about one of his or her conditions while hoping that the physician will allow him or her the opportunity of talking about the *real* problem that is often nonmedical in the strictest sense. Unconscious transference of symptoms to another system leads in many cases to a so-called psychosomatic disorder or to depression, thus concealing the real problem, which is often a dilemma that the patient and family do not know how to solve. The patient will often complain of a minor problem because he or she does not know how the physician will react to the real worry (often involving sexual or other intimate problems).
3. Complaints presented through a second person. Often a spouse or child will bring out the major problem that the patient may deny or belittle at first. In those instances in which the elderly person is incapable of presenting a history, this information will, of necessity, come from an intimate associate.
4. Complaints presented by another patient of the same family. Occasionally, the entire family system is disrupted by an elderly person and the presenting patient may not even be the aged one but rather another member of the family. Examples include a daughter who is the main caretaker of her disabled father and who presents with severe headaches; a son-in-law who develops a recurring duodenal ulcer attack; a grandchild with a behavioral problem who in reality is the scapegoat for family conflict due to the activities of a demented grandmother.

### *Characteristics of Disease Presentation*

Multiple pathologic processes in multiple systems are characteristic in the elderly patient. Various studies have found three to four conditions in the ambulatory aged and five to nine among institutionalized elderly.[22] A corollary of this is that there are often multiple complaints without necessarily a major complaint. Despite the universal acceptance of this characteristic, today as many as 10 per cent of the elderly do not have a chronic disorder (distinct from age-related changes) discernible at checkups.

The chronic conditions usually have a prolonged onset. In addition, owing to their altered physiologic conditions and reactions, the elderly have many conditions with unusual presentations compared with those in younger adults. For example, in the elderly, painless myocardial infarctions are very frequent and account for approximately 30 per cent of reported infarcts as found by Medalie and Goldbourt.[23] In Rodstein's series[24] of elderly patients, 31 per cent of myocardial infarctions were silent and 40 per cent were atypical.[24] The atypical presentation is often increased dyspnea rather than pain. In my own practice, I have had three patients over 70 years old with perforated duodenal ulcers, two of which were painless and caused acute fatigue. Similarly, tuberculosis, multiple pulmonary embolism, thyrotoxicosis, pneumonia, and appendicitis are some of the diseases that often present without the typical symptoms, thus obscuring diagnosis. Acute confusion can signal pneumonia or a urinary tract infection. An elderly man with a fractured clavicle and wrist may have fallen as a result of arrhythmia and not by tripping on the carpet.

Difficulties are often caused by an altered clinical course or unusual response to illness. Examples include acute infections with no rise in temperature, acute appendicitis with no localizing right iliac fossa pain, depression masking a myocardial infarct, and, very commonly, confusion produced by transferring an elderly patient to the hospital.

Conditions peculiar to this age group (e.g., cataracts, prostatic hypertrophy, nocturia, and unstable gait) are commonly seen, whereas hyperosmolar nonketotic diabetic coma and hypothermia are occasionally seen.

Because of reduced reserves, elderly patients often experience heart failure following relatively minor conditions or become very anxious and confused following minor surgical operations. Drug-induced conditions are very common, and other iatrogenic disorders are precipitated, for example, by restricted mobility.

## COMMON SYMPTOMS, PROBLEMS, AND DISEASES IN PRIMARY CARE

The number of consultations that physicians have with members of the 65 and over age group varies considerably in different parts of the country and from country to country. In the United Kingdom, with its National Health Service, every person is on a panel of a general practitioner, and the average number of annual contacts between physicians and patients 65 years and older is 6.3. To compare this average with that in the United States, one has to add up the contacts of the elderly with general or family physicians (2.1), medical specialists (1.3), and surgical specialists (1.3). This gives a figure of 4.7 (National Ambulatory Medical Survey, 1973 to 1974) per annum.[25] A recent report from the Johnson Foundation points out that 20.9 per cent of all family practice encounters are with patients aged 65 and over.[26] In my own practice, over a 6-year period, my annual average number of contacts per patient was 3.2, but the majority of these patients were young elderly.

### *Diseases (Diagnostic Categories) Seen in Primary Care*

There are a number of good, current studies of primary care practitioners in the United States. In combination these studies give an accurate picture of the most common illnesses seen among the elderly. These studies include the following.

In the National Ambulatory Medical Care Survey, approximately 1000 office-based physicians are surveyed over a week's period each year. Their response rate is over 75 per cent, and the personal and practice information collected has become a valuable source of valid and reliable data.[25]

A national study of medical activities and a manpower project done by the University of Southern California consisted of a stratified sample of all medical specialties. Physicians filled out a week-long log diary and a detailed questionnaire of all activities during a 3-day period. The data of the general practitioners and the family physicians were analyzed in a separate study.[26] The Virginia study is an analysis of a 2-year, continuous survey of 36 family physicians and 92 family practice residents.[27] The Wisconsin study collected and analyzed the contacts of 109 family physicians one day each week for 4 weeks and various reports of individual practices.[28]

There are some aspects of these studies that make comparison difficult. For example, in their analyses the Virginia and Wisconsin studies utilized up to six diagnoses for each encounter, whereas the University of Southern California study used only the principal diagnosis. All in all, these studies do highlight some important dissimilarities among different areas of the country. However, they also show striking similarities, particularly in relation to the most common major diagnoses.

There are four conditions or diagnostic clusters that always appear to be among the top five on ambulatory lists and account for a large percentage of the patients hospitalized by primary care physicians. These are (1) hypertension, (2) cardiovascular conditions (especially ischemic heart disease), (3) diabetes mellitus, and (4) arthritis and rheumatism. Other common reasons for office visits are (1) general medical examinations, (2) mental or emotional problems, variously classified as depression, anxiety, or neuroses, (3) surgical (and medical) aftercare, and (4) injuries (sprains, fractures, dislocations).

The following conditions, although not occurring as frequently as the preceding disorders, are common: urinary tract infections, cerebrovascular conditions, dermatitis, diseases of the eye, lower back pain, diseases of the digestive system, respiratory infections, emphysema, chronic obstructive pulmonary disease, neoplasms, ear conditions, and obesity (see Tables 6-1 and 6-2).

## *Symptoms and Symptom Complexes among the Elderly*

It appears logical that the symptoms of the diseases or conditions listed previously would be the most common complaints or symptoms brought to the physician. However, some of the common diseases have no specific early symptoms (e.g., hypertension), whereas others can present in many different ways. Therefore, the common symptoms of the elderly do not appear to have a close association with the diseases diagnosed.

In addition, I have found from my own experiences that as my knowledge, understanding, and relationship with my patients improved (similarly their understanding of me), there was an increase of complaints regarding their life in general, with decreasing emphasis on bodily symptoms that were "medically acceptable." A 6-year analysis of our small group practice revealed that of the total complaints, 44.7 per cent were disease-oriented and 55.3 per cent were not disease-oriented.[29] Of the latter group, 22.9 per cent were related to social adjustment problems, 17.4 per cent to finances and occupation, and 15.0 per cent to problems related to the family (children). Other experienced family physicians with whom I have discussed this issue agree that their patients bring these types of complaints to them. However, the physicians, for reasons related to the diagnostic classification of diseases, their own medical education, and/or the reimbursement policies of third-party payers, rarely include these complaints in the problem list!

Hull[30] studied a group of general practitioners over a 6-month period and found that in patients over 65 years the major symptoms in order of frequency were musculoskeletal pain, skin-related disorders, general feeling of poor health, diarrhea and vomiting, "lumps," cough, abdominal pain, ear and eye symptoms, depression, and injury-related complaints.[30] Many of these complaints were significantly related to marital status and socioeconomic class; for example, the frequency of musculoskeletal pain was inversely related to social class, whereas eye

**Table 6-1.** MOST COMMON DIAGNOSES IN THE ELDERLY (65 YEARS AND OVER)

| U.S. California Study (1977)[26] | % of All Diagnoses | Wisconsin Study (1978)[29] | % of All Diagnoses |
|---|---|---|---|
| 1. Hypertension | 15.1 | 1. All cardiovascular disorders | 14.4 |
| 2. Ischemic heart disease | 9.8 | 2. Hypertension | 8.9 |
| 3. General medical examination | 8.1 | 3. Diabetes | 5.5 |
| 4. Degenerative joint disease | 6.5 | 4. Arthritis of all types | 4.8 |
| 5. Diabetes | 5.0 | 5. General medical examinations | 3.1 |
| 6. Depression/anxiety | 2.9 | 6. Surgical aftercare | 2.8 |
| 7. Soft tissue injuries | 2.3 | 7. Neuroses, etc. | 2.0 |
| 8. Urinary tract infection | 2.2 | 8. Obesity | 1.8 |
| 9. Emphysema | 2.0 | 9. Emphysema | 1.3 |
| 10. Acute upper respiratory infection | 1.9 | 10. Cerebrovascular disorders | 1.3 |
| 11. Fractures/dislocations | 1.5 | | 45.9% |
| 12. Acute sprains/strains | 1.3 | | |
| 13. Dermatitis/eczema | 1.2 | | |
| 14. Acute lower respiratory infections | 1.0 | | |
| 15. Bursitis, etc. | 1.0 | | |
| | 61.8% | | |

**Table 6–2.** MOST COMMON DIAGNOSES BY CATEGORIES*

| Diagnosis Category | Condition |
|---|---|
| 1. Communicable diseases | Diarrhea and or vomiting; intestinal infectious disease<br>Pyrexia of unknown origin<br>Tuberculosis |
| 2. Neoplasms, including reticuloses | Breast (Category 2—benign)<br>Skin (Category 2—benign)<br>Leukemia, all types<br>All other malignant neoplasms |
| 3. Allergic, endocrine, metabolic, and nutritional disorders | Diabetes mellitus<br>Obesity<br>Asthma |
| 4. Diseases of blood and blood-forming organs | Iron deficiency (hypochromic) anemia (male and female)<br>Other specific anemias (male and female)<br>Pernicious (megaloblastic) anemia |
| 5. Mental illness, personality disorders, and psychoneurosis | Depressive neurosis<br>Anxiety neurosis<br>Tension headache<br>Abuse of alcohol |
| 6. Diseases of nervous system and sense organs | Otitis media, acute<br>Vascular lesions<br>Otitis externa<br>Conjunctivitis and ophthalmia |
| 7. Diseases of the circulatory system | Benign or unspecified hypertension, with or without heart and/or renal disease<br>Arteriosclerosis (including cardiovascular disease)<br>Congestive heart failure<br>Other ischemic heart disease |
| 8. Diseases of the respiratory system | Pharyngitis (including febrile sore throat and tonsillitis)<br>Bronchitis, acute<br>Coryza (nonfebrile common cold)<br>Sinusitis (acute) |
| 9. Diseases of the digestive system | Abdominal pain other than colic<br>Acute gastritis or duodenitis<br>Other diseases of intestines and peritoneum |
| 10. Diseases of the genitourinary system | Vulvitis, vaginitis, and cervicitis (nonvenereal)<br>Urinary infection (cystitis)<br>Other infections of urinary system, including prostatitis |
| 11. Pregnancy disorders | |
| 12. Diseases of skin and cellular tissue | Dermatitis, contact<br>Other local infections of skin and subcutaneous tissue<br>Rash |
| 13. Diseases of bones and joints | Other forms of arthritis and rheumatism<br>Osteoarthritis<br>Back pain alone<br>Rheumatoid arthritis |
| 14. Congenital malformation | |
| 15. Certain diseases of early infancy | |
| 16. Symptoms and ill-defined conditions | Headache<br>Weight loss<br>Debility or fatigue |
| 17. Accidents, poisoning, and violence | Lacerations, amputations, contusions, and abrasions<br>Sprains and strains<br>Foreign body |
| 18. Prophylactic procedures | Other medical examinations for preventive and presymptomatic purposes<br>Cervical smear<br>Other prophylactic procedures |
| 19. Other procedures | |
| 20. Problems other than specific diagnostic/symptomatic | Family relationship problems |
| 21. Family history of selected diseases | Hypertension<br>Carcinoma<br>Anemia (including hemoglobinopathies)<br>Diabetes |
| 22. Selective therapeutic index | Other psychotropic drugs<br>Thiazide diuretics<br>Other cardiac drugs |

* Data from Marsland DW, Wood M, and Mayo F: The content of family practice. J Fam Pract 3:37, 1976.

**Table 6–3.** SYMPTOMS ASSOCIATED WITH ADJUSTMENT TO LIVING SITUATION*

| Symptoms Described by Patient | Symptoms Described by Closest Associate |
|---|---|
| Lonely, isolated | Is a nuisance |
| Can't cope | Can't cope with him/her |
| Don't want to go on like this | Can't take it anymore |
| Can't afford heating | Incontinent |
| Bored—nothing to do | Prowls at night and we can't sleep |
| Afraid to go out | |
| No respect from children | Smokes in bed and we're scared of fires |
| The world has changed | |
| Don't seem to have any friends | Unstable walk—falls a lot |
| | Doesn't remember anything |
| Family fighting over inheritance before I'm dead | Is sometimes completely nuts and other times is fine! |
| None of my children want me for more than a few days | |

and gynecologic symptoms were directly related.

In an attempt to summarize the major symptoms and symptom complexes of the elderly population, I have organized them into four tables, with the last one listing the traditional medical complaints (Tables 6–3 to 6–6).

The majority of these symptom complexes are dealt with directly in various chapters. However, to provide an example of a differential diagnostic approach appropriate for a geriatric physician, dizziness will now be discussed. The reader is also referred to Chapter 26.

## *Differential Diagnosis of Dizziness*

Webster defines dizzy as "a whirling sensation in the head with a tendency to fall," and its importance is that it is a very common symptom or complaint among the elderly. Estimates of its prevalence vary from 19 to 57 per cent in the 65 and over age group. In the United Kingdom, the complaint is referred to as "giddiness," whereas in other countries the term used often means "head going round."[31] Kennie and colleagues[32] also point out that dizziness usually indicates serious, underlying disease; commonly results in decreased mobility, and patient and caretaker anxiety; and is a factor in many falls. As a result, unrelieved dizziness usually leads to requests for institutionalization.

It is difficult to classify the causes of dizziness, but attempts have been made by Drachman and Hart,[33] Kennie,[32] Daroff,[34] and Lassiter[35] to evolve a clinically relevant differentiation. Building on their suggestions, I propose the following classification outlined in Table 6–7 based on the answers to two basic questions.

1. *When you are dizzy, do you feel any movement (falling, going around)?*
2. *Is the dizziness accompanied by fainting or loss of consciousness?*

### Dizziness with a Sensation of Movement

The patient experiences a sensation of movement either of himself or of his surroundings.

**Table 6–4.** SYMPTOMS RELATED TO LIFE-CYCLE CHANGES

| |
|---|
| Menopause |
| Retirement |
| Terminal illness of friends |
| Death of spouse or others |

**Table 6–5.** SYMPTOMS RELATED TO PERIODIC CHECKUPS AND GENERAL MEDICAL EXAMINATIONS

| |
|---|
| Diminution of strength |
| Decreased sleep |
| Diminished libido |

**Table 6–6.** SYMPTOMS AND SYMPTOM COMPLEXES*

| | |
|---|---|
| Confusion | Chapter 20 |
| Related to hypertension | Chapter 32 |
| Dizziness: falls, syncope, vertigo | |
| Musculoskeletal pain or discomfort: lower extremity, lower back, upper extremity | Chapter 36 |
| Chest pain and abdominal pain | Chapters 29, 46 |
| Fatigue | |
| Depression/anxiety | Chapter 17 |
| Change in bodily functions: postmenopausal bleeding, rectal bleeding, shortness of breath, difficulty in walking, severe constipation, dribbling, dryness of skin | Chapters 22, 24, 25, 29, 30, 33, 35, 36, 41, 46 |
| Problems with vision | Chapter 24 |
| Problems with hearing | Chapter 25 |
| Reactions to drugs and medicine | Chapter 12 |
| Related to alcoholism | |

* Further discussion of individual symptoms and symptom complexes can be found in the chapters listed.

**Table 6–7.** THE CLASSIFICATION OF DIZZINESS

| |
|---|
| **Dizziness with Sensation of Movement** |
| A definite sensation or illusion of movement, usually, but not necessarily, rotatory. This group is invariably vertigo. |
| **Dizziness Without Sensation of Movement** |
| Dizziness/lightheadedness with occasional or frequent fainting or loss of consciousness |
| Dizziness without fainting |
| Dysequilibrium, including instability of gait and fear of falling |
| Associated principally with malaise and weakness |
| Lightheadedness |
| **Mixed or Ill-Defined Types of Dizziness** |

This type of dizziness is considered true vertigo. Generally vertigo may result from pathologic conditions involving the vestibulolabyrinthine system and its nerves, or the vestibular nuclei. In the elderly, cerebrovascular arterial insufficiency of one type or another is the most common cause.

**Etiology**

***Cerebrovascular causes.*** Cerebrovascular causes include vertebrobasilar insufficiency. The vast majority of patients with this condition have dizziness as one of their major symptoms. Movements of the head and neck often contribute to this insufficiency owing to cervical arthritis. Sometimes the subclavian steal syndrome can produce dizziness on the side of the pulseless limb when the latter is exercised.

***Disorders of the Ear.*** The following conditions are associated with vertigo:

1. Impaction of the *external canal* with wax.
2. *Otitis media* (especially if there has been a large perforation of the drum).
3. Disorders affecting the *vestibulolabyrinthine apparatus.* These include benign paroxysmal positional vertigo, associated with the position of the head; labyrinthitis (infective etiology); damage caused by ototoxic agents (e.g., quinidine, streptomycin, gentamycin, salicylates, alcohol), and often associated with diminished hearing and tinnitus; and Meniere's disease, which occurs mainly in the second half of life and results in recurrent, severe vertigo with nausea, vomiting, hearing loss, and tinnitus.

***Cerebral conditions.*** Cerebral conditions that may cause vertigo include the following:

1. Acoustic neuroma of the eighth cranial nerve may cause vertigo, unilateral nerve deafness, and tinnitus. A most important early sign is diminished corneal sensation.
2. Cerebellar tumors.
3. Multiple sclerosis.

***Trauma to Head and Neck***

***Positional Vertigo.*** This type of vertigo is common when looking down from heights and is a complaint of some elderly when their sensory organs are not functioning as well as previously (e.g., diminished eyesight due to cataracts).

### DIZZINESS WITHOUT SENSATION OF MOVEMENT

**With Occasional or Frequent Fainting or Loss of Consciousness**

*Cerebrovascular* disease can produce this type of dizziness. An example is transient ischemic attacks. Other causes are vasovagal attacks; severe orthostatic (postural) changes; and cardiovascular disorders, e.g., arrhythmias such as heart block, bradycardia, and severe aortic stenosis. Less common causes can include micturition syncope, especially of males during the night, which can be helped by convincing these patients to urinate while sitting; attacks of coughing or, occasionally, partial choking on food, which can cause the elderly to faint; and tight collars.

**Without Sensation of Movement or Fainting Attacks**

*Dysequilibrium* or loss of balance is usually a disorder of motor control or instability of gait and is often accompanied by complaints of dizziness. Causes of dysequilibrium include the following:

1. Parkinsonism.
2. Ataxia due to cerebellar lesions or alcoholism.
3. One-sided weakness following a stroke.
4. Fractures of the hip or other parts of lower limb.
5. Painful arthritis, causing difficulty in walking.
6. Unfamiliar surroundings when the patient does not see too well, especially following a cataract operation.
7. Precarious or hazardous surroundings, e.g., moving stairs, uneven surfaces, dimly lit places.
8. Anxiety state, e.g., fear of falling.

*Malaise and weakness* may be associated with dizziness without sensation of movement or fainting. Elderly patients with chronic conditions who also have inadequate nutritional intake often complain of dizziness attacks, which can be associated with anemia, postural hypotension, and other reasons. Patients included in this category are those with chronic infections, carcinoma, or heart failure.

*Lightheadedness* or the sensation of faintness is a common symptom and is associated with various emotional and pathophysiologic organic changes. Examples include the following:

1. Postural hypotension.
2. Cardiac arrhythmias of various types.
3. Emotional problems such as insoluble conflicts often related to family problems, as well as anxiety states due to fear for security.
4. Rapid changes in glucose level in uncontrolled diabetics (hypoglycemia) may produce dizziness as a chief complaint.
5. Mild cerebrovascular arterial insufficiency.
6. Anemic states, e.g., polycythemia or sickling might result in enough interference with blood flow in the brain to produce symptoms.
7. Postoperative procedures of almost any type but especially after cataract or prostate surgery.
8. Occasionally, *dysfunctioning thyroid.*
9. Malnutrition.

### Mixed Types of Dizziness

Mixed or ill-defined types of dizziness may also occur, particularly with the multiple pathologic conditions that are so common in the elderly.

In differentiating the preceding types of dizziness, a detailed, accurate biopsychosocial history is the sine qua non. This should be followed by a careful clinical examination of the cerebrovascular, cardiovascular, and neurologic systems, supplemented by special tests for posture (head and neck), ears (hearing), eyes (vision, nystagmus), and gait. The basic laboratory investigation should include complete blood count; determination of erythrocyte sedimentation rate, blood urea nitrogen and electrolytes, and blood sugar level; thyroid function tests; electrocardiogram; and chest x-ray. Other procedures such as audiometry or computed axial tomography scan of the brain are done when indicated.

## References


1. Brocklehurst JC, Hanley T: Geriatric Medicine for Students. London, Churchill-Livingstone, 1976.
2. Adams GF: Essentials of Geriatric Medicine. 2nd ed. New York, Oxford University Press, 1981.
3. Burnet FM: An immunological approach to aging. Lancet 2:358, 1970.
4. Hayflick L: The cell biology of human aging. N Engl J Med 295:1302, 1976.
5. Levinson DJ, Darrow CN, Klein EB, et al: The Season's of a Man's Life. New York, Alfred A. Knopf, 1978, pp. 33–39.
6. Bachrach LL: Assessment of outcomes in community support systems. Schizophrenia Bull 8:39, 1982.
7. Erikson EH, Erikson JM: Reflections on aging. *In* Spicker SF, Woodward KF, Van Tassel DD (eds.): Aging and the Elderly. New Jersey, Humanities Press, 1978, pp. 1–8.
8. Walsh F: The family in later life. *In* Carter EA, McGoldrick M (eds.): The Family Life Cycle. New York, Gardner Press, 1980, pp. 197–220.
9. Duvall EM: Marriage and Family Development. 5th ed. New York, Harper and Row, 1977, pp. 385–408.
10. Mossey J, Shapiro E: Self-rated health: A predictor of mortality among the elderly. Am J Public Health 72:800, 1982.
11. The well-being of older people in Cleveland, Ohio. Comptroller's General Report to Congress. General Accounting Office, Washington, DC, April 19, 1977.
12. Linn MW, Hunter KI, Linn BS: Self-assessed health, impairment and disability in Anglo, Black and Cuban elderly. Med Care 18:282, 1980.
13. Engel GL: The need for a new medical model. Science 196:129, 1977.
14. Kleinman A, Eisenberg L, Good B: Culture, illness and care. Ann Intern Med 88:251, 1978.
15. Medalie JH, Kitson GC, Zyzanski SJ: A family epidemiological model. J Fam Pract 12:79, 1981.
16. Steel K: Evaluation of the geriatric patient. *In* Reichel W (ed.): Clinical Aspects of Aging. Baltimore, Williams and Wilkins, 1978, pp. 3–12.
17. Kerzner LF, Greb L, Steel K: History-taking forms and the care of geriatric patients. J Med Educ 57:376, 1982.
18. Cutler P: Special aspects of problem solving in the geriatric patient. *In* Cutler P (ed.): Problem Solving in Clinical Medicine. Baltimore, Williams and Wilkins, 1979, pp. 359–364.
19. Nowlin JB, Busse EW: Psychosomatic problems in the older person. *In* Witthower ED, Warnes H (eds.): Psychosomatic Medicine: Its Clinical Applications. New York, Harper and Row, 1977, pp. 325–334.
20. Kennie DC, Kane WJ, and Moore JT: The Aging Process I: Monograph No. 10. American Academy of Family Physicians Home Study Program. Kansas City, Missouri, 1979.
21. Schneiderman LJ: Preventive health care in older adults. *In* Schneiderman LJ (ed.): The Practice of Preventive Health Care. Menlo Park, California, Addison-Wesley Co., 1981.
22. Green, MF: Geriatric medicine. Br J Hosp Med 10:672, 1973.
23. Medalie JH, Goldbourt U: Unrecognized myocardial infarction: Five-year incidence, mortality, and risk factors. Ann Intern Med 84:526, 1976.
24. Rodstein M: The characteristics of non-fatal myocardial infarction in the aged. Arch Intern Med 98:84, 1956.
25. National Ambulatory Medical Survey (NAMS), 1973–1974.
26. Mendenhall RC, et al: Medical practice in the United States. Special report of the Robert Wood Johnson Foundation. Princeton, New Jersey, 1981.
27. Marsland DW, Wood M, Mayo F: The content of family practice. J Fam Pract 3:37, 1976.
28. Silvertson SE: Common problems of ambulatory geriatric patients. Postgrad Med 64:83, 1978.

29. Mann KJ, Medalie JH, Lieber E, et al: Visits to Doctors. Jerusalem, Israel, Academic Press, 1970.
30. Hull FM: M.D. Doctoral Dissertation. London, University of Cambridge, 1975.
31. Mackenzie I: Vertigo. *In* Hart FD (ed.): French's Index of Differential Diagnosis. 11th ed. Bristol, England, John Wright, 1979, pp. 817–819.
32. Kennie DC, Kane WJ, Moore JT: The Aging Process I: Monograph No. 21. American Academy of Family Physicians Home Study Program. Kansas City, Missouri, 1980.
33. Drachman DA, Hart CW: An approach to the dizzy patient. Neurology 22:323, 1972.
34. Daroff RB: Vertigo. Am Fam Physician 16:143, 1977.
35. Lassiter WB: Dizziness. *In* Medley ES (ed.): Common Health Problems in Medical Practice. Baltimore, Williams and Wilkins, 1982, pp. 240–249.

## Chapter 7

# Screening the Elderly

Mark J. Magenheim

*The Queen gives leave that . . . a Publick Brothel should be set up at Avignon . . . that on every Saturday the Women in the House should be singly examined by the Abbess and a Surgeon appointed by the Directors and if any of them have contracted any Illness by their Whoring that they be separated from the rest and not suffer to prostitute themselves for fear the Youth who have to do with them should catch their Distempers.*

(OLD STATUTES OF THE STEWS OF AVIGNON, 1347).[1]

Although the idea of screening is not new, scientific interest in screening has developed only within the past 25 years, and research within the past decade. As a point of reference, screening can be defined generally as "the *presumptive* identification of *unrecognized* disease or defect by the application of tests, examinations, or other procedures which can be applied rapidly to sort out apparently well persons who *probably* have a disease from those who *probably do not.* A screening test is *not* intended to be diagnostic. Persons with positive or suspicious findings must be referred to their physicians for diagnosis and necessary treatment."[2]

Two distinct forms of screening programs are commonly recognized: (1) screening programs (epidemiologic surveys) primarily aimed at identifying or describing a population that has *not* sought medical assistance and (2) screening aimed at case-finding among people who *have* sought medical assistance. Within the category of case-finding, there are two broad types: those interventions incidentally provided for individuals who have *not* sought screening services directly (such as checking the blood pressure of every adult at each office visit) and those interventions aimed at populations who *have* sought screening assistance for self-identified purposes of maintaining or improving personal health status (such as those individuals who believe that an annual "physical check-up" will be of value to them). One difference between these two forms of case-finding is that the first is generated in the office by a *provider* of health services whereas the second is initiated directly by the *consumer* of services.

In any discussion of screening, it is worth noting that the strategies, benefits, costs, and outcomes of screening vary depending on the different objectives, test features, and points of view of the screening program and participants. In this chapter we will focus on screening in the form of case-finding for functional impairments or diseases among elderly individuals. This office-based *prescriptive screening* is aimed at early detection of important conditions or diseases amenable to efficacious and efficient therapy to prevent or postpone disability and premature death. For the elderly especially, prescriptive screening aims to improve the *quality of life* by enhancing functional capacity.

Although there has been considerable screening of the elderly during the past 20 years, most work has focused on community surveys rather than on office-based case-finding.[3-16] In general, findings have failed to show sufficient benefits to justify mass screening, even when screening services are conducted in homes of the elderly by nonphysician assessors with back-up laboratory services.[17-20] Lowther concluded that "the end result of all our early diagnostic activities has thus been an improvement in 67 patients—that is, 23 per cent of the whole group, and . . . it is unlikely that many general practitioners will be able to accept this further burden in the near future."[6] Similarly, Currie reported that "the results of the (Glasgow) survey were perhaps incommensurate with the effort expended since most of the unreported morbidity was trivial, and . . . community health screening of the elderly may be very time-consuming and expensive in time and money."[9]

Research on office-based and special population case-finding among the elderly has also been reported,[21-25] but, again, results have been largely unimpressive, often owing to major methodologic flaws. Even in well-designed studies, findings have been weak. Freedman and associates reported a very low incidence (2.8 per cent) of serious illness among 682 patients screened in Freedman's general practice in Newcastle and "analysis revealed that the vast majority of positive symptoms and physical signs were either already known to the patient's general practitioner or were of no real significance to the health and well-being of the patient . . . including previously undiagnosed mental and emotional illness."[24]

The randomized controlled trial reported by Tulloch and Moore in 1979 was a rigorous evaluation of screening among 295 elderly patients over a 2-year period. They reported that "in both screened and unscreened groups, patients were well adapted in most cases to their problems so that the quality of life of these old people was relatively unimpaired." They commented that screening had made no significant impact on socioeconomic, functional, and medical disorders affecting health, that risk rating in the two groups differed only marginally, and that screening and surveillance appeared to have made little impact on health status or vulnerability to stress (represented by risk rating).[25]

Among recent work in North America, probably the most useful projects reported to date have been the studies of Somers and associates,[26] Frame and co-workers,[27-29] and the Canadian Task Force on the Periodic Health Examination.[30] These researchers conducted rigorous and comprehensive evaluations of screening and periodic health assessments, and their conclusions on screening emphasize a selective age-related approach targeted to specific high-risk groups and conditions. In the form of "Health Protection Packages," the recommendations of the Canadian Task Force[30] combine sound theoretic and scientific criteria with practical clinical sense. The work of Frame and associates[27-29] focuses even further on the need to identify explicit health goals for each age group and to apply sound methodologic criteria for evaluating screening decisions in terms of these goals in primary care. For the elderly, screening goals are not yet sufficiently precise or operational, although in recent years, a number of useful proposals have been introduced.

## GOALS OF SCREENING THE ELDERLY

With respect to screening the elderly, what might be considered reasonable goals and approaches for office-based preventive geriatrics? From the United Kingdom, Anderson[31] advocates screening the elderly to try to preserve physical health, to maintain mental health, and to preserve social standing and circumstance, although these goals are not operationally defined. Thomas[5] stresses geriatric screening to discover minor disabilities that can limit coping ability and enjoyment of life. Barber and Wallis[14] suggest that goals for screening the elderly include (1) establishing comprehensive baselines, (2) devising forms and systems to promote periodic assessments as integral elements of office practice, (3) enabling team approaches to be fostered and used, and (4) developing information on problems and needs of the elderly for planning community services.

Williamson[32] submits that screening may be used to detect problems at an early stage to prevent or reduce deterioration. High-risk groups suggested for this special observation are those with locomotor difficulties, those recently discharged from hospitals, and those who are socially isolated.[32] To this group, could be added those living alone and those recently bereaved,[33] those with financial difficulties,[34] and those over 80 years of age, regardless of health status.[35]

The World Health Organization has taken a position that defines the purpose of screening in geriatrics as preventive care "to keep the elderly in good health and happiness in their own houses for as long as this is possible."[36] More recently, Breslow and Somers have proposed health goals for the elderly in the form of a global lifetime health-monitoring program: In those 60 to 74 years old, the goals should be to prolong optimum physical/mental/social activity, minimize handicapping from chronic conditions, and prepare for retirement; in those older than 75 years, the goals should be to prolong effective activity and ability to live independently, avoid institutionalization so far as possible, minimize inactivity and discomfort from chronic conditions, and, when illness is terminal, assure as little physical and mental distress as possible and provide emotional support to patient and family.[37]

Although no one would dispute the laudatory nature of all these goals, it is difficult to define and to justify precise screening activities that health professionals, elderly patients, and health care systems should undertake to achieve these goals. At this point, probably the most useful approach for office-based geriatric case-finding is to start from general principles that pertain to all screening programs regardless of population or condition of interest and then to formulate, adapt, and evaluate specific recommendations concerning screening among the elderly. Details of this approach are presented below.

## METHODOLOGIC CRITERIA FOR SCREENING

Standards for screening were proposed more than 25 years ago,[38] and in 1968 the World Health Organization proposed a comprehensive set of general principles regarding screening.[39] These principles were adopted by the World Health Assembly in 1971,[40] and in the past 15 years practical, methodologic criteria have been developed for making decisions about screening.[41–61]

### Burden of Disease or Disability

1. *Is the condition of interest an important health problem for the individual and the community? (What is the prevalence of the problem? What is the type and magnitude of suffering among those affected?)*

### Etiology and Clinical Course

2. *What is the natural history of the condition, including its development from latent to declared disease or disability? (Is there a recognizable latent or early symptomatic stage?)*
3. *Will early detection alter prognosis of the condition of interest?*
4. *Is there efficacious treatment for the condition of interest?*

### Efficacy of Screening

5. *Is there a suitable screening test for detecting the condition of interest at the latent or early symptomatic stage?*
6. *Is the screening test likely to do more good than harm?*
7. *Is the test valid for the condition of interest?*
8. *What is the effect of prevalence of the condition of interest on the predictive value (yield) of the screening test?*
9. *Is the screening test acceptable to both consumer (the individual patient or client) and provider (the health professional or the health care system)?*
10. *What is the effect of labeling from a positive test result?*
11. *What is the level of compliance with screening among patients, providers, and the health system? (For example, do patients and health professionals follow recommended screening procedures? Do third-party insurers reimburse for such services? Do incentives for prevention exist, and do they work?)*

### Community Effectiveness

12. *Are* diagnostic *facilities available and accessible for persons with positive screening results for the condition of interest?*
13. *Is treatment* available *and* accessible *to those in need?*
14. *What is the level of* compliance *with treatment (among both patients and providers of care)?*
15. *Is there suitable* coverage? *(Are those in need of care receiving effective services and treatment?)*
16. *What is the* impact *of effective diagnosis and treatment upon the burden of suffering?*

### Efficiency (Economic Evaluation)

17. *Is screening cost-effective when compared with other means of diagnosis and treatment for the condition of interest? (What is the relative benefit of preventing, arresting, or curing the problem early?)*
18. *Is screening for Condition A cost-effective compared with screening for Condition B in terms of criteria for screening efficacy and effectiveness?*
19. *Is diagnosis and treatment for Condition A cost-effective compared with diagnosis and treatment for Condition B in terms of community effectiveness and the total population burden of suffering?*
20. *What are the results of cost-utility analyses of screening and treatment alternatives? (For example, does screening and early detection lead to an improvement in end-results when measured in quality-adjusted life-years?)*

Attention to these questions enables rational evaluation of screening and can promote effective clinical practices and policies. Although the full range of questions listed previously covers a "spectrum of evidence"[62] that will inevitably remain incomplete for the foreseeable future, critical assessment of information and practice according to scientific principles and methods is particularly useful when making decisions about screening tests and programs.

Among the important issues concerning screening recommendations for the elderly, questions about burden of suffering, natural history (etiology and clinical course), and the efficacy and effectiveness of early detection maneuvers are necessary and feasible to consider. Questions dealing with community effectiveness and economic analysis (efficient allocation of scarce resources) are also germane, but these are complex issues to address in a limited review and they will not be considered in detail here.

## APPLICATION OF SCREENING RECOMMENDATIONS

For purposes of illustration, let us review essential hypertension as an example for applying rules of evidence to screening recommendations. Steps required in this analysis are presented below.

### *Step One: Burden of Disease or Disability*

Approximately 5 to 35 per cent of North American adults have elevated diastolic and/or systolic blood pressure, depending on age, sex, and race.[63-67] (The wide range of prevalence is itself a useful measure of the difficulty in determining the true burden of disability.) Among both men and women, diastolic blood pressure peaks in late middle age (55 to 64 years) and then drops with advancing years (75+). By contrast, mean systolic blood pressure rises steadily with age in both sexes. The peak prevalence of diastolic hypertension (≥ 95 mm Hg) is 16 per cent in males and 19 per cent in females at 55 to 64 years, and the peak of isolated systolic hypertension (≥ 160 mm Hg) occurs in about 28 per cent of males and 33 per cent of females aged 75 to 79.[68] Data are not available for those over 80 years.

Determining the true prevalence of both diastolic and systolic hypertension among those over 65 years is difficult owing to frequent misreporting and misclassification in elderly populations and to inadequate data on this population generally. The burden of suffering among the elderly *with* hypertension is also problematic owing to the generally asymptomatic nature of the condition and the adverse side effects of treatment. Overall, however, target organ damage, which can occur as a consequence of untreated hypertension, poses an enormous burden to society, to individual patients and their families, and to the health care system. As such, disability and premature death from congestive heart failure, myocardial infarction, coronary heart disease, cerebrovascular accident, and atherothrombotic brain infarction due to untreated hypertension constitute major public health problems that warrant concerted action.

### *Step Two: Etiology and Clinical Course*

Information on the etiology of essential hypertension is limited, but data on the clinical course of the condition are substantial. Increased risks of serious outcomes associated with untreated moderate diastolic (≥ 105 mm Hg) and systolic (≥ 160 mm Hg) hypertension have been well documented.[69-73] Among those aged 65 to 74, data consistently show significantly higher rates for congestive heart failure and death from cardiovascular disease in men with moderate diastolic hypertension and for myocardial infarction, stroke, and death from cardiovascular disease in diastolic hypertensive women compared with nonhypertensives matched for age and sex. Risks associated with isolated systolic hypertension have not yet been fully evaluated in those aged 65 to 79, and there is no evidence about risks associated with hypertension in those over 80 years.

Efficacy studies on treated hypertension with compliant patients have shown an 83 per cent reduction in mortality and a 92 per cent reduction in morbidity among severe diastolic hypertensives (≥ 115 mm Hg before treatment),[74] a 67 per cent reduction in events among moderate diastolic hypertensives (95 to 114 mm Hg),[75] and a 17 per cent mortality reduction in mild hypertensives (90 to 104 mm Hg),[66] among those *under* 65 years of age. Treatment programs have shown that optimal control can be achieved after 5 years for over 65 per cent of those adults requiring antihypertensive therapy,[66] but information about control among the elderly is not available.

Both the Veterans Administration Cooperative Study and the Hypertension Detection and

Follow-up Program (HDFP) included elderly patients, and results unequivocally demonstrated benefits of therapy for those aged 60 to 74 with moderate (105 to 114 mm Hg) or severe diastolic hypertension ($\geq$ 115 mm Hg). However, efficacy of treatment was *not* demonstrated among those over age 60 with *mild* diastolic hypertension ($\leq$ 104 mm Hg) or with isolated systolic hypertension, and no information has been reported for patients aged 75 and over.[65,66,74,75]

In addition, the positive outcomes of step-care treatment of hypertension are often compromised by problems associated with treatment. Among the elderly, negative side effects include postural hypotension, abrupt changes in blood pressure, hypokalemia, mental depression, sedation, urinary incontinence, fatigue, weakness, anorexia, and confusion. Thus, the case for treatment needs to be established clearly before subjecting an elderly patient to the rigors of daily antihypertensive therapy. Although there is a high burden of suffering among untreated moderate and severe diastolic hypertensives ($\geq$ 105 mm Hg), there is not yet compelling evidence for an altered clinical course among those with mild diastolic hypertension or isolated systolic hypertension.[76-80] As these are the most common forms of hypertension among those over 65 years of age, definitive treatment recommendations must await outcomes of further research, and screening recommendations must be tempered accordingly.

## *Step Three: Efficacy of Screening*

With respect to the technical aspects of screening (which determine efficacy), it is of foremost importance to establish test *validity* before undertaking large-scale programs or specific interventions. Validity here refers to the degree to which the test correctly identifies individuals *with* the condition (sensitivity) and the degree to which the test correctly identifies those *without* the condition (specificity). The extent to which the screening test results conform to those derived from an acknowledged "gold standard" of diagnostic accuracy provides a measure of sensitivity, specificity, and test validity. Table 7–1 illustrates these concepts, from which algebraic values for various measures of the validity of a screening test can be calculated.

As we see from Table 7–1, it is possible to place each screened individual into one of the cells (a), (b), (c), or (d) and to compute the relative percentages in each cell. In our example, let us look at a hypothetical screening program for hypertension in a community of 1000 adults where population screening has not previously been available. We will assume that the measuring devices are reliable and that the blood pressure readings obtained are diagnostically accurate. Given the suitability of the screening test and previously established information on the benefits of early detection and treatment, we now wish to determine if our test program is valid.

Ideally, in the perfect screening test (i.e., 100 per cent sensitivity, 100 per cent specificity, and no false-positive or false-negative results) all diseased subjects would be in cell (a) and all nondiseased subjects in cell (d). In actual practice, however, this is neither attainable methodologically nor desirable administratively. (To achieve "perfection," tests would necessarily become exceedingly cost-ineffective and potential benefits to be derived from screening would be lost.)

Instead of seeking perfection, the goal of

**Table 7–1.** RESULTS OF SCREENING TEST ILLUSTRATING SENSITIVITY AND SPECIFICITY

| *Results of Screening Test* | "True" Condition or Disease State | | |
|---|---|---|---|
| | *Condition or Disease (+)* | *No Condition or Disease (−)* | *Total Number Screened* |
| Positive (+) | True positive (TP) (a) | False positive (FP) (b) | Total positive (a + b) |
| Negative (−) | (c) False negative (FN) | (d) True negative (TN) | Total negative (c + d) |
| | TP + FN* (a+c) | TN + FP† (b+d) | Total screened (a + b + c + d) |

* Sensitivity $= \frac{TP}{TP + FN} = \left(\frac{a}{a + c}\right) \times 100.$

† Specificity $= \frac{TN}{TN + FP} = \left(\frac{d}{b + d}\right) \times 100.$

screening for case-finding is to achieve the highest levels of both sensitivity and specificity consistent with other essential elements of screening for the given condition. To achieve this balance, the approach that is taken in screening for case-finding is to "trade off" the sensitivity and the specificity of a test. Operationally this is done in part by setting a level in advance that must be met for a test outcome to be deemed "positive."[81] This "criterion of positivity"[82] is determined clinically and statistically as that point on the spectrum of measurement (from "definite health" to "definite disease") that affords optimal sensitivity and specificity for the condition in question, at the lowest cost, pain, inconvenience, and risk.[39] Among the many factors affecting this criterion of positivity are value preferences for "health" and "acceptable risk," cost-benefit ratios for different points on the spectrum of measurement, and the prevalence of the condition of interest. As we will see below, differences in the cutoff level chosen can lead to substantial variation in screening results obtained.[38]

From standards validated elsewhere[65,66,83] we will use in our example (see Table 7–2) a fifth-phase Korotkoff level of 105 mm Hg as the cutoff point for diastolic hypertension. Those patients identified as "hypertensive," with a diastolic reading of 105 mm Hg or greater on screening, would then be referred for definitive diagnosis and treatment (the "gold standard"). Suppose the results of our screening program are those as noted in Table 7–2.

From these results we conclude that the screening program for hypertension appears to be very good at correctly identifying individuals without diastolic hypertension (specificity = 95.0 per cent) and with diastolic hypertension (sensitivity = 95.0 per cent). At this cutoff level of 105 mm Hg in an unselected population, it also shows very good *predictive value* for both positive test results (88.0 per cent) and for negative test results (98.0 per cent). This means that the post-test likelihood of actually being hypertensive or nonhypertensive based on this screening test alone is quite high. Furthermore, we conclude that the prevalence of diastolic hypertension (≥ 105 mm Hg) in this population of 1000 persons is 280/1000 or 28 per cent, which is within the expected range from other surveys. We might well conclude that our screening test is valid on the basis of these results.

Let us now apply the same screening test to a population of 1000 persons over age 65 who live in a retirement community in the Sun Belt. With our results from Table 7–2, we determined that the sensitivity of diastolic hypertension screening was 95 per cent and the specificity was 95 per cent, with a prevalence of 28 per cent in a general unselected population. Assuming that the sensitivity and specificity of the test remain the same in different settings (which is to

**Table 7–2.** EXAMPLE FOR CALCULATING SCREENING TEST SENSITIVITY AND SPECIFICITY FOR DIASTOLIC HYPERTENSION (≥ 105 mm Hg)

| *Result of Blood Pressure Screening Test* | True Disease State: *Disease (+) Hypertensive* | True Disease State: *Disease (−) Not Hypertensive* | *Total No. Screened* |
|---|---|---|---|
| Positive test (≥ 105 mm Hg) | 266 (a) | 36 (b) | 302 (a+b) |
| Negative test | (c) 14 | (d) 684 | (c + d) 698 |
| (< 105 mm Hg) | (a + c) 280 | (b + d) 720 | (a+b+c+d) 1000 |

Percentage sensitivity $= \frac{a}{a+c} = \frac{266}{280} \times 100 = 95.0\%$

Percentage specificity $= \frac{d}{b+d} = \frac{684}{720} \times 100 = 95.0\%$

Post-test likelihood of a positive test (positive predictive value) $= \frac{a}{a+b} = \frac{266}{302} \times 100 = 88.0\%$

Post-test likelihood of a negative test (negative predictive value) $= \frac{d}{c+d} = \frac{684}{698} \times 100 = 98.0\%$

Prevalence of diastolic hypertension $= \frac{a+c}{\text{Total}} = \frac{280}{1000} \times 100 = 28.0\%$

be expected), what is the effect of prevalence on test validity?

First, we begin with previous information that prevalence of diastolic hypertension among those over age 65 is approximately 8 per cent.[84,85] Using this figure with our test sensitivity of 95 per cent and specificity of 95 per cent, we would expect the screening results noted in Table 7–3.

Working "backwards," we start with a total population of 1000 and an expected prevalence of 8 per cent in the population of interest. The resulting a + c (prevalence) equals 80 (8 per cent of 1000). The total population (a + b + c + d) of 1000 less expected prevalence a + c (80) equals 920 nondiseased (or b + d). Using our known percentages for sensitivity (95 per cent) and for specificity (95 per cent), we can then calculate values for all remaining cells. From Table 7–2, we know that the sensitivity and specificity remain unchanged, and thus, the percentages of false-negative and false-positive results will also remain the same. However, when we compare the "predictive value" of the same hypertension screening test in these two settings with disease prevalences of 28 per cent and 8 per cent, respectively, the results are quite different.

The predictive value of a screening test refers to the likelihood that the subject with a positive test result actually has the disease or condition (positive predictive value) or that a subject with a negative test result does not have the disease or condition in question (negative predictive value). The calculation of predictive value is derived by computing the ratio of true outcomes to all outcomes for both negative and positive test results, based on Bayes' probability theorem.[86] Expressed mathematically, the predictive value of a positive test is $\frac{TP}{TP + FP}\left(\text{or } \frac{a}{a+b}\right)$ and the predictive value of a negative test is $\frac{TN}{TN + FN}$ $\left(\text{or } \frac{d}{c+d}\right)$. From Table 7–2, the positive predictive value is $\frac{266}{302} \times 100$ or 88.0 per cent, and the negative predictive value is $\frac{684}{698} \times 100$ or 98.0 per cent. From Table 7–3, the positive predictive value is $\frac{76}{122} \times 100$ or 62.3 per cent, and the negative predictive value is $\frac{874}{878} \times 100$ or 99.5 per cent.

Comparing these values shows us that a difference in prevalence can have a major impact on the predictive value of a screening test result. In the first example (see Table 7–2), the predictive value of a positive test result was over 88 per cent. This means that 88 people out of each 100 with a positive test result would be true positives

**Table 7–3.** CALCULATION OF EXPECTED DIASTOLIC HYPERTENSION SCREENING OUTCOMES (PREVALENCE OF 8%, TEST SENSITIVITY OF 95%, AND SPECIFICITY OF 95%)

| | True Disease State | | |
|---|---|---|---|
| ***Result of Blood Pressure Screening Test*** | ***Disease (+) Hypertensive*** | ***Disease (−) Not Hypertensive*** | ***Total No. Screened*** |
| Positive test (≥105 mm Hg) | 76 (a) | 46 (b) | 122 (a+b) |
| Negative test (<105 mm Hg) | (c) 4 | (d) 874 | (c+d) 878 |
| | (a+c) 80 | (b+d) 920 | (a+b+c+d) 1000 |

Given Sensitivity: $95\% = \frac{a}{a+c} = \frac{a}{80}$

then: $a = 0.95 \times 80 = 76$

Given Specificity: $95\% = \frac{d}{b+d} = \frac{d}{920}$

then: $d = 0.95 \times 920 = 874$

Positive Predictive Value $= \frac{a}{a+b} = \frac{76}{122} = 62.3\%$

Negative Predictive Value $= \frac{d}{c+d} = \frac{874}{878} = 99.5\%$

(and that 12 individuals with positive test results would *not* be true positives). In Table 7–3, the predictive value of a positive test result was less than 63 per cent. Thus, only 62 elderly persons out of each 100 with a positive test result would be true positives, and 38 elderly individuals with positive test results would in fact *not* be hypertensive.

This problem of limited predictive value is even greater when prevalence is very low. As Vecchio[87] has shown, the predictive value of a single diagnostic test in unselected populations is markedly affected by the prevalence of the condition and by the pretest "likelihood of positivity." Thus, even when test sensitivity and specificity are high, there may still be an unacceptably large number of false-positive results when prevalence is low. This relationship is displayed graphically in Figure 7–1, and it has been well-elucidated for many disorders, including diabetes mellitus, lung cancer, breast cancer, and cervical cancer.[88–91]

In addition to these concerns, there are many biases to which the screening process in general is susceptible.[92] These include unmasking (signal detection) bias; diagnostic suspicion bias; lead-time (starting time) bias; exposure-suspicion bias; volunteer bias; diagnostic access bias; mimicry bias; previous opinion bias; and Neyman (prevalence-incidence) bias. All these biases (and others) can produce screening results that differ systematically from the truth,[93] and the extent to which bias is controlled affects the overall validity of the screening process and its results.

In summary, the overall efficacy of a screening procedure or diagnostic test is influenced by many factors. Although most of these are outside the control of the individual medical practitioner, all of them determine the ultimate value of screening in the form of case-finding in office-based practice.

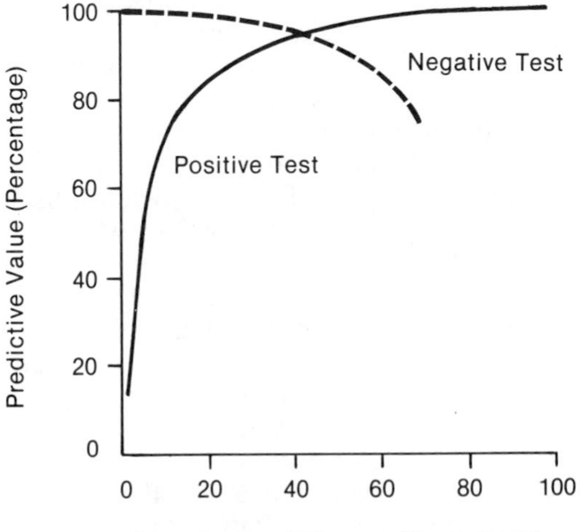


**Figure 7–1.** Relationship between prevalence of disease and predictive value, with sensitivity held constant at 95 per cent and specificity held constant at 95 percent. (Adapted from Vecchio TJ: Predictive value of a single diagnostic test in unselected populations. N Engl J Med, 274:1171, 1966.)

## *Step Four: Effectiveness of Screening*

With respect to blood pressure screening, there is considerable evidence that the procedure is well accepted by patients, providers, and the health care system generally. However, evidence is mounting that the labeling of an individual as "hypertensive" can often lead to unanticipated negative outcomes, including lowering of self-esteem, higher rates of absenteeism, lower work productivity, and "sick-role" behavior.[94,95] These phenomena have been shown to occur not only among untreated hypertensives but also among mislabeled normotensives. Such problems can thus be attributed to the labeling process itself and are not necessarily consequences of the disease process of "hypertension" (which is asymptomatic in the great majority of patients) or to side effects of treatment.[96] These recent findings yield considerable information on the human behavioral responses to medical diagnostic labeling, and this area warrants special consideration in the context of screening among the elderly.

The issue of compliance has also emerged as a major area of concern in clinical practice and research in recent years.[97] The rate of compliance with preventive regimens (such as attending screening clinics or keeping appointments following screening for blood pressure or glaucoma) has ranged from 50 to 83 per cent.[98] Factors affecting compliance with screening recommendations include demographic features of the patient, features of the screening test or procedure, setting of the clinical encounter, features of the condition of interest, features of the perceived therapeutic regimen, features of the patient-therapist interaction, and sociobehavioral features of the patient and of the therapist.[99] Thus, even the most rigorous and valid screening test (with high sensitivity, high specificity, and high predictive value) may lack adequate effectiveness if the test is unacceptable or if compliance with the test requirements is too low to achieve the screening goal.

### *Step Five: Community Effectiveness*

Here we are concerned with the availability, accessibility, and validity of definitive diagnostic services and with efficacy and effectiveness of therapeutic regimens for conditions identified among individuals with positive screening test results. For hypertension, interobserver and intraobserver variations in blood pressure measurement limit diagnostic accuracy for this condition,[69,100,101] and there continues to be controversy about what constitutes hypertension warranting treatment, especially among the elderly. Although efficacy of treatment for hypertension is well established for some elevations of blood pressure in some populations, the problems of diagnostic inaccuracy, clinical disagreement, and lack of patient and provider compliance markedly reduce the effective coverage and impact of appropriate services and treatment for hypertension. These problems have been reported to be especially relevant among elderly hypertensives, and the issues of community effectiveness for hypertension in this population deserve full and careful consideration.

### *Step Six: Efficiency (Economic Evaluation)*

The last step in analysis of evidence on screening, and probably the most difficult to conduct, is often concerned with the evaluation of cost-effectiveness. For hypertension, comprehensive analysis of cost-effectiveness has been undertaken by Weinstein and Stason.[102-104] In their work, they estimated that the cost of hypertension screening and care per year of increased quality-adjusted life expectancy (impact) is lowest when services are provided in the form of office-based case-finding as opposed to complete community screening. Logan[105] compared the cost-effectiveness of nurse practitioner care for hypertensives at the work site with physician care and found that nurse care was both more effective and less costly. Neither the cost-benefit nor the cost-utility of treating hypertension has been analyzed, nor has the cost-effectiveness of treating hypertension been compared with that of treating other disorders.

Economic analysis of screening and/or care for hypertension among the elderly has not yet been thoroughly evaluated, although Weinstein and Stason's work did comment on this issue. They pointed out, for example, that different blood-pressure cutoff levels markedly affect cost-effectiveness results and that what is cost-effective in screening 30 year olds is not cost-effective in screening 60 year olds. They concluded that "these analyses underline the principle that even though screening (for hypertension) is relatively inexpensive, the large attrition between detection and ultimate blood-pressure control severely compromises its cost-effectiveness . . . Programs to screen for hypertension are indicated, on cost-effectiveness grounds, only if adequate resources are available to ensure that detection is translated into effective long-term blood-pressure control."[103]

## SPECIFIC RECOMMENDATIONS

In the analysis of screening for hypertension, we have shown that important methodologic criteria affect decision-making about screening and case-finding. From general principles, we recognize the need to focus only on major health problems and to undertake only those tests and procedures of sufficient validity that are acceptable and likely to make a difference to overall health status. We also recognize that scientific evidence to make fully informed decisions on behalf of individual patients seen in the office is often lacking. Thus, numerous decisions about screening and case-finding remain problematic, and for many conditions among the elderly, definitive recommendations must await further research.

Given current gaps in our knowledge about office-based case-finding among the elderly, many of the recommendations that follow are necessarily limited. In categories in which information is incomplete, recommendations are based on best available current data, with appropriate notations and references. When a firm recommendation is either absent or when the recommendation is equivocal, the reader is advised to combine sound clinical judgment with an appreciation of these general guidelines.

The figure and tables that follow present current recommendations for periodic health assessment and health maintenance activities for the elderly. Table 7–4 displays 20 conditions for which direct intervention and follow-up are judged to be warranted. Many of the suggested interventions can be efficiently and effectively conducted in the office by nonphysician health personnel. Follow-up in the home (often in association with other community resources) is necessary and appropriate in many instances.

**Table 7-4.** RECOMMENDED HEALTH ASSESSMENT AND HEALTH MAINTENANCE ACTIVITIES FOR ELDERLY PATIENTS

| Condition | Recommended Intervention | Follow-up Action | References |
|---|---|---|---|
| Accidents | Careful history in the office once between ages 65-70 years, then every 2 years to age 75, and then annually in home visits | With positive history, monitor very closely; conduct comprehensive history and physical examination as appropriate | 111-114 |
| Alcohol abuse or dependency | Careful history/review in the office once between age 65-70 years and once between 70-75 years and then regularly during home assessments | Nutrition review and assessment of social supports and personal status to link with community resources as needed | 115-120 |
| Breast cancer | Annual office examination and teaching/reinforcement of self-breast examination regularly at home | Refer for mammography if clinically indicated or if previously equivocal between ages 50-59 years | 121-133 |
| Colorectal cancer | Flexible sigmoidoscopic examination in the office every 3-5 years to age 80; annual stool examination for occult blood to age 80 | Depending on clinical findings, monitor and assess closely; refer as indicated | 134-156 |
| Depression | Careful history at least once between ages 65-70 and 70-75 and then annually during home assessments; monitor closely after loss; anticipate risk of self-harm and/or suicide | Home assessment and review when findings indicate closer attention warranted; brief therapy with drugs and possibly counseling is useful in some cases | 157-165 |
| Drug hazards | Comprehensive review of all drugs prescribed and taken from all sources at every visit from age 65 years, plus annual home assessments from age 75 years; periodic tests of renal function are useful | Monitor drug actions, interactions, and adverse reactions on regular basis and seek to reduce type, number, and dosages to bare minimum | 166-180 |
| Falls | Detailed history at least once between ages 65-70 years, then every 2 years to 75 years, and then annually | Monitor closely with history of one fall; investigate when history is positive for two | 181-185 |
| Foot care | Assess once by history and inspection between ages 65-70 years, then every 2 years to age 75, and then annually during course of regular home assessments | Regular assessments during visits for blood pressure and weight checks in the office; refer for chiropody or orthopedics as indicated | 186-191 |
| Hearing impairment | Discretionary assessment in office once between ages 65-70 years and 70-75 years, and then every 2 years or more often if high-risk or previous history of loss | Office audiometry and/or referral for tests or aids/enhancements; office procedures such as syringing of canals frequently sufficient | 192-200 |
| Hypertension | Blood pressure check yearly in office and discretionary during visits for other reasons, annually during regular home assessments after age 75 | Monitor according to step-care protocols and consider carefully before instituting drug therapy in this group | 201-218 |
| Immunization status | History of previous immunizations and documentation in office chart; for high-risk patients, immunize for influenza annually to age 75, and then annually for all over 75; | Tetanus booster every 10 years; polio (Salk) vaccine discretionary every 10 years; influenza annual vaccine for some to age 75, and for all over 75 years; pneumonia vaccine once every 5 years only | 219-232 |

*Table continued on following page*

**Table 7-4.** RECOMMENDED HEALTH ASSESSMENT AND HEALTH MAINTENANCE ACTIVITIES FOR ELDERLY PATIENTS *(Continued)*

| Condition | Recommended Intervention | Follow-Up Action | References |
|---|---|---|---|
| | discretionary for international travelers, BCG test,* and diphtheria immunizations | | |
| Impaired mobility | Careful history in the office once between ages 65–70 years, then every 2 years to age 75, and then each year in home assessments and in office for other reasons | Careful review of all medications, social situation, nutritional status, musculoskeletal system; investigate and treat as appropriate | 233–240 |
| Loss and bereavement | Comprehensive history and inspection during course of office visits for other reasons to age 75 and then annually at home also; short-term drug therapy or counseling can help | Special attention to hidden "signals" during office visits; monitor closely after death of spouse or pets or change in status, e.g., income or residence | 241–254 |
| Obesity | Weight check during physical examination once from ages 65–70 and with every blood pressure check in office; annually at home during assessments after 75 years | Diet counseling can help in some patients; food purchase/ preparation assistance; exercise and peer support useful for some patients | 255–264 |
| Periodontal disease and dental caries; oral cancer | History and inspection of oral cavity discretionary to age 75 years and then each year in home assessments in reference to dentures/oral cancer or for dental care needs | Investigate if suspicious lesions seen; refer for proper assessment of dentures; link patient to community resources in reference to nutrition if indicated or for dental restoration | 265–275 |
| Progressive incapacity with advanced age | Annual office visits for review of functional status, abilities, and impairments; home assessments at least once yearly for all patients over age 75 years | Depending on level of abilities and extent of support system, refer to community resources when appropriate | 276–301 |
| Stature/height | Check height during examination in office once between ages 65–70 years with weight check, and then every 3–5 years in the office; reassess annually at home at each assessment in patients over 75 years | Monitor weight for height and document shortening of stature and development of any obesity, kyphosis, knee and/or hip flexion, and spinal osteoporosis with or without neurologic deficits; investigate/refer/treat with diet, analgesics, other medications, braces and supports, walkers, and/or rehabilitation as appropriate | 302–305 |
| Urinary incontinence | Establish trusting rapport with patients over time; obtain careful history in office at least once between ages 65–70 and 70–75 and then follow closely each year at home assessments; anticipate problem in high-risk patients or circumstances | Investigate reversible causes such as urinary tract infection, stress, detrusor instability; organize support in community to maintain person at home as long as possible with treatment/ referral as needed | 306–313 |
| Victimization and abuse | Careful history in office at any time when suspicion index is high or when clinical evidence suggests physical, psychologic, or material abuse, nutritional deprivation, or intentional over-medication (chemical strait-jacketing); regular review during annual home | Thorough documentation to identify and distinguish areas of intentional and unintentional neglect, misinformation, ignorance, or direct/indirect abuse; development of personal advocacy role to counsel caregivers; referral to self-help and support groups, | 314–322 |

**Table 7-4.** RECOMMENDED HEALTH ASSESSMENT AND HEALTH MAINTENANCE ACTIVITIES FOR ELDERLY PATIENTS *(Continued)*

| Condition | Recommended Intervention | Follow-Up Action | References |
|---|---|---|---|
| | assessments in patients after 75 years in all settings; use of home safety and medication check lists is often helpful in monitoring | information and education source, and community liaison | |
| Visual impairments | Obtain history of visual function and refractive corrections during visits for other reasons up to age 70 years and then follow more closely, with annual review during assessments at home after age 75 years. For diabetic patients, do fundoscopic exam with dilatation in office every year. | Office examinations and/or referral as indicated; Glaucoma tonometry may be warranted; monitor all previously diagnosed patients; marshal community resources, e.g., special visual aids. Refer all diabetics to ophthalmologist annually. | 323–328 |

* BCG = Bacille Calmette-Guerin: Immunization for *Mycobacterium tuberculosis* administered to select populations at special risk.

**Table 7-5.** CONDITIONS REQUIRING FURTHER RESEARCH TO DETERMINE APPROPRIATENESS OF SCREENING AND CASE-FINDING IN ASYMPTOMATIC ELDERLY

**A. Conditions for which periodic assessment *may* be warranted in the asymptomatic elderly***

| *Condition* | *Suggested Approach* | *References* |
|---|---|---|
| Anemia, iron-deficiency type; malnutrition | Periodic hemogram (every 2–5 years) with follow-up and treatment PRN | 329–338 |
| Glaucoma, chronic open-angle type | Ocular tonometry or tonography every 3–5 years with referral PRN *may* be useful despite low sensitivity, low specificity, and diagnostic inaccuracy | 339–353 |
| Gynecologic neoplasia<br>Cervical<br>Endometrial<br>Ovarian | Pap smears are *not* warranted after age 60 when previously negative; pelvic examination every 2 years potentially useful for uterine or ovarian enlargement; jet washings and biopsy only for high-risk women with postmenopausal bleeding | 354–395 |
| Hyperglycemia | Fasting serum glucose (or 2-hour postcibal) at 2–5 year intervals | 396–406 |
| Prostatic carcinoma | Rectal palpation annually at time of assessment for colorectal carcinoma; urinary cytology and serum acid phosphatase levels are *not* warranted | 383, 407–414 |
| Renal impairment | For monitoring—creatinine clearance useful (if obtainable); chemical urinalysis, blood urea nitrogen, and serum creatinine (every 2–5 years) at time of hemogram and serum glucose determinations | 415–429 |
| Tuberculosis | Intradermal PPD-Tween (5 T.U.) tuberculin sensitivity testing every 5 years in two-step procedure (7–10 days apart, although 10–20% of elderly will have anergy); sputum staining. Culture. Chest x-ray as appropriate; treatment PRN | 430–442 |

**B. Conditions that do *not* presently warrant periodic assessment in the asymptomatic elderly†**

| *Condition* | *References* |
|---|---|
| Confusion/dementia | 443–455 |
| Hyperlipidemia | 456–463 |
| Hypothyroidism | 464–471 |
| Lung cancer | 472–480 |
| Osteoporosis | 481–489 |
| Skin cancer | 490–496 |

* However, data are equivocal or insufficient for definitive recommendations at this time.
† Based on established scientific principles and screening criteria.

For elderly patients, the medical practitioner's role must include a large element of coordination of services for health maintenance and preservation of independent functioning.

Table 7 – 5 contains a list of 15 conditions that require further research to determine if screening or case-finding among the elderly is warranted and, if so, in what form, frequency, and duration. Ten problem areas are listed in Part A that may warrant periodic assessment, and five

Name of Patient: ____________

Birthdate: ____________

Sex: Male ___ Female ___

MARK AN "X" OVER EACH BOX WHEN ASSESSMENT IS DONE

| Date day/month/year | | | | | | | | | | | | | | | | | | | | | | | | | | |
|---|---|---|---|---|---|---|---|---|---|---|---|---|---|---|---|---|---|---|---|---|---|---|---|---|---|---|
| Age at this Assessment | 65 | 66 | 67 | 68 | 69 | 70 | 71 | 72 | 73 | 74 | 75 | 76 | 77 | 78 | 79 | 80 | 81 | 82 | 83 | 84 | 85 | 86 | 87 | 88 | 89 | 90 |
| RECOMMENDED INTERVENTION | | | | | | | | | | | | | | | | | | | | | | | | | | |
| Comprehesive Functional Assessment in the Office | ○ | | ○ | | ○ | | ○ | | ○ | | ○ | ○ | ○ | ○ | ○ | ○ | ○ | ○ | ○ | ○ | ○ | ○ | ○ | ○ | ○ | ○ |
| Full Medication Review | ○ | ○ | ○ | ○ | ○ | ○ | ○ | ○ | ○ | ○ | ○ | ○ | ○ | ○ | ○ | ○ | ○ | ○ | ○ | ○ | ○ | ○ | ○ | ○ | ○ | ○ |
| Blood Pressure Check | ○ | ○ | ○ | ○ | ○ | ○ | ○ | ○ | ○ | ○ | ○ | ● | ● | ○ | ● | ○ | ● | ● | ● | ● | ● | ● | ● | ● | ● | ● |
| Weight Check | ○ | ○ | ○ | ○ | ○ | ○ | ○ | ○ | ○ | ○ | ○ | ● | ● | ○ | ● | ○ | ● | ● | ● | ● | ● | ● | ● | ● | ● | ● |
| Influenza Immunization | ○ | ○ | ○ | ○ | ○ | ○ | ○ | ○ | ○ | ○ | ○ | ● | ● | ○ | ● | ○ | ● | ● | ● | ● | ● | ● | ● | ● | ● | ● |
| Breast Examination | ○ | ○ | ○ | ○ | ○ | ○ | ○ | ○ | ○ | ○ | ○ | ● | ● | ○ | ● | ○ | | | | | | | | | | |
| Stools for Occult Blood | ○ | ○ | ○ | ○ | ○ | ○ | ○ | ○ | ○ | ○ | ○ | ○ | ○ | ○ | ○ | ○ | | | | | | | | | | |
| Prostatic Examination (*) | ○ | ○ | ○ | ○ | ○ | ○ | ○ | ○ | ○ | ○ | ○ | | | | | | | | | | | | | | | |
| Pelvic Examination (*) | ○ | | ○ | | ○ | | ○ | | ○ | | ○ | | | | | | | | | | | | | | | |
| Pneumonia Immunization | ○ | | | | | | | | | | ○ | | | | | | | | | | ○ | | | | | |
| Tetanus (Td) Booster | ○ | | | | | | | | | | ○ | | | | | | | | | | ○ | | | | | |
| Poliomyelitis Booster | ○ | | | | | | | | | | ○ | | | | | | | | | | ○ | | | | | |
| Comprehensive Phys. Exam. | ○ | | | | | | | | | | ○ | | | | | | | | | | | | | | | |
| Home Assessment | ● | | | | | | | | | | ● | ● | ● | ● | ● | ● | ● | ● | ● | ● | ● | ● | ● | ● | ● | ● |
| Accident Prevention | ○ | | | | | | ○ | | ○ | | ○ | ● | ● | ● | ● | ○ | ● | ● | ● | ● | ○ | ● | ● | ● | ● | ● |
| Alcohol Dependency Review | ○ | | | | | | ○ | | ○ | | ○ | ● | ● | ● | ● | ○ | ● | ● | ● | ● | ○ | ● | ● | ● | ● | ● |
| Depression Review | ○ | | | | | | ○ | | ○ | | ○ | ● | ● | ● | ● | ○ | ● | ● | ● | ● | ○ | ● | ● | ● | ● | ● |
| Falls and Gait Review | ○ | | | | | | ○ | | ○ | | ○ | ● | ● | ● | ● | ○ | ● | ● | ● | ● | ○ | ● | ● | ● | ● | ● |
| Foot Care/Podiatry Check | ○ | | | | | | ○ | | ○ | | ○ | ● | ● | ● | ● | ○ | ● | ● | ● | ● | ○ | ● | ● | ● | ● | ● |
| Loss/Bereavement Review | ○ | | | | | | ○ | | | | ○ | ● | ● | ● | ● | ○ | ● | ● | ● | ● | ○ | ● | ● | ● | ● | ● |
| Psychosocial Review | ○ | | | | | | ○ | | | | ○ | ● | ● | ● | ● | ○ | ● | ● | ● | ● | ○ | ● | ● | ● | ● | ● |
| Urinary Continence Review | ○ | | | | | | ○ | | | | ○ | ● | ● | ● | ● | ○ | ● | ● | ● | ● | ○ | ● | ● | ● | ● | ● |
| Victimization/Abuse Check | ○ | | | | | | ○ | | | | ○ | ● | ● | ● | ● | ○ | ● | ● | ● | ● | ○ | ● | ● | ● | ● | ● |
| Vision Assessment | ○ | | | | | | ○ | | | | ○ | ● | ● | ● | ● | ○ | ● | ● | ● | ● | ○ | ● | ● | ● | ● | ● |
| Mental Status Examination | ○ | | | | | | ○ | | | | ○ | | ● | | ● | ○ | ● | ● | ● | ● | ○ | ● | ● | ● | ● | ● |
| Hearing Assessment | ○ | | | | | | ○ | | | | ○ | | ● | | ● | ○ | | ● | | ● | ○ | ● | | ● | | ● |
| Periodontal/Oral Check | ○ | | | | | | ○ | | | | ○ | | ● | | ● | ○ | | ● | | ● | ○ | ● | | ● | | ● |
| Hemogram Check (*) | ○ | | | | | | ○ | | | | ○ | | | ○ | | | | | | | | | | | | |
| Fasting Serum Glucose (*) | ○ | | | | | | ○ | | | | ○ | | | ○ | | | | | | | | | | | | |
| BUN/Serum Creatinine (*) | ○ | | | | | | ○ | | | | ○ | | | ○ | | | | | | | | | | | | |
| Chemical Urinalysis (*) | ○ | | | | | | ○ | | | | ○ | | | ○ | | | | | | | | | | | | |
| Tuberculin Sensitivity (*) | ○ | | | | | | ○ | | | | ○ | | | | | ○ | | | | | | | | | | |
| Measurement of Height (*) | ○ | | | | | | ○ | | | | ○ | | | | | ○ | | | | | | | | | | |
| Glaucoma Assessment (*) | ○ | | | | | | ○ | | | | ○ | | | | | ○ | | | | | | | | | | |
| Flexible Sigmoidoscopy (*) | ○ | | | | | | ○ | | | | ○ | | | | | ○ | | | | | | | | | | |

○ = Office ● = Home Address ____________ Telephone ____________

(*) Research is needed to determine the validity and appropriate frequency of this intervention; use individual discretion for patients in advanced years.



**Figure 7 – 2.** Health maintenance flow sheet for older adults (65 to 90 years of age).

problems are shown in Part B that do not presently warrant either screening or case-finding.

Figure 7-2 is presented in the form of a health maintenance flow sheet for older patients. The recommended schedule of preventive interventions is based on current knowledge and principles consistent with methodologic criteria for case-finding and screening in general. Modifications and revisions of Tables 7-4 and 7-5 and Figure 7-2 are expected as more information from primary care research becomes available, and contributions from users are encouraged.

## CONCLUSION

Key principles and proposals in screening of the elderly can be summarized as follows:

1. The use of nonphysician health personnel is key to a sound program of health screening and surveillance in the elderly.
2. Screening the elderly is acceptable and preferable when conducted in the office and in the home rather than in the community-at-large.
3. Regular episodic "health maintenance" to preserve function and to prevent or reduce impairment is more appropriate than an exhaustive, expensive, and often ineffective search for new disease or diagnoses.
4. Systematic check lists and office chart flow sheets are expeditious methods for monitoring and recording screening results and health status of elderly patients.
5. Modern technology offers considerable promise to meet the requirements of screening programs for the elderly, but invalidated procedures or methods are unwarranted in any event.
6. The periodic health examination has a relatively low sensitivity for the detection of major disorders that have lethal outcomes, and extensive surveillance programs in the elderly are not justifiable at this time.
7. With respect to the frail elderly in the community, the "inverse care law" may apply in that those in greatest need of screening and surveillance may well be those most likely to be missed or to default. Thus, active case-finding and follow-up of special high-risk groups (the lonely, the bereaved, the poor) are important.
8. The concept of lifetime health-monitoring is a useful step in the development of risk-based screening and surveillance, and extension of this approach among the elderly is worthwhile.
9. The paucity of strong evidence concerning efficacy and effectiveness of screening in the elderly indicates the need for a major commitment in support of sound clinical epidemiologic research to address important questions in this field.
10. The ultimate dictum of "primum non nocere" is especially germane to screening the elderly. As Holland wrote in 1974, "In the middle aged and elderly . . . simple tests for vision and hearing, and tests to identify people in need of chiropody or walking aids, may be far more effective than more complex biochemical and laboratory-oriented procedures in improving the 'quality of life'."[49]

There is a growing body of literature concerning recommendations for or against screening the elderly for various conditions,[106-110] but the quality of the evidence remains inadequate in many cases to justify rigorous intervention. There is a real risk in screening the elderly that apparently clinically or biochemically unexplainable "abnormalities" will lead to overzealous investigation and treatment, which in turn can lead to "overtreatment" of the elderly and to an *increased* burden of disease and disability. Counsel in the direction of prudence and critical assessment of recommendations for case-finding and screening among the elderly is therefore advised.

### References

1. Schneiderman LJ (ed.): The Practice of Preventive Health Care. Menlo Park, CA, Addison-Wesley Publishing Company, 1981.
2. Commission on Chronic Illness: Chronic Illness in the United States. Vol. 1. Prevention of Chronic Illness. Cambridge, MA, Harvard University Press, 1957, p. 45.
3. Anderson WF, Cowan NR: A consultative health centre for older people. Lancet 2:239, 1955.
4. Williams EI: A follow-up of geriatric patients after socio-medical assessment. J R Coll Gen Pract 24:341, 1974.
5. Thomas P: Experiences of two preventive clinics for the elderly. Br Med J 2:357, 1968.
6. Lowther CP, MacLeod RDM, Williamson J: Evaluation of early diagnostic services for the elderly. Br Med J 3:275, 1970.
7. Dunn TB: The Redbridge scheme for routine medical examination of elderly people. Mod Geriatr 1:261, 1970.
8. Hiscock E, Prangnell DR, Wilmot JF: A screening survey of old people in a general practice. Practitioner 210:271, 1973.
9. Currie G, MacNeil RM, Walker JG, et al: Medical and social screening of patients aged 70-72 by an urban general practice health team. Br Med J 2:108, 1974.
10. Akhtar AJ, Broe GA, Crombie A, et al: Disability and dependence in the elderly at home. Age Ageing 2:102, 1973.
11. Pike LA: Screening the elderly in general practice. J R Coll Gen Pract 26:698, 1976.
12. Milne JS, Maule M, Williamson J: Method of sam-

pling in a study of older people with a comparison of respondents and non-respondents. Br J Prev Soc Med 25:37, 1971.
13. Powell C, Crombie A: The Kilsyth questionnaire: A method of screening elderly people at home. Age Ageing 3:23, 1974.
14. Barber JH, Wallis JB: Assessment of the elderly in general practice. J R Coll Gen Pract 26:106, 1976.
15. Williamson J, Stokoe IH, Gray S, et al: Old people at home: Their unreported needs. Lancet 1:1117, 1964.
16. Williamson J, Lowther CP, Gray S: The use of health visitors in preventive geriatrics. Gerontol Clin 8:362, 1966.
17. Meyrick RL, Cox A: A geriatric survey repeated. Lancet 1:1146, 1969.
18. Burns C: Geriatric care in general practice. A medico-social survey of 391 patients undertaken by health visitors. J R Coll Gen Pract 18:287, 1969.
19. Tomlinson JM: Setting up a geriatric survey in general practice. Update Feb:277, 1976.
20. Taylor GF: Eddy TP, Scott DL: A survey of 216 elderly men and women in general practice. J R Coll Gen Pract 21:267, 1971.
21. MacLennan WJ: Screening procedures for the geriatric outpatient. Mod Geriatr 3:253, 1973.
22. Steel K, Williams F, Fairbank M, Knox K: Laboratory screening in the evaluation and placement of geriatric patients. J Am Geriatr Soc 22:538, 1974.
23. Brocklehurst JC, Carty MH, Leeming JT, Robinson J: Medical screening of old people accepted for residential care. Lancet 2:141, 1978.
24. Freedman GR, Charlewood JE, Dodds PA: Screening the aged in general practice. J R Coll Gen Pract 28:421, 1978.
25. Tulloch AJ, Moore V: A randomized controlled trial of geriatric screening and surveillance in general practice. J R Coll Gen Pract 29:733, 1979.
26. Somers AR, Bruch TL, Frame PS, et al: Lifetime health monitoring: A whole life-plan for well-patient care. Patient Care 13:160, 1979; 13:201, 1979; 13:83, 1979; and 13:120, 1979.
27. Frame PS, Carlson SJ: A critical review of periodic health screening using specific screening criteria. J Fam Pract 2:29, 123, 189, 283, 1975.
28. Frame PS: Periodic health screening in a rural private practice. J Fam Pract 9:57, 1979.
29. Frame PS, Kownlich B: Stool occult blood screening for colorectal cancer. J Fam Pract 15:1071, 1982.
30. Spitzer W: Report of the Canadian Task Force on the Periodic Health Examination. Can Med Assoc J 121:1193, 1979.
31. Anderson F: The effect of screening on the quality of life after seventy. J R Coll Physicians 10:161, 1976.
32. Brocklehurst JC (ed.): Textbook of Geriatric Medicine and Gerontology. 2nd ed. London, Churchill Livingstone, 1978, p. 783.
33. Macmillan D: Preventive geriatrics: Opportunities of a community mental health service. Lancet 2:1439, 1960.
34. Jones RVH: Recognition of geriatric problems in general practice. Update 13:643, 1976.
35. Andrews GR, Cowan NR, Anderson WF: The practice of geriatric medicine in the community. In McLachlan G (ed.): Problems and Progress in Medical Care: Essays on Current Research. London, Oxford University Press, 1971.
36. World Health Organization: Planning and organization of geriatric services. Technical Report Series, No. 548. Geneva, World Health Organization, 1974.
37. Breslow L, Somers AR: The lifetime health-monitoring program: A practical approach to preventive medicine. N Engl J Med 296:601, 1977.
38. Thorner RM, Remein QR: Principles and Procedures in the Evaluation of Screening for Disease. U.S. Public Health Service, Division of Chronic Diseases. Monograph No. 67. Publication No. 846. Government Printing Office, Washington, DC, 1961.
39. Wilson JMG, Jungner G: Principles and practice of screening for disease. Public Health Papers, No. 34. Geneva, World Health Organization, 1968.
40. Wilson JMG, Hilleboe HE: Mass health examinations as a public health tool. Technical Report Series, No. A24. Public Health Papers, No. 45. Geneva, World Health Organization, 1971.
41. Blumberg MS: Evaluating health screening procedures. Operations Res 5:351, 1967.
42. Cohen, Lord, Williams ET, McLachlan G (eds.): Screening in Medical Care: Reviewing the Evidence. Published for the Nuffield Prov Hospitals Trust. London, Oxford University Press, 1968.
43. Zelen M, Feinleib M: On the theory of screening for chronic diseases. Biometrika 56:601, 1969.
44. Feinleib M, Zelen M: Some pitfalls in the evaluation of screening programs. Arch Environ Health 19:412, 1969.
45. Sackett DL: Can screening programmes for serious disease really improve health? Sci Forum 15:9, 1970.
46. Cochrane AL, Holland WW: Validation of screening procedures. Br Med Bull 27:3, 1971.
47. Cochrane AL: Effectiveness and Efficiency: Random Reflections on Health Services. Published for the Nuffield Prov Hospitals Trust. London, Oxford University Press, 1972.
48. Sackett DL: The usefulness of laboratory tests in health-screening programs. Clin Chem 19:366, 1973.
49. Holland WW: Screening for disease. A series of articles in Lancet from Oct 1974 to Dec 1974 (Issues 7884–7895).
50. Sackett DL, Holland WW: Controversy in the detection of disease. Lancet 2:357, 1975.
51. Sackett DL: Screening for early detection of disease: To what purpose? Bull NY Acad Sci 51:3, 1975.
52. Spitzer WO, Brown BP: Unanswered questions about the periodic health examination. Ann Intern Med 83:257, 1975.
53. Delbanco TL: The periodic health examination for the adult: Waste or wisdom? Primary Care 3:205, 1976.
54. Prorok PC: The theory of periodic screening. I. Lead time and proportion detected. Adv Appl Probl 8:127, 1976.
55. Prorok PC: The theory of periodic screening. II. Doubly bounded recurrence times and mean lead time and detection probability estimation. Adv Appl Probl 8:460, 1976.
56. Ryan JGP: Periodic health examination of the elderly. Aust Fam Physician 7:285, 1978.
57. Ransohoff DF, Feinstein, AR: Problems of spectrum and bias in evaluating the efficacy of diagnostic tests. N Engl J Med 299:926, 1978.
58. Day E: Is the periodic health examination worthwhile? Cancer 1:1210, 1981.
59. Charap MH: The periodic health examination: Genesis of a myth. Ann Intern Med 95:733, 1981.
60. American College of Physicians, Medical Practice Committee: Periodic health examination: A guide for designing individualized preventive health care in the asymptomatic patient. Ann Intern Med 95:729, 1981.
61. Tugwell P, Bennett KJ, Sackett DL, Haynes RB: Rel-

ative risks, benefits and costs of intervention. *In* Warren KS and Mahmoud AAF (eds): Tropical and Geographical Medicine. New York: McGraw-Hill, 1984.
62. Haynes RB: Evidence and quality of decisions in health care. *In* Squires B (ed.): Proceedings of the Conference on Health in the '80's and '90's: Its Impact on Health Sciences Education, Montebello, Quebec, 1982. Toronto, Council of Ontario Universities, 1983.
63. National Center for Health Statistics: Blood Pressure of Adults by Age and Sex: United States 1960–1962. Series 11. No. 4, Washington, DC, U.S. Dept. of Health, Education and Welfare, 1964.
64. Bergland G, Anderson D, Wilhelmsen L: Prevalence of primary and secondary hypertension. Studies in a random population sample. Br Med J 2:554, 1976.
65. Hypertension Detection and Follow-up Program Cooperative Group: Blood pressure studies in 14 communities: A two-stage screen for hypertension. JAMA 237:2385, 1977.
66. Hypertension Detection and Follow-up Program Cooperative Group: Five-year findings of the Hypertension Detection and Follow-up Program. I. Reduction in mortality of persons with high blood pressure, including mild hypertension. JAMA 242:2562, 1979.
67. Chobanian AV: Hypertension. *In* Wilkins RW, Levinsky NG (eds.): Medicine: Essentials of Clinical Practice. 3rd ed. Boston, Little Brown and Company, 1982.
68. Hutchison B: Hypertension in the elderly. Can Fam Physician 27:1579, 1981.
69. Shurtleff D: Some characteristics related to the incidence of cardiovascular disease and death: Framingham Study, 18-year follow-up. *In* Kannel WB, Gordon T (eds.): The Framingham Study. DHEW Publication No. (NH-1) 74-559. Washington DC, U.S. Government Printing Office, 1974.
70. Kannel WB, Gorgon T, Schwartz MJ: Systolic versus diastolic blood pressure and risk of coronary heart disease: The Framingham Study. Am J Cardiol 27:335, 1971.
71. Kannel WB, Castelli WP, McNamara PM, et al: Role of blood pressure in the development of congestive heart failure: The Framingham Study. N Engl J Med 287:781, 1972.
72. Kannel WB, Dawber TR, Sorlie P, et al: Components of blood pressure and risk of atherothrombotic brain infarction: The Framingham Study. Stroke 7:327, 1976.
73. Shekelle RB, Ostfeld AM, Klawans HL Jr: Hypertension and risk of stroke in an elderly population. Stroke 5:71, 1974.
74. Veterans Administration Co-operative Study Group on Antihypertensive Agents: Effects of treatment on morbidity in hypertension. I. Results in patients with diastolic blood pressures averaging 115 through 129 mm Hg. JAMA 202:1028, 1967.
75. Veterans Administration Co-operative Study Group on Antihypertensive Agents: Effects of treatment on morbidity in hypertension. II. Results in patients with diastolic blood pressures averaging 90 through 114 mm Hg. JAMA 213:1143, 1970.
76. Peart WS, Miall WE: Hypertension and special clinics. Br Med J 280:180, 1980.
77. Moser M: "Less severe" hypertension: Should it be treated? Am Heart J 101:465, 1982.
78. Freis ED: Should mild hypertension be treated? N Engl J Med 307:306, 1982.
79. Kaplan NM: Therapy for mild hypertension: Toward a more balanced view. JAMA 249:365, 1983.
80. McAlister NH: Should we treat "mild" hypertension? JAMA 249:379, 1983.
81. Galen RS, Gambino SR: Beyond Normality: The predictive value and efficiency of medical diagnoses. New York, John Wiley and Sons, 1975, pp. 141–146.
82. Cole P, Morrison A: Basic issues in population screening for cancer. JNCI 64:1263, 1980.
83. Joint National Committee on Detection, Evaluation, and Treatment of High Blood Pressure: Report of the Joint National Committee on Detection, Evaluation, and Treatment of High Blood Pressure: A Co-operative Study. JAMA 237:255, 1977.
84. National Center for Health Statistics: Blood Pressure of Persons 18–74 Years: United States 1971–1972. Series 11, No. 150. Washington, DC, U.S. Dept of Health, Education and Welfare, 1975.
85. Stamler J, Stamler R, Riedlinger WF, et al: Hypertension screening of 1 million Americans: Community Hypertension Evaluation Clinic (CHEC) Program, 1973 through 1975. JAMA 235:2299, 1976.
86. Colton T: Statistics in Medicine. Boston, Little Brown and Company, 1974, pp. 71–74.
87. Vecchio TJ: Predictive value of a single diagnostic test in unselected populations. N Engl J Med 274:1171, 1966.
88. Orchard TJ, Daneman D, Becker D, et al: Glycosylated hemoglobin: A screening test for diabetes mellitus? Prev Med 11:595, 1982.
89. Fontana RS, Taylor WF: Screening for lung cancer: The Mayo Lung Project. *In* Miller AB (ed.): Screening in Cancer. Technical Report Series, Volume 40. Geneva, Union Internationale Controllé du Cancer, 1978, pp. 233–253.
90. Shapiro S. Evidence on screening for breast cancer from a randomized trial. Cancer 39:2772, 1977.
91. Clarke EA, Anderson TW: Does screening by "Pap" smears help prevent cervical cancer? Lancet 2:1, 1979.
92. Sackett DL: Bias in analytic research. J Chronic Dis 32:51, 1979.
93. Murphy EA: The Logic of Medicine. Baltimore, Johns Hopkins University Press, 1976.
94. Haynes RB, Sackett DL, Taylor DW, et al: Increased absenteeism from work after detection and labeling of hypertensive patients. N Engl J Med 299:741, 1978.
95. Soghikian K, Fallick-Hunkeler EM, Ury HK, Fischer AA: The effect of high blood pressure treatment and awareness on emotional well-being. J Clin Invest Med 4:191, 1981.
96. Macdonald LA, Sackett DL, Haynes RB, Taylor DW: Hypertension: The effects of labelling on behavior. Qual Life Cardiovasc Care Jan/Feb, 129–139, 1985.
97. Sackett DL, Haynes RB: Compliance with Therapeutic Regimens. Baltimore, Johns Hopkins University Press, 1976.
98. National Heart, Lung, and Blood Institute, Working Group on Compliance in Hypertension: Management of patient compliance in the treatment of hypertension. Hypertension 4:415, 1982.
99. Haynes RB, Taylor DW, Sackett DL (eds.): Compliance in Health Care. Baltimore, Johns Hopkins University Press, 1979.
100. Lew EA: High blood pressure, other risk factors and longevity: The insurance viewpoint. Am J Med 55:281, 1973.
101. Department of Clinical Epidemiology and Biostatistics, McMaster University: Clinical disagreement. I.

How often it occurs and why. Can Med Assoc J 123:499, 1980.
102. Weinstein MC, Stason WB: Hypertension: A Policy Perspective. Cambridge, MA, Harvard University Press, 1976.
103. Stason WB, Weinstein MC: Allocation of resources to manage hypertension. N Engl J Med 296:732, 1977.
104. Weinstein MC: Stason WB: Economic considerations in the management of mild hypertension. Ann NY Acad Sci 340:424, 1978.
105. Logan AG, Milne BJ, Achber C, et al: Worksite treatment of hypertension by specially trained nurses. A controlled trial. Lancet 2:1175, 1979.
106. Avron J: Benefits and cost analysis in geriatric care: Turning age discrimination into health policy. N Engl J Med 310:1294, 1984.
107. Cadman D, Chambers LW, Feldman W, Sackett DL: Assessing the effectiveness of community screening programs. JAMA 251:1530, 1984.
108. Kaplan EB, Sheiner LB, Boeckmann AJ et al: The usefulness of preoperative laboratory screening. JAMA 253 (24):3576, 1985.
109. Prorok PC, Hankey BF, Bundy BN: Concepts and problems in the evaluation of screening programs. J Chron Dis 34:159, 1982.
110. Williams ME, Retchin SM: Clinical geriatric research: Still in adolescence. J Am Geriatr Soc 32:851, 1984.
111. Rodstein M: Accidents among the aged: Incidence, causes, and prevention. J Chronic Dis 17:515, 1964.
112. Anand MP: Accidents in the home. *In* Anderson WF, Isaacs B (eds.): Current Achievements in Geriatrics. London, Cassell, 1964.
113. Agate J: Accidents to old people in their homes. Br Med J 2:785, 1966.
114. Rodstein M: Accidents among the aged. *In* Reichel W (ed.): Clinical Aspects of Aging. Baltimore, Williams and Wilkins, 1978.
115. Rosalki SB, Rau D, Lehmann D, et al: Gammaglutamyltranspeptidase in chronic alcoholism. Lancet 2:1139, 1970.
116. Bailey A: Is pre-employment medical examination of value? The validity of a computerized health questionnaire. Proc R Soc Med 67:180, 1974.
117. Busse EW, Pfeiffer E: Functional psychiatric disorders in old age. *In* Busse EW, Pfeiffer E (eds.): Behavior and Adaptation in Late Life. Boston, Little, Brown and Company, 1975.
118. Droller H: Some aspects of alcoholism in the elderly. Lancet 2:137, 1964.
119. Gaitz CM, Baer PE: Characteristics of elderly patients with alcoholism. Arch Gen Psychiatry 24:372, 1971.
120. Rosin AJ, Glatt MM: Alcohol excess in the elderly. Qu J Stud Alcohol 32:53, 1971.
121. Thier SO: Breast cancer screening: A view from outside the controversy. N Engl J Med 297:1063, 1978.
122. Pomerance W, Connor RJ, Fink DJ, et al: Screening for breast cancer. Lancet 1:143, 1976.
123. Shapiro S: Evidence on screening for breast cancer from a randomized trial. Cancer 39:2772, 1977.
124. Kirch RL, Klein M: Prospective evaluation of periodic breast examination programs. Cancer 38:265, 1976.
125. Irwig LM: Breast cancer. Lancet 2:1305, 1974.
126. Hutchinson GB, Shapiro S: Lead time gained by diagnostic screening for breast cancer. JNCI 41:665, 1968.
127. Strax P, Venet L, Shapiro S: Value of mammography in reduction of mortality in mass screening. AJR 117:686, 1973.
128. Chamberlain J, Ginks S, Rogers P, et al: Validity of clinical examination and mammography as screening tests for breast cancer. Lancet 2:1026, 1975.
129. MacMahon B, Cole P, Brown J: Etiology of human breast cancer: A review. JNCI 50:21, 1973.
130. Moskowitz M, Russell P, Fidler J, et al: Breast cancer screening. Preliminary report of 207 biopsies performed in 4128 volunteer screenees. Cancer 36:2245, 1975.
131. Devitt JE: Screenings for breast cancer: Current status, problems, prospects. Can Fam Phys 31:85, 1985.
132. Frank JW, Mai V: Breast examination in young women: More harm than good? Lancet 8456, 2:654, 1985.
133. Skrabanek P: False premises and false promises of breast cancer screening. Lancet 8450, 2:316, 1985.
134. Elwood TW, Erickson A, Lieberman S: Comparative educational approaches to screening for colorectal cancer. Am J Public Health 68:135, 1978.
135. Winawer SJ, Miller DG, Schottenfeld D, et al: Feasibility of fecal occult-blood testing for detection of colorectal neoplasia. Cancer 40:2616, 1977.
136. Dutton JJ: Sigmoidoscopy as a periodic screening test. J Fam Pract 7:1041, 1978.
137. Bolt RJ: Sigmoidoscopy in detection and diagnosis in the asymptomatic individual. Cancer 28:121, 1971.
138. Sangster JF, Gerace TM: Screening for carcinoma of the colon: A family practice perspective. Can Fam Physician 28:1599, 1982.
139. Diehl A: Screening for colorectal cancer. J Fam Pract 12:625, 1981.
140. Hoogewerf P, Cleator I, Elwood M, et al: Early detection of colorectal cancer: Second feasibility study. Can Fam Physician 26:1145, 1980.
141. Winawer S, Schottenfeld D, Sherlock P (eds.): Colorectal Cancer: Prevention, Epidemiology, and Screening. New York, Raven Press, 1980, pp. 181–187.
142. Calkins WG: Pre-malignant gastrointestinal lesions. Geriatrics 19:707, 1964.
143. Morrow G, Way J, Hoagland A, Cooper R: Patient compliance with self-directed Hemoccult testing. Prev Med 11:512, 1980.
144. Frame PS, Kowulich BA: Stool occult blood screening for colorectal cancer. J Fam Pract 15:1071, 1982.
145. Gilbertsen VA, McHugh R, Schuman L, et al: The earlier detection of colorectal cancers. Cancer 45:2899, 1980.
146. Ahlquist DA, McGill DB, Schwartz S, et al: Fecal blood levels in health and disease: A study using HemoQuant. N Engl J Med 312:1422, 1985.
147. Applegate WB, Spector MH: Colorectal cancer screening. J Comm Health 7:138, 1981.
148. Frank JW: Routine Hemoccult screening: The current evidence. Can Fam Phys 31:99, 1985.
149. Frank JW: Occult-blood screening for colorectal carcinoma: The benefits. Am J Prev Med 1:3, 1985.
150. Frank JW: Occult-blood screening for colorectal carcinoma: The risks. Am J Prev Med 1:25, 1985.
151. Frank JW: Occult-blood screening for colorectal carcinoma: The costs. Am J Prev Med 1:18, 1985.
152. Kristein MM: The Economics of screening for colorectal cancer. Soc Sci Med 14C:275, 1980.
153. Neuhauser D, Lewicki AM: What do we gain from the sixth stool guaiac? N Engl J Med 293:226, 1975.
154. Peterson WJ, Fordtran JS: Quantitating the occult. N Engl J Med 312:1448, 1985.

155. Simon JB: Occult blood screening for colorectal carcinoma: A critical review. Gastroenterology 88:820, 1985.
156. Winamer SJ, Fleischer M: Sensitivity and specificity of the fecal occult blood test for colorectal neoplasia. Gastroenterology 82:986, 1982.
157. Busse EW, Blazer D (eds.): Handbook of Geropsychiatry. New York, Van Nostrand Reinhold Company, 1980.
158. Whanger AD, Verwoerdt A: Management of affective disorders. *In* Verwoerdt A (ed.): Clinical Geropsychiatry 2nd ed. Baltimore, Williams and Wilkins, 1983.
159. Busse EW, Pfeiffer E: Behavior and Adaptation in Late Life. Boston, Little, Brown and Company, 1975.
160. Isaacs AD, Post F: Studies in Geriatric Psychiatry. New York, John Wiley and Sons, 1978.
161. De Alarcón R: Hypochondriasis and depression in the aged. Gerontol Clin 6:266, 1974.
162. Carroll BJ, Feinberg M, Greden JF, et al: A specific laboratory test for the diagnosis of melancholia. Arch Gen Psychiatry 38:15, 1981.
163. Levy MT: Psychiatric assessment of elderly patients in the home: A survey of 176 cases. J Am Geriatr Soc 33:9, 1985.
164. Reifler B, Raskind M, Kethley A: Psychiatric diagnoses among geriatric patients seen in an outreach program. J Am Geriatr Soc 31:530, 1982.
165. Schmidt GL: Depression in the elderly. Wisc Med J 82:25, 1983.
166. Hall MRP (ed.): Symposium on evaluation of drug therapy in the elderly. Gerontol Clin 15:1, 1973.
167. Oliver MF: Risks of correcting the risks of coronary disease and stroke with drugs. N Engl J Med 306:297, 1982.
168. Williamson J: Prescribing problems in the elderly. Practitioner 220:749, 1978.
169. Hurwitz N: Admissions to hospital due to drugs. Br Med J 1:539, 1969.
170. Hansen JM, Kamponaur J, Lauren H: Renal excretion of drugs in the elderly. Lancet 1:1170, 1970.
171. Davison W: Drug hazards in the elderly. Br J Hosp Med 6:83, 1971.
172. Crooks J, O'Malley K, Stevenson IH: Pharmacokinetics in the Elderly. Clin Pharmacokinet 1:280, 1976.
173. Judge TG, Caird FI: Drug Treatment of the Elderly Patient. London, Pitman Medical Publishing Company, 1978.
174. Williamson J: Adverse reactions to prescribed drugs in the elderly. *In* Crooks J, Stevenson IH (eds.): Drugs and the Elderly. London, MacMillan, 1979.
175. Stanaszek WF: Drug interactions in the elderly patient. Pharmacy Times 54, January 1979.
176. Lawson IR, Chapron DA: Basic pharmacopoeia for geriatric practice. *In* Reichel W (ed.): Clinical Aspects of Aging. Baltimore, Williams and Wilkins, 1978.
177. Hall MRP: Use of drugs in elderly patients. NY State J Med 75:67, 1975.
178. Anderson WF: Administration, labellings, and general principles of drug prescription in the elderly. Gerontol Clin 16:4, 1974.
179. Freeman JT: Clinical Principles and Drugs in the Aging. Springfield IL, Charles C Thomas, 1963.
180. Conrad K, Bressler R: Drug Therapy for the Elderly. St. Louis, C.V. Mosby Company, 1982.
181. Gordon M: Occult cardiac arrhythmias associated with falls and dizziness in the elderly. J Am Geriatr Soc 2:418, 1978.
182. Sheldon JH: On the national history of falls in old age. Br Med J 4:1685, 1960.
183. Clark AWG: Falls in old age. Mod Geriatr 2:332, 1973.
184. Rodstein M: Falls by the Aged. *In* Cape R, Coe R, Rassman J (eds.): Fundamentals of Geriatric Medicine. New York, Raven Press, 1983.
185. Overstall PW, Johnson AL, Exton-Smith AN: Instability and falls in the elderly. Age Aging 7:(Suppl) 92, 1978.
186. Lapidus PW, Guidotti FP: Painful heel: Report of 323 patients with 634 painful heels. Clin Orthop 39:178, 1965.
187. Woodhouse NJY: Clinical applications of calcitonin. Br Hosp Med 11:677, 1974.
188. Locke KR, Menneli J, Sgarlato TH: Foot complaints: "Doctor, my feet are killing me." J Pract Fam Med 9:20, 1975.
189. DuVries HL: Disorders of the skin and toenails. *In* Inman VT (ed.): DuVries' Surgery of the Foot. 3rd ed. St. Louis, C.V. Mosby Company, 1973.
190. Helfand AE: Reflections on "Keep them walking." Geriatr Institutions 16:20, 1969.
191. Werter H, Helfand AE, Margolis E: Disorders of the foot. *In* Libow L, Sherman F (eds.): The Core of Geriatric Medicine. St. Louis, C.V. Mosby Company, 1981.
192. Richards S: Deafness in the elderly. Gerontol Clin 13:350, 1971.
193. Cooper AF, Curry AR: The pathology of deafness in the paranoid and affective psychoses of later life. J Psychosom Res 20:97, 1976.
194. Hazell JWP: Vestibular problems of balance. Age Aging 8:258, 1979.
195. Hinchcliffe R: The threshold of hearing as a function of age. Acoustica 9:303, 1959.
196. Stevenson PW: Responses to speech audiometry and phonemic discrimination patterns in the elderly. Audiology 14:185, 1975.
197. Schow RL, Christensen JM, Hutchinson JM, Nerbonne MA: Communication Disorders of the Aged: A Guide for Health Professionals. Baltimore, University Park Press, 1978.
198. Corso JF: Presbycusis: Hearing loss and aging. Audiology 16:146, 1977.
199. Alberti PW: Hearing aids and aural rehabilitation in a geriatric population. J Otolaryngol (Suppl) 6 (4):1–50, 1977.
200. Klotz RE, Kilbane M: Hearing in an aging population: Preliminary report. N Engl J Med 266:177, 1962.
201. Colandrea MA, Friedman GD, Nachman MZ, Lynd CM: Systolic hypertension in the elderly: An epidemiologic assessment. Circulation 41:239, 1970.
202. Hypertension in the Elderly. Lancet 1:684, 1977.
203. Jackson G, Pierscianowski TA, Mahon W, Condon J: Inappropriate antihypertensive therapy in elderly patients. Lancet 1:731, 1965.
204. Koch-Weser J: Arterial hypertension in old age. Herz 3:235, 1978.
205. Miall WE, Chinn S: Screening for hypertension: Some epidemiologic observations. Br Med J 3:595, 1974.
206. Tarazi RC, Gifford RW Jr: Clinical significance and management of systolic hypertension. *In* Oresti G, Brest AN (eds.): Hypertension: Mechanisms, Diagnosis, and Treatment. Philadelphia: F.A. Davis Company, 1978.
207. Kannel WB, Brand F, McGee D: Hypertension in

the Elderly. *In* Cape R, Coe R, Rassman I (eds.): Fundamentals of Geriatric Medicine. New York, Raven Press, 1983, pp. 275–285.
208. Tarazi RC: Should you treat systolic hypertension in elderly patients? Geriatrics 33:25, 1978.
209. Brest AM, Haddad M: Should systolic hypertension be treated? Controversies in Cardiology 8:217, 1977.
210. Jones JV, Graham DI: Hypertension and the cerebral circulation—its relevance to the elderly. Am Heart J 96:270, 1978.
211. Jones JV: Hypertension in the elderly. Lancet 1:684, 1977.
212. Ostfeld AH: Elderly hypertensive patients. NY State J Med 78:1125, 1978.
213. Caird FI, Dall JLC, Kennedy RD: Cardiology in Old Age. NY: Plenum Publishing Company, 1976.
214. Koch-Weser J: The therapeutic challenge of systolic hypertension. N Engl J Med 289:481, 1973.
215. Fry J: Natural history of hypertension. A case for selective non-treatment. Lancet 2:431, 1974.
216. Dyer AR, Stamler J, Skekelle RB, et al: Hypertension in the elderly. Med Clin North Am. 61:513, 1977.
217. Amery A et al: Mortality and morbidity results from the European Working Party on high blood pressure in the elderly trial. Lancet 1:1349, 1985.
218. Dustan HP (Chairman): The 1984 Report of the Joint National Commission on Detection, Evaluation, and Treatment of High Blood Pressure, Special Report. Arch Intern Med 144:1045, 1984.
219. Gladstone JL, Recco R: Host factors and infectious diseases in the elderly. Med Clin North Am 60:1225, 1976.
220. Phair JP: Aging and infection: A review. J Chronic Dis 32:535, 1979.
221. Austrian R: Prevention of pneumoccal infection by immunization with capsular polysaccharides of *Streptococcus pneumoniae:* Current status of polyvalent vaccines. J Infect Dis 136(Suppl):S38, 1977.
222. Barker WH, Mullooly JP: Influenza vaccination of elderly persons. JAMA 244:2547, 1980.
223. Centers for Disease Control: Influenza vaccines 1982–1983. MMWR 31:350, 1982.
224. Ruben FL: Prevention of influenza in the elderly. Am J Geriatr Med 30:577, 1982.
225. Schoenbaum SC: A perspective on the benefits, costs, and risks of immunization. *In* Weinstein L, Fields BN (eds.): Semin Infect Dis 3:294, 1980.
226. Bentley DW: Pneumococcal vaccine in the institutionalized elderly: Review of past and recent studies. Rev Infect Dis 3(Suppl):S61, 1981.
227. Schwartz JS: Pneumococcal vaccine: Clinical efficacy and effectiveness. Ann Intern Med 96:208, 1982.
228. Centers for Disease Control: Pneumococcal polysaccharide vaccine. MMWR 30:410, 1981.
229. Smit P, Oberholzer D, Hayden-Smiths S, et al: Protective efficacy of pneumococcal polysaccharides vaccines. JAMA 238:2613, 1977.
230. Public Health Service Advisory Committee on Immunization Practices: Pneumococcal polysaccharides. MMWR 27:25, 1978.
231. Ammann AJ, Schiffman G, Austrian R: The antibody responses to pneumococcal capsular polysaccharides in aged individuals. Proc Soc Exp Biol Med 164:312, 1980.
232. Recommendations of the Public Health Service Advisory Committee on Immunization Practices: Influenza vaccine. MMWR 26:193, 1977.
233. Steinberg FU: Gait disorders in old age. Geriatrics 22:134, 1966.
234. Barron RD: Disorder of gait related to the aging nervous system. Geriatrics 22:113, 1967.
235. Garn SM: Bone loss and aging. *In* Goldman R, Rockstein M (eds.). The Physiology and Pathology of Human Aging. New York, Academic Press, 1975.
236. Carter AB: The neurologic aspects of aging. *In* Rossman I (ed.): Clinical Geriatrics. 2nd ed. Philadelphia, J.B. Lippincott Company, 1979.
237. Chamberlain J: Evaluation of screening tests for unreported disability in the elderly. Br J Prev Soc Med 26:55, 1972.
238. Fitzgerald JAW, Newman PH: Degenerative spondylolisthesis. J Bone Joint Surg 58:184, 1976.
239. Wilcock GK: Benefits of total hip replacement to older patients and the community. Br Med J 2:37, 1978.
240. Azar GJ, Lawton AH: Gait and stepping as factors in the frequent falls of elderly women. Gerontologist 4:83, 1964.
241. Moore JT, Whanger AD: Functional psychiatric disorders. *In* Cape R, Coe R, Rassman I (eds.): Fundamentals of Geriatric Medicine. 1983, pp. 129–137.
242. Levenson AJ, Tollett SM: Rapid psychiatric assessment of the geriatric patient for immediate psychiatric referral. Geriatrics 35:113, 1980.
243. Wilson FG: Social isolation and bereavement. Lancet 2:1356, 1970.
244. Rowland KF: Environmental events predicting death for the elderly. Psychol Bull 84:349, 1977.
245. Jeffers FC, Verwoerdt A: How the old face death. *In* Busse EW, Pfeiffer E (eds.): Behavior and Adaptation in Late Life. Boston, Little, Brown and Company, 1968, pp. 163–181.
246. Feifel H, Jones R: Perception of death as related to nearness of death. Proceedings of the 76th Annual Convention of the American Psychological Association 3:545, 1968.
247. Glaser BG: The social loss of aged dying patients. Gerontologist 6:77, 1966.
248. Kalish RA: Death and dying in a social context. *In* Binstock R, Shanas E (eds.): Handbook of Aging and the Social Sciences. New York, Van Nostrand Reinhold, 1976.
249. Feifel H, Branscomb AB: Who's afraid of death? J Abnorm Psychol 81:282, 1973.
250. Swenson WM: Attitudes toward death in an aged population. J Gerontol 16:49, 1961.
251. Cartwright A, Hockey L, Anderson JL: Life Before Death. London, Routledge and Kegan Paul, 1973.
252. Parkes CM, Brown RJ: Health after bereavement: A controlled study. Psychosom Med 34:449, 1972.
253. Rees WD, Lutkins SG: Mortality of bereavement. Br J Med 4:13, 1967.
254. Schoenberg B, Gerber I, Wiener A, et al (eds.): Bereavement, Its Psychological Aspects. New York, Columbia University Press, 1975.
255. Behnke JA, Finch CE, Moment GB: The Biology of Aging. New York, Plenum Press, 1978.
256. Shock NW: Systems physiology and aging. Fed Proc 38:161, 1979.
257. Carlson L: Nutrition of Old Age. Stockholm, Almqvist and Wiksell, 1972.
258. Association of Life Insurance Medical Directors of America, Philadelphia, and Society of Actuaries, Chicago: Report of the Ad Hoc Committee of the New Build and Blood Pressure Study. 1980.
259. Pooling Project Research Group: Relationship of blood pressure, serum cholesterol, smoking habit,

relative weight and ECG abnormalities to incidence of major coronary events: Final report of the Pooling Project. J Chronic Dis 31:201, 1978.
260. Mann GV: The influence of obesity on health. N Engl J Med 291:178, 226, 1974.
261. Exton-Smith AN: Nutrition of the elderly. Br J Hosp Med 5:639, 1971.
262. Ross MH, Bras G: Dietary preference and disease of age. Nature 250:263, 1974.
263. Hawkins WW: Nutrition of the Aged. Quebec City, The Nutrition Society of Canada, 1978.
264. Hickler RB, Wayne KS: Nutrition and the elderly. Am Fam Phys 29:137, 1984.
265. Anderson JN, Storer R: Immediate and Replacement Dentures. Oxford, Blackwell Scientific Publications, 1973.
266. Storer R: Oral cancer. Lancet 1:430, 1972.
267. Hartles RL, Harrand RB: The etiology of dental caries. Br Dent J 126:136, 1969.
268. Sheiham A: The prevention and control of chronic periodontal disease. Dent Health 10:1, 1971.
269. Hobdell MH: Epidemiology of the impaired dentition. Proc R Soc Med 66:589, 1973.
270. Jackson D, Murray J: The loss of teeth in dentate populations. Dent Pract Rec 22:186, 1972.
271. Manson JD: The elderly dental cripple. Proc R Soc Med 66:597, 1973.
272. Bolden TE: Factors related to oral cancer. *In* Caldwell RC, Stallard RE (eds.): A Textbook of Preventive Dentistry. W.B. Saunders Company, Philadelphia, 1977, p. 102.
273. Mandel ID: Effects of dietary modifications on caries in humans. J Dent Res 49:1201, 1970.
274. Sheiham A: Is there a scientific basis for six-monthly dental examinations? Lancet 2:442, 1977.
275. Suomi JD: Prevention and control of periodontal disease. J Am Dent Assoc 83:1271, 1971.
276. Hodkinson HM, Exton-Smith AN: Factors predicting mortality in the elderly in the community. Age Aging 5:110, 1976.
277. Sheldon JH: The Social Medicine of Old Age. London, Oxford University Press, 1948.
278. Exton-Smith AN: Functional consequences of Aging: Clinical manifestations. *In* Exton-Smith AN, Grimley Evans J (eds.): Care of the Elderly: Meeting the Challenge of Dependency. London, Academic Press, 1977.
279. Heron A, Chown S: Age and Function. London, Churchill Livingstone, 1967.
280. Hayflick L: The cell biology of human aging. N Engl J Med 295:1302, 1976.
281. Kemp R: The diagnosis of old age. Lancet 2:515, 1962.
282. Busse EW: The early detection of aging. Bull NY Acad Med 41:1090, 1965.
283. Clarke M: Problems of the elderly: an epidemiological perspective. J R Coll Phys Lond 18:128, 1984.
284. Fisk AA: Comprehensive health care for the elderly. JAMA, 249:230, 1983.
285. Frame PS, Kowulich BA, Llewellyn AM: Improving physician compliance with a health maintenance protocol. J Fam Pract, 19:341, 1984.
286. Grundy E: Mortality and morbidity among the old. Br Med J 288:663, 1984.
287. Herbert CP, Moore D: A study of health maintenance protocols in family practice. Can Fam Phys 31:47, 1985.
288. Keller GC: Cancer detection in the periodic physical examination. Cancer 51:2446, 1983.
289. Kelley BC: Planning for aging in the twenty-first century. Am J Prev Med 1:18, 1985.
290. Kennie DC: Good health care for the aged. JAMA 249:770, 1983.
291. Kennie DC: Health maintenance of the elderly. J Amer Geriatr Soc 32:316, 1984.
292. Khoury MJ, Newill CA, Chase GA: Epidemiologic evaluation of screening for risk factors. Am J Pub Health 75:1204, 1985.
293. Kimber J, Silver PC: Home visiting by a geriatric department. Royal Coll Gen Pract 31:41, 1981.
294. Morrison A: Screening in Chronic Disease. New York: Oxford University Press, 1985.
295. Nelson E, Conger B, Douglass R, et al: Functional health status levels of primary care patients. JAMA, 249:3331, 1983.
296. Periodic health examination: A guide for designing individualized preventive health care in the asymptomatic patient. Report of the Medical Practice Committee, American College of Physicians. Ann Intern Med 95:729, 1981.
297. Rowe JW: Health care of the elderly. N Engl J Med 312:827, 1985.
298. Szekais B: Adult day centers: Geriatric day health services in the community. J Fam Pract 20:157, 1985.
299. The Use of Epidemiology in the Study of the Elderly. Report of a WHO Scientific Group on the Epidemiology of Aging. WHO Technical Report Series, 706, 1984.
300. Williams ME, Hadler NM: The illness as the focus of geriatric medicine. N Engl J Med 308:1357, 1983.
301. Zimmer JG, Groth-Juncker A, McCusker J: A randomized controlled study of a home health care team. Am J Pub Health, 75:134, 1985.
302. Miall WE, Ashcroft MT, Lovell HG, Moore F: A longitudinal study of the decline of adult height with age in two Welsh communities. Hum Biol 39:445, 1967.
303. Dequeker JV, Baeyens JP, Claessens J: The significance of stature as a clinical measurement of aging. J Am Geriatr Soc 17:169, 1969.
304. Master AN, Lasser RP, Beckman G: Tables of average weight and height of Americans, aged 65 to 94 years. JAMA 172:658, 1960.
305. Garn SM: Bone-loss and aging. *In* Goldman R, Rockstein M (eds.): The Psychology and Pathology of Human Aging. New York, Academic Press, 1975.
306. Willington FL (ed.): Urinary Incontinence in the Elderly. London, Academic Press, 1976.
307. Sourander L: Urinary tract infection in the aged: An epidemiological study. Ann Intern Med Fenn 55:7, 1966.
308. Williams MD, Pannill FC: Urinary incontinence in the elderly: Physiology, pathophysiology, diagnosis, and treatment. Ann Intern Med 97:895, 1982.
309. Yarnell JWG, St. Leger AS: The prevalence, severity, and factors associated with urinary incontinence in a random sample of the elderly. Age Aging 8:81, 1979.
310. Wells TJ, Brink CA: Urinary continence: Assessment and management. *In* Burnside IM (ed.): Nursing and the Aged. 2nd ed. New York, McGraw Hill Book Company, 1981.
311. Mandelstam D: Incontinence. London, Disabled Living Foundation, 1977.
312. Vetter NJ, Jones DA, Victor CR: Urinary incontinence in the elderly at home. Lancet 2:1275, 1981.
313. Freedman LR: Urinary-tract infections in the elderly. N Engl J Med 309:1451, 1983.
314. Beck C: Abuse in the elderly. Paper presented at the

Western Gerontological Society meeting. Seattle, Washington, April 1981.
315. Brenton M: The Runaways. Boston, Little, Brown and Company, 1978.
316. Butler RN: Why Survive? Being Old in America. New York, Harper and Row, 1975.
317. Kimsey LR, Tarbox AR, Bragg DF: Abuse of the elderly—the hidden agenda. I. The caretakers and the categories of abuse. J Am Geriatr Soc 29:465, 1981.
318. Renvoize J: Web of Violence: A Study of Family Violence. London, Routledge and Kegan Paul, 1978.
319. Steinmetz SK: Battered parents. Society 15:54, 1978.
320. Warshaw BA, Moore JT, Friedman SW, et al: Functional disability in the hospitalized elderly. JAMA 248:847, 1982.
321. Moore JT: Abuse of the elderly. *In* AFP Family Practice Annual, 1983. Kansas City, American Academy of Family Physicians, 1983, pp. 79–89.
322. Salend E, Kane RA, Satz M, Pynoos J: Elder abuse reporting: Limitations of statutes. Gerontologist 24:61, 1984.
323. Kini MM, Liebowitz HM, Cotton T, et al: Prevalence of senile cataract, diabetic retinopathy, senile macular degeneration, and open angle glaucoma in the Framingham Eye Study. Am J Ophthalmol 85:28, 1978.
324. Fozard JL, Wolf E, Bell B, et al: Visual perception and communication. *In* Birren JE, Schaie KW (eds.): Handbook of the Psychology of Aging. New York, Van Nostrand Reinhold, 1977.
325. Gordon DM: Visual impairment in the older patient. J Am Geriatr Soc 15:1025, 1967.
326. Kasper RL: Eye problems of the aged. *In* Clinical Aspects of Aging, 2nd ed. Reichel, WM (ed.): Baltimore, Williams & Wilkins, 1983, pp. 479–497.
327. Kornzweig AL: Ocular conditions of the aged. Geriatrics 19:24, 1964.
328. Kornzweig AL, Feinstein M, Schneider J: The eye in old age. Am J Ophthalmol 22:29, 1957.
329. MacLennan WJ, Andrews GR, MacLeod C, Caird FI: Anemia in the elderly. Q J Med 42:1, 1973.
330. Leask RGS, Andrews GR, Caird FI: Normal values for 16 blood constituents in the elderly. Age Aging 2:14, 1973.
331. Sackett DL: The usefulness of laboratory tests in health screening programs. Clin Chem 19:336, 1973.
332. Brunning RD: Differential diagnosis of anemia. Geriatrics 29:52, 1974.
333. Elwood PC, Waters WE, Greene WJ, Wood MM: Evaluation of a screening survey for anaemia in adult non-pregnant women. Br Med J 4:714, 1967.
334. Elwood PC, Shinton NK, Wilson CID, et al: Haemoglobin, vitamin $B_{12}$ and folate levels in the elderly. Br J Haemat 21:557, 1971.
335. Hallberg L, Hogdahl AM: Anemia and old age. Gerontol Clin 13:31, 1971.
336. Evans DMD, Pathy MS, Sanerkin NG, Deeble TJ: Anemia in geriatric patients. Gerontol Clin 10:228, 1968.
337. Ehtisham M, Cape RDT: Protocol for diagnosing and treating anemia. Geriatrics 32:91, 1977.
338. Canton AM: A study of pernicious anemia in elderly patients. Gerontol Clin 5:23, 1963.
339. Williams MT: Community screening for glaucoma and diabetes. Sight Sav Rev 44:79, 1974.
340. Williams MT, Hayakawa J, Vaughan DG, et al: Evolution of a prevention of blindness program in Santa Clara County. Special emphasis on glaucoma detection (1960–1970). JAMA 219:737, 1972.
341. Turnbull CJ: Screening for glaucoma in a geriatric unit: Report of a pilot study. Age Aging 10:169, 1981.
342. Phillip MA: Early detection of chronic simple glaucoma in general practice. J R Coll Gen Pract 27:601, 1977.
343. Abrahamson IA Jr: Intraocular pressure tonometry. Am Fam Physician 17:75, 1978.
344. Graham PA: Screening for chronic glaucoma. Proc R Soc Med 59:1215, 1966.
345. Kornzweig AL: Ocular conditions of the aged. Geriatrics 19:24, 1964.
346. Anderson DR, Hoskins HD: The management of elevated intraocular pressure with normal optic discs and visual fields. I. Therapeutic approach based on high risk factors. II. An approach to early therapy. Surv Ophthalmol 21:479, 1977.
347. Graham PA: Epidemiology of simple glaucoma and ocular hypertension. Br J Ophthalmol 56:223, 1972.
348. Kitazawa Y, Horie T, Aoki S, et al: Untreated ocular hypertension. A long-term prospective study. Arch Ophthalmol 95:1180, 1977.
349. Pollack IP: The challenge of glaucoma screening. Surv Ophthalmol 13:4, 1968.
350. Shaffer R: 'Glaucoma suspect' of 'ocular hypertension'? Arch Ophthalmol 95:588, 1977.
351. Wilensky JT, Podos SM: Prognostic parameters in primary open angle glaucoma. *In* Anderson DR, Drance SM, Galin MA, et al (eds.): Symposium on Glaucoma (Transactions of the New Orleans Academy of Ophthalmology). St. Louis, C.V. Mosby, 1975, p. 7.
352. Bankes JLK, Perkins ES, Tsolakis S, Wright JE: Bedford glaucoma survey. Br Med J 1:791, 1968.
353. Morin JD: Screening for glaucoma in family practice. Can Fam Phys 31:113, 1985.
354. Cervical Cancer Screening Programs: The Walton Report. Task Force of the Conference of Deputy Ministers of Health. Can Med Assoc J 114:2, 1976.
355. Clarke EA, Anderson TW: Does screening by "Pap" smears help prevent cervical cancer? Lancet 2:1, 1979.
356. NIH Consensus Development Conference on Cervical Cancer Screening: Consensus—more or less—on the Pap smear. Science 209:672, 1980.
357. Seeley TJ: Cancer of the cervix uteri: An epidemiological survey. Clin Radiol 27:43, 1976.
358. Dickinson L, Mussey ME, Soule EH, et al: Evaluation of the effectiveness of cytologic screening for cervical cancer. I. Incidence and mortality trends in relation to screenings. Mayo Clinic Proc 47:534, 1972.
359. Foltz AM, Kelsey JL: The annual Pap test: A dubious policy success. Milbank Mem Fund Q 56:427, 1978.
360. Frame PS, Carlson SJ: A critical review of periodic health screening using specific screening criteria. Part 3. Genitourinary systems. J Fam Pract 2:189, 1975.
361. Frost JK: Diagnostic accuracy of cervical smears. Obstet Gynecol Surv 24:893, 1969.
362. Gad C, Koch F: Population screening for cervical carcinoma in Fredricksberg Borough—results of second and third rescreenings, 1966–1972. Dan Med Bull 20:141, 1973.
363. Gardner JW, Lyon JL: Efficacy of cervical cytologic screening in the control of cervical cancer. Prev Med 6:487, 1977.
364. Guzick DS: Efficacy of screening for cervical cancer: A review. Am J Public Health 68:125, 1975.
365. Miller AB: Screening for cancer of the cervix in Canada, Post Walton. *In* Miller AB (ed.): Screening in Cancer: A Comprehensive Report Commissioned by

the UICC Technical Report Series, Vol. 40, Geneva, UICC, 1978, pp. 73–92.
366. Periodic Cancer Screening for Women. Chicago, American College of Obstetrics and Gynecology, 1980.
367. Richard RM: Current concepts in obstetrics and gynecology. The patient with an abnormal Pap smear—screening techniques and management. N Engl J Med 302:332, 1980.
368. Sandmire HF, Austin SD, Bechtel RC: Experience with 40,000 Papanicolaou smears. Obstet Gynecol 48:56, 1976.
369. Terris M, Oalmann MC: Carcinoma of the cervix: Epidemiologic study. JAMA 174:1847, 1960.
370. Walton RJ: Cervical cancer screening programs. I. Epidemiology and natural history of carcinoma of the cervix. Can Med Assoc J 114:1003, 1976.
371. Wright VC, Riopelle MA: Age at time of first intercourse vs. chronological age as a basis for Pap smear screening. Can Med Assoc J 127:127, 1982.
372. Bean HA: Carcinoma of the Endometrium in Saskatchewan 1966 to 1971. Gynecol Oncol 6:503, 1978.
373. Bibbo M, Shanklin DR, Wied GL: Endometrial cytology on jet wash material. J Reprod Med 8:90, 1972.
374. Burk JR, Lehman HF, Wolf FS: Inadequacy of the Papanicolaou smear in the detection of endometrial cancer. N Engl J Med 291:191, 1974.
375. Creasman WT, Weed JC: Screening techniques in endometrial cancer. Cancer 38:436, 1976.
376. Periodic Cancer Screening for Women. Chicago, American College of Obstetrics and Gynecology, June 1980.
377. Anderson JE, Meltzer HD, Scarborough JE, et al: Adenocarcinoma of the endometrium. Cancer 18:955, 1965.
378. Gravelee LC: Jet irrigation method for the diagnosis of endometrial adenocarcinoma. Obstet Gynecol 34:168, 1968.
379. Horwitz RI, Feinstein AR: Alternative analytic methods for case-control studies of estrogens and endometrial cancer. N Engl J Med 299:1089, 1978.
380. Chandrabrant AS, Green TH: Evaluation of the current management of endometrial carcinoma. Obstet Gynecol Surv 27:803, 1972.
381. Hibbard LT, Schwinn CE: Diagnosis by endometrial jet washings. Am J Obstet Gynecol 11:1039, 1971.
382. Chatfield WR, Bremmer AD: Intrauterine sponge biopsy. Obstet Gynecol 39:323, 1972.
383. Frame PS, Carlson SJ: A critical review of periodic health screening using specific screening criteria. Part 3. Selected diseases of the genitourinary system. J Fam Pract 2:189, 1975.
384. Clark DG, Hilaris BS, Ochoa M: Treatment of cancer of the ovary. Clin Obstet Gynecol 3:159, 1976.
385. Fox H, Agrawal K, Langley FA: A clinico-pathological study of 92 cases of granulosa cell tumour of the ovary with specific reference to factors influencing prognosis. Cancer 35:231, 1975.
386. Graber EA: Early diagnosis of ovarian cancer. Clin Obstet Gynecol 12:958, 1961.
387. Parker RT, Parker CH, Wilbanks GD: Cancer of the ovary. Am J Obstet Gynecol 108:878, 1970.
388. Barber HRK, Graber EA: The PMPO syndrome (post-menopausal palpable ovary syndrome). Clin Obstet Gynecol 38:921, 1971.
389. American Cancer Society: Guidelines for the cancer-related check-up. Cancer 30:194, 1980.
390. Cutler SJ, Myers MH, Green SB: Trends in survival rates of patients with cancer. N Engl J Med 293:122, 1975.
391. Fuller AF: Role of the primary physician in the detection and treatment of gynecologic cancer. Primary Care 8:1, 111, 1981.
392. Boone MI, Calvert JC, Gates HS: Uterine cancer screening by the family physician. Am Fam Phys 30:157, 1984.
393. Cramer JH, Osborne RJ: Endometrial neoplasia—screening the high-risk patient. Am J Obstet Gynecol 139:285, 1981.
394. Koss LG, Schreiber K, Oberlander SG, et al: Screening of asymptomatic women for endometrial cancer. Obstet Gynecol 57:681, 1981.
395. Parkin DM, Leach K, Cobb P, Clayden AD: Cervical cytology screening in two Yorkshire areas: Results of testing. Publ Health (Lond) 96:3, 1982.
396. Andres P: Aging and diabetes. Med Clin North Am 55:835, 1971.
397. Siperstein MD, Foster DW, Knowles HC, et al: Control of "blood" glucose and diabetic vascular disease. N Engl J Med 296:1060, 1977.
398. Malins JM: Diabetes. Lancet 2:1367, 1974.
399. Working Party of the College of General Practitioners. Br Med J 1:1497, 1962.
400. Bailey A: Biochemistry of well populations. Lancet 2:1436, 1974.
401. Marble A, White P: Joslin's Diabetes Mellitus. Philadelphia, Lea and Febiger, 1971.
402. Frame PS, Carlson ST: A critical review of periodic health screening using specific screening criteria. Part II. J Fam Pract 2:123, 1975.
403. Stamler R, Stamler J (eds.): Asymptomatic hyperglycemia and coronary heart disease. J Chronic Dis 32:683, 1979.
404. Soerjodibroto WS, Hearn CR, Exton-Smith AN: Glucose tolerance, plasma insulin levels and insulin sensitivity in elderly patients. Age Aging 8:65, 1979.
405. Denham MJ: The value of random blood glucose determinations as a screening method for detecting diabetes mellitus in the elderly patient. Age Aging 1:55, 1972.
406. Tokuhata GK, Miller W, Digon E, Hartman T: Diabetes mellitus: An underestimated public health problem. J Chronic Dis 28:23, 1975.
407. Patterson WB: Management of cancer in the elderly. *In* Cape RDT, Coe RM, Rossman I (eds.): Fundamentals of Geriatric Medicine. New York, Raven Press, 1983.
408. Herman JR: Carcinoma of the prostate. NY State J Med 72:841, 1972.
409. Byer DP: The Veterans Administration cooperative urological research group's studies of cancer of the prostate. Cancer 32:1126, 1973.
410. Coune A: Carcinoma of the prostate. *In* Staquet JJ (ed.): Randomized Trials in Cancer: A Critical Review by Sites. New York, Raven, 1978, p. 389.
411. Rotkin ID: Studies in the epidemiology of prostatic cancer: Expanded sampling. Cancer Treat Rep 61:173, 1977.
412. Schuman LM, Mandel J, Blackard C, et al: Epidemiologic study of prostatic cancer: Preliminary report. Cancer Treat Rep 61:181, 1977.
413. Fott AG, Cooper JF, Herschman H, et al: Detection of prostatic cancer by solid-phase radioimmunoassay of serum prostatic acid phosphatase. N Engl J Med 297:1357, 1977.
414. Owen WL: Cancer of the prostate: A literature review. J Chronic Dis 29:89, 1976.
415. Goldman R: Aging of the excretory system: Kidney

and bladder. *In* Finch CE, Hayflick L (eds.): Handbook of the Biology of Aging. New York, Van Nostrand Reinhold Company, 1977.
416. Lindeman RD: Age changes in renal function. *In* Goldman R, Rockstein M (eds.): The Physiology and Pathology of Human Aging. New York, Academic Press, 1975.
417. Dunnill MS, Halley W: Some observations on the quantitative anatomy of the kidney. J Pathol 110:113, 1973.
418. Darmady EM, Offer J, Woodhouse MA: The parameters of the aging kidney. J Pathol 109:195, 1973.
419. Rowe JW, Andres R, Tobin JD, et al: The effect of age on creatinine clearance in man: A cross-sectional and longitudinal study. J Gerontol 31:155, 1976.
420. Hollenberg NK, Adams DF: Senescence and the renal vasculature in normal man. Circ Res 34:309, 1974.
421. Papper S: The effects of age in reducing renal function. Geriatrics 28:83, 1973.
422. Brod J: Changes in renal function with age. Scr Med Fac Med Brun 41:223, 1968.
423. Davies DF, Shock NW: Age changes in glomerular filtration rate, effective renal plasma flow and tubular excretory capacity in adult males. J Clin Invest 29:496, 1950.
424. Dontas AS, Papanayiotou P, Marketos S, Papanicolaou N: The effect of bacteriuria on renal functional patterns in old age. Clin Sci 34:73, 1968.
425. Geill T: Genito-urinary disturbances in old age. Gerontol Clin 1:153, 1959.
426. Lewis WH Jr, Alving AS: Changes with age in the renal function in adult men: I. Clearance of urea. II. Amount of urea nitrogen in the blood. III. Concentrating ability of the kidneys. Am J Physiol 123:500, 1938.
427. Shock NW: Kidney function tests in aged males. Geriatrics 1:232, 1946.
428. Sourander LB: Urinary tract infection in the aged. An epidemiological study. Ann Med Intern Fenn 5(Suppl 45):1, 1966.
429. Woodford-Williams E: Renal function in the aged. Br J Clin Pract 14:351, 1960.
430. Horwitz O: Long-range evaluation of a mass screening. Am J Epid 100:20, 1974.
431. Colley JRT: Diseases of the lung. Lancet 2:1125, 1974.
432. Seaton A: Today's treatment: Tuberculosis. Br Med J 1:701, 1978.
433. Kasik JE, Schuldt S: Why tuberculosis is still a health problem in the aged. Geriatrics 32:63, 1977.
434. Edsall J, Collins G: Routine follow-up of inactive tuberculosis: A practice to be abandoned. Am Rev Resp Dis 107:850, 1973.
435. Myers JA: Tapering off of tuberculosis among the elderly. Am J Public Health 66:1101, 1976.
436. Glassroth JL, White MC, Snider DE Jr: An assessment of the possible association of isoniazid with human cancer deaths. Am Rev Resp Dis 116:1065, 1977.
437. Ten Dam HG, Toman K, Hitze KL, et al: Present knowledge of immunization against tuberculosis. Bull WHO 54:255, 1976.
438. American Thoracic Society: The tuberculin skin test. Am Rev Resp Dis 124:356, 1981.
439. American Thoracic Society and Centers for Disease Control: Treatment of tuberculosis and other mycobacterial diseases. Am Rev Resp Dis 127:790, 1983.
440. American Thoracic Society and Centers for Disease Control, USPHS: Control of tuberculosis. Am Rev Resp Dis 128:336, 1983.
441. Reichman LB, Farer LS, Chaparas SD, et al: Guidelines for the Diagnosis of Tuberculosis Infection (Symposium Monograph). New York: Audio-Visual Medical Marketing, Inc., 1984.
442. Stead WW: TB among elderly persons: An outbreak in a nursing home. Ann Intern Med 94:606, 1981.
443. Bowen DM, Davison AN: Biochemical changes in the normal aging brain and in dementia. *In* Isaacs B (ed.): Recent Advances in Geriatric Medicine. Edinburgh, Churchill Livingstone, 1978.
444. Hachinski VC, Iliff LD, Zilkha E, et al: Cerebral blood flow in dementia. Arch Neurol 32:632, 1975.
445. Marsden CD, Harrison MJG: Outcome of investigation of patients with presenile dementia. Br Med J 2:249, 1972.
446. Pitt B: Psycho-geriatrics: An introduction to the Psychiatry of Old Age. Edinburgh, Churchill Livingstone, 1974.
447. Roth M, Myers DH: The diagnosis of dementia. Br J Hosp Med 2:705, 1969.
448. Hakim AM, Mathieson G: Basis of dementia in Parkinson's disease. Lancet 2:729, 1978.
449. Levenson AJ, Tollett SM: Rapid psychiatric assessment of the geriatric patient for immediate psychiatric referral. Geriatrics 35:113, 1980.
450. Smith WL, Kinsbourne M: Aging and Dementia. New York, Spectrum Publications, 1977.
451. Libow LS: Pseudo-senility: Acute and reversible organic brain syndromes. J Am Geriatr Soc 21:112, 1973.
452. Irving G, Robinson RA, McAdam W: The validity of some cognitive tests in the diagnosis of dementia. Br J Psychiatry 117:149, 1970.
453. Benson DF, Blumer D (eds.): Psychiatric Aspects of Neurologic Disease. New York, Grune and Stratton, 1975.
454. Gilmore A: Brain failure at home. Age Ageing 6:56, 1977.
455. Freeman FR: Evaluation of patients with progressive intellectual deterioration. Arch Neurol 33:658, 1976.
456. Kannel WB, Dawber TR, Glennon WE, Thorne MC: Preliminary report: The determinants and clinical significance of serum cholesterol. Mass J Med Technol 4:11, 1962.
457. Oliver MF, Heady JA, Morris JN, Cooper J: A co-operative trial in the primary prevention of ischaemic heart disease using clofibrate. Report from the Committee of Principal Investigators. Br Heart J 40:1069, 1978.
458. Sackett DL: Clinical diagnosis and the clinical laboratory. Clin Invest Med 1:37, 1978.
459. Glasunov IS, Dowd JE, Jaksić Z, et al: Bull WHO 49:423, 1973.
460. Mann GV: Diet-heart: End of an era. N Engl J Med 297:644, 1970.
461. Stamler J: Research related to risk factors. Circulation 60:1575, 1979.
462. Hodkinson HM: The interpretation of biochemical data. *In* Isaacs B (ed.): Recent Advances in Geriatric Medicine. Edinburgh, Churchill Livingstone, 1978.
463. Davis CE, Havlik RJ: Clinical trials of lipid lowering and coronary artery disease prevention. *In* Rifkind BM, Levy RI (eds.): Hyperlipidemia: Diagnosis and Therapy. New York, Grune and Stratton, 1977, p. 79.
464. Burrows AW, Shakespear RA, Hesch RD, et al: Thyroid hormones in the elderly sick: T4 euthyroidism. Br Med J 4:437, 1975.
465. Bahemuka M, Hodkinson HM: Screening for hypothyroidism in elderly patients. Br Med J 2:601, 1975.
466. Murphy EA: A scientific viewpoint on normalcy. Perspect Biol Med 9:333, 1966.
467. Epstein KA, Schneiderman LJ, Bush JW, et al: The

"abnormal" screening serum thyroxine (T4): Analysis of physician response, outcome, cost and health effectiveness. J Chronic Dis 34:175, 1982.
468. Dales LG, Friedman GD, Collen MF: Evaluating periodic multiphasic health check-ups: A controlled trial. J Chronic Dis 32:385, 1979.
469. Hodkinson HM, Denham MJ: Thyroid function tests in the elderly in the community. Age Ageing 6:67, 1977.
470. Jeffreys PM, Farran HEA, Hoffenberg R, et al: Thyroid function tests in the elderly. Lancet 1:924, 1972.
471. Davis PJ, Davis FB: Hyperthyroidism in patients over the age of 60 years. Medicine 83:161, 1974.
472. Brett GZ: The value of lung cancer detection by six monthly chest radiographs. Thorax 23:414, 1968.
473. Cochrane AL, Elwood PC: Screening—the case against it. Med Officer 53-57, 1969.
474. Fontana RS, Taylor WF: Screening for lung cancer: The Mayo Clinic Project. *In* Miller AB (ed.): Screening in Cancer. Geneva, UICC Technical Report Series. 40:73, 1978.
475. Boucot KR, Weiss W: Is curable lung cancer detected by semiannual screening? JAMA 224:1361, 1973.
476. Carbone PP, Frost JK, Feinstein AR, Higgins GA, Selawry OS: Lung cancer: Perspectives and prospects. Ann Int Med 73:1003, 1970.
477. Paulson DL, Reisch JS: Long-term survival after resection for bronchogenic carcinoma. Ann Surg 184:324, 1976.
478. Melamed M, Flehinger B, Miller D, et al: Preliminary report of the lung cancer detection program in New York. Cancer 39:369, 1977.
479. Miller AB: Recent trends in lung cancer mortality in Canada. Can Med Assoc J 116:28, 1977.
480. Porter AMW, McCullough DM: Counselling against cigarette smoking: A controlled study from a general practice. Practitioner 209:688, 1972.
481. Nordin BEC: Clinical significance and pathogenesis of osteoporosis. Br Med J 1:571, 1971.
482. Guggenheim K, et al: An epidemiological study of osteoporosis in Israel. Arch Environ Health 22:259, 1971.
483. Bollet AJ, Engh G, Parson W: Epidemiology of osteoporosis. Arch Intern Med 116:191, 1965.
484. Newton-John HF, Morgan DB: Osteoporosis: Disease or senescence? Lancet 1:232, 1968.
485. Avioli LV: Postmenopausal osteoporosis prevention versus cure. Fed Proc 40:82, 1981.
486. Dent CE, Watson L: Osteoporosis. Postgrad Med J 42(Suppl):583, 1966.
487. Garn SM, Rohmann CF, Wagner B: Bone loss as a general phenomenon in man. Fed Proc 26:1729, 1967.
488. Heaney RP: A unified concept of osteoporosis. *In* Barzel US (ed.): Osteoporosis. New York, Grune and Stratton, 1970.
489. Shapiro JR, Moore WT, Jorgensen H, Reid J, Epps CH, Whedon D: Osteoporosis: Evaluation of diagnosis and therapy. Arch Intern Med 135:563, 1975.
490. Verbov J: Skin Diseases in the Elderly. London, William Heinemann Medical Books, 1974.
491. Gilchrest BA: Age-associated changes in the skin: Overview and clinical relevance. J Am Geriatr Soc 30:139, 1982.
492. Montagna W, Kligman AM, Wuepper KD, Bentley JP: Special issue on aging. J Invest Dermatol 73:1, 1979.
493. Emmett EA: Occupational skin cancer: A review. J Occup Med 17:44, 1975.
494. Mihm MC Jr, Fitzpatrick TB: Early detection of malignant melanoma. Cancer 37(Suppl):597, 1976.
495. Weary PE: A two-year experience with a series of rural skin and oral cancer detection clinics. JAMA 217:1862, 1971.
496. Zagula-Mally ZW, Rosenberg EW, Kashgarian M: Frequency of skin cancer and solar keratoses in a rural southern county as determined by population sampling. Cancer 34:345, 1974.

*Chapter 8*

# *Comprehensive Assessment of Frail Elderly in Relation to Needs for Long-Term Care*

*T. Franklin Williams*

## THE NEED FOR COMPREHENSIVE ASSESSMENT

As is well documented in other chapters in this text (see Chapters 4 and 14), many older people acquire chronic diseases that in turn result in varying degrees of disability. This is clearly not true for all elderly people; some in their 80s and 90s continue to be vigorous in all aspects of life. However, the number of elderly who have some degree of impairment in carrying out usual functions does increase with later years, with approximately 60 per cent of those aged 85 and older reporting some limitation in activity.[1] Such older people may be referred to as "frail elderly"; it is they who are likely to need some form of long-term assistance or care in order to continue to maintain as much independence in living as possible.

In order to determine and help make arrangements for the types of assistance needed by frail elderly people, the physician and other health professionals must conduct a comprehensive diagnostic evaluation or assessment that is fully analogous to the careful diagnosis that must precede any type of treatment decisions. The medical conditions that underlie and contribute to the functional losses must be identified and appropriately treated, but this is only a part of the necessary effort: The types and degrees of functional losses themselves must be carefully addressed, as well as the extent of family and other social supports available to help meet the needs.

Unfortunately, careful functional and social assessments as steps in decision-making for long-term care have often been neglected, with the result that inappropriate types of long-term care have often been provided.[2,3] Without such efforts, frail elderly people may end up in nursing homes when it might have been possible for them to live in less confining settings or at home with support services. Conversely, the patient with unassessed needs may not be provided with the type or intensity of long-term care that he or she requires, resulting in accelerated disability or accelerated burn-out on the part of family care-givers.

By contrast, careful use of comprehensive assessment and recommendations and assistance in arranging for long-term care has been shown to result in care that is more appropriate to the needs of the person and in less use of institutional care, e.g., nursing homes.[3,4] Functional assessment is also essential as a basis for choosing rehabilitative therapies (see Chapter 14) and for following the progress of patients with chronic disabilities.

In this chapter the following aspects of assessment are addressed:

1. Special features of assessment relevant to long-term decisions (i.e., the multiple domains that must be assessed, the need for multidisciplinary comprehensive efforts, and the need for consistency)

2. Settings in which assessments may be or need to be carried out

3. Translation of the identified needs into appropriate services and appropriate settings for care.

## SPECIAL FEATURES OF ASSESSMENT RELEVANT TO LONG-TERM CARE DECISIONS

The domains or areas that are most important and that must be considered when making decisions about long-term care include (1) needs for chronic medical treatment, (2) physical functioning, (3) mental functioning, (4) family and social supports available, and (5) environmental features. These areas of assessment are discussed in relation to the approaches that may be taken and methods that may be used in clinical practice; more detailed analyses, including critical comparisons of different methods and discussion of other uses of assessment, are available.[5-9]

### *Assessment of Needs for Chronic Medical Treatment*

A patient's need for certain modalities of chronic treatment may call for very specific equipment and trained services, which will, in turn, have a major impact on the care plan, on who will provide the care, and on where the care can be given. For example, a patient may need management of a tracheostomy or other type of ostomy, oxygen, intravenous fluids or medications, traction, frequent treatments by a respiratory therapist, physical therapist, occupational therapist, or speech therapist, or specialized nursing treatment, such as for the care of a major pressure ulcer. In some instances, it may be possible to train family care-givers to provide such treatment. In other instances, it will be important to recognize that family members are not capable of carrying out these modalities and that they must be provided through professional home support services or in an institution. In any event, it is necessary that these treatment needs be fully specified in the assessment process.

### *Assessment of Physical Functioning*

Limitations of a person's ability to carry out ordinary daily physical activities are the most common causes of the need for long-term care assistance. It may appear to be an unnecessary tautology to say that a person who cannot carry out one or another ordinary daily activity that is necessary for independent living must have some assistance or service; however, diagnostic assessment of such functional characteristics has been neglected so often that the need for it must be emphasized. The therapeutic goal is to provide assistance to compensate for the functional disability or disabilities that have been identified and, by this means, assure continued independent living to the maximum extent possible.

The assessment of physical (and mental) functioning is a part of the diagnostic work-up of a frail older patient and is distinct from and only secondarily related to the diagnosis of specific disease entities that may cause loss of function. That is, it is necessary to determine the functional characteristics of a patient and address these specifically in the therapeutic plan, no matter what their underlying causes are. Proper treatment of the latter may, of course, and hopefully will, contribute to improved function, but some degree of functional loss may continue to be present even with optimal treatment of diseases.

The development of consistent, useful approaches to assessment of physical functioning owes much to the original work of Katz and colleagues[10] in defining activities of daily living (ADL) and Lawton and colleagues[11,12] in defining so-called instrumental activities of daily living (IADL). Tables 8-1 and 8-2 list the key elements in these assessments.

It may be seen that carrying out ordinary activities of daily living can be analyzed in terms of personal self-care (e.g., feeding oneself, bathing, dressing, toileting), ability to move around in-

**Table 8-1.** ASSESSMENT OF ACTIVITIES OF DAILY LIVING

Assess whether the person can accomplish each activity independently, whether he or she needs partial supervision or assistance or whether he or she is fully dependent on others.

| | |
|---|---|
| Personal self-care | Feeding oneself |
| | Bathing |
| | Toileting |
| Mobility | Able to move from bed to a standing position or to a chair |
| | Able to walk (with or without assistive devices) or use a wheelchair |
| Continence | Continent of urine: always, or rarely incontinent, or frequently or usually continent |
| | Continent of feces |

**Table 8-2.** ASSESSMENT OF INSTRUMENTAL ACTIVITIES OF DAILY LIVING

Assess whether the person can accomplish each activity necessary to manage his or her living environment independently or whether he or she is dependent on others?

| | |
|---|---|
| Within the home | Cooking |
| | Housecleaning |
| | Laundry |
| | Management of medications |
| | Management of telephone |
| Outside the home | Shopping for food, clothing, drugs, etc. |
| | Use of transportation traveling to necessary and desired activities (e.g., physician's appointments, religious and social events) |

dependently (e.g., move from bed to a walking position or wheelchair, locomotion), and control of one's bladder and bowel function. A person who can carry out all these functions for himself or herself does not need the personal assistance of anyone else. Conversely, a lack of ability to perform any of these activities does mean that some external assistance must be provided. Some help with bathing and dressing, if this is all that is required, can usually be provided by a family member or staff of a minimum-care domiciliary facility once or twice a day. On the other hand, a person needing regular help with ambulation, incontinence, or feeding obviously requires almost constant attendance.

The IADL has to do with the ability of the person to manage his or her living environment, that is, to procure and prepare food, manage laundry and house cleaning, and travel to necessary or desirable activities outside the home. Any lack of the ability to carry out these functions for oneself means that some type of assistance or service is needed; services to compensate for IADL problems may be more varied and may not need to be as personal as those required to address ADL needs.

To document the ADL and IADL status of patients, numerous protocols and scales have been developed with the aim of consistency in information, which may be communicated between health care providers and may also be useful in documenting change over time. Such protocols are also useful as a consistent basis on which decisions may be made by those who provide and pay for services. Certain scales or protocols have been found to be useful in particular situations; for example, the Barthel Index[13-15] is extensively used in rehabilitative services for monitoring progress; Kane and Kane[7] have published a comprehensive summary and critical review of the forms of ADL and IADL data recording in current use and include examples of common forms.

In regular medical practice, it is highly desirable to select a format for recording the functional assessment information routinely and consistently as a part of the medical record. An example is the patient assessment form (PAF) of the ACCESS long-term care program in Monroe County, New York (see Fig. 8-1); it has been found to serve well in making assessment decisions for home care as well as for institutional care. The precise details of any functional limitation should be noted because such details serve as a basis for planning specific supportive services. A total score or scale, in an attempt to summarize an overall impression of degree of disability, serves no useful purpose in guiding specific therapeutic plans.

## *Assessment of Mental, Emotional, and Psychobehavioral Functioning*

Limitations in mental function can result in as severe losses of autonomy, as do problems in physical functioning, and can of course contribute to limitations in ADL and IADL. Losses of mental function often require different types of assistance from those needed to supplement physical needs.

Methods for assessing the mental, emotional, and psychobehavioral status of frail elderly people in ways that are useful for determining needs for long-term care services are not as adequately developed as is desirable. With regard to mental or cognitive functioning, several relatively short tests have been developed and widely used, each of which includes questions on orientation, short- and longer-term memory, arithmetic, and ability to reproduce a geometric design. Examples of the most commonly used tests are given in the work of Kane and Kane.[7] These tests identify the presence of a significant degree of decline in mental or cognitive functioning. However, they do not correlate well with what a patient can actually do or not do in his or her daily living activities. For example, a patient with considerable loss of memory (typically the first sign of dementia) may perform very poorly on such tests—e.g., the patient may be oriented only to people and have no ability to answer the other questions correctly—and yet may still function satisfactorily and independently in his or her familiar home environment. Conversely,

## NURSING ASSESSMENT

### I - ACTIVITIES OF DAILY LIVING

| SELECT CORRECT NUMBER OR NUMBER/LETTER COMBINATION | DATE | INITIAL | UPDATE | UPDATE | DISCH. | COMMENTS (SHORT TERM GOALS, REHAB POTENTIAL, PROBLEMS) ESP. AT TIME OF DISCHARGE |
|---|---|---|---|---|---|---|
| **AMBULATION** | 1. Independence w/wo assistive device<br>2. Walks with supervision<br>3. Walks with continuous physical support<br>4. Bed to chair (Total Help)<br>5. Bedfast | 61 | | | | |
| **TRANSFER** | 1. No assistance<br>2. Equipment only<br>3. Supervision only<br>4. Requires transfer w/wo equipment<br>5. Bedfast | 62 | | | | |
| **WHEEL CHAIR USE** | 1. Independent<br>2. Assistance in difficult maneuvering<br>3. Wheels a few feet<br>4. Unable<br>☐ NA | 63 | | | | |
| **BLADDER CONTROL** | 1. Continent<br>2. Rarely eg. h.s.<br>3. Occasional - once/week or less<br>4. Frequent - up to once a day<br>5. Total incontinence<br>6. Catheter - indwelling | 64 | | | | ☐ self-care |
| **BOWEL CONTROL** | 1. Continent<br>2. Rarely<br>3. Frequent - once a week or more<br>4. Total incontinence<br>5. Ostomy | 65 | | | | ☐ self-care |
| **BATHING** | 1. No assistance<br>2. Supervision only<br>3. Assistance in shower/tub<br>4. Is bathed in shower/tub<br>5. Is bathed - bed bath procedure | 66 | | | | |
| **DRESSING** | 1. Dresses self<br>2. Minor assistance<br>3. Partial help, completes ½ dressing<br>4. Has to be dressed | 68 | | | | |
| **TOILETING** | 1. No assistance<br>2. Assistance to/from & transfer<br>3. Help in clothes adjustment/personal hygiene<br>4. Toileting at bedside commode - nighttime | 69 | | | | |
| **FEEDING** | 1. No assistance<br>2. Minor assistance - needs tray set up only<br>3. Help in feeding/encouraging<br>4. Is fed | 71 | | | | |
| **ENDURANCE** | 1. Tolerates distances (250 Ft. +) / Sustained activity<br>2. Needs intermittent rest<br>3. Barely tolerates short activities<br>4. No tolerance | 72 | | | | |

### II - SENSORY IMPAIRMENTS - COMMUNICATION

| | | INITIAL | DISCH. | AID/PROSTHESIS |
|---|---|---|---|---|
| **SIGHT** | 1. Good<br>2. Vision adequate - Unable to read/see details<br>3. Vision limited - Gross object differentiation<br>4. Blind | 73 | | |
| **HEARING** | 1. Good<br>2. Hearing slightly impaired<br>3. Limited hearing (e.g. — must speak loudly)<br>4. Virtually/completely deaf | 74 | | |
| **SPEECH** | 1. Speaks clearly with others of same language<br>2. Some defect - usually gets message across<br>3. Unable to speak clearly or not at all | 75 | | |
| **COMMUNI-CATION** | 1. Transmits messages/receives information<br>2. Limited ability<br>3. Nearly or totally unable | 76 | | |

### III - SKIN CONDITION

COMMENT ON GENERAL SKIN CONDITION AND PROBLEMS - I.E. AREA, SIZE AND CONDITION OF DECUBITUS

INITIAL DATE:

DISCH. DATE:

### IV - TREATMENTS AND THERAPIES

CHECK TREATMENT OR THERAPY INDICATED AND TIMES NEEDED.
COMMENT ON (ESP. AT TIME OF DISCHARGE) FREQUENCY, DESCRIPTION OF THERAPY AND POTENTIAL FOR REHAB.

| DATE | INITIAL | DAYS | EVES NIGHTS | DISCHARGE UPDATE | DAYS | EVES NIGHTS | |
|---|---|---|---|---|---|---|---|
| INHALATN RX | 3 8 | | | | | | |
| OXYGEN | 9 | | | | | | |
| SUCTIONING | 10 | | | | | | |
| PARENTERAL FLUIDS | 11 | | | | | | |
| TUBE FEEDINGS | 12 | | | | | | |
| ASEPTIC DRESSING | 13 | | | | | | |
| LESION IRRIG. | 14 | | | | | | |
| DECUBITUS CARE | 15 | | | | | | |
| SP. SKIN CARE SP. FOOT CARE | 16 | | | | | | |

| DATE | INITIAL | DAYS | EVES NIGHTS | DISCHARGE UPDATE | DAYS | EVES NIGHTS | |
|---|---|---|---|---|---|---|---|
| SK. OBSERV. | | | | | | | |
| CATH. IRRIG. | 17 | | | | | | |
| OSTOMY CARE | 18 | | | | | | |
| BOWEL-BLAD. REHAB | 19 | | | | | | |
| PAREN. MEDS | 20 | | | | | | |
| P.T. | 21 | | | | | | |
| O.T. | 22 | | | | | | |
| S.T. | 23 | | | | | | |
| MEDS. REQ'G. ADJ. | | | | | | | |

**ACCESS ORIGINAL COPY**

**Figure 8-1.** Relevant portions of the pre-admission assessment form. (From the Monroe County Long-Term Care Program, Rochester, New York. Reproduced with permission.)

*Illustration continued on following page*

**PSYCHO-SOCIAL ASSESSMENT**

**I - PSYCHO-BEHAVIORAL CONDITIONS**

1. NO/MINIMAL PROBLEM - LITTLE OR NO EFFECT ON CARE PLAN
2. MODERATE FREQUENCY/INTENSITY - ENOUGH TO CONSTITUTE CONSIDERATION IN PLANNING CARE
3. FREQUENT (OVER ONCE/WK.) OR SPECIAL PROBLEM - REQUIRING CONSTANT OR ACTIVE CONSIDERATION

DIAGNOSED PSYCH DISORDER? ☐ YES ☐ NO 28

COMMENT:

| Condition | | Description | INITIAL | UPDATE | UPDATE | DISCH. | ✓ IF REHAB. POTENTIAL COMMENTS: |
|---|---|---|---|---|---|---|---|
| LEVEL OF CONSCIOUSNESS | 29 | Unaware, clouding of consciousness, unable to perceive/react to significant environmental stimulus. | | | | | ☐ |
| IMPAIRED JUDGMENT | 30 | Unsafe self direction - unable to accept or weigh advice, may be confused, bewildered or forgetful. | | | | | ☐ |
| HALLUCINATES | 32 | Subjectively perceives what does not exist. | | | | | ☐ |
| DEPRESSED | 33 | Persistent feeling of hopelessness, withdrawn, dejected, suicidal. | | | | | ☐ |
| AGITATION | 34 | Hyperactivity, anxiety; unstable - fluctuates emotionally. | | | | | ☐ |
| REGRESSION | 36 | Temporary stress reaction - eg. - refuses to participate in voluntary incontinency, Bizzare acts - hoards, undressing, etc. | | | | | ☐ |
| WANDERS | 37 | No concern for territorial constraints or outside conditions | | | | | ☐ |
| ABUSIVE | 38 | Threatens, berates, uses foul language | | | | | ☐ |
| ASSAULTIVE | 39 | Strikes, uses force or violence | | | | | ☐ |
| RESTRAINTS | 40 | Physically attached or put about patient | | | | | ☐ |

**II - PSYCHO-SOCIAL FUNCTIONS AND ADAPTATION**

**EMOTIONAL STRENGTH AND MOTIVATION**

1. INDEPENDENT, CONFIDENT, HIGHLY MOTIVATED
2. GOOD EMOTIONAL STRENGTHS, MOTIVATED WITH SUPPORT
3. POORLY, UNREALISTICALLY MOTIVATED, REQUIRES REG. GUIDANCE
4. PASSIVE, AFRAID OR INSECURE, NEEDS MUCH SUPPORT
5. ACTIVELY RESISTIVE, NEGATIVE OR HOSTILE
6. UNRESPONSIVE, CANNOT RATE

INITIAL ☐ 41 UPDATE ☐ COMMENTS:

**RESPONSE TO ILLNESS**

1. ACCEPTS CHANGE - ACTIVELY ADAPTING
2. ACCEPTS BUT NEEDS HELP ADAPTING
3. NEUTRAL OR PASSIVE
4. WITHDRAWING
5. DENIAL, ANGER OR OTHER OVERT REACTION
6. UNRESPONSIVE, CANNOT RATE

INITIAL ☐ 42 UPDATE ☐ COMMENTS:

COMMENT ON RECENT TRAUMAS AND ON SPECIAL INTERESTS/ COPING MECHANISMS: ____

**III - DOMESTIC EVALUATION OF PATIENT AND SUPPORTS**

CODE:
1. COMPLETELY ABLE TO PERFORM
2. LIMITED, MODIFIED ABILITY
3. COMPLETELY UNABLE OR UNWILLING

| | | CAN HELP WITH: BATHING | TOILETING | TRANSFER | HOUSE WORK | LAUNDRY | SHOPPING | TRAVEL | FINANCE | MEDS | MEALS | PHONE USE | ON SITE ATTEN. | PLEASE COMMENT ON AVAILABILITY (HRS.), RELIABILITY, LIMITATIONS OF SUPPORT PERSONS | |
|---|---|---|---|---|---|---|---|---|---|---|---|---|---|---|---|
| PATIENT | | 43 | 44 | 45 | 46 | 47 | 48 | 49 | 50 | 51 | 52 | 53 | 54 | | |
| SUPPORT PERSON | 55 | 56 | 57 | 58 | 59 | 60 | 61 | 62 | 63 | 64 | 65 | 66 | 67 | 68 | 69, 70, 71, 72 |
| SUPPORT PERSON 4 | 8 | 9 | 10 | 11 | 12 | 13 | 14 | 15 | 16 | 17 | 18 | 19 | 20 | 21 | 22, 23, 24, 25 |

SUGGESTED LIMITATIONS OF SUPPORT PERSON
1. WORK — JOB RESPONSIBILITIES
2. FAMILY RESPONSIBILITIES
3. OTHER SICKNESS
4. PT. NEEDS ARE HEAVY PHYSICAL BURDEN
5. POOR ACCOMMODATIONS
6. POOR FINANCES
7. SUPPORTS ARE EMOTIONALLY —MENTALLY INCAPABLE
8. PT. WANTS INDEPENDENCE/NOT TO BE BURDEN
9. DISRUPTIVE TO FAMILY LIFESTYLE
10. PT. USED TO INSTITUTION

RELIABILITY OF SUPPORT PERSON: VR R S/WR UR

**Figure 8-1.** *Continued*

a person may score well on a number of items, such as the arithmetic and geometric questions and some features of memory, and yet be quite confused when carrying out ordinary daily activities and need almost constant supervision. Furthermore, we do not yet know enough to relate specific segments of such cognitive testing to specific anatomic or physiologic abnormalities in the central nervous system.

Despite such limitations, it is probably still helpful to choose and employ one of the commonly used tests as a regular part of the work-up of an elderly frail patient to identify any gross evidence of dementia and to provide a baseline for future comparisons for evidence of change. A test may be chosen from those reviewed in Kane and Kane[7] and those discussed in Chapter 18. The identification of any evidence of dementia by such tests should call for a thorough work-up to determine the extent and nature of the dementia and to identify potentially modifiable functional disorders, whatever their causes (see Chapter 18). More research and development is needed to provide more refined and useful techniques for measuring and following mental status.

Other mental disorders in the elderly that may have major effects on functioning include depression, delirium, and paranoid psychotic states. Depression occurs so commonly and is so often not recognized or is passed off as dementia that special attention needs to be paid to detecting its presence. In the regular work-up of the patient, the observations of the physician, nurse, or social worker should provide clues to this problem. In addition, one of the standardized short depression tests may be used as a screening test to identify the need for more intensive work-up and possible treatment.[7,16] However, as with the mental status tests, the results of these depression tests cannot be used as a quantitative reflection of the degree of loss of daily functioning due to depression.

When any features that suggest delirium are present, including hallucinations and paranoid tendencies, one should always look for possible causes, such as use of drugs or alcohol or metabolic disorders.

Psychobehavioral problems impose severe burdens on those who are providing care to ill elderly people, whether at home or in institutions, and the presence or absence of any of these types of problems (see Fig. 8 – 1) should be ascertained from the care-givers. The following are psychobehavioral problems that may be present: (1) wandering, (2) agitation, (3) abusive or assaultive behavior, (4) fluctuating emotional state, (5) bizarre actions (e.g., hoarding, undressing), (6) hallucinations, (7) impaired judgment, and (8) depression and suicidal tendencies. A person who wanders unpredictably or who has unpredictable explosive episodes of antagonism or assault toward others tests the physical and emotional reserves of families and of staff members at long-term care institutions. Approaches to management are addressed in Chapter 18; here it is important to note that the assessment of such features should be a part of the regular functional assessment of frail elderly persons.

## *Assessment of Social Supports and Environmental Characteristics*

The characteristics of the environment in which the frail elderly person is currently living, including both the social and physical environments, often have contributed, positively or negatively, to the clinical conditions for which the patient is being seen and are always important in making plans for long-term care. The degree of support that the patient is receiving and can expect to receive from family and friends is often the deciding factor in determining whether institutional care is necessary. The capabilities and desires of family members must be assessed, as well as the extent of burn-out from current care burdens. Information is also needed on the present and potential availability of services from supportive agencies. The social worker member of the assessment team should be involved with family, agencies, and patient and should play a role from the earliest stages of the assessment consultation in obtaining essential information.[17]

Standardized questionnaires and scales for documenting the social information have been developed (see Kane and Kane[7] for a review). In general, these instruments are geared for research rather than for use in regular practice. Information on the extent of social support is included in the assessment form illustrated in Figure 8 – 1. (See also the comments that follow on comprehensive multidisciplinary assessment instruments.)

The physical environment of the patient's home and surroundings should be assessed by a visiting or community health nurse or by a member of the assessment team. This is an essential step in determining both the likelihood that the patient, with his or her functional limitations, can continue to function safely and effectively in that setting and the actions that might be taken to modify the home to make it more satisfactory, such as the installation of handrails, raised toilet seats, or widened doors for wheelchair use. In order to make precise recommendations, it is often necessary for an occupational therapist or a specially trained community health or visiting nurse to visit the home.

## *Comprehensive Assessment Instruments*

Because most of the elements of assessment described in the preceding section are essential parts of the diagnostic work-up and the decision-making processes for determining what types of long-term supportive services are needed, a number of comprehensive, multidisciplinary assessment guides or protocols have been developed. These have been used primarily by community-based agencies in their roles as decision-makers, that is, in determining the types of services needed. However, the information that is collected in this way can be very helpful to the physician and other members of the assessment team in their diagnostic work-up of a patient and in following the course of the patient.

In particular, in communities where community-wide long-term care service systems are evolving, such comprehensive assessment forms are becoming a regular part of the diagnostic work-up and decision-making processes for frail elderly patients. Examples of forms that are in general use are the PAF form of the ACCESS program of Monroe County Long-Term Care, Rochester, New York, the assessment instrument of TRIAGE (now Connecticut Community Care, Hartford, Connecticut), and the Philadelphia Geriatric Center multilevel assessment instrument of Lawton and associates.[8] Portions of the PAF form are illustrated in Figure 8-1. Other comprehensive assessment instruments, which have been designed primarily for research purposes, such as the OARS instrument of Duke University[18] and the comprehensive assessment and referral evaluation (CARE) instrument,[19] can also be used, with some modifications.

Although the information that may be made available to the assessment team from such instruments can be quite helpful, it does not take the place of careful review and, when indicated, further exploration of each of the areas of assessment described previously.

## SETTINGS OR CIRCUMSTANCES IN WHICH ASSESSMENTS MAY BE NEEDED

Assessments of frail elderly people may be needed for any one of a variety of purposes: (1) for screening for early detection of potential disabilities, (2) for case-finding in order to offer relevant care to those identified as needing it, (3) for comprehensive diagnostic work-up, as a necessary part of developing a plan of therapy, (4) for monitoring progress, (5) for determining the level or setting of long-term care required by a patient, and (6) for determining the appropriateness of utilization of long-term care services and facilities.

The approach to assessment and methods to be used must be modified according to which one of the preceding purposes is to be served. Unfortunately, there has been a tendency to attempt to apply a method or protocol that was developed for one purpose to another use or in different circumstances, with unsatisfactory results. This chapter deals primarily with comprehensive assessment as a necessary part of the diagnostic work-up of individual frail elderly people; reference to the other purposes served by assessments is made simply to serve as a reminder that caution must be exercised in considering the use of guides or protocols that have been developed for other purposes.

The most important use of assessment as a part of the diagnostic work-up of a frail elderly person is in the evaluation of a patient whose physical, mental, or social condition is changing, most likely resulting in an increasing need for long-term services. Such a person may present to a physician in his or her office; may be referred to a health or social agency, which in turn seeks comprehensive diagnostic assessment; or may be referred to a geriatric evaluation clinic or inpatient unit. Such clinics and units are well-established parts of the geriatric care system in the United Kingdom and other Western countries. Our own experience in Rochester, New York, has illustrated the value of such settings for comprehensive multidisciplinary assessment of the needs of more complexly ill or frail older persons. These people are reaching, or have reached, a critical point because of changing functional status or changes in the family supports available and are often facing a decision about continuing at home with increased support services or entering a long-term care institution.

Essential components of such specialized geriatric units and clinics are regular participation in the diagnostic evaluation by physicians, nurses, and social workers with special competence in this arena; accessibility of consultants in other specialties, such as psychiatry, neurology, and rehabilitation medicine, and occasionally other fields, such as arthritis, endocrinology, physical therapy, occupational therapy, and speech therapy; ready availability and appropriate use of diagnostic radiologic and laboratory procedures; development of consistent data bases; and establishment of regular team conferences for review of all information and a system for transmittal of findings and recommendations to other professionals for follow-up.

## TRANSLATING IDENTIFIED NEEDS INTO APPROPRIATE SERVICES AND SETTINGS FOR LONG-TERM CARE

Once the information described previously has been gathered, the physician and other health professionals must work with the patient, family members, and any relevant agency personnel to develop a plan of care appropriate to the identified needs of the patient. This plan should include specification of the types of services required and the options for settings in which these services may be appropriately provided.

Development of such a plan of care usually requires the expert knowledge and participation of others in addition to the physician — that is, a community health or visiting nurse, a social worker, and often others, such as an occupational or physical therapist. In other words, a true team effort, involving patient and family as well as professionals, is usually necessary in establishing a sound care plan (see Chapter 3). Although members of such a "team" may be dispersed in various community agencies, the goals may be accomplished through consultative relationships.

It should be kept in mind that the entire process of assessment and decision-making about long-term care is, in itself, a stressful experience for the frail older person. There should always be a trusted personal advocate, who is a source of personal support, accompanying and helping to sustain the older person through this process. This person can be a family member, close friend, or representative of a social agency.[17]

It is possible and useful to organize one's thinking about this translation of identified needs into service plans around some form of decision sequence. Approaches of this type have been published.[20,21]

The following series of questions may serve the same purpose. These questions, which are based on assessment data, are to be considered in arriving at long-term care plans:

1. *Does this person need further specialized diagnostic work-up and/or intensive rehabilitation treatment before a long-term care plan can be developed?*

   **If so,** such steps should be taken first on an outpatient or inpatient basis.

2. *Is this person physically and mentally capable of managing independently all activities of daily living (ADL) and instrumental activities of daily living (IADL)?*

   **If so,** no special long-term care plans or living arrangements are needed. However, this person should undergo appropriate periodic checkups for chronic conditions, and arrangements should be made to ensure that this person is in regular contact with a supportive network.

   **If not:**

3. *Can this person manage all personal and instrumental activities of daily living within his or her home? That is, does he or she simply need assistance in traveling to and from necessary or desirable activities outside the home, such as shopping, visits to physicians, or social and religious activities?*

   **If so,** help in transportation or provision of shopping services should suffice; however, such a person is at high risk for social isolation, and there should be positive attention to maintaining or adding social activities, including day programs.

4. *Does this person have regular and adequate meals prepared and other household chores performed (e.g., cleaning, laundry) by himself or herself, his or her spouse, or other housemate?*

   **If not,** these housekeeping functions must be provided through help from nearby family members, use of Meals-on-Wheels or housekeeper services, or similar help from staff members of a domiciliary facility in which the person may live.

5. *Does the person maintain adequate personal hygiene (e.g., bathe himself or herself) and dress and undress adequately?*

   **If not,** some help or supervision is needed, probably twice daily, from a family member or home health aide, or a similar staff member of a congregate living institution, such as an immediate-care facility.

6. *Can the person ambulate independently with or without mechanical assistive devices, such as canes or walkers, and manage any necessary stairs in his or her dwelling?*

   **If not,** can the person transfer to and operate a wheelchair without assistance? Any limitation in locomotion or transfer may require a different living environment (e.g., a one-floor dwelling or a congregate living facility) or personal assistance several times daily by a family member or health aide for toileting, coming to meals, and so forth.

7. *Is the person sufficiently oriented and mentally and emotionally competent to manage being alone all day or for hours at a time?*

   **If not,** constant or almost constant supervision by a family member, companion, or health aide is necessary in the home, or residence in a facility that has a restricted environment area or constantly supervising staff may be needed.

8. *Is the person usually continent of urine and feces?*

   **If not,** thorough evaluation and efforts to treat any identifiable causes are indicated and, if not successful, frequent daily personal care by family members or personal care aides in the home or in an institution is necessary.

9. *Can the person feed himself or herself?*

   **If not,** assistance in eating at every mealtime by family or personal care aides at home or in an institution is necessary.

10. *Does the person have some disability that*

*requires regular nursing or rehabilitative therapy, such as care for pressure ulcers, ostomy care, respiratory treatments, or physical or occupational therapy?*

**If so,** this care must be provided through visiting home health care services or in an institution staffed to provide these services.

## THE NEED FOR CONTINUING REVIEW OF ASSESSMENT FINDINGS

This chapter has focused on the importance of and approach to functional assessment as an essential part of initial decision-making about long-term care. The findings must be incorporated into the ongoing care activities of the primary physician, the other professionals involved in the care of the patient, and family members and must be reviewed regularly inasmuch as further changes in functional status of the patient are likely.

### References

1. Rice DP, Feldman JJ: Demographic changes and health needs of the elderly. Presented at the annual meeting of the Institute of Medicine, National Academy of Sciences, Washington, DC, Oct. 20, 1982.
2. Wenkert W, Hill J, Berg RL: Health care of the aged. Report of Ford Foundation Study. Rochester, NY, University of Rochester, Department of Preventive and Rehabilitation Medicine, 1968.
3. Williams TF, Hill JC, Fairbank ME, Knox KG: Appropriate placement of the chronically ill and aged: A successful approach by evaluation. JAMA 226:1332, 1973.
4. Eggert GM, Bowlyow JE, Nichols CW: Gaining control of the long-term care system: First returns from the ACCESS experiment. Gerontologist 20:356, 1980.
5. Lawton MP, Klaven MH: Assessment: The concept and prospects. Rockville, MD, National Institute of Mental Health, 1979.
6. Hedrick SC, Katz S, Stroud MW III: Patient assessment in long-term care: Is there a common language? Aged Care and Services Review 2:1, 1980–1981.
7. Kane RA, Kane RL: Assessing the Elderly: A Practical Guide to Management. Lexington, MA, Lexington Books (D.C. Heath), 1981.
8. Lawton MP, Moss M, Fulcomer M, Kleban MH: A research and service oriented multi-level assessment instrument. J Gerontol 37:91, 1982.
9. Williams TF: Assessment of the elderly in relation to needs for long-term care: An emerging technology. Paper presented at Conference on Long-Term Care sponsored by Office of Technology Assessment, Millwood, VA, Jan. 25, 1983.
10. Katz S, Ford AB, Moskowitz RW, et al: Studies of illness in the aged. The index of ADL: A standardized measure of biological and psychosocial function. JAMA 185:94, 1963.
11. Lawton MP, Brody E: Assessment of older people: Self-maintaining and instrumental activities of daily living. Gerontologist 9:179, 1969.
12. Lawton MP: Assessing the competence of older people. *In* Kent D, Kastenbaum R, Sherwood J (eds.): Research, Planning and Action for the Elderly. New York, Behavioral Publications, 1972.
13. Mahoney FI, Barthel DW: Functional evaluation: The Barthel index. MD State Med J 14:61, 1965.
14. Granger CV, Dewis LS, Peters NC, et al: Stroke rehabilitation: Analysis of repeated Barthel index measures. Arch Phys Med Rehabil 60:14, 1979.
15. Gresham GE, Phillips TF, Labi MLC: ADL status in stroke: Relative merits of three standard indexes. Arch Phys Med Rehabil 61:355, 1980.
16. Brink TL, Yesavage JA, Lum O, et al: Screening test for geriatric depression. Clin Gerontol 1:37, 1982.
17. Silverstone B, Burack-Weiss A: The social work function in nursing homes and home care. J Gerontological Social Work 5:7, 1982.
18. Duke University Center for the Study of Aging and Human Development: Multi-Dimensional Functional Assessment: The OARS Methodology. Durham, NC, Duke University, 1978.
19. Gurland G, Kuriansky J, Sharpe L, et al: The comprehensive assessment and referral evaluation (CARE)—rationale, development and reliability. Part II. A factor analysis. Int J Aging Hum Dev 8:9, 1977.
20. Williams ME, Williams TF: Assessment of the elderly for long term care. J Am Geriatr Soc 30:71, 1982.
21. Williams TF: Assessment of the geriatric patient in relation to needs for services and facilities. *In* Reichel W (ed.): Clinical Aspects of Aging. 2nd edition. Baltimore, MD, Williams & Wilkins, Co., 1983.

Chapter 9

# Ethical Dilemmas in the Clinical Care of the Elderly

Christine K. Cassel

*"Medicine is at heart a moral enterprise. All its efforts converge ultimately on decisions and actions which are presumed to be good for some person in need of help and healing."*

PELLEGRINO

The discipline of biomedical ethics came into its own in the 1970s. No longer considered by either philosophers or clinicians to be an irrelevant or irreverent meddling of outsiders or an immiscible mixture of "philosophy" and "practicality," [1,2] it has emerged rather as a new discipline forged from the perspective and expertise of philosophers, theologians, health care professionals, legal scholars, and social scientists.[3] These diverse specialists offer both data and methodologies that contribute to the formulation of ethical questions and resolution of ethical dilemmas in modern medicine. Like geriatrics, bioethics has to be interdisciplinary if it is to be effective. The need for a systematic analytic methodology in medical decision-making became increasingly clear as diagnostic and therapeutic technologies became more complex, more potent, and more potentially risky.

In both practice and policy arenas, geriatric medicine is dense with ethical issues.[4] This will be obvious to people who work with the elderly in the helping professions, especially those in a primary care relationship.[5] Elderly persons are at greater risk for life threatening and severely disabling conditions, raising questions concerning how extensively or aggressively to treat.[6,7] In the last year of life, more expensive medical resources are consumed than any other, except for certain episodes in the first year of life in the care of high-risk premature infants.[8] Patients themselves often find life-prolonging technologies objectionable, and yet physicians' fears of litigation for acts resembling "euthanasia" are not totally unfounded. The per capita health care expenditures for the population over the age of 65 is three times greater than that for people in younger age brackets. Should we therefore be responding to cost containment constraints by limiting the resources available to this high-utilization group?[9] The issue of informed consent, whether it be for conventional or experimental procedures, is sometimes complicated by disorders of cognition or communication, such as Alzheimer's disease or aphasia.[10]

Ethical dilemmas are not rare or esoteric events. One cannot take every ethical problem to court (even it if were desirable to do so), to a hospital ethician, or to an ethics committee (even if every health care institution were so fortunate to have such a resource). Day-to-day decisions must be made as they arise. Therefore, in addition to technical competence in medicine, one must also attain a certain level of ethical competence.

What does this mean? Being a moral or religious person is not enough. Moral values and standards are often thought to be simple immutable personal beliefs, learned at the mother's knee or its equivalent. Indeed, we all do have moral beliefs that are personal and individual. It is one of the basic principles of our culture that people should respect each other's right to hold different beliefs, as long as those beliefs do not infringe on the rights of others. Although we live in a culture of religious pluralism, most of our basic values have grown out of a shared cultural heritage. The goal of moral behavior is to protect important values, such as the quality of life for individuals or for the community as a whole, or a liberty or freedom. We try to act in accordance with these values in our daily personal and professional lives. However, there are occasions when the moral course of action is not obvious, and reflection upon a situation may raise more questions than it solves. In such cases a process begins of weighing the alternatives, trying to arrive at the "most correct" of several less than optimal solutions, trying to ascertain if a feeling of discomfort signals that a clinical decision may not have been the most ethical one, trying to resolve a strong disagreement among several health professionals regarding decisions about a certain patient.

Ethics, like medicine, is both an art and a science. It is that part of philosophy that deals with systematic approaches to these kinds of problems.[11] The approach of an ethicist includes knowledge of the philosophic principles involved[12] and their origins in cultural traditions,[13] the analysis of risk,[14] and the decision process.[15] Much of this knowledge is within the reach of all health professionals and should be a part of their basic competence.[16,17] There are ethical dilemmas that are so difficult or complex that one must turn to an expert—either an ethicist or ethics committee or to the courts. The level of basic competence includes knowing when to ask for consultation.

## ANALYSIS OF AN ETHICAL DILEMMA

The basic elements of analysis of an ethical dilemma can be outlined as follows:

**Factual Data and Conceptual Clarity.** Who is involved? What information is available and relevant? What missing information would make a significant difference if it were known? Is it possible to know it?

**Examination of Motives.** Are the motives clear? What conscious or unconscious motives may be at work in the patient, the family, and the involved health professionals?

**Application of Rules or Principles.** How are they selected? Can they be placed in order of priority? What are the associated assumptions? Are they controversial or broadly applicable?

**Examination of All Possible Consequences.** How will it affect the patient, the family, the decision-makers? Any others? Are there generalizable consequences to society?

**Making the Decision.** Not to act is also to take a stance. Once one decides what to do, one must also consider how to do it.

In the following case study, this framework will be applied in order to demonstrate its use and also to elucidate some basic principles, which will be summarized in the conclusion.

**Case Study.** Mr. James is an 86 year old man who was quite an accomplished pianist and had stayed active during his retirement. Among other things, he belonged to a senior center and would often volunteer his time at nursing homes, playing music for the elderly people who were less fortunate than himself. One summer he suffered a sizeable anterior myocardial infarction and, at the hospital, had a cardiac arrest with a successful resuscitation. He then spent several weeks recovering and was just about to go home when he had a left brain cerebrovascular accident, which left him aphasic and hemiplegic. As his insurance benefits dwindled and it was obvious his hospitalization would be prolonged, he was transferred to the Veterans Hospital for stroke rehabilitation. In spite of the vigorous and skillful efforts of the rehabilitation service, he did not do well. He had several bouts of pneumonia, probably related to aspiration, since his swallowing was also impaired. He stopped eating and refused to get out of bed or cooperate with therapy. It seemed likely that he was depressed. He was started on antidepressants and transferred to the geriatrics service, since in his present condition he was not benefiting from rehabilitation efforts. They decided to feed him using a nasogastric tube while he was being evaluated by the interdisciplinary team and while the team waited for his son and daughter to arrive from Colorado. He seemed to understand what the tube was for but would not cooperate in placing it. Once it was down, he would pull it out, which meant that the nurses had to use soft restraints to tie his one good hand to the bed rail.

In this case, the obvious question is whether to continue aggressive efforts at nutrition. Should the patient's apparent wish to die be respected? If he develops another pneumonia, should it be treated with intravenous antibiotics? If he becomes sick enough to require intensive care, is such an investment of resources warranted? If he suffers another cardiac arrest, should he be resuscitated?

All the members of the team were extremely uncomfortable in this situation. Discomfort is a fairly reliable sign of a significant ethical uncertainty. Some team members argued in favor of ceasing the struggle and letting the patient die peacefully. Others believed a more aggressive rehabilitation effort was warranted but were uncertain about how long it should be maintained.

## THE APPROACH TO PROBLEM SOLVING

### *Collect Data*

Often what is perceived as an ethical dilemma turns out to be a problem of insufficient information. Is Mr. James clinically depressed? Is that depression treatable? How much does he understand of what is said to him? How reliable are his answers? Speech pathologists and neuropsychologists were able to tell that he could understand most significant content of spoken communication, although his dense expressive aphasia persisted. When asked if he wanted to die, he would nod yes. When asked if he wanted to get better, he would nod yes. When told "we must insert this tube," he would shake his head angrily.

Stroke rehabilitation in the elderly is a long and slow process; full potential is often not achieved until as long as a year or more after the acute event. The patient might still recover significantly. With Mr. James it seemed that the ethical dilemma was centered on the role of depression.[18]

When the patient's son and daughter arrived, they said that he had often stated that he did not want to be kept alive by extraordinary means when "his time had come." They were sure he would not want to live as a cripple in a nursing home, but they would be willing to care for him if he was able to improve enough to go home.

The patient's spirits improved considerably in the presence of his children. The wards of any hospital can be extremely depressing even for one not critically ill. Mr. James had been in a room with patients who were either severely demented or moribund. Moving him from that room, encouraging visits from his children, and establishing continuity of the primary professionals caring for him made it possible for him to overcome his depression enough to learn swallowing, resume therapy, and begin to interact meaningfully with people.

The following information was needed to solve the ethical dilemma: (1) What was his rehabilitation potential? (2) Was he suffering from a treatable depression? (3) What were his own expressed wishes in regard to the different possible outcomes? Discovering the answers to the first two questions took the expertise of certain professionals and enough time for intensive trials of therapy. Since he was aphasic, his children were important sources of information concerning the third question. Their appropriate role in this context was to help to inform the physicians as to the patient's expressed wishes or his attitudes and values relevant to decisions about life-prolonging therapy in the face of severe disability.[19]

Having reviewed the factual data needed for these decisions and how that data might be obtained, the third question could be restated as follows: "Is it ethical to feed this patient against his will in order to find out if added strength will change his mind and give him the will to live?"

## *Examine Motives*

In making an ethical decision, those persons whose motives are relevant are the patient, the family, and the involved health care professionals.

**The Patient.** Obviously the consideration of depression is a major one, as well it should be in this case. We often consider depression because people facing severe disability at any age, and especially toward the end of life, are more likely to respond in a positive way to antidepressive therapy. We must always be cautious, however, not to dehumanize the very real suffering of people in this condition by making their despair clinical and impersonal with the diagnosis of depression.[20] Confronting the end of one's life is sometimes, although not always, a deeply saddening experience. Thus, a trial of antidepressant therapy is appropriate, but the symptoms of depression should still be treated as a human expression of a human experience. If the patient does not respond to antidepressants, the despair must be treated as real and the patient's decisions that are made in the context respected.

**The Family.** In this case, the family seemed very loving and supportive. If the family members urge that everything be done to keep the elderly person alive, it is important to find out from them if that is their perception or their actual report of the patient's wishes as expressed to them before he became ill or whether it is their own desires they are reporting. Unless the children have been made legal guardians of the patient, their desires as regards medical decisions are not legally binding.[21] This distinction is frequently misunderstood by medical professionals. The appropriate role of the spouse and the children is to help the health professional to understand what the wishes of the patient are or would have been. It is a situation that must be handled with some delicacy because it is neither respectful nor compassionate to pressure family members to make a life or death decision about their loved ones. Sometimes they will request that everything possible be done to keep the old person alive out of a sense of guilt for their neglect. Often their motivations are based on family dynamics of much longer duration. Although they are an important part of the decision-making process, they should not be made to feel that their decision alone determines the outcome. To do so would place on them an unrealistic and heavy burden of responsibility. Obviously, one must also be alert to more overt and destructive motives in family members, such as desire to acquire the elderly person's property in the event of his or her death. The contribution of social work professionals can be invaluable in sorting out this important information.

**The Involved Health Professionals.** Here we find relevant motives at many different levels. One must examine in oneself feelings about death, about the dying process, and about aging and disability.[22] One should not exercise one's own raging against mortality at the cost of the gentle death of a patient. On the other hand, one should not abandon the caring role because one cannot face for oneself the specter of continued life with severe disability.[23] These are important and ongoing challenges to every person who works in the health professions and in clinical geriatrics. Baser motivations must also be mentioned in this context. Such things as socioeconomic prejudices,[24] financial gain, fatigue, having a weekend off, or getting rid of a troubling patient are obviously not appropriate or relevant to a sound clinical and ethical decision.[25]

## *Application of Rules or Principles*

The principles of ethical action are shaped by one's cultural context within the tradition of Western culture. Traditions of Judaism and Christianity and secular, political, and social philosophies all contribute somewhat different perspectives. However, there is a remarkably broad commonality among them. Scholars looking at ethical problems in medicine over the last two decades have established a framework, which includes these fundamental principles.

**Respect for People.** Respect for people is a principle on which our legal system of rights and constitutional entitlements is based. It operates toward ensuring harmonious interactions in the human community. In medical care, it has major implications for disclosure of information, informed consent, and self-determination.[26] One should, in most cases, be frank with patients about their diagnosis and about what is known and not known about that diagnosis and enlist them as partners when decision-making of any ambiguous nature needs to be done.[27] The exceptions to this are the few cases when it seems truly medically or psychiatrically dangerous to give the information to the patient or, as sometimes happens, when the patient requests not to be told and asks that the doctor make all decisions for him. It becomes difficult in cases of cognitive disorder or, as in the case of Mr. James, in aphasia, in which it is difficult to know how much the patient is understanding. Still, the effort must be made, and it is often surprising how much is understood in either case. With people who have memory deficits, one must be prepared to patiently repeat the information sometimes many times over. Informed consent is often an ongoing process of communication rather than a single encounter focused on the signing of a piece of paper.[28]

Another aspect of this principle is self-determination, which is basically that the patient be allowed to decide for himself or herself what is the most favorable course, according to his or her own value system. It is a common pitfall for health professionals to judge a patient's decisions by their own value system rather than by that of the patient.[29] Classically, we explain that a patient is making a wrong decision because he or she does not understand enough or does not have the medical knowledge that we have. It is incumbent upon us, as much as is possible, to give that patient that knowledge but then to accept his or her decision. It is often difficult in cases of implied, possible, or mild cognitive impairment to sort out whether the patient is, in fact, mentally incompetent or is simply making a decision that is not consistent with the value system of the health professionals. Some investigators have noted that with psychiatric patients the question of mental competence almost never arises except in cases when the patient's decision conflicts with that of the physician.[30] Decision theory analysts have demonstrated that patients may have value systems that are very different from those held by physicians.[31,32] A 72-year-old woman who refused amputation for a gangrenous leg was thought to be incompetent by the surgeons who believed that she would surely die without the operation and therefore should "rationally" agree to accept the risk of surgery. A court found that she was competent and that her decision was consistent with her value system as reflected by her entire life.[33] She would rather have died than have had the amputation and the likely subsequent dependency. In many states, such a decision cannot even be brought to a court for a test of competency except under laws that apply only to the elderly. That is, if this woman had been 42- or even 59-years-old, barring obviously distorted perceptions of reality and a history of mental illness, there would have been no basis on which to question her refusal, and in fact, any decision to proceed would have been legally constituted battery. One must listen to what it is the patient is saying and distinguish what the words mean to him or her from what they mean to you.

A third aspect of respect for people is constituted by respectful action. If a patient is not aware enough to engage in meaningful dialogue about the nature and prognosis of his or her disease, one must take care to treat that patient respectfully. This includes a whole range of concerns having to do with how the patient is addressed, handled, clothed, and treated during the course of hospitalization. Our actions toward those who are most vulnerable not only reflect our attitudes toward ourselves as members of the human community but also may strengthen or instill those attitudes in others.

One also shows respect for people in one's ambulatory practice by doing what is possible to ensure that patients do not have a long wait in an uncomfortable situation, that they have ample time with the health care provider, that there is acoustic as well as visual privacy for the interaction, and finally that, whenever possible, the patient and the physician can openly discuss the patient's concerns and wishes about his or her death and aggressiveness of therapy in the event of severe incapacity.

**Beneficence.** Beneficence simply means doing good. It has a corollary that is an often quoted Hippocratic statement: "Do no harm." Often the two aspects of this principle come into conflict with each other. The most obvious example of this is when a very risky or painful therapy has a chance of benefiting a patient: One wants to do good but wonders if the decision to follow the more conservative route of doing no harm is not, in fact, the most ethical.[34] In this particular conflict it is, whenever possible, the patient's own decision to make.[35] In the case of an incommunicative, comatose, or severely demented person, one is helped enormously by prior knowledge of the patient, his or her life's values and plans, and contributing information from family and friends.

It is important in understanding the principle of beneficence to distinguish doing what is best for the patient from paternalistic action. Paternalism is a stance in which one makes decisions on behalf of another, as a parent would for a child, when that person can either not decide for himself or herself or when it is believed that he or she is making the wrong decision.[36] The history of medicine is largely one of paternalistic attitudes toward patients. It is only recently that health professionals have begun a serious attempt to share medical information with their patients. The image of the caring family physician who takes all the troubles of the patient on his or her shoulders and makes all the hard decisions and simply tells the patient not to worry or that "I did everything I could" is fading from view. However, we should not reject all the qualities of that era, for there is a great deal of caring concern that emerges from such an image. In the new model of collaborative decision-making, it is possible to lose the caring and beneficent aspect of health care practice in a colder and more impersonal negotiated contract. This risk is increased by physicians' fear of litigation.

In the name of beneficence, we sometimes make decisions about letting a patient die to put an end to needless suffering that cannot be relieved. Merciful and compassionate treatment of the dying is a very important part of any medical practice.[32] The skills and knowledge in this area include courage and sensitivity needed to make the ethical decisions involved and these ought to be a part of the training of every health care professional.

In ethical dilemmas concerning elderly patients, one often encounters the issue of "quality of life." Decisions made on the basis of "quality of life" considerations must be examined scrupulously because there is significant risk of generalizing one's own values in such an assessment. This is a time when the golden rule must be viewed in the complexity added by the concept of respect for others.[38] This caveat is clearly exemplified by consideration of a patient with dementia. One often hears it said that a person who is demented, particularly one who is in a nursing home, has such a poor quality of life that it is not worth living. Clinical decisions may be made on this basis. Medical care is not given to many of these people, e.g., fevers are not evaluated or treated.[39] Although we may not explicitly acknowledge this, there is often an assumption that such people ought to be mercifully allowed to die.

Before such decisions are made and acted on, it is useful to examine the following issues. First, decisions that are made to relieve the suffering of the patient must take into account whether or not that patient is actually suffering. In fact, one of the most disconcerting aspects of dementing syndromes is that the patient loses insight about his or her own condition. If they are well cared for, patients with dementia often do not appear to suffer. The care-givers may suffer, seeing a potential future self reflected in the patients.[40] Physicians in particular find the prospect of developing a dementing illness to be fearful and abhorrent. Physicians sometimes seem to value intelligence more highly than almost any other human characteristic. But not everyone shares this value system. There may be a significance to life that goes beyond one's cognitive ability. It is interesting that we have not seen fit to refuse medical treatment to retarded children, even though their cognitive function may not be any greater than that of a moderately demented elderly person.[41] Secondly, part of our worry about their suffering is justified by the realities of acute and long-term care facilities. If we must place patients in institutions where they are given poor care, are neglected, and may even be mistreated, then concern for suffering is certainly warranted. But how can we justify a decision based on the miserable quality of life in the nursing home if, in fact, that is amenable to change? The moral obligation here is to take socially responsible action toward changing these conditions rather than to let the patient die because the conditions are so poor.

**Justice.** The third major principle is that of justice. Simply stated, the resources (material and otherwise) of human society should be distributed as fairly as possible. Philosophers have found this subject a fascinating one because it seems to be an ideal that is quite appealing to most people but not one that is easy to describe in terms of how it might actually be arrived at or carried out. Its most direct application to health care involves deliberations about allocation of scarce resources.[42]

Currently, there is a great deal of discussion about the high cost of medical care and about the physician's role in keeping unnecessary costs down. These are complex issues and critically important ones for our society but they should not be directly incorporated into a caring physician's decision about his or her individual patient.[43] Obviously one should not needlessly waste scarce resources in medicine any more than in any other sphere. Nor should one use expensive technology on a patient who has asked to be allowed to die or for whom medical care cannot help. Except for those two situations, a physician who is making a decision for any patient on the basis of how much the treatment will cost is not acting strictly in the medical role. What one is really saying is that if the cost of care is the determining factor in a medical decision, then the value of this patient to society does not warrant the expenditure of medical resources. This is a social perspective, and one in which our institutions should carefully weigh the fairness of distributive policies. However, the physician has not been trained as an arbiter of justice, nor is he or she the appropriate person to take that role.[44] Except in wartime, overwhelming disasters, and other instances of dire scarcity, the rationing of health care resources must occur at the level of social policy. The relationship between the physician and the patient is a fiduciary one, implying trust that the physician is acting first and foremost as the advocate of the patient. Health professionals should participate in the formation of that policy, but as individuals their primary concern should be that of loyalty toward each patient.

What does it mean to say that we are spending too much for health care in this country? That statement is often made and yet the question has not been carefully examined. Some other developed Western countries spend more on health care than the United States.[45] We have not carefully examined the components of the health care budget and the forces that determine its magnitude. Although we have a very expensive health care system, it is not necessarily very efficient nor does it supply the basic resources that might be most effective in caring for great numbers of people. For example, although chronic renal dialysis is severely limited in the United Kingdom under the National Health Service, a spectrum of home care services enables elderly people to remain at home in spite of significant disabilities. The use of resources in this manner is based on social decisions, and not on choices that are made by individual physicians for their individual patients.

The elderly are often spotlighted when concern about rising medical costs are discussed. If it is true that the elderly account for a greater share of health costs, is this necessarily wrong? Many of these people are, in fact, in greater need of health care. Is health care not a good of our society that should be distributed according to what one needs rather than to some more mathematical distribution? Don't we all want medical care to be available if we need it?

It is important for physicians who feel pressured about resource utilization to consider that the dollars that are saved in withholding resources from the care of a particular patient will not necessarily be translated into care for more needy patients or food for hungry children. These trade-offs, which are often used in a rhetorical sense, are not trade-offs over which the physician has any power. Thus, it seems important to keep in perspective one's primary relationship with the patient and make decisions accordingly.

## *Examination of Consequences*

This analytic process is one that is familiar to clinicians. However, it is one that is important to reassess using insights gained from the other steps. Here we have a chance to use sensitivity testing, an aspect of decision analysis.[46] The risks and benefits of a given decision are compared, and then changes are made in critical elements within the facts of the case to see whether those changes would significantly affect one's decision in such a situation. It is more useful (and most realistic) to test the aspects of the case that are the most uncertain, such as the prognosis of this patient with stroke. If one had implemented aggressive treatment for Mr. James and after 2 months he was not significantly better, would the decision be considered poor? The answer to that particular question is probably no, as long as the patient's discomfort during that time had been minimized. At that point, then, one could proceed anew with the results of the therapeutic trial as part of the relevant data. One very useful form of sensitivity testing to use in ethical dilemmas with elderly patients is to imagine a similar situation in a younger patient. If one can critically examine the case of the same patient at the age of 45 or 55 or 65 and reach the same decision, one can be fairly sure that the influence of age is not predominant.

The microcommunity of the health care team should be considered in the analysis of consequences. Including the feelings and ideas of several relevant care-givers in the decision process is not always simple but has the advantage of requiring clarification of ethical reasoning. A common example of a practice in which the feelings of others are too easily overlooked is tube feeding.[47] Often, a physician will decide not to institute tube feeding in an elderly mentally disabled patient in a long-term care facility because of the potential discomfort to the patient and because the physician feels some uneasiness with the level of aggressiveness that even tube feeding represents. Instead, in a patient who is not taking nourishment, the physician will write an order to the nursing staff to feed the patient aggressively. The people who actually have to carry out this order are generally nurses' aides who may spend most of their day trying to feed patients who do not want to eat or who cannot eat. Often it seems to hurt the patient or causes choking. The patient may become combative, distressed, or frightened when a bolus of food is placed inside an unwilling mouth. For nurses' aides who must go through this with several patients day after day, distancing and dehumanization are probably the defenses that make it endurable. These psychologic consequences of the decision may therefore contribute to poor care of other and future patients.

In patients with severe terminal disease and those who are unresponsive, there may be a time when aggressive feeding measures are not indicated, especially if they interfere with the attentive care of the staff.[48] But in our case study it is clearly too soon to give up the therapeutic effort, which must include adequate (if possible, optimal) nutrition, if any accurate conclusions are to be drawn about the patient's rehabilitation potential. Intravenous hyperalimentation for a defined period may be more acceptable to patient and staff. Feeding gastrostomy should also be considered. It is up to the physician to provide leadership in finding solutions to the problem of how to manage this feeding. Such leadership may, for example, involve exerting administrative pressure to allow nurses, dieticians, psychologists, and rehabilitation therapists to perform their work in a humane context.

Finally, one must always consider consequences to society. In fact, those who argue against the legalization of active euthanasia, even for terminal patients in extreme suffering, often state that it would erode the moral fiber of the profession and of society to allow physicians to actually administer a lethal dose of a drug to a patient. This is the same argument that is used against having physicians involved in capital punishment even though the form of death thereby may be more merciful. One may counter this argument with the claim that compassionate care of the dying may have to include instances of assisted voluntary suicide, but the influence on society could be positive because responsible caring for the dying deepens our sense of humanity.

## *Making the Decision*

Once a decision is made, in particular a decision to withdraw or not to institute an aggressive therapy, the ethical context includes the enactment of the decision. These actions take extraordinary sensitivity and extreme responsibility.[49] The less dramatic, more intimate details of caring for a patient can and should continue and perhaps even intensify in that situation.[50] Alternatively, if one decides an all out effort is appropriate and the patient is apparently depressed and is resisting help, how one goes about that aggressive effort is critically important.[51] The temptation to be angry with an uncooperative ("noncompliant") patient must be resisted. Persistent sympathy must be cultivated.[52] Anger directed toward the patient, however sublimated, will only make one's job more difficult and defeat the most caring of ethical decisions.

This brief analysis of one case study is intended to demonstrate a method for approaching an ethical dilemma. It is equally important that one develop a sensitivity to the occurrence of ethical problems and the signs of discomfort that they produce in oneself or in colleagues. Sometimes there will simply be a perception that nothing seems to be going well or that communication is inadequate. Attending to values and value conflicts may significantly clarify many of these situations.

## References


1. Clouser KD: What is medical ethics? Ann Intern Med 80:657, 1974.
2. Clouser KD: Medical ethics: Some uses, abuses and limitations. N Engl J Med 293:384, 1975.
3. Pellegrino ED: Ethics and the moral center of the medical enterprise. Bull NY Acad Med 54:625, 1978.
4. Dervin J, Dervin P, Jonsen AR: Eldercare: A Practical Guide to Clinical Geriatrics. *In* O'Hara-Devereaux M, Andrus LH, Scott CD, Gray MI (eds.): New York, Grune & Stratton, 1981.
5. Libow LS: The interface of clinical and ethical decisions in the care of the elderly. Mt Sinai J Med 48:480, 1981.
6. Goldman R: Ethical confrontations in the incapacitated aged. J Am Geriatr Soc 29:241, 1981.
7. Cryer PE, Kissane JM (ed.): Clinicosociologic conference: Decisions regarding the provision or withholding of therapy. Am J Med 61:915, 1976.
8. Medical Staff Conference, University of California at San Francisco: The ailing health care system. West J Med 128:512, 1978.
9. Fried C: Rights and health care—beyond equity and efficiency. N Engl J Med 293:241, 1975.
10. Faden AL, Faden RR: Informed consent in medical practice with particular reference to neurology. Arch Neurol 35:761, 1978.
11. Gorowitz, SA et al: Moral Problems in Medicine, 2nd ed., Englewood Cliffs, NJ, Prentice-Hall, 1983.
    *A collection of excerpts and essays, with coherent introductions to each subject area by the editors. One of the best of its kind.*
12. Beauchamp TL, Childress JF: Principles of Biomedical Ethics. New York, Oxford University Press, 1979.
    *A clearly written explanation of basic ethical principles, showing how they are applied to issues such as informed consent, risk-benefit assessment, confidentiality, and decisions to terminate therapy.*
13. Veatch RM: A Theory of Medical Ethics. New York, Basic Books, 1981.
14. McNeil BJ, Weichselbaum R, Panku SG: Fallacy of the five-year survival in lung cancer. N Engl J Med 299:1397, 1978.
15. Brody DS: The patient's role in clinical decision making. Ann Intern Med 93:718, 1980.
16. Purtilo RB, Cassel CK: Ethical Dimensions in the Health Professions. Philadelphia, W.B. Saunders Co., 1981.
    *A short clearly written textbook strongly oriented toward clinical realism and including consideration of interdisciplinary issues.*
17. Jonsen AR, Siegler M, Winslade W: Clinical Ethics: A Practical Approach to Ethical Decisions in Clinical Medicine.
    *A small, concise handbook that delineates the major issues in common clinical situations and provides guidelines to decision-making.*
18. Weitzel WD, Purtilo RB: Aggressive treatment of geriatric depression: What limits on intervention? Psych Opinion 16:9, 1979.
19. Cassel CK: Ethical and legal dilemmas in treatment of psychiatric illness in the elderly. *In* Abrahams JP, Crooks V (eds.): Geriatric Mental Health: A Clinical Guide. New York, Grune & Stratton (in press).
20. Hauerwas S: Reflections on suffering, death and medicine. Ethics Sci Med 6:229, 1979.
21. Annas G: The Rights of Hospital Patients: ACLU Handbook. New York, Avon Books, 1975.
    *Readable guide intended for lay audiences. Should be owned by every clinician.*
22. Cassem NH: Being honest when technology fails. Harvard Medical School Alumni Bulletin 53:23, 1978.
23. Cassel CK, Jameton AL: Dementia in the elderly: An analysis of medical responsibility. Ann Intern Med 97:426, 1982.
24. Eisenberg JM: Sociological influences on decision making by clinicians. Ann Intern Med 93:354, 1980.
25. Meier D, Cassel CK: Euthanasia in old age: A case study and ethical analysis. J Am Geriatr Soc 31:294, 1983.
26. Annas GJ: Informed consent. Annu Rev Med 29:9, 1978.
27. Cassileth BR: Information and participation preferences among cancer patients. Ann Intern Med 92:832, 1980.
28. Cassileth BR: Informed consent—why are its goals imperfectly realized. N Engl J Med 302:896, 1980.
29. Abernathy V, Lundin K: Competency and the right to refuse medical treatment. *In* Abernathy V (ed.): Frontiers in Medical Ethics: Application in a Medical Setting. Cambridge, MA, Ballinger, 1980.
30. Roth L, Meisel A, Lidz CW: Tests of competency to consent to treatment. Am J Psychiatry 134:279, 1977.
31. McNeil BJ, Weichselbaum R, Parker SG: Speech and survival: Tradeoffs between quality and quantity of life in laryngeal cancer. N Engl J Med 305:982, 1981.
32. Coles R: Medical ethics and living a life. N Engl J Med 301:444, 1979.
33. In the matter of Mary C. Northern: Application for Stay of Mandate of Tennessee Court of Appeals. 434 U.S. 1090, February 22, 1978.
34. Lo B, Jonsen AR: Clinical decision to limit treatment. Ann Intern Med 93:764, 1980.
35. Bok S: Personal directions for care at the end of life. N Engl J Med 297:308, 1977.
36. Suber DG, Tabor WJ: Law and medicine. Withholding of life-sustaining treatment from the terminally ill, incompetent patient: Who decides? JAMA 248:2250, 1982.
37. Buchanan A: Medical paternalism. Philos Publ Affairs 7:725, 1977.
38. Dunphy JE: Annual discourse—on caring for the patient with cancer. N Engl J Med 295:313, 1976.
39. Bromberg S, Cassel CK: Suicide in old age: A case study and ethical analysis. J Am Geriatr Soc 31:698, 1983.
40. Brown NK, Thompson DJ: Non-treatment of fever in extended-care facilities. N Engl J Med 300:1246, 1979.
41. Poe W: Marantology, a needed speciality. N Engl J Med 286:102, 1972.
42. Wikler D: Paternalism and the mildly retarded. Philos Publ Affairs 8:373, 1979.
43. Outka G: Social justice and equal access to health care. *In* Reiser SJ, Dyck AJ, Curran WJ (eds.): Ethics in Medicine: Historical Perspectives and Contemporary Concerns. Cambridge, MA, MIT Press, 1977, pp. 593–597.
44. Hiatt HH: Protecting the medical commons: Who is responsible? N Engl J Med 293:235, 1975.
45. Veatch RM: Voluntary risks to health: The ethical issues. JAMA 243:50, 1980.

46. Purtilo R: Justice, Liberty, Compassion—"Humane" Health Care and Rehabilitation in the U.S.: Some Lessons from Sweden. New York, World Rehabilitation Fund, Monograph No. 8, 1981.
47. Weinstein MC, Fineberg HV: Clinical Decision Analysis. Philadelphia, W.B. Saunders Co., 1980.
48. Bexell G, Norberg A, Norberg B: Ethical conflicts in long-term care of aged patients: Analysis of the tube-feeding decision by means of a technological ethical model. Ethics Sci Med 7:141, 1980.
49. Swiss Academy of Sciences: Guidelines concerning assistance to the dying. Reprinted in Hastings Center Report. 7:30, 1977.
50. Cassem N, Hackett T: Massachusetts General Hospital Handbook of General Hospital Psychiatry. St. Louis, C.V. Mosby, 1978, pp. 573–574.
51. Burnam JF: The scientific value of personal care. Ann Intern Med 91:643, 1970.
52. Woolf V: The Moment and Other Essays. New York, Harvest Books, 1974.

Chapter 10

# Principles of Care in the Nursing Home

Robert N. Butler

Rosemary Stevens[1] has observed that the development of pediatrics in the United States was stimulated in part by the "clean milk movement" on behalf of children. She suggested that geriatrics would be similarly stimulated by a "clean up the nursing home movement." As she predicted, the recent evolution of nursing homes has had some effect on the development of geriatrics as well as on broad principles of care for older people in and out of nursing homes.

In 1958 when I first began visiting nursing homes for professional purposes, I found that they rarely had registered nurses and hardly qualified for the use of the word "home." Following the passage of Medicare and Medicaid (new titles to the Social Security Act) in 1965, came the rapid growth of nursing homes. By 1980 some 20,000 nursing homes containing about 1.5 million people existed in the United States (Table 10–1). Annual nursing home costs were over $20 billion.[2] At present there are 1.3 nursing home beds for every acute care bed in this country.[3]

In part a reflection of the socioeconomic impact of these institutionalized elderly, a growth of interest in both gerontology and geriatrics began to emerge. The Research on Aging Act, calling for the creation of the National Institute on Aging at the National Institutes of Health, was passed in 1974 and implemented by 1976. The National Institute on Aging stimulated the development of geriatric programs in some of the nation's 127 medical schools. Several endowed chairs in geriatrics were founded. Pioneering geriatricians such as Leslie S. Libow and T. Franklin Williams devoted their energies to improving the care of patients in the nursing home environment and to catalyzing educational and research programs in medical schools.

Long-term care is now emerging as a critical health issue in the 1980s. Increasing public demands and government concern, high costs, altered reimbursements, and growing knowledge, combined with the increasing maturity of the nursing home industry and the expansion of nursing home chains, all point toward change in the approach to and delivery of long-term care. This chapter will discuss some basic principles of care in the nursing home that have gained prominence in the last two decades. It will also suggest some future trends.

## CATEGORIES OF NURSING HOMES

There are two major types of long-term care institutions for the aged: the skilled nursing facility (SNF) and the intermediate-care facility (ICF). Detailed sets of standards and reimbursement systems distinguish between these "levels of care." In general, skilled nursing care refers to those services that must be performed under the supervision of professional registered nurses. Intermediate care is "more than room and board, but less than skilled nursing." Because these terms are not altogether clear to health professionals or to the public, the blanket term "nursing home" is used.

The fact that nursing home residents are not a homogeneous group has been noted by Keeler and associates.[4] They placed nursing home admissions into two categories. Between one third and one half of admissions, the "short stayers,"

**Table 10–1.** NUMBER AND FINANCING OF NURSING HOME BEDS, 1980*

| Type of Facility | Number of Beds | Financing |
|---|---|---|
| Intermediate care facilities | 905,000 | Medicaid only beds |
| Skilled nursing facilities | 43,715 | Both Medicaid and Medicare beds |
| | 144,000 | Medicaid only beds |
| | 27,000 | Medicare only beds |
| *Total* | 1,119,715 | |

* Data from Department of Health and Human Resources, Health Care Finance Administration, 1980. There may be an additional 700,000 beds in other facilities for long-term care, mainly residential beds in domicilary or personal care homes that are not federally certified.

either die within the first 3 months (8 per cent of admissions) or are discharged. For the most part, these are patients who are admitted from acute care hospitals for a period of convalescence following acute illness (Table 10–2). The other group consists of those, usually of advanced age and often with mental problems, who are no longer able to live outside the institution. As seen in Table 10–3, some form of cognitive impairment constitutes the majority of mental disturbances. The primary diagnoses of nursing home residents have been listed by a number of investigators. Although frequency estimates for specific diagnoses differ, Table 10–3 lists representative data.

## PRINCIPLES OF CARE

### *Proper Placement and Assessment*

The first and quintessential principle of care in the nursing home is proper placement of the patient.[5] This in turn depends on effective, prompt, and comprehensive assessment (see Chapter 8).

Those patients deemed suitable for placement into long-term care institutions constitute

**Table 10–2.** LENGTH OF STAY OF NURSING HOME RESIDENTS, 1977*

| Distribution of Length of Stay | % of Residents |
|---|---|
| Less than 3 months | 13 |
| 3–6 months | 10 |
| 6–12 months | 14 |
| 1–3 years | 32 |
| 2-plus years | 31 |
| Median length of stay: 582 days or 1.6 years | |

* Data from U.S. Public Health Service, National Center of Health Statistics, Washington, DC, 1977.

**Table 10–3.** PRIMARY DIAGNOSIS AT LAST EXAMINATION

| *Diseases of the Circulatory System* | Number | Percentage |
|---|---|---|
| Total | 1,303,100 | 100 |
| Congestive heart failure | 52,800 | 4.1 |
| Arteriosclerosis | 264,400 | 20.3 |
| Hypertension | 47,700 | 3.7 |
| Stroke | 103,500 | 7.9 |
| Heart attack, ischemic heart disease | 22,500 | 1.7 |
| Other circulatory system diseases | 25,800 | 2.0 |
| ***Mental Disorders and Senility Without Psychosis*** | | |
| Total | 266,100 | 20.4 |
| Senile psychosis | 21,200 | 1.6 |
| Other psychosis | 57,400 | 4.4 |
| Chronic brain syndrome | 96,400 | 7.4 |
| Senility without psychosis | 26,600 | 2.0 |
| Mental retardation | 42,400 | 3.3 |
| Alcoholism | 6,800 | 0.5 |
| Other mental disorders | 15,300 | 1.2 |
| ***Other Diagnoses*** | | |
| Total | 429,700 | 33.0 |
| ***Diseases of the Musculoskeletal System*** | 56,200 | 4.3 |
| ***Diseases of the Nervous System and Sense Organs*** | | |
| Blindness | 5,100 | 0.4 |
| Multiple sclerosis | 7,300 | 0.6 |
| Epilepsy | 6,800 | 0.5 |
| Parkinson's disease | 23,300 | 1.8 |
| ***Accidents, Poisonings, and Violence*** | | |
| Hip fracture | 29,300 | 2.2 |
| Other bone fracture | 10,600 | 0.8 |
| ***Endocrine, Nutritional, and Metabolic Diseases*** | | |
| Diabetes | 71,700 | 5.5 |
| ***Neoplasms*** | | |
| Cancer | 28,900 | 2.2 |
| ***Diseases of the Respiratory System*** | | |
| Emphysema | 8,000 | 0.6 |
| Pneumonia* | | |
| Other respiratory diseases | 18,500 | 1.4 |
| ***Diseases of the Digestive System*** | | |
| Ulcers | 8,600 | 0.7 |
| ***Diseases of the Blood and Blood-Forming Organs*** | | |
| Anemia | 7,300 | 0.6 |
| ***Diagnosis Unknown*** | 90,500 | 6.9 |

Data from U.S. Public Health Service National Center for Health Statistics, 1977.
* No data provided for pnemonia.

a diverse group. Unfortunately, accurate assessment of a patient's needs and long-term goals are often lacking prior to placement. The misplacement of the patient in the nursing home is most unfortunate for the individual and for society, since it may obviate the provision of a "lower" (i.e., less intensive and less expensive) level of care to patients who might, with a properly designed therapeutic regimen, achieve a greater degree of independence.

A number of studies support the observation that there are many people in nursing homes who do not belong there. It is my impression and that of other gerontologists that there may be an equal number of people who are left stranded and unprotected in the community who should be in nursing homes. In any case, there is an irreducible minimum of individuals suffering from severe disabling cerebrovascular disease, arthritis, and other disorders who can no longer maintain themselves in their homes.

The assessment of the individual must not only specify medical and nursing factors but must also provide a portrait of psychologic and social status and functions. In addition, socioeconomic data, pension and legal rights, recreational interests of the patient, and other information must be gathered. Most importantly, the assessment must include an appraisal of possible intervention.

## *Proactive Intervention*

The second principle of nursing home care, then, is proactive, dynamic intervention. Every effort must be made to intervene through a diagnostic approach that seeks treatment possibilities. For example, in the care of mental impairments in older persons, the assessment procedure should identify those instances of intellectual confusion that are potentially reversible. It is imperative that an older person not be stereotyped "senile" or be told "this is what you have to expect at your age." This principle of proactive intervention must continue even after admission to the nursing home in order to prevent further debilitation (e.g., muscle contracture).

Both the procedure of assessment and the efforts at intervention must focus on the functional status of the individual. The nursing home staff, for instance, must be presented with an individual portrait of the sensory- and motor-impaired person and, simultaneously, be taught techniques for moderating such impairments.

Although active rehabilitative efforts are essential to good nursing home care,[6] it should be appreciated that a significant number of nursing home residents have limited capacity for rehabilitation. Such individuals must not be regarded as of secondary importance compared with residents provided rehabilitative efforts. Quality of life is very important and more dominant in the lives of long-term patients than in those suffering from acute illness. Even in these patients, active intervention may still positively affect quality of life and morbidity and mortality. Quality of life issues include social factors as well as efforts at prevention of "medical complications" such as pressure sores. For example, several investigators have demonstrated that efforts to enhance the sense of control by nursing home residents over aspects of their environment have a positive impact on patient satisfaction, level of physical activity, and overall mortality.[7-9] Active participation by family members in nursing home activities, including specific caring tasks, also has a positive impact on life satisfaction and morale of nursing home patients.[10]

## *Avoidance of Iatrogenic Illness*

Apart from underlying disease and social milieu, the outcome of nursing home residents may be adversely affected by iatrogenic illness. Of particular importance is overmedication by physicians and the attendant adverse drug reactions.

In one study, the average number of drugs prescribed for each nursing home resident was 7.06,[11] with 43 of 50 patients studied receiving neuroleptics. Fifty-eight per cent of nursing home patients receive laxatives.[12] In part, this multiplicity of drugs reflects the fact that many elderly people have four or five concurrent diseases. In addition, especially in nursing homes, many drugs are prescribed without clear indication.[11] PRN orders are especially apt to be inappropriate and indiscriminately followed.[13] Overprescription of drugs increases the likelihood of adverse drug reactions. It also contributes to added cost, not only for the drugs actually taken but also for the drugs discarded unused. In one 100-bed nursing home, it was estimated that the annual cost of discarded drugs was in excess of $1600.[14]

*Nonpharmacologic* therapy may also be of harm to nursing home patients. For example, excessive use of physical restraints may lead to serious medical complications.[15] Appropriate emphasis on reality orientation, remotivation, attitude therapy, and sensory stimulation may obviate the need for use of restraints or chemical sedation. Thus, the third principle of care in the nursing home is that the physician and other care providers should do no harm.

### *Interdisciplinary Care*

The fourth principle is the sophisticated utilization of the interdisciplinary or team approach, particularly the collegial collaboration of the nurse and the social worker. Since this subject is discussed elsewhere in this book (see Chapter 3), it will not be repeated here.

### *Improving the Relationship with the Acute Hospital*

The fifth principle of care requires the formalization and strengthening of the relationship between long-term care institutions and acute hospitals. About 30 per cent of all nursing home discharges comprise individuals who are transferred to acute hospitals for a variety of reasons, including bowel obstruction, psychiatric emergencies, and fractures. An absolute number of 340,000 such patients were transferred in 1980. The Medicare legislation required transfer agreements between nursing homes and hospitals.

The factors relating to transfers to and from nursing homes have been examined by Stark and associates.[16] Not surprisingly, patients without support at home are more apt to be institutionalized than those who enjoy a strong family and home support system. Nearly one quarter of individuals admitted to nursing homes require readmission to an acute care hospital within the first year. All too often patients are transferred to acute hospitals that are not prepared to deal sensitively with the special problems of the older patient. Following hospitalization, 50 per cent of the residents are readmitted to the same long-term care institution and at the same level of care.

### *Involving the Family*

The importance of family participation constitutes the sixth principle of nursing home care. Because women tend to outlive their husbands, the bulk of nursing home residents (approximately 75 per cent) are women. A significant number of women are childless. Thus, some 50 per cent of present day nursing home residents do not have significant family members. When there is a family, every effort must be made to involve them in the direct care of the institutionalized family member. From the point of view of the family, the admission to the nursing home is the first of two "deaths." The first death is psychologic and concerns the leaving of the home for "the last refuge." This psychologic death is eventually followed by the somatic death. A family's frequency of visits usually falls after admission unless the nursing home finds ways to effectively encourage continuing family participation. The physician and staff should be prepared to help the family make decisions, such as when the patient's home can be closed or sold.

### *Providing a Prognosis*

This brings us to the last of the basic principles: providing the older person and the family with a prognosis. This can be exceedingly difficult. However, data are beginning to emerge that elucidate the prognostic indicators of residents of nursing homes and long-term care facilities. Goldfarb and associates[17] evaluated prognostic indicators in nursing homes, "old age homes," and state mental hospitals. Factors indicative of a poor prognosis included severe senile dementia, physical dependence (i.e., poor capacity to perform activities of daily living), and incontinence. Brauer and associates[18] have also emphasized the adverse prognostic implications of fecal and urinary incontinence. Recent data concerning outcomes of patients admitted to nursing homes have been presented by Kane and associates.[19]

When the patient and family are given a reasonable estimate of prognosis, they feel greater control over the situation. A prognosis allows the patient and family to make plans and initiate actions.

## THE ROLE AND RESPONSIBILITY OF THE PHYSICIAN

At present, only a minority of American physicians visit nursing homes. Mitchell[20] found that in a sample of 3482 physicians in 15 specialties, 72.4 per cent saw no nursing home patients. The majority of nursing home visits were made by cardiologists, general practitioners, and internists, in that order. In the future, it is to be hoped and expected that many more physicians will be participating regularly in the care of nursing home residents, either as medical directors or attending physicians.

Other chapters of this book cover assessment and the treatment of various conditions common in nursing homes, ranging from incontinence (see Chapter 33) to swallowing difficulties (Chapters 13 and 46). The names and addresses of major nursing home associations are listed in Table 10–4. The physician and other health providers have a responsibility to stay abreast of the growing corpus of geriatric knowledge.

In addition to understanding and addressing these issues, the nursing home physician must appreciate the many problems faced by nursing homes today. High interest rates have stifled necessary construction. Fragmented and limited funding has constricted efforts to increase quality. Medicare and Medicaid cutbacks since 1980 have further compromised the need for improvement within nursing homes. There have been recent federal pressures toward "deregulation" and the reduction in frequency of inspections. In addition, a limited curriculum in nursing and medical schools has contributed to the low numbers of physicians and nurses interested in working in nursing homes.

In order to enhance our understanding of the many problems confronting nursing homes and their residents and professional staff and to stimulate greater involvement by medical schools and other health science schools, this author has proposed the creation of a long-term care counterpart to the teaching hospital: the teaching nursing home.[21] The structure and behavior of contemporary nursing homes are similar to that of general hospitals at the turn of the century, prior to the medical school reforms introduced by the Flexner Report. Establishment of a limited number of teaching nursing homes would provide an educational base for medical, nursing, social work, and allied health students and nursing home administrators. It would help to clarify issues of misplacement and aid in the development of various forms of home care.* Senile dementia of the Alzheimer's type, recurrent falling disorders, decubitus ulcers, and incontinence are among conditions that have not been subject to significant scientific study elsewhere; these could be studied conveniently and constructively in an academic nursing home environment. At their best, clinical services, education, and research go together.

The development of academic programs of this sort would not be necessary or desirable for all nursing homes. Just as some 400 teaching hospitals exist at present among approximately 7000 general hospitals, the establishment of 127 teaching nursing homes, one for each medical school, might be appropriate.

**Table 10–4.** MAJOR ASSOCIATIONS OF NURSING HOMES AND HOMES FOR THE AGING

**American Association of Homes for the Aging (AAHA)**
1050 17th St., N.W., Suite 770, Washington, DC 20005
*Membership*—represents nonprofit community-sponsored housing, homes for the aging, and health-related facilities serving older people. Homes are sponsored by religious, fraternal, labor, civic, and county organizations.

**American Health Care Association***
1200 15th St., N.W. Washington, DC 20005
*Membership*—federation of state associations of commercial homes in 49 states (Oklahoma not included). Some 200 nonprofit homes also belong, usually small homes with about 60 beds. This is a nonprofit organization.

**National Council of Health Centers***
1200 15th St., N.W. Washington, DC 20005
*Membership*—voluntary association of proprietary health care companies. Members own and manage nursing homes, hospitals, psychiatric facilities, clinics, home health agencies, and child day-care centers. Members must meet accreditation standards of the Joint Commission on Accreditation of Hospitals. Membership is open to any private company owning and operating three or more medical facilities with a minimum of 300 beds.

* In the process of merger.

## CONCLUSION

It is easy to be critical of the nursing home. It is a relatively new instrument of care and is under substantial public and private pressure. This pressure will continue. Patients entering nursing homes are older and sicker than they used to be. The average age on admission has increased to 80 years. Older people do not fall neatly into institutional categories. A wide spectrum of services and facilities, including the nursing home, will continue to evolve to effectively meet the diverse needs of older people.

### References

1. Stevens R: Presentation, National Institute on Aging. Bethesda, Maryland. March 1977.
2. Libow LS: Geriatric medicine and the nursing home: A mechanism for mutual excellence. Gerontologist 22:134, 1982.

* Day hospitals, homemakers, day care, etc., could create a spectrum of facilities and services more in keeping with the nature and needs of old age. These types of alternatives to nursing homes are believed to constitute the wave of the future.

3. Campion E, Bang A, May MI: Why acute care hospitals must undertake long-term care. N Engl J Med 308:71, 1983.
4. Keeler EB, Kane RL, Solomon DH: Short- and long-term residents of nursing homes. Med Care 19:363, 1981.
5. Kane RL, Rubenstein LZ, Brook RH, et al: Utilization review in nursing homes: Making implicit level-of-care judgments explicit. Med Care 19:3, 1981.
6. Hefferin EA: Rehabilitation in nursing home situations: A survey of the literature. J Am Geriatr Soc 15:296, 1968.
7. Elias JW, Phillips ME, Wright LL: The relationship of perceived latitude of choice to morale in nursing home environment. Exp Aging Res 6:357, 1980.
8. Morganti JB, Nehrke MF, Hulicka I: Resident and staff perceptions of latitude of choice in elderly institutionalized men. Exp Aging Res 6:367, 1980.
9. Beck P: Two successful interventions in nursing homes: The therapeutic effect of cognitive activity. Gerontologist 22:378, 1982.
10. Shuttlesworth GE, Rubin A, Duffy M: Families versus institutions: Incongruent role expectations in the nursing home. Gerontologist 22:200, 1982.
11. Segal JL, Thompson JF, Floyd RA: Drug utilization and prescribing patterns in a skilled nursing facility: The need for a rational approach to therapeutics. J Am Geriatr Soc 27:117, 1979.
12. Lamy P, Krug BH: Review of laxative utilization in a skilled nursing facility. J Am Geriatr Soc 26:544, 1978.
13. Howard JB, Strong KE, Strong KE Jr: Medication procedures in a nursing home: Abuse of PRN orders. J Am Geriatr Soc 25:83, 1977.
14. Howard JB, Strong KE, Strong KE Jr: Nursing home medication costs. J Am Geriatr Soc 26:228, 1978.
15. Covert A, Rodrigues T, Solomon K: The use of mechanical and chemical restraints in nursing homes. J Am Geriatr Soc 25:85, 1977.
16. Stark AJ, Gutman GM, McCashin B: Acute-care hospitalizations and long-term care: An examination of transfers. J Am Geriatr Soc 30:509, 1982.
17. Goldfarb AL, Finch M, Gerber IE: Predictions of mortality in the institutionalized aged. Diseases of the nervous system. Dis Nerv Syst 27:21, 1966.
18. Brauer E, Mackeprang B, Bentzon MW: Prognosis of survival in a geriatric population. Scand J Soc Med 6:17, 1978.
19. Kane RL, Bell R, Riegler S, et al: Predicting the outcomes of nursing home patients. Gerontologist 23:200, 1983.
20. Mitchell JB: Physician visits to nursing homes. Gerontologist 22:45, 1982.
21. Butler RN: The teaching nursing home. JAMA 245:1435, 1981.

## *Additional Reading*

Butler RN: Why Survive? Being Old in America. New York, Harper and Row, 1975.

Morris RA: Proposal—Alternatives to Nursing Home Care. U.S. Senate Special Committee on Aging. Washington, DC, U.S. Government Printing Office, 1971.

Vladek B: Unloving Care: The Nursing Home Tragedy. New York, The Twentieth Century Fund, 1980.

## Chapter 11

# Home Care

*J. Andrew Billings*
*Fred Rubin*
*John D. Stoeckle*

Until this century, the vast majority of encounters between physicians and patients occurred in the home. Even in the 1930s, house calls accounted for 50 per cent of the physician's workload; now they amount to 3 per cent or less. Home attending today consists largely of advice over the telephone. The home, however, remains the principal site of care for the ill. Patients and families usually manage this care with only occasional help from physicians and nurses.

The practice of home visiting may be returning. Physicians are now making house calls for the following reasons: (1) to provide more appropriate care for the "homebound"; (2) to assess the needs of patients and families in the context of their daily living; (3) to participate in the multidisciplinary teams that support ill people in the home; (4) to reduce medical costs, especially by promoting home care as an alternative to long-term institutionalization; and (5) to provide more personal care. Moreover, physicians who are in relatively greater supply and find themselves not fully occupied by office or hospital work may offer house calls in order to attract patients or keep them in the practice.

Home visiting may be viewed as a "procedure"—a special contribution of expertise and service in the care of the elderly. The contemporary geriatrician must advise about the scope, limits, and details of home care, make appropriate referrals to community agencies, and certify patients for needed home services. Besides personally attending the homebound patient, the physician collaborates in team care—coordinating, supporting, and supervising the multiple providers of home care services. Many of the physician's duties in the home can be delegated to nurses, nurse-practitioners, or physicians' assistants, although licensing and reimbursement schemes often prevent such a rational allocation of tasks.[1]

Regardless of any revival of house calls, home visits are no longer an automatic response to the patient's request to see a physician. This chapter describes contemporary indications for house calls and their use for the promotion of home care.

## WHY MAKE HOUSE CALLS?

Home visits are recommended to fill the needs of special patients and to perform special clinical tasks. Three categories of patients and five clinical tasks are described.

### *The Psychologically Homebound Patient*

Some patients cannot visit the physician's office because their psychologic impairments are so great. This category of patients includes agoraphobics, "eccentrics," reclusives, and other psychiatric patients who will not seek out or accept medical care unless visited at home. This group also includes the demented or retarded who show such marked anxiety or regression when removed from their familiar surroundings that they are better seen at home.

### *The Physically Homebound Patient*

Many patients have disabilities, either transient or chronic, that make travel to the office or hospital costly, uncomfortable, risky, or, at least, very inconvenient. The patient's environment, such as physical barriers to getting out of the house or lack of public transportation, may also prevent travel to the physician.

In addition to allowing for the evaluation of acute and chronic medical problems, the house call enables the physician to observe the patient's functioning and to assess the support received from the family, social network, and community agencies.[2] Home visits often provide invaluable personal attention to an isolated individual, although they can be a disservice to patients who, despite many problems getting to the office, find such appointments a welcome escape from the house and an enjoyable opportunity for social interaction with staff and other patients.

Transient conditions associated with immobility include trauma, being "too sick to move," convalescence (e.g., after myocardial infarction),[3] acute episodes of chronic illness (e.g., podagra), the onset of probable chronic conditions (e.g., stroke), and temporary barriers to coming to the office (e.g., snowstorms or lack of usual transportation).

Among the chronic conditions for which home visits may be indicated are major neurologic deficits (e.g., hemiparesis, paraplegia, dementia, and other degenerative diseases of the central nervous system), musculoskeletal diseases (e.g., severe rheumatoid or degenerative arthritis, prolapsed disc, and muscular dystrophy), amputation, end stage organ failure (e.g., renal, cardiac, respiratory, and hepatic), multiple severe sensory deficits, and advanced stages of terminal cancer.[4]

## *Terminally Ill Patients*

A physician may offer to make house calls to terminally ill patients in deference to their wishes to be at home with family and friends (and perhaps to die there) and to provide assurance of continuing medical supervision as the illness progresses. Hospice programs, whose publicity initially focused on specialized inpatient units for the dying and on the intelligent use of narcotics to control chronic cancer pain, have recently emphasized home care.[4] Cardinal features of a hospice program are careful attention to the palliation of symptoms, provision of multidisciplinary, family-oriented medical and psychosocial support during the terminal period and the time of bereavement, 24-hour availability of services, coordinated outpatient and inpatient care, the use of volunteers as "friendly visitors," and the development of staff training and support, which includes attention to the emotionally difficult task of working with the dying.

## *Attending a Death*

The pronouncement of death is the most common emergency and late night indication for a home visit. Tasks of the visit include confirming that the patient is dead; preparing the death certificate; helping with decisions about an autopsy and with the funeral arrangements; advising on the disposal of medications, equipment, and supplies; answering the family's questions about the illness and death; facilitating the process of bereavement; and, if necessary, arranging for ongoing support of the bereaved.[4]

## *Home Evaluation of Functional Status*

Neuropsychologic problems and impaired mobility are often best assessed in the home setting. For instance, a demented patient's disorientation is often exaggerated in the unfamiliar medical office, whereas the patient's functioning, as assessed in the home, will appear to be satisfactory. Conversely, subtle losses of mental and physical abilities are often most evident in the home where the physician may observe deterioration in the handling of minor household tasks.[5]

## *Psychosocial Evaluation and Management*

Many visits to homebound people are necessary not only to provide medical evaluation but also to respond to acute concerns of the family and to help them to cope with home care.[6] In order to prevent "breakdown" of the home care plan, the physician must continuously assess the adequacy of support systems. Periodic visits from the physician and home care team can provide the expertise, reassurance, and support that help to keep a family together and prevent institutionalization.[2,7]

Additional common psychosocial reasons for visiting include the following:

- To assess and promote compliance with medications, diet, or physical therapy, e.g., a review of medication containers and of the procedures of administering drugs.
- To meet the primary caretakers and other

members of the home care team (family, friends, volunteers and professional workers), review home care directions, and establish relationships that can facilitate later communications.

- To exchange information at family gatherings, e.g., to share upsetting news, assess family dynamics, provide counseling and support, plan caretaking chores, and evaluate the impact of the illness and burdens of home care on the household.
- To establish a closer therapeutic alliance by joining the patient in the "natural habitat," e.g., sharing a meal, learning firsthand about the patient's activities, hobbies, and interests, and gaining an overall feeling for the home and neighborhood.
- For the convenience of the physician, e.g., the physician can see patients at night or on weekends who live near his or her residence or who are otherwise easy to visit.
- For personal rewards, e.g., to fulfill curiosity about how patients live by seeing them in the home, to appreciate the inspirational volunteerism of families and friends, or to manage care by using bedside clinical skills unaided by complicated technology.[8,9]

### *Home Medical Management*

A wide range of diagnostic and therapeutic interventions can be carried out in the home. Many common laboratory tests are readily obtained there, whereas treatments might include intramuscular administration of diuretics, intravenous fluid and electrolyte therapy, or thoracentesis for symptomatic relief from a malignant pleural effusion. With adequate training and supervision, patients may receive renal dialysis, long-term intravenous antibiotic treatment, and hyperalimentation in the home setting.

### *Administrative Evaluation and Coordination of Home Care*

For the physician to function as manager or consultant of a home care team, house calls may be needed to assess the services of various home health agencies and community supports, especially when new adjustments are required of patients, family, and staff (e.g., after hospitalization) and when new problems arise in longstanding home care arrangements.[10]

### *Why Not to Make Home Visits*

When the patient and family are committed to home care and when basic home services are available, almost any chronic illness can be managed, largely or entirely, at home.[11] Home care should not be encouraged if (1) the patient is too sick, i.e., needs frequent or continuous nursing care that cannot be organized in the community; (2) the patient needs prompt diagnostic and/or therapeutic procedures not readily available at home; (3) the demands of care exceed the tolerance of home health supports (most commonly because of emotional distress and fatigue of the family); or (4) the patient or family strongly favor institutional care for the relief of their physical, emotional, social, or economic burdens.

## HOW TO CONDUCT HOME VISITS

The essentials of a house call are well known to practicing physicians. These include telephoning the home ahead of time; obtaining good, precise directions, including how to enter the house; becoming familiar with the medical record; and providing oneself with examination tools, paper for recording notes, prescription blanks, and whatever special supplies may be required, such as equipment for blood and urine specimens, dressing changes, or catheterization.

The visit usually begins with the identification of acute problems or with a general discussion of the living situation. What does the patient do all day? What is the quality of his or her life? What most impedes him or her from doing what he or she would like to be able to do? Does the patient require assistance with any of the activities of daily living—bathing, feeding, dressing, toileting, or ambulating? Are family members or neighbors helpful? Who takes primary responsibility for supervising care at home? How does the patient obtain help in an emergency?

What medications are present? Ask to see the medicine cabinet and all the medication containers. Review the medication schedule. Who supervises and administers the medication?

The condition of the house or apartment and its neighborhood should be noted. A tour of the house can be requested or access to other rooms may be gained by requesting the use of a bathroom for hand-washing. Where does the patient stay during the day? Where is the television? What cooking facilities are available?

**Table 11-1.** HOME CARE: A CHECKLIST FOR ASSESSMENT OF THE PHYSICAL SETTING AND TASKS OF HOME CARE

**Housing (Satisfactory physical setting for care)**
Comfort, cleanliness, spaciousness
Safety and comfort of the neighborhood
Access for patient, family, friends
Consider housing assistance programs (e.g., mortgage maintenance and rental supports)
Consider special housing (for independent or assisted living)
- Handicapped housing
- Senior citizen housing
- Foster homes

**Room**
Where will patient be? Consider rearranging rooms.
Where will others sleep and carry on their lives?

**Bed (Rent, buy, or borrow bed for special needs)**
Elevated, adjustable (mechanical or electrical adjustments)
Side rails, trapeze
Mattress (foam, air, water, or regular)
Bedding (e.g., sheepskin, plastic sheets, underpads)
- Changing bedding
- Moving, turning
- Washing
- Special skin care (preventing and treating decubitus ulcers)

**Mobility**
Transfer techniques (e.g., lifting, mechanical devices)
Special chairs, couches
Assistance in ambulation (e.g., canes, walkers, wheelchairs, rails, ramps, bars)
Check for safety hazards (e.g., loose rugs, obstructions)
Exercise (active and passive), physical therapy

**Dressing**
"Bedclothes" and normal clothes
Laundry

**Grooming**
Hair and nails
Makeup

**Bathing**
Aids (e.g., flexible shower heads, long-handled brushes, adhesive strips to prevent slipping, safety bars)

**Bowel and Bladder Function**
Continent
- Use of bedpan, urinal, bedside commode, elevated toilet seat
- Access to the bathroom
- Bowel regimens, suppositories

Incontinent
- Underpads, plastic sheets, towels, hampers, diaper service
- External or indwelling urinary catheter
- Drainage systems and their management

**Feeding**
Shopping or ordering food; Meals-on-Wheels
Preparation
- Soft and liquid diets
- Tube feedings
- Assistance in eating
- Bedside fluids, snacks
- Special utensils, straws

Alcohol
Food stamps and other nutritional support programs

**Medication**
Purchase and delivery
Storage and safety
Refilling
Monitoring
Recording
Adjusting
Self-administered vs. given by family member
Aid in swallowing (e.g., mashing pills, mixing with food, liquid preparations)
Suppositories
Topical treatments
Injections

**Supplies and Equipment**
Purchasing, borrowing, or renting
Delivery
Storage and safety
Proper use of gloves, syringes, needles, sterile dressings, solutions
Catheter equipment
Oxygen, suction equipment
Intravenous therapy, hyperalimentation
Dialysis

**Attending**
Professional "skilled" help vs. "unskilled" help
- Visiting nurses
- Physical therapy, speech therapy, occupational therapy
- Home health aides
- Homemakers, chore services
- Companions and volunteer services

Training nonprofessional helpers (e.g., to change dressing, give injections, monitor vital signs)
Constant vs. intermittent availability of help
Regular, anticipated chores (e.g., dressing changes, meals, skin care, medications) vs. intermittent needs (e.g., snacks, "as needed" medications, some transfers)
Night call
Methods for calling for help (e.g., phones, buzzers, bells, intercoms)
What to do when questions arise? Caretakers absent? Emergencies?

**Diversions, Entertainment, Recreation**
Hobbies, books, television, radio, tapes, records
Personally important objects (e.g., photographs, paintings, gifts, souvenirs, and mementos)
Family access and visitors
Excursions

**Pastoral Care**

**Legal Aid**

**Financial Aid**
Knowledge of the availability of and eligibility requirements for services and the process of obtaining help
- Hospital-based and community-based social service agencies

Sources
- Third-party health insurance (e.g., Blue Cross/Blue Shield, Medicare, Medicaid, and other private insurers)

Social Security, general relief
Area agency on aging
United Way and other community charities
Special funds (e.g., American Cancer Society, local and national philanthropic organizations, hospital funds)

**Out of Home Help**
Senior citizens' center for meals, recreation
Day care
Respite care
Rehabilitation services
Transportation

Where does the patient sleep? What hazards exist? Frequent dangers are scatter rugs, electric cords, thresholds, and shag rugs. Is the home secure from outsiders? Is there adequate heat? What physical barriers limit the patient's function? Are stairs necessary to reach the bathroom, bedroom, or street? The bathroom is frequently the site for falls and fractures. Is it safe and accessible? Are grab-bars or a raised toilet seat indicated? How does the patient bathe?

The physical examination may be carried out with the family absent, allowing for a confidential exchange in which the patient may be able to speak more freely. Later, the entire family can be involved in the presentation of findings and decisions about management. Allow time for discussion. Before leaving, the physician should be sure that the family knows how to reach him or her by telephone and understands about night-time, weekend, and emergency coverage.

Even if a patient's physical status cannot be changed, his or her functional abilities and quality of life can be improved by judicious environmental modification, use of adaptive equipment, and family counseling. Specific home services are regularly required and are reviewed in the following section.

Table 11-1 contains a list of considerations in the evaluation and promotion of home care. Social workers, the local visiting nurse association, and the area agency on aging should be familiar with community resources. Inseparable from the management of physical and social problems is the provision of psychologic support, particularly dealing with insecurity (see Psychologic Issues, page 113).

## COMMUNITY RESOURCES

In most communities, the following services are available to homebound patients:

- The Visiting Nurse Association (VNA) and licensed home care agencies can provide registered nurses, occupational, physical and speech therapists, homemakers (to clean the house and prepare meals), and home health aides (to help with the patient's personal care). Typically, a patient might be seen by a nurse once every 2 weeks, by an aide once or twice a week, and by a homemaker daily on weekdays. Chore services do occasional heavy cleaning.[2]
- Meals-on-Wheels can supply one or two hot meals daily.
- Day care, usually with transportation service included, provides diversion and supervision for the patient and respite for the family.
- Mental health services, social services, nutritional counseling, physical therapy, occupational therapy, and speech therapy may be available in the home through local hospitals or neighborhood health centers.[7]
- Home dentistry, optometry, and podiatry may be arranged through local practitioners.
- Hospice programs have trained volunteers to make home visits to families with a terminally ill patient. Friendly visiting programs for the elderly are available in some communities.
- Special equipment (wheelchairs, walkers, electric beds, and adaptive services for people with impaired use of their extremities) is available through surgical supply companies and drugstores. Consultation with a physical or occupational therapist may be helpful. The Lifeline, an electronic beeper that can summon emergency help, may particularly aid those impaired elderly who live alone and might be unable to reach a phone after a fall.
- Commercial laboratories may collect laboratory specimens in the home and obtain electrocardiograms and some x-ray studies.
- State agencies may offer special programs for the deaf, the blind, the handicapped, and the elderly. They may provide rehabilitation, transportation, fuel assistance, and housing.
- Legal advice is often needed in dealing with landlords, housing authorities, tenants, utility companies, and social service agencies (especially Medicaid), for handling medical and other debts, and for answering questions about guardianship, conservatorship, and wills.
- Many health centers and hospitals employ fulltime coordinators for the elderly—a friendly, accessible ombudsperson who becomes a familiar social contact for older patients and who acts, for both professionals and patients, as a source of practical advice about housing, transportation, medical insurance, and community services.[12]

If enough resources are expended and the patient and family are committed to home care, virtually anyone can be maintained in the community, no matter how impaired, although the technical care may not be optimal. Well-organized, comprehensive services can often prevent a frustrating hospital or nursing home admission, precipitated by lack of adequate home support. A brief "respite admission" to the hospital (or, ideally, a nursing home) may provide valuable relief for the family. The prospect of enjoying such respite care a few times each year may make the family's fulltime duties seem more manageable.

A break-even point exists beyond which the cost and complexity of home services and the family burden become excessive.[11] A thorough review of the patient's physical status, home supports, and available community resources is required for making the difficult decision to either continue care at home or to find suitable temporary or permanent institutional care.

## PSYCHOLOGIC ISSUES

### *Dealing with Insecurity*

Sick people and their families are often worried about the inevitable medical uncertainties in their future.[4] The responsibility for handling crises, real or imagined, rests on those at home. When such concerns are not addressed, anxiety escalates and the burdens of care may appear to be overwhelming. Frequent phone calls, emergency room visits, or demands for hospitalization follow. For instance, when a patient with advanced chronic lung disease is managed at home, the patient or family may harbor fears about choking, suffocation, severe pain, or bizarre behavior. Such fears become apparent to the physician after careful listening and by direct questioning; for example:

- *What kinds of problems do you think might arise in the next few weeks?*
- *Have you had any particular worries?*
- *What have you heard about other people with this kind of condition?*

Unrealistic fears can be handled with careful reassurance, whereas realistic concerns need to be addressed with concrete plans:

- If he becomes more short of breath, you can put the oxygen up to 5 L per minute. Call me if he is not getting better within 15 minutes, and I'll tell you what to do next.
- If her weight goes up to 132 lb, you should give her an extra Lasix tablet at midday. If her weight goes above 138 lb, you should notify the nurse.
- We are expecting him to die quietly in the next few days. He will just fall asleep and eventually stop breathing. He won't suffer. When he dies, call me. Don't call the police. I'll come by and help.

### *Psychologic Support*

Even if the burden of physical care is manageable and the patient and family feel secure facing the uncertainties of illness, a host of psychologic issues may present barriers to successful home care. Longstanding family tensions often emerge, exacerbated by such factors as the increasing needs of the patient or personal reactions to illness and anticipated loss.

Families that functioned satisfactorily during periods of physical well-being may become incompatible when a family member is sick. For instance, some patients will have difficulty accepting dependence on their family, saying they do not want to "impose." Exploration of the past relationships of the family members may reveal that a commitment to care for each other and to make personal sacrifices was never present or that a husband or wife "never could stand being around someone who is sick." Sanford[13] has also described "intolerable" conditions in a geriatric population, particularly sleep disorders and incontinence, which, if not properly treated, are likely to lead the family to give up home care. All disturbing symptoms—pain, disorderly behavior, vomiting—must be managed aggressively.

## CONCLUSION

Clinicians should remember that there are rewards to patient, family, and physician from care at home, although its burdens fall largely on the family. The physician and nurse can assist the family by delegating chores and by setting limits on each member's responsibilities. If the family feels overwhelmed, the physician can also arrange for additional help—registered nurses, homemakers, home health aides, Meals-on-Wheels, day care respite admission—to make the burden more tolerable. Finally, the physician's regular presence in the home, "making sure that everything is being done right," is an important reassurance. Professional recognition and praise for the patient, family, and other caretakers about the quality of their care can help to sustain these essential efforts.

## References


1. Master RJ, et al: A continuum of care for the inner city. N Engl J Med 302:1434, 1980.
*An urban academic group of primary care physicians and midlevel practitioners describe their experiences in caring for elderly patients in health centers, homes, nursing homes, and hospitals. Issues for discussion include physician recruitment, program costs, and possible reduction in hospitalization.*
2. Brickner PW: Home Health Care for the Aged. New York, Appleton-Century-Crofts, 1978.
*A detailed description of an urban community home care program, and thoughtful advice from a veteran clinician.*
3. Mather HG, Morgan DC, Pearson NG, et al: Myocardial infarction: A comparison between home and hospital care for patients. Br Med J 1:925, 1976.
*A landmark, randomized study comparing home care with hospital care for patients with acute uncomplicated myocardial infarction. Mortality was lower at home for patients aged 60 to 70.*
4. Billings JA: Palliative Care in Advanced Cancer. Philadelphia, J.B. Lippincott, 1984.
*A review of symptom control and home support in terminal illness.*
5. Currie CT, et al: Assessment of elderly patients at home. A report of fifty cases. J Am Geriatr Soc 24:398, 1981.
*In-home consultations by academic geriatricians regularly identified new diagnoses and suggested more effective home supports.*
6. Bailey AJM: Home visiting: The part played by the intermediary. JR Coll Gen Pract 29:137, 1979.
*A perceptive analysis of the family dynamics behind the request for a physician house call.*
7. Butler RN, Lewis MI: Aging and Mental Health. 2nd ed. St. Louis, C.V. Mosby Co., 1977, pp. 211–235.
*A very readable discussion of the formal supports that can be mobilized to keep elders at home.*
8. Lawson IR: The teaching of chronic illness and aging in home care settings. *In* Clark DW, Williams TF (eds.). Teaching of Chronic Illness and Aging. U.S. Government Printing Office, Publication No. 75-876, 1975, pp. 33–41.
*Through the experience of home visiting with faculty clinicians, medical students learn about chronic illness.*
9. Williams WC: The Farmer's Daughters: Collected Stories of William Carlos Williams. New York, New Directions Publishing Corp., 1961.
*William Carlos Williams was a poet, short story writer, and practicing physician who describes some of his house call experiences in these stories.*
10. U.S. Department of Health, Education, and Welfare: A Guide for Development and Administration of Coordinated Home Care Programs. Public Health Service Publication No. 1579, 1966.
*A dated, but still useful, review of organizational problems.*
11. Comptroller General of the United States: Home Health—The Need for a National Policy to Better Provide for the Elderly. General Accounting Office, HRD-78-19, December 30, 1979.
*A federal study of homebound elders, which developed a methodology for measuring the direct and "hidden" costs of maintaining an elder at home and which proposed a "break-even point" of impairment beyond which institutionalization would be less expensive than home care.*
12. Silverstone B, Hyman HK: You and Your Aging Parent. 2nd ed. New York, Pantheon Books, 1982.
*An excellent handbook of practical information for the supporters of vulnerable elders.*
13. Sanford JRA: Tolerance of debility in elderly dependents by supporters at home: Its significance for hospital practice. Br Med J 3:471, 1975.
*Article identifies the factors that lead family supporters to feel overwhelmed and to institutionalize their elderly dependents. Frequent critical impairments include sleep disturbances, incontinence, and falls.*


## *Additional Reading*


1. Elford RW, et al: A study of house calls in the practices of general practitioners Med Care. 10:178, 1972.
*Interesting data on a series of 703 house calls.*
2. U.S. General Accounting Office: The Elderly Should Benefit From Expanded Home Health Care but Increasing These Services Will Not Insure Cost Reductions. Report to the Chairman, Committee on Labor and Human Resources, U.S. Senate, December 7, 1982.
*A review of the current status of demonstration home health care projects.*

## Chapter 12

# Clinical Pharmacology: Special Considerations in the Elderly

*Barry J. Cusack*
*Robert E. Vestal*

The elderly form an important segment of the drug industry market. Because the prevalence of symptomatic disease is high in those over 65 years of age, drug expenditure by this population accounts for about 25 per cent of the total in developed countries.[1] There is also evidence that within this age group, drug consumption increases with age[2] and is higher in females than in males.[3] At this level of drug consumption, close cooperation between physician and patient is necessary to obtain maximum benefit with minimum risk. The unfortunate paradox is that the elderly who need such cooperation most, probably receive it least. Such patients are often less alert, more forgetful, and suffer from poor vision, deafness, or physical frailty. They often live alone, and social isolation attends their increasing disability and age. As their dependency increases, the ability of elderly patients to maintain communication with health care providers frequently deteriorates. Attitudes concerning aging also affect therapeutics in the elderly. Many aged patients attribute disease symptoms and drug-induced adverse effects to old age. The temptation to treat symptoms with drugs frequently produces polypharmacy. Added to this is the problem of age-associated change in drug kinetics and effects that may alter dose requirements. The end result is often inappropriate drug therapy and poor patient management, with frequent iatrogenic illness.

This chapter discusses particular problems related to drug prescribing for the elderly, with a view to developing a more rational basis for safe, effective therapy. Information accrued from pharmacologic research is outlined, and findings of clinical or methodologic significance are discussed. Methods of improving drug compliance are considered in some detail. The chapter also emphasizes that prescribing drugs is only a part of the therapeutic approach in geriatric medicine.

## ADVERSE DRUG REACTIONS

It is widely stated that adverse drug reactions (ADR) occur most commonly in the elderly,[4] but this statement needs careful analysis to determine both its validity and clinical significance.[5] The initial evidence indicating a higher incidence of adverse drug reactions in the aged came from prospective hospital studies.[4,6] Incidence of reactions increased with age in elderly patients so that in those over 80 years, the incidence was approximately twice as high as in those under 65. The rate of adverse reactions was also higher in patients receiving many drugs and in those who had suffered from previous adverse reactions. Unfortunately, neither of these factors (nor that of illness severity), which might have influenced the apparent age effect, were taken into account in these studies. It is significant that a more recent report showed that the increase in incidence of drug reactions with age reflected disease patterns rather than age per se.[7] The elderly in that study suffered more frequently from severe illness. In addition, data from other inpatient series have shown that there was no difference between the mean ages of those who did and those who did not suffer adverse drug reactions.[8-10] Thus, the evidence concerning the effect of aging on adverse drug reactions in hospital patients is inconclusive. Furthermore, many of these hospital-based studies included many mild reactions that were not of major clinical significance.

Reports of adverse drug reactions in community subjects indicate that iatrogenic disease is an important cause of hospital admission. Caranasos and associates[11] showed that 40 per cent of patients with adverse reactions to drugs causing hospitalization were elderly, and they suggested that such reactions occurred more frequently in this age group. Alternatively, their findings may simply reflect greater drug consumption or more serious disease in the aged than in the younger adults in their study population. Other reports also suggest that adverse reactions significantly contribute to hospitalization of elderly patients. Learoyd[12] reported that 16 per cent of 236 consecutive admissions to a psychogeriatric unit were due to adverse drug reactions mainly causing neurologic and somatic disturbances and that these patients responded to withdrawal of the offending therapy. In a large multicenter study of almost 2000 admissions to British geriatric units, adverse reactions were considered the sole cause for admission in 1.8 per cent and a contributing cause in 7.7 per cent.[13] Extrapolation of these figures to the country at large suggests that during each year in the United Kingdom, about 4000 admissions are solely and a further 11,000 partly due to adverse drug reactions. Over 5000 of these people would not be expected to make a full recovery from drug effects. Although the group was a biased selection from the general population, the report does strongly suggest that adverse reactions represent serious economic and health problems in the aged in the community.

The more common and important drug reactions that occur in the elderly in our experience are listed in Table 12–1. It should be noted that many drugs produce similar symptoms. Therefore, a drug history should always be taken in elderly patients, particularly when dealing with symptoms such as staggering gait, falls, confusion, urinary retention, incontinence, and hypothermia.

Some factors are associated with particular risk of adverse drug reactions in old age. Reports indicate that polypharmacy, previous adverse reactions, and prolonged exposure to drugs are associated with a higher reaction rate.[4] Certain drugs, such as antihypertensive, antiparkinson, hypnotic, and sedative agents, are associated with more severe reactions.[13] Patients with certain diseases also appear to be at greater risk. Demented patients, especially if they live alone, are apt to become confused by anticholinergic, antiparkinson, and psychotropic drugs. In our experience, anticholinergic agents, which include tricyclic antidepressants, certain antihistamines, major tranquilizers, and disopyramide, can cause urinary retention, which may be irreversible in those with prostatism. In those with open angle disease, precipitation of acute glaucoma appears to be unusual and may not be

**Table 12–1.** ADVERSE DRUG REACTIONS IN THE ELDERLY

| Type of Drug | Adverse Reactions |
|---|---|
| Aminoglycosides | Tinnitus, deafness, renal impairment |
| Analgesics | |
| Aspirin | Anemia |
| Nonsteroidal anti-inflammatory drugs | Anemia, fluid retention, confusion |
| Opiates | Drowsiness, respiratory depression, confusion, constipation |
| Anticholinergics | Glaucoma, urinary retention, constipation, visual hallucinations, confusion |
| Antidepressants (tricyclics) | Postural hypotension, drowsiness, confusion, anticholinergic effects, hypothermia, falls |
| Antihypertensives | Postural hypotension, falls |
| Barbiturates | Drowsiness, confusion, ataxia, falls, excitement, hypothermia |
| Beta-blockers | Peripheral cyanosis, cold extremities, dyspnea, wheezing |
| Corticosteroids | Peptic ulcer, diabetes mellitus, osteoporosis, poor wound healing, decreased resistance to infection, activation of tuberculosis |
| Digoxin | Arrhythmias, nausea, vomiting |
| Diuretics | Dehydration, hypokalemia, hyponatremia, postural hypotension, carbohydrate intolerance, hyperuricemia |
| Levodopa | Confusion, postural hypotension, dyskinesias |
| Hypnotics/sedatives | Drowsiness, confusion, ataxia, falls |
| Major tranquilizers | Drowsiness, postural hypotension, hypothermia, tardive dyskinesias, anticholinergic effects |

so catastrophic; if it is dealt with quickly, eyesight may not be lost and attention will have been brought to bear on the presence of this insidious disorder. Drug-induced postural hypotension occurs more commonly in patients with a pre-existing orthostatic defect. Therefore, in order to minimize the risk of causing adverse reactions, careful drug selection is required, considering both drug effects and the patient's susceptibilities. When possible, such as in some nursing homes, pharmacist drug surveillance helps to reduce the incidence of adverse reactions[14] and draws attention to such events to expedite appropriate changes of medication.[15]

Drug interactions probably occur more commonly as more drugs are used. One must be aware in particular of additive effects of drugs in causing adverse reactions in the elderly. Examples include antiparkinson agents and diuretics, causing postural hypotension; antidepressants and disopyramide, producing urinary retention; and potassium-sparing diuretics and potassium salts, causing hyperkalemia.

Over-the-counter drugs are widely used by the elderly[3] and may be the cause of adverse reactions. In particular, anemia may be caused by aspirin derivatives and drowsiness by antihistamine preparations.

In conclusion, drug reactions are a common and important source of morbidity in the elderly person, and their effects may lead to hospitalization, permanent disability, or death. Care must be taken not to compromise the frail elderly by misguided therapy.

## DRUG COMPLIANCE

Drug compliance should be regarded as a means to a therapeutic goal rather than as an end in itself. Thus, noncompliance is probably best considered as a level of nonadherence to drug therapy that interferes with attainment of the therapeutic goal. Although endeavors to maintain full compliance are justifiable, attempts to detect minor deviations may be of little clinical importance, since therapeutic effectiveness may not have been significantly diminished. Thus, the statement that compliance in adult groups with long-term medication is on the average only 50 per cent does not necessarily imply inadequate therapy in 50 per cent of patients.[16]

It is difficult, therefore, to precisely define and measure significant noncompliance. Measurement of steady-state plasma concentrations of a drug with a long half-life is the best available method at present, but this approach is not always applicable. Statements regarding the effect of aging on drug compliance must be viewed with some circumspection. It is widely said that aging alters drug compliance,[17] but there is no good evidence that this is so. Taggart and colleagues[18] observed no effect of age on compliance, as measured by plasma digoxin concentrations. A large community study in France indicated that compliance (measured by tablet count) was not affected by age, but increased risk of noncompliance appeared to be related to other factors, such as low memory score.[19] Polypharmacy with complex drug regimens is associated with reduced compliance in younger adults[20] as well as in the elderly.[21]

Although aging per se does not appear to compromise compliance significantly, clinical experience suggests that there is a subgroup of elderly patients who are less likely to adhere to therapeutic drug regimens. Those with poor vision, physical disability with subsequent difficulty in taking medication, and impaired mental function are indeed at risk, particularly when living alone. Attention must be directed toward patients with these disabilities.

Many methods of enhancing compliance have been attempted. Instructions and training in drug compliance should be regarded as part of the general rehabilitation program.[22,23] A short period of instruction in drug taking,[24] tear-off calendars, or use of simple explanatory drug regimen cards are useful.[25] Surprisingly, education of the elderly patient about his or her disease and its treatment does not enhance compliance.[26] Use of special color-coded packs can help compliance,[27] and it is our experience that multicompartment drug boxes are also useful. Since elderly patients have difficulty with label instructions and bottle tops,[28] clear labeling of bottles and use of easily opened containers should make compliance easier for those with poor vision, weak hands, or stiff fingers.

## PATTERNS OF DRUG PRESCRIBING FOR THE ELDERLY

In developed countries drug prescribing for the elderly is disproportionately high compared with the rest of the adult population. Despite differences in health care systems, there is a broadly similar rate of prescribing for the elderly in the United States,[29] Canada,[2,30] and the United Kingdom.[1] In these countries, the elderly constitute between 10 and 14 per cent of the total population but receive between 25 and

33 per cent of total drug prescriptions. Not only do more elderly people take drugs but also each individual consumes more drugs. One study cited that the average drug prescription rate rose from 3.0 drugs per patient in those aged 35 to 54 up to 4.5 drugs in those aged over 85.[2] There is good evidence that drug use increases with age in patients living in the community not only in North America[2,31] but also in the United Kingdom[32] and Sweden.[33] Use of over-the-counter drugs must also be considered. More than two thirds of elderly people of either sex in the United States[3] and a higher proportion of females in Canada[30] use over-the-counter drugs. In many cases, this higher rate of drug use may be warranted and appropriate, commensurate with the higher prevalence of chronic disease among the elderly.[34]

It is of interest to analyze the patterns of prescriptions for the elderly in order to consider what groups of drugs are more commonly prescribed and to whom they are given. This type of knowledge helps to pinpoint areas where habits of drug prescribing may not be optimal. It is apparent that among ambulatory patients, the use of both psychotropic and nonpsychotropic drugs increases with age in the United States. According to one report the most commonly prescribed drugs include analgesics (with codeine), methyldopa, furosemide, indomethacin, triamterene, hydrochlorothiazide, potassium chloride, chlorpropamide, thioridazine, and digoxin, in that order.[31]

Elderly institutionalized patients are expected to be more frail and more commonly subject to chronic disease. Consequently, it is not surprising that drug use is higher in this group than in those in the community. Use of psychotropics is considerably higher in nursing home patients than in community patients or in those attending day care.[31] In contrast with their findings in the community as mentioned previously, Zawadski and co-authors[31] reported that thioridazine, Hydergine, furosemide, digoxin, potassium chloride, chloral hydrate, haloperidol, analgesics (with codeine), and amitriptyline were the most commonly prescribed drugs in elderly patients in institutions.

Although greater use of psychotropics may be justifiably related to a higher incidence of psychiatric symptoms in nursing home patients, reviews of prescribing in nursing homes indicate that this is simply not the case. One report suggests that rural family practitioners with large nursing home practices are likely to prescribe more antipsychotic medicines than any other group of physicians.[35] Such drugs are most frequently prescribed in large nursing homes and in homes with one physician who provides the majority of care.

Examples are also cited of undefined criteria for pro re nata (p.r.n.) drug prescription, use of nonrecommended drugs,[36] use of drugs without proper indication, or in circumstances in which the action of drugs was judged to be unnecessary or ineffective.[37] Polypharmacy[38] and poorly supervised repeat drug prescription habits[36] have been other criticisms of prescribing in nursing homes.

The overall level of prescribing to the elderly in the community does not appear inordinately high, but analysis of individual drug use reveals some disquieting evidence of questionable prescribing practices. Thus, one would question the widespread use demonstrated in California of codeine, methyldopa, indomethacin, and thioridazine[31] because they may produce susceptibility to adverse reactions such as constipation, postural hypotension, depression, and confusion, respectively. Other drugs could be used that would tend to produce fewer adverse reactions. Second, although treatment of hypertension is of some value in patients under 75 years,[39] the widespread use of antihypertensive agents is not warranted in more elderly subjects in whom treatment has not yet been shown to be of value.[40] Third, it is surprising that major tranquilizers appear to be much more commonly prescribed than antidepressant drugs. This suggests underdiagnosis or mistreatment of depression in the elderly, a finding that has been noted elsewhere.[41]

In Saskatchewan, other questionable prescribing habits were reported, such as greater use of methyldopa and reserpine in the elderly, in whom the risk:benefit ratio of such antihypertensive treatment is high. Use of diazepam and flurazepam was also greater in the elderly despite their higher risk of adverse reactions.[42,43] Another particularly disappointing finding in the Saskatchewan report was a three- to fourfold increase in the number of prescriptions for phenobarbital and other barbiturates for aged patients, although it has been suggested for quite some time that they may cause paradoxical reactions, such as excitement,[44] and are associated with falls and fractures.[45] These adverse effects have not been observed in all studies, however.[46,47] Similarly, overprescription of iron to elderly patients has been reported in Sweden.[48] Unnecessary repeat prescribing for geriatric patients commonly occurs in family practices in the United Kingdom.[49]

It is apparent that elderly patients receive more drugs than the rest of the adult population. Also prescribing habits indicate many practices of polypharmacy and unnecessary or inappropriate prescribing with poor long-term follow-up of therapy. Elimination of such practices would both benefit the patient and reduce health care costs considerably.

## DRUG KINETICS

Pharmacokinetics is the study of the fate of a drug in the body, measuring, when possible, drug absorption, distribution, and elimination by hepatic and/or renal mechanisms. Such data are necessary in calculating dose requirements for therapeutic effect, and this knowledge is especially useful for prescribing drugs with a low therapeutic index (i.e., drugs in which there is a small difference between therapeutic and toxic dose).

Absorption refers to the passage of a drug from the site of administration, such as bowel or muscle sites. There are two independent aspects of absorption to consider—rate and extent of absorption. The rate of absorption of a drug is a major determinant of the time of onset of pharmacologic activity. Thus, rapid absorption is a useful property for analgesic and hypnotic drugs. Extent of absorption describes the amount of drug that passes through the absorptive surface into the body. It is not synonymous with the term "bioavailability," which denotes the fraction of administered drug that enters the systemic circulation. After oral drug administration, bioavailability is determined not only by the extent of absorption through bowel mucosa but also by presystemic drug elimination in the liver as the drug passes from the portal circulation. This distinction is important for some drugs, as is discussed later.

After absorption, the plasma concentration of a drug chiefly depends on the extent to which the drug distributes in the body—the wider the distribution, the lower the plasma level. The space in which a drug distributes is termed the apparent volume of distribution ($V_d$) and is a guide to loading dose requirements (the higher the $V_d$, the greater the dose required).

Drugs are chiefly eliminated by the hepatic or renal routes. Fat-soluble drugs cannot be cleared efficiently by the kidney because they are reabsorbed in the kidney tubule. These drugs are metabolized in the liver, and the more water-soluble metabolites (similar to water-soluble drugs) are then excreted through the kidney. The most definitive term describing drug elimination is clearance (Cl), which is the volume of plasma or blood cleared of drug per unit time. Plasma elimination half-life ($T_{½}$) is the time required for plasma drug concentration to fall to one half of the initial value during the phase of drug elimination. Half-life depends not only on clearance but also on volume of distribution. Hence, half-life is not necessarily an accurate index of rate of drug elimination.

Drugs administered on a chronic basis attain steady-state concentrations, which are directly related to the extent of drug absorption and inversely related to drug clearance. Since the extent of absorption of many drugs may not vary much among individuals, clearance is the important variable that determines individual steady-state concentrations. Elimination half-life is not related to steady-state concentration but is an index of the time required for drug concentration to attain steady-state concentration after inception of chronic therapy and also for drug elimination after cessation of chronic dose administration. In each case the time equals approximately four half-lives.

It is pertinent to consider the changes in human physiology and body composition in old age (Table 12–2) that indicate a basis for altered drug kinetics. Some of these changes do indeed effect a change in drug kinetics, such as renal drug excretion, but in other instances do not appear to alter the relevant kinetic parameter in any consistent way. It should also be remembered that most studies on changes in body physiology with age and, indeed, on drug pharmacokinetics with age are cross-sectional. True longitudinal studies would provide a more accurate picture of the aging process, but their prohibitive cost and the administrative difficulties of such studies preclude their widespread use.

### *Absorption of Drugs*

It has been reported that basal and peak gastric acid output declines with age, particularly in

**Table 12–2.** AGE-RELATED CHANGES IN BODY COMPOSITION AND PHYSIOLOGY

| Parameter | Change |
|---|---|
| Total body water[50] | ↓ |
| Lean body mass[51] | ↓ |
| Total body potassium[52] | ↓ |
| Total body fat[51] | ↑ |
| Serum albumin[53] | ↓ |
| Splanchnic blood flow[54] | ↓ |
| Small bowel surface area[55] | ↓ |
| Liver mass[56] | ↓ |
| Renal plasma flow[57] | ↓ |
| Creatinine clearance[58] | ↓ |
| Renal tubular function[59,60] | ↓ |

females.[61] Changes in gastric pH alter the lipid solubility of some drugs and hence absorption. However, the net effect of alterations in gastric pH is unpredictable, since a rise in pH may hasten gastric emptying, which in some cases enhances absorption.[62] The decline in splanchnic blood flow[54] and in small bowel surface area[55] with advancing age would lead one to consider that absorption might be delayed or reduced. However, it is apparent from Table 12–3 that age has little or no effect on drug absorption. In particular the rate of absorption of many drugs has been studied. Cusack and co-workers,[91] demonstrated a delay in digoxin absorption. Contrary findings have been observed in cases of metoprolol[89] and temazepam.[90] Extent of absorption appears to be unaffected by age.

The bioavailability of certain drugs such as lidocaine[74] and propranolol[80,96] (drugs that have high intrinsic clearance; see Hepatic Metabolism of Drugs, page 121) is greater in the elderly, reflecting less presystemic uptake of the drug. However, the opposite has been shown in the case of prazosin.[98] It is not clear, therefore, what effect age has on bioavailability of such drugs.

**Table 12–3.** EFFECT OF AGING ON DRUG ABSORPTION

| No Change | Increase | Decrease |
|---|---|---|
| | ***Rate of Absorption*** | |
| Acetaminophen[63,64] | Metoprolol[89] | Digoxin[91] |
| Ampicillin[65] | Temazepam[90] | |
| Antipyrine[66] | Chlordiazepoxide[92] | |
| Aspirin[66–69] | Chlormethiazole[93] | |
| Azapropazone[70] | | |
| Clobazam[71] | | |
| Diclofenac[72] | | |
| Levodopa[73] | | |
| Lidocaine[74] | | |
| Lormetazepam[75] | | |
| Mecillinam[76] | | |
| Oxazepam[77] | | |
| Practolol[78] | | |
| Propicillin K[79] | | |
| Propoxyphene[66] | | |
| Propranolol[80,81] | | |
| Propylthiouracil[82] | | |
| Quinine[69] | | |
| Sotalol[83] | | |
| Sulfamethiazole[63] | | |
| Temazepam[85] | | |
| Tetracycline[86] | | |
| Theophylline[87,88] | | |
| | ***Extent of Absorption or Bioavailability*** | |
| Acetaminophen[84] | Labetalol[97*] | Prazosin[98*] |
| Atenolol[94] | Lidocaine[74*] | |
| Cimetidine[95] | Propranolol[80*] | |
| Digoxin[91] | | |
| Lormetazepam[75] | | |
| Propranolol[96*] | | |
| Propylthiouracil[82] | | |
| Ranitidine[99] | | |
| Sotalol[83] | | |
| Sulfamethiazole[63] | | |

* Bioavailability influenced by presystemic extraction.

## *Distribution of Drugs*

The distribution of drugs is considered to be largely determined by physicochemical properties. Fat-soluble (nonpolar) drugs cross membranes more easily and spread widely, with particular uptake in adipose tissue. Water-soluble (polar) drugs tend to cross barriers less easily and are largely confined to lean body tissue. Thus, since body fat in man tends to rise and lean body mass to fall with age, one would expect that fat-soluble drugs distribute more widely and polar drugs less widely in the elderly. According to expectations, the volume of distribution of most fat-soluble drugs, such as diazepam,[126,129] thiopental,[133,134] chlordiazepoxide,[92,123] and chlormethiazole,[102] increases with age (Table 12–4). However, for other fat-soluble drugs such as amobarbital,[102] lorazepam,[112,113] and lormetazepam,[75] volume of distribution is not greater in old age. There is therefore a tendency, albeit with some exceptions, for more extensive distribution of fat-soluble drugs in the elderly. With regard to water-soluble drugs, such as cimetidine,[95,139] digoxin,[91] ethanol,[140] and antipyrine,[119,136,138] volume of distribution declines with age. These findings show a good accord with predictions, but again, of course, there are some exceptions, such as pancuronium[117,118] and tobramycin.[121]

There appears to be a tendency toward lower protein binding of drugs in old age (Table 12–5), related to the decline in serum albumin concentrations.[53]* However, lidocaine, which is bound primarily to alpha-1-acid-glycoprotein (AGP), shows higher protein binding in the elderly.[74] Changes in protein binding with resultant shifts in free drug concentration are of particular importance in acute drug administration. On the other hand, with chronic dosing, free-drug concentrations tend to "renormalize," and age changes in drug binding may not be as important in this situation.

* This decline appears to be related to factors such as the presence of disease rather than to advanced age per se.

**Table 12-4.** RELATIONSHIP BETWEEN VOLUME OF DISTRIBUTION AND AGING

| No Change | Increase | Decrease |
|---|---|---|
| Acetaminophen[63,100] | Acetaminophen[64] | Antipyrine[119,136–138] |
| Acetanilid[101] | Aspirin[68] | Cimetidine[95,139] |
| Ampicillin[65] | Chlordiazepoxide[123] | Digoxin[91] |
| Amobarbital[102] | Chlormethiazole[124] | Ethanol[140] |
| Antipyrine[103] | Clobazam[71] | Gentamycin[141] |
| Aspirin[69] | Desmethyldiazepam[125] | Kanamycin[141] |
| Atenolol[94] | Diazepam[126–129] | Lorazepam[113] |
| Azapropazone[70] | Lidocaine[130] | Meperidine[142] |
| Carbenoxolone[104] | Midazolam[131] | Phenytoin[119*] |
| Desmethyldiazepam[105,106] | Oxazepam[132] | Propicillin K[79] |
| Diazepam[107] | Prazosin[98] | Quinine[69] |
| Digitoxin[108] | Thiopental[133,134] | Sotalol[83] |
| Diphenhydramine[109] | Tolbutamide[135] | Theophylline[143*] |
| Flurazepam[110] | | |
| Heparin[111] | | |
| Labetalol[97] | | |
| Lidocaine[74] | | |
| Lorazepam[112,113] | | |
| Lormetazepam[75] | | |
| Meperidine[114] | | |
| Nitrazepam[115] | | |
| Oxazepam[96,116] | | |
| Pancuronium[117,118] | | |
| Phenylbutazone[63] | | |
| Phenytoin[119†] | | |
| Propranolol[80] | | |
| Propylthiouracil[82] | | |
| Quinidine[120] | | |
| Sulfamethiazole[63] | | |
| Temazepam[85] | | |
| Theophylline[87] | | |
| Tobramycin[121] | | |
| Warfarin[122] | | |

* For free drug.
† For total drug.

**Table 12-5.** EFFECT OF AGING ON PLASMA PROTEIN BINDING OF DRUGS

| No Change | Increase | Decrease |
|---|---|---|
| Etomidate[152] | Lidocaine[74†] | Cimetidine[139] |
| Haloperidol[153,154] | | Carbenoxolone[104] |
| Meperidine[142] | | Chlormethiazole[93] |
| Phenytoin[146] | | Furosemide[144] |
| Quinidine[120] | | Meperidine[145] |
| Warfarin[122,155] | | Penicillin G[146] |
| | | Phenobarbital[146] |
| | | Phenylbutazone[147*] |
| | | Phenytoin[119,148,149] |
| | | Salicyclic acid[147*] |
| | | Sulfadiazine[147*] |
| | | Theophylline[143] |
| | | Thiopental[134] |
| | | Tolbutamide[135,150] |
| | | Warfarin[151] |

* No difference as a result of age was observed in those on no drugs, but binding in elderly on multidrug therapy was less than in drug-free young adults.
† Bound to $\alpha$-1-acid glycoprotein.

## *Hepatic Metabolism of Drugs*

The effect of aging on liver function has been examined in some detail. Routine liver function tests are relatively crude and show no age relationship.[156] Some investigators have demonstrated altered bromosulphthalein (BSP) retention[156] and indocyanine green (ICG) clearance[157] in the elderly. These changes may reflect changes in hepatic blood flow rather than in liver function[157] and are consistent with findings of reduced splanchnic blood flow in older patients.[54]

Hepatic drug metabolism follows two physiologic patterns.[158] For drugs that are metabolized relatively slowly by the liver (low intrinsic clearance), the rate-limiting step in their clearance is the rate of metabolism. Such metabolism is said to be capacity-limited. For drugs with a very rapid rate of metabolism (high intrinsic clearance), the rate-limiting step in metabolism is the speed of delivery of the drug to the liver, namely hepatic blood flow. This latter form is described as flow-limited metabolism. In addition, bioavailability of such drugs is limited because of presystemic hepatic metabolism. Finally, other drugs such as propranolol have intermediate properties, with metabolism that is partly dependent on both physiologic parameters. This discussion is relevant to the consideration of age-related drug metabolism. Since biochemical evidence does not demonstrate any particular change in hepatic function with age, one might expect insignificant alterations in capacity-related drug metabolism. Second, the demonstrated fall in splanchnic blood flow with age[54] would predict slower elimination in the elderly of drugs with metabolism that is flow-limited. Finally, for drugs with intermediate properties, any changes in rate of elimination in the elderly would depend on the age dependence of the physiologic parameter with overriding influence on metabolism.

Effects of increasing age on half-life and clearance of metabolized drugs are shown in Tables 12–6 and 12–7, respectively. Antipyrine is regarded as a model drug, which undergoes capacity-limited metabolism by the hepatic microsomal enzyme system. Initial findings with this drug demonstrated an age-dependent decline in the rate of metabolism.[160] Some[119,136,138] but not all[162] further studies confirmed this observation. Clearance of other drugs metabolized by microsomal systems, such as diazepam,[107,126,127,129] desmethyldiazepam,[71,105] and lorazepam,[112,113] shows no definite trend with age. Similarly, rates of elimination of drugs metabolized by nonmicrosomal systems, such as acetaminophen,[63,64,84,100] carbenoxolone,[104] isoniazid,[159] and ethanol,[140] do not show age dependence. It is interesting that in some studies, clearance of phenytoin[148] and tolbutamide[135] appears to be greater in old age, but this may be related to lower protein binding[135,148] rather than altered metabolism per se. Therefore, the current impression is that aging appears to have no clear-cut influence on drug metabolism.

**Table 12–6.** EFFECT OF AGING ON HALF-LIFE OF METABOLIZED DRUGS

| No Change | Increase |
|---|---|
| Acetaminophen[63,64,86] | Acetaminophen[100] |
| Acetanilid[101] | Acetanilid[159] |
| Antipyrine[162] | Amobarbital[102] |
| Antipyrine[137]† | Antipyrine[103,119,136,160] |
| Chlordiazepoxide[92] | Antipyrine[137]* |
| Chlorpropamide[165] | Carbenoxolone[104] |
| Diazepam[107] | Clobazam[71] |
| Digitoxin[108] | Chlordiazepoxide[123] |
| Diphenhydramine[109] | Chlormethiazole[93] |
| Flunitrazepam[110] | Desmethyldiazepam[71,105] |
| Heparin[111] | Desmethylimipramine[161] |
| Imipramine[161] | Diazepam[126–129] |
| Isoniazid[159] | Indocyanine green[162] |
| Lorazepam[112,113] | Labetalol[97] |
| Lormetazepam[75] | Lignocaine[74,130] |
| Meperidine[142] | Meperidine[114] |
| Metoprolol[89] | Nitrazepam[163] |
| Midazolam[131] | Nortriptyline[164] |
| Morphine[166] | Prazosin[98] |
| Nitrazepam[115] | Propranolol[80] |
| Oxazepam[77,116,132] | Salicylate[68] |
| Phenylbutazone[63,160] | Thiopental[133,134] |
| Phenytoin[119] | |
| Propranolol[96] | |
| Quinine[69] | |
| Temazepam[85,90] | |
| Theophylline[87,143] | |
| Tobutamide[167,168] | |
| Warfarin[122] | |

* Comparison of young and elderly healthy volunteers.
† Comparison of young volunteers with elderly patients.

Many of these investigations were not carefully controlled to exclude the effects of environmental factors, such as smoking, environmental pollution, and diet, which can alter drug metabolism. In addition, many studies compared young healthy adults with elderly patients, hence not accounting for any effect of disease and medications on drug metabolism.

Some of these investigations examined the effects of certain environmental factors and age on drug metabolism. Vestal and associates[96,162] and Wood and associates[162] investigated the relationship of smoking and age with metabolism of drugs having low (antipyrine), intermediate (propranolol), and high (indocyanine green) intrinsic clearance. The rate of metabolism of antipyrine did not change with age in nonsmokers but fell with age in smokers. This suggested that smoking produced an enzyme induction effect, with an enhanced rate of metabolism, in the young but not in the elderly. Flow-related metabolism (indocyanine green) declined with age in smokers and nonsmokers alike, reflecting lower apparent hepatic blood flow in the elderly. Clearance of the drug with intermediate metabolism (propranolol) was not age-related in nonsmokers but in smokers did show a slower rate of metabolism in old age. These and other findings[69] suggest that smoking produces a response of enzyme induction in young adults, which is blunted in elderly subjects. However, there is evidence to the contrary suggesting that smoking may indeed affect enzyme induction in old age.[87]

Swift and colleagues[137] examined the effect of aging and hospitalization on antipyrine metabolism. Comparison of clearance of antipyrine in

**Table 12–7.** CHANGES IN CLEARANCE OF METABOLIZED DRUGS IN THE ELDERLY

| No Change | Increase | Decrease |
|---|---|---|
| Acetaminophen[63,64,100] | Phenytoin[148] | Acetaminophen[84] |
| Acetanilid[101] | Theophylline[88] | Antipyrine[119,136,138] |
| Antipyrine[136†] | Thiopental[133] | Antipyrine[137**] |
| Antipyrine[162‖] | Tolbutamide[135] | Carbenoxolone[104] |
| Aspirin[68,69] | | Clobazam[71*] |
| Diazepam[107,126] | | Chlordiazepoxide[92,123] |
| Diclofenac[72] | | Chlormethiazole[93] |
| Digitoxin[108] | | Desmethyldiazepam[71*] |
| Diphenhydramine[109] | | Desmethyldiazepam[105] |
| Ethanol[140] | | Diazepam[127,129‡] |
| Flunitrazepam[110] | | Diazepam[128] |
| Heparin[111] | | Indocyanine green[162] |
| Labetalol[97] | | Lorazepam[113] |
| Lidocaine[74,130] | | Meperidine[114] |
| Lorazepam[112] | | Norepinephrine[169] |
| Lormetazepam[75] | | Nortriptyline[164] |
| Midazolam[131] | | Phenytoin[119‡] |
| Nitrazepam[163] | | Propranolol[80] |
| Oxazepam[77,116,132] | | Quinidine[170] |
| Phenytoin[119§] | | Quinine[69] |
| Prazosin[98] | | Theophylline[171] |
| Propranolol[81,96] | | Theophylline[143‡] |
| Propylthiouracil[82] | | |
| Temazepam[85] | | |
| Theophylline[87,172] | | |
| Thiopental[134] | | |
| Tolbutamide[167] | | |
| Warfarin[122,155] | | |

* In males only; no change in females.
† In elderly hospitalized patients compared with a healthy young control group.
‡ Free clearance.
§ Total clearance.
‖ In nonsmokers only.
** In healthy subjects only.

groups of healthy young and elderly ambulant volunteers showed that clearance was lower in the elderly group. However, mean clearance in a group of elderly hospital patients was similar to that in the young volunteers and was significantly greater than the value in elderly healthy volunteers. These observations suggested an induction effect on antipyrine metabolism in the elderly patients, possibly related to hospitalization or due to other drugs.

It is apparent from these studies that the effect of environmental factors may obscure any possible modification of drug metabolism caused by age. Subjects must be selected carefully in an attempt to limit environmental effects in these cross-sectional studies. Since few investigations performed to date adequately meet such standards, our knowledge of the influence of age on drug metabolism is still not adequate. It appears that capacity-related metabolism is variably and not greatly altered by age, whereas flow-related metabolism declines with age.

## *Renal Elimination of Drugs*

Both glomerular and tubular renal function declines with age, as shown in Table 12–2. One would therefore expect renal elimination of drugs to show a similar change. It is significant that mean rate of elimination of drugs that are cleared by the kidney is consistently lower in aged subjects (Table 12–8). This is also true of drugs such as penicillin,[182,183] which depend on tubular function for elimination. However, it must be remembered that these studies compare mean values in groups of individuals. When any one study is considered, it is apparent that there is wide interindividual variation in the rate of renal elimination of drugs in the elderly group. This consideration must be borne in mind when prescribing drugs for elderly patients. As a group, the elderly require a lower average dose; in a given patient, the dose may need to be adjusted, depending on the individual renal function of that patient.

**Table 12-8.** CHANGES IN RENAL ELIMINATION OF DRUGS IN OLD AGE*

| No Change | Decrease |
|---|---|
| | Acetylprocainamide[173] |
| Practolol[78] | Ampicillin[65] |
| Tobramycin[121] | Atenolol[81] |
| | Azapropazone[70] |
| | Cefuroxime[174] |
| | Cephradine[175] |
| | Cimetidine[95,139] |
| | Digoxin[91,176] |
| | Dihydrostreptomycin[177] |
| | Doxycycline[178] |
| | Gentamycin[141] |
| | Kanamycin[179] |
| | Lithium[180,181] |
| | Pancuronium[117,118] |
| | Penicillin[182,183] |
| | Phenobarbital[184] |
| | Procainamide[173] |
| | Propicillin[79] |
| | Sotalol[83] |
| | Sulfamethiazole[63] |
| | Tetracycline[86,177] |

* Indicated by changes in elimination half-life and/or systemic clearance.

**Table 12-9.** RELATIONSHIP OF AGING TO STEADY-STATE DRUG CONCENTRATIONS IN PLASMA

| No Change | Increase | Decrease |
|---|---|---|
| Nortriptyline[163] | Amitriptyline[161] | Diazepam[192] |
| Propranolol[96,189*] | Desipramine[161] | Phenytoin[193] |
| Warfarin[155,194] | Diazepam[129] | |
| | Hydroxydesipramine[185] | |
| | Imipramine[161] | |
| | Insulin[186] | |
| | Mianserin[187] | |
| | Phenytoin[188†] | |
| | Propranolol[96,189‡] | |
| | Salicylate metabolites[190] | |
| | Theophylline[191] | |

* In nonsmokers.
† Serum phenytoin concentrations measured.
‡ In cigarette smokers only.

## *Steady-State Drug Kinetics*

Evaluation of the effect of aging on steady-state drug concentrations in plasma with chronic dose administration is of particular clinical applicability, since most drugs are given in this way. As previously discussed, steady-state drug concentrations are primarily determined by two variables, bioavailability and systemic drug clearance. Both of these parameters can be estimated from single-dose studies, but the conclusions may not be capable of extrapolation to the chronic dosing situation. Hence, the importance of examining steady-state kinetics is readily apparent.

A number of drugs have been studied and are listed in Table 12-9. Generally, higher plasma concentrations are found in older subjects, and certain examples are of particular interest because they raise issues of importance in the interpretation of these data. In an investigation of the effect of aging on antidepressant drug concentrations,[161] the authors reported significantly higher plasma concentrations of imipramine and its active metabolite desipramine in elderly patients. Amitriptyline plasma concentrations were also higher, but values for its metabolite, nortriptyline, were not age-dependent. The authors concluded that, with the exception of nortriptyline, doses of these drugs ought to be reduced in the elderly. The study also emphasizes the importance of considering age-related kinetics of active or toxic metabolites when deciding drug dosage. Imipramine has another active metabolite called hydroxydesipramine, which attains higher steady-state concentrations, probably due to lower renal clearance in aged patients.[185] Likewise, although kinetics of nortriptyline do not warrant dose amendment, possible lower renal elimination of its active metabolite 10-hydroxynortriptyline[195] may necessitate dose reduction in elderly patients.

It is difficult to explain the disparate results of the two reports of diazepam concentrations in relation to age.[129,192] However, these studies highlight the need to control other variables. Most subjects were outpatients, and good compliance was not documented. Second, smoking and concomitant drug ingestion in these patients may have confounded results.

Two groups of workers have demonstrated that propranolol steady-state concentrations are higher in elderly smokers but not in nonsmokers.[96,189] Both groups concluded that aging had no direct effect on steady-state kinetics of propranolol but that it did attenuate the acceleration of metabolism due to smoking. Feeley and associates[189] also reported that a disease state, such as hyperthyroidism, can have an age-dependent inducing effect on propranolol kinetics.

Although findings of steady-state kinetic studies are useful from a clinical perspective, they must be interpreted with caution because they are more frequently performed in patients rather than in healthy subjects, and the effects of other variables, such as disease, compliance, concomitant drug therapy, and smoking, are generally not adequately accounted for. Nevertheless, these reports contain some guidelines that help in selection of a starting dose level in patients. Common sense would dictate that the dose must be subsequently adjusted according to the patient's progress.

## PHARMACODYNAMICS

The study of pharmacodynamics refers to measurement of the effect of drugs in the body. The effect of a given dose of drug may vary among different individuals, depending on the sensitivity of each individual to the drug. This section examines the results of investigations designed to measure the influence of aging on drug sensitivity. Reports concerning drug toxicity that yield indirect evidence of altered drug sensitivity are not included because much of this information is dealt with elsewhere in this book and because conclusions regarding dynamics based on indirect evidence may not be quite accurate. Examination of Table 12–10 indicates that cardiovascular drugs, sedatives, anticoagulants, and analgesics are the drug classes that have been most frequently studied. This is because these drugs have readily measurable effects. Reports have also indicated an apparently higher risk of adverse reactions in aged patients to some of these drugs, such as benzodiazepines,[42] digoxin,[4] beta-blockers,[214] and anticoagulants.[215]

Studies comparing drug dynamics between groups should measure plasma drug concentrations or pharmacokinetic parameters in the individuals examined. Unless this is done, it cannot be certain whether any observed difference in pharmacologic effect is due to altered sensitivity in itself or to altered drug kinetics. It should be noted that many studies in Table 12–10 are deficient in this respect.

In addition, it sometimes can be difficult to evaluate the importance of drug concentrations in plasma, especially in relation to an acute drug effect. For example, the two investigations of the acute sedative effect of diazepam in patients

**Table 12–10.** PHARMACODYNAMICS AND AGING

| Drug | Plasma Levels Measured | Age Change In Dynamics | Method of Measurement of Effect |
|---|---|---|---|
| Antidepressants[211†] | No | ↔ | Systolic-time intervals |
| Chlormethiazole[94] | Yes | ↔ | Psychomotor function, postural sway |
| Chlormethiazole[196] | Yes | ↑ | Choice reaction time, flicker-fusion threshold, postural sway |
| Coumarins[197*] | No | ↑ | Prothrombin time |
| Deslanoside[198] | No | ↔ | Systolic time intervals |
| Diazepam[199] | Yes | ↑ | Sedation for endoscopy |
| Diazepam[200] | Yes | ↑ | Sedation for cardioversion |
| Diazepam[201] | No | ↑ | Postural sway |
| Dichloralphenazone[196] | Yes | ↑ | Postural sway |
| Diphenhydramine[109] | Yes | ↔ | Psychomotor function |
| Heparin[202] | Yes | ↔ | Activated partial thromboplastin time |
| Isoproterenol[203] | No | ↓ | Chronotropic effect |
| Isoproterenol[204] | No | ↓ | Forearm blood flow, chronotropic effect, renin-output response |
| Isoproterenol[205] | No | ↓ | Chronotropic effect |
| Levodopa[206] | No | ?↑ | Dose limitation due to side effects |
| Morphine[207] | No | ↑ | Analgesic effect |
| Morphine[208] | No | ↑ | Extent and duration of pain relief |
| Nitrazepam[115] | Yes | ↑ | Psychomotor function, sedation |
| Pentazocine[207] | No | ↑ | Analgesic effect |
| Propranolol[205] | Yes | ↑ | Chronotropic effect |
| Temazepam[94] | Yes | ↔ | Psychomotor function, postural sway, electroencephalogram |
| Temazepam[209] | Yes | ↑ | Postural sway, flicker-fusion threshold, choice-reaction time, sedation |
| Tolbutamide[210] | No | ↓ | Hypoglycemic effect |
| Warfarin[212] | No | ↑ | Thrombotest |
| Warfarin[122] | Yes | ↑ | Prothrombin time, clotting factor synthesis |
| Warfarin[213‡] | No | ↑ | Prothrombin time |

* Including warfarin, phenoprocoumarin, bishydroxycoumarin.
† Including amitriptyline, trimipramine, imipramine, maprotiline, and mianserin.
‡ Only in patients treated for thromboembolic disease and coronary artery disease and not in patients with peripheral vascular disease or valvular heart disease.

showed that plasma concentrations at which standard sedation was achieved were lower in the elderly.[199,200] This suggests a greater effect of diazepam in old age; however, this response could also be due to more rapid distribution of the drug to the brain. Thus, although they are obviously of clinical value, the merit of such studies in elucidating the mechanisms of age differences in pharmacologic responses is limited.

Elderly subjects appear to be more sensitive to depressant effects of neuroactive drugs such as diazepam,[199,200] nitrazepam,[113] and morphine.[207,208] Results of some of these studies are open to question. For example, Giles and coworkers[199] noted that the effect of diazepam was less evident in those on chronic diazepam therapy. Inclusion of this factor in the age analysis renders the age effect insignificant. Again this is an illustration of the fact that careful subject selection is required when performing a study. Similarly, diseases may alter the influence of age on drug sensitivity. A retrospective study indicated that lower doses of warfarin were required to produce standard anticoagulation in old age.[212] When indications for anticoagulants were considered in a subsequent report, this age relationship was true for patients treated for thromboembolic disease and coronary artery disease but not for those given warfarin for peripheral arterial disease or valvular heart disease.[213]

One must also be cautious in interpreting studies showing no difference between young and elderly subjects. For instance, the report of Briggs and associates,[90] showing no age difference in effects of temazepam and chlormethiazole has been criticized by others on the grounds of insufficiently sensitive techniques for measuring drug effects[201] and small sample size, together with suboptimal study design and data analysis.[216]

Drugs acting on the sympathetic nervous system have been investigated in vivo and in vitro. In vivo sensitivity of the cardiac beta-adrenergic receptor to propranolol[205] and isoproterenol[203,205] appears to decline with age. In vitro studies of activation by isoproterenol of lymphocyte beta-adrenoceptors (as measured by cyclic adenosine monophosphate [AMP] response) have confirmed these observations,[217,218] albeit with some dissent.[219] Some authors ascribed this change in beta-receptor sensitivity to lower receptor density in target organs or to lesser agonist affinity,[221,222] but these findings were later disputed.[220,226] Furthermore, it has been demonstrated that stimulation of lymphocyte cyclic AMP by prostaglandin $E_1$ (which is independent of adrenoceptor mechanisms) is less in the elderly.[218] These workers later demonstrated that the probable mechanism of attenuated cyclic AMP response in lymphocytes of elderly subjects to beta-adrenoceptor stimulation is due to alteration of cell membranes rather than to an intrinsic receptor change in itself.[223] The impact of aging on alpha-adrenoceptor sensitivity has also been examined. Studies performed on isolated perfused arteries[224,225] and veins[225] showed no age dependence.

Although Jick and associates[215] reported an increasing frequency of heparin toxicity with age (especially in females), more recent evidence[202] indicates that the heparin effect is not age-dependent. The apparent age relationship noted by Jick and colleagues may have been due to possible epiphenomena, such as age-related changes in serum protein concentrations or coagulation factors, which are good predictive indices of heparin requirements.

Information on drug effects in old age is still patchy and at times unclear. More extensive investigation is required to provide the clinician with a more rational basis for therapeutic decision-making. A better knowledge of the quantitative effect of dynamic interactions of drugs in the elderly would also be of value to the clinician.

## IMPROVEMENT OF DRUG PRESCRIBING TECHNIQUES

Many authors have written on the subject of prescribing, and we shall attempt to combine what we consider to be their most helpful suggestions with practices we have found beneficial in our own clinical experience.

### *Know the Drug*

"Know the drug" is an often repeated statement that is certainly germane to geriatric medicine. There is no doubt that it is better to be familiar with a few rather than slightly acquainted with many drugs. A physician who uses many drugs is not necessarily better than the physician who uses a small select number of drugs. It is important to know the general pharmacology of the drugs one uses, including potential for drug interactions. This latter skill is vital when prescribing many drugs for one patient, a common occurrence in geriatric practice.

Knowledge of age-related pharmacology helps one to select an appropriate dose for an elderly patient. In the case of a drug excreted by the kidney, one should use a dose that is one third to one half less than the standard adult dose. In the case of metabolized drugs, the same general rule of thumb applies at least for initial prescribing. This guideline is especially important for drugs having a narrow therapeutic index, such as aminoglycosides, digoxin, lithium, antiarrhythmic drugs, theophylline, and major tranquilizers. Initial maintenance doses may require subsequent adjustment in light of the patient's progress. For many other drugs with a higher therapeutic index, such as penicillins, the average adult dose may not need amendment. However, when there is an indication to use maximal doses of any drug, such as penicillins, a lower maximum dose should always be used in elderly patients. It is also important to realize that certain drugs, such as digoxin and diazepam, that have particularly long half-lives in the elderly may only achieve steady-state plasma concentrations well after 1 week of use, when maximum effect is achieved or adverse reactions become apparent.

## *Encourage Compliance*

In our experience one of the most important aspects of therapy in the elderly is promotion of compliance. Many old patients will present no problem, but special care and arrangements are required for mildly demented or frail patients, especially those living alone. One should endeavor to prescribe as few drugs as possible. This reduces the risk not only of poor compliance but also of adverse drug reaction. Schedules of drug dosage should be simplified to a once or twice daily regimen if possible. Easily opened containers should be used and should be labeled with large type outlining the drug regimen. These arrangements can be made simply by contacting local pharmacists. It is advisable to ensure that the patient receives simple, clear instructions concerning the drug regimen. Instruction cards and other educational devices are useful but obviously less so than aid and supervision provided by relatives, friends, or neighbors, whose help should be actively recruited. On occasion a patient may manage a multicompartment pill tray filled once weekly by a responsible caretaker, such as a relative or visiting nurse. Thus, one adapts the compliance-aid technique to the individual needs of the patient. At subsequent visits, one must always avail of the opportunity to check that the patient still understands the regimen and is adhering to it. A simple and effective way to do this is to insist that each patient brings in all medications at each visit. The patient can then be questioned about how often pills are taken from each bottle; this is a simple way to check the patient's understanding of the regimen. One can also reiterate what each type of medication is for and emphasize the importance of correct compliance with more essential medication. This also helps to prevent patients from taking some pills for wrong indications, such as digoxin for pain. Occasional spot checks by pill count can also be used to check compliance with the drug regimen. One can also check to see if the patient can open the container. This procedure is time-consuming but useful and can be fitted in by good management. For instance, most of this compliance evaluation and prevention procedure can be conducted by a clinic or visiting nurse. It must also be established whether the patient is taking other pills without the physician's knowledge. If possible, a responsible person should check the home for other hoarded medications. Over-the-counter medications must be considered in this search. Noncompliance may also be due to drug interaction or other adverse complications.

## *Monitor and Review Therapy Periodically*

In reviewing therapy one should not only monitor the efficacy and potential hazards of the regimen but also question the indication for each component of that regimen. For instance, one may be able to reduce or stop the use of hypnotics, diuretics, antihypertensive agents, or tranquilizers, to name a few examples. The use of digoxin can be frequently stopped in patients with sinus rhythm, without any adverse effect.

Careful scrutiny for presence of adverse drug reactions is also necessary. In the elderly, one should always consider drugs in the differential diagnosis of any new symptoms, especially falls, confusion, forgetfulness, and incontinence. Of course, geriatric patients also suffer from specific adverse reactions.

Finally, it is worth remembering that *non-drug therapy is not therapeutic nihilism.* Many conditions such as stroke, frailty with poor mobility, or dementia are not indications for drug therapy unless attended by complicating factors. The art of medicine is still extant in these situations. Such patients can respond to caring attitudes, discussion, and emotional support.

One ought to remember the words of the bard in these situations: "A body yet distemper'd which to his former strength may be restored with good advice and little medicine."[226] It is certainly true that good advice regarding self-care, good use of social facilities, and appropriate recruitment of paramedical therapeutic skills can greatly improve the quality of life of many elderly patients. Geriatric therapeutics is a sophisticated, comprehensive program that entails more than simply prescribing pills. One must always regard drug prescribing as only one facet of patient management.

### Acknowledgments

The authors are grateful to June Bush, Gayle Cory, and Patricia Martinez for their assistance with the preparation of the manuscript.

### References

1. Vestal RE: Pharmacology and aging. J Am Geriatr Soc 30:191, 1982.
   *This review discusses many of the problems of drug therapy in the aged.*
2. Skoll SL, August RJ, Johnson GE: Drug prescribing for the elderly in Saskatchewan during 1976. Can Med Assoc J 121:1074, 1979.
   *A large community survey of habits of drug prescribing for the elderly. Contains useful age-related comparative data.*
3. Guttmann D: Patterns of legal drug use by older Americans. Addict Dis Int J 3:337, 1978.
4. Hurwitz N: Predisposing factors in adverse reactions to drugs. Br Med J 1:536, 1969.
5. Klein LE, Gedman PS, Levine DM: Adverse drug reactions among the elderly: A re-assessment. J Am Geriatr Soc 29:525, 1981.
   *A very good review of adverse drug reactions.*
6. Seidl LG, Thornton GF, Smith JW, Cluff LE: Studies on the epidemiology of adverse drug reactions. 3. Reactions in patients in a general medical service. Bull Johns Hopkins Hosp 119:299, 1966.
7. Steel K, Gertman PM, Crescenzi C, Anderson J: Iatrogenic illness on a general medical service at a university hospital. N Engl J Med 304:638, 1981.
   *The report documents adverse effects due to procedures as well as due to drugs.*
8. Smith JW, Seidl LG, Cluff LE: Studies on the epidemiology of adverse drug reactions. V. clinical factors influencing susceptibility. Ann Intern Med 65:629, 1966.
9. Schimmel EM: The hazards of hospitalization. Ann Intern Med 60:100, 1964.
10. Ogilvie RI, Ruedy J: Adverse drug reactions during hospitalization. Can Med Assoc J 97:1450, 1967.
11. Caranasos GJ, Stewart RB, Cluff LE: Drug induced illness leading to hospitalization. JAMA 228:713, 1974.
12. Learoyd BM: Psychotropic drugs and the elderly patient. Med J Aust 1:1131, 1972.
13. Williamson J, Chopin JM: Adverse reactions to prescribed drugs in the elderly. A multicentre investigation. Age Ageing 9:73, 1980.
   *This is a survey of admissions of patients to geriatric units in the United Kingdom as a result of adverse drug reactions. A large number of subjects were included.*
14. Mutnick AH, Swanson LN: Clinical pharmacist intervention in an extended care facility, using an individualized method for digoxin dosing. Drug Intell Clin Pharm 14:507, 1980.
15. Segal JL, Thompson JF, Floyd RA: Drug utilization and prescribing patterns in a skilled nursing facility: The need for a rational approach to therapeutics. J Am Geriatr Soc 27:117, 1979.
16. O'Hanrahan M, O'Malley K: Compliance with drug treatment. Br Med J 283:298, 1981.
   *A good, well-argued review of drug compliance.*
17. Blackwell B: Drug therapy. Patient compliance. N Engl J Med 289:249, 1973.
18. Taggart AJ, Johnson GD, McDevitt DG: Does the frequency of daily dosage influence compliance with digoxin therapy? Br J Clin Pharmacol 11:31, 1981.
19. Spriet A, Beiler D, Dechorgrat J, Simon P: Adherence of elderly patients to treatment with pentoxifylline. Clin Pharmocol Ther 27:1, 1980.
20. Weintraub M, Au WY, Lasagna L: Compliance as a determinant of serum digoxin concentrations. JAMA 224:481, 1973.
21. Hemminki E, Heikkila J: Elderly people's compliance with prescriptions and the quality of medication. Scand J Soc Med 3:87, 1975.
22. Baxendale C, Gourlay M, Gibson JM: A self-medication retraining program. Br Med J 2:1278, 1978.
23. Libow LS, Mehl B: Self administration of medications by patients in hospitals or extended care facilities. J Am Geriatr Soc 18:81, 1970.
24. McDonald ET, McDonald JB, Phoenix M: Improving drug compliance after hospital discharge. Br Med J 2:618, 1977.
25. Wandless I, Davie JW: Can drug compliance in the elderly be improved? Br Med J 1:359, 1977.
26. Klein LE, German PS, McPhee SJ, et al: Aging and its relationship to health knowledge and medication compliance. Gerontologist 22:384, 1982.
27. Martin DC, Mead K: Reducing medication errors in a geriatric population. J Am Geriatr Soc 30:258, 1982.
28. Kendrick R, Bayne JRD: Compliance with prescribed medication by elderly patients. Can Med Assoc J 127:961, 1982.
29. Robinson H: Drugs and the elderly. U.S. Congressional Record. October 11, 1974.
30. Chaiton A, Spitzer WO, Roberts RS: Patterns of medical drug use—a community focus. Can Med Assoc J 114:33, 1976.
31. Zawadski RT, Glazer GB, Lurie E: Psychotropic drug use among institutionalized and non-institutionalized medical aged in California. J Gerontol 33:825, 1978.
32. Skegg DCG, Doll R, Perry J: Use of medicines in general practice. Br Med J 1:1561, 1977.
33. Boethius G, Westerholm B: Is the use of hypnotics, sedatives and minor tranquillizers really a major health problem? Acta Med Scand 199:502, 1976.
34. Wilson LA, Lawson IR, Braws W: Multiple disorders in the elderly. A clinical and statistical study. Lancet 2:841, 1962.
35. Ray WA, Federspiel CF, Schaffner W: A study of antipsychotic drug use in nursing homes: Epidemiologic evidence suggesting misuse. Am J Pub Health 70:485, 1980.
36. Ingman SR, Lawson IR, Pierpaoli PG, Blake P: A survey of the prescribing and administration of drugs

in a long-term care institution for the elderly. J Am Geriatr Soc 23:309, 1975.
37. Bergman HD: Prescribing of drugs in a nursing home. Drug Intell Clin Pharm 9:365, 1975.
38. Kalchthalter T, Coccaro E, Lichtiger S: Incidence of polypharmacy in a long-term care facility. J Am Geriatr Soc 25:308, 1977.
39. Koch-Weser J: Treatment of hypertension in the elderly. *In* Crooks J, Stevenson IH (eds.): Drugs and the Elderly. New York, Macmillan, 1979, pp. 247–266.
40. O'Malley K, O'Brien E: Management of hypertension in the elderly. N Engl J Med 302:1397, 1980.
41. Achong MR, Bayne JRD, Gerson LW, Golshoni S: Prescribing of psychoactive drugs for chronically ill elderly patients. Can Med Assoc J 118:1503, 1978.
42. Boston Collaborative Drug Surveillance Program: Clinical depression of the central nervous system due to diazepam and chloriazepoxide in relation to cigarette smoking and age. N Engl J Med 288:277, 1973.
43. Marttila JK, Hammel RJ, Alexander B, Zustiak R: Potential untoward effects of long-term use of flurazepam in geriatric patients. J Am Pharm Assoc 17:692, 1972.
44. Exton-Smith AN: The use and abuse of hypnotics. Gerontol Clin 9:264, 1967.
45. MacDonald JB, MacDonald ET: Nocturnal femoral fractures and continued widespread use of barbiturate hypnotics. Br Med J 2:483, 1977.
46. Brocklehurst JC, Exton-Smith AN, Lempert Barber SM, Palmer MK: Barbiturates and fractures. Br Med J 2:669, 1977.
47. Miller RR, Greenblatt DJ: Experiences of the Boston Collaborative Drug Surveillance Program, 1966–1975. New York, Wiley, 1976.
48. Reizenstein P, Liunggren G, Smedby B, et al: Overprescribing iron tablets to elderly people in Sweden. Br Med J 2:962, 1979.
49. Tulloch AJ: Repeat prescribing for elderly patients. Br Med J 1:1669, 1981.
50. Edelman IS, Leibman J: Anatomy of body water and electrolytes. Am J Med 27:256, 1959.
51. Forbes GB, Reina JC: Adult lean body mass declines with age: Some longitudinal observations. Metabolism 19:653, 1970.
52. Novak LP: Aging, total body potassium, fat-free mass, and cell mass in males and females between 18 and 85 years. J Gerontol 27:438, 1972.
53. Greenblatt DJ: Reduced serum albumin concentration in the elderly: A report from the Boston Collaborative Drug Surveillance Program. J Am Geriatr Soc 27:20, 1979.
54. Sherlock S, Bearn AG, Billing BH, Paterson JCS: Splanchnic blood flow in man by the bromosulfalein method: The relation of peripheral plasma bromosulfalein level to the calculated flow. J Lab Clin Med 35:923, 1950.
55. Warren PM, Pepperman MA, Montgomery RD: Age changes in small intestinal mucosa (letter). Lancet 2:849, 1978.
56. Calloway NO, Foley CF, Lagerbloom P: Uncertainties in geriatric data. II. Organ size. J Am Geriatr Soc 13:20, 1965.
57. Davies DF, Shock NW: Age changes in glomerular filtration rate, effective renal plasma flow and tubular excretory capacity in adult males. J Clin Invest 29:496, 1950.
58. Rowe JW, Andres R, Tobin JD, et al: The effect of age on creatinine clearance in man: A cross-sectional and longitudinal study. J Gerontol 31:155, 1976.
59. Miller JH, McDonald RK, Shock NW: Age changes in the maximal rate of renal tubular reabsorption of glucose. J Gerontol 7:196, 1952.
60. Rowe JW, Shock NW, DeFronzo RA: The influence of age on renal response to water deprivation in man. Nephron 17:270, 1976.
61. Baron JH: Studies of basal and peak acid output with an augmented histamine test. Gut 4:136, 1963.
62. Richey DP, Bender AD: Pharmacokinetic consequences of aging. Annu Rev Pharmacol Toxicol 17:49, 1977.
63. Triggs EJ, Nation RL, Long A, Ashley JJ: Pharmacokinetics in the elderly. Eur J Clin Pharmacol 8:55, 1975.
64. Divoll M, Ameeer B, Abernathy DR, Greenblatt DJ: Age does not alter acetaminophen absorption. J Am Geriatr Soc 30:240, 1982.
65. Triggs EJ, Johnson JM, Learoyd B: Absorption and disposition of ampicillin in the elderly. Eur J Clin Pharmacol 18:195, 1980.
66. Melander A, Bodin NO, Danielson K, et al: Absorption and elimination of D-propoxyphene, acetyl salicylic acid, and phenazone in a combination tablet (Doleron). Comparison between young and elderly subjects. Acta Med Scand 203:121, 1978.
67. Castleden CM, Volans CN, Raymond K: The effect of ageing on drug absorption from the gut. Age Ageing 6:138, 1977.
68. Cuny G, Royer RJ, Mur JM, et al: Pharmacokinetics of salicylates in the elderly. Gerontology 25:49, 1979.
69. Salem SAM, Stevenson IH: Absorption kinetics of aspirin and quinine in elderly subjects (abstract). Br J Clin Pharmacol 4:397P, 1977.
70. Ritch AES, Perera WNR, Jones CJ: Pharmacokinetics of azapropazone in the elderly. Br J Clin Pharmacol 14:116, 1982.
71. Greenblatt DJ, Divoll M, Puri SK, et al: Clobazam kinetics in the elderly. Br J Clin Pharmacol 12:631, 1981.
72. Willis JV, Kendall MJ: Pharmacokinetic studies on diclofenac sodium in young and old volunteers. Scand J Rheumatol Suppl 22:36, 1978.
73. Evans MA, Triggs EJ, Bore GA, Saines N: Systemic availability of orally administered L-dopa in the elderly parkinsonian patient. Eur J Clin Pharmacol 17:215, 1980.
74. Cusack B, Kelly JG, Lavan J, et al: Pharmacokinetics of lignocaine in the elderly (abstract). Br J Clin Pharmacol 9:293P, 1980.
75. Hümpel M, Nieuweboer B, Milius W, et al: Kinetics and biotransformation of lormetazepam. II. Radioimmunologic determinations in plasma and urine of young and elderly subjects: First-pass effect. Clin Pharmacol Ther 28:673, 1980.
76. Ball AP, Viswan AK, Mitchard M, Wise R: Plasma concentrations and excretion of mecillinam after oral administration of pivmecillinam in elderly patients. J Antimicrob Chemother 4:141, 1978.
77. Greenblatt DJ, Divoll M, Harmatz JS, Shader RI: Oxazepam kinetics: Effects of age and sex. J Pharmacol Exp Ther 215:86, 1980.
78. Castleden CM, Kaye CM, Parsons RL: The effect of age on plasma levels of propranolol and practolol in man. Br J Clin Pharmacol 2:303, 1975.
79. Simon C, Malerezyk V, Müller U, Müller G: Zur Pharmakokinetik von Propicillin bei geriatrischen Patienten in Verglich zu jüngeren Erwachsenen. Dtsch Med Wochenschr 97:1999, 1972.
80. Castleden CM, George CF: The effect of ageing on the hepatic clearance of propranolol. Br J Clin Pharmacol 7:49, 1978.

81. Barker HE, Hawksworth GM, Petrie JC, et al: Pharmacokinetics of atenolol and propranolol in young and elderly subjects (abstract). Br J Clin Pharmacol 12:118P, 1981.
82. Kampmann JP, Mortensen HB, Bach B, et al: Kinetics of propylthiouracil in the elderly. Acta Med Scand (Suppl) 624:93, 1979.
83. Ishizaki T, Hirayama H, Tawara K, Pharmacokinetics and pharmacodynamics in young normal and elderly hypertensive subjects: A study using sotalol as a model drug. J Pharmacol Exp Ther 212:173, 1980.
84. Fulton B, James O, Rawlins MD: The influence of age on the pharmacokinetics of paracetamol (abstract). Br J Clin Pharmacol 7:418P, 1979.
85. Divoll M, Greenblatt DJ, Harmatz JS, Shader RI: Effect of age and gender on disposition of temazepam. J Pharm Sci 70:1104, 1981.
86. Kramer PA, Chapron DJ, Benson J, Mercik SA: Tetracycline absorption in elderly patients with achlorhydria. Clin Pharmacol Ther 23:467, 1978.
87. Cusack B, Kelly JG, Lavan J, et al: Theophylline kinetics in relation to age: The importance of smoking. Br J Clin Pharmacol 10:109, 1980.
88. Fox RW, Samaan S, Bukantz SC, Lockey RF: Theophylline kinetics in a geriatric group. Clin Pharmacol Ther 34:60, 1983.
89. Quarterman CP, Kendall MJ, Jack DB: The effect of age on the pharmacokinetics of metoprolol and its metabolites. Br J Clin Pharmacol 11:287, 1981.
90. Briggs RS, Castleden CM, Kraft CA: Improved hypnotic treatment using chlormethiazole and temazepam. Br Med J 280:601, 1980.
91. Cusack B, Kelly JG, O'Malley K, et al: Digoxin in the elderly: Pharmacokinetic consequences of old age. Clin Pharmacol Ther 25:772, 1979.
*This study is one of the few that showed an age-related difference in rate of drug absorption.*
92. Shader RI, Greenblatt DJ, Harmatz JS, et al: Absorption and disposition of chlordiazepoxide in young and elderly male volunteers. J Clin Pharmacol 17:709, 1977.
93. Nation RL, Vine J, Triggs EJ, Learoyd B: Plasma levels of chlormethiazole and two metabolites after oral administration to young and aged human subjects. Eur J Clin Pharmacol 12:137, 1977.
94. Rubin PC, Scott PJW, McLean K, et al: Atenolol disposition in young and elderly subjects. Br J Clin Pharmacol 13:235, 1982.
95. Somogyi A, Rohner HG, Gugler R: Pharmacokinetics and bioavailability of cimetidine in gastric and duodenal ulcer patients. Clin Pharmacokinet 5:84, 1980.
96. Vestal RE, Wood AJJ, Branch RA et al: Effects of age and cigarette smoking on propranolol disposition. Clin Pharmacol Ther 26:8, 1979.
*A sophisticated examination of the relationship of aging and smoking to pharmacokinetics.*
97. Kelly JG, McGarry K, O'Malley K, O'Brien ET: Bioavailability of labetalol increases with age. Br J Clin Pharmacol 14:304, 1982.
98. Rubin PC, Scott PJW, Reid JL: Prazosin disposition in young and elderly subjects. Br J Clin Pharmacol 12:401, 1981.
99. Young CJ, Daneshmend TK, Roberts CJC: Pharmacokinetics of ranitidine in hepatic cirrhosis and in the elderly (abstract). Br J Clin Pharmacol 14:152P, 1982.
100. Briant RH, Dorrington RE, Cleol J, Williams FH: The rate of acetaminophen metabolism in the elderly and the young. J Am Geriatr Soc 24:359, 1976.
101. Playfer JR, Baty JD, Lamb J, et al: Age-related differences in the disposition of acetanilide. Br J Clin Pharmacol 6:529, 1978.
102. Ritschel WA: Age-dependant disposition of amobarbital: Analog computer evaluation. J Am Geriatr Soc 26:540, 1978.
103. Liddell DE, Williams FM, Briant RH: Phenazone (antipyrine) metabolism and distribution in young and elderly adults. Clin Exp Pharmacol Physiol 2:481, 1975.
104. Hayes MJ, Sprackling M, Langman MJS: Changes in plasma clearance and protein binding of carbenoxolone with age, and their possible relationship with adverse drug effects. Gut 18:1054, 1977.
105. Klotz U, Muller-Seydlitz P: Altered elimination of desmethyldiazepam in the elderly. Br J Clin Pharmacol 7:119, 1979.
106. Shader RI, Greenblatt DJ, Ciraulo DA, et al: Effect of age and sex on disposition of desmethyldiazepam formed from its precursor clorazepate. Psychopharmacology 75:193, 1981.
107. Macleod SM, Giles HG, Bengert B, et al: Age and gender-related differences in diazepam pharmacokinetics. J Clin Pharmacol 19:15, 1979.
108. Donovan MA, Castleden CM, Pohl JEF, Kraft CA: The effect of age on digoxin pharmacokinetics (letter). Br J Clin Pharmacol 11:401, 1981.
109. Berlinger NJ, Goldberg MJ, Spector R, et al: Diphenhydramine: Kinetics and psychomotor effects in elderly women. Clin Pharmacol Ther 32:387, 1982.
110. Kanto J, Kangas L, Aaltonem L, Hilke H: Effect of age on the pharmacokinetics and sedative effect of flunitrazepam. Int J Clin Pharmacol Ther Toxicol 19:400, 1981.
111. Cipolle RJ, Seifert RD, Neilan BA, et al: Heparin kinetics: Variables related to disposition and dosage. Clin Pharmacol Ther 29:387, 1982.
112. Kraus JW, Desmond PV, Marshall JP, et al: Effects of aging and liver disease on disposition of lorazepam. Clin Pharmacol Ther 24:411, 1978.
113. Greenblatt DJ, Allen MD, Locniskar A, et al: Lorazepam kinetics in the elderly. Clin Pharmacol Ther 25:103, 1979.
114. Holmberg L, Odar-Cederlof I, Boreus LO, et al: Comparative disposition of pethidine and norpethidine in old and young patients. Eur J Clin Pharmacol 22:175, 1982.
115. Castleden CM, George CF, Marcer D, Hallet C: Increased sensitivity to nitrazepam in old age. Br Med J 1:10, 1977.
*An important study in that it was one of the first to show that drug sensitivity varies with age.*
116. Murray TG, Chiang ST, Koepke HH, Walker BR: Renal disease, age and oxazepam kinetics. Clin Pharmacol Ther 30:805, 1981.
117. McLeod K, Hull CJ, Watson MJ: Effects of ageing on the pharmacokinetics of pancuronium. Br J Anaesth 51:435, 1979.
118. Duvaldestin P, Saada J, Berger JL, et al: Pharmacokinetics, pharmacodynamics and dose relationship of pancuronium in control and elderly subjects. Anaesthesiology 56:36, 1982.
119. Bach B, Hansen MJ, Kampmann JP, et al: Disposition of antipyrine and phenytoin correlated with age and liver volume in man. Clin Pharmacokinet 6:389, 1981.
120. Ochs HR, Greenblatt DJ, Woo E, Smith TW: Reduced quinidine clearance in elderly subjects. Am J Cardiol 42:481, 1978.
121. Bauer LA, Blouin RA: Influence of age on tobramycin pharmacokinetics in patients with normal renal

function. Antimicrob Agents Chemother 9:587, 1981.

122. Shepherd AMM, Hewick DS, Moreland TA, Stevenson IH: Age as a determinant of sensitivity to warfarin. Br J Clin Pharmacol 4:315, 1977.
*A good study in which warfarin effect was examined in detail.*

123. Roberts RK, Wilkinson GR, Branch RA, Sheuker S: Effect of age and parenchymal liver disease on the disposition and elimination of chlordiazepoxide (Librium). Gastroenterology 75:479, 1978.

124. Nation RL, Learoyd B, Barber J, Triggs EJ: The pharmacokinetics of chlormethiazole following intravenous administration in the aged. Eur J Clin Pharmacol 10:407, 1976.

125. Allen MD, Greenblatt DJ, Harmatz JS, Shader RI: Desmethyldiazepam kinetics in the elderly after oral prazepam. Clin Pharmacol Ther 28:196, 1980.

126. Klotz U, Avant GR, Hoyampa A, et al: The effects of age and liver disease on the disposition and elimination of diazepam in adult man. J Clin Invest 55:347, 1975.
*A very good detailed study that showed prolonged half-life but unaltered clearance of diazepam in the elderly.*

127. Macklon AF, Barton M, James O, Rawlins MD: The effect of age on the pharmacokinetics of diazepam. Clin Sci 59:479, 1980.

128. Kanto J, Mäempaä M, Mäntylä R, et al: Effect of age on the pharmacokinetics of diazepam given in conjunction with spinal anesthesia. Anesthesiology 51:154, 1979.

129. Greenblatt DJ, Allen MD, Harmatz JS, Shader RI: Diazepam disposition determinants. Clin Pharmacol Ther 27:301, 1980.

130. Nation RL, Triggs EJ, Selig M: Lignocaine kinetics in cardiac patients and aged subjects. Br J Clin Pharmacol 4:439, 1977.

131. Collier PS, Kawar P, Gamble JAS, Dundee JW: Influence of age on the pharmacokinetics of midazolam (abstract). Br J Clin Pharmacol 13:602P, 1982.

132. Shull HJ, Wilkinson GR, Johnson R, Schenker S: Normal disposition of oxazepam in acute viral hepatitis and cirrhosis. Ann Intern Med 84:420, 1976.

133. Christensen JH, Andreasen F, Jansen JA: Influence of age and sex on the pharmacokinetics of thiopentone. Br J Anaesth 53:1189, 1981.

134. Jung D, Mayersohn M, Perrier D, et al: Thiopental disposition as a function of age in female patients undergoing surgery. Anesthesiology 56:263, 1982.

135. Miller AK, Adir J, Vestal RE: Effect of age on the pharmacokinetics of tolbutamide in man (abstract). Pharmacologist 19:128, 1977.

136. Vestal RE, Norris AH, Jordan D, et al: Antipyrine metabolism in man: Influence of age, alcohol, caffeine and smoking. Clin Pharmacol Ther 18:425, 1975.
*This was the first paper to indicate that environmental factors are important to consider in age-related kinetic research.*

137. Swift CG, Homeida M., Halliwell M, Roberts CJC: Antipyrine disposition and liver size in the elderly. Eur J Clin Pharmacol 14:149, 1978.
*This study demonstrated that elderly patients metabolize drugs at a rate different from that of healthy elderly controls.*

138. Greenblatt DJ, Divoll M, Abernathy DR, et al: Antipyrine kinetics in the elderly: Prediction of age-related changes in benzodiazepine oxidizing capacity. J Pharmacol Exp Ther 220:120, 1982.

139. Redolfi A, Borgogelli E, Lodola E: Blood level of cimetidine in relation to age. Europ J Clin Pharmacol 15:257, 1979.

140. Vestal RE, McGuire EA, Tobin JD, et al: Aging and ethanol metabolism. Clin Pharmacol Ther 21:343, 1977.

141. Lumholtz B, Kampmann J, Siersback-Nielsen K, Molholm-Hansen J: Dose regimen of kanamycin and gentamycin. Acta Med Scand 190:521, 1974.

142. Chan K, Mitchard M: Elevated plasma pethidine levels in elderly patients after intravenous administration. Proc Br Pharmacol Soc Meet, Feb 1978. C33.

143. Antal EJ, Kramer PA, Mercik SA, et al: Theophylline pharmacokinetics in advanced age. Br J Clin Pharmacol 12:637, 1981.

144. Andreasen F, Husted S: The binding of furosemide to serum proteins in elderly patients: Displacing effect of phenprocoumarin. Acta Pharmacol Toxicol 47:202, 1980.

145. Mather LE, Tucker GT, Pflug AE, et al: Meperidine kinetics in man: Intravenous injection in surgical patients and volunteers. Clin Pharmacol Ther 17:21, 1975.

146. Bender AD, Post A, Meier JP, et al: Plasma protein binding of drugs as a function of age in adult human subjects. J Pharmacol Sci 64:1711, 1975.

147. Wallace S, Whiting B, Runcie J: Factors affecting drug binding in plasma of elderly patients. Br J Clin Pharmacol 3:327, 1976.
*This paper indicated that drug-displacing effects may be important in old age.*

148. Hayes MJ, Langman MJS, Short AH: Changes in drug metabolism with increasing age. Phenytoin clearance and protein binding. Br J Clin Pharmacol 2:73, 1975.

149. Patterson M, Hegelwood R, Smithurst B, Eadie MJ: Plasma protein binding studies of phenytoin in the aged: In vivo studies. Br J Clin Pharmacol 13:423, 1982.

150. Adir J, Miller AK, Vestal RE: Effects of total plasma concentration and age on tolbutamide plasma protein binding. Clin Pharmacol Ther 31:488, 1982.

151. Hayes MJ, Langman MJS, Short AH: Changes in drug metabolism with increasing age. Warfarin binding and plasma proteins. Br J Clin Pharmacol 2:69, 1975.

152. Carlos R, Calvo R, Erill S: Plasma protein binding of etomidate in different age groups and in patients with chronic respiratory insufficiency. Int J Clin Pharmacol Toxicol 19:171, 1981.

153. Rowell FJ, Hiu SM, Fairbairn AF, Eccleston D: Total and free serum haloperidol levels in schizophrenic patients and the effect of age, thioridazine and fatty acids on haloperidol serum protein binding in vitro. Br J Clin Pharmacol 12:401, 1981.

154. Tedeschi G, Bianchetti G, Henry JF, et al: Influence of age and disease states on the plasma protein binding of haloperidol (abstract). Br J Clin Pharmacol 11:430P, 1981.

155. Routledge PA, Chapman PH, Davis DM, Rawlins MD: Pharmacokinetics and pharmacokdynamics of warfarin at steady state. Br J Clin Pharmacol 8:243, 1979.

156. Thompson EN, Williams R: Effect of age on liver function with particular reference to bromosulphalein excretion. Gut 6:266, 1965.

157. Kitani K: Functional aspects of the ageing liver. *In* Platt D (ed.): Liver and Aging. New York, Schattaner Verlag, 1977, pp. 5–19.

158. Nies AS, Shand DG, Wilkinson GR: Altered hepatic blood flow and drug disposition. Clin Pharmacokinet 1:135, 1976.

159. Farah F. Taylor W, Rawlins MD, James O: Hepatic drug acetylation and oxidation: Effects of aging in man. Br Med J 2:155, 1977.
160. O'Malley K, Crooks J, Duke E, Stevenson IH: Effect of age and sex on human drug metabolism. Br Med J 3:607, 1971.
*An important landmark paper that was the first clinical study of drug metabolism in old age.*
161. Nies A, Robinson DS, Friedman MJ, et al: Relationship between age and tricyclic antidepressant plasma levels. Am J Psychiatry 134:790, 1977.
162. Wood AJ, Vestal RE, Wilkinson GR, et al: Effect of aging and cigarette smoking on antipyrine and indocyanine green elimination. Clin Pharmacol Ther 26:16, 1979.
*A very good study that demonstrated the value of a physiologic approach to drug kinetic studies.*
163. Kangas L, Iisalo E, Kanto J, et al: Human pharmacokinetics of nitrazepam: Effect of age and diseases. Eur J Clin Pharmacol 15:163, 1979.
164. Dawling S, Crome P, Braithwaite RA, Lewis RR: Nortriptyline therapy in elderly patients: Dosage prediction after single dose pharmacokinetic study. Eur J Clin Pharmacol 18:147, 1980.
165. Sartor C, Melander A, Scherster B, Waklin-Boll E: Influence of food and age on the single-dose kinetics and effects of tolbutamide and chlorpropramide. Eur J Clin Pharmacol 17:285, 1980.
166. Berkowitz BA, Ngai SH, Yang JC, et al: The disposition of morphine in surgical patients. Clin Pharmacol Ther 17:629, 1975.
167. Scott J, Poffenbarger PL: Pharmacokinetics of tolbutamide metabolism in humans. Diabetes 28:41, 1979.
168. Sontaniemi EA, Huhti E: Half-life of intravenous tolbutamide in the serum of patients in medical wards. Ann Clin Res 6:146, 1974.
169. Esler M, Skews H, Leonard P, et al: Age-dependance of noradrenaline kinetics in normal subjects. Clin Sci 60:217, 1981.
170. Drayer DE, Hughes M, Lorenzo B, Reidenberg MM: Prevalence of high (3s) -3-hydroxyquinidine/quinidine ratios in serum, and clearance of quinidine in cardiac patients with age. Clin Pharmacol Ther 27:72, 1980.
171. Jusko WJ, Gardner MJ, Mangione A, et al: Factors affecting theophylline clearances: Age, tobacco, marijuana, cirrhosis, congestive heart failure, obesity, oral contraceptives, benzodiazepines, barbiturates and ethanol. J Pharm Sci 68:1358, 1979.
172. Bauer L, Blouin RA: Influence of age on theophylline clearance in patients with chronic obstructive pulmonary disease. Clin Pharmacokinet 6:469, 1981.
173. Reidenberg MM, Comacho M, Kluger J, Drayer DE: Aging and renal clearance of procainamide and acetylprocainamide. Clin Pharmacol Ther 28:732, 1980.
174. Brockhuysen J, Deger F, Douchamps J, et al: Pharmacokinetic study of cefuroxime in the elderly. Br J Clin Pharmacol 12:801, 1981.
175. Simon C, Malerczyk V, Tenschert B, Mohlenbeck F: Die geriatrische Pharmakologic von Cefazolin, Cefradin and Sulfisomidin. Arzneim Forsch 26:1377, 1976.
176. Ewy GA, Kapadia GC, Yao L, et al: Digoxin metabolism in the elderly. Circulation 39:449, 1969.
177. Vartia KO, Leikola E: Serum levels of antibiotics in young and old subjects following administration of dihydrostreptomycin and tetracycline. J Gerontol 15:392, 1960.
178. Simon C, Malerczyk V, Engelke H: Die Pharmakokinetik von Doxycyclin bei Niereninsuffizienz und geriatrischen Patienten in Vergleich zu jüngeren Erwachsenen. Schweiz Med Wochenschr 105:1615, 1975.
179. Kristensen M, Molholm-Hansen J, Kampmann J, et al: Drug elimination and renal function. J Clin Pharmacol 14:307, 1974.
180. Hewick DS, Newbury P, Hopwood S, et al: Age as a factor affecting lithium therapy. Br J Clin Pharmacol 4:201, 1977.
181. Lehmann K, Merten K: Die Elimination von Lithium in Abhängigkeit vom Lebensalter bei Gesunden and Niereninsuffizienten. Int J Clin Pharmacol 10:292, 1974.
182. Kampmann J, Molholm-Hansen J, Siersback-Nielsen K, Laursen H: Effect of some drugs on penicillin half-life in blood. Clin Pharmacol Ther 13:516, 1972.
183. Leikola E, Vartia KO: On penicillin levels in young and geriatric subjects. J Gerontol 12:48, 1957.
184. Traeger A, Kiesewetter R, Kunze M: Zur Pharmakokinetik von Phenobarbital bei Erwachsenen und Greisen. Dtsch Ges Wesen 29:1040, 1974.
185. Kitanka I, Ross RJ, Cutler NR, et al: Altered hydroxydesipramine concentrations in elderly depressed patients. Clin Pharmacol Ther 31:51, 1982.
186. Reaven GM, Greenfield MS, Wondon CE, et al: Does insulin removal rate from plasma decline with age? Diabetes 31:670, 1982.
187. Montgomery S, McAuley R, Montgomery DB: Relationship between mianserin plasma level and antidepressant effect in a double-blind trial comparing a single night time and divided daily dose regimens. Br J Clin Pharmacol 5:71S, 1978.
188. Houghton GW, Richens A, Leighton M: Effect of age, height, weight and sex on serum phenytoin concentration in epileptic patients. Br J Clin Pharmacol 2:251, 1975.
189. Feely J, Crooks J, Stevenson IH: The influence of age, smoking and hyperthyroidism on plasma propranolol steady-state concentration. Br J Clin Pharmacol 12:73, 1981.
*This study demonstrated that aging alters the effect of smoking and hyperthyroidism on propranolol kinetics.*
190. Montgomery PR, Sitar DS: Increased serum salicylate metabolites with age in patients receiving chronic acetylsalicylic acid therapy. Gerontology 27:329, 1981.
191. Ramsay LE, Mackay A, Eppel ML, Oliver JS: Oral sustained release aminophylline in medical inpatients: Factors related to toxicity and plasma theophylline concentration. Br J Clin Pharmacol 10:101, 1980.
192. Rutherford DM, Okoko A, Tyrer PJ: Plasma concentrations of diazepam and desmethyl-diazepam during chronic diazepam therapy. Br J Clin Pharmacol 6:69, 1978.
193. Bauer LA, Blouin RA: Age and phenytoin kinetics in adult epileptics. Clin Pharmacol Ther 31:301, 1981.
194. Hotraphino K, Triggs EJ, Maybloom B, Maclaine-Cross A: Warfarin sodium: Steady-state plasma levels and patient age. Clin Exp Pharmacol Ther 5:143, 1978.
195. Bertilsson L, Mellstrom B, Sjoqvist F: Pronounced inhibition of noradrenaline uptake by 10-hydroxymetabolites of nortriptyline. Life Sci 25:1285 1979.
196. Hockings N, Stevenson IH, Swift GC: Hypnotic response in the elderly-single dose effects of chlormethiazole and dichloralphenazone. Br J Clin Pharmacol 14:143P, 1982.

197. Husted S, Andreasen F: The influence of age on the response to anticoagulants. Br J Clin Pharmacol 4:559, 1977.
198. Cokkinos DV, Tsartsalis GD, Heimonas ET, Gardikas CD: Comparison of inotropic action of digitalis and isoproterenol in younger and older individuals. Am Heart J 100:802, 1980.
199. Giles HG, MacLeod SM, Wright JR, Sellers EM: Influence of age and previous use on diazepam dosage required for endoscopy. Can Med Assoc J 118:513, 1978.
200. Reidenberg MM, Levy M, Warner H, Coutinho CB, et al: Relationship between diazepam dose, plasma level, age and central nervous system depression. Clin Pharmacol Ther 23:371, 1978.
201. Swift GC, Haythorne JM, Clarke P, Stevenson IH: Chlormethiazole and temazepam (letter). Br Med J 280:1322, 1980.
202. Whitfield LR, Schentag JJ, Levy G: Relationship between concentration and anticoagulant effect of heparin in plasma of hospitalized patients: Magnitude and predictability of interindividual differences. Clin Pharmacol Ther 32:503, 1982.
203. Bertel O, Buhler FR, Kiowski W, Lutold BE: Decreased beta adrenoceptor responsiveness as related to age, blood pressure and plasma catecholamines in patients with essential hypertension. Hypertension 2:103, 1980.
204. Van Brummelen P, Buhler FR, Kiowski W, Amann FW: Age-related decrease in cardiac and peripheral vascular responsiveness to isoprenaline: Studies in normal subjects. Clin Sci 60:571, 1981.
205. Vestal RE, Wood AJJ, Shand DG: Reduced $\beta$-adrenoceptor sensitivity in the elderly. Clin Pharmacol Ther 26:181, 1979.
*This study demonstrated impaired sensitivity to propranolol and isoproterenol in old age.*
206. Grad B, Wener J, Rosenberg G, Wener SW: Effects of levodopa therapy in patients with Parkinson's disease: Statistical evidence for reduced tolerance to levodopa in the elderly. J Am Geriatr Soc 22:489, 1974.
207. Bellville JW, Forrest WH, Miller E, Brown BW: Influence of age on pain relief from analgesics. A study of postoperative patients. JAMA 217:1835, 1971.
208. Kaiko RF: Age and morphine analgesia in cancer patients with postoperative pain. Clin Pharmacol Ther 28:823, 1980.
*This large study indicated that morphine analgesia is greater in old age.*
209. Swift CG, Haythorne JM, Clarke P, Stevenson IH: The effect of ageing on measured responses to single doses of oral temazepam (abstract). Br J Clin Pharmacol 11:413P, 1981.
210. Swerdloff RS, Pozefsky T, Tobin JD, Andreas R: Influence of age on the intravenous tolbutamide response test. Diabetes 16:161, 1967.
211. Burckhardt D, Raeder E, Muller V, et al: Cardiovascular effects of tricyclic and tetracyclic antidepressants. JAMA 239:213, 1978.
212. O'Malley K, Stevenson IH, Ward CA, et al: Determinants of anticoagulent control in patients receiving warfarin. Br J Clin Pharmacol 4:309, 1977.
213. Routledge PA, Chapman PH, Davies DM, Rawlins MD: Factors affecting warfarin requirements. A prospective study. Eur J Clin Pharmacol 15:319, 1979.
214. Greenblatt DJ, Koch-Weser J: Adverse reactions to propranolol in hospitalized medical patients: A report from the Boston Collaborative Drug Surveillance Program. Am Heart J 86:478, 1973.
215. Jick H, Stone D, Borda IT, Shapiro S: Efficacy and toxicity of heparin in relation to dose and sex. N Engl J Med 279:284, 1968.
216. Oswald I, Adam K: Chlormethiazole and temazepam (letter). Br Med J 860, 1980.
217. Dillon N, Chung S, Kelly J, O'Malley K: Age and beta adrenoceptor-mediated function. Clin Pharmacol Ther 27:769, 1980.
218. Doyle VM, O'Malley K, Kelly JG: Lymphocyte cyclic AMP production in the elderly: The effects of prostaglandin $E_1$ (letter). Br J Clin Pharmacol 12:597, 1981.
219. Kraft CA, Castleden CM: The effect of aging on B-adrenoreceptor-stimulated cyclic AMP formation in human lymphocytes. Clin Sci 60:587, 1981.
220. Abrass IB, Scarpace PJ: Human lymphocyte beta-adrenergic receptors are unaltered with age. J Gerontol 36:298, 1981.
221. Schocken DD, Roth GS: Reduced beta-adrenergic receptor concentrations in aging man. Nature 267:856, 1977.
*A widely referenced paper that was the first to suggest altered receptor density in old age.*
222. McAllister RG, Boldt DH, Tan TG: Alterations in lymphocyte $\beta$-adrenergic receptors associated with aging in normal men (abstract). Clin Res 29:705A, 1981.
223. Doyle VM, O'Malley K, Kelly JG: Lymphocyte adenylate cyclase activity and sodium flouride sensitivity in relation to age (abstract). Br J Clin Pharmacol 13:582P, 1982.
*An important report that suggests that altered beta-adrenoceptor sensitivity may be due to membrane changes rather than to receptor changes.*
224. Scott PJW, Reid JL: The effect of age on the responses of human isolated arteries to noradrenaline (letter). Br J Clin Pharmacol 13:237 1982.
225. Stevens MJ, Lipe S, Moulds RFW: The effect of age on the responses of human isolated arteries and veins to noradrenaline (letter). Br J Clin Pharmacol 14:750, 1982.
226. Shakespeare W, Henry IV, Act 2.

## *Additional Reading*

1. Crooks J, O'Malley K, Stevenson IH: Pharmacokinetics in the elderly. Clin Pharmcokinet 1:280, 1976.
*One of the better earlier reviews of pharmacokinetics. Contains some useful diagrams and tables.*
2. Greenblatt DJ, Sellers EM, Shader RI: Drug disposition in old age. N Engl J Med 306:1081, 1982.
*A short review, which contains a useful introductory discussion on pharmacokinetics in the elderly.*
3. Norman TR, Burrows GD, Scoggins BA, Daines B: Pharmacokinetics and plasma levels of antidepressants in the elderly. Med J Aust 1:273, 1979.
*A short but useful guide to the kinetics of this important group of drugs in old age.*
4. O'Malley K, Judge TG, Crooks J: Geriatric clinical pharmacology and therapeutics. *In* Avery G (ed.): Drug Treatment 2nd ed. Sydney and New York, Avis Press, 1980, pp. 158–181.
*This chapter contains a common sense appraisal of drug therapy in the elderly.*
5. O'Malley K, Laher M, Cusack B, Kelly JG: Clinical pharmacology and the elderly patient. *In* Denham MJ (ed.): Drug Treatment of Medical Problems in the Elderly. Lancaster, MTP Press, 1980, pp. 1–33.

*A good general monograph reviewing pharmacologic aspects of drug treatment of geriatric patients.*

6. Ouslander JG: Drug therapy in the elderly. Ann Intern Med 95:711, 1981.
   *Written by a physician, this discussion is good and has a different approach to that found in many of the other reviews.*
7. Plein JB, Plein EM: Aging and drug therapy. Am Rev Gerontol Geriat 2:211, 1981.
   *An excellent comprehensive review that contains detailed tables of age-related pharmacokinetic parameters.*
8. Richey DP, Bender AD: Pharmacokinetic consequences of aging. Am Rev Pharmacol Toxicol 17:49, 1977.
9. Schmucker DL: Age-related changes in drug disposition. Pharmacol Rev 30:445, 1979.
   *A good guide to animal pharmacology in particular.*
10. Shand DG: Biological determinants of altered pharmacokinetics in the elderly. Gerontol 28 (Suppl 1) 8, 1982.
   *This presentation is interesting in that it is followed by a good discussion of aspects of drug metabolism.*
11. Thompson TL, Moran MG, Nies AS: Psychotropic drug use in the elderly. N Engl J Med 308:134, 1983.
   *A good recent review with up-to-date references.*
12. Vestal RE: Drug use in the elderly: A review of problems and special considerations. Drugs 16:358, 1978.
   *A very good discussion of clinical pharmacology in the elderly. Also, some approaches to drug prescribing are outlined.*
13. Vestal RE: Aging and pharmacokinetics: Impact of altered physiology in the elderly. Physiology and cell biology of aging. *In* Cherkin A (ed.): Aging. New York, Raven Press, 1979, pp. 185–201.
   *Chapter provides an interesting discussion of a physiological orientation towards metabolism drugs in old age.*

## Chapter 13

# Nutritional Assessment

*Robert M. Russell*
*Nadine R. Sahyoun*
*Rosalind Whinston-Perry*

Knowledge of the nutritional needs of the elderly and the evaluation of nutritional status of this age group has not kept pace with the increasing number and proportion of elderly people in the United States. Malnutrition in the aged can result from degenerative disease states or decreased dietary intake due to problems such as physical disabilities, restricted income, health problems, dental problems, drug reactions, malabsorption, faddish diets, lack of appetite, depression, loneliness, and social isolation. Some symptoms of subclinical nutrient deficiencies (e.g., fatigue, irritability, anxiety, decreased appetite) are inaccurately attributed to the normal aging process itself. Many age-related changes, however, are not completely understood. When evaluating the elderly individual, questions arise as to whether subnormal measures of nutrient status reflect dietary lack or physiologic changes in the digestion, absorption, or utilization of nutrients. The establishment of improved standards which reflect the nutritional needs of the elderly and which can be used for evaluating the nutritional status of elderly populations, depends on answers to these questions.

The present Recommended Daily Allowances (RDAs*)[1] used for aged adults are based on the needs of younger adults, which are assumed, with few exceptions, to be the same as the needs of the elderly. However, age-related changes affecting absorption, metabolism, and excretion of most nutrients indicate the need for age-specific standards for the elderly. For example, one question of current interest concerns whether elderly people require decreased levels of some nutrients because of diminished utilization by the aging tissue. Age- and sex-specific anthropometric standards must be defined further for the elderly so that appropriate clinical evaluations can be conducted.

In addition, further data are required relative to the assessment of the nutritional status of hospitalized elderly. The demands placed on health care services as a result of chronic degenerative diseases in the elderly population have grown at a disproportionate rate (see Chapters 1, 5, and 16). Yet, only in recent years have the implications of malnutrition of the hospitalized patient begun to be fully recognized. With the development of improved clinical indicators of nutritional status, a high frequency of previously unrecognized malnutrition among hospitalized patients has been reported.[2,3] Downward trends in nutritional parameters during hospitalization have been documented, resulting in increased operative morbidity and mortality and length of hospital stay. Whether the prevalence of these findings can be altered by nutritional intervention requires further research.

Thus, despite the uncertainties due to our lack of knowledge, evaluation of the nutritional status of the elderly is an important part of the clinical assessment and should become a routine hospital procedure. A thorough evaluation should address not only the nutritional implications of medications prescribed (see page 148) but also the specific individual needs of the patient that may interfere with his or her nutritional status. A list of key questions to be asked as part of a nutritional assessment of the elderly individual is presented in Table 13-1. This chapter addresses both the practical difficulties that arise when evaluating the malnourished elderly patient and the most up-to-date normative values recommended for use by the health practitioner for nutritional assessment.

* Throughout this chapter, RDA refers to the 1980 RDA.

**Table 13-1.** LIST OF KEY QUESTIONS IN NUTRITIONAL ASSESSMENT OF THE ADULT

1. Is there recent weight gain or weight loss?
2. Are there changes in appetite?
3. Are there changes in sense of smell or taste?
4. Are there problems with chewing or swallowing?
5. Does the individual have poor dentition or poorly fitting dentures?
6. Are there symptoms of gastrointestinal disorders: diarrhea, constipation, nausea, vomiting?
7. Does the individual live alone? If not, who prepares meals? Does he or she know how to cook?
8. Are there adequate cooking facilities and refrigeration in the person's home?
9. Is the individual financially able to buy an adequate variety of food?
10. Are one or more meals eaten outside of the home?
11. Is the person handicapped? Does this prevent the individual from shopping, cooking, or feeding herself or himself?
12. Does the person take any dietary supplements (e.g., vitamins)?
13. How much alcohol does the individual consume?
14. Does the person use prescription or nonprescription drugs?
15. Are there any religious beliefs, food allergies, or ethnic beliefs that prevent adequate food intake?
16. Does the person follow a dietary restriction? Is it doctor-prescribed or self-imposed?
17. Is the individual depressed?

## CLINICAL PRESENTATION OF MALNUTRITION IN THE ELDERLY

Three caveats, which apply to both young and old, should be recognized when discussing the clinical presentation of malnutrition: (1) The earliest clinical signs of malnutrition are relatively nonspecific (e.g., lassitude, irritability, loss of appetite), (2) single nutrient deficits rarely occur alone, and (3) specific signs of malnutrition (e.g., impaired dark adaptation) can be caused by deficits of several individual nutrients (e.g., vitamin A, zinc, protein, and calories).[4-6] Thus, the diagnosis of specific nutrient deficiencies based on clinical signs and symptoms alone is frequently uncertain. Clinical data should be corroborated with dietary, anthropometric, or biochemical data in order to make a definite judgment as to nutritional adequacy or inadequacy.

The use of clinical signs to diagnose malnutrition may be less applicable in the elderly than in younger age groups in that several of the bodily changes that accompany aging mimic specific signs of malnutrition. For example, the dry flaking skin of old people may look like the skin changes seen in protein-calorie and zinc malnutrition. Bleeding gums may be the result of ill-fitting dentures rather than of vitamin C deficiency. Sparse hair is also a sign associated with protein-calorie malnutrition. In the national Health and Nutrition Examination Survey (HANES*),[7] clinical signs of niacin deficiency (e.g., tongue fissures) were seen in about 15 per cent of white and black elderly. However, tongue fissures were seen more frequently in upper-income groups than in lower-income groups for both races, which casts doubt on the utility of this sign in the diagnosis of niacin deficiency in the elderly. Similarly, bleeding gums were found to have no correlation with vitamin C dietary intakes. The clinical signs suggesting malnutrition that were present most frequently among the elderly (in greater than 5 per cent of those examined) were atrophy and fissuring of the tongue (niacin), absence of ankle and knee jerks (thiamin), bowing of the legs (vitamin D), follicular hyperkeratinosis of the upper arms (vitamin A), and bleeding or swollen gums (vitamin C). However, corroborative evidence was lacking that these signs actually represented malnutrition of specific nutrients. Studies are needed to correlate specific clinical signs with biochemical, dietary, and functional tests of malnutrition so that reliable clinical signs of malnutrition for the older person can be defined.

There are many causes of malnutrition in the elderly. The effects that depression and loneliness may have on one's appetite and the desire to cook and care for oneself are obvious. Chronic illness and medication usage may affect appetite as well as the absorption and metabolism of many nutrients. In our experience, patients with chronic obstructive pulmonary disease or cancer are the most poorly nourished of any patient group.[8,9] The large number of medications prescribed to patients with these diseases probably plays a contributing role. Unfortunately, relatively little is known about drug-nutrient interaction in the elderly (see page 148). For example, the long-term effects of diuretic usage on micronutrient metabolism have not been extensively studied. Changes in gastrointestinal and liver functions with age could affect the body's ability to absorb and utilize nutrients, but these functions have also not been investigated carefully in the elderly. Other factors that may enter into the pathogenesis of malnutrition in the elderly are the decline in taste and smell acuity with age, ill-fitting dentures, difficulty in swallowing, neurologic disabilities (e.g., Parkinson's disease), pseudobulbar palsy, and occult thyrotoxicosis.

It is clear that most malnutrition in the United States is subclinical. In our own experi-

* Throughout this chapter HANES refers to HANES I.

ence among hospitalized patients, physicians failed to recognize moderately or severely malnourished patients about 50 per cent of the time, the diagnosis of malnutrition having been made on the basis of severely substandard anthropometric values.[10] Functional tests are often useful in detecting previously unsuspected cases of malnutrition. For example, dark adaptation testing has been shown to be of use in the diagnosis of subclinical vitamin A and zinc deficiency.[4,5] Many patients who have abnormal dark adaptation test results do not complain of night blindness or show other physical signs of hypovitaminosis A. Nevertheless, the results of the dark adaptation test returns to normal with vitamin A or zinc treatment. This test, however, is not completely specific, and the use of such a test in elderly subjects is confounded by the fact that age alone affects the test results due to lens and retinal changes.[11] Taste testing is one other example of a functional test that could be used to diagnose malnutrition (e.g., zinc deficiency).[12,13] Taste function is also affected by age itself, and the usefulness of taste testing in the elderly for nutritional diagnosis remains uncertain.[14-16] Norms for results of functional tests need to be developed for the elderly, but to date this has not been achieved.

The usual clinical signs and symptoms of malnutrition are listed in Table 13-2. The health provider should continue to look for these classic clinical signs until more sensitive indices for the diagnosis of malnutrition in the elderly are available. It should be recognized that when most of these signs and symptoms occur, the deficit is usually quite profound.

More sensitive means of detecting nutritional deficits (e.g., biochemical, anthropometric, functional tests) should be applied if the health provider suspects subclinical malnutrition, so that the deficit can be corrected at an early stage. For example, if a dietary or social history reveals heavy use of alcohol, the health provider may wish to go ahead with nutritional, biochemical, and anthropometric tests to diagnose nutritional inadequacy, even though no specific clinical sign of malnutrition listed in Table 13-2 is present. Obvious predisposing causes of malnutrition should be sought and corrected when possible (e.g., poor-fitting dentures). Patients whose eating habits are poor should be referred to a nutritionist/dietitian for specific counseling. At times, specific supplemental foods or preparations may be indicated. Social or group eating activities should be encouraged. Finally, the possibility of drug-nutrient interactions should be kept in mind, even if only to the extent of recognizing unpleasant gastrointestinal side effects of many preparations, which could depress appetite.

## *Anthropometric Evaluation*

The lack of established standards upon which to base nutritional assessment of the elderly is a

**Table 13-2.** CLINICAL SIGNS AND SYMPTOMS OF MALNUTRITION

| Nutrient Deficiency | Sign or Symptom* |
|---|---|
| Calorie† | Wasting, emaciation; flaking dermatitis; muscle wasting; weakness of extremities |
| Protein† | Flaking dermatitis; sparse, thin hair (easy to pull out); parotid enlargement (of neck); edema of extremities; transverse lines on nails; muscle wasting; weakness of extremities |
| Vitamin A | Xerophthalmia; follicular hyperkeratosis; history of night blindness (especially impaired visual recovery after glare); photophobia; blurring; conjunctival inflammation; keratomalacia; Bitot's spots |
| Thiamin | Beriberi: muscle tenderness, muscle pain of extremities; paresthesias; loss of reflexes; wrist drop; foot drop; edema of extremities |
| Riboflavin | Bruising; scrotal dermatosis; photophobia; blurring; conjunctival inflammation; glossitis; cheilosis; hypogeusia; tongue atrophy |
| Niacin | Pellagra; skin pigmentation changes; flaking dermatitis; glossitis of oral mucous membranes; tongue fissuring; tongue atrophy; dementia; disorientation |
| Folic Acid | Glossitis; macrocytic anemia; gastrointestinal disturbances; pallor of skin |
| Vitamin $B_{12}$ | Pernicious anemia; pallor of skin; glossitis of oral mucous membranes; loss of vibratory and position sense |
| Vitamin C | Scurvy; perifollicular petechiae; bruising; bleeding gums; bone ache; joint pain of extremities |
| Vitamin D | Rickets; osteomalacia; bone tenderness; muscle wasting and weakness |
| Iron | Anemia; pallor of skin; spooning of nails; tongue atrophy |
| Zinc | Flaking dermatitis; hypogeusia |
| Iodine | Goiter |

* Specific signs and symptoms of malnutrition may be caused by several nutrients.

† Signs associated with protein-calorie malnutrition include loss of appetite, changes in pigmentation of skin, temporal muscle wasting, distention of abdomen, and hepatomegaly.

factor affecting not only clinical measures but also the interpretation of dietary information and anthropometric measurements. Significant changes in body composition, characterized by the loss of lean body mass, the increase in proportion of body fat, and known height and weight changes, occur with the aging process. These changes indicate the need for age-specific standards for evaluation of the elderly population. To date, most anthropometric standards for the elderly have been estimated by extrapolation from research conducted on a young adult population and thus do not account for the confounding changes that occur with age. Research is needed to provide age-, sex-, and race-specific values that will adequately assess the elderly population. Until such standards are established, use of estimated anthropometric, dietary, and biochemical values must be applied to the aged for nutritional assessment.

The anthropometric assessment[17] is a direct evaluation tool of little cost that requires minimal time of the health provider. Measurements for anthropometric evaluation include height, weight, triceps, skinfold, and midarm circumference. These assessment modalities are based on evidence indicating that when the body is nutritionally deprived, it utilizes its nutritional stores in the form of muscle protein and fat. Anthropometric measurements can be of use for initial assessment of nutritional status, for evaluation of therapeutic progress, and as a screening device used in conjunction with dietary and biochemical information.

## Height and Weight

Various studies have indicated that the average lifetime height loss is about 2.9 cm for men and 4.9 cm for women.[18] In addition, HANES found that the body weight increases consistently with age for both males and females, reaching a maximum between ages 35 to 55 for men and ages 55 to 65 for women. Thereafter, weight appears to decrease in both sexes, although more slowly for women than men. Since weight tends to increase after growth in stature has ended, weight standards that account for the changes that occur with aging need to be determined.

These documented height and weight trends, which are now known to accompany aging, are not apparent in the height and weight tables derived from life insurance data. The Metropolitan Life Insurance values are limited as a reference for the elderly because they are based on actuarial tables from a younger population, are not age-specific, and do not account for the diverse socioeconomic and ethnic differences that characterize the United States population. The values derived from the HANES survey (Table 13–3), in contrast, are normative values that include a wider cross section of minority and socioeconomic groups, are age-specific, and include data from elderly groups up to the age of 74 years. However, the HANES values, are probably too high to use as a reference standard, since the accumulation of weight with age, as reflected in these normative values, may not be desirable. The "ideal" body weight for older Americans remains controversial, particularly in light of reports of lower mortality among mildly or moderately obese elderly persons.[19,20]

For evaluation of elderly individuals, two measures are recommended. The health practitioner should compare individual weight-for-height measurements with the average weight-for-height value of people with a medium-sized frame (Tables 13–4 and 13–5) derived from 1983 life insurance tables. Although these values are flawed because they are not age-specific, they are currently the most appropriate values available. In addition, a record of both rate and amount of weight loss or gain can be used to further reflect the nutritional status of the individual patient. A loss of over 10 per cent

**Table 13–3.** AVERAGE WEIGHT FOR HEIGHT FOR PEOPLE AGES 65 TO 74 FROM THE HEALTH AND NUTRITION EXAMINATION SURVEY*

| Height | | Weight | | | |
|---|---|---|---|---|---|
| | | *Male* | | *Female* | |
| *(in.)* | *(cm)* | *(lb)* | *(kg)* | *(lb)* | *(kg)* |
| 57 | 144.8 | — | — | 130 | 59.0 |
| 58 | 147.3 | — | — | 133 | 60.3 |
| 59 | 149.9 | — | — | 137 | 60.1 |
| 60 | 152.4 | — | — | 138 | 62.1 |
| 61 | 154.9 | — | — | 144 | 62.6 |
| 62 | 157.5 | 148 | 67.2 | 146 | 65.3 |
| 63 | 160.0 | 146 | 66.2 | 149 | 66.2 |
| 64 | 162.6 | 147 | 66.7 | 152 | 67.6 |
| 65 | 165.1 | 155 | 70.3 | 153 | 69.0 |
| 66 | 167.6 | 160 | 72.5 | 162 | 69.4 |
| 67 | 170.2 | 167 | 75.8 | 173 | 78.5 |
| 68 | 172.7 | 169 | 76.7 | 168 | 76.2 |
| 69 | 175.3 | 172 | 78.0 | — | — |
| 70 | 177.8 | 181 | 82.1 | — | — |
| 71 | 180.3 | 188 | 85.3 | — | — |
| 72 | 182.9 | 183 | 83.0 | — | — |
| 73 | 185.4 | 190 | 86.2 | — | — |
| 74 | 188.0 | 194 | 88.0 | — | — |

* Adapted from Abraham S, Johnson L, Najjar M: Weight by Height and Age for Adults 18–74 Years: United States, 1971–1974. National Center for Health Statistics 14:1. DHEW Publ. No.(PHS) 79-1656, 1979.

of original weight within 6 months or weights falling below 80 per cent of the actuarial reference weight may indicate a need for nutritional support.[21]

### MIDARM MUSCLE CIRCUMFERENCE (MAMC)

Estimates of somatic muscle protein are derived by measures of midarm muscle circumference. Average values from HANES for MAMC for white older adults have been compiled by Frisancho[22] and are provided in Table 13–6. Similar values based on a cross-sectional population from the HANES data have also been compiled for MAMC.[23] These values do not show significant decreases between the ages of 30 and 70 years and thus are not consistent with our knowledge of the decrease in lean body mass that occurs with age. For the elderly population, it may be that sites other than midarm circumference may be more accurate measures for assessment of nutritional status. Further research is needed to determine other anthropometric measurements that may accurately assess the nutritional status of the elderly individual. In the meantime, the standards derived from HANES by Frisancho[22] are recommended for evaluation of MAMC in the elderly.

**Table 13–4.** 1983 WEIGHT FOR HEIGHT FOR MALES FROM LIFE INSURANCE DATA*

| Height | | Weight† | |
|---|---|---|---|
| *(in.)* | *(cm)* | *(lb)* | *(kg)* |
| 58 | 147.3 | — | — |
| 59 | 149.9 | — | — |
| 60 | 152.4 | — | — |
| 61 | 154.9 | — | — |
| 62 | 157.5 | 133.0 | 60.3 |
| 63 | 160.0 | 135.0 | 61.2 |
| 64 | 162.6 | 137.5 | 62.4 |
| 65 | 165.1 | 140.0 | 63.5 |
| 66 | 167.6 | 143.0 | 64.9 |
| 67 | 170.2 | 146.0 | 66.2 |
| 68 | 172.7 | 149.0 | 67.6 |
| 69 | 175.3 | 152.0 | 68.9 |
| 70 | 177.8 | 155.0 | 70.3 |
| 71 | 180.3 | 158.5 | 71.9 |
| 72 | 182.9 | 162.0 | 73.9 |
| 73 | 185.4 | 166.0 | 75.3 |
| 74 | 188.0 | 169.5 | 76.9 |
| 75 | 190.5 | 174.0 | 78.9 |

* These values correct the 1983 Metropolitan tables of weights and heights of unclothed people.

† These are the average weights of people with a medium-sized frame.

**Table 13–5.** 1983 WEIGHT FOR HEIGHT FOR FEMALES DERIVED FROM LIFE INSURANCE DATA*

| Height | | Weight† | |
|---|---|---|---|
| *(in.)* | *(cm)* | *(lb)* | *(kg)* |
| 58 | 147.3 | 114.0 | 51.7 |
| 59 | 149.9 | 116.5 | 52.8 |
| 60 | 152.4 | 119.0 | 53.9 |
| 61 | 154.9 | 122.0 | 55.3 |
| 62 | 157.5 | 125.0 | 56.7 |
| 63 | 160.0 | 128.0 | 58.0 |
| 64 | 162.6 | 131.0 | 59.4 |
| 65 | 165.1 | 134.0 | 60.8 |
| 66 | 167.6 | 137.0 | 62.1 |
| 67 | 170.2 | 140.0 | 63.5 |
| 68 | 172.7 | 143.0 | 64.9 |
| 69 | 175.3 | 146.0 | 66.2 |
| 70 | 177.8 | 149.0 | 67.6 |
| 71 | 180.3 | 152.0 | 69.0 |
| 72 | 182.9 | — | — |
| 73 | 185.4 | — | — |
| 74 | 188.0 | — | — |
| 75 | 190.5 | — | — |

* These values correct the 1983 Metropolitan Tables of weights and heights of unclothed people.

† These are the average weights of people with a medium-sized frame.

### TRICEPS SKINFOLD (TSF)

Triceps skinfold measurements provide an estimate of fat stores as measured by a skinfold caliper. The deltoid triceps is the ideal site for skinfold measurements, since this area is usually absent of edema. The skinfold measurements appear most appropriate as an anthropometric measurement for the elderly because they are less affected by state of hydration than is weight and are relatively independent of height (which may be difficult to measure in bedridden patients or because of postural changes).[24] However, TSF measurements are variable from study to study, and few measurements have been reported upon which a standard may be based. Results from the Ten-State Nutrition Survey (TSNS) suggest that the TSF is relatively independent of age in men but affected by age in women. This trend was also observed by Bishop and associates[23] when examining triceps skinfold measurements from cross-sectional data collected by HANES. Norms for triceps skinfold thickness have been compiled by Frisancho[22] from the HANES data and are provided in Table 13–6. For practical purposes, the 50th percentile value corresponding to the age range of 24 to 35 years should be used as a standard for people under 65 years of age; for people over the age of 65, the 50th percentile value correspond-

**Table 13-6.** AVERAGE VALUES FROM THE HEALTH AND NUTRITION EXAMINATION SURVEY FOR TRICEPS SKINFOLD THICKNESS AND MID-UPPER ARM MUSCLE CIRCUMFERENCE FOR OLDER ADULTS*

| Age group (yr) | Triceps Skinfold (mm) | Mid-arm Muscle Circumference (cm) |
|---|---|---|
| *Men* | | |
| 25-34.9 | 12 | 27.9 |
| 35-44.9 | 12 | 28.6 |
| 45-54.9 | 12 | 28.1 |
| 55-64.9 | 11 | 27.8 |
| 65-74.9 | 11 | 26.8 |
| *Women* | | |
| 25-34.9 | 21 | 21.2 |
| 35-44.9 | 23 | 21.8 |
| 45-54.9 | 25 | 22.0 |
| 55-64.9 | 25 | 22.5 |
| 65-74.9 | 24 | 22.5 |

* From Frisancho A: New norms for upper arm limb fat and muscle areas for assessment of nutritional status. Am J Clin Nutr 34:2450, 1981. Reproduced with permission.

ing to the age range of 65 to 75 years should be applied.

### Interpretation of Anthropometric Measurements

Generally, interpretation of anthropometric measurements is achieved by relating measurements to a percentile derived from a standard population. Bishop[23] and Frisancho[22] provide age-specific percentiles for MAMC and TSF derived from HANES. Although there are arguments against using a single value rather than a range as a standard,[25] in the elderly population, norms and ideal values may approach one another, since the survivors make up the norm and represent an "ideal" healthy value. For the elderly population, mean values may provide the most practical measure for establishment of an ideal standard. However, these values have yet to be derived. One criterion used to rank the severity of malnutrition and obesity is presented in Table 13-7. This classification is based on median values from HANES for TSF, MAMC and the 1983 Metropolitan Life Insurance data for weight-for-height.

Many questions still exist concerning the interpretation of anthropometric measurements in the elderly. Changes in body composition resulting from the aging process may resemble protein-calorie malnutrition (i.e., redistribution of body fat, increase in skin laxity, changes in lean body mass and compressibility). These changes are difficult to distinguish and should not be confused when using anthropometric measurements for assessment, particularly in the elderly. To date, no standards are available that adequately reflect the entire elderly population. Data from HANES are the most appropriate data available for evaluation of people up to the age of 74 years. Because the variance among aged people is greater than among younger adults, there exists a need for age-, race-, and sex-specific normative data reflective of each age decade through the age of 90 years.

## *Laboratory Assessment*

A diet may appear to be adequate when assessed according to present dietary standards; yet a change in metabolism and decreased absorption of nutrients may lead to biochemical deficiencies. Interpretation of biochemical results is limited for some of the same reasons found when interpreting dietary and anthropometric parameters. Not only might the aging process itself affect the metabolism of nutrients, resulting in altered biochemical values as well as an altered ability to utilize nutrients, but standards and results that are used for interpretation of biochemical values vary from study to study.

### Serum Protein

Reports on serum protein values in the elderly adult population are conflicting. The TSNS reported that the prevalence of low values of serum protein appeared to increase with age. Reduced organ function associated with aging may result in low serum protein among the elderly.

There have been a number of reports of lower serum albumin values in elderly subjects than in younger controls.[21,26] One study reported serum albumin values to be approximately 0.4 gm/dl lower in people over the age of 80, as compared with people under the age of 40. In this study, it appeared that the lower albumin level could not be pushed higher with dietary protein, indicating that a lower set point for albumin synthesis may occur with the aging process.[26] Serum albumin or prealbumin may be the best predictor of malnutrition, but no normative values are presently available that apply specifically to the elderly population. In the meantime, each laboratory should derive mean ranges of serum albumin for the elderly population and establish a cut-off point of 20 per cent below the lower limit as an indication of malnutrition.

**Table 13-7.** SUGGESTED CRITERIA TO JUDGE MALNUTRITION AND OBESITY IN THE UNITED STATES ADULT POPULATION

| | Malnutrition | | Obesity | |
|---|---|---|---|---|
| | *% Standard* | *Percentile* | *% Standard* | *Percentile* |
| Wt/Ht | <80 | 5th* | >120 | 75* |
| TSF† | <40 | 5th | >190 | >90th |
| MAMC‡ | <80 | 5th | NA | NA |

* Criteria for evaluating weight for height are based on comparison of Metropolitan 1983 data of HANES I percentiles.
† TSF = Triceps skinfold.
‡ MAMC = Midarm muscle circumference.

### Creatinine/Height Index

The creatinine/height index is influenced by declining creatinine clearance with age. In addition, this measure is affected by the decline in physical activity, decrease in muscle mass, and height decreases that accompany aging. Standards are needed that can control for these factors before the index can be applied to the elderly population. Although arm length may be used to replace the uncertainty of height measures, problems of renal clearance still confound these measures when applied to the elderly.[21]

### Hematologic Indices

There is evidence indicating both a reduction in hematopoiesis and an increased incidence of anemia in the aged (see Chapter 43). Whether these lower hematologic values reflect effects of the aging process remains controversial. In addition, the cause of anemias observed in the elderly population remains unclear. As a result, the interpretation of hematologic findings remains complex.

Yearick and associates[27] reported low levels of folate among elderly subjects, but these findings did not appear to correlate with any hematologic parameters. In another study, 60 per cent of aged low-income black and Spanish Americans surveyed were reported at a high risk of folate deficiency based on red blood cell folacin concentration.[28] Gershoff and associates,[29] conducting an iron fortification study on 200 elderly subjects with initial low hemoglobin values, reported a high prevalence of low serum folate[29]; however, the low folate values did not appear to correlate with low hemoglobin values.

Two separate studies have reported adequate mean hemoglobin and hematocrit values among elderly subjects but have indicated that over 20 per cent of males and under 11 per cent of females were found with low hemoglobin and hematocrit values.[30,31] In both studies, the cause of the anemias was uncertain. Among nursing home residents, low mean hemoglobin and hematocrit values were observed in patients with adequate mean folic acid, plasma iron, and transferrin saturation.[32]

Both the TSNS and HANES reported a high prevalence of low hemoglobin and hematocrit levels among the elderly subjects. Although low levels of serum iron were marked in the TSNS, HANES reported a low prevalence of decreased serum iron and serum transferrin. The results of the TSNS were interpreted as reflecting a high prevalence of iron deficiency anemia in the elderly population. However, in contrast, the results of HANES left the etiology of anemia in the elderly unexplained, excluding iron deficiency as its cause. These findings are confirmed in a study of the effect of age and sex on nutritional assessment measures.[21] Both hemoglobin and hematocrit values for healthy elderly males and females were significantly lower than values found in the younger adult group. At present, it is unclear what the low hematologic values indicate in elderly subjects, i.e., whether they can be attributed to the aging process and, if so, whether these changes have a nutritional basis. Until appropriate hematologic ranges are available, each laboratory should establish its own sex- and age-specific normal ranges and determine a value of 20 per cent below the lower limit for diagnostic purposes.

### Immunologic Tests

Lymphocyte counts are applicable as a test of nutriture in the elderly, since no known decreases in lymphocyte counts occur with age. Cell function, however, does decrease with age. The utility of skin sensitivity testing in the elderly is uncertain.[31]

## DIETARY REQUIREMENTS OF THE ELDERLY

Several surveys have been conducted that assess the nutritional needs of the elderly, but only limited information can be inferred from these studies. Limitations result from variation in methodologic design from one survey to another, the application of different methodologies used for the collection of dietary information, and the use of varying standards for interpretation of information obtained. Confounding factors such as socioeconomic status of survey participants, rural versus urban populations, life-style setting of participants (for example, nursing home residents versus noninstitutionalized subjects), age, and sample size of survey populations limit the ability to compile and compare the results from the different studies. These problems are a sampling of the difficulties that confront researchers in the field of nutrition research today. There is a need for more standardized procedures to help resolve some of these uncertainties.

The dietary needs of the elderly may vary widely because of individual differences in the rate of aging, differences in levels of physical activity, the presence of a range of degenerative diseases, and the effects of drugs on nutrient utilization. In addition, it is possible that nutrient needs may vary from one age decade to another, independent of the previously mentioned factors. The outstanding problem in assessing the nutritional status of the elderly remains the lack of established and agreed-upon nutrient guidelines. The most frequently used standards for estimating the adequacy of nutrient intake are the Recommended Dietary Allowances (RDAs). The RDAs for adults, however, may not be an appropriate standard for the elderly population. The 1980 RDAs established standards for a combined age group of 51 years and older.[1] These recommendations for the aged are based on extrapolations from the needs of younger adults and are therefore only an estimate of the true dietary needs of the elderly.

### *Calories*

Evidence exists indicating an age-related decrease in energy intake associated with decreases in basal metabolism and physical activity. Low mean caloric intakes in the elderly population were reported in two national surveys (TSNS and HANES). A recommendation based on calories per kilogram of body weight for differing levels of activity may prove to be the most useful guide for evaluation of the elderly.

The RDA for energy is the only category in which the standard is established at the lowest value considered adequate (other nutrient recommended intakes are set high enough to meet the upper limits of variability). In the ninth edition of the RDA (1980),[1] the recommendation for calories for older adults is divided into two age groups: 51 to 75 years and 76 years and older. Although these values have taken into account an age-related decrease in energy intake associated with decreases in both basal metabolic rate and physical activity,[33] individual caloric needs depend on body size and levels of activity.

### *Vitamin A*

Some studies have indicated that the diets of a large number of elderly subjects supplied less than the RDA for vitamin A, even though mean intakes of the survey populations were adequate.[27,32,34–36] Although vitamin A intake was reportedly low in HANES among many elderly people, these low dietary values did not correlate well with deficient biochemical values. The functional significance of reported low intakes of vitamin A in the elderly is unclear, since vitamin A is stored in the liver throughout life. As a result, dietary information alone is not adequate for determining vitamin A deficiency in the elderly.

### *Vitamin C*

Mean values of vitamin C intake were found to meet two thirds of the RDA and, in many studies, intake values were much higher. A correlation between levels of serum vitamin C and intake in the diet has been reported.[27,32,37] TSNS concluded that the correlation was due more to quality differences of food intake than to quantity.[37] A study performed in 1982 that evaluated the vitamin C status of noninstitutionalized, middle class, elderly men and women from New Mexico reported dietary intakes of ascorbic acid among this group to be 2.4 times the 1980 RDA.[38] In addition, saturated blood levels were achieved with an average daily intake of 75 mg for women and 150 mg for men, suggesting increased sex- and age-specific requirements for vitamin C for the elderly.[38]

## *B Vitamins*

Of all the B vitamins, thiamin is most frequently reported to be at low levels in the diets of the elderly. In one study, 47 per cent of older women were reported to have thiamin values less than two thirds of the RDA.[36] Similarly, nursing home residents were reported to have a mean intake of thiamin below two thirds of the RDA.[39,40]

Riboflavin intake was reported to meet two thirds of the RDA in all surveys reviewed. Preformed niacin was reported by some studies to be inadequate, and when compared with the current RDA, these values fell below the standard.[36,37,39] A closer look, however, revealed adequate protein intake, suggesting that the formation of niacin from the amino acid tryptophan could decrease the risk of a deficiency.

Urine analysis of the B vitamins provides a rough estimate of body reserves. Therefore, decreased intake may result in decreased output, as reflected in the urine. However, declining renal function with aging makes interpretation of urinary vitamin levels uncertain. Among elderly women, urinary riboflavin and thiamin were reported to be low in 15 and 17 per cent of the surveyed subjects, respectively.[36] Among institutionalized residents, high percentages of low urinary thiamin, riboflavin, and pyridoxine values were reported.[41,42] In a study that compared values of vitamins $B_2$ and $B_6$ in both institutionalized and noninstitutionalized subjects, lower urinary values of these vitamins were reported among institutionalized residents.[30] In addition, this study suggested that aging was associated with a significant decline in urinary riboflavin and pyridoxine values. A more sensitive biochemical assessment of B vitamin status can be obtained from a blood sample.

## *Calcium*

An increased prevalence of lactose intolerance among the elderly and the notion that calcium is no longer necessary beyond the ages of growth and development have contributed to a decline in the intake of milk and milk products among the elderly. This trend is apparent in the results of a number of surveys.

The calcium standard set by the TSNS for elderly males and females is one half of the current RDA. The HANES standard is slightly above two thirds the RDA for females and one half the RDA for males. The results from both the TSNS and HANES reported mean calcium dietary values that appeared adequate when compared with their own standards for all elderly population subgroups, with the exception of elderly black females. When compared with the RDA, a different interpretation of results is apparent. All groups from the TSNS and HANES are found to have mean calcium values falling below the RDA standard but above the two-thirds standard, except for the black female subgroup, whose mean intake fell below two thirds of the RDA. Many of the smaller studies reviewed confirm these findings (i.e, a mean calcium intake between the two-thirds standard and the full RDA standard) among both noninstitutionalized subjects[27,35,39] and nursing home residents.[32,39,40]

Further research is needed to determine if a decrease in calcium intake affects physiologic function in the elderly population. One area of current investigation involves the possibility of an increased calcium requirement greatly exceeding the present RDA for middle-aged and elderly women[43,44] (see Chapter 39). With the high incidence of osteoporosis found among middle-aged and older women, these findings could have their strongest impact on both the treatment and prevention of the disease.

## *Iron*

Iron standards used in the national surveys are similar to the current RDAs. The TSNS and HANES reported mean values of iron intake that fell below the RDA but above the two-thirds standard for all elderly female groups. Low dietary intake of iron was also reported among elderly females residing in nursing homes.[32,40] These low values are not, however, necessarily associated with anemia.

## *Dietary Supplements*

Intake of dietary supplements among the elderly has become very popular, particularly as a compensation for decreased appetite and, possibly, due to inadequate knowledge of dietary needs. Several studies investigating the use of dietary supplements indicate that only a small number of people using supplements chose them wisely and appropriately.[27,32,34] In fact, all three studies reviewed concluded that the intake of dietary supplements was frequently inappropriate or superflous. A large number of people who took supplements were found to have adequate diets, while others used nutrient supplements that did not match the deficient nutrients required. Consideration of dietary supplements is an important aspect of dietary assessment of any population group.

## CONCLUSION

At the present time the prevalence of malnutrition among the elderly is uncertain. From the information available, it would appear that the noninstitutionalized elderly in the United States are adequately nourished with regard to most nutrients, when using standards derived from younger populations. However, much more information is needed before final conclusions can be drawn, and the sick, institutionalized, or drug-taking elderly must be considered as special populations who appear to be at greater risk for malnutrition.

### References


1. Food and Nutrition Board: National Research Council Recommended Dietary Allowances. 9th rev. ed. Washington, DC, National Academy of Sciences, 1980.
2. Weinser RL, Hunker EM, Krumdieck CL, Butterworth CE: Hospital malnutrition. A prospective evaluation of general medical hospitalization. Am J Clin Nutr 32:418, 1979.
3. Mullen JL, Gertner MH, Buzby GP, et al: Implications of malnutrition in the surgical patient. Arch Surg 114:121, 1979.
4. Russell RM, Multack R, Smith V, et al: The use of dark adaptation as a reversible indicator of subclinical vitamin A deficiency in patients with chronic small intestinal disease. Lancet 2:1161, 1973.
5. Morrison SA, Russell RM, Carney EA, Oaks EV: Zinc deficiency: A cause of abnormal dark adaptation in cirrhotics. Am J Clin Nutr 31:276, 1978.
6. Dutta SK, Russell RM, Lakhanpal V: Abnormal dark adaptation associated with low plasma levels of vitamin A transport proteins: Correction by protein repletion. Nutr Res 1:443, 1981.
7. Lowenstein FW: Nutritional status of the elderly in the United States of America, 1971 – 1974. J Am Coll Nutr 1:165, 1982.
8. Kelly K. Russell RM, Greenberg L, et al: Nutritional status of adult patients in two acute care hospitals: A University Hospital and an affiliated Veterans Administration Medical Center. Nutr Res 2:213, 1982.
9. Hynak MT, Al-Ibrahim MS, Russell RM, et al: Nutritional and pulmonary function assessment in patients with chronic obstructive lung diseases. Nutr Res 1:461, 1981.
10. Bushman L, Russell RM, Warfield RD, et al: Malnutrition among patients in an acute care veterans facility. J Am Diet Assoc 77:462, 1980.
*This paper presents a prototype of a nutritional status survey conducted on patient populations at many hospitals. Although the standards used are now outdated, the findings of this survey are in keeping with the high prevalence of unrecognized hospital malnutrition found at many health care institutions in the United States.*
11. Carney EA, Russell RM: Correlation of dark adaptation test results with serum vitamin A levels in diseased adults. J Nutr 110:552, 1980.
*This article examines the relationship between serum vitamin A and vitamin A-dependent rod function (dark adaptation). An increase in the rod final threshold was found with advancing age. Further, in chronically ill patients, a high serum-vitamin level (up to 40 mg/dl) was required to insure normal rod function.*
12. Henkin RI, Bradley DF: Hypogeusia corrected by $Ni^{++}$ and $Zn^{++}$. Life Sci 9:701, 1970.
13. Schechter PJ, Friedewald WT, Bronzert DA, et al: Idiopathic hypogeusia: A description of a single blind study with zinc sulfate. *In* Pfeiffer CC (ed.): International Review of Neurobiology (Suppl). New York, Academic Press, 1972, pp. 125 – 140.
14. Schiffman SS, Hornack K, Reilly D: Increased taste thresholds of amino acids with age. Am J Clin Nutr 32:1622, 1979.
15. Nilsson B: Taste acuity of the human palate. III. Studies with taste solutions on subjects in different age groups. Acta Odontol Scand 37:235, 1979.
16. Grzegorczyk PB, Jones SW, Mistretta CM: Age-related differences in salt taste acuity. J Gerontol 34:834, 1979.
17. Russell RM, Jacob R, Greenberg L. Clinical assessment of the nutritional status of adults. *In* Linder M (ed.): Nutritional Biochemistry and Metabolism. New York, Elsevier Science Publishing Co., 1985, pp. 285 – 308.
18. Rossman I: Anatomic and body composition changes with aging. *In* Finch C, Hayflick L (eds.): Handbook of the Biology of Aging. New York, Van Nostrand Reinhold, 1977, pp. 189 – 221.
19. Butler RN: Diet related to killer disease. VII. Nutrition: Aging and the elderly. Hearing before the Select Committee on Nutrition and Human Needs of the United States Senate. September 23, 1977, p. 30.
20. Andres R: Influence of obesity on longevity in the aged. Adv Pathobiol 7:238, 1980.
*This report summarizes findings from several surveys that seem to show a mild advantage in terms of longevity to having a weight 10 per cent or greater than the 1959 Metropolitan Life Insurance Standards.*
21. Mitchell CO, Lipschitz DA: The effect of age and sex on the routinely used measurements to assess the nutritional status of hospitalized patients. Am J Clin Nutr 36:340, 349, 1982.
22. Frisancho AR: New norms of upper limb fat and muscle areas for assessment of nutritional status. Am J Clin Nutr 34:2540, 1981.
*Anthropometric norms for people ages 1 to 74 from HANES data are provided and are recommended to replace older standards based on TSNS data.*
23. Bishop CW, Bowen PE, Ritchey SJ: Norms for nutritional assessment of American adults by upper arm anthropometry. Am J Clin Nutr 34:2530, 1981.
24. Bowman BB, Rosenberg IH: Assessment of the nutritional status of the elderly. Am J Clin Nutr 35:1142, 1982.
25. Gray G, Gray LK: Validity of anthropometric norms used in the assessment of hospitalized patients. JPEN 3:366, 1979.
26. Greenblatt DJ: Reduced serum albumin concentration in the elderly: A report from the Boston Collaborative Drug Surveillance Program. J Am Geriatr Soc 27:20, 1979.

*The trend for decreased serum albumin levels with advancing age is presented. This trend has implications concerning the differences in drug disposition among the elderly and also in the assessment of the nutritional status of the elderly.*

27. Yearick ES, Wang ML, Pisias SJ: Nutritional status of the elderly: Dietary and biochemical findings. J Gerontol 35:663, 1980.
28. Baily LB, Wagner PA, Christakis GJ, et al: Folacin and iron status and hematologic findings in predominantly black elderly persons from urban low-income households. Am J Clin Nutr 32:2346, 1979.
29. Gershoff SN, Brusis OA, Nino HV, Huber AM: Studies of the elderly in Boston. I. The effects of iron fortification on moderately anemic people. Am J Clin Nutr 30:226, 1977.
*Iron fortification was used to correct anemia in elderly subjects. Over 6 to 8 months later, the hemoglobin level was found to rise in two groups of elderly: those receiving iron fortification and those receiving the same food without fortification. This study points out the pitfalls of nutrition intervention studies in that the rise in hemoglobin was due to an ill-defined intervention effect.*
30. Chen LH, Fan-Chiang WL: Biochemical evaluation of riboflavin and vitamin $B_6$ status of institutionalized and noninstitutionalized elderly in Central Kentucky. Int J Vitam Nutr Res 51:232, 1981.
31. Kohrs MB, O'Neal R, Preston A, et al: Nutritional status of elderly residents in Missouri. Am J Clin Nutr 31:2186, 1978.
32. Justice CL, Howe JM, Clark HE: Dietary intakes and nutritional status of elderly patients. J Am Diet Assoc 65:639, 1974.
33. McGandy RB, Barrows CH, Spanias A, et al: Nutrient intakes and energy expenditure in men of different ages. J Gerontol 21:581, 1966.
*The results from this study show a relative decrease in caloric intake with age, accounted for by a decrease in the amount of calories expended per day by activity rather than basal caloric output.*
34. Reid DL, Miles JE: Food habits and nutrient intakes of non-institutionalized senior citizens. Can J Public Health 68:154, 1977.
35. Grotkowski ML, Sims LS: Nutritional knowledge, attitudes, and dietary practices of the elderly. J Am Diet Assoc 72:499, 1978.
36. Harrill I, Cervone V. Vitamin status of older women. Am J Clin Nutr 30:431, 1977.
37. Center for Disease Control: Ten-State Nutrition Survey, 1968–1970. V. Dietary (DHEW Pub. No. (HMS) 72-8133). Atlanta, GA, U.S. Department of Health, Education and Welfare, 1972.
38. Garry PJ, Goodwin JS, Hunt WC, Gilbert BA: Nutritional status in a healthy elderly population: Vitamin C. Am J Clin Nutr 36:332, 1982.
39. Brown PT, Bergan JG, Parsons EP, Krol I: Dietary status of elderly people. J Am Diet Assoc 71:41, 1977.
40. Stiedmann M, Jansen C, Harrill I: Nutritional status of elderly men and women. J Am Diet Assoc 73:132, 1978.
41. Pollitt NT, Salkeld RM: Vitamin B status of geriatric patients. Nutr Metab 21(Suppl I):24, 1977.
42. Vir SC, Love AH: Nutritional evaluation of B groups of vitamins in institutionalized aged. Int J Vitam Nutr Res 47:211, 1977.
43. Heaney RP, Recher RR, Saville PD: Calcium balance and calcium requirements in middle-aged women. Am J Clin Nutr 30:1603, 1977.
*The mean intake required for zero calcium balance for postmenopausal women was reported as 1.504 gm/day. For premenopausal women, the mean intake for zero calcium balance was 0.989 gm/day. Both values are in excess of the current RDA for calcium for female adults.*
44. Heaney RP, Recker RR, Saville PD: Menopausal changes in calcium performance. J Lab Clin Med 92:953, 1978.

### *Additional Reading*

1. Munro HN: Nutrition and Aging. Br Med Bull 37:83, 1981.
2. Third Ross Roundtable on Medical Issues: Assessing the Nutritional Status of the Elderly—State of the Art. Report of the Third Ross Roundtable on Medical Issues. Columbus, OH, Ross Laboratories, 1982.

# *Special Issues in Nutrition*

## *Protein-Calorie Malnutritional Therapy*

*Paul Katz*
*David Dube*
*Evan Calkins*

The hazards and uncertainties incident to clinical assessment of nutritional deficiency have been cited in detail in Chapter 13. However, sufficient data are available to indicate that severe protein-calorie malnutrition is evident in many elderly patients at the time of entry into the hospital. In one study, 61 per cent of men 65 years of age and older who were admitted to a general hospital were found to have significant malnutrition.[1] Estimates of the frequency of protein-calorie malnutrition among the hospitalized elderly have ranged from 17 to 44 per cent for general medical patients[1,2] to 30 to 65 per cent for patients on the general surgical services.[3-7] Numerous studies have shown that patients with severe protein-calorie malnutrition exhibit decreased immune competence,[1,8-13] poor wound healing,[14,15] and other complications leading to increased duration of hospital stay and higher mortality.[16,17]

Although progressive malnutrition is frequently concomitant with hospitalization, the fact that many patients on both medical and surgical services already evidence malnutrition at the time of admission reinforces the importance of the determination of the weight of elderly patients as a routine part of every office visit. Loss of significant weight (10 to 20 per cent of a person's total weight) over the course of a few months clearly demands careful evaluation and initiation of appropriate therapy.

The history should include a thorough search for symptoms of associated disease, such as hyperthyroidism, neoplasm, or maldigestion (e.g., secondary to anatomic lesion, enzyme deficiencies, or mucosal defects). In addition, careful attention should be directed toward delineating psychologic or social problems with a potential impact on food consumption and availability (e.g., depression, change in social support system). A careful nutritional history should always be obtained. The examination should focus on the extent of nutritional deficits (e.g., through anthropometry) and on clues to possible underlying disease. If the history suggests dysphagia, the patient should be observed in the process of deglutition.

Important laboratory tests include complete blood count; estimations of total serum protein and albumin concentrations and triiodothyronine ($T_3$) and thyroxine ($T_4$) uptake; examination of stool for blood, fat, and undigested muscle fibers; and, if appropriate, determination of serum vitamin $B_{12}$ and folate concentrations. Further details concerning evaluation of the gastrointestinal system are provided in Chapter 46.

In many elderly patients, especially of very advanced age, it is not possible to attribute weight loss to any single cause, and one is forced to conclude that it is due to a combination of factors, many of which are referred to elsewhere in this book (e.g., loss of sense of taste and smell, ill-fitting dentures, poor oral hygiene, depression, social isolation and failure of social support system). Although difficulties in swallowing are not uncommon in the elderly, the cause remains obscure. The dysfunction may be attributable to a specific identifiable cause, such as Parkinson's disease, pseudobulbar palsy, or esophageal diverticulum, or may be associated with other factors not fully understood.

In seeking to reverse malnutrition of unknown etiology in a person living at home, an attempt should first be made to remedy or lessen each of the many factors that might contribute to the problem. Efforts should be made to ensure the preparation of good food, the presence of cheerful company while the elderly person is eating, optimal oral and dental hygiene, and the reduction of other apparently unrelated symptoms that might distract the patient, such as urinary retention. Selection of food should cater, insofar as is possible, to the patient's individual desires. Total calorie count should be ascertained.

If food consumption cannot be brought to a point that is judged to be adequate, the physician, patient, and family must decide whether enteral alimentation by way of gastric intubation is warranted. Before reaching this point, the physician often resorts to the use of oral nutritional supplements. Several formulations are currently available, differing in caloric source and content, including concentrations of vitamins and minerals. Russell, however, in Chapter 13, admonishes that "only a small number of people using supplements choose them wisely and appropriately" (see Chapter 13, references 27, 32, and 34). Several reviews conclude that "the intake of dietary supplements is frequently inappropriate and superfluous." Clearly, the physician must use this form of nutritional support with discretion, paying attention not only to efficacy but also to cost.

## TUBE FEEDING

If it proves impossible to maintain appropriate nutrition by the oral route, use of the nasal gastric feeding tube should be considered. This may be employed for months or years in patients both at home or in acute and long-term care institutions. However, this procedure does carry with it the hazards of aspiration and must be used with care. The appropriateness of maintaining patients on this form of alimentation for indefinite periods raises certain ethical considerations (see Chapter 9). Nevertheless, in hospitalized patients who are receiving the benefit of sophisticated and expensive medical and surgical management, to ignore the needs of nutritional support is illogical and seriously lessens the chances of ultimate success. Therefore, vigorous nutritional supplementation should, in our view, become much more widely used for elderly hospitalized patients than is currently the case in most institutions.

In the presence of a functional gastrointestinal tract, enteral alimentation allows repletion of lost calories by a means that most closely approximates the natural physiologic state. In general, feeding tubes should be pliable, of small caliber, and weighted for easy passage into the proximal small intestine, thus assuring patient comfort and decreasing the risk of aspiration. Tube insertion may be facilitated by the use of rigid "stylets." A conventional nasal gastric tube can be used to carry down a smaller feeding tube, with the use of an empty gelatin capsule holding both ends in place.

Once the enteral route has been selected for alimentation, selection of the proper feeding mixture is essential.[18] In the presence of a normally functioning gastrointestinal tract, without evidence of maldigestion, a polymeric formula is well tolerated. Such formulas (e.g., Isocal, Ensure, Osmolite) are generally lactose free and have the advantage of relatively low osmolality and cost. In contrast, monomeric formulas (e.g., Vivonex, Travasorb) must be utilized in the presence of abnormal digestive processes. Such mixtures tend to have higher osmolalities and are expensive. Both feeding mixtures usually provide one calorie per milliliter. In the presence of underlying cardiac, renal, or hepatic disease, special formulations may be warranted for salt or protein restrictions. Amino acid repletion may also be helpful in selected cases.[18]

Administration of the selected feeding mixture is easily accomplished using a constant infusion pump, with the head of the bed elevated approximately 30 degrees. Such precautions are taken to avoid problems such as aspiration or gastric distention. Initial rates and formula strengths should be low and gradually increased as tolerated. A daily multivitamin and mineral supplement may be given by way of the feeding tube. Monitoring of weight gain and other nutritional indices allows a reassessment of caloric needs on a continuing basis.

Complications are not uncommon but are often easily remedied. In the presence of diarrhea, a decrease in the feeding rate and/or concentration of the feeding mixture is usually helpful. Intercurrent illness with gastrointestinal manifestations must always be ruled out. If symptoms persist, the addition of an antidiarrheal agent, such as Lomotil, to the formula may be necessary.

If there is clinical evidence for gastric distention, retention may be confirmed by way of aspiration of gastric contents approximately 1 hour following feeding. If anatomic obstruction is not apparent, a decrease in the rate of formula administration and/or metaclopramide hydrochloride may alleviate the problem. For suspected aspiration, in addition to comprehensive medical management, one must confirm adequate tube placement by x-ray studies and assure proper head elevation throughout the day. Gastrostomy and/or jejunostomy may be required for recurrent aspiration.

## GASTROSTOMY/ JEJUNOSTOMY

For those patients intolerant of the nasal gastric tube or who suffer recurrent bouts of aspiration pneumonia, consideration must be given to feeding gastrostomy/jejunostomy. The risk of aspiration is inversely proportional to the distance of the ostomy site from the stomach.[19] Thus, jejunostomy would be preferable to gastrostomy for those patients still plagued by reflux of food into the esophagus with its attendant pulmonary complications. Jejunostomy, however, often requires the use of the more expensive monomeric formulas.

## PARENTERAL ALIMENTATION

Details of parenteral alimentation have been described in several recent publications.[20] This form of nutritional support is particularly suited to those patients whose gastrointestinal tract is non functional and in whom enteral alimentation is contraindicated, for example, as a result of gastrointestinal bleeding or obstruction. In addition, parenteral alimentation may have a role in the treatment of elderly patients with severe protein-calorie malnutrition, in the preparation for major cardiac surgery, or during the course of intensive medical treatment. However, in view of potential complications, it is our belief that in older people, nutritional therapy is best initiated by the oral or enteral route if at all possible.

### References

1. Bienia R, Ratcliff S, Barbour GL, Kummer M: Malnutrition in the hospitalized geriatric patient. J Am Geriatr Soc 30:433, 1982.
2. Bistrian BR, Blackburn GL, Vitale J, et al: Prevalence of malnutrition in general medical patients. JAMA 235:1567, 1976.
3. Bistrian BR, Blackburn MD, Hallowell E, Heddle R: Protein status of general surgical patients. JAMA 230:858, 1974.

4. Hill GL, Bowen JC, Copeland EM, et al: Malnutrition in surgical patients. Lancet 1:689, 1977.
5. Dionigi R, Ariszonta, Dominioni L, et al: The effects of total parenteral nutrition on immunodepression due to malnutrition. Ann Surg 185:467, 1977.
6. Willicutts HD: Nutritional assessment of one thousand surgical patients in an affluent suburban community hospital. JPEN 1:25, 1977.
7. Young GA, Hill GL: Assessment of protein calorie malnutrition in surgical patients from plasma proteins and anthropometric measurements. Am J Clin Nutr 31:429, 1978.
8. Buzby GP, Mullen JL, Matthews DC, Hobbs CL, Rosato EF: Prognostic nutritional index in gastrointestinal surgery. Am J Surg 139:160, 1980.
9. Mullen JL, Gertner MH, Buzby GP, et al: Implications of malnutrition in the surgical patient. Arch Surg 114:121, 1979.
10. Mullen JL: Reduction of operative morbidity and mortality by combined preoperative and post-operative nutritional support. Ann Surg 192:604, 1980.
11. Bistrian BR, Blackburn GL, Scrimshaw NS, et al: Cellular immunity in semistarved states in hospitalized adults. Am J Clin Nutr 28:1148, 1975.
12. Spanier AH, Pletsch JB, Meakins JL, et al: The relationship between immune competence and nutrition. Surg Forum 27:332, 1976.
13. Copeland EM, Daly JM, Guinn E, et al.: Effects of protein malnutrition on cell mediated immunity. Surg Forum 27:340, 1976.
14. Bozzetti F, Terno G, Longoni C: Parenteral hyperalimentation and wound healing. Surg Gynecol Obstet 141:712, 1975.
15. Irvin TT: Effects of malnutrition and hyperalimentation on wound healing. Surg Gynecol Obstet 146:33, 1978.
16. Blackburn GL, Bistrian BR, Maini BS, et al: Nutritional and metabolic assessment of the hospitalized patient. JPEN 1:11, 1977.
17. Roberts-Thompson IC, Whittingham S, Youngchaiyud U: Ageing, immune response, and mortality. Lancet 2:368, 1974.
18. Heymsfield SB, Bethel RA, Ansley JD, et al: Enteral hyperalimentation: An alternative to central venous hyperalimentation. Ann Intern Med 90:63, 1979.
19. Torosian MH, Ranbeau JL: Feeding by the tube enterostomy. Surg Gynecol Obstet 150:918, 1980.
20. Phillips GD, Odgers CL: Parenteral nutrition: Current status and concepts. Drugs 23:276, 1982.


# *Drug-Nutrient Interrelationships*

*Jeffrey Blumberg*

The effect of drug exposure on nutritional status and, conversely, the effect of nutrient intake on the fate and effectiveness of drugs are potentially serious problems for the geriatric patient. Although substantial data have been generated in animal species, only limited information exists in humans as to the clinical significance and the frequency of occurrence of these interactions (see references[1–5] for reviews). In this brief discussion, these interrelationships are presented as they have been demonstrated in elderly people and categorized by their principal locus in drug disposition or utilization processes.

## ABSORPTION

Changes in intestinal motility, intraluminal pH, mucosal cell morphology, enzyme kinetics, and bacterial flora and the presence of chelators represent the principal mechanisms whereby drugs may interfere with the absorption and availability of essential nutrients. The age-related physiologic changes of the gastrointestinal tract that could affect drug absorption, such as decreases in splanchnic blood flow, gastric acidity, and intestinal motility, appear to be overcome to a considerable degree by the very large capacity of the system for absorption of small molecular-weight compounds. There are, however, numerous examples of drug-induced malnutrition syndromes. No general set of rules or comprehensive hypothesis, however, serves to categorize or predict their occurrence. Examples of commonly used drugs that may affect absorption include antacids, laxatives, anti-inflammatory drugs, cardiovascular agents, and certain antibacterials.

### *Antacids*

Antacids usually contain aluminum and/or magnesium hydroxide, which combines with dietary phosphate to form insoluble salts. Symptoms of phosphate depletion, such as proximal limb muscle weakness, malaise, paresthesias, and anorexia, are most likely to occur in patients with low phosphate diets who use antacids habitually. The elevation of gastric pH by antacids also decreases the solubility and absorption of iron and destroys thiamin.

### *Laxatives*

Laxative abuse is common in the elderly. Stool softeners, such as mineral oil, if taken at mealtime or in the postprandial absorptive period, prevent the absorption of carotene and the fat-soluble vitamins by way of solubilization. Use of mineral oil should be avoided near or during mealtimes and in food preparation. Overuse of diphenylmethane derivatives, including phenolphthalein (ExLax) and bisacodyl (Dulcolax), has resulted in severe malabsorption, with steatorrhea, decreased glucose, calcium, and vitamin D absorption, and protein-losing enteropathy.[6] Daily consumption of milk or milk products is recommended to counter the phenolphthalein effects (if lactose intolerant, use fermented dairy products) and increased potassium, protein, and carbohydrate intake should accompany chronic use of bisacodyl. Laxatives such as dioctylsulfosuccinate (Colace, Doxinate), which alter electrolyte transport, are commonly associated with potassium deficiency; this hypokalemia is most likely to develop in geriatric patients with marginal potassium intake and in those receiving prescriptions for potassium-losing diuretics.

### *Anti-inflammatory Drugs*

Anti-inflammatory drugs, such as aspirin and indomethacin (Indocin), produce multiple small hemorrhages of the gastrointestinal mucosa, leading to iron deficiency anemia and decreased absorption of vitamin C. Chronic aspirin therapy is also associated with folacin deficiency and macrocytic anemia, with the greatest risk occurring in patients with low folacin intake.[7] Colchicine has been noted to decrease the absorption of protein, fat, lactose, carotene, vitamin $B_{12}$, sodium, potassium, and bile acids as a result of villous damage. For patients using these drugs, nutritional recommendations indicate a low fat diet, including low fat yogurt and cheese, with no whole milk.

### *Antibiotics*

Neomycin administration may be associated with a malabsorption syndrome, with reduced absorption of xylose, glucose, cholesterol, carotene, iron, and vitamin $B_{12}$ and increased fecal loss of fat, nitrogen, sodium, postassium, and calcium.[8] The tetracycline antibiotics decrease the absorption of iron, calcium, magnesium, amino acids, fats, and fat soluble vitamins. Cycloserine (Seromycin) decreases the absorption of calcium, magnesium, folic acid, and vitamins $B_6$ and $B_{12}$.

The presence of food in the gastrointestinal tract may delay gastric-emptying time, increase gastric pH, and alter drug stability and solubility. The clinical significance of altered therapeutic efficacy due to food-induced changes in drug bioavailability occurs principally with drugs that have low therapeutic indices, steep dose-response curves, or narrow divisions between therapeutic and toxic blood levels. Extensive lists have been published concerning when to administer drugs before, during, or after meals.[9]

The risk of drug-induced nutritional deficiencies is greatest for individuals who are on marginal diets and are using high doses of drugs over long periods and whose nutritional status is compromised by the physiologic stress of preexistent disease. Appropriately selected nutritional diets and/or daily vitamin and mineral supplementation to provide 100 per cent of the United States Department of Agriculture's Recommended Dietary Allowance (RDA) is sufficient in many cases to overcome decreased nutrient absorption induced by drug therapy. However, it is necessary to appreciate that for the elderly, the RDAs of some nutrients, such as calcium, may themselves be inadequate.

## DISTRIBUTION

Nutritional influences on drug distribution appear limited to the large reduction of plasma albumin seen in poorly nourished geriatric patients. Even in well-nourished, healthy elderly people, albumin concentrations have been found, in some studies, to be lower than in young adults.[10*] Thus, for extensively protein-bound drugs, such as diazepam and warfarin, whose binding may be reduced in old age and whose free fraction is therefore increased, lower ranges of therapeutic and toxic plasma concentrations may be seen.[12]Dietary fats may modify drug distribution; free fatty acids compete for anionic binding sites on plasma albumin, increasing the pharmacologic activity of the displaced drug.

## METABOLISM

Rates of drug metabolism decrease with age, and this change may be altered by nutritional status or diet.[13] High protein diets increase and low protein–high carbohydrate diets decrease the rate of drug metabolism.[14] The indolic com-

* Other studies have shown that healthy noninstitutionalized elderly people have normal concentrations of serum albumin.[11]

pounds present in vegetables of the Brassica family, such as cabbage and Brussels sprouts, appear to stimulate drug metabolism pathways. Charcoal-broiling of food can promote hepatic drug metabolism. Alterations of intestinal microflora produced by changes in the dietary level or source of protein or fiber may influence intestinal drug metabolism.

Several clinically significant effects of nutrient abundance on drug metabolism have been documented. Diet supplementation with vitamin $B_6$ blocks the therapeutic effectiveness of L-dopa by serving as coenzyme for L-dopa decarboxylase, thereby converting the drug to dopamine, which does not readily cross the blood-brain barrier. High doses of vitamin K ingested by way of foods such as spinach, cheese, or liver are contraindicated for patients receiving coumarin or indanedione anticoagulants because it can negate the drug's action of inhibiting regeneration of vitamin K from the hepatic 2,3-epoxide storage form. Megadoses of vitamin E in addition to a therapeutic regimen of warfarin sodium result in severely depressed levels of vitamin K–dependent coagulation factors and a hemorrhagic syndrome. Evaluation of altered rates of drug metabolism in the elderly is complicated by a reduced enzyme induction response, e.g., smoking increases drug metabolism in young adults but this effect is diminished or lost in the elderly.[15] Also, the metabolism of nutrients may be altered by drug-stimulated enzyme induction, resulting in an increased requirement for nutrients. Correctable pyridoxine-deficiency peripheral neuropathies have resulted during hydralazine antihypertensive therapy, although the mechanism of the interaction is not clear.

## EXCRETION

As noted in Chapter 31, a general reduction in total clearance of drugs is associated with old age.[16] This reduction is due, in part, to the declines in the glomerular filtration rate and the function of hepatic microsomal enzymes responsible for phase I oxidative drug metabolism (principally hydroxylation and N-dealkylation). Protein malnutrition, if present, further diminishes the gastrointestinal absorption and renal excretion of drugs, owing to the presence of edema, and impairs drug metabolism in the liver. The increased loss of nutrients consequent to drug administration has been documented in several cases.[10] Stimulation of sodium and potassium loss in the urine occurs as a result of thiazide or furosemide diuretic therapy; supplemental potassium is often necessary to replace the loss. The possibility of this excessive urinary output increasing the loss of trace metals and water-soluble vitamins has not been closely examined. Isoniazid and penicillamine form water-soluble complexes with pyridoxal phosphate, which is excreted by the kidneys, resulting in neurologic manifestations of vitamin $B_6$ deficiency.

## PHARMACODYNAMIC CONSIDERATIONS

The drug-nutrient interactions discussed previously occur on a pharmacokinetic level and influence the amount of drug that can be made available to a given receptor. Pharmacodynamic alterations in response are attributable to changes in the activity or number of receptor sites, mechanical limitations imposed by pathologic lesions, and the loss of coordinated homeostatic responses of systems that in the younger patient are sufficiently integrated to minimize the secondary actions of drugs. Several such adverse drug reactions, such as those resulting from interactions between monoamine oxidase inhibitors and tyramine-containing foods and between aldehyde dehydrogenase inhibitors and ethanol, have been clearly documented.[2] However, the influence of nutrition on age-related parameters affecting drug action, such as the loss of betaadrenoceptors, central nervous system neurons, and pancreatic beta cells, is, at present, only speculative.

## APPETITE

Although drugs may induce hyperphagia or hypophagia, drug effects on appetite are strongly influenced by situational factors.[16] Appetite in debilitated elderly patients may be stimulated by cyproheptadine (Periactin), an antagonist of both histamine and serotonin.[17] Psychotropic agents, such as the phenothiazines and benzodiazepines, appear to increase food intake in some individuals, although high doses in elderly patients, whose rate of drug metabolism is slow, may induce somnolence and indifference to food. Amitriptyline and related tricyclic antidepressants stimulate appetite but sometimes cause behavioral agitation, which may interfere with eating.[18] The oral hypoglycemic agents, such as tolbutamide and chlorpropamide, may stimulate appetite by way of pancreatic release of insulin. Anabolic steroids and glucocorticoids also appear to increase food intake. Brief or prolonged periods of anorexia associated with pharmacologic therapy are often due to effects on the gastrointestinal tract. Antineoplastic drugs, such as *cis*-platinum and methotrexate, induce nausea, vomiting, and aversion to food.[19] Chelation of zinc or copper by thiol-containing drugs, such as d-penicillamine, griseofulvin, lincomycin, and thiamazole, appears to reduce taste acuity.[20] The cardiac glycosides produce anorexia accompanied by nausea; high-dose treatment may result in digitalis cachexia.[21] Although alcohol abuse can cause anorexia, among the elderly, even social drinkers tend to have lower food intake than age-matched nondrinkers.

## CONCLUSION

Drugs may influence the dietary intake of nutrients, their disposition within the body, and their rates of elimination. Conversely, the nutritional status of the patient can influence both the efficacy and toxicity of drug treatment. The physiologic changes in organ function that occur with aging further complicate these interrelationships in assessing the geriatric patient. These interrelationships often appear to be subtle but significant. However, they have only recently begun to be studied clinically. Awareness of these situations can alert the practicing physician to potential problems and practical remedies.

### References


1. Mueller JF: Drug-nutrient interactions. *In* Afin-Slater RB, Kritchevsky D (eds.): Human Nutrition: A Comprehensive Treatise. Vol. 3B. New York, Plenum Press, 1980, pp. 351–365.
   *This chapter presents an overview of drug-nutrient interactions, with an emphasis on drug metabolism in animal studies.*
2. Hathcock JN, Coon J: Nutrition and Drug Interactions. New York, Academic Press, 1978.
3. Parke DV, Ioannides C: The role of nutrition in toxicology. Ann Rev Nutr 1:207, 1981.
   *A review of the influence of nutrition on the detoxication and activation of xenobiotics, with an emphasis on microsomal mixed function oxidase systems.*
4. Roe DA: Drug-Induced Nutritional Deficiencies. Westport, CT, Avi Publishing Co., 1976.
   *The only full textbook to date covering basic nutritional and pharmacologic concepts, with critical reviews of relevant literature.*
5. Hartshorn EA: Food and drug interactions. J Am Diet Assoc 70:15, 1977.
6. Levine D, Goode AW, Wingate DL: Purgative abuse associated with reversible cachexia, hypogammaglobulinaemia, and finger clubbing. Lancet 1:919, 1981.
7. Weiss HJ: Aspirin—a dangerous drug? JAMA 229:1121, 1974.
8. Jacobson ED, Prior JT, Faloon WW: Malabsorptive syndrome induced by neomycin: Morphologic alterations in the jejunal mucosa. J Lab Clin Med 56:245, 1960.
9. Toothaker RD, Welling PG: The effect of food on drug availability. Annu Rev Pharmacol Toxicol 20:173, 1980.
   *This is a review, with extensive tabulated data, of the effects of food and fluid volumes on the rate and extent to which oral dosage forms are absorbed.*
10. Greenblatt DJ, Sellers EM, Shader RI: Drug disposition in old age. N Engl J Med 306:1081, 1982.
    *A concise review of age-related pharmacokinetic changes and discussion of methodologic pitfalls.*
11. MacLennan WJ, Martin P, Mason BJ: Protein intake and serum albumin levels in the elderly. Gerontology 23:360, 1977.
12. Richey DP, Bender AD: Pharmacokinetic consequences of aging. Annu Rev Pharmacol Toxicol 17:49, 1977.
13. O'Malley K, Crooks J, Duke E, Stevenson IH: Effect of age and sex on human drug metabolism. Br Med J 3:607, 1971.
14. Alvares AP, Anderson KE, Cooney AH, Kappas A: Interactions between nutritional factors and drug biotransformations in man. Proc Natl Acad Sci USA 73:2501, 1976.
15. Vestal RE, Norris AH, Tobin JD, et al: Antipyrine metabolism in man: Influence of age, alcohol, caffeine, and smoking. Clin Pharmacol Ther 18:425, 1975.
16. Pawan GLS: Drugs and appetite. Proc Nutr Soc 33:239, 1974.
17. Stiel JN, Liddle, GW, Lacy WW: Studies on the mechanism of cyproheptadine-induced weight gain in human subjects. Metabolism 19:192, 1970.
18. Paybel PS, Mueller PS, DeLa Vergne PM: Amitriptyline weight gain and carbohydrate craving: A side effect. Br J Psychiatr 123:501, 1973.
19. Morrison SD: Origins of anorexia in neoplastic disease. Am J Clin Nutr 31:1104, 1978.
20. Hanlon DP: Interaction of thiamazole with zinc and copper. Lancet 1:929, 1975.
21. Banks T, Ali N: Digitalis cachexia. N Engl J Med 290:746, 1974.


### *Additional Reading*


1. Molleson AL, Gallagher-Allred CR: Nutrient and Drug Interactions. Nutrition in Primary Care Series, Ohio State University, 1980.
   *This resource book presents tables of drug-nutrient interactions and related information, such as tyramine content of foods and sodium content of drugs.*
2. Roe DA (ed.): Drug-Nutrient Interactions. New York, Alan R. Liss.
   *The only periodical devoted exclusively to drug-nutrient interactions and reporting both experimental and clinical data. Volume 1 was published 1981 to 1982.*

Chapter 14

# Rehabilitation for the Elderly

Carl V. Granger

On the basis of data from the National Center for Health Statistics,[1] it has been determined that being older, of low income, female, or of a racial minority are factors associated with a higher probability of having limitations in activity, that is, of having a disability. The figures presented in Table 14-1 reflect the increasing prevalence of disability with age. A widely held tenet is that early identification of disability is more likely to result in successful management. On the other hand, early identification of disability is not common in medical practice. A survey performed in Atlanta showed that 25 per cent of physicians from specialties likely to see patients with physical impairments reported seeing no patients who were in need of rehabilitation services over the 6-month period prior to the survey.[2]

This chapter addresses the issue of disability and its amelioration through rehabilitation. Disability is most frequently experienced by those of our population who are disadvantaged in other ways, including the frequent failure of physicians to incorporate a functional perspective in providing their health care. The discussion to follow covers theoretic conceptualization and terminology of disablement, consideration of the combination of factors that contribute to disability, and methods of functional assessment. Rehabilitation is the discipline that combines the functional perspective with efforts to ameliorate functional limitations, whether caused by disease, environment, or the aging process. Aging is not an inexorable march, year-by-year, toward progressive functional decline. Aging is not one thing but many, and there are large differences among aged individuals in both the kinds of components and the rates at which they change. As a result, selective rehabilitative interventions may improve important abilities. Strategies for including rehabilitation or the functional perspective in the care of elderly patients, for early identification of disability, and for approaching severe disability, as well as factors important to geriatric inpatient rehabilitation, are discussed.

In 1980, two publications addressed the issues of theoretic conceptualization, development of a glossary and refinement of definition, unification of the terminology of disablement, and exploration of social policy toward disablement. These publications are the International Classification of Impairments, Disabilities, and Handicaps (ICIDH)[3] and the monograph People With Disabilities—Toward Acquiring Information Which Reflects More Sensitively Their Problems and Needs.[4] The aim of both publications was to overcome the constraints of the medical model by extending beyond disease per se to concepts and classification schemes for the consequences of disease, namely, impairment, disability, and handicap. The important concepts and definitions include the following: (1) Impairments are the anatomic, physiologic, mental, and psychologic deficits that represent the organic dysfunctions that are coded in the *International Classification of Disease—9th Edition—Clinical Modification* (ICD—9—CM).[5] (2) Disabilities are deficits in performance (resulting from impairment) that represent restrictions in the manner or range of activities considered normal within the context of the physical and social environments. (3) Handicaps (resulting from impairment and disability or impairment alone) are the social disadvantages that an individual experiences in fulfilling roles that are considered normal, depending upon the age and sex of the

**Table 14-1.** PERCENTAGE OF POPULATION WITH FUNCTIONAL LIMITATIONS BY TYPE OF LIMITATION, DATA SOURCE, AND AGE GROUP*

| | Functional Limitation (%) | | | |
|---|---|---|---|---|
| | *Personal Care* | | *Personal Care and/or Mobility* | |
| **Age Group** | *HIS*† | *SIE*‡ | *HIS*† | *SIE*‡ |
| Adults under 45 | 0.2 | 0.5 | 0.5 | 0.5 |
| 45–64 | 1 | 2 | 2 | 3 |
| 65–74 | 4 | 5 | 7 | 8 |
| 75–84 | 12 | 14 | 20 | 21 |
| 85 plus | 38 | 40 | 53 | 50 |

* Modified from 1980 Data Coverage of the Functionally Limited Elderly. Report of the Interagency Statistical Committee on Long-Term Care for the Elderly, U.S. Office of Management and Budget.

† 1977 Health Interview Survey plus 1977 National Nursing Home Survey.

‡ 1976 Survey of Income and Education plus 1977 National Nursing Home Survey.

individual as well as social and cultural factors. Since handicaps are influenced by social role norms and social policy, problems related to social disadvantages should be distinguished from problems related to activity restrictions (disability) or problems related to organic dysfunction (impairment). Examples of disability are activity restrictions in performing toileting, ambulation, or household chores, maintaining person-to-person contacts, carrying out the tasks of an assigned job, and using transportation resources to travel from place to place. Examples of handicaps are the social stigma, disadvantage, and restrictions imposed by social policy when one is deviant from the norm in either appearance, demeanor, or performance, or even by virtue of certain diagnostic labels. There are negative attitudes felt toward the elderly that constitute a major barrier to securing adequate physical and mental health care and appropriate rehabilitative care for many people over the age of 65 years.

A major reason for distinguishing the consequences of chronic illness from those of acute illness is that the burdens placed by each on the individual, family members, and society in general are different, both qualitatively and quantitatively. In particular, the strategy of treatment of chronic illness is directed not toward cure but toward optimal case management. In order to respond more appropriately to the burdens of disablement, data on impairment, disability, and handicap must be collected. In analyzing the data, three factors that differentiate acute from chronic disorders must be recognized: In chronic illness, (1) the time scale is such that the importance of the initial pathologic process becomes dwarfed by consequent health and psychosocial considerations, (2) clinical outcomes are variable and less finite, calling for repeated assessments over time, and (3) solutions to clinical problems extend beyond the usual medical interventions and must incorporate a range of other professional disciplines and include use of physical aids, physical and psychologic treatments, and social support.

## THE FUNCTIONAL PERSPECTIVE

Rehabilitation in the health care setting, along with usual medical and surgical care, means maximizing the individual's abilities and functions in physical, mental, emotional, social, and vocational terms. A rehabilitation (or functional) perspective requires not only that priority be given to matters of controlling and stabilizing medical problems but that priorities for treatment be balanced to support needs for both the health and the personal well-being of the individual. Particularly for those whose conditions are noncurable and are therefore chronic, the end-points of treatment can be evaluated in terms of the outcomes in personal functioning and quality of life. The specific domains are discussed later in this chapter.

The idea of assessing a patient's need for treatment on the basis of accurate diagnosis and understanding of the pathophysiologic processes is well embedded in the traditional medical education and systems of practice. Less traditional, but sometimes more appropriate to the situation, is a specific analysis of the degree to which organic, psychologic, and social circumstances in combination account for limitations in function and how these limitations can be reduced to preserve the range of normal activities through medical and physical restoration, psychologic training, or boosting of social supports.

This kind of analysis is especially appropriate for the elderly person who becomes ill because the organic, psychologic, and social factors often become inextricably intertwined. The fact that the symptom complexes and signs of illness may be much less dramatic in the elderly person adds confusion to the processes of diagnosis and treatment. Too often the analysis of a patient's problems stops before consideration is given to issues related to disability and handicap. Although the knowledge of the pathologic state and its etiology aid the physician in understanding the nature of disease and its prognosis, there are limits to the value of this kind of information in the patient with chronic disease. Sometimes the impairment is more apparent through loss of function than it is by anatomic changes, such as in visual or hearing loss or loss of muscle strength. In addition, cognitive and affective disorders are notable as a result of functional changes rather than as a result of the presence of particular types of pathologic conditions. One of the important reasons for using functional assessment in the care of the elderly is that "diagnoses alone present an inadequate index of health because the range of severity within a diagnosis is often greater than that among diagnoses."[6,7] Since there may be more variation in functional capacity among individuals with the same diagnosis than among people with different diagnoses, it can be expected that traditional medical factors alone would not explain status or outcomes in the broader dimensions of functional activities. Therefore, it is necessary to know the psychosocial characteristics of the elderly patient and to be able to integrate this information with that which is known about the organic impairments. Doing this in a timely, comprehensive, and continuous fashion will result in enhancement of health status and psychosocial well-being, which is the goal of rehabilitation.

## FUNCTIONAL ASSESSMENT

Given that (1) activity restrictions (disability) become more common with advancing age; (2) health care providers are not inclined toward early recognition of functional deficits nor toward management of patients from the perspective of enhancing functional status by a combination of treatment interventions; (3) the time scale of disability is such that the initial pathologic process becomes dwarfed by the consequent health and psychosocial circumstances; (4) clinical outcomes are not finite in people with disability; (5) solutions to clinical problems must incorporate a range of sociomedical approaches; and (6) the aged and aging individuals represent a wide scatter of abilities, limitations and circumstances, then, clinicians require a data base and guidance system that acknowledges factors that are important to well-being that extend beyond just biomedical concerns. Functional assessment is a method for describing abilities and limitations in order to measure an individual's performance of the activities that are necessary for daily living. The technique includes coding selected categories of impairment, certain behavioral responses, levels of social support, and the degree to which social role expectations are being met.

One of the earliest definitions of functional assessment was provided by Lawton.[8] He stated that it "means any systematic attempt to measure objectively the level at which a person is functioning, in any of a variety of areas such as physical health, quality of self-maintenance, quality of role activity, intellectual status, social activity, attitude toward the world and self, and emotional status." He listed these reasons for using functional assessment: (1) All areas of functioning are considered in treating the patient, (2) a more complete picture of the person is obtained, (3) objective evidence is developed to support the clinical impression, (4) communication to others is facilitated, (5) the results of treatment are more easily assessed, and (6) functional assessment helps the practitioner to monitor the results of professional techniques employed in treatment.

Historically, functional assessment has evolved from the measurement of single body functions, such as posture, range of joint motion, muscle strength, or intelligence, to the measurement of composite behaviors within various environmental contexts. Earlier tools for functional assessment yielded poor measurement characteristics. Very few of the many scales that now exist have been tested with any rigor regarding reliability, validity, precision, or feasibility. The index of the activities of daily living, developed by Katz,[9] was one of the first to emphasize the functioning of the person as a whole rather than the measurement of pieces. Because of the multidimensional nature of data being collected through periodic assessments of the same individuals, modern methods of functional assessment incorporate computer technology for systematic storage and retrieval of the information in order to facilitate long-term tracking of patients in the clinical setting. An excellent compendium of functional assessment instruments has been written by Kane and Kane[6] (see Chapter 8 for an alternative strategy for functional assessment).

The clinician who is proficient in using functional assessment will have a performance-oriented data base that can be analyzed along with the patient's known diagnostic and impairment conditions in order to produce a complete profile on how effectively the person interacts with the environment. Equipped with this dynamic profile, the clinician will improve case management by focusing on problems and needs quickly and accurately. Thus, appropriate intervention and coordination of services can be developed to optimize clinical outcomes and quality of life.

Much of what is known and understood about functional assessment instruments has been derived from research and demonstration projects. Despite the greater complexities involved in caring for the elderly, clinicians generally resist using systematic assessment of function in practice. Reasons for this are complex but probably are related to over-reliance on diagnostically related data, a sense that using functional assessment checklists is too "cookbookish," and a poor understanding of the relationships of functional behaviors to overall well-being. Yet, the core of geriatric practice is case management, and a case manager needs to use the most pertinent information—which in the case of nonacute geriatric care relates to the results of the assessment of the patient's functional status. Some crucial concepts covered by Kane and Kane include the following:[6]

1. The case manager is responsible for decisions about the way resources are allocated to an individual patient on the basis of the patient's needs; the presumed effects of various management strategies on the patient's well-being; and of course, the availability of resources across the total community.
2. A physician may not necessarily make all of the assessments that lead to the service prescription, but it is argued that he serves a coordinating role.
3. Although cutoff scores on such scales could hardly be used as mechanical guides to specific actions, they can assist a case manager in reviewing the amount of care required by an individual, translating his functional limitations into practical factors relating to his capacity for self-care, considering the individual's affective state and social circumstances, and eventually reaching recommendations. Multidimensional assessments have also been used as tools to predict who will be able to remain in the community; to the extent that such scales have prognostic capability, they can be used to establish norms for the kinds and numbers of long-term care services needed.
4. Furthermore, measures of functional status may also be used as an indicator of the quality of care received.[6]

In terms of practical utility, although an infinite number of variables may be collected, decisions have to be made concerning what to measure or not measure. On the other hand, documentation of small gains in ability to handle tasks of daily living can have enormous quality benefits for the patient and mean relief of a considerable burden of care for a family member and for the community. Because they do not understand comprehensive assessment well, many clinicians adopt the "cafeteria" approach to measurement, picking and choosing assessment instruments based upon what strikes the fancy. Also, lured by a false sense of economy, clinicians may compile meaningless data that not only cannot be interpreted but also cannot be communicated to other clinicians and investigators who are working with the same or similar problems.

## VITALITY AND AGING VERSUS THE SLOW EPIDEMIC OF DISABILITY

According to Strehler[10] and to Fries and Crapo,[11] a person's life span is fixed at an average age of 85 years, with an absolute limit of 115 years even when the person is free of diseases and accidents. By plotting "percentage survival" against "age at death" from ancient times to 1980, they estimate that 80 per cent of premature death has been eliminated (Fig. 14–1). Thus, "most remaining premature death is concentrated in the years over age 60 and is due to the chronic illnesses."[11] They propose a health strategy involving removal of the risk factors associated with acceleration of these disease processes. By such a strategy, the time of clinical threshold is delayed to a point in time that projects beyond the finite life span, which allows the chronic disease process to appear as if it were actually prevented. If such a strategy was successful, the implication would be that infirmity and incapacity would be compressed against a fixed life span, so that as the age of manifestation of illness is extended, the period of illness must become shorter and less lingering. "With chronic illness delayed—in some cases, so delayed that the illness will not occur within the life span—the period of adult vigor is prolonged."[11] One beneficial effect of this "rectangularization of the survival curve" would be to cause a decline in overall health care costs per person by as much as 20 per cent.

In contrast to this picture of what may occur with the strategy of delaying the manifestation of chronic diseases[10] is a projection of current trends by Wylie[12]: (1) From 1953 to 1978, the population aged 65 and older rose by 76 per cent, twice as fast as the total population, creating large demands on hospital and health services. If death rates continue to fall, that population will remain the fastest growing segment. Should death rates remain constant, the elderly population would reach 32 million by 2003, compared with 23 million at the present time. Constant death rates would double the population aged 85 and over, whereas falling death rates would cause the advanced age group to

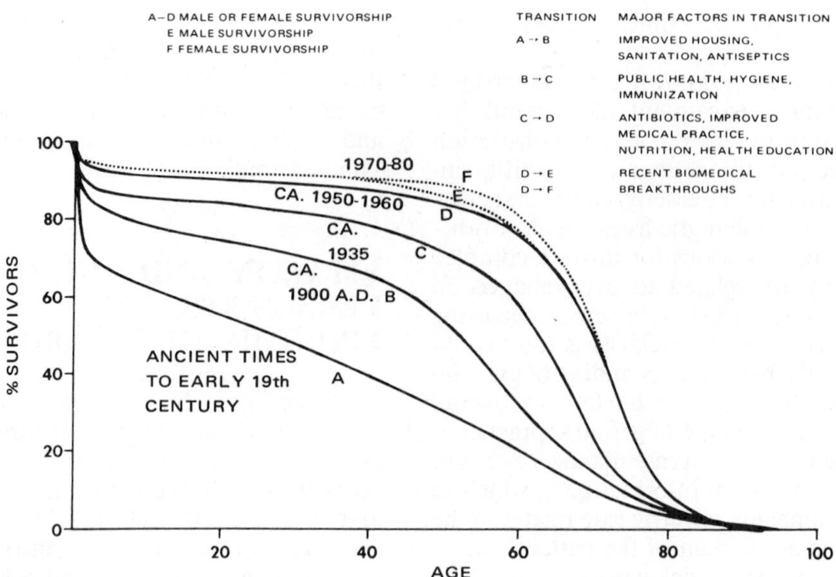


**Figure 14–1.** Human survivorship trends from ancient times to the present. These idealized curves illustrate the rapid approach to the limiting rectangular curve that has occurred during the last 150 years. The inset on the upper right lists major factors responsible for these transitions. Note that life expectancy for males has not changed since 1950 in the 50+ age group but that female survivorship has improved during this period, partially, at least, because of better treatment of reproductive system malignancies. (From Strehler BL: Implications of aging research for society. *In* Thorbecke GJ (ed.): Biology of Aging and Development. Bethesda, FASEB and New York and London, Plenum Press, 1975. Reproduced with permission.)

triple in number.[2] Since disease-related problems rise with age, both the expanding size and the advancing average age of the future population will have a multiplicative effect on the use of health services. On the basis of responses to the question obtained from the National Health Interview Survey,[13] "Does your health limit your ability to work, participate in leisure activities, perform household chores, move about or perform selfcare?" it was projected that between now and the year 2003, there will be 11 to 15 million more people with activity limitations than there are at present. Such people make high demands on the health services, not just because of their functional limitations but also because more new illnesses of all kinds develop in them than in the nonlimited population.[3] By 2003, about 40 per cent of hospital days of care will be delivered to the population aged 65 and over, compared with 37 per cent at the present time. Even greater will be the increase in nursing home residents from 1.3 million in 1973 to probably 2.8 million in 2003.

Shock[14] showed that many important physiologic functions decline with age (Fig. 14–2). Since these data were obtained from healthy subjects, the observed decline does not depend on disease. However, this decline erodes excess organ reserve that is beyond immediate functional needs, except under circumstances of unusual stress. In spite of these physiologic measures of decline in organ function, chronologic age is at best a rough approximation of these changes, and there is a wide range of differences in performance of age-related functions for any single-age cohort.[15] Costa and McCrae[15] stated the following:

> Chronological age is indeed a dummy variable, and research should attempt to replace it in every case with an account of the real etiology of age-related changes. . . . The changes which occur with time do not march arm-in-arm toward death to the drumming of 'functional age' but rather execute a more subtle and complicated dance which only painstaking and systematic research will uncover.[15]

Fries and Crapo[11] observed that none of the anatomic or physiologic changes is a satisfactory marker of aging, and the "scatter" around the average or variability actually increases with age, such that the differences between individuals grow with aging. They noted that aging is not one process but many; therefore, approaches to modification of aging must focus on the particular attribute to be changed. They predict that markers such as "graying of hair, the

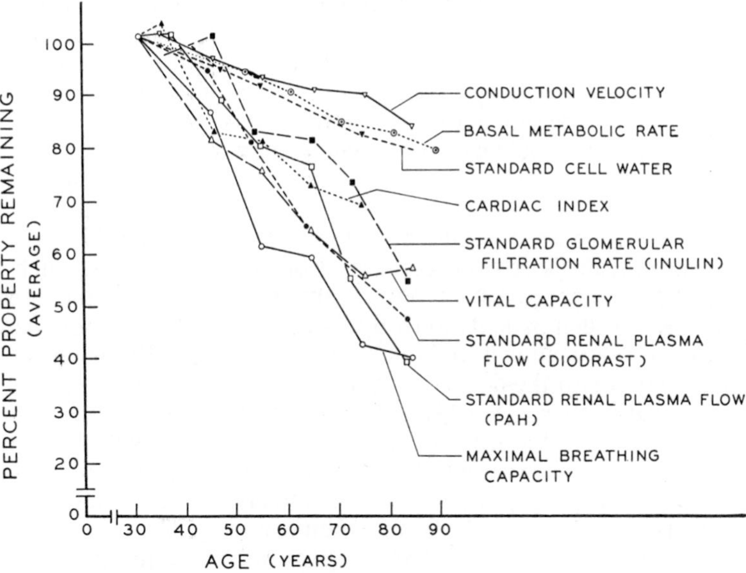


Fig. 4. Decline in Various Human Functional Capacities and Physiological Measurements with Age

**Figure 14-2.** Decline in various human functional capacities and physiologic measurements with age. (From Shock NW: Discussion on mortality and measurement in aging. *In* Strehler BL, Ebert SD, Glass HR, Shock NW (eds.): The Biology of Aging: A Symposium. Washington, DC, American Institute of Biological Sciences, 1960. Reproduced with permission.)

elasticity of skin, the rigidity of the arteries, the kidney function and the opacification of the lens of the eye cannot be changed." On the other hand, "exercise tolerance,[16] maximal breathing capacity,[17,18] cardiac reserve, reaction time,[19-21] physical strength, short-term memory,[22] intelligence as measured by intelligence tests,[23,24] ambulatory activities, and social abilities[25] can be maintained or even improved with advancing age." These latter functions are the specific targets of selective rehabilitation interventions.

A philosophic point about rehabilitation intervention should be made here concerning the school of thought that suggests that "we can't do much to rehabilitate the elderly, but we can do a great deal to modify the environment in which the elderly find themselves." On the one hand, environmental adaptation and psychologic adjustment are important forms of rehabilitation intervention for long-term disability. On the other hand, rehabilitation intervention also calls for pharmacologic, surgical, or physical treatment or other means to restore or improve important functions. As mentioned previously, such functions include exercise tolerance, physical strength, short-term memory, and ambulatory activities. Not to distinguish those patients and circumstances for whom physiologic functioning can be improved is to treat aging as a disease rather than as a part of human development and to negate the effects that training has on human performance, regardless of age.

Hunt[26] states that the aim of geriatric medicine is the maintenance of fitness and the support of independent living. He offers this list of general guidelines for rehabilitation of the aged: (1) set realistic goals with the patient, (2) allow for temporary relocation confusion, (3) restore and maintain the patient's water and electrolyte balance, (4) arrange priorities for drugs and schedules to suit needed activity, (5) search for treatable causes for instability and falls and provide stable walking aids, (6) always aim for early mobilization, (7) take immediate measures to offset incontinence, (8) use special care in assessing pain, (9) prevent overheating, (10) schedule activity-concentrated therapy for the morning, (11) keep assistive devices simple, and (12) promote community support services.

## STRATEGIES FOR INCLUDING REHABILITATION IN CARE OF THE ELDERLY

Rehabilitation should be included in the pattern of care of elderly patients in order to achieve the following:

1. Reversible functional limitations consequent to acute illness will be prevented or else promptly identified and corrected.
2. Patients with neurologic or musculoskeletal impairments or functional limitations that

are not readily reversible will be referred to a medical rehabilitation facility or team.

3. Patients in an ambulatory medical care setting who are experiencing early functional limitations will be systematically identified and their disability problems appropriately managed.

With regard to point one, patients with severe or prolonged acute illnesses are commonly on prolonged periods of bed rest. In the past, abnormal responses in such patients were ascribed to the illness. It is now known that many of these effects were due to the deconditioning effects of bed rest rather than to the disease. For example, in patients with myocardial infarction, bed rest has been shown to result in intolerance to change to an upright posture.[27] Additionally, circulating blood volume, plasma volume, and red cell mass are decreased, as are lung volume, vital capacity, and serum proteins. A poorer contractile state of body musculature and a negative nitrogen balance also occur during periods of bed rest. Saltin and associates[28] had five healthy normal young men exercise twice daily after 20 days of bed rest. Pre-bed rest condition returned in the poorly conditioned men after 10 days, whereas 29 and 43 days were required for the two better-conditioned young men to reach their previous state of training. Thus, with respect to recovery from acute illness, efforts should be made to encourage early ambulation and reconditioning to prevent adverse responses to bed rest. To accomplish this, as early as the patient's medical condition permits, range of motion movements of major joints must be performed to prevent contractures; strength of antigravity muscles of the trunk and lower limbs must be restored and/or maintained so that the patient is able to rise up from a low seat, climb a flight of stairs, and walk the length of the hospital corridor; cardiopulmonary function must be restored and/or maintained to a level to sustain at least 3 to 4 METs of energy output for periods of up to 5 minutes at a time; and the patient must have sufficient judgment and, if necessary, training in safety techniques to minimize hazards of falling.

Hospitalized patients should be referred to a medical rehabilitation team or facility if they have neurologic or musculoskeletal impairments or functional limitations not readily reversible owing to major involvement of organ systems that result in any of the following: paresis, multiple or complex fractures of the lower limb, amputation, incapacitating pain, or poor stamina or other condition that significantly interferes with ability to function independently. Patients cared for in an ambulatory medical setting who are experiencing difficulties and lack of ease in performing activities in personal care, household chores, social interactions, occupational pursuits, and traveling should be identified systematically and their disability problems managed. This may require consultation with a physiatrist or a referral made to a rehabilitation therapist, such as a physical, occupational, or speech therapist, a professional counselor, or other home-based care provider.

By assessing patients who are experiencing disability in the outpatient or office setting, the physician not only is able to identify areas of unmet need and then refer the patient to a resource for help but also is given the opportunity to formulate a functional prognosis. For example, it is possible to identify groups of patients with different probabilities for short-term outcomes (over a period of 15 to 18 months), such as death or need for supports from the public service system, whether institutional or home-based. These services may include transportation, personal care, housekeeping, social activities, emergency assistance, food shopping, and food preparation.

Data from a demonstration project in Wood River, Rhode Island,[29] identified levels of "risk" related to patients' functional status. From a study group of 323 patients aged 60 years and older who were followed by personnel in a community health facility, 103 were categorized as being at high risk because of dependency needs (i.e., needing help from another person) in self-care and mobility, and 132 were categorized as at physiologic risk, not because of dependency in personal care functions but because of limitations in walking outdoors or in climbing stairs. During a study interval of 18 months, 33 people died, 22 from the high-risk group and 10 from the physiologic-risk group. Of 10 patients who were placed in nursing homes during the 18-month interval, eight were from the high-risk group and one was from the physiologic-risk group.

The studies suggest that categorization of the elderly based upon analysis of functional status can be useful for estimating prognosis in case management, program planning, and allocation of scarce and expensive resources. Resources should be allocated where the need is greatest and the results are likely to be most effective. Vulnerability can be considered high for elderly people who are dependent in one or more areas of personal care (e.g., feeding, grooming, bathing, dressing, sphincter control, transferring, ambulation, and stair climbing). The strategy of care for this group would be a comprehensive rehabilitation evaluation, with appropriate prescription of restorative exercise or adaptive devices intended to reduce the burden of care on the patient, family members, and support agencies. Vulnerability can be considered "physiologic" when there are no personal care dependency needs but the individual is limited in walking 50 yards outdoors or in climbing stairs. This limitation may be because of discomfort, slowness, or need for an ambulatory support device. Such patients should be evaluated to assure that the devices being used are optimal and that cardiopulmonary and musculoskeletal functioning permits expenditures of at least 3 to 4 METs of energy output for up to 5 minutes. These patients may benefit from conditioning exercises in particular and also from psychosocial and financial counseling. Vulnerability that is not caused by anatomic and physiologic factors can be an indication for psychosocial and financial evaluation, and some patients with this vulnerability may benefit from recreational and financial counseling as well as from prescription of general conditioning exercises.

Except for those aged 85 years and older, many of the elderly are not functionally limited (see Table 14–1) and, therefore, are not at short-term risk of becoming so. There is an unfortunate tendency to discourage activity, particularly exercise, in the elderly. Jokl[30] noted that in 1952 at the National Gymnastic Festival at Marburg, there was a wide age range in the several hundred trained participants: 50 to 59 years (men), on the side horse; 60 to 84 years (men), on parallel bars; and 32 to 52 years (women), on the horizontal bar. He concluded that the degree of neuromotor differentiation required from these older gymnasts was such that healthy young men and women between 18 and 22 years of age would be unable to perform these exercises unless they had practiced regularly for prolonged periods; therefore, training is a more potent determinant of neuromuscular fitness than is age.

A prognosis established through functional assessment should not be considered a self-fulfilling prophesy; rather, through appropriate intervention, the outcome may be improved from what might have been otherwise expected. The functional assessment categorization allows the physician to direct the patient toward rehabilitation, treatment, and social support systems in a more systematic and effective manner than is possible when the physician only knows the diagnosis and related medical treatments.

## A METHOD FOR IDENTIFICATION OF EARLY DISABILITY

Having completed the organ-centered medical history and the physical and laboratory examinations, the physician should interview the patient specifically to explore the his or her expected and hoped-for status with regard to the six major "survival roles" noted by the World Health Organization (WHO)[3]: (1) orientation to one's surroundings, (2) self-sufficiency in maintaining an independent existence, (3) mobility for effectively moving about in one's surroundings, (4) social integration, with participation in customary social relationships, (5) occupation, that is, utilizing time appropriately during the working day, and (6) economic resources sufficient to meet one's needs. This exploration, coupled with the previously obtained social data covering the patient's habits and opportunities for social interactions, residential arrangements, family membership, and vocational and avocational interests, will reveal any deficits in fulfilling expected social roles that are not balanced with available social supports. The next task is to document the functional status through use of a "screening" questionnaire that very briefly specifies key items inferred by the National Health Interview Survey question, "Does your health limit your ability to work, participate in leisure activities, perform household chores, move about or perform selfcare?" The 15 questions taken from the Functional Assessment Screening Questionnaire (FASQ)[31] serve to screen for difficulty with (1) *p*ersonal activities of daily living, (2) *i*nstrumental activities of daily living, (3) social activities and active use of *l*eisure time, (4) *o*ccupational activities, and (5) *t*raveling activities. (The italicized letters spell the mnemonic PILOT.) The patient may report having difficulty with a task for different reasons, such as pain, fatigue, weakness, need of a device, or need for assistance of another person. A patient who reports having some or much difficulty or who is unable to perform four or more task items should be considered to be in need of closer evaluation by a physiatrist or a rehabilitation therapist. The questionnaire also identifies nine "functional systems" for examination, i.e., upper limbs and neck, manual dexterity, lower limbs and trunk, speaking and writing, seeing and reading, hearing, stamina (cardiopulmonary), cognition, and affective (emotional) adaptability, and their presumed relationship to the "functional activity history."

In using the form, the physician may indicate from examination those functional examination systems that are contributing to the patient's difficulties. The systems that contribute to disability would then become targets for more refined evaluation by the physiatrist or a rehabilitation therapist as well as targets for restorative or adjustment treatment efforts.

By conducting a systematic inventory of what task items are performed and how they are performed, the person carrying out the functional assessment collects information to represent the individual's experience of living with disability. Analysis at this level may reveal reversible disability and indications for restorative therapy or for psychologic adjustment and behavior modification. Analysis may also reveal disability that cannot be accounted for by the identified impairment; therefore, additional evaluation is needed in order to determine the presence of another impairment or else social, environmental, or psychologic factors that may be at work. The goal of functional analysis of task performance is to discover the presence of unmet needs at all levels—medical, restorative, psychosocial, and environmental—in order to develop appropriate interventions with the intent of achieving optimal functioning. With this comprehensive assessment, plans for further management may include: (1) investigation of unresolved issues, (2) amelioration of treatable impairment, (3) a rehabilitation medicine consultation if disability significantly impedes life-roles, and/or (4) preparation of the patient and family members for any needed long-term personal adjustments and mobilization of appropriate community supports. The plan should recognize unrealistic expectations, problems in compliance, overutilization or underutilization of health care resources, and possible reasons for stress among family members.

## APPROACHES TO MANAGING SEVERE DISABILITY

In the Handbook of Severe Disability, three important characteristics of disability are described:

> (1) There is no one-to-one correlation between a disease and the spectrum of associated disability problems. The same disease can produce separate sets of disability problems in different individuals. (2) There is no one-to-one relationship between a disease and the amount of residual disability. Disability problems can be removed even though the disease is unchanged. (3) The ability of a patient and the total health care team to remove disability in the face of chronic disease is dependent upon the patient's residual capacity for physiological and psychological adaptation. Residual strength must be evaluated and enhanced to "work around" an impairment in order to remove disability.[32]

A therapeutic approach to severe disability in the geriatric patient is best accomplished in a medically directed comprehensive inpatient rehabilitation setting. There are programs in alternative settings that may also be effective, such as home-care programs, outpatient rehabilitation programs, and skilled nursing facility programs. However, these tend to lack a great deal of medical input and the intensity of services of a hospital setting and may take an extremely long time to obtain results. Comparison studies between various alternative settings for treating severe disability are not common. However, Smith and associates[33] report a controlled study in which patients with neurologic impairment who were rehabilitated in stroke units were compared with patients with similar impairment rehabilitated in medical units. A higher proportion of those rehabilitated in stroke units achieved independence.

A consensus does not exist with regard to how extensively rehabilitation services should be provided in skilled nursing homes. Reimbursement at fixed and rather low rates and a chronically short supply of qualified personnel are but two major factors that perpetuate problems that make efficient rehabilitation programs an impossibility for many homes.

> However, the universal feasibility of comprehensive rehabilitation programs in nursing homes will not be attained until there is also a universal coordination of extra-hospital with intra-hospital services. This should be accomplished in one or more of the following ways: through extensive affiliations with hospital extended-care facilities, through use of multidisciplinary rehabilitation teams offering a community-wide coverage, or through intensive and continuing training of all nursing home personnel in rehabilitation principles and techniques.[34]

Bringing the talents of several health-care professionals together to identify and solve problems in concert provides the patient in the inpatient setting with a unity of direction and an intensity of services that cannot be achieved by having the professionals working separately. Participation in case conferences is an important technique for facilitating interdisciplinary collaboration. Communication among rehabilitation team members is enhanced and program effectiveness is increased when a standard measurement of ability and disability is used. In contrast to the outpatient who may be experiencing disability to varying degrees in several or only one of the areas of major life activities (e.g., personal care, household tasks, socialization, occupation, or traveling), the inpatient has marked losses in self-sufficiency to the point of needing the help of another person for from 2 to 24 hours per day. When dependency in personal care is extreme, other life activities are usually also compromised severely. Therefore, since ability to perform one's personal care activities independently is an important determinant of ability to perform other life activites, it is very useful to incorporate a measure of personal care status into the rehabilitation process.

A number of different measures are used by different workers, which for the most part measure similar phenomena. Of these, the Barthel index has been tested extensively.[35-40] The Barthel index measures independence in the basic tasks of feeding, dressing, toileting, and mobility. Scoring for the modified form is shown in Table 14-2. The Barthel index is reliable and easy to administer and has been used to monitor progress in rehabilitation medicine.[35-37,40] It is also useful for making placement decisions and designing continuing care services.[38,39] Assessing the patient's personal care status periodically during the rehabilitation process with the Barthel index provides a valid measure of the progress to date and the residual needs and also facilitates communication among rehabilitation team members.

An additional measure, the ESCROW profile,[39] incorporates six factors of social support: (1) *e*nvironment (suitability of housing location and arrangement), (2) *s*ocial interaction (person-to-person contacts versus reliance on social agency supports), (3) *c*luster of family members (availability of competent others in the household), (4) *r*esources (financial situation), (5) *o*utlook (general ability to make decisions based on intellectual and emotional adaptability), and (6) *w*ork (vocational or other participatory status in the community if the individual is retired for age). These describe the situation in the community that the patient will encounter upon completion of the intensive rehabilitation process (see Appendix II).

In 1962, Steinberg[41] noted the following:

The average family and household can accept and manage a disabled patient if the following conditions can be met:

1. He must be able to walk, or at least transfer himself from bed to chair, or from chair to wheelchair, without having to be lifted.
2. He must have normal or near normal control of his excretory functions.
3. He should be able to take care of all, or at least an essential part, of his personal needs, such as eating, bathing, and dressing.
4. His mental condition should be adequately clear.

**Table 14-2.** MODIFIED BARTHEL INDEX SCORING*

| **Independent** | | **Dependent** | | |
|---|---|---|---|---|
| ***Intact*** | ***Limited*** | ***Helper*** | ***Null*** | **Self-care and Mobility** |
| 10 | 5 | 3 | 3 | Drink from cup; feed from dish |
| 5 | 5 | 3 | 0 | Dress upper body |
| 5 | 5 | 2 | 0 | Dress lower body |
| 0 | 0 | −2 | NONE | Don brace or prosthesis |
| 5 | 5 | 0 | 0 | Grooming |
| 4 | 4 | 0 | 0 | Wash or bathe |
| 10 | 10 | 5 | 0 | Bladder continence |
| 10 | 10 | 5 | 0 | Bowel continence |
| 4 | 4 | 2 | 0 | Care of perineum, clothing at toilet |
| 15 | 15 | 7 | 0 | Transfer, chair |
| 6 | 5 | 3 | 0 | Transfer, toilet |
| 1 | 1 | 0 | 0 | Transfer, tub or shower |
| ( ) | ( ) | ( ) | ( ) | Transfer, automobile |
| 15 | 15 | 10 | 0 | Walk on level 50 yards or more |
| 10 | 10 | 5 | 0 | Up and down stairs for 1 flight or more |
| ( ) | ( ) | ( ) | ( ) | Walk outdoors 50 yards or more |
| 15 | 5 | 0 | NONE | Wheelchair/50 yds—*Only if not walking* |
| ____ | ____ | ____ | ____ equals | ____ TOTAL |

* Criteria for assessment are in Granger CV: Health accounting—functional assessment of the long-term patient. *In* Kottke FJ, Stillwell GK, Lehmann JF (eds.): Krusen's Handbook of Physical Medicine and Rehabilitation. 3rd ed. Philadelphia, W. B. Saunders Co., 1982, pp. 259-261.

5. His medical care should be adapted in such a way that it can be handled in a home environment.

From a practical point of view, use of the Barthel index provides a quantitative measure of these five concerns. First, patients with more favorable prognoses tend to gain at a rate of 5 or more points per week during the course of intensive rehabilitation, for a total of 20 or more points. Second, a Barthel index score of 61 points or more is desirable at the time of discharge from the inpatient setting to the home setting. A Barthel score level of around 61 means that the patient is at the level of "assisted independence," at which the burden of care on family members is estimated to be not more than 2 hours per day, a level of support that most families are able to absorb on a consistent basis. It can be expected that over the weeks and months that the patient is in the home setting, improvement will continue[38,40] and that a score of 75 or better may be attained. At this score level, no more than 1 hour per day of direct care would be required. This assistance would be provided throughout the day, but chiefly in the morning and evening. After the patient's discharge from a rehabilitation inpatient setting, the health care worker should reinforce the expectation of the patient and family that improvement in performance of everyday activities will continue. This improvement should be facilitated through provision of rehabilitation services after discharge by way of either home care or outpatient therapies. It is useful to reassess functional status using the Barthel index and ESCROW profile at about 3 to 6 months after inpatient discharge and at annual intervals thereafter.

It is not unusual for an aging couple to consider a change in residence (not necessarily a geographic change) because the present residence is inconveniently located in relation to shopping, transportation, or relatives and associates, because of difficulties of upkeep of an older or larger home, because of financial considerations, or because the presence of disability in one or both has changed what used to be a hospitable environment into one that is difficult and even possibly hostile. Through the course of rehabilitation and follow-up, the rehabilitation professional can help the patient to prepare for decisions about how best to satisfy future housing needs by helping the older patient keep in touch with how his or her functional needs may be helped or hindered by conveniences or inconveniences in his or her housing environment. In order to better understand the degree to which housing (in this case, adapted housing or housing that includes case management and other services) can be a therapeutic tool that is important to the lives of disabled and elderly people, the reader is referred to the volume *An Alternative to Institutionalization: The Highland Heights Experiment.*[7] The conclusions include the observation that "severely impaired persons functionally eligible for intermediate care facilities (ICF) or skilled nursing facilities (SNF) who moved to Highland Heights from a long-term care institution can indeed function successfully in this type of community living arrangement." With respect to death the authors state that "experimentals (those living in Highland Heights) were significantly less likely to die, at least for the first four years of the impact study" and that "death is related to vulnerability, and it is for the most vulnerable ones that Highland Heights appeared most useful in prolonging life."

## FACTORS IMPORTANT TO GERIATRIC INPATIENT REHABILITATION

### Orientation of the Rehabilitation Program

The rehabilitation inpatient unit must have a distinct geographic location in the facility and 24-hour coverage by rehabilitation nurses. It is the attitudes and special skills of the nursing staff that provide the distinctive therapeutic milieu and sustain and reinforce the gains directed by the physician and established by the therapists. The nurses monitor the patient's reserve of energy, motivation, mood, and ability to cooperate, follow orders, learn instructions, observe safety precautions, and avoid skin breakdown. In the final analysis, the nurses permit and encourage the patient to practice and utilize the skills being taught by the therapists. The managing physician, with advice from the rehabilitation team, must have the final say as to which patients are suitable for admission to the unit. Not all disabled patients are able to be helped significantly by intensive rehabilitation. Some patients should be in a slower-paced program.

Members of the medical rehabilitation team usually include a physiatrist, rehabilitation nurse, physical therapist, occupational therapist, speech therapist, clinical psychologist, social worker, and others as appropriate, such as a recreational therapist, dietitian, vocational counselor, and orthotist/prosthetist. The physiatrist assesses the extent of the impairment and the degree to which the patient's functioning can be improved and coordinates the treatment plan. The nurse performs a variety of care tasks and is most responsible for establishing the rehabilitation treatment milieu in which the patient can learn to help himself or herself. The physical therapist emphasizes strengthening of muscles and learning and relearning movement patterns and corrective postures and administers various physical treatment modalities. The occupational therapist emphasizes kinesiologic principles of the upper limb and hand and the use of splints and adaptive devices for self-help and trains patients with perceptual-motor deficits. The speech therapist, using knowledge of physiologic and neurologic principles, works to improve the patient's communication processing. The clinical psychologist uses principles of human behavior and tests of mental status, intelligence, neuropsychologic functioning, and perception to counsel the patient and advise other team members how to overcome difficulties in treatment and management. The social worker identifies interactions in the family dynamics, social policy, and community resources and advises the patient, family members, and other team members regarding optimal lifestyle adaptations.

### Medical Stability

Patients should be referred into rehabilitation early, as soon as medical stability is established, rather than later; however, patients who are too ill to be mobilized are not suitable for a rehabilitation unit. Medical stability means that the patient is able or is expected to be able to tolerate at least 3 to 4 METs of energy output sustained for at least 5 minutes.

### Physiologic Deconditioning

Since deconditioning from bed rest occurs rapidly and is repaired slowly, the patient must exercise frequently for short periods throughout the day in order to build stamina. This may be accomplished by performance of exercises with ropes and pulleys or weights for the upper limbs and through a pedal exerciser rigged to the bed for the lower limbs. Similarly, the patient must rest periodically during the day; often this is convenient after lunch.

### Mental Status

Dementia definitely impedes rehabilitation and, if severe enough, blocks rehabilitation. In the case of dementia of significant degree, if the family members are committed to providing care for the patient at home and they clearly understand that the patient is unlikely to change (if that is truly the case), the patient may be admitted to rehabilitation for purposes of training the family members in providing care in the most effective and efficient manner. Too often family members, sometimes misinformed by acute care personnel, misinterpret admission to rehabilitation as a cue that miraculous changes are about to occur. It sometimes happens that a patient is mistakenly identified as severely demented because an overlay of anxiety or depression has masked remaining cognitive ability. In this case, the reassurances that are received in the rehabilitation setting may allay the anxiety or lift the depression sufficiently to reveal more cognitive ability than was first appreciated. In a study by Schuman and associates,[42] the outcomes of elderly patients with intellectual dysfunction in a medical rehabilitation program are documented. They concluded that patients over 65 years of age "with intellectual impairment should be treated in programs designed specifically for them rather than in standard rehabilitation programs."

### Emotional Status

Almost every patient undergoing rehabilitation manifests some degree of anxiety, depression, and denial — the degrees of which may flucuate over time. For the elderly, in particular, much of the anxiety is based on a fear of the consequences of losing independence in mobility and having to rely on someone else for help or else having to be placed in a long-term care institution. This sense of helplessness, if severe, can lead to hopelessness. Helplessness can be learned through misdirected "helping" by the staff, as is suggested in a study by Avorn and Langer.[43] Depression may have preceded the illness event and be based on a troubled life situation that preceded the need for rehabilitation or it may be an expected (or grief) reaction to the disabling circumstances. Denial may be an adaptive adjustment if it does not interfere with accomplishment of rehabilitation goals or with realistic planning for life after inpatient discharge. Usually recognition of these symptoms and use of cognitive direction are helpful techniques for management. Patients with lesions in the right cerebral hemisphere (usually with left-sided hemiparesis) often exhibit an "organic" denial syndrome, the deficit being an inability to relate visual-spatial with visual-motor events. Anosognosia is the lack of awareness or denial of existence of a functional limitation. True anosognosia is associated with a lesion of the inferior parietal lobe in the region of the supramarginal gyrus.[44]

## CONCLUSION

Medical rehabilitation is composed of paradoxes:

1. It is medically directed but is activity-behavior-oriented rather than impairment-pathology-oriented.
2. It is not cure-oriented but is care-oriented, with the main theme being that of management of interacting problem-sets.
3. Although many principles of rehabilitation are useful and applicable throughout the lifetime of the individual, either for prevention of disability or for maximizing activity and quality of life when disability exists, the intensive, interdisciplinary phase of medical rehabilitation is structured around goal-setting and goal-attainment and is time-limited.
4. Although the treatment model of rehabilitation is important, the teaching model of rehabilitation is necessary for enduring benefit.
5. Despite advanced years and fixed organic impairments, many elderly patients can benefit from an appropriately designed and applied medical rehabilitation program, provided that the patient is behaviorally flexible and that conditions are conducive to effecting and maintaining behavioral change.
6. Rehabilitation is not intended to remove the symptoms of a chronic disorder but rather enhances the individual's ability to cope with functional limitations through compensatory physical and psychosocial mechanisms.
7. Rehabilitation is expensive, but it is often the most cost-effective method for reducing the burden of care that results from disability.

Rehabilitation is a necessary part of social policy if we are to maintain as many elderly as possible at home with family members or within appropriate community settings in preference to custodial institutional placement. There are a number of ways in which this policy may be implemented:

1. by controlling the number of people discharged from hospital settings to intermediate-care facilities, particularly those for whom home care alternatives may have been feasible;
2. by developing effective discharge planning in hospitals that incorporate reliable and valid measures of functional status;
3. by utilizing recognized medical rehabilitation units and hospitals to improve functional status and enable more patients to return to community settings after acute hospitalization;
4. by avoiding prolonged stays in acute hospitals;
5. by maintaining the levels of independence of people who have been discharged from inpatient medical rehabilitation programs; and
6. by identifying the indicators of disability early in ambulatory patients and incorporating the functional (rehabilitation) perspective into their medical care.

It is important to keep in mind that if a person experiencing disability does not use residual abilities and skills, they are likely to be lost.

### References

1. Rudov MH, Santangelo N: Health status of minorities and low-income groups. DHEW Publication No. (HRA) 79-627, Washington DC, U.S. Government Printing Office, 1979.
2. Brogan DR: Rehabilitation service needs: Physician's perceptions and referrals. Arch Phys Med Rehabil 62:215, 1981.
3. World Health Organization: International Classification of Impairments, Disabilities, and Handicaps (ICIDH). Geneva, World Health Organization, 1980.
4. Wood PHN, Badley EM: People with Disabilities—Toward Acquiring Information Which Reflects More Sensitively Their Problems and Needs. International Exchange of Information in Rehabilitation Fund, 400 East 34th Street, New York, NY, 10016, 1980.
5. Commission on Professional and Hospital Activities: International Classification of Disease—9th Edition—Clinical Modification (ICD-9-CM). Ann Arbor, MI, 48105, July 1978.
6. Kane RA, Kane RL: Assessing the Elderly: A Practical Guide to Measurement. Lexington, MA, Lexington Books, 1981, pp. 4, 5, 31.
7. Sherwood S, Greer DS, Morris JN, Mor V: An Alternative to Institutionalization: The Highland Heights Experiment. Cambridge, MA, Ballinger Publishing Co., 1981, pp. 86–87.
8. Lawton MP: The functional assessment of elderly people. J Am Geriatr Soc 19:465, 1971.
9. Katz S, Downs TD, Cash HR, et al: Progress in development of the Index of ADL. Gerontologist 10:20, 1970.
10. Strehler BL: Implications of aging research for society. *In* Thorbecke GJ (ed.): Biology of Aging and Development. Bethesda, MD, FASEB, and New York and London, Plenum Press, 1975.
11. Fries JF, Crapo LM: Vitality and Aging. San Francisco, W. H. Freeman and Co., 1981.
12. Wylie CM (ed.): PAS Reporter, Special Issue, The Elderly: Selected Studies on the Health Condition and Hospital Care of Geriatric Patients. Commission on Professional and Hospital Activities, 1968 Green Road, Ann Arbor, MI, 48106, Vol. 16, No. 18, August, 1979.
13. National Center for Health Statistics: Limitation of Activity and Mobility Due to Chronic Conditions: United States, 1972. Rockville, MD, National Center for Health Statistics, DHEW Publicaton No. (HRA) 75-1523, 1974.

14. Shock NW: Discussion on mortality and measurement in aging. *In* Strehler BL, Ebert SD, Glass HR, Shock NW (eds.): The Biology of Aging : A Symposium. Washington, DC, American Institute of Biological Sciences, 1960, pp. 22, 23.
15. Costa PT, McCrae RR: Functional age: A conceptual and empirical critique. *In* Haynes SG, Feinleib M (eds.): Second Conference on the Epidemiology of Aging. U.S. Dept. Health and Human Services, NIH Publication No. 80-969, July, pp. 23–50.
16. Pollock ML, Miller HS, Wilmore J: Physiological characteristics of champion American track athletes 40 to 75 years of age. J Gerontol 29:645, 1974.
17. Dehn MM, Bruce RA: Longitudinal variations in maximal oxygen uptake with age and activity. J Appl Physiol 33:805, 1972.
18. DeVries H: Physiologic effects of an exercise training regimen upon aged men aged 52–88. J Gerontol 25:325, 1970.
19. Spirduso WW: Reaction and movement time as a function of age and physical activity level. J Gerontol 30:435, 1975.
20. Spirduso WW: Physical fitness, aging and psychomotor speed: A review. J Gerontol 35:850, 1980.
21. Spirduso WW, Clifford P: Replication of age and physical activity effects on reaction and movement time. J Gerontol 33:26, 1978.
22. Langer EJ, et al: Environmental determinants of memory improvement in late adulthood. J Pers Soc Psychol 37:003, 1979.
23. Nesselroade JF, Schaie KW, Baltes PB: Ontogenetic and generational components of structural and quantitative change in adult behavior. J Gerontol 27:222, 1972.
24. Plemons JK, Willis SL, Baltes PB: Modifiability of fluid intelligence in aging: A short-term longitudinal training approach. J Gerontology, 33:224, 1978.
25. Langer EJ, Rodin J: The effects of choice and enhanced personal responsibility for the aged: A field experiment in an institutional setting. J Pers Soc Psychol 34:191, 1976.
26. Hunt TE: Practical considerations in the rehabilitation of the aged. J Am Geriatr Soc 28:59, 1980.
27. Wenger NK: Coronary Care, Rehabilitation after Myocardial Infarction. New York, American Heart Association, 1973, p. 5.
28. Saltin B, Blomquist G, Lamb LE, et al: Response to exercise after bed rest and after training. Circulation 38:Suppl 7:1, 1968.
29. Department of Elderly Affairs, State of Rhode Island; Family and Community Support Systems (final report). December, 1982, AoA Grant #01-AM-00009.
30. Jokl E: Physiology of Exercise. Springfield, IL, Charles C Thomas, 1971, pp. 32–33.
31. Seltzer GB, Granger CV, Wineberg D: Functional assessment: Bridge between family and rehabilitation medicine within an ambulatory practice. Arch Phys Med Rehabil 63:453, 1982.
32. Stolov WC, Clowers MR (eds.): Handbook of Severe Disability. USDE/RSA. Washington DC, Superintendent of Documents, U.S. Government Printing Office, Stock No. 017-090-00054-2, 1981, p. 2.
33. Smith ME, Garraway WM, Smith DL, Akhtar AJ: Therapy impact on functional outcome in a controlled trial of stroke rehabilitation. Arch Phys Med Rehabil 63:21, 1982.
34. Hefferin EA: Rehabilitation in nursing home situations. A survey of the literature. J Am Geriatr Soc 16:296, 1968.
35. Donaldson SW, Wagner CC, Gresham GE: A unified ADL evaluation form. Arch Phys Med Rehabil 54:175, 1973.
36. Granger CV, Dewis LS, Peters NC, et al: Stroke rehabilitation: Analysis of repeated Barthel index measures. Arch Phys Med Rehabil 60:14, 1979.
37. Gresham GE, Phillips TF, Labi MLC: ADL status in stroke: Relative merits of three standard indexes. Arch Phys Med Rehabil 61:355, 1980.
38. Eggert GM, Granger CV, Morris R, Pendleton SF: Caring for the patient with long-term disability. Geriatrics 32:102, 1977.
39. Fortinsky RH, Granger CV, Seltzer GB: The use of functional assessment in understanding home care needs. Med Care 19:489, 1981.
40. Granger CV, Albrecht GL, Hamilton BB: Outcome of comprehensive medical rehabilitation: Measurement by PULSES profile and the Barthel index. Arch Phys Med Rehabil 60:145, 1979.
41. Steinberg FU: Rehabilitation and restoration of the chronically ill geriatric patient. J Am Geriatr Soc 10:618, 1962.
42. Schuman JE, Beattie EJ, Steed DA, et al: Geriatric patients with and without intellectual dysfunction: Effectiveness of a standard rehabilitation program. Arch Phys Med Rehabil 62:612, 1981.
43. Avorn JL, Langer EJ: Inducing disability in nursing home patients: A controlled trial. J Am Geriatr Soc 30:397, 1982.
44. Mayo Clinic: Clinical Examinations in Neurology. 3rd ed. Philadelphia, W. B. Saunders Co., 1971, p. 214.

## Chapter 15

# Assistive Devices for the Elderly

*John B. Redford*

The past two decades have seen a proliferation of assistive devices and other appliances to provide more independence to people with physical disability. These devices range from modified standard objects for daily use (e.g., spoons with built-up handles, elastic shoelaces, door knobs with rubber levers) to complex electrically activated environmental control devices, such as powered wheelchairs controlled by tongue and lip movements. For handicapped elderly people, such living aids—often rather simple ones—may mean the difference between totally independent living and partial or complete reliance on others to assist in performing activities of daily living.

Appliances and equipment for the physically disabled take many forms, such as exercise equipment, prosthetic and orthotic appliances, and wheelchair and automobile modifications. Proper selection of these items often requires rather specialized knowledge; this can be accomplished by referral to a rehabilitation facility. However, primary care physicians should be aware that a large number of items are easily available from such sources as the Sears, Roebuck, and Company catalogue, which do not require any referral to a rehabilitation facility or special patient training. These devices can generally be classified as living aids or self-help aids. The greatest concern of most elderly people, even those with minimal impairments, is how to maintain independence at home and stay out of institutions. The family physician, therefore, should be prepared to give advice, particularly about living aids or home modifications, to elderly people who have this concern.

Prescriptions for an elderly patient who needs special assistive devices may require full rehabilitation assessment to integrate the device effectively into the patient's total rehabilitation program. However, because rehabilitation medicine physicians are not always available for consultation, the attending physician, with advice from the staff who nursed the patient, may have to choose the most suitable equipment. Several textbooks that describe such equipment are available.[1-5]

Some points are worth considering before prescribing *any* equipment. First, careful attention should be given to the patient's functional disability and proposed living arrangements. If the patient can function reasonably well without the aid or if he or she rejects the idea of accepting the impairment, the equipment may never be used. Furthermore, if much training is needed to use the device, the equipment will likely be discarded unless the training is readily available. Costs are always a factor; therefore, simple aids are better than complex ones. In addition, the less conspicuous the aid, the more acceptable it will be. Unfortunately, the walking cane, one of the most effective and cheapest aids, is the most conspicuous and thus is often discarded. In a lament over this situation, a well-known orthopedic surgeon wrote a memorable editorial: "Don't throw away the cane."[6]

The *Directory of Living Aids for the Disabled Person,*[7] recently published by the United States Veterans Administration, classifies aids into eight major categories: mobility, eating, dressing, hygiene, communication, recreation, and maintenance. This classification is used for the headings in this chapter, except for the last category—really a miscellaneous grouping that includes items and equipment for exercises, home care, and so forth. This directory provides names and addresses of vendors of rehabilitation equipment and also includes lists of books and other literature that can be a further source of practical information. Another excellent guide with outstanding illustrations is *The Sourcebook for the Disabled,*[8] available at most book stores. This book ends with eight pages and almost 400 references to resources for the disabled, including national organizations, reading material, and sources of special supplies.

## MOBILITY AIDS

Most patients with lower limb disorders benefit from a cane, crutches, or walker for ambulation. Usually, the more disabled the individual, the more complex the walking device required. A cane can transmit up to 25 per cent of body weight away from the lower limb; crutches or walkers can improve balance more effectively and reduce weight bearing on both limbs by 50 per cent. Details of different designs of walking aids and methods of gait training are widely available.[1,4,5] The most useful aid for most elderly hemiplegics is the four-legged or quad cane or the hemiwalker, which combines features of the walker and the quad cane (Fig. 15–1).

An important aspect of mobility is the ability to transfer in and out of beds and chairs. A patient who is able to walk may not be able to get up without help. Simple aids such as bed rails, an overhead trapeze, a rope ladder, or a braided bedpull attached to the foot of the bed may be all that is needed for improved bed mobility (Fig. 15–2). For the elderly patient with arthritic knees or other disorders that make it difficult to rise from low chairs, recessed wooden blocks may be placed under the feet of furniture to elevate them several inches. Chairs are also available with either a spring or motor-driven rising seat. Some elderly patients have found that these chairs aid them in getting up and are well worth the additional cost. To make dressing simple and safe, the elderly person's bedroom should have chairs with arm supports for stability and firm seats that are not lower than the height of the knees.

A wheelchair to suit the individual's lifestyle is often the key element in maintaining independence. Physicians should realize that a wheelchair is more than "a chair with wheels." For the patient unable to walk, his or her whole life and contact with the environment will revolve around the wheelchair. It is an independence-giving, energy-saving substitute, essential for disabled people to participate in the world around them. Wheelchairs come in a bewildering variety of models and sizes; few of these can be reviewed here. Therefore, any patient with special problems who requires a permanent wheelchair should be referred to rehabilitation programs for advice, not simply advised to go to the nearest wheelchair dealer for an opinion and, perhaps, a needlessly expensive solution. However, hospital equipment dealers can be very helpful as they all can give information about prescribing wheelchairs and advise physicians of the various features available.

For the elderly person who needs a wheelchair mainly as an accessory aid to mobility, the basic rear-wheel drive or standard wheelchair with a seat that allows at least 2 in. of clearance on either side should be adequate. This chair may be selected with a standard adult, 18-in.-wide seat, or a narrow adult, 16-in.-wide seat, depending on the build of the patient. The chair should be as narrow as possible, as every inch saved is important in entering doorways. The

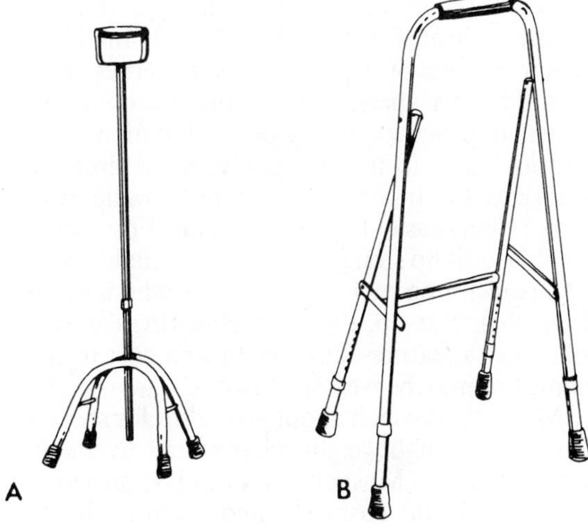


**Figure 15–1.** Walking aids. *A,* Four-legged or quad cane. *B,* Hemiwalker or walk cane. (From Varghese G: Crutches, canes and walkers. *In* Redford JB (ed): Orthotics, Etcetera. 2nd ed. © 1980, the Williams and Wilkins Co., Baltimore. Reproduced with permission.)

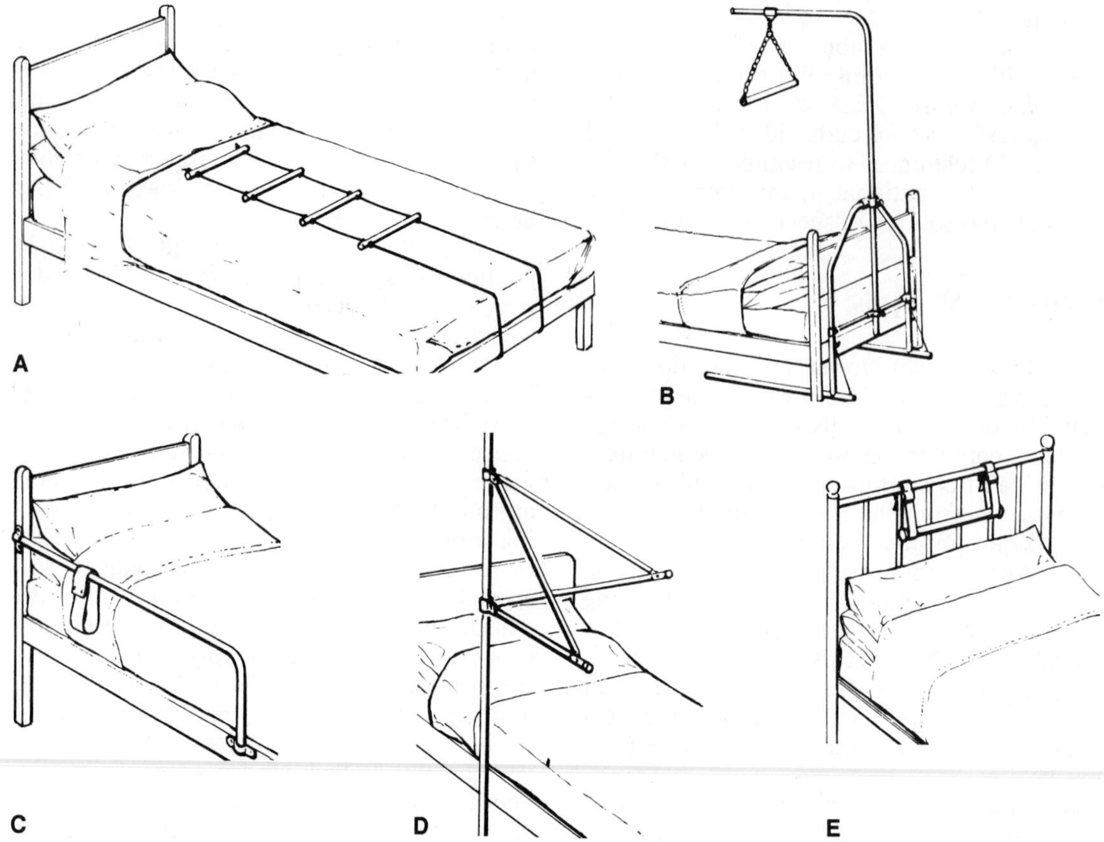


**Figure 15–2.** Bed aids. *A*, Rope ladder. *B*, Free-standing trapeze. *C*, Handrail with leather loop. *D*, Swivel bar assembly with upright that attaches to floor and ceiling. *E*, Bed bar. (From Hale G (ed.): The Source Book for the Disabled. Philadelphia, WB Saunders Co., 1979.)

standard wheelchair has 8-in. casters in the front, a straight back, brakes, and fixed or removable footrests (Fig. 15–3). The arms should be padded. In some wheelchairs, the arms can be stepped down, thus allowing the chair to slide under a desk. The arms can also be removed to permit sideways transfer to a bed, toilet, or commode, with or without the help of a transfer board. A transfer or sliding board, made of heavy plastic or polished wood, serves as a bridge from a wheelchair to another surface and assists in moving a heavy or weak patient who cannot stand to transfer easily. Solid tires are standard for indoor use but pneumatic tires make chairs easier to propel outside. For people unable to sit up straight, a chair is available with a fully reclining back, and for those who need to keep their legs up, there are elevating legrests. Each extra feature adds weight and cost to the chair but may be well worthwhile.

Most chairs weigh about 40 lb, but for special cases, very lightweight chairs are available weighing 24 lb. Most chairs should be provided with wheelchair cushions, and foam cushions are generally sufficient. However, special cushions to minimize pressure over bony points, whether filled with air, water, or special gels, are absolutely essential for patients with poor sensation or limited sitting tolerance. Many other wheelchair features and accessories are available, with special forms for prescribing them. Information on wheelchairs is readily obtained from rehabilitation equipment catalogs, from local dealers, or from textbooks.[1,9,10,11]

If a person must be confined to a wheelchair in his or her home, there are a few general considerations regarding home arrangements. Ramps for entrances should be at least 36 in. wide (surfaced with nonskid materials) and rise no more than 1 ft in height for every 12 ft in length. Handrails are also very helpful on ramps and should be alongside all outside entrances of the home of an elderly person to assist in stair climbing. For wheelchairs, the area at the top of the ramp should be at least 5 ft in depth if the door opens outward. Portable ramps are available but are quite heavy and so are not very practical. For special situations in which the ele-

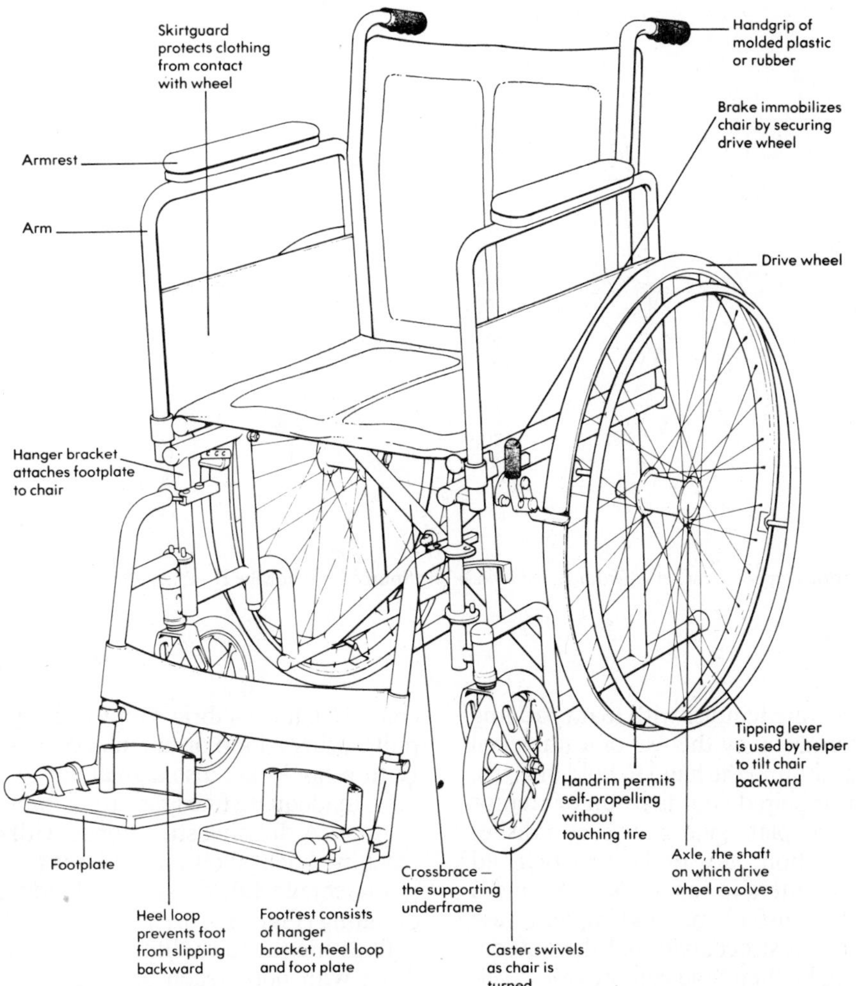


**Figure 15–3.** Features of a standard wheelchair. (From Hale G (ed.): The Source Book for the Disabled. Philadelphia, WB Saunders Co., 1979.)

vation is too high, precluding even a double ramp, outdoor self-operating elevators can be substituted but are more expensive. Further information on home modifications is found in the references.[3,4,8,12]

Doorways should be at least 30 in. but preferably 36 in. wide. Door knobs and locks can be fitted with levers for those with poor grasp or limited reach. Indoor stair lifts are available but are very expensive; it is usually cheaper for the family to modify the house so that the disabled adult can live on the main floor. Floors should be smooth and kept in good repair and, if carpeted, should have minimal pile. Mossy carpet or loose throw rugs are not only difficult for the wheelchair user but may create problems even for elderly people able to walk unaided.

In a wheelchair, a person's standing height is decreased by one third and his or her width is doubled. Therefore, wheelchairs need a circumference of at least 5 ft to turn. This merits consideration, particularly in the kitchen, bedrooms, and bathrooms. Reach from a wheelchair is very limited and usually done from the side, although forward reach can be aided by removable foot pedals. A variety of reachers are available, especially for wheelchair users and others with limited mobility (Fig. 15–4). Length, width of opening, and degree of grasp required should all be considered in advising potential users about reachers.

## EATING AIDS

Many attractive and durable mealtime aids are available from medical supply houses for those with poor grasp, impaired coordination, and disorders affecting the shoulder or elbow. Poor grasp can readily be improved, either by

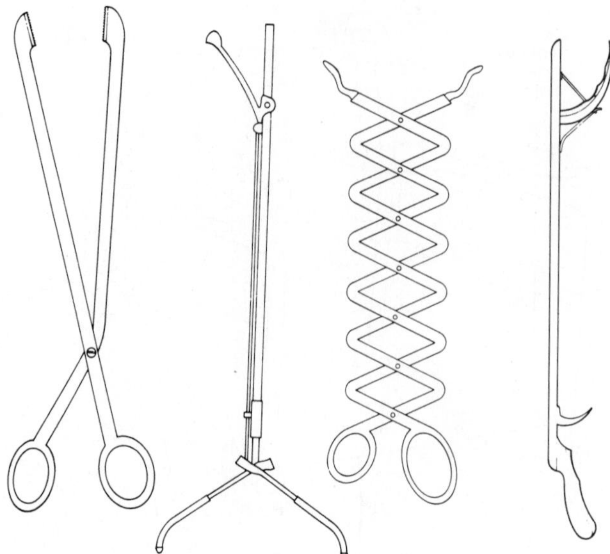

**Figure 15–4.** Various types of reachers. (From Hale G (ed.): The Source Book for the Disabled. Philadelphia, WB Saunders Co., 1979.)

enlarging silverware handles with foam padding or other materials or by the use of a universal cuff that straps around the hand to hold utensils. Patients with impaired coordination or tremor may be aided by plate guards or scoop dishes (Fig. 15–5), suction cups or Dycem twin lid openers, pizza cutters to replace knives, and a Crock-pot, which usually proves simpler to use than the oven. Most occupational therapy departments have kitchens and can provide excellent advice to families about meal preparation and special equipment. An excellent description of mealtime aids and food preparation as well as general advice on housekeeping for a handicapped person is found in the book by Hale.[8]

## DRESSING AIDS

Clothing for the disabled elderly should be adjustable and expandable, easily put on and taken off, and reinforced against wear by braces and crutches. Above all, it should look attractive. With today's informal fashions of stretchable fabrics, well-chosen garments can enhance physical attributes and conceal flaws. As expressed by a patient who has written a self-help guide for those with amyotrophic lateral sclerosis, "To feel good, you need to look good."[13]

Easy-to-fasten garments that open in the front provide freedom of movement and eliminate the need to reach upward (for example, front-fastening brassieres).[14] Velcro closures are excellent substitutes for buttons and can be purchased at most fabric shops. Enlarging zipper pulls, using a loop or tab, makes closure easier. Button hooks are also a great aid to those who have inadequate fine grasp to manipulate small buttons. A dressing stick tipped with foam or a reaching stick allows an elderly person to remain seated while dressing and reduces the risk of falling (Fig. 15–6).

Dressing the lower limbs is often difficult for those with poor reach or balance. A stocking gutter of stiff plastic with pull tabs makes it possible to don stockings without bending. Shoes can be converted to slip-ons with elastic shoelaces, or zippers or Velcro closures can be stitched in by any shoemaker.

Ideas for aids to dressing and adaptive clothing are readily available in any occupational therapy department. Information is also available in texts on activities of daily living or general rehabilitation[15,16] and are illustrated in many manuals distributed by voluntary health organizations.[17] The Veterans Administration Directory[7] lists 30 sources of dressing aids. Sears, Roebuck, and Company now publishes a home health catalog, which features clothing as well as many health care aids. Several companies have specialized in designing clothing for the disabled and elderly.*

* Fashion Able Self-Help Items, Rocky Hill, New Jersey 08553; Betty Butler, Inc., P.O. Box 51, Tenafly, New Jersey 07670; Geri Fashions, 301 E. Illinois Street, Newberg, Oregon 97132.

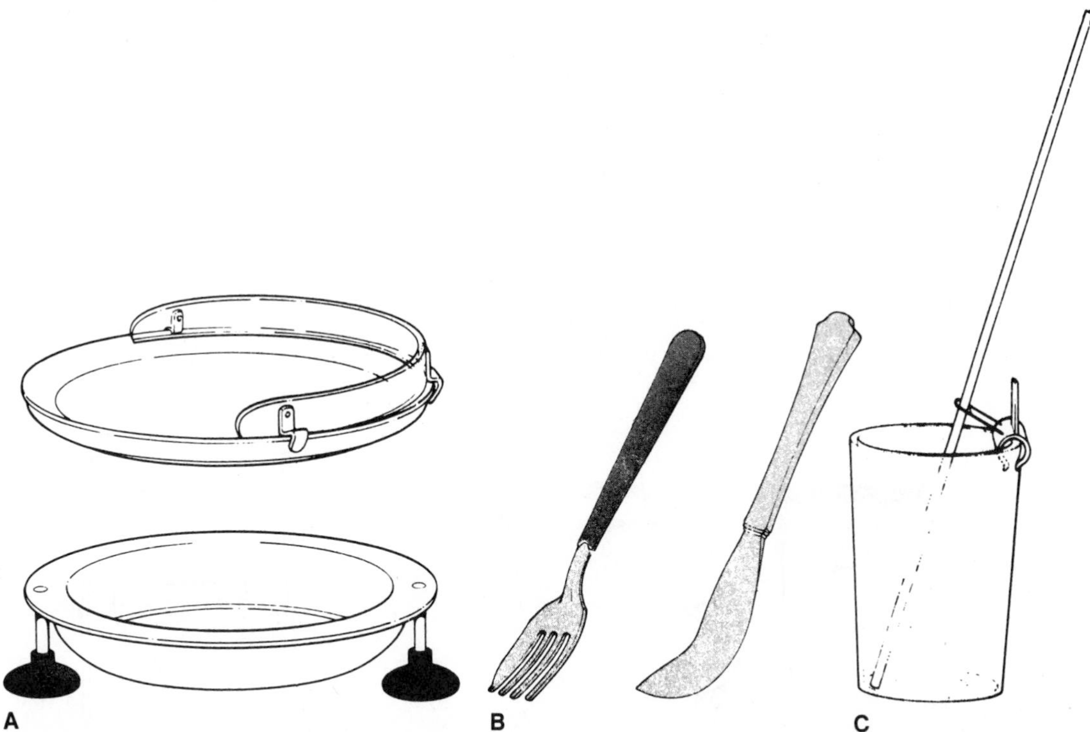


**Figure 15-5.** Mealtime aids. *A*, Plates with plate guards and suction cups. *B*, Side cutter fork and rocker knife. *C*, Plastic straw with bulldog clip attached to side of glass. (From Hale G (ed.): The Source Book for the Disabled. Philadelphia, WB Saunders Co., 1979.)

## HYGIENE AIDS

The bathroom, with its slippery floors and narrow spaces, is the most dangerous place in the home for anyone with impaired balance, joint limitation, or slowness of movement. A call for help may be unheeded, especially when water is running or the bathroom door is closed. Thus, the bathroom should be made as safe as possible and equipment provided to increase ease of bathing and grooming without mishap.

Grab bars should be placed where needed around tubs, showers, and toilets. Nonskid strips should be attached to the tub or shower floor or rubber mats placed on such surfaces. Raised toilet seats for persons with weakness or stiffness of the lower limbs are readily available in many medical supply stores. Seats for the bathtub or shower, and bath lifters are also widely available (Fig. 15-7). Those with restricted lower limbs who cannot actually sit down in the bottom of a tub will benefit from a hand-held shower. Washing aids include wash mitts, soap on a rope, brushes with suction

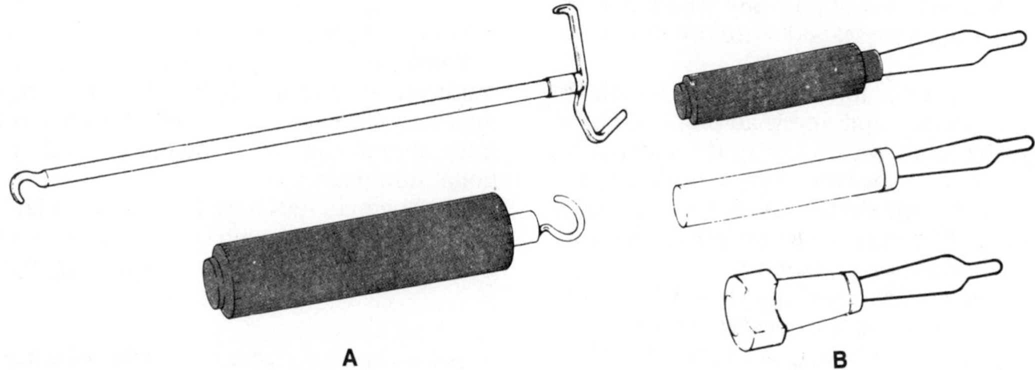


**Figure 15-6.** Dressing aids. *A*, Dressing stick and zipper pull. *B*, Various button hooks. (From Hale G (ed.): The Source Book for the Disabled. Philadelphia, WB Saunders Co., 1979.)

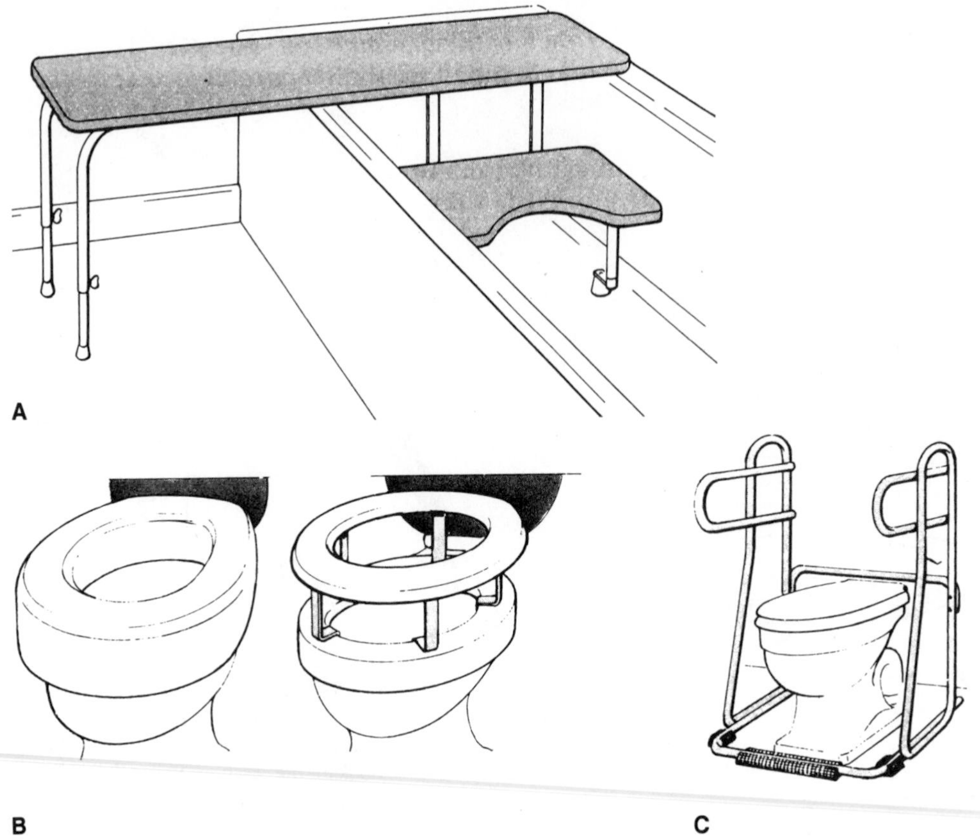


**Figure 15–7.** Bathroom devices. *A*, Bath bench and tub seat. *B*, Two types of removable elevating toilet seats. *C*, Grab bars that fit any toilet. (From Hale G (ed.): The Source Book for the Disabled. Philadelphia, WB Saunders Co., 1979.)

backs, and long-handled sponges. If the individual cannot walk into the bathroom (for anyone permanently in a wheelchair, bathroom entrances are usually hopeless), a bedside commode may have to be substituted for the bathroom toilet. It should be a sturdy structure, with side-arms, and should be arranged to permit the feet to touch the floor. Of course, the bathroom doorway can be widened, but this may be very costly. As an alternative, a wheelchair narrower fits almost any wheelchair; its crank squeezes the seat sidewards by almost 3 to 5 in.[10]

To compensate for limited grasp, handles of combs, brushes, and fingernail files can be enlarged by foam padding or other material, as previously described for eating utensils. Electric toothbrushes and electric razors are much easier to use than manual ones for individuals with hand coordination problems.[8]

Equipment for bowel and bladder incontinence is beyond the scope of this chapter. However, patients with such problems should be aware that there are many types of collecting devices for bladder care and bowel care* that make it possible for them to lead a normal life. Primary care physicians should make themselves familiar with the various forms of pads and urinary collecting devices currently on the market and advise an individual, depending on special physical or social requirements.

## COMMUNICATION AIDS

Many elderly people with motor or sensory impairment have very limited ability to communicate. As a result, their isolation increases, their safety is endangered, and they are cut off from normal sources of intellectual and emotional stimulation.

Reading materials have been widely adapted for the handicapped, with large print books, special magnifiers, and even special magnifying

* Hollister Inc., 2000 Hollister Drive, Libertyville, Illinois 60048.

television screen systems. If the main problem is to hold reading matter in a comfortable position, help is readily obtained by a variety of aids. The simplest reading aids are angled bookstands that can be placed on tables, over beds, or even on the floor like a music stand. People with difficulty in turning pages can use rubber thimbles or rubber-tipped pencils to grip the pages. Although they cost several hundred dollars, electric page turners are available for the severely handicapped, and these serve a special need for avid readers.[8]

Prismatic glasses make it possible to see objects at right angles, and they aid with reading if a person must lie flat. They can reduce eye strain and neck pain, particularly when neck motion is limited. For those unable to read even books with large print or using special magnifying devices, but who still wish to keep up with the world, there are now many "talking books." Services are available by contacting the local National Federation for the Blind, and the Library of Congress, Division of Blind and Physically Handicapped, will send information on reading aids and the availability of "talking books." *

Aids can be used to help those with problems of grip or coordination to write. Handles of writing implements can be enlarged by rubber bands or by foam rubber, attached by glue, or one may even enlarge the handle of a pen by sticking it through a plastic golf ball. Occupational therapy departments feature plastic pencil holders with Velcro closures, which strap the implement to the fingers. Note pads are usually easier to use than loose sheets, and clipboards are often helpful to stabilize the paper if one hand is weak, as in hemiplegia. Various types of reading stands can double as writing stands for those who are too seriously disabled to write at a table or desk.

Many elderly people cannot write easily; for them the electric typewriter has been a great benefit, especially if they lack strength and coordination to use the controls on a manual typewriter. An electric typewriter can be operated by a hand-held stick or even a stick attached to a mouthpiece. Advice concerning how to learn to type either with the right or left hand is provided by Richardson.[18] For those who find both writing and typing a problem, a cassette tape recorder is a useful substitute. In selecting such a recorder, one should consider how difficult it is to operate and select only one that has simple controls.

* An excellent library of "talking books" is available from Books on Tape, Newport Beach, California 92660.

There is little doubt that the telephone is the most vital tool of communication, especially for elderly people who live alone. Advances in telephone design have made it much easier for the disabled to send or receive calls. Obviously the telephone should be positioned for the most efficient and comfortable use, especially if reach is limited. For dialing the telephone, simple dialing aids such as a pencil or dialing tool can solve coordination problems, but for some, it is probably easier to use the touch-tone type of telephone. Giant push button telephone adaptors are currently available to make these phones easier to use. A Call-maker completely eliminates the need to dial by calling automatically at the press of a button or insertion of a card into a slot. If a person has limited arm strength, having the telephone mounted on a gooseneck arm or using headsets can eliminate holding it for any length of time. As an alternative, the conventional telephone can be replaced entirely by a dial, microphone, and speaker set in a special boxed unit. A call to the telephone company is the easiest way for a handicapped person to be advised of the various options available.

There are many other types of communication aids, such as sophisticated electronic devices that even provide vocal responses to those without speech. Whenever a serious communication problem develops, the physician is well advised to consult a speech pathologist, whose primary purpose is to develop communication skills in patients. The local chapter of the American Speech and Hearing Association can suggest where to turn for consultation.

## RECREATION AIDS

The easiest and perhaps the only way an elderly disabled person may become part of the community, make new friends, or escape from an institutional setting is through participation in recreational activities. Physicians, therefore, should encourage elderly handicapped people to participate not only in group exercises or in outdoor sports but in any recreational activity that interests them. Handicapped elderly people can find many indoor sports and games that have been adapted for various disabilities. For example, special playing-card-holders and battery-powered card shufflers are now available. Special tools for indoor gardening and shop work have been developed for specific handicaps. The section on leisure and recreation in the book by Hale[8] is an excellent guide, and the book also lists various organizations promoting leisure activities for the handicapped.

## CONCLUSION

The aim of this chapter has been to provide a short guide to resources for the elderly disabled. A complete list of resources would be impossible to summarize in any meaningful fashion but the Veterans Administration Directory[7] can largely serve this purpose. The Publications Office of the Institute of Rehabilitation Medicine* will send, on request, a list of commercial sources for adaptive equipment. Another source of such information is the Buyer's Guide from Accent on Living.†

The newest attempt to assist handicapped people and others in obtaining information about commercially available rehabilitation equipment and aids is the ABLEDATA System. This is a computer-based information program accessible anywhere in the United States to people with subscriptions and approved passwords through special telecommunication lines such as TELENET or TYMNET. At present direct access is limited to "information brokers," who are trained to search the database and provide interface between the computer hardware and the person needing information. Therefore, if a patient requires a specific rehabilitation product, local information brokers may provide this information free of charge. Names of information brokers may be obtained from the State Vocational and Rehabilitation Division or by contacting the National Rehabilitation Information Center.‡

It is planned that the system will also be compatible with many rehabilitation product information systems that are being developed internationally.

The Yellow Pages of the telephone directory may be consulted for volunteer health organizations or social service agencies that assist people with handicaps or various diseases. If a person has a specific, chronically disabling disease, a call to the local branch of the national organization will usually provide information about assistive devices. Information is also available from some large department stores. Local medical supply dealers generally carry a large line of rehabilitation equipment. They have salespeople who are often very well informed about living aids or equipment and the options available for different disabling conditions. Finally, exhibitions are held annually in large cities to show handicapped people, vendors, and other rehabilitation personnel the latest equipment and devices to aid the disabled.

* 400 E. 34th Street, New York, New York 10016.

† Accent Special Publications, Box 700, Bloomington, Illinois 61701

‡ National Rehabilitation Information Center, 4407 8th Street N.E., Washington, DC 20017–2299.

### References

1. Kottke JF, Stillwell GK, Lehmann JF: Krusen's Handbook of Physical Medicine and Rehabilitation. 3rd ed. Philadelphia, W.B. Saunders, 1982.
2. Lawton EB: Activities of Daily Living for Rehabilitation. McGraw-Hill, New York, 1963.
3. Nichols JR (ed.): Rehabilitation Medicine: The Management of Physical Disabilities. 2nd ed. London, Boston, Butterworth's, 1980.
4. Redford JB (ed.): Orthotics Etcetera, 2nd ed. Baltimore, Williams & Wilkins, 1980.
5. Rusk HA, Taylor EJ: Rehabilitation Medicine. 4th ed. St. Louis, C.V. Mosby, 1977.
6. Blount WP: Don't throw away the cane. J Bone Joint Surg (Am) 38:695, 1956.
7. United States Veterans Administration: Directory of Living Aids for the Disabled Person. Washington, DC, Superintendent of Documents, U.S. Government Printing Office (undated).
8. Hale G (ed.): The Source Book for the Disabled. Philadelphia, W.B. Saunders, 1979.
9. American Academy of Orthopedic Surgeons: Atlas of Orthotics. St. Louis, C.V. Mosby, 1975.
10. Kamenetz HL: Wheelchairs and other indoor vehicles for the disabled. *In* Redford JB (ed.): Orthotics Etcetera, 2nd ed. Baltimore, Williams & Wilkins, 1980.
11. Lee MHM, Pazen KDP, Dacso MM: Wheelchair Prescription: Public Health Service Publication #1666, Washington, DC, Superintendent of Documents (undated).
12. May EE, Waggoner NR, Hotte EB: Independent Living for the Handicapped and the Elderly. Boston, Houghton Miflin, 1974.
13. Hamilton MR: Why Didn't Somebody Tell Me About These Things? Amyotrophic Lateral Sclerosis Society of America. 15300 Ventura Blvd., Sherman Oaks, CA 91403, 1985.
14. Hoffman AM: Clothing for the Handicapped, Springfield, Illinois, C.C. Thomas, 1979.
15. Brown ME: Self-Help Clothing. *In* Redford JB (ed): Orthotics Etcetera. 2nd ed. Baltimore, Williams & Wilkins, 1980.
16. Willard HS, Spackman CS: Occupational Therapy. 4th ed. Philadelphia, J.B. Lippincott, 1971.
17. Robinson MB: Aids, Equipment and Suggestions to Help the Patient with Parkinson's Disease in the Activities of Daily Living, The American Parkinson Disease Association. 116 John St., New York, N.Y. (undated).
18. Richardson NK: Type With One Hand. New Rochelle, South-Western Publishing Co., 1959.

## Chapter 16

# Issues in Paying for Health Care of the Aged

C. Carl Pegels

On the average and in the aggregate, Americans spend about 10 per cent of the gross national product on health care. However, the expenditures of older Americans for health care services have been estimated to be as high as 30 per cent of their income. With declining incomes during the later years of life, a single expenditure of 30 per cent imposes a considerable burden on the elderly.

The government has responded to the considerable health care needs of the elderly by providing several government funded mechanisms for health care cost reimbursement. The most important one of these is Medicare. Medicare is a form of national health insurance for the elderly, that is, for those 65 years and older. In comparison with national health insurance programs in other countries, Medicare is not comprehensive. It covers only scant amounts of ambulatory care, requires that patients pay the approximate equivalent of their first day in the hospital, and provides virtually no coverage for nursing home care.

Elderly patients unable to pay for nursing home care usually become eligible for Medicaid. Medicaid is a federal government–sponsored program of health care cost reimbursement for the needy that is administered by the state governments, which also share in its cost.

Home health care and home care consisting of the services of home health aids, homemaker services, home meals, and transportation are partially funded by Title XX funds of the Social Security Administration, another federally funded program administered by the state governments.

Many elderly also purchase private health insurance for health costs not covered by governmental health insurance. However, even with the several forms of coverage itemized previously, the elderly, on average, still spend 30 per cent of their income on personal health care needs.

## MODALITIES OF CARE AND PAYMENT MECHANISMS

Health care for the elderly can be segmented into five modalities: ambulatory care, hospital care, nursing home care, home care, and day care. Some of these health care modalities overlap to an extent, but virtually all care can be included in these five categories. Health-related services, such as the filling of prescriptions, dental care, and hearing and vision services, are included in the category of ambulatory care.

Payment to finance the health care supplied through these five modalities can similarly be segmented into five payment mechanisms: Medicare, Medicaid, supplementary health insurance, self pay, and funds available through Title XX of the Social Security Act. These five financing sources are fairly complete. One could argue that there is a sixth source: When none of the other five is able to pay, the provider essentially absorbs the cost of providing that care.

Figure 16–1 shows how the five care modalities and the five payment mechanisms interact. An estimate of the amount of funds provided by the respective payment mechanism is provided for each interaction (each cell). For instance, home care is heavily funded through Title XX funds; some funding comes through self pay by the care recipients, and only small amounts of

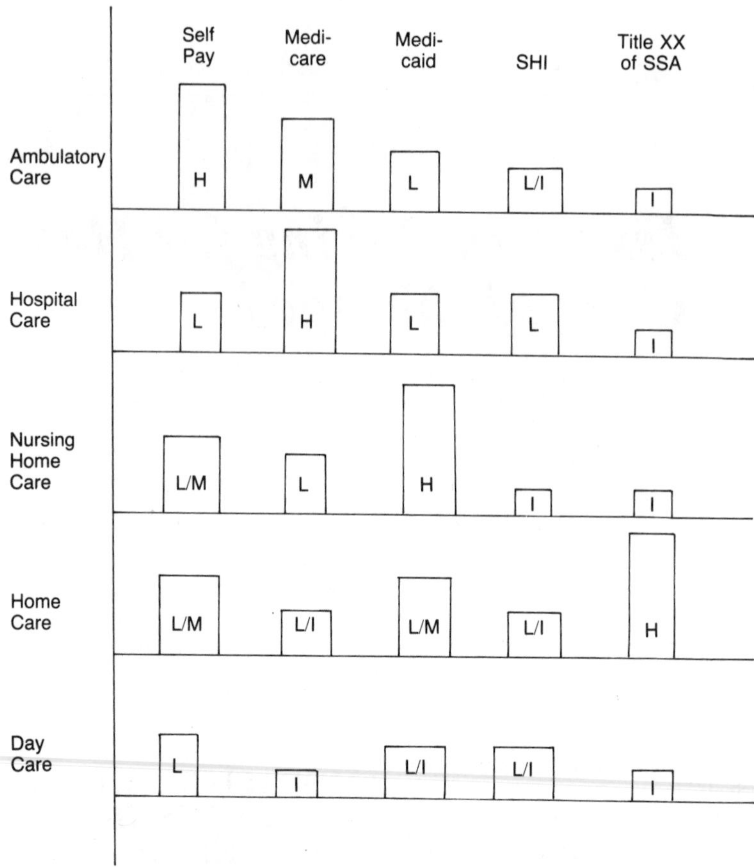


**Figure 16–1.** Payment mechanisms and level of payment for health care modalities. H = significant amount; M = a fair amount; L = a small amount; I = an insignificant amount or none; SSA = Social Security Administration; SHI = supplementary health insurance.

financing of home care are provided by Medicare and Medicaid funds.

## *Mechanisms of Health Care Financing*

### Medicare and Medicaid Programs—The Primary Mechanisms of Financing

The Medicare and Medicaid programs have helped the elderly to carry much of the burden of health care costs. Government expenditures for these two programs have increased substantially since their introduction in the late 1960s. Together, the two programs provide approximately $2000 per elderly person per year, i.e., about two thirds of the average per capita health care costs incurred by the elderly. The remaining one third, or over $1000 per person, is the responsibility of the elderly themselves. Actual payment comes from self pay and private supplementary health insurance.

The preceding figures are only average figures; however, not all older individuals are eligible for both Medicare and Medicaid. Medicaid is available only to those senior citizens whose incomes fall below the poverty line. Individuals with incomes above the poverty line (i.e., about four of five seniors) are generally not eligible for Medicaid. For these people, on the average, Medicare covers only 38 per cent of the yearly health care bill.

Medicaid is generally considered a welfare program by most of the population. As a result, being forced to accept Medicaid can be traumatic for many senior citizens who have grown up with the ethic that one must care for oneself and not be dependent on governmental handouts. Interestingly enough, having to accept government help through Medicare is considered quite acceptable. Medicare reimbursement, with all its limitations, is considered to be a civil right, and one seldom hears of concern by individuals about having health care costs reimbursed by Medicare.

## Supplementary Health Insurance and Self Pay

In order to offset the ever-escalating cost of health care, senior citizens are buying private health insurance policies to supplement their Medicare coverage. Two thirds, or 15 million of 23 million older Americans, have at least one such policy. These policies are often called wraparound (around Medicare) health insurance or also "medigap" insurance. The main purpose of these policies is to provide coverage for those areas where Medicare by itself does not suffice. Senior citizens often acquire more than one such policy and often as many as four or five. As of 1978, there were an estimated 19 million health insurance policies in effect for the elderly.

An average of $200 in annual premiums was paid for each policy for a total expenditure of $3.8 billion. The policyholders received an estimated $1.3 billion in benefits. This amounts to less than 35 per cent or premiums collected on average.

The low return of these health insurance policies is, in part, caused by the many multiple policies often held by the elderly. In order to maximize protection, many of the elderly buy more than one policy. However, in most instances, when they become sick they can only claim benefits from one policy. Thus, the real beneficiaries of this wasteful practice are the private insurance companies. These private health insurance companies "cover" about 50 per cent of the elderly health insurance market and Blue Cross/Blue Shield and Health Maintenance Organizations cover the balance. None of the practices described herein are attributed to the latter organizations. According to a congressional investigation examining this situation, the root of the problem lies in the limited coverage that Medicare provides and in the lack of knowledge that many older Americans have concerning what Medicare covers.

It is well known to critics of supplemental health insurance, especially of private health insurance plans, that no insurance policy will cover all expenses that Medicare does not cover. Items that are frequently excluded from supplemental policies are private duty nursing, routine checkups, eyeglasses, hearing aids, dental work, cosmetic surgery, custodial care in nursing homes, psychiatric care, and self-administered drugs. Most supplemental policies also follow Medicare guidelines, thus further limiting the coverage that is provided. This fact probably more than anything else causes one to question the need for such policies in the first place.

Senior citizens, often acting with the assurance of insurance agents that their policy will cover all of the medical expenses that Medicare will not pay, naively purchase these supplementary policies. In reality, however, the holder of numerous policies often discovers, when it is too late, that the policies do not provide the security that they sought when they originally subscribed or were enlisted.

Although this situation paints a shady view of the insurance industry as a whole, most experts agree that there is good economic value and financial risk protection in the purchase of one supplementary health insurance policy, particularly from reputable organizations such as Blue Cross/Blue Shield. Blue Cross/Blue Shield and other reputable private insurance companies return, in some cases, in excess of 90 per cent of the premiums collected to the insured in the form of claims paid. On the other hand, there are many other private insurance companies that sell policies which return as little as 20 per cent of premiums collected.[1]

Based on the preceding, one can see that a good portion of what the elderly pay for supplementary health insurance could better be saved and, if necessary, used for self pay of health care services. A good part of health care for the elderly is still covered through self pay, especially in those areas that are not covered by any insurance. The areas of dental care, vision care, hearing aids, drugs, and sundry appliances are usually financed through self pay by the elderly. In addition, a good part of ambulatory medical visits are paid directly by the elderly. Hence, health care, even with Medicare and supplementary health insurance, is still a heavy economic burden on the elderly.

## Title XX of the Social Security Act

Federal funds made available under Title XX of the Social Security Act[2] provide much of the support for home health aids and homemaker support services for the elderly. The federal funds do not go directly to the elderly but are provided to states as block grants based on state populations. The states are paid a large portion of social service program costs, up to the Title XX ceilings, which vary depending on the type of program supported. A wide variety of services are available under the program. By providing home support services for the elderly who are medically needy, the program seeks to prevent inappropriate institutional care.

The eligibility criteria vary from state to state. Payments are usually made to Area Offices of the Aging or to subcontractors of the area offices. The sum spent for health aide and homemaker services amounts to about 10 to 15 per cent of total Title XX funds.[3] Average expenditure per beneficiary amounted to about $1000 in 1977 dollars. Approximately one-half million people were served by Title XX funds in 1977. California had the highest proportion of expenditures of Title XX funds for home services, amounting to about 30 per cent of total health care costs. In addition to Title XX funds, considerable amounts of private funds are also utilized for home health aides and homemaker services.

## *Modalities of Care*

### AMBULATORY CARE

Ambulatory care of the elderly provided by the physician is financed largely by Medicare if the attending physician accepts assignment of claims. By accepting assignment of claims, the physician agrees to accept Medicare's allowed charge as full payment.[4] This acceptance of assignment of claims is of considerable importance in relieving the elderly's burden of the costs of medical care services. If the physician does not accept assignment of claims, the Medicare patient is liable for the difference between the amount charged and the amount Medicare allows. If this difference is large, the liability of the elderly patient can be substantial. Hence, the decision of the physician to accept or not accept assignment can be of considerable consequence to the out-of-pocket costs of the elderly.

For example, suppose a Medicare beneficiary has met the fixed dollar deductible and is charged $90 for a physician service. Fixed dollar deductible is the amount of the medical bill the patient must pay before Medicare reimbursement can begin. If the Medicare-allowed charge is $50, and if the physician accepts assignment, Medicare will reimburse the physician 80 per cent of the allowed charge or $40. The Medicare beneficiary then owes the physician the difference ($10). If the physician does not accept assignment of claims, the Medicare beneficiary owes the physician the $10 plus the difference between the $90 physician fee and the $50 allowed charge, for a total out-of-pocket cost of $50. Hence, in this example, the elderly person has a larger out-of-pocket cost than the Medicare reimbursement.

In the United States during 1975, assignment of claims was accepted by physicians for about one half of physician charges covered by Medicare. The rate of acceptance varies considerably by region. For instance, in New England nearly two thirds of the physician charges were covered by assignment, whereas on the West coast the acceptance rate was just over one third of all charges.

There are two reasons why physicians accept assignment of claims. One is concern for the financial burden of the elderly as a result of substantial out-of-pocket medical bills. The other reason is that, if assignment is not accepted, payment may not be made at all if the patient is financially unable to pay and if the patient does not claim for reimbursement from Medicare for the portion of the medical bill covered by Medicare. Assignment of claims is, as a result, accepted more readily for larger than for smaller medical bills.

Alternatively, the physician may not consider the burden imposed on the elderly by refusing assignment of claims to be significant. On the basis of typical middle-class income, his or her assumption may be correct. Unfortunately, many elderly must subsist on much lower than middle-class incomes, and physician charges may thus impose a considerable financial burden.

Some of the additional physician charges may be covered by private supplementary health insurance. Unfortunately, most supplementary health insurance plans primarily cover hospital-based medical services, including surgery. Ambulatory care, on the other hand, is seldom covered by supplementary health insurance, and ambulatory care provides the setting in which the primary contact between the elderly person and the physician is established. The barriers to care should be minimal at this point of contact. Unfortunately, imposing the need for considerable out-of-pocket charges can impose an undesirable barrier to care at this point. In addition, as noted previously, few of the miscellaneous health-related expenditures, such as for dental care, hearing aids, eyeglass prescriptions, and prescription drugs, are covered by Medicare or supplementary insurance. As a result, these expenditures are usually paid for by the elderly.

### HOSPITAL CARE

During 1979, approximately $85 billion was spent on hospital care in the United States.[5] About 25 per cent of the total amount ($21.6 billion) was paid by Medicare. Although the elderly are not the only beneficiaries of Medicare, they are by far the largest group. Thus, the percentage of Medicare costs relating to hospitalization of the elderly is more than twice the percentage of the population made up by the elderly. In addition, Medicare does not pay for all hospital care. There is an initial co-payment for each hospitalization equal to about the first day of hospitalization, and for long hospital stays, there are limits on hospital stay coverage.

Nursing home stays are practically excluded from coverage by Medicare. Medicare coverage only applies under restricted conditions. As a result, elderly people admitted to nursing homes either pay for it themselves, if they have the assets to do so, or apply for Medicaid. These nursing home stays provide additional institutionalization for the elderly but are not included in the hospital expenditure figures shown previously. Hence, the 25 per cent spent by Medicare on hospitalization for the elderly should be augmented by those funds spent on nursing home stays in order to obtain true cost of institutionalization for the elderly.

To obtain a different perspective, figures derived from a study carried out by the Health Systems Agency of Western New York[6] showed that hospitalization for patients 65 years and older amounted to 4138 days per 1000 people. Hospitalization amounted to 487 days per 1000 people for individuals between 15 and 44 years of age and to 1371 days per 1000 people for those between 45 and 64 years of age. Hospitalization for children between 0 and 14 years of age is even lower (326 days per 1000 children). Hence, the rate of hospitalization for individuals 65 years and older is three times the rate of those 45 to 64 years of age, 8.5 times the rate of those 15 to 44 years of age, and 12.7 times the rate of those 0 to 14 years of age.

These high expenditures from Medicare for hospitalization of elderly people have led to increased attention by policymakers in the federal government to cost containment for in-hospital care. One of the ways to slow down cost increases is through the medium of "prospective reimbursement." Prospective reimbursement compensates hospitals on the basis of prior year patient loads, on the basis of diagnosis, or on other bases. Over the past several years, a number of prospective hospital reimbursement plans have been under investigation and several have been adopted. Hospital reimbursement plans on the basis of diagnostic related groups (DRGs) have also been adopted. It appears that the government will continue experimentation with these and other reimbursement plans in the future. Although hospital cost increases cannot be entirely eliminated, it is anticipated that prospective reimbursement plans are able, at least, to stem the escalating hospital cost spiral so that it will remain close to changes in the consumer price index.

Cost containment of all health care, but especially of hospitalization, is critically important to the provision of health care for the elderly. With such a large percentage of reimbursement coming from the Medicare fund, the pressure for benefit reductions is directly proportional to increases in health care expenditure. Any success in curbing increases in health care costs will therefore indirectly benefit the availability and financing of health care to the elderly.

## Nursing Homes

There are basically two levels of care provided by a nursing home; skilled care and intermediate care. Skilled care is that level of nursing home care nearest to hospital care. Intermediate care facilities are, as the name suggests, intended to help those who do not need around-the-clock nursing care or other mandatory services provided by a skilled nursing facility. In some states, the term "health related facility" is used instead of intermediate care facility. Federal financing under Medicare was originally available for only skilled nursing care. However, in 1967, an amendment to the Social Security Act made possible direct payments to recipients in intermediate care facilities.*

An increasing proportion of the nation's health dollar is being allotted to long-term care administered through nursing homes. In 1960,

---

* The intermediate care facility is currently referred to in the Medicare Handbook as a skilled nursing facility. A skilled nursing facility is defined as a specially qualified facility that has the staff and equipment to provide skilled nursing care or rehabilitation services, as well as other related health services. According to the Medicare Handbook, Medicare hospital insurance can help pay for inpatient care in a participating skilled nursing facility after the patient has been in a hospital. Specifically, to qualify for Medicare coverage, the following five conditions must be satisfied:

1. A 3-consecutive-day stay in a hospital before transfer to the skilled nursing facility.
2. Treatment for the same condition as in the hospital.
3. Hospital stay of 3 consecutive days must have occurred within 14 days of admission to the skilled nursing facility.
4. Certification by a physician that care in a skilled nursing facility is needed and provided.
5. A utilization review committee does not disapprove of the patient's stay.

In each benefit period, Medicare hospital insurance pays for all covered services for the first 20 days the patient is in a skilled nursing facility. After 20 days, Medicare hospital insurance pays for all covered services from the 21st through the 100th day, except for a daily co-payment ($22.50 per day in 1980 and higher in subsequent years). After 100 days, the patient must pay all charges or apply for Medicaid coverage.

this amount accounted for a little more than 1 per cent, growing to 4 per cent in 1970, and to over 5 per cent at present. In 1972, Medicaid expenditures for nursing home care exceeded expenditures for surgical and general hospitals for the first time. Assistance by various government agencies has been given to nursing homes through numerous programs.

**Who Are the Nursing Home Residents?**

Of all people age 65 years and older, 1 in 18 (5.6 per cent) is in an institution.[7] The number of people over 65 years in the United States has increased 600 per cent since the turn of the century. One third of these people are over 75. Surveys have revealed that only one in 18 seniors is in a nursing home or related facility on any given day, but one of five seniors will eventually spend some time in a nursing home.

According to data collected by the National Center for Health Statistics,[8] approximately 75 per cent of the 1,027,850 people over 65, living in institutions in 1976, were in nursing homes; 11 per cent were in mental hospitals; and 14 per cent were in all other types of institutions. Eighty-nine per cent of nursing home patients and 28 per cent of patients in mental hospitals were over 65 years of age.

It is apparent that the typical nursing home resident needs help of some kind. Less than one half of the patients can walk. About 55 per cent require assistance in bathing, 47 per cent need help in dressing, 11 per cent need help in eating, and 33 per cent are incontinent.[9]

## Home Health Care Programs

Home health care, as an alternative to providing long-term institutional care, has become a valuable and important resource in many communities. It provides needed services to many people but especially to the elderly ill who are functionally impaired. Although many of these ill elderly are provided with needed emotional and physical support by relatives or friends, the professional assistance provided through these home care programs is an important ingredient in avoiding the need for institutionalization of many of the elderly.

The presence of a chronic condition such as arthritis or diabetes is a cause of functional impairment but usually is not a sufficient or the sole determinant of the need for institutional long-term care. Individuals who are functionally disabled are often bedridden, need help with dressing and bathing, or need help moving around outside the home. These people are candidates for home health care and do not necessarily need to be institutionalized. Availability or lack of institutional facilities, willingness of family or friends to care for the person, costs of care, reticence on the part of the elderly person to enter an institution, and availability of home care are all important variables that determine whether or not an individual enters an institutional facility.

Generally, home health care is provided or subsidized through a governmental program. The programs usually operate under federal, state, or county sponsorship and support. The programs provide a gamut of home services, such as diagnostic health care, therapeutic health care, nutrition, transportation, and recreation.

**Cost Effectiveness and Social Appropriateness of Home Care**

The cost effectiveness, quality, and cost of home health care, including homemaker services, have been debated for some years. Interest in the savings potential of this service stems from the combined pressures of the "geriatric boom," rising expenditures of health care, and a concern for overall quality of care for the aged.

A review of the literature to determine under which conditions home health care is both cost effective and socially appropriate has failed to produce an analysis that combined both the social and economic aspects. In addition, interviews of social workers, nursing home administrators, home health agency workers, and other professionals in the health care field revealed that they believed that home health care is justified from the perspective of need rather than cost effectiveness.

Widely divergent views exist as to what policies are desirable and possible when considering home health care as an alternative to institutionalization. There is unanimous agreement that two variables, family support and degree of functional impairment, are the key factors in determining the use of home health care. Whether implicitly or explicitly stated, the availability of family support is the determining factor in prescribing or advocating home health care services instead of institutionalization.

Despite the continuing importance and willingness of families to support the aged, historical changes have created new constraints on families, which must be taken into account in policy decisions. More and more women are leaving the home environment to enter the work force, thus shrinking the pool of families that is able to support the aged in a home environment.

An abundance of recent literature on intergenerational relationships addresses various aspects of this issue and should be integrated into the cost-effectiveness debate. Although the methodologic problems in such studies are still in need of refinement, they do substantiate the need for caution in assuming the continued existence or desirability of the extensive family support suggested in the cost-effectiveness studies. The difficulty of determining "true" costs is indeed a complex problem. According to the Comptroller General's 1977 GAO Report,[10] the true costs of maintaining the elderly and sick in their homes have been largely hidden because the greatest portion of such costs represents the services provided by families and friends rather than those provided at public expense. The social and policy implications based on such an assumption are exhaustive, and further interdisciplinary knowledge is crucial.

It has been suggested that just as the Medicare-Medicaid programs were created by pressures from providers (physicians and hospitals who were not receiving payment), new approaches to dealing with the "geriatric problem" might well evolve from pressures of families. Future policy recommendations will require consideration of changing characteristics of both older populations and other segments of the population in regard to needs, attitudes, and other social changes. In other words, a long-term policy is indicated; however, it is unlikely that such a program will be accomplished easily.

## Day Health Care Programs

In comparison with nursing home residency and home health care, day care programs for senior adults are probably the least developed modality of care for the elderly. However, there are strong indications that day care programs will become increasingly common. There are basically two reasons for providing day care. The first and most common reason is the avoidance or prevention of admittance to nursing homes for patients who can live at home but need a variety of health-related services for their health maintenance and rehabilitation. The second reason for provision of day care services to the frail elderly is to assist them in achieving a better quality of life.

Day care programs should not be confused with senior citizen centers, which provide companionship, crafts, lectures, subsidized lunches, and referral services. They should also be differentiated from home health care, which is for those frail elderly who are physically or emotionally unable to participate in normal everyday activities. Day care emphasizes health maintenance, health promotion, health restoration, and rehabilitation of physical ailments. Services in a day care center are provided by a team of health care providers, such as occupational therapists, social workers, and nursing personnel. A senior adult day care program[11] must be able to provide some basic services, including a bright and protective environment with generous opportunities for socializing with other senior adults and staff members. For each participant, the basic minimum service should also include one nutritious meal per day, a rest period, social activities, arts and crafts, appropriate exercises, and transportation to and from his or her home. Participants should be ambulatory or able to operate their wheelchairs, and they should be able to administer their own medications with a minimum of supervision.

Day care programs should be able to provide personal care services, family and professional counseling, training in the activities of daily living, and rehabilitative therapy. Personal care services as part of a day care program include such routine activities as personal hygiene, taking baths, cutting nails, meal preparation, exercising, and routine health maintenance activities. Family and professional counseling includes help with legal services, bill paying, making arrangements for the provision of routine services, health education, and other group activities. Training in the activities of daily living is especially important to those senior adults who need assistance after having become disabled. This includes training in the use of crutches, wheelchairs, and prosthetic devices. Rehabilitative therapy includes treatments provided by physical, occupational, and speech therapists in order to enable the disabled senior adult to go back to living as normal a life as is possible.

A model day care program, such as the one outlined previously may be located in a rehabilitation-oriented nursing home or in a hospital-sponsored facility. The purpose of the program is to return the clients to a normal environment, living on their own or with close relatives, such as adult children.

## Costs of Day Care Versus Costs of Nursing Home Care

The analysis that follows is based on a brief article by Grimaldi,[12] which commented on a more extensive and earlier journal article by Weissert.[13] Weissert's thesis, supported by findings, is that adult day care is less costly than nursing home care. Therefore, Weissert argues, adult day care should be expanded in order to reduce nursing home care. Grimaldi questions Weissert's conclusion because he believes that it is based on several unrealistic assumptions. For example, Grimaldi argues that patients in intermediate care facilities would be more likely candidates for day care than patients in skilled nursing facilities, and since per diem costs of intermediate care facilities generally are less than those of skilled nursing facilities, the case Weissert makes is thereby weakened. Grimaldi also argues that estimating the costs of day care is considerably more difficult than estimating the costs of care in skilled nursing facilities or intermediate care facilities. Furthermore, in estimating the costs of day care, the patient's cost or the relatives' cost of maintaining the patient in a home environment is usually not included or is significantly understated. Obviously, the cost of transportation must also be included. Finally, Grimaldi argues that it is unlikely that adult day care centers would furnish all needed medical services. The costs for these additional required services need to be included in a reasonable cost comparison. There is general agreement that increased availability of day care will cause an increase in total adults applying for services. People with less severe debilitating problems would probably not enter a nursing home but most likely would take advantage of a day care program in their community. Hence, even if costs by case load were comparable, the total expenditures for day care would most likely be higher. Therefore, one must reach the conclusion that, on strictly an aggregate cost basis, day care is not necessarily less costly than nursing home care. However, the quality of life for many of our elderly can be considerably enhanced by a well-thought-out and well-managed day care program.

## HEALTH CARE EXPENDITURES—THE PRESENT AND FUTURE

### *The Present*

Health care expenditures for personal care for the entire population of this country amounted to $203 billion during the 1980 year ending in June.[14] Of this amount, about $59 billion was expended for health care for those 65 years and older; the remaining $144 billion, for health care for those under 65 years of age.

On a population base of about 222 million people, which includes about 24 million (10.8 per cent) elderly, the per capita personal health care expenditure for the elderly was $2458, compared with $727 for those under 65 years of age. Thus, we find that the cost of personal health care for those 65 years of age and over is about 3.4 times greater than the costs of personal health care for those under 65 years of age. In Table 16–1 these statistics are itemized in detail.

### *The Future*

In Table 16–2 we have projected the costs derived in the previous section to the year 2030. We have projected 2030 costs in 1980 dollars to obtain a useful comparison.

The population is projected to increase by 26 per cent, from 222 million in 1980 to 280 million in 2030. In 2030 the population will consist of 51 million (18.2 per cent) 65 years of age and older, and 229 million people under 65 years of age.[15] Per capita health care expenditures for those 65 years and over and those under 65 are projected to remain unchanged at $2458 and $727, respectively.

With the increase in population, total personal health care expenditures will increase from $144 billion to $166 billion for those under 65 and from $59 billion to $125 billion for those 65 years and over. The total annual dollar expenditure in 2030 will reach $291 billion, an increase of $88 billion over the 1980 figures. The percentage expenditure increase for those under 65 amounts to 15.3 per cent ($22 billion), whereas for those 65 years and over, the percentage expenditure increase amounts to 112 per cent ($66 billion).

Adjusting the 2030 health care expenditures for the increase in population from 222 million in 1980 to 280 million in 2030 results in an increase in annual per capita personal health care expenditures from $914 in 1980 to $1039 in 2030. The $125 per capita increase (14 per cent) over the 1980 figure is entirely due to the increase in the elderly population from 24 billion (10.8 per cent) to a projected 51 billion (18.2 per cent) of the total population.

## CONCLUSION

The cost of providing health care to those 65 years of age and over is considerable now but will increase even further in the future as the percentage of people 65 years and older increases from 10.8 per cent in 1980, to 12.6 per cent in 1990, and to 18.2 per cent in 2030.[16]

The modalities of health care in serving the elderly have been segmented into ambulatory

**Table 16-1.** HEALTH CARE EXPENDITURES FOR 1980 (YEAR ENDING IN JUNE)

| | Population (<65 years) | Population (≥ 65 years) | Total Population |
|---|---|---|---|
| Personal health care expenditures | $144 billion | $59 billion | $203 billion |
| Proportion of total | 71 | 29 | |
| Population numbers | 198 million | 24 million | 222 million |
| Proportion of total | 89.2 | 10.8 | |
| Per capita expenditures | $727 | $2458 | $914 |
| Ratio to 65 and under population | 1.0 | 3.4 | 1.26 |

care, hospital care, nursing home care, home care, and day care. These five modalities have then been related to five care payment mechanisms consisting of Medicare, Medicaid, supplementary health insurance, self pay, and Title XX funding. The five modalities of care and the five payment mechanisms can be shown to be related through a matrix model.

The issue of who pays for the health care of the elderly in the future is critical because of the enormous size of the personal health care expenditures. Assuming that the relative health care costs remain the same as indicated in this chapter, in the year 2030, the personal health care expenditures for those 65 years and older will amount to $125 billion in 1980 dollars, 43 per cent of total national personal health care expenditures.

To assume that government will pay for these expenditures is unrealistic. Medicare, instituted in the late 1960s, was an honest attempt to do just that. It failed. Medicare currently only pays slightly more than one third of the health care costs of the elderly. Medicaid as a source of funds is not the answer either because it, after all, obtains its funds from the same source as Medicare, the government, and ultimately the taxpayer.

There is a need to look for alternatives. The most desirable alternative is to search for different and less expensive ways of providing personal health care. Can technologic breakthroughs and radical discoveries in drug therapy keep personal health care costs down? If these breakthroughs and discoveries do not materialize, our society will have to give up many amenities we now enjoy to pay for the health care of our elderly citizens. On the other hand, if breakthroughs and discoveries do materialize, new priorities will need to be established.

## References


1. Gaines P Jr: 77 claims favored. The National Life Underwriter, Life and Health Insurance Edition, No. 24. Washington, DC: Life and Health Insurance Institute, June 17, 1978, p. 1.
2. Callahan JJ Jr, Diamond LD, Giele JZ, Morris R: Responsibilities of families for their severely disabled elders. Health Care Financing Review 1:29, 1980.
3. Kane RL, Kane RA: A guide through the maze of long-term care. West J Med 135:503, 1981.
4. Ferry FP, Gornick M, Newton M, Hockerman C: Physicians' charges under medicare: Assignment rates and beneficiary liability. Health Care Financing Review 1:49, 1980.
5. Health Care Financing Administration: Hospital Reimbursement. *In* Research and Demonstrations in Health Care Financing 1980–1981, Washington, DC: U.S. Dept. of Health and Human Services, p. 3.
6. Health Systems Agency of Western New York: Acute care bed need projections according to Part 709.2 of the New York state hospital code. Health Systems Agency of Western New York, Buffalo, NY, November 1981.


**Table 16-2.** HEALTH CARE EXPENDITURES FOR 2030 (IN 1980 DOLLARS)*

| | Population (<65 years) | Population (≥ 65 years) | Total Population |
|---|---|---|---|
| Personal health care expenditures | $166 billion | $125 billion | $291 billion |
| Proportion of total | 57 | 43 | |
| Population numbers | 229.0 million | 51.0 million | 280.0 million |
| Proportion of total | 81.8 | 18.2 | |
| Per capita expenditures | $727 | $2458 | $1039 |

* Total personal health care expenditures increased from $203 billion to $291 billion, an increase of 43 per cent. However, total population also increased from 222 million to 280 million, an increase of 26 per cent. Hence, the aggregate per capita expenditure increased from $914 to $1039, an increase of 14 per cent.

7. Statistical Abstracts of the United States, Washington, DC, U.S. Government Printing Office, 1978, p. 113.
8. National Center for Health Statistics: Health U.S. Washington, DC, U.S. Government Printing Office, 1978.
9. Subcommittee on Long-Term Care, Special Senate Committee on Aging: Nursing Home Care in the United States: Failure in Public Policy. Washington, DC, U.S. Government Printing Office, 1975.
10. General Accounting Office Report to the Congress: Home Health—The Need for National Policy to Better Provide for the Elderly. Washington, DC, U.S. Government Printing Office. December 30, 1977.
11. Brickner P, Scharer LK: Hospital provides home care for elderly at one-half nursing home cost. Forum Health Care Financing Administration of HEW, Washington, DC, Nov.–Dec., 1977, p. 6.
12. Grimaldi PL: The costs of adult day care and nursing home care: A dissenting view. Inquiry 16:162, 1979.
13. Weissert WG: Costs of adult day care: A comparison to nursing homes. Inquiry 15:10, 1978.
14. Waldo DR (comp.): Health Care Financing Trends. Health Care Financing Administration Office of Research, Demonstrations, and Statistics, Baltimore, MD. Vol. 2, No. 1, Fall, 1980.
15. Pegels CC: Health Care and the Elderly. Rockville, MD, Aspen Systems, 1981.
16. Freeland MS, Schendler CE: National health expenditures: Short-term outlook and long-term projections. Health Care Financing Review 2:97, 1981.

## Section II

# PSYCHIATRIC, NEUROSENSORY, AND RELATED DISORDERS

## Chapter 17

# Depression

Donna Cohen
Carl Eisdorfer

Depression is a serious national health problem, affecting people of all ages. As many as 50 per cent of the population may have a significant depressive episode during their lifetime.[1] The term depression describes a continuum of complex behavior.[2] The word may refer to a perfectly appropriate mood state in the lives of healthy people, characterized by feelings of sadness and social withdrawal. Depression may also refer to an acute situational disturbance that occurs for a short period of time and appears to be related to recent psychosocial stress, e.g., loss of status, restricted income, and death of a spouse, child, or friend. Finally, depression is a major psychiatric disorder characterized by sadness or dysphoric mood and a wide range of physical and psychologic symptoms.

Accurate prevalence and incidence data are needed.[3,4] Estimates for the prevalence of depressive symptoms in the aged range as high as 44 per cent, but the prevalence of unipolar depressive disorders ranges from 1 to 3 per cent.[3-6] In a classic survey, Blazier and Williams[5] evaluated 997 people over age 65 living in the community and reported that 14.7 per cent had significant depressive symptoms (4.5 per cent had dysphoric symptoms, 1.8 per cent manifested symptoms of a primary depressive disorder, 1.9 per cent had a secondary depression disorder, and 6.5 per cent had depressive symptoms associated with poor physical health). The overall rate of depression in this population was 8.2 cases per 100 persons aged 65 and older, a rate no different than that for major depressive disorders at any other stage of the life cycle.[3,7]

## CLINICAL MANIFESTATIONS

Late-onset depression often appears similar to depression in younger persons. However, it may present a diagnostic challenge to the clinician because of its atypical expression in the aged. For example, it may be characterized by lack of clearly distinct episodes of depression; by cognitive impairment, neurotic symptoms, prominent anxiety, somatization, and high bodily concern; and by a past history of diagnostic confusion. Since depressive disorders are not always obvious to the observer, they are, perhaps, the most poorly recognized and therefore untreated psychiatric disturbances in the aged. Older people may complain about physical problems but say little about their feelings. Often sadness is denied at the same time the person reports apathy or emptiness, mood statements that often reflect clinical depression. Physical disorders, personal losses, use of drugs, and other psychiatric disorders can also produce depressive symptoms, further complicating the differential diagnosis.

Symptoms of depressive illnesses may range in severity from mild to incapacitating, reflecting disturbances in at least four major areas: affective, somatic, behavioral, and psychological.[8] Affective states that involve dysphoric mood, associated with sad, mournful facial expressions and blunted emotional expression, are characteristic of depression in young adults. Depressed facial features may coincide with reports of depressed mood or despondent feelings in the aged. However, the older patient often denies or is unaware of such moods.

Although behavioral manifestations may be the first sign of a major affective disturbance, they are not always easily recognized. Easy fatigability due, perhaps, to a coincidental medical disorder, may produce apathy, social withdrawal, and loss of interest in previously pleasurable activities. Some patients manifest psychomotor retardation, such as slowing of speech and body movements. In severe cases, this may result in social withdrawal, neglect of self-care, and even refusal to eat or speak. Other patients may display psychomotor activation, characterized by agitation, hand-wringing, obsessive worrying, compulsive behavior, or restlessness. Marked *changes* in an individual's normal behavior or level of activity or behavior should alert the clinician to the possibility of a depressive illness.

The *confusion, memory impairment,* and *attentional disturbances* commonly seen in late-onset depression can easily be mistaken for dementia. Cognitive dysfunction, such as disturbances of memory, attention, and orientation, rarely seen in young depressives, is often a prominent feature of late-onset depression. These symptoms are reversible when the underlying depression is treated. Some clinicians suggest that the history of an obvious precipitant, the presence of depressive mood preceding intellectual impairment, or the absence of progressive intellectual decline may help distinguish pseudodementia from dementia.[9] However, the two conditions may also be quite difficult to separate clinically. The fact that the cognitive impairment is potentially reversible underscores the need for clinical awareness that a primary affective disturbance may mimic dementia. As many as 20 to 40 per cent of patients with cognitive disturbances may have a treatable depression disorder.[10,11]

The *somatic signs* of depression may be the most common symptoms of an affective disturbance in late life. Sleep disturbances, in particular, appear to be one of the earliest signs of depression. Other "vegetative" signs, so-called because they characterize a somatic wasting or deterioration, may include fatigue, a loss of libido, and weight changes. Anorexia with weight loss is seen in 85 per cent of patients, whereas weight gain occurs in about 15 per cent. The direction of weight changes appears to be related to circulating levels of norepinephrine. Gastrointestinal complaints, particularly constipation, are also common. Somatic preoccupations (e.g., multiple vague complaints of physical discomfort or pain, unrelated to physical causes) may approach hypochondraisis at times. This high bodily concern may explain why depressed older people are often seen initially by nonpsychiatric physicians providing primary or specialty care to the patient.

*Psychologic symptoms* are commonly seen in depressed older people, including feelings of despair, pessimism, inadequacy, helplessness, hopelessness, worthlessness. The severely depressed patient may exhibit bizarre delusions of worthlessness, guilt, or self deprecation. Somatic delusions, particularly involving gastrointestinal function, are common in the severely depressed patient.

## DIFFERENTIAL DIAGNOSIS

Among the major affective disorders manifested by older persons (Table 17-1) are unipolar depression, bipolar illness, schizoaffective disorder, and adjustment disorder.[3,8] The differential diagnosis in older adults also includes depression induced by physical disease and medications, depression coexisting with other

**Table 17-1.** DIFFERENTIAL DIAGNOSIS OF DEPRESSIVE DISORDERS AND SYMPTOMS IN THE AGED

I. Major affective disorders
   A. Major depressive disorders
      1. Single episode
      2. Recurrent episodes
   B. Bipolar disorders
   C. Schizoaffective disorders
   D. Adjustment disorder with depressed mood
II. Psychiatric disorders in which depression may coexist
   A. Alzheimer's disease and related disorders
   B. Late-onset paranoid disorders
   C. Anxiety disorders
   D. Somatoform disorders
      1. Psychogenic pain
      2. High bodily concern
   E. Sleep disorders
III. Physical illness accompanied by depression
IV. Medication and substance abuse accompanied by depression
   A. Antihypertension medication
   B. Barbiturate intoxication
   C. Alcohol intoxication
V. Adult Adjustment Reaction
   A. Bereavement
   B. Marital conflict
   C. Parent-child problem
   D. Other family conflict
   E. Other interpersonal problem
   F. Life crisis
VI. Existential sadness

psychiatric disorders, reactive depression, and existential sadness (see also Table 17–1).

The diagnostic criteria for major unipolar depression, according to the Diagnostic and Statistical Manual of the American Psychiatric Association (DSM-III)[12] are given in Table 17–2. This table also specifies the DSM-III criteria for bipolar illness, which must include a manic phase marked by symptoms of elevated mood, irritability, hyperactivity, and pressured speech. The bipolar affective disorders are those in which patients exhibit both periods of mania and episodes of depression, although not necessarily in any predictable cyclic manner. Unipolar disorders are those in which patients have single or recurrent episodes of depression without evidence of a manic phase to their illness. Since the bipolar disorder may not be distinguishable from the unipolar affective disorder during the depressive phase, a careful history is important.

A number of medical diseases produce symptoms that mimic the vegetative symptoms of depression.[13,14] Table 17–3 highlights some of the most common medical conditions to be considered in a differential diagnosis of a depressed older patient. Prominent among these conditions are metabolic and endocrine disturbances, many of which can produce apathy, anorexia, malaise, decreased energy, and somatic preoccupation, easily mistaken for depression.

The *number of medications* taken by adults increases with age,[15] and older people are also more sensitive to the adverse side effects of medication.[16] These issues may be particularly relevant for the depressed patient, since many drugs can exacerbate underlying depressive conditions or produce depression-like symptoms.

Since some drugs, such as certain antihypertensives, are more commonly used by the aged, the differential diagnosis of depression should include an evaluation of all medicines. It is often

**Table 17–2.** DIAGNOSTIC CRITERIA FOR MAJOR DEPRESSIVE DISORDERS*

I. Dysphoric mood, that is, the loss of interest or pleasure in all or almost all usual activities, is present. Dysphoric mood is characterized by depressed symptoms such as sadness, blue feelings, hopelessness, and irritability. The disturbance must be prominent and relatively persistent but not necessarily the most dominant symptom. It does not include momentary shifts from one dysphoric mood to another (e.g., anxiety to depression to anger), such as are seen in states of acute psychotic turmoil.

II. The illness must have a duration of at least 2 weeks, during which, for most of the time, at least four of the following symptoms have persisted and been present to a significant degree.
   A. Poor appetite or significant weight loss (when not dieting), or increased appetite or significant weight gain.
   B. Insomnia or hypersomnia.
   C. Loss of energy, fatigability, or tiredness.
   D. Psychomotor agitation or retardation (but not subjective feelings of restlessness or of being slowed down).
   E. Loss of interest or pleasure in usual activities, or decrease in sexual drive (not included if limited to a period when patient is delusional or hallucinating).
   F. Feelings of self-reproach or excessive or inappropriate guilt (either may be delusional).
   G. Complaints or evidence of diminished ability to think or concentrate, such as slowed thinking or indecisiveness (not associated with obvious formal thought disorder).
   H. Suicidal ideation, desire to die, or any suicide attempt.

III. The depressive symptoms cannot be superimposed on either schizophrenia, schizophreniform disorder, or a paranoid disorder.

IV. None of the following should dominate the clinical picture for more than 3 months after the onset of the depressive episode.
   A. Preoccupation with a delusion or hallucination.
   B. Marked formal thought disorder.
   C. Bizarre or grossly disorganized behavior.

* From Diagnostic and Statistical Manual of Mental Disorders (DSM-III). Washington, DC, American Psychological Association, 1980.

**Table 17–3.** MEDICAL DISEASES THAT MAY EXACERBATE OR PRODUCE DEPRESSIVE SYMPTOMS*

**Metabolic**

Abnormalities of serum glucose, potassium, and calcium and of blood urea nitrogen
Hepatic dysfunction

**Endocrine**

Hypothyroidism
Hyperthyroidism
Diabetes
Hypoparathyroidism
Hyperparathyroidism
Cushing's disease
Addison's disease

**Central Nervous System**

Tumors and other mass lesions
Parkinson's disease
Multiple sclerosis
Alzheimer's disease
Vascular disease

**Miscellaneous**

Pernicious anemia
Pancreatic disease
Carcinoma
Systemic lupus erythematosus
Infectious disease
Congestive heart failure
Porphyria

* Adapted from Eisdorfer C, Cohen D, Veith R: Psychopathology of Aging, Kalamazoo, Michigan, Scope, 1981.

valuable to request that the patient show the clinician all drugs prescribed, as well as those bought over-the-counter. Since older persons tend to share drugs among friends and neighbors in congregate housing settings, attention should not be restricted to prescription drugs ordered for the specific patient.

Given the multiple problems and losses of the aged, it seems reasonable that a certain degree of existential sadness will be normal and that it may vary from one occasion to another. Unfortunately, "normal" sadness is rather difficult to quantify. Thus, although the clinician must be sensitive to the existential human qualities, it would be tragic to assume that the aged are *supposed* to be depressed as a natural reaction to or as a natural consequence of aging. A careful monitoring of a patient's mood, somatic signs, and elements of dysphoria is important.

## CLINICAL EVALUATION

The focus of the clinical evaluation and subsequent intervention should be to identify and evaluate those medical, psychosocial, and environmental factors contributing to depression. Special attention should be directed to determining the availability and effectiveness of the psychosocial support system, which includes family, friends, neighbors, and the community. Recent changes in living arrangements, finances, and the health (or death) of friends or loved ones should also be noted, since these events are frequent precipitants of stress and depression.

Since suicide may be a significant risk factor among depressed patients, particularly among Caucasian men, probing for self-destructive ideas is warranted.[17] When this is a problem, hospitalization may be necessary for adequate evaluation of the patient's clinical condition and for initiation of treatment. If the depressive episode is severe or suicide risk high, or if medical illness complicates the picture, evaluation and initiation of treatment within the hospital may be more appropriate than outpatient treatment.

The older, depressed patient deserves a thorough *medical evaluation* to determine if the depressive syndrome is produced or exacerbated by reversible medical conditions. This workup should include a physical and neurologic examination, with appropriate laboratory studies; it may be helpful diagnostically to reduce or discontinue all drugs that are not life-sustaining. Not infrequently, this produces dramatic clinical improvement.

New laboratory tests are being developed, and one in particular, the dexamethasone suppression test, may be useful in the differential diagnosis of the older patient. It has been proposed that the failure of a 1.0 or 2.0 mg dose of dexamethasone, administered at 11.00 P.M., to suppress corticosterone plasma levels to 5.0 mg per dl or less on the day after administration is a specific and reasonably sensitive biological indicator of unipolar depression.[18–20] Approximately 50 per cent of patients with a DSM-III diagnosis of unipolar depression show an abnormal early escape from suppression compared with 4 per cent of patients with other psychiatric disorders. However, the utility of the dexamethasone depression test in the diagnosis of older persons with depression remains to be demonstrated. Therefore, the results of this test should be interpreted very cautiously when used as a diagnostic tool for older patients suspected of having dementia and depression.[21]

## TREATMENT APPROACHES

Unipolar depression may be responsive to a range of pharmacologic and nonpharmacologic therapies. Tricyclic antidepressants[22–24] and monoamine oxidase inhibitors[25] are now well studied. Newer medications have also been introduced, although there is still a paucity of data on their effects on older patients.[26] Cognitive therapy,[27,28] interpersonal therapies,[29] multicomponent behavioral therapy,[30] and social skills training[31] are among the psychotherapeutic approaches that have been employed. Often, a combination of drugs and psychotherapy are used effectively in the treatment of unipolar depression.

Conceptualizing depressive disorders on a continuum of reactive versus endogenous has been useful for deciding between psychologic or drug interventions. In general, the more sudden, milder depressions, commonly called situational, reactive, or neurotic, are often characterized by an obvious precipitant, are short-lived, and are not perceived as "inappropriate" by the patient or the family. Treatment with environmental manipulation and supportive psychotherapy or counseling is usually effective. The endogenous depression is more severe and prolonged and is often pervasive. It may or may not have obvious precipitants and is notable for the presence of the vegetative symptoms of depression and, perhaps, diurnal variation, i.e., the individual feels worse in the morning.

A recent investigation by Hirschfeld[32] has raised questions about the validity of the concept of situational depression, at least in young and middle-aged adults. No differences were observed in the number of psychosocial stresses and upsetting life events prior to the depression in situational depressive disorders compared with that prior to nonsituational major depressive disorders. The average age of these patients from the National Institute of Mental Health Collaborative study was in the mid-thirties. Situational depression may in fact be a more valid concept when applied to the older population.

Although both "reactive" and "endogenous" depressive syndromes may be quite distressing, the latter interferes more significantly with normal functioning. Depressions that more closely approximate the "endogenous" symptom pattern are more likely to require and to respond to treatment with the tricyclics or electroconvulsive therapy. The constellation of endogenous symptoms, not the presence or absence of an obvious precipitant, should be the criterion for consideration of somatic interventions.

A combination of pharmacologic and psychosocial or psychologic therapies is the most effective treatment for clinical depression. One of the most significant challenges in geriatric psychiatry may be to develop an improved understanding of the psychosocial and cognitive dynamics of depressive behavior. A promising investigation demonstrated that social skills training plus placebo was the only treatment (of four) that resulted in improvement of more than 50 per cent of patients with unipolar (nonpsychotic) depressive disorders (compared with the use of amitriptyline alone, social skills training plus amitriptyline, and psychotherapy plus placebo).[31]

The aged are excellent candidates for psychotherapy.[33,34] Individual therapy can be useful for identifying interpersonal assets and coping skills that will assist patients in adapting to different situations in later life. It may also be useful to facilitate processes-of-life review in dealing with losses as well as anticipatory grieving for inevitable losses. Older patients exhibit a directness and a perspective on life not usually encountered in the young; this can provide an intense and gratifying experience for both the patient and the therapist.

For a reactive depression secondary to a major loss, the availability of a confidante or a support group is salutary. Bereavement counseling and post-stroke groups are examples of interactions that help socialize individuals to their new situation, provide role models and practical help with coping, and facilitate the grieving process. The clinician's role is to facilitate the patient's contact with such people or groups and to become more actively involved if the reactive depression does not resolve itself within a reasonable period of time and if significant weight changes are observed.

## *Pharmacotherapy*

### TRICYCLIC ANTIDEPRESSANTS

The most common drugs chosen for treatment of depression unresponsive to environmental manipulation or psychotherapy are the tricyclic antidepressants.[35] Although few clinical studies have investigated the use of these drugs exclusively in aged populations,[22] these agents are widely used and are effective in appropriately selected patients. In a recent review of the literature, Bielski and Friedel[25] determined that insidious onset of depression and disturbances of sleep, appetite, and psychomotor activity level are the symptoms that best predict a therapeutic response to tricyclic or tetracyclic antidepressants. Tricyclic anti-depressants appear to block presynaptic reuptake of serotonin and/or norepinephrine in selected neurons. Identification of this mechanism of action provided support for the biogenic amine hypothesis of depression. This proposed that deficiencies of one or both of these neurotransmitters are responsible for depressive illness.[36]

Individual agents exhibit variable selectivity in the ability to block reuptake of norepinephrine and serotonin (5-HT).[37] Clinical studies of depressed patients involving measurement of urinary 3-methoxy-4-hydroxyphenylglycol (MHPG) and 5-hydroxyindoleacetic acid (5-HIAA) (the biogenic amine metabolites thought to reflect central nervous system turnover of norepinephrine and serotonin, respectively) suggest that distinct biologic subtypes of depression may exist. Recent studies suggest that it may be possible to predict tricyclic response based on these biochemical measurements. Although exciting, these findings are controversial and preliminary.[36] They have not, however, been applied specifically to the aged.[37,38]

Although these findings suggest that selection of tricyclics may become more specific in the future, at present, in the absence of a history of therapeutic response to a particular drug, the *choice of an individual agent* is generally determined by the adverse effects likely to be produced. Differences among these drugs, in their propensity to produce sedation or anticholinergic effects (dry mouth, blurred vision, constipation, and urinary hesitancy) can be useful in their selection (Table 17–4). For example, the

**Table 17-4.** COMMONLY PRESCRIBED TRICYCLIC AND OTHER ANTIDEPRESSANTS*

| Tricyclic Antidepressants | Usual Dose Range (mg/day) *Young Adult* | *Older Adult* | Sedative Property | Anticholinergic Property |
|---|---|---|---|---|
| ***Tertiary Amines*** | | | | |
| Amitriptyline (Elavil) | 100–300 | 25–150 | +++ | ++++ |
| Imipramine (Tofranil) | 100–300 | 25–150 | ++ | +++ |
| Doxepin (Sinequan) | 100–300 | 25–150 | +++ | ++++ |
| ***Secondary Amines*** | | | | |
| Nortriptyline (Aventyl) | 50–100 | 10–50 | + | +++ |
| Desipramine (Norpramin) | 100–300 | 25–150 | 0 | ++ |
| Protriptyline (Vivactil) | 20–60 | 5–30 | 0 | +++ |
| ***Triazolopyridine*** | | | | |
| Trazodone (Desyrel) | 150–400 | 50–300 | +++ | + |
| ***Tetracyclic Agent*** | | | | |
| Maprotiline (Ludiomil) | 100–300 | 25–150 | ++ | +++ |

* Adapted from Eisdorfer C, Cohen D, Veith R: Psychopathology of Aging. Kalamazoo, Michigan, Scope, 1981.

choice of a tricyclic with sedative properties, such as amitriptyline, may be more appropriate for the agitated patient with pronounced sleep disturbance than for a withdrawn, apathetic patient, in whom sedation may aggravate the condition. The selection of the least anticholinergic tricyclics, desipramine and nortriptyline, may offer an advantage for older men in whom prostate enlargement may increase susceptibility to development of urinary obstructive symptoms. Individuals with orthostatic hypertension appear to respond well to nortriptyline, which causes fewer changes in blood pressure than the other tricyclics.[39]

Regardless of which agent is selected, all tricyclics must be used in doses less than those usually prescribed for the young and middle-aged adult.[35,40] A typical starting dose (except for the more potent nortriptyline and protriptyline) is 25 to 50 mg orally at bedtime. This dose can be increased gradually in 25 mg increments, at 4 to 5 day intervals, until a therapeutic effect is achieved, prohibitive side effects occur, or a daily dose of 150 mg is reached. Exceeding a total daily dose of 150 mg, without obtaining plasma drug levels, should be done cautiously. When a daily dose of 100 mg is exceeded, administration of the drug in divided doses instead of a large bedtime dose will reduce the likelihood of postural hypotension. Patients and family caregivers should be informed that several weeks may be required to achieve a maximal therapeutic effect, although individual symptoms, such as sleep disturbance, may respond rapidly. If a therapeutic response is obtained, the dose should be maintained for at least 6 months and then tapered gradually as the symptoms dictate. Patients should not be given large quantities of a tricyclic, since these drugs can be lethal in an overdose.

Recent research activity has focused on determining the relationship between plasma levels of tricyclics and therapeutic effects.[40] The issue is far from resolved and is reviewed elsewhere.[41–43] At present, it appears that plasma tricyclic levels are a rough gauge of absorption. This may be clinically useful in those patients who are not responding to usual therapeutic doses or for those patients who experience unusually prominent adverse effects on low doses.

The adverse effects of tricyclics often complicate their use in the aged, who appear to be more sensitive to these agents than are younger patients.[44] They may cause sedation; anticholinergic effects; and signs of adrenergic hyperactivity, such as tremulousness, sweating, and cardiovascular effects. The cardiovascular effects are complex.[45] The atropine-like anticholinergic effect of these medications routinely produces tachycardia, and postural hypotension may occur, particularly in the older patient receiving high doses. A recent review of a large number of patients receiving imipramine suggests, however, that postural hypotension during treatment is best predicted by the degree of pretreatment hypotension and is independent of age and plasma tricyclic level.[39] The tricyclics also produce a quinidine-like membrane-stabilizing effect. This may be reflected electrocardiographically by nonspecific ST-T changes and T-wave flattening.[35] With increasing doses, progressive prolongation of conduction reflected in increasing P-R, QRS and Q-T interval prolongation may also develop. Owing to their tendency to produce conduction disturbances, these drugs should be used cautiously in patients with evidence of pre-existing conduction abnormalities and in patients receiving antiarrhythmic drugs with quinidine-like properties.[46,47]

Tricyclics should not be used within 2 months following a myocardial infarction. Poorly compensated congestive heart failure, a history of sensitivity to tricyclics, and significant pretreatment postural hypotension are also contraindications. These agents should be used cautiously in patients with narrow-angle glaucoma, urinary obstructive symptoms, or a history of seizures. Tricyclics also block the effect of guanethidine and antagonize the effects of clonidine and methyldopa, frequently used to treat hypertension in the elderly.

Used alone, tricyclics may be ineffective in treating severely depressed patients who also have delusions. Some authors suggest that delusionally depressed patients simply require the use of higher doses of the tricyclic agent.[48] Delusional patients may respond best to the use of a low-dose of a potent neuroleptic medication such as perphenazine, either alone or in combination with a tricyclic.[49]

### Monoamine Oxidase (MAO) Inhibitors

Although the MAO inhibitors have received increased attention in the treatment of atypical depression,[50,51] their use in treating older persons is limited by the adverse effects that they produce. Few older patients can tolerate the dietary restrictions necessitated by these drugs. Tyramine-containing foods in conjunction with MAO inhibitors can produce hypertensive crisis, hyperpraxia, seizures, and death. MAO inhibitors can also produce postural hypotension, a particular problem for the older patient.

### Stimulants

Stimulant drugs such as dextroamphetamine and methylphenidate may be useful as antidepressant agents for symptomatic relief, when used in selected patients over brief periods of time.[52] However, they are rarely effective for any significant length of time and tend to produce adverse effects such as anorexia. Long-term use has also been associated with dysphoria.[53]

Newer antidepressant agents, with different biochemical structures, appear to have diminished anticholinergic properties, according to their manufacturers. However, presently there is limited evidence that these drugs have greater effectiveness.[54,55] There is as yet no data base to enable us to judge their value for use among the aged.

## Electroconvulsive Therapy (ECT)

ECT has been somewhat controversial in recent years and has been the subject of a major study by the American Psychiatric Association.[56] Historically, there was excessive zeal in its use, and confusion existed regarding the value of the resulting convulsive episode. Early practitioners did not order the use of the muscle relaxants or sedatives with ECT; respiratory complications were common, and the subjective experience was sometimes frightening. These factors, along with the widespread use of this procedure and the lack of guidelines limiting the number of treatments per patient resulted in considerable criticism of this technique.

It seems clear at this time, however, that ECT is the treatment of choice for severely depressed patients who fail to respond to other treatment modalities or who are poor candidates for tricyclics. ECT may also be rapidly effective in treating acutely suicidal patients or patients facing imminent death from starvation who may be unable to tolerate the 3 to 4 week delay for a tricyclic response.

As currently practiced, with the use of muscle relaxants and anesthesiologic assistance, ECT is as safe and effective for older persons as are the other biogenic treatments. Its use is not recommended, however, in older people with dementia of the Alzheimer type, in whom it frequently exacerbates confusion associated with this disease. Its use among older persons *without* signs of irreversible dementing illness, however, should not produce long-term untoward effects.[56] There is also some evidence of the value of ECT, when used with a single electrode on the nondominant lobe, in treatment of the depression of patients with multi-infarct dementia. Nondominant single electrode treatment may be of value in all patients, but long-term outcome data are still forthcoming.

## References

1. Lewinsohn PM, Hoberman HM: Depression. *In* Bellcek AS, Heven M, Kazdin AE (eds.): International Handbook of Behavior Modification and Therapy. New York, Plenum Press (in press).
2. Craighead WE: Away from a unitary model of depression. Behav Ther 11:122, 1980.

3. Blazier D: The epidemiology of late life depression. J Am Geriatr 30:587, 1982.
4. Weissman MM, Myers JK, Thompson WD: Depression and its treatment in a United States urban community. Arch Gen Psychiatry 38:417, 1981.
5. Blazier D, Williams CD: Epidemiology of dysphoria and depression in an elderly population. Am J Psychiatry 137:439, 1980.
6. Gurland B, Dem L, Cross P, Golden R: The epidemiology of depression and dementia in the elderly: The use of multiple indicators of these conditions. *In* Cole J, Barrett J (eds.): Psychotherapy in the Aged. New York, Raven Press, 1980.
7. Weissman MM, Myers JK: Affective disorders in a U.S. urban community: The use of research diagnostic criteria in an epidemiology survey. Arch Gen Psychiatry 35:1304, 1978.
8. Eisdorfer C, Cohen D, Veith R: Psychopathology of Aging. Kalamazoo, Michigan, Scope, 1981.
9. Wells C (ed.): Dementia. 2nd ed. Philadelphia, F.A. Davis Company, 1977.
10. National Institute on Aging Task Force: Senility reconsidered: Treatment possibilities for mental impairment in the elderly. JAMA 244:259, 1980.
11. Reifler BV, Kethley A, O'Neill P, et al: Five year experience of a community outreach program for the elderly. Am Psychiatry 139:220, 1982.
12. Diagnostic and Statistical Manual of Mental Disorders (DSM-III). Washington, DC, American Psychological Association, 1980.
13. Ouslander J: Physical illness and depression in the elderly. J Am Geriatr Soc 30:593, 1982.
14. Salzman C, Shader RI: Clinical evaluation of depression in the elderly. *In* Raskin A, Jarvik CF (eds.): Psychiatric Symptoms and Cognitive Loss in the Elderly. Washington, DC, Hemisphere, 1979.
15. Parry HJ, Balter MB, Mellinger GD, et al: National patterns of psychotherapeutic drug use. Arch Gen Psychiatry 28:769, 1973.
16. Salzman C: A primer on geriatric psychopharmacology. Am J Psychiatry 139:67, 1982.
17. Resnick H, Cantor J: Suicide and aging. J Am Geriatr Soc 18:152, 1970.
18. Carroll BJ, Feinberg M, Greden JF, et al: A specific laboratory test for the diagnosis of melancholia. Arch Gen Psychiatry 38:15, 1981.
19. Brown WA, Shuey I: Response to dexamethasone and subtype of depression. Arch Gen Psychiatry 37:747, 1980.
20. Schlesser MA, Winokur G, Sherman BM: Hypothalamic-pituitary-adrenal axis activity in depressive illness. Arch Gen Psychiatry 37:737, 1980.
21. Spar JE, Gerner R: Does the dexamethasone suppression test distinguish dementia from depression? Am J Psychiatry 139:238, 1982.
22. Veith RC: Treatment of psychiatric disorders. *In* Vestal R (ed.): Drug Therapy in the Elderly. Aukland, New Zealand, ADIS Press (in press).
23. Grof P: Continuation and maintenance antidepressant drug treatment. *In* Ayd FJ (ed.): Clinical Depressions: Diagnostic and Therapeutic Challenges. New York, Ayd Medical Communications, 1980.
24. Ravaris CL, Robinson DS, Ives JO, et al: Phenelzine and amitriptyline in the treatment of depression, a comparison of present and past studies. Arch Gen Psychiatry 37:1075, 1980.
25. Bielski RJ, Friedel RO: Prediction of tricyclic antidepressant response: A critical review. Arch Gen Psychiatry 33:1479.
26. Gershon S, Georgotas A, Newton R, Bush D: Clinical evaluation of two new antidepressants. *In* Costa E, Racagni G (eds.): *Typical and Atypical Antidepressants.* New York, Raven Press, 1982.
27. Beck A: Cognitive Therapy and the Emotional Disorders. New York, International Universities Press, 1976.
28. Rush AJ, Beck AT, Kovacs M, et al: Comparative efficacy of cognitive therapy and pharmacotherapy in the treatment of depressed outpatients. Cognitive Ther Res 1:17, 1977.
29. Weissman MM, Prusoff BA, Dimascio A, et al: The efficacy of drugs and psychotherapy in the treatment of acute depressive episodes. Am J Psychiatry 136:555, 1979.
30. McLean PD, Hakstian L: Clinical depression: Comparative efficacy of outpatient treatments. J Consult Clin Psychol 47:818, 1979.
31. Bellack AS, Hersen M, Himmelhoch J: Social skills training compared with pharmacotherapy and psychotherapy in the treatment of unipolar depression. Am J Psychiatry 138:1562, 1981.
32. Hirschfeld RA: Situational depression: Validity of the concept. Br J Psychiatry 139:297, 1981.
33. Blum JE, Tross S: Psychodynamic treatment of the Elderly: A review of issues in theory and practice. *In* Eisdorfer C (ed.): Annual Review of Geriatrics and Gerontology. New York, Springer Publishing Company, 1980.
34. Eisdorfer C, Cohen D, Preston C: Behavioral and psychological therapies in the older patient with cognitive impairment. In Miller N, Cohen D (eds.): Clinical Aspects of Senile Dementia. New York, Raven Press, 1981.
35. Veith RC: Cardiac effects of tricyclic antidepressants: Clinical implications for treating the elderly. *In* Eisdorfer C, Fann W (ed.): Psychopharmacology and the Aging Patient. New York, Springer Publishing Company, 1982.
36. Schildkraut JT: Current status of the catecholamine hypothesis of affective disorders. *In* Lipton MA, Dimascio A, William KF (eds.): Psychopharmacology: A generation of progress. New York, Raven Press, 1978.
37. Maas JW: Biogenic amines and depression: Biochemical and pharmacological separation of two types of depression. Arch Gen Psychiatry 32:1357, 1975.
38. Goodwin FK, Cowdry RW, Webster MH: Predictors of drug response in the affective disorders. *In* Lipton MA, Dimascio A, Killam KF: (eds.): Psychopharmacology: A Generation of Progress. New York, Raven Press, 1978.
39. Glassman AH, Bigger JT: Cardiovascular effects of therapeutic doses of the tricyclic antidepressants. Arch Gen Psychiatry 38:815, 1981.
40. Vestal R: Drug use in the elderly: A review of problems and special considerations. Drugs 16:358, 1978.
41. Hollister L: Plasma concentrations of tricyclic antidepressants in clinical practice. J Clin Pract 43:66, 1982.
42. Usdin E (ed.): Symposium on plasma level monitoring of tricyclic antidepressants. Common Psychopharmacology 2:371, 1978.
43. Risch SC, Huey LY, Janowski DS: Plasma levels of tricyclic antidepressants and clinical efficacy: Review of the literature. Part I. J Clin Psychiatry 40:4, 1979.
44. Davies RK, Tucker GD, Hanow M, Detre TP: Confusion episodes and antidepressant medication. Am J Psychiatry 128:95, 1971.
45. Donlon PT: Cardiac effects of antidepressants. Geriatrics 37:53, 1982.
46. Bigger JT, Giardina EGV, Perel JM, et al: Cardiac antiarrhythmic effects of imipramine hydrochloride. N Engl J Med 296:206, 1977.

47. Veith RC, Reskind MR, Caldwell J, et al: Cardiovascular effects of the tricyclic antidepressants in depressed patients with heart disease. N Engl J Med 306:954, 1982.
48. Quitkin F, Rifkin A, Kein DF: Imipramine response in deluded depressive patients. Am J Psychiatry 135:806, 1978.
49. Nelson JC, Bowers MG: Delusional uinpolar depression. Arch Gen Psychiatry 35:1321, 1978.
50. Ashford W, Ford CV: Use of MAO inhibitors in elderly patients. Am J Psychiatry 136:1466, 1979.
51. Quitkin F, Rifkin A, Klein DF: Monoamine oxidase inhibitors. Arch Gen Psychiatry 36:749, 1979.
52. Katon W, Raskind MR: Treatment of depression in the medically ill elderly with methylphenidate. Am J Psychiatry 137:963, 1980.
53. Raskind MA, Eisdorfer CE: Psychopharmacology of the aged. *In* Simpson LL (ed.): *The Use of Psychotherapeutic Drugs in the Treatment of Mental Illness.* New York, Raven Press, 1975.
54. Borrome A: A new antidepressant agent: Amitriptyline-*N*-oxide. *In* Costa E, Racagni G (eds.): Typical and Atypical Antidepressants. New York, Raven Press, 1982.
55. Sebjanic V, Grombein S: Viloxazine (Vivalen ICl) in depression: Results of a field trial of 276 patients in neuropsychiatric practice. *In* Costa E, Racagni G (eds.): Typical and Atypical Antidepressants. New York, Raven Press, 1982.
56. American Psychiatric Association Task Force on ECT: No. 14. Washington, DC, American Psychiatric Association, 1979.

## *Chapter 18*

# *Dementing Disorders*

*Donna Cohen*
*Carl Eisdorfer*

Cognitive impairment is not the inevitable consequence of the process of aging. During the course of adult development and aging, a proportion of the population fail to develop their genetic intellectual potential due to such factors as poor nutrition, inadequate education, lack of motivation, or lack of opportunities. Furthermore, with the passage of time, any number of biological, psychosocial, and cultural factors may have an impact on cognitive functioning, e.g., head trauma, alcohol and drugs, sensory and intellectual deprivation, inadequate nutrition, changes in motivation, and lack of involvement in cognitive activities. A variety of physical and psychiatric conditions and disorders may be the basis for cognitive dysfunction as well as for personality changes: These include hypertension, strokes and other forms of cardiovascular disease, pulmonary disease, medications, infections, electrolyte imbalance, depression, and situational disturbances, as well as central nervous system disorders. Thus, although cognitive impairment is observed in middle-aged and older adults, age per se is not an antecedent condition or an explanatory variable.[1,2]

It is estimated that 10 to 20 per cent of the population over age 65, more than 3 million individuals, manifest significant cognitive dysfunction or dementia.[3-5] The estimated prevalence increases from 1 per cent in people under age 60 to 5 per cent in those age 65, 20 per cent in people age 80, and 50 per cent in those age 90.[3,6]

## TYPES OF DEMENTIA

### *Reversible Dementia*

A proportion of the cognitively impaired aged have a reversible dementia, e.g., depression, metabolic toxic reaction, medication-induced toxicity, and vitamin deficiency (Table 18–1). It is estimated that 30 to 40 per cent of individuals referred with memory disturbances have a reversible and, therefore, treatable dementia.[8-10] Most of these patients also have physical disorders, but psychiatric disturbances such as depression are a significant challenge in the differential diagnosis. Whereas treatment of conditions such as depression, drug-induced delirium, infections, and metabolic disturbances leads to a complete restoration of functioning, the reversibility of cognitive function after treatment for such conditions as vitamin deficiency, hypertension, and chronic disease, is an important area of research. In many instances, prompt diagnosis and appropriate treatment will reverse the dementia. Delay increases the probability that the patient may not fully recover some of the lost functions.

### *Nonreversible Dementias*

When no reversible cause of intellectual impairment can be identified, the presumptive clinical diagnosis is a nonreversible dementia. There are a host of diseases that can produce a progressive and irreversible dementia.[11,12] Most of these are quite rare or readily diagnosed in adults of all ages. The more frequent nonreversible dementias, which account for virtually all the clinical problems, can be classified as primary neuronal degeneration of the Alzheimer's type, multi-infarct dementia, mixed dementia, and other dementias that may be associated with Parkinson's disease, multiple sclerosis, Huntington's disease, Creutzfeldt-Jakob disease, Pick's disease, syphilis, and alcohol abuse.[13,14]

Many of these disorders may have similar

**Table 18-1.** POTENTIALLY REVERSIBLE CAUSES OF COGNITIVE DYSFUNCTION

I. Structural causes
  A. Subdural hematoma (secondary to head trauma)
  B. Tumors
  C. Normal pressure hydrocephalus
  D. Sensory disturbances
II. Infectious disorders
  A. Acute and Subacute systemic (febrile) infections of any etiology, e.g., pneumonia
  B. Chronic infectious illness, e.g., abscess
III. Metabolic disorders
  A. Electrolyte disturbance, hyponatremia and hypernatremia, e.g., secondary to diuretic therapy, dehydration
  B. Thyroid disorders, hypothyroidism and hyperthyroidism
  C. Diabetes mellitus, hypoglycemia and hyperglycemia
  D. Hypocalcemia and hypercalcemia
  E. Toxic substances
IV. Nutritional disorders
V. Circulatory diseases
VI. Pulmonary diseases
VII. Medications
  A. Improper use of over-the-counter medications
  B. Alcohol
  C. Use of illicit drugs
  D. Misuse of prescribed medications
    1. Self-medication or failure to use as prescribed
    2. Use of multiple drugs from multiple physicians without adequate communication among physicians
    3. Drug-drug interactions
VIII. Psychiatric disorders
  A. Depression
  B. Mania
  C. Anxiety
  D. Paranoia
  E. Situational disturbances

* Modified from Eisdorfer C, Cohen D, Veith R: Psychopathology of Aging. Kalamazoo, Michigan, Scope, 1981.

symptoms at the outset, but they have different etiologies, courses, and responses to intervention. It is important to note, too, that many of the problems that cause a transient (reversible) cognitive disturbance in older people can also affect individuals who already have a nonreversible dementia. The clinician is thus challenged to identify and treat both the physical and the psychiatric disorders that accompany the dementias. Such intervention may give months or even years of adaptive capacity to the patient, despite progressive brain degeneration.

Among the aged, the most common form of irreversible dementing illness (found in 50 to 70 per cent of all persons with dementia) is primary neuronal degeneration of the Alzheimer type.[15] Multi-infarct or vascular dementias account for approximately 15 to 25 per cent of the dementias. Other irreversible dementias, often called "mixed" dementias, result from a combination of vascular injury and primary neuronal damage and account for the remaining dementias found.

### Alzheimers Disease

The cause of Alzheimer's disease is unknown, although several etiologic factors are being investigated.[16,17] These include alterations in the cholinergic neurotransmitter system, accumulation of deposits of aluminum and other metals in neuronal nuclei, immunologic changes, active and latent viruses or viroids (prions), and genetic influences. The genetics of the disease is a mystery. If a family member has Alzheimer's disease of early onset, first-degree relatives may be at slightly increased risk of becoming affected by the disorder. In some families, there is clearly an autosomal dominant mode of transmission. At present no tests are available to allow prediction of who will be afflicted.

Recent evidence indicates that trisomy 21 (Down's) syndrome and Alzheimer's disease may occur more frequently in the same family than would be expected by chance alone.[18] In addition, it has been suggested that maternal age may be a risk factor in Alzheimer's disease, i.e., children born to older mothers may be at an increased risk to develop this adult-onset condition, perhaps due to an increased mutation rate in parents.[19] Alterations in the immune system are seen in Alzheimer's patients and may be associated with increases in autoimmune reactions.[20] As the disease progresses, the patient's immune system appears to become more impaired, and the most common causes of death for Alzheimer patients are pneumonia and infection. Individuals with dementia of the Alzheimer type appear to have a reduced life expectancy compared with age-matched normal controls.[21] Although the course is progressive, the rate of cognitive deterioration is variable because it depends on neuronal integrity, somatic decompensation, and the adequacy of environmental, social, and medical supports available to the patient.[4,22]

### Multi-Infarct Dementia

The course of multi-infarct dementia is reported to be stepwise deterioration, in contrast to the progressive gradual decline seen in Alzheimer's disease.[33] Focal neurologic signs are typically elicited in addition to the cognitive impairment. The individual frequently has a history of hypertension, strokes, periodic blackouts, diabetes mellitus, and hyperlipidemia;

other cardiovascular illness may also be present in such patients. Table 18-2 provides a 10-point check list adapted from Hachinski for the clinical evaluation of multi-infarct dementia.[2] The higher the total score, the higher the probability that the individual has a multi-infarct dementia. A modification of this scale has been validated by neuropathologic studies.[24]

There are probably many forms of multi-infarct dementia,[25] but it is generally thought that there are three clinical types: large-vessel, middle-vessel, and small-vessel disease. Large-vessel disease is due to multiple strokes caused by the blockage of large- or medium-sized blood vessels. High blood pressure is the cause of about 50 per cent all strokes.[26] The cause of the remainder is unknown.

The second group of patients are those with lacunae strokes, often showing brain lacunae upon autopsy. These lacunae appear as small (less than 0.5 cm in diameter) holes, attributed to emboli and to the pathologic consequences of hypertension in the smaller blood vessels of the brain. Patients with a history of arrhythmias may be particularly vulnerable.

The third form of multi-infarct disease affects even smaller blood vessels and is known as microinfarct dementia. This is a rare and difficult disease to diagnose. Patients may not be hypertensive or manifest arrhythmias, and their blood vessels may not show clear evidence of arteriosclerosis.

### Diagnostic Criteria for Nonreversible Dementia

The clinical diagnosis of dementing illness of the Alzheimer type is necessarily presumptive because a confirmatory diagnosis can only be made on the basis of neuroanatomic features

**Table 18-2.** TEN-POINT CHECKLIST FOR THE EVALUATION OF MULTI-INFARCT DEMENTIA (Scores are assigned on the basis of a medical history and examination).*

| Signs and Symptoms | Score |
|---|---|
| 1. Abrupt onset | 2 |
| 2. Step-by-step deterioration | 1 |
| 3. Fluctuating course | 2 |
| 4. Emotional liability | 1 |
| 5. Anxiety or depression | 1 |
| 6. History of high blood pressure | 1 |
| 7. History of strokes | 2 |
| 8. Evidence of associated atherosclerosis | 1 |
| 9. Focal neurologic symptoms | 2 |
| 10. Focal neurologic signs | 2 |

* From Eisdorfer C, Cohen D: Research diagnostic criteria for primary neuronal degeneration of the Alzheimer type. J Fam Pract 11:553, 1980.

observable only on post-mortem evaluation. Figure 18-1 presents strict research and clinical diagnostic criteria for assessing clinical features of the early and middle stages of the disease.[2] Table 18-3 presents the criteria cited in the Diagnostic and Statistical Manual of Mental Disorders (DSMIII).[7]

Although the onset of SDAT (Senile Dementia of the Alzheimer Type) is often gradual, the course is progressive. The rate of degeneration is variable, depending not only upon the neuronal loss and somatic decompensation but also upon the adequacy of the medical and social support systems. Some patients decline abruptly and then plateau; others remain relatively stable, with only small declines before rapid deterioration. In some patients, deterioration is gradual, whereas in others the course of the disease fluctuates. These different patterns accentuate the possibility that SDAT is a heterogeneous disorder, representing no one disease entity but very possibly a cluster of several different disorders.

In later stages of the disease, patients may show marked restlessness, aphasia, perseveration, and emotional lability. The patient's knowledge regarding self and interpersonal relationships becomes compromised. It is important to note that although the affected individual becomes more disoriented and activities of daily living and self-care become progressively more difficult, there may be marked differences in the type and extent of cognitive deficits.

The most prominant sign of Alzheimer's disease and multi-infarct dementia is cognitive dysfunction, including deficits in attention, learning, memory, and expressive and receptive language skills. Additionally, impairment in focal skills such as calculation, judgment, abstraction, and orientation is frequently reported. Social skills, including the ability to communicate effectively, and relationships with family and friends, become impaired. Inept social behavior and personality changes occur, including paranoid ideation, aggressiveness, and alterations in sexual behavior.

Several mental status examinations can be used to diagnose dementia and to evaluate the strengths and weaknesses of the patient.[27,28] The brief Mental Status Questionnaire (Fig. 18-2)[29] provides a quick assessment of the moderate and severe dementias, but it is of little value in the assessment of mild dementias. The Mini-Mental State Examination (Fig. 18-3)[30] is a useful instrument in the diagnosis and evaluation of older patients in a clinical interview.*

* The Short Portable Mental Status Questionnaire (SPMSQ) is reproduced in Chapter 20.

The development of a broadly applicable instrument, with guidelines that can be used uniformly by clinicians, remains to be developed.[31]

The loss of specific cognitive skills is an important factor that determines the relative ability of impaired adults to function in their environment (see Chapters 4, 5, 8, and 14).[32] Accurately assessing functional cognitive abilities is helpful for diagnostic purposes; it is also used to help families manage the dementia. Traditional orientation questions are not particularly effective in evaluating cognitive status. For example, many patients who appear poorly oriented in time, person, and place are readily manageable in the home. Gaining insight into the skills an individual retains during phases of illness can provide guidelines for cognitive retraining as well as supply families or caregivers with a realistic baseline for performance.[33]

During the diagnostic examination computerized tomography (CT) can be used to identify potentially reversible disorders, such as trauma, mass lesions, and hydrocephalus.[34,35] When the CT scan reveals no abnormality in a person presenting with dementia, the physician should search for other reversible causes, such as hypothyroidism and pernicious anemia. Although CT can demonstrate cerebral atrophy by help-

**University of Washington Research Diagnostic Criteria for Primary Neuronal Degeneration of the Alzheimer's Type**

**Clinical Features for Inclusion**

A deterioration of general cognitive functions from a previously higher performance level compromising the ability to adapt to the environment, including:

| A. Onset | Yes | No |
|---|---|---|
| 1. Gradual progression | ___ | ___ |
| 2. Duration of at least 6 months | ___ | ___ |

B. Impairment of at least *two* of the following abilities (on the basis of performance on the Mini-Mental Status, the Wechsler Adult Intelligence Scale).

| | Absent | Mild | Moderate | Severe |
|---|---|---|---|---|
| 1. Learning | ___ | ___ | ___ | ___ |
| 2. Attention | ___ | ___ | ___ | ___ |
| 3. Memory | ___ | ___ | ___ | ___ |
| 4. Orientation | ___ | ___ | ___ | ___ |

C. Impairment on at least one of the following cognitive skills (on the basis of performance on the WAIS and Mini-Mental Status).

| | Absent | Mild | Moderate | Severe |
|---|---|---|---|---|
| 1. Calculation | ___ | ___ | ___ | ___ |
| 2. Abstraction and judgment | ___ | ___ | ___ | ___ |
| 3. Comprehension | ___ | ___ | ___ | ___ |

D. Problems in at least one of the following areas (on the basis of the psychosocial examination.

| | Absent | Mild | Moderate | Severe |
|---|---|---|---|---|
| 1. Ability to work | ___ | ___ | ___ | ___ |
| 2. Ability to relate to family | ___ | ___ | ___ | ___ |
| 3. Ability to relate to peers | ___ | ___ | ___ | ___ |
| 4. Ability to function socially | ___ | ___ | ___ | ___ |

E. Indication of cerebral dysfunction on at least one of the following:

| | Yes | No |
|---|---|---|
| 1. Cerebral atrophy on CT scan<br>2. Abnormal EEG (see also exclusion criteria) | ___ | ___ |

F. Ischemic Score ≤ 4 (modified from Hachinski, 1978)

| Feature | Possible Score | Real Score |
|---|---|---|
| 1. Abrupt onset | 2 | ___ |
| 2. Stepwise deterioration | 1 | ___ |
| 3. Fluctuating course | 2 | ___ |
| 4. Nocturnal confusion | 1 | ___ |
| 5. Emotional lability | 1 | ___ |
| 6. History of hypertension | 1 | ___ |
| 7. History of strokes | 2 | ___ |
| 8. Evidence of associated atherosclerosis | 1 | ___ |
| 9. Focal neurologic symptoms | 2 | ___ |
| 10. Focal neurologic signs | 2 | ___ |

**Figure 18-1.** University of Washington research diagnostic criteria for primary neuronal degeneration of the Alzheimer type. (From Eisdorfer C, Cohen D: Research diagnostic criteria for primary neuronal degeneration of the Alzheimer type. J Fam Pract 11:553, 1980. Reproduced with permission.)

*Illustration continued on following page*

| University of Washington Research Diagnostic Criteria for Primary Neuronal Degeneration of the Alzheimer's Type (Continued) | | |
|---|---|---|
| **Medical Exclusion Criteria** | Yes | No |
| A. Focal neurologic signs (including EEG foci) | ___ | ___ |
| B. Medical history of: | | |
| 1. Myocardial infarction or chronic cardiovascular disease | ___ | ___ |
| 2. Cardiovascular accident | ___ | ___ |
| 3. Alcoholism or substance abuse | ___ | ___ |
| 4. Chronic psychiatric illness | ___ | ___ |
| 5. Syphilis | ___ | ___ |
| 6. Brain damage sustained earlier from a known cause, eg, hypoxia | ___ | ___ |
| 7. Chronic renal, hepatic, pulmonary, or endocrine disease | ___ | ___ |
| 8. Parkinson's disease, Huntington's chorea, Pick's disease, or related neurologic disorders selectively affecting specific brain regions | ___ | ___ |
| 9. Multi-infarct dementia | ___ | ___ |
| 10. Hypertensive cardiovascular disease | ___ | ___ |
| C. Pseudodementias | | |
| 1. Primary manic disorder | ___ | ___ |
| 2. Primary depressive disorder | ___ | ___ |
| 3. Physical disorders, metabolic intoxicity, drug interaction | ___ | ___ |

**Figure 18-1.** *(continued)*

**Table 18-3.** DIAGNOSTIC CRITERIA FOR DEMENTIA

A. A loss of intellectual abilities of sufficient severity to interfere with social or occupational functioning.
B. Memory impairment.
C. At least one of the following:
   1. Impairment of abstract thinking, as manifested by concrete interpretation of proverbs, inability to find similarities and differences between related words, difficulty in defining words and concepts, and other similar tasks
   2. Impaired judgment
   3. Other disturbances of higher cortical function, such as aphasia (disorder of language due to brain dysfunction), apraxia (inability to carry out motor activities despite intact comprehension and motor function), agnosia (failure to recognize or identify objects despite intact sensory function), "constructional difficulty" (e.g., inability to copy three-dimensional figures, assemble blocks, or arrange sticks in specific designs)
   4. Personality change, i.e., alteration or accentuation of premorbid traits
D. State of consciousness not clouded (i.e., does not meet the criteria for delirium or intoxication, although these may be superimposed).
E. Either (1) or (2):
   1. Evidence from the history, physical examination, or laboratory tests of a specific organic factor that is judged to be etiologically related to the disturbance
   2. In the absence of such evidence, an organic factor necessary for the development of the syndrome can be presumed if conditions other than organic mental disorders have been reasonably excluded and if the behavioral change represents cognitive impairment in a variety of areas

* From Diagnostic and Statistical Manual of Mental Disorders (DSM-III). Washington, DC, American Psychological Association, 1980.

ing to document the presence of Alzheimer's disease (because gross atrophy of the brain with widening of the cortical sulci and enlargement of the ventricles is a characteristic feature), it should be noted that cortical and ventricular atrophy are also seen in CT scans of the normal elderly.

The examination of the patient should include a careful medical history and physical examination, including a drug inventory; an evaluation of the sensorium; a neurologic evaluation; a psychiatric interview; a psychosocial assessment of the patient's environment; and various laboratory tests, including hematologic studies, urinalysis, serology, and chest x-ray. A minimum number of screening tests necessary for the evaluation of dementia has been recommended by the National Institute on Aging.[8] From the information gained from these tests, it is possible to establish a presumptive diagnosis of dementing illness secondary to nonreversible changes in the brain.[14] A diagnosis of dementia of the Alzheimer type has profound physical, emotional, and financial consequences for the patient and family.

## PHARMACOLOGIC APPROACHES TO DEMENTIA

There are no medications available today that reverse the primary characteristic of dementia —progressive intellectual loss.[36,37] However,

**Mental Status Questionnaire (29)**

| | Question | Response | Incorrect Responses(✓) |
|---|---|---|---|
| 1. | What is the name of this place? | ______ | ______ |
| 2. | Where is it located (address)? | ______ | ______ |
| 3. | What is today's date (day of month)? | ______ | ______ |
| 4. | What month is it? | ______ | ______ |
| 5. | What is the year? | ______ | ______ |
| 6. | How old are you? | ______ | ______ |
| 7. | When is your birthday? | ______ | ______ |
| 8. | When were you born (year)? | ______ | ______ |
| 9. | Who is president of the U.S.? | ______ | ______ |
| 10. | Who was president before him? | ______ | ______ |
| | | TOTAL INCORRECT: | ______ |

**Figure 18-2.** Mental status questionnaire. (From Kahn RL, Goldfarb AI, Pollack KM, et al: Brief objective measures for the determination of mental states in the aged. Am J Psychiatry 117:326, 1960. Reproduced with permission.)

Patient ______
Examiner ______
Date ______

**"MINI-MENTAL STATE"**

**Score** **Orientation**

( ) What is the (year) (season) (date) (day) (month)?
( ) Where are we: (state) (county) (town) (hospital) (floor).

**Registration**

( ) Name 3 objects: 1 second to say each. Then ask the patient all 3 after you have said them. Give 1 point for each correct answer. Then repeat them until he learns all 3. Count trials and record.
Trials ______

**Attention and Calculation**

( ) Serial 7's. 1 point for each correct. Stop after 5 answers. Alternatively spell "world" backwards.

**Recall**

( ) Ask for the 3 objects repeated above. Give 1 point for each correct.

**Language**

( ) Name a pencil, and watch (2 points)
Repeat the following "No ifs, ands or buts." (1 point)
Follow a 3-stage command:
"Take a paper in your right hand, fold it in half, and put it on the floor" (3 points)
Read and obey the following:

Close your eyes (1 point)

Write a sentence (1 point)
Copy design (1 point)
Total score
ASSESS level of consciousness
along a continuum ______
Alert Drowsy Stupor Coma

**INSTRUCTIONS FOR ADMINISTRATION OF MINI-MENTAL STATE EXAMINATION**

**Orientation**

(1) Ask for the date. Then ask specifically for parts omitted, e.g., "Can you also tell me what season it is?" One point for each correct.

(2) Ask in turn "Can you tell me the name of this hospital?" (town, county, etc.). One point for each correct.

**Figure 18-3.** Mini-mental state examination. (From Folstein MF, Folstein SE, McHugh PR: "Mini-mental state," a practical method for grading the cognitive state of patients for the clinician. J Psychiatr Res 12:189, 1975. Copyright Pergamon Press, Ltd. Reproduced with permission.)

*Illustration continued on following page*

**Registration**

Ask the patient if you may test his memory. Then say the names of 3 unrelated objects, clearly and slowly, about one second for each. After you have said all 3, ask him to repeat them. The first repetition determines his score (0-3) but keep saying them until he can repeat all 3, up to 6 trials. If he does not eventually learn all 3, recall cannot be meaningfully tested.

**Attention and calculation**

Ask the patient to begin with 100 and count backwards by 7. Stop after 5 subtractions (93, 86, 79, 72, 65). Score the total number of correct answers.

If the patient cannot or will not perform this task, ask him to spell the word "world" backwards. The score is the number of letters in correct order. E.g. dlrow = 5, dlorw = 3.

**Recall**

Ask the patient if he can recall the 3 words you previously asked him to remember. Score 0-3.

**Language**

*Naming:* Show the patient a wrist watch and ask him what it is. Repeat for pencil. Score 0-2.

*Repetition:* Ask the patient to repeat the sentence after you. Allow only one trial. Score 0 or 1.

*3-Stage command:* Give the patient a piece of plain blank paper and repeat the command. Score 1 point for each part correctly executed.

*Reading:* On a blank piece of paper print the sentence "Close your eyes", in letters large enough for the patient to see clearly. Ask him to read it and do what it says. Score 1 point only if he actually closes his eyes.

*Writing:* Give the patient a blank piece of paper and ask him to write a sentence for you. Do not dictate a sentence, it is to be written spontaneously. It must contain a subject and verb and be sensible. Correct grammar and punctuation are not necessary.

*Copying:* On a clean piece of paper, draw intersecting pentagons, each side about 1 in., and ask him to copy it exactly as it is. All 10 angles must be present and 2 must intersect to score 1 point. Tremor and rotation are ignored.

Estimate the patient's level of sensorium along a continuum, from alert on the left to coma on the right.

**Figure 18–3.** *(continued)*

drugs are frequently used to treat the behavioral disturbances that accompany dementia—violent behavior, agitation, depression, paranoia. These psychiatric problems are often a challenge to the family, the physician, and the nursing home. In order to manage behavioral disturbances, psychotropic drugs are prescribed, but even in the most competent hands, these drugs can lead to complications. Since these are often powerful drugs, their use can lead to side effects, which may create new problems. Drugs should be employed very cautiously and carefully in patients with dementing disorders.

## *Antipsychotic Medications*

Antipsychotic medications are used to treat a number of serious psychiatric conditions, including bizarre behavior, severe delirium, schizophrenia, and paranoid states. Antipsychotic medications are also useful in the treatment of hallucinations and delusions. In small doses they may be used to treat delirium, which is noticed in some patients with Alzheimer's disease in the early evening. This is frequently called the sundown syndrome. The restlessness, agitation, irritability, and hostility frequently seen in patients with dementia may subside if treated effectively.

Although these medications are effective and helpful when used properly, psychotropic drugs should only be considered after a careful and thorough evaluation. It is also worth remembering that when patients with dementia develop medical problems, they are more likely to develop metabolic or toxic conditions that affect their behavior, causing them to "act crazier." Environmental disruptions with which patients cannot cope also exacerbate the dementia. It is important, therefore, that the patient is carefully evaluated for a medical, environmental, or psychosocial problem and that it is not assumed that the dementia is simply worsening. A thorough evaluation of current medications should be carried out prior to changes in treatment. In addition, psychologic interventions should be used in conjunction with drugs or as alternatives to drugs.

Antipsychotic drugs are not always successful in treating the irritability and agitation associated with dementia. The regulation of dosage may be difficult in older persons. Often the doses are set so high that they have a sedative rather than an antipsychotic effect. Starting doses of one fourth to one third of that used for middle-aged adults should be considered. Much still remains to be done to determine the efficacy of these drugs in very low dosages. It must be kept in mind that there is no evidence that the drugs will improve or reverse the intellectual impairment, which is the primary characteristic of Alzheimer's disease or multi-infarct dementia. However, they may help a great deal with the management of problem behaviors.

The selection of an antipsychotic drug must be tailored to the patient. Consideration should be given to whether the person has other physical problems or is taking other medications. Once a therapeutic response is seen, it is necessary to determine the lowest effective dose and the maintenance dose for the patient. This is done by gradually lowering the daily dose to the lowest effective amount. The antipsychotic drug should also be withdrawn at regular intervals to determine whether it is necessary to continue treatment. If the patient does not show a therapeutic response or if the maintenance dose becomes ineffective, the drug should be withdrawn.

The antipsychotics all seem to work equally well, but they do differ in the side effects they produce. Therefore, the choice of drug is usually made on the basis of the side effects produced. Short-term side effects are not universal, but they are not rare. Common side effects include sedation, dry mouth, constipation, blurred vision, and urinary retention, i.e., anticholinergic effects. Patients may also show extrapyramidal symptoms such as stiffness, rigidity, and drooling, which are characteristic of Parkinson's symptomatology. Cardiovascular side effects may also occur, including arrhythmias and postural hypotension.

Oral doses of some drugs (such as chlorpromazine and thioridazine) appear to be more sedating than the other antipsychotics. This may be useful to the clinician who can then treat the sleep disturbance of an agitated patient with dementia by using only one medication instead of two. However, because sedation leads to clouded consciousness, this may, in some patients, cause more confusion and disorientation.

Chlorpromazine and thioridazine reportedly lead to anticholinergic effects more frequently than other medications. These effects—dry mouth, blurred vision, delirium—often make it difficult to reach an effective dose. In some patients a paradoxical effect may occur with antipsychotic medication. A patient who is agitated and already taking antipsychotic medication will become more and more agitated. If the dose is increased to calm the agitation, the patient will only become worse. The increased agitation is caused by the toxic effects of the drug.

The extrapyramidal side effects can be a major problem. The use of the antipsychotics will often be accompanied by the very gradual development of increasing stiffness and slowing of movement. This may cause the loss of the ability of individuals to take care of themselves beyond that caused by dementia. Haloperidol, thiothixene, and trifluoperazine are most often associated with side effects. When such problems occur, as they may in 25 or 30 per cent of patients, the use of antiparkinsonian drugs can be helpful. Although thioridazine and chlorpromazine have strong anticholinergic effects, they are less likely to cause the extrapyramidal effects. Therefore, it should be clear that using drugs requires the clinician to make a series of decisions, for example: which drug will cause the least harm and provide the best treatment for the particular patient?

There is one long-term effect that deserves serious attention—tardive dyskinesia. This disorder, associated with the long-term use of antipsychotic drugs, affects up to 15 per cent of patients. After several years on regular doses of antipsychotic medication, patients display obvious movements of the mouth, tongue, and lower facial area that they are unable to control. At the moment, the only treatment is to recognize the problem early, usually by examining the tongue for fasciculations, and to stop the use of the drugs. The disorder can best be prevented by employing the smallest amount of medication required to accomplish the clinical purpose.

## *Antidepressant Medications*

Depression is a common occurrence in persons with nonreversible dementias, occurring in 20 per cent more of dementia victims.[9] As discussed earlier, depression is also the most common psychiatric disturbance in the older population. And, of course, depressive symptoms affect many family members caring for a relative with Alzheimer's disease or a related disorder.

The recognition of depression in the older patient with a dementia may be difficult, since these patients are less able to act and communicate effectively. The intellectual losses of dementia are debilitating and progressive in themselves. The effect of a major depression will make the individual act even more "demented." Since the major treatment objective is to maintain the highest possible level of functioning, successfully treating the concomitant depression will usually reduce the apathy, inattention, irritability, blunted affect, and social withdrawal of the patient. The difficulty, apart from the possible side effects of the medication, may be in the undue optimism of the family that the patient is "cured." Although this is indeed the case in instances in which the depression alone caused the dementia (sometimes referred to as pseudodementia), it is not to be confused with a "cure" for all dementia. Those families still denying the presence of a confirmed Alzheimer's or multi-infarct dementia grasp at straws and, inevitably, become disappointed and reactively depressed themselves.

The tricyclic antidepressants are the drugs most often used to treat a major depression in patients with dementia. The tricyclic antidepressants have adverse side effects, and the older patient with dementia is more at risk for side effects. Therefore, as described earlier, lower doses of these drugs are appropriate.

However, drugs are not necessary for all forms of depression. Reactive depressions occur in the face of many major losses. In these instances, supportive psychotherapy and social interventions are appropriate; drugs are not. Alzheimer patients are still fully human beings, who may grieve over their loss of control or the death of relatives when they attend a funeral.

It is almost never appropriate to give the patient more than one drug in a major psychotropic drug class at one time. This means that a person should not receive two or more antidepressant or antipsychotic drugs at once. It may be appropriate to administer an antipsychotic drug along with an antidepressant when the individual with depression also has delusions or hallucinations, but even this intervention should be evaluated with great caution.

Some patients will not be able to tolerate tricyclics or they may not respond to treatment, especially as the dementia progresses. In the early and middle stages of dementia, supportive psychotherapy, maintaining a supportive and stimulating environment, or changing the environment consistent with the needs and preferences of the patient should be considered and implemented.

If tricyclics are used to treat the depression in a cognitively impaired patient, which ones are probably useful? As mentioned previously, the choice is often determined by the tolerance of the patient for the medication, the patient's other medical conditions, other medications the patient may be taking, and the side effects associated with a particular tricyclic agent. For example, a tricyclic with sedative effects such as amitriptyline or doxepin may be useful in low doses for a demented patient who is very agitated and has obvious sleep disturbances. These sedative tricyclics would probably not be useful in a demented patient who is more apathetic and withdrawn.

Whenever a tricyclic drug is used, the doses should be low, following the principles outlined previously (see Chapter 12). As described earlier, these medications also increase the likelihood of a range of side effects, which may be exaggerated in this group of patients. In a cognitively impaired person, postural hypotension can cause falls and injury, further impairing the physical activity that is a source of great satisfaction for many patients. Careful monitoring is thus indicated.

## *Antianxiety Medications*

Anxiety has not been well studied in either the aged or those with dementia.[9] Certainly, anxiety is a frequent feature in dementia. It may also be caused by medical disorders or drugs, which in turn aggravate the dementia.

Anxiety may refer to a "normal" state of tension and expectation in response to life situations. The appropriateness of the anxiety and the severity of the symptoms and the degree to which they disrupt a person's effectiveness define anxiety as either a psychologic symptom or a psychiatric disorder. It is sometimes difficult to diagnose anxiety in the older patient with dementia. At other times, the hyperactivity, apprehensiveness, and agitation are easy to recognize.

The usefulness of antianxiety medications in patients with dementia is not well studied. Nondrug interventions can be useful in the reduction of the anxiety of dementia patients. Here we must confront the need to construct a supportive and nourishing environment for afflicted individuals and to encourage activities appropriate to the level of impairment. Supportive psychotherapy helps provide confidence and recognition that the person is coping successfully. Patients may be aware of their dementia, at least until the later stages of the disorder, and may be highly anxious about it. The loss of the mind before physical death is a profound tragedy and legitimate cause for anxiety. This anxiety must be recognized and dealt with supportively when the patient is ready to handle it.

### *Sleep Medications*

Sleep disturbances of one sort or another are commonly seen in the aged patient with dementia, and they often become more severe as the dementia progresses.[38] The problems attendant on a person's sleep problem are usually decisive in the prevention of nursing home placement.

The benzodiazepines may have some value if used for brief periods but may not be helpful in the long-term management of the dementia patient. Long-term use of these drugs may lead to effects that make the sleep problem worse. In addition dependence on sedative-hypnotics can create psychologic problems for members of the family who may get caught up in the conflict of providing or not providing such medication. Behavioral approaches are the treatment of choice. Simple strategies such as rising at the same time each morning, eliminating or minimizing afternoon naps, regular exercise, proper nutrition, and a carefully planned day can go a long way. At least through the early and middle stages of dementia, patients whose days are meaningful and reasonably active will tire in the evening and sleep at night.

### *Principles of Drug Management in Patients with Dementia*

Drugs should be used cautiously in the cognitively impaired older adult. The following principles are important to keep in mind:

1. Start with low doses and increase gradually if necessary.
2. A drug should be given for the patient's benefit.
3. Drugs have side effects that can make the patient uncomfortable and aggravate the dementia. The risks must be evaluated along with the benefits.
4. When a drug regimen is begun, plans should also be made for withdrawing the drug.
5. A patient's physical condition affects the way a drug acts.
6. Drugs interact with each other and can cause serious problems.
7. Drugs should never be used alone. They should be used in conjunction with psychological, social, and environmental therapies.
8. Drugs can hurt the patient if not used appropriately.
9. Drugs may not work at all.

## NONPHARMACOLOGIC MANAGEMENT OF THE PATIENT WITH DEMENTIA

At least within certain limits, the stronger the social and medical support systems, the higher the level of functioning (of both patient and family) during the course of illness. Management then involves direct service to the patient and family.[4,22,39] As previously stated, recognition and treatment of any ancillary disorder (depression, anxiety, paranoia, or medical disease) may improve the adaptive functioning of the patient. The family can be counseled and guided, for example, to change the interior physical environment of the house to accommodate to the patient's needs. Also beneficial to the patient are regular daily routines of physical exercise, a routine schedule of activities, and socialization outside the home. If employment is no longer possible, work in and around the home helps the patient maintain a sense of social participation and usefulness. Identifying simple tasks that the patient can master proves very helpful in this regard.

Patients with dementia undergo a series of changes and losses throughout the course of the illness, but the natural history of the disease is largely undocumented. The challenge for both health professionals and family members is to recognize and maximize remaining strengths, as well as weaknesses in the patient.

Table 18–4 lists the areas to be considered in the management of the patient.[4] It should be noted that medical care, although crucial, cannot stand alone. The physician will need to assist

**Table 18–4.** ISSUES IN CLINICAL MANAGEMENT

- Provision of information
- Clinical care of concurrent disorders
- Referral to medical specialists
- Referral for community social services
- Institutionalization
- Referral for legal and financial counseling
- Counseling or psychotherapy
- Home visits and environmental modifications
- Ongoing evaluations of cognitive status
- Therapeutic family intervention
- Referral to self-help organizations

the family in identifying social, financial, legal, and psychiatric assistance early in the illness before the family itself pays a heavy toll for its caring responsibilities.

Early and careful financial planning is very important and cannot be overstressed. States vary in the legal obligations of spouses, children, and others in the care of the patient. Legal issues involving competence, estate planning, and fiscal management are frequent concerns at some point during the course of the disease. The patient can play a major role early in the illness, and often a subsequent conflict among other family members can be avoided if early planning is undertaken.

Active efforts to maximize whatever remains of the mental and physical capacities of patients, in conjunction with family counseling and guidance, can do much to improve or maintain the functional effectiveness of patients and to relieve undue stress on the caregivers. Patients with dementia deserve the opportunity to be active and to remain in the community for as long as possible. Over time, the losses associated with dementia force the patients to redefine their self-identity. The physician, by establishing open communication channels with patients and their families, can win their trust and respect. This physician-patient-family relationship can be an extremely valuable asset in the months and years ahead. Furthermore, an active program of patient and family management can have a profound impact on the quality of life of all concerned. However, such a program rests upon a careful and thorough appreciation of the clinical manifestations of the dementia throughout the course of illness.[40]

## References


1. Cohen D, Wu S: Language and cognition during aging. *In* Eisdorfer C (ed.): *Annual Review of Geriatrics and Gerontology*. New York, Springer Publishing Company, 1980.
2. Eisdorfer C, Cohen D: Research diagnostic criteria for primary neuronal degeneration of the Alzheimer type. *J Fam Pract* 11:553, 1980.
3. Kay DWK: The epidemiology of brain deficit in the aged: Problems in patient identification. *In* Eisdorfer C, Friecleh RO (eds.): The Cognitively and Emotionally Impaired Elderly. Chicago, Yearbook Medical Publications, 1977.
4. Eisdorfer C, Cohen D: Management of the patient and family coping with dementing illness. J Fam Pract 12:831, 1981.
5. Mortimer JA: Epidemiologic aspects of Alzheimer's disease. *In* Maletta G, Pirozzolo F (eds.): Advances in Neurogerontology. Vol. 1. The Aging Nervous System. New York, Praeger, 1980.
6. Jarvik LF, Ruth V, Matsnyama S: Organic brain syndromes and aging: A six year follow-up of surviving twins. Arch Gen Psychiatry 37:280, 1980.
7. Diagnostic and Statistical Manual of Mental Disorders (DSM-III). Washington, DC, American Psychological Association, 1980.
8. National Institute on Aging Task Force: Senility reconsidered: Treatment possibilities in the elderly. JAMA 244:259, 1980.
9. Eisdorfer C, Cohen D, Keckich W: Depression and anxiety in the cognitively impaired aged. *In* Klein D, Rabkin J (eds.): Anxiety, New Research and Changing Concepts. New York, Raven Press, 1981.
10. Smith JS, Kiloh LG: The investigation of dementias: Results in 200 consecutive admissions. Lancet. 1:824, 1981.
11. Katzman R, Karasu TB: Differential diagnosis of dementia. *In* Fields WS (ed): Neurological and Sensory Disorder in the Elderly. New York, Grune and Stratton, 1975.
12. Wells C (ed.): Dementia 2nd ed. Philadelphia, F. A. Davis, 1977.
13. Wells C: Chronic brain disease: An update on alcoholism, Parkinson's disease and dementia. Hosp Community Psychiatry. 33:111, 1982.
14. Gustafson L, Nilsson L: Differetial diagnosis of presenile dementia on clinical measures. Acta Psychiatr Scand 65:194, 1982.
15. Tomlinson BE, Blessed G, Roth M: Observations on the brains of demented old people. Neural Sci 11:205, 1970.
16. Brody J: An epidemiologist views senile dementia—facts and fragments. Am J Epidemiol 115:155, 1982.
17. Schneck M, Reisberg B, Ferris S: An overview of current concepts of Alzheimer's disease. Am J Psychiatry 139:165, 1982.
18. Heston L, Mastri, AR: The genetics of Alzheimer's disease. Arch Gen Psychiat 28:1085, 1980.
19. Cohen D, Eisdorfer C, Leverenz J: A Hypothesis: Maternal age and Alzheimer's Disease. J Am Geriatr Soc 30:656, 1982.
20. Henschke PD, Bell DA, Cape RDT: Immunologic indices in Alzheimer dementia. J Clin Exp Gerontol 1:23, 1979.
21. Vitaliano PP, Peck A, Johnson D, et al: Dementia and other competing risks for mortality in the institutionalized aged. J Am Geriatr Soc 29:513, 1981.
22. Blumenthal M: Psychosocial factors in reversible and irreversible brain failure. J Clin Exp Gerontol 1:93, 1979.
23. Hachinski V, Lassen NA, Marshall J: Multi-infarct dementia. Lancet 2:207, 1974.
24. Rosen WG, Terry RD, Fuld P, et al: Pathological verification of ischemic score in differentiation of dementia. Ann Neurol 7:486, 1980.
25. Ladurner G, Iliff L, Lechnec H: Clinical factors associated with dementia in ischaemic stroke. J Neurol Neurosurg Psychiatry 45:97, 1982.
26. Birkett DP, Raskin A: Arteriosclerosis, infarct, and dementia. J Am Geriatr Soc 30:261, 1982.
27. Cohen D, Eisdorfer C, Holm CL: The mental status examination in aging. *In* Albert ML (ed.): Clinical Neurology of Aging. New York, Oxford University Press, 1984.
28. Reisberg B, Ferris S: Diagnosis and assessment of the older patient. Hosp Community Psychiatry 33:104, 1982.
29. Kahn RL, Goldfarb AI, Pollack KM, et al: Brief objective measures for the determination of mental states in the aged. Am J Psychiatry 117:326, 1960.
30. Folstein ME, Folstein SF, McHugh PR: "Minimental state," a practical model for grading the cognitive

states of patients for the clinician. J Psychiatr 12:189, 1975.

31. Cohen D, Eisdorfer C: Cognitive theory and the assessment of change in the cognitively impaired aged. *In* Raskin A, Jarvik LF (eds.): Psychiatric Symptoms and Cognitive Loss in the Elderly. Hemisphere, Washington, DC, 1980.
32. Cohen D: Psychological issues in the diagnosis and management of the cognitively impaired aged. *In* Eisdorfer C, Fann E (eds.): Clinical Psychopharmacology of Aging. New York, Springer Publishing Company, 1982.
33. Eisdorfer C, Cohen D, Preston C: Behavioral and psychological therapies for the older patient with cognitive impairment. *In* Miller N, Cohen D (eds.): Clinical Aspects of Senile Dementia. New York, Raven Press, 1981.
34. DeLeon MJ, Ferris SH, George AE, et al: Computed tomography evaluation of brain-behavior relationships in senile dementia of the Alzheimer's type. Neurobiol Aging 1:69, 1980.
35. Soininen H, Puranen M, Riekkinen PJ: Computed tomography findings in senile dementia and normal aging. J Neurol, Neurosurg Psychiatry 45:50, 1982.
36. Eisdorfer C, Fann WE: Psychopharmocology of Aging. New York, Springer Publishing Company, 1982.
37. Eisdorfer C, Cohen D, Veith R: Psychopathology of Aging. Kalamazoo, Michigan, Scope, 1981.
38. Prinz PN, Raskind M: Aging and Sleep Disorders. *In* Williams RL, Karacan I, (eds.): Sleep Disorders: Diagnosis and Treatment. New York, John Wiley, 1978.
39. Cohen D, Coppel D, Eisdorfer C: Management of the family: Psychotherapeutic issues. *In* Reisberg B (ed.): Alzheimer's Disease and Senile Dementia. New York, Macmillan Publishing Company, 1983.
40. Cohen D, Shapiro J: Clinical manifestations of nonreversible dementia. Geriatr Med Today 1:68, 1982.

## Chapter 19

# Paranoia

*Donna Cohen*
*Carl Eisdorfer*

## SCHIZOPHRENIC AND PARANOID STATES

Empirical data about the paranoid disorders of later life—etiology and pathophysiology as well as diagnosis and treatment—are limited. The older patient may display symptoms ranging from mild suspiciousness to a well-defined delusional system with hallucinations. The essential feature of paranoid disorders is the presence of false beliefs or delusions, which are held despite logical information to the contrary. The delusions are grandiose or persecutory; they are sometimes accompanied by auditory hallucinations, which lead to disturbing alterations in an individual's behavior and affect. Paranoid patients are suspicious and distrustful in their relationships with others. They may try to conceal their bizarre ideas unless they believe that they have found a sympathetic confidant or are confronted by their apparent beliefs. If threatened, paranoid patients may be prone to both verbally and physically attack. These attacks can be very frightening to the patient and bystanders alike and may serve to enhance the patient's conviction that the paranoid beliefs are real, especially when there is retaliation.

Paranoia may emerge as the predominant symptom in many physical and psychiatric disorders. Paranoid thoughts may occur in *delirium** caused by toxic metabolic states, e.g., infections (subacute bacterial endocarditis, pneumonia, urinary infections), systemic illness (congestive heart failure, uremia), dehydration, and electrolyte imbalance. These symptoms may also be a troublesome accompaniment to the progressive cognitive deterioration in Alzheimer's disease and related disorders. Onset of paranoia may be one of the earliest symptoms of Alzheimer's disease, as a patient tries to make sense of his or her intellectual losses.[1,2] Acute and fluctuating paranoid symptoms in the individual with severe cognitive impairment may herald the worsening of the disease or the onset of another physical illness. Indeed, the sudden appearance of psychiatric symptoms may be the only observable sign of an acute physical illness in an already cognitively compromised frail elderly person. Paranoid symptoms may also appear in the aftermath of cerebral damage related to a stroke or trauma. It may be virtually impossible at times to differentiate the paranoia that may emerge from physical disorders from that related to a major depressive disorder in a stroke victim.[3]

Older patients may also exhibit paranoid symptoms from use of medications such as propranolol, cimetidine, antiparkinson agents, anticonvulsants, steroid preparations, amphetamines, and nasal decongestants. It is essential that a physician thoroughly evaluate the drug history of any patient with acute paranoid symptoms.

Paranoia may be observed in several psychiatric disorders. Usually there is a previous history to suggest its origin. It may be an important symptom in the major affective disorders, including both unipolar depressive illness as well as the manic phase of bipolar illness. Self-reproach may accompany paranoid suspicions in depression and is not characteristic of other paranoid states. Paranoid ideation may also emerge in the acute psychotic episodes of an older chronic schizophrenic patient.[4]

* For further discussion of delirium, see Chapter 20.

Some elderly patients develop de novo a paranoid state called *paraphrenia* or late paraphrenia. This is unrelated to a deteriorating cognitive status or physical illness.[4-6] Late paraphrenia is characterized by a persecutory delusional system, but the cognitive and affective changes commonly associated with chronic schizophrenic patients are not observed. In fact, patients often remain remarkably alert and function well within the constraints of their bizarre belief system. Whether late-onset paranoia represents a separate entity or is in reality part of the spectrum of schizophrenic illness requires scientific investigation.

## Etiology of Late-Life Paranoid States

The etiology of these conditions is poorly understood. There is limited evidence of familial risk.[7-9] Other predisposing factors include a premorbid distrustful personality associated with declining sensory capacities, increasing social isolation, and other environmental stresses.[9-12] Women with these disorders outnumber men approximately seven to one, and most are unmarried or living alone. Many appear to have lifelong coping mechanisms of suspiciousness, leading to a lifelong degree of social isolation. Many women exhibiting late-life paranoia have often experienced significant environmental stresses and losses (death of family members, reduced economic resources, relocation), which exacerbate the degree of isolation. A significant proportion of older people with paranoia manifest an appreciable degree of hearing impairment, which can lead to further isolation and impaired communication skills.[10]

Diminution in communication skills, combined with reduced social contact, may result in the development of bizarre ideation, with projection and paranoia, particularly in predisposed individuals.[13] The multiple losses sustained by the aged (e.g., impaired sight and hearing, physical changes, loss of income secondary to inflation) often occur slowly, and the impact of many losses may result in beliefs or attributions that the world is outside of the individual's range of control. In the absence of clear targets, premorbidly suspicious individuals may regress to a primitive interpretation of their environment to reduce the ambiguity. In essence, paranoid thinking may emerge as a defense to enable individuals to regain control of their environment.

## Differential Diagnosis of Paranoid States

We propose that the paranoid states of later life are best understood as a set of disorders ranging from maladaptive suspiciousness to schizophreniform illness.[5]

### Suspiciousness

Significant suspiciousness may occur in some older people who become concerned about external forces or individuals controlling their life. These individuals may display a generalized suspiciousness, or they may focus upon a few targets, usually persons in the patient's immediate environment who emerge as malevolent, e.g., landlords, bosses, children or their spouses. Generalized feelings of desertion may emerge, and the individual may complain of abuse by the younger generation, the government, or negative outside forces. The symptoms are usually poorly formed, and they are troublesome rather than disabling. They do not involve subjective perceptions of influence over the patient's body or mind. They are not accompanied by hallucinations, and they do not involve outside organizations in any systematic pattern. The complaints tend to be narrowly focused and may be transient if treatment is implemented. The individual will usually resort to someone for help. Clinical studies of this troublesome disturbance do not exist.

### Transient Paranoid Reaction

Post[14] described paranoid hallucinosis as a condition in which individuals exhibit focal severe paranoid thinking. Distortions are easily related to the immediate environment. They are often persecutory, and they are disturbing to patients and to others around them. These reactions may be accompanied by hallucinations, which often are directly related to the focal delusion, e.g., people talking about the patient to get them to move. The external focus is usually a neighbor, landlord, or relative. Delusions of grandeur are not reported, nor is there evidence for feelings of possession by spirits or extraterrestrial forces.

Social isolation is a conspicuous feature in this form of paranoia. Hearing or other communication impairments may also be observed. In many instances, the patient has recently moved or is separated from friends, relatives, and neighbors. The nature of the transient paranoid behavior typically exacerbates interpersonal problems and isolates the individual even more.

**Management**

Environmental manipulation is usually effective to reduce cognitive and social isolation.[4] Indeed, restoring opportunities for social communication often ameliorates transient symptoms. Correcting auditory loss and/or increasing social contacts may also be helpful. The establishment of a good interpersonal relationship between the patient and someone prepared to remain in contact with the patient through brief scheduled visits is valuable in maintaining and monitoring the patient's progress.

Although paranoid symptoms may clear without further treatment subsequent to social intervention, in those instances in which delirium or dementia exists, the possibility of some physical or metabolic etiology should be considered.[2] Short-term psychopharmacologic treatment with small doses of antipsychotic medications is often effective.[15,16] However, drugs are an adjunctive therapy, not an alternative to psychosocial intervention strategies.

### Paraphrenia and Late-Life Schizophrenia

Delusional ideation and hallucinations are prominent in paraphrenia; cognitive deficits, affective blunting, and the more bizarre personality attributes of schizophrenia are not present. Furthermore, the deterioration that typifies schizophrenics does not occur. Clinical investigations are needed to identify those features that distinguish between *paraphrenia with onset in later adult life* and *paranoid schizophrenia or schizophreniform illness of late onset.*

Aged patients with schizophrenia and schizophreniform illnesses typically present with hallucinations and a reasonably organized delusional system.[4] Delusions in older patients are often banal in comparison with those of younger schizophrenic patients. Grandiosity and persecution may appear in more seriously impaired patients, and persons in close proximity are often accused of interfering in patients' lives. These individuals often have a well-developed delusional system with auditory hallucinations. Post[14] observed that older patients (with initial onset of schizophrenia) only manifest some of the Schneiderian first-rank symptoms, e.g., thought intrusions, depersonalization, experiences of influence, and voices discussing him or her in the third person.[17]

## *Management and Treatment*

Effective treatment or management of severe schizophrenia and paranoid symptoms in the aged depends on careful evaluation of the quality and intensity of the symptoms.[18] For any type of paranoid disturbance, five types of intervention should be considered: (1) identification and/or substitution of losses, (2) environmental manipulations, (3) observation and monitoring, (4) psychotherapies, and (5) psychopharmacologic strategies.[18]

Premorbid personality aside, the development of suspiciousness may be a function of the physical and social context in which individuals find themselves. Precipitating events may include a subtle perception of physical and object loss and a feeling of an increasing lack of control over the environment. Significant strategies in the appropriate care of these patients include dealing with the perceived losses and helping patients regain greater mastery over their lives.[19] In long-term care institution, investing residents with decision-making control often proves effective, e.g., opportunities to select and structure visiting hours, choices concerning activities, as well as other options that restore dignity to the individual. Counseling the family and staff about the fears and needs of the patient may be helpful for patients at home as well as in institutions.

The restoration and prevention of losses are extremely important treatment strategies.[20] The use of appropriate hearing aids, in conjunction with individual counseling, may be crucial in helping a person deal with hearing loss.[12] Counseling should cover issues including the patient's attitudes and feelings about the appliance, the distorted quality of the amplified sounds, and the concerns and feelings attendant on impaired hearing. Maintaining social interventions and active normal participation is an important component of the management strategy. In view of the potential impact of the patient's improved behavior on others in the immediate community, the clinician may need to find a way to inform others that the patient has recovered.

Major environmental changes, particularly when they are accompanied by other traumas (e.g., moving from home following the death of a spouse, being moved into an institution or from one nursing home to another) are typically accompanied by heightened anxiety and stress and may initiate suspiciousness and/or transient paranoia. Supportive environmental manipulation has been reported to be beneficial in cases of even severe paranoid ideation.[8]

Although psychopharmacologic treatment with antipsychotic medication is not indicated for the mildly suspicious person, it is effective for the paraphrenic patient. Herbert and Jacobsen[7] and Post[8] have reported success in treating some paraphrenic patients with phenothiazines. Raskind and colleagues[20] reported the increased effectiveness of very low doses of intramuscular depot medication, (prolixine enanthate) in paraphrenic outpatients. Social interventions were also used to decrease patients' social isolation and diminish the existing concerns of immediate neighbors (many of whom were targets of patients' suspicion and accusations).

Our knowledge base about paranoid disorders is still limited, and clinical research studies are lacking. Thus, the confusing diagnostic nomenclature and the limited number of outcome studies have done little to help the clinician. Variables such as genetic vulnerability, multiple age-related losses, social isolation, and sensory impairments all appear to play a role in the etiology of paranoia, although their specific influences are not clearly defined. Further investigations are needed to improve our knowledge of the diagnosis and treatment of paranoid and schizophrenic states in older adults.

## References


1. Katzman R, Karasu TB: Differential diagnosis of dementia. *In* Fields WS (ed.): Neurological and Sensory Disorders in the Elderly. New York, Grune and Stratton, 1975.
2. Manshreck TC: The assessment of paranoid features. Comprehensive Psychiatry 20:370, 1979.
3. Ross ED, Rush A: Diagnosis and neuroanatomical correlates of depression in brain-damaged patients. Arch Gen Psychiatry 38:1344, 1981.
4. Post F: Paranoid, schizophrenia-like, and schizophrenic states in the aged. *In* Birren JE, Sloan RB (eds.): Handbook of Mental Health and Aging. Englewood Cliffs, NJ, Prentice-Hall Inc, 1980, 591–615.
5. Eisdorfer C: Paranoid states in later life. *In* Busse E, Blazier D (eds.): Handbook of Geriatric Psychiatry. New York, Van Nostrand Reinhold, 1980.
6. Fish FJ: Senile paranoid states. Gerontol Clin I, 1959.
7. Herbert ME, Jacobsen S: Late paraphrenia. Br J Psychiatry 113:461, 1967.
8. Post F: Persistent Persecutory States of the Elderly. England, Pergamen Press, 1966.
9. Kay DWK, Roth M: Environmental and hereditary factors in the schizophrenias of old age ("late paraphrenia") and their bearing on the general problems of causation in schizophrenia. J Ment Sci 107:699, 1961.
10. Cooper AF, Kay DWK, Curry AR, et al: Hearing loss in paranoid and affective psychoses of the elderly. Lancet 2:851, 1974.
11. Cooper AF, Garside RF, Kay DWK: A comparison of deaf and non-deaf patients with paranoid and affective psychoses. Br J Psychiatry 129:532, 1976.
12. Eastwood R, Corbin S, Reed M: Hearing impairment and paraphrenia. J Otalaryngol 10:306, 1981.
13. Sparacino J: An attributional approach to psychotherapy with the aged. Am Geriatr Soc 26:9, 1978.
14. Post F: Paranoid disorders in the elderly. Postgrad Med 53:52, 1973.
15. Langley GE: Functional psychoses. *In* Howells JG (ed.): Modern Perspectives in the Psychiatry of Old Age. New York, Brunner/Mazel, 1975.
16. Branchley MH, Lee JH, Amin R, Simpson GM: High- and low-potency neuroleptics in elderly psychiatric patients. JAMA 239:1860, 1978.
17. Schneider K: Primäre und sekundäre Symptoms bei Schizophrenie. Fortsch Neurol Psychiatr 25:487, 1957.
18. Eisdorfer C, Cohen D, Veith R: Psychopathology of Aging. Kalamazoo, Michigan, Scope, 1981.
19. Eisdorfer C, Cohen D, Preston C: Behavioral and psychological therapies in the older patient with cognitive impairment. *In* Miller N and Cohen G (eds.): Clinical aspects of senile dementia. New York, Raven Press, 1981.
20. Raskind, M, Alvarez, C, Herlin, S: Fluphenazine enanthate in the outpatient treatment of late paraphrenia. J Am Geriat Soc 27:451, 1979.

# Chapter 20

# Confusion (Delirium)

*Jack H. Medalie*
*H. Reddy Pasem*
*Evan Calkins*

Confusion, characterized by memory loss; disorientation in time, place, and person; and an inability to think clearly, may be acute or chronic. *Acute* confusion or delirium, often accompanied by fluctuating levels of consciousness, develops over the course of days or weeks; *chronic* confusion or dementia, which develops over a course of months or years, is, primarily, a reflection of brain damage. Elderly patients with varying amounts of brain damage are also susceptible to acute confusional states. Acute confusion or delirium is, in most instances, due to an underlying condition that may be reversible. If uncorrected, the condition may lead to death. Therefore, the presence of this disorder should be regarded as a medical emergency. It is essential that the physician accurately identify the presence of delirium and be aware of the conditions that may cause it.

The prevalence of confusion depends on the observer, i.e., the primary care practitioner, geriatrician, or psychiatrist. Lipowski[1] has estimated that between 5 and 10 per cent of hospitalized medical-surgical patients will exhibit an acute confusional reaction or delirium at one time or another during an inpatient stay; for hospitalized *geriatric* patients, the prevalence may be closer to 40 per cent.[2]

## APPROACH TO DIAGNOSIS

The diagnostic criteria for delirium, as recorded in the Diagnostic and Statistical Manual of Mental Disorders (DSM-III) of the American Psychiatric Association[3], are provided in Table 20-1. There are several scales that are used to determine the level of orientation, memory, and cognitive ability. The most commonly used scales are the Short Portable Mental Status Questionnaire (SPMSQ) by Pfeiffer,[4] the "Mini-Mental State" by Folstein and associates,[5] and the Mental Status Questionnaire by Kohn and associates.[6] An additional scale has been developed by Hodkinson.[7] Several of these scales are reproduced in Chaper 18.

The questions most commonly employed in these scales refer to (1) the patient's age, (2) the patient's date of birth, (3) today's date, (4) where the interview is taking place (name of place or location), (5) the time (day of week or actual time), (6) the name of current President (two authors ask for name of the preceding President), (7) the address or telephone number of patient, (8) where the patient was born,[6] (9) the maiden name of the patient's mother,[4] and (10) the year of World War I.[7] The patient may be asked to (11) count backwards from 20 to 1,[7] (12) subtract 3 from 20 and keep going,[4] and (13) recognize two people known to patient.[7]

One of us, JHM, recommends that any 10 of these questions could be used, although his preference is always to include number 13 (recognition of two people, one of whom is the physician) and exclude 12. Pfeiffer believes that eight to ten errors on ten questions reveal severe intellectual impairment; up to two errors still indicate intact intellectual functioning.

In addition to determining the degree of orientation (or lack of same) and cognitive deficit, it is important to inquire, carefully, whether the patient is experiencing hallucinations. These may be visual (spiders or other insects, or people, large or small) or auditory (voices, music, bells). Hallucinations, infrequently present in dementia, are especially characteristic of delirium. Patients do not mind being questioned in

**Table 20-1.** DIAGNOSTIC CRITERIA FOR DELIRIUM*

A. Clouding of consciousness (reduced clarity of awareness of the environment), with reduced capacity to shift, focus, and sustain attention to environmental stimuli.
B. At least two of the following:
   1. Perceptual disturbance: misinterpretations, illusions, or hallucinations
   2. Speech that is at times incoherent
   3. Disturbance of sleep-wakefulness cycle, with insomnia or daytime drowsiness
   4. Increased or decreased psychomotor activity
C. Disorientation and memory impairment (if testable).
D. Clinical features that develop over a short period of time (usually hours to days) and tend to fluctuate over the course of a day.
E. Evidence, from the history, physical examination, or laboratory tests, of a specific organic factor judged to be etiologically related to the disturbance.

* From American Psychiatric Association: Diagnostic and Statistical Manual of Mental Disorders. 3rd ed. Washington, DC, American Psychiatric Association, 1980. Reproduced by permission.

this regard, and the physician should not neglect to do so.

Once it has been determined that the patient is exhibiting evidence of confusion, the next step is to determine the course of its development. This is an essential ingredient in the differential diagnosis. How fast did this confusion develop? Did the patient change from being sensible to confused in a matter of hours, days, or weeks, or did the process evolve gradually over months or even years? Was it an acute change in an otherwise normal person, or was it an acute change on top of an already existing deterioration of mental and social abilities? Is this patient exhibiting an acute, a chronic, or an acute-on-chronic condition? Questions concerning the nature and course of the problem should be directed both to the patient and to a family member or someone who has been closely associated with the patient. In directing questions to the patient it is usually advisable to repeat the questions either the same day or the next day. In cases of patients who answer that they "don't know" or "don't care," or "ask my son or daughter," the primary care physician has to rely on the family or his or her perception of the change in the patient in order to differentiate confusion from depression, paranoia, or, occasionally, a mixture of these conditions, which is not uncommon in the elderly.

Delirium characteristically develops over the course of days or weeks, rarely longer. The history of an alteration in the patient's *medical* status, pharmacologic management, social support system, or environment antedating the development of an acute confusional process provides additional support to the diagnosis of delirium. Another hallmark of delirium is variability from one time of day to another. Symptoms frequently become worse at night.

## *Etiology*

Causes of delirium can be classified as (1) most common, (2) common, and (3) rare.

Most common causes include the following:

1. Drugs. Drug toxicity and drug-drug interaction commonly occur in the elderly owing in part to multiple drugs required for multiple illnesses and also to errors in the medication program (see Chapter 12). In many instances, these adverse reactions are manifested by acute delirium. Use of hypnotic sedatives, tranquilizers, antihypertensive agents, antiparkinsonian drugs, analgesics, digitalis, and cimetidine (Tagamet) is particularly apt to be accompanied by delirium.
2. Location change: It is not uncommon that elderly persons are shifted from one setting to another, without adequate preparation. This often leads to acute confusion, sometimes accompanied by severe agitation.
3. Fecal impaction or urinary retention. If allowed to continue for a long time without intervention, these conditions may lead to acute confusion, readily reversible following disimpaction or catheterization.
4. Infections (especially pneumonia and urinary tract infection).
5. Cardiovascular causes (myocardial infarction, congestive heart failure, arrhythmia, varying degrees of heart block, and pulmonary emboli).
6. Metabolic/endocrine factors. The following may induce delirium: hypoglycemia, hyperglycemia, hypothyroidism, liver failure, and fluid/electrolyte imbalance.
7. Neoplasia, either primary in the brain or secondary from another site, or severe unrelieved pain.

The following are common causes of delirium:

1. Emotional factors, notably depression. Depression, one of the most common psychiatric problems in the elderly, may at times be manifested by confusion; in this case it is called pseudodementia.

2. Alcohol. Alcohol abuse is frequent among the elderly. Confusion may be due to alcohol withdrawal and the Wernicke-Korsakoff syndrome, or Korsakoff's psychosis, a complication of chronic alcohol intake.
3. Anesthesia and surgery. It is not clear whether the confusion is due to the procedure itself, the anesthesia, the lack of proper preparation of the patient (patient education), or a little of each.
4. Cerebral infarction or hemorrhage.

Rarer causes of acute confusional states are as follows:

1. Anemia, which may be acute, as in bleeding duodenal ulcer, or chronic, as a result of conditions such as uremia, neoplasia, or pernicious anemia.
2. Malnutrition due to deficiencies of various vitamins, including vitamins $B_1$, $B_{12}$, C, and niacin.
3. Head injury or other injury, such as hip fracture.
4. Epilepsy and periarteritis nodosa.

### *Diagnostic Procedures*

In addition to a history and a complete physical examination, the following procedures should be carried out:

1. Urinalysis, urine culture, and antibiotic sensitivity.
2. Complete blood cell count and differential leukocyte count. Note that infection in the elderly often occurs without leukocytosis.
3. Erythrocyte sedimentation rate (ESR). Determination of the ESR may provide a clue to unsuspected infection or malignancy; bear in mind, however, that the ESR in normal elderly persons is usually higher than that in young individuals.
4. Screening for occult blood in stool.
5. Electrocardiogram, with reference to possible myocardial infarction or arrythmia.
6. Chest x-ray (look for evidence of infection, emboli, or neoplasm).
7. Blood chemistry (glucose, potassium, and sodium chloride; blood urea nitrogen (BUN) and/or creatinine; serum calcium and phosphorus; triiodothyronine ($T_3$) and thyroxine ($T_4$); and vitamin $B_{12}$ and serum folate concentration). In special cases, as it seems appropriate, a serologic test for syphilis, liver function tests, and serum acid phosphatase determination should be obtained. In patients who enter the hospital from home, serum drug level and x-ray of the skull may also be indicated.

## MANAGEMENT OF DELIRIUM

First priority should go to identification of the underlying cause and initiation of appropriate medical treatment. In most cases, this will be accompanied by a return of the patient's cognitive and behavioral function to the baseline level. Although remission of the delirium may occur over the course of a few days, it may require a longer period, sometimes extending for several weeks. During this interval, careful symptomatic treatment of the delirium per se is an essential requisite for a good outcome.

Careful attention should be given to the patient's environment. The patient should be placed in a private room, away from the confusion of an active ward. If possible, a family member should be present in the room at all times, including the night, especially during the period of severe confusion. If this is not possible, an attendant should be assigned to stay in the room at all times. Every person who comes into contact with the patient should convey a spirit of reassurance and should emphasize patient orientation by appropriate reference to regularly scheduled events, such as breakfast, lunch, and so on. Family members should be encouraged to bring in family photographs, which help convey a sense of continuity of interpersonal relationships. The presence of a television set will help provide sensory stimulation.

Lighting should be adequate. A light should be left on during the night. The patient should be encouraged to obtain adequate sleep. Unnecessary interruptions, such as recording of nighttime vital signs, should be avoided insofar as possible.

Although the preceding measures will usually contribute greatly to lessening the symptoms of delirium, sedation may be necessary. This is best accomplished through use of one of the high potency neuroleptics, such as haloperidol (Haldol). Initial dosage should be low (for example 2 mg intramuscularly or orally three times a day). Doses of 2 mg per hour may be given if the patient is highly agitated.

The use of physical restraints should be avoided if at all possible. Restraints usually increase agitation and do not contribute to its alleviation. Repeated reassurance, in the environment described previously, coupled with use of appropriate sedation provides a better avenue of therapy.

## References


1. Lipowski ZJ: Delirium. Springfield, Ill., Charles C Thomas, 1980, p. 219.
2. Robinson WR: Toxic delirium. *In* Kaplan AJ (ed.): Mental Disorders in Older Life. Stanford, Calif., Stanford University Press, 1950.
3. American Psychiatric Association: Diagnostic and Statistical Manual of Mental Disorders. 3rd ed. Washington, DC, American Psychiatric Association, 1980.
4. Pfeiffer E: A short portable mental status questionnaire for assessment of organic brain deficit in elderly patients. J Am Geriatr Soc 23:433, 1975.
5. Folstein MF, Folstein EE, McHugh PR: "Mini-mental state." A practical method for grading the cognitive state of patients for the clinician. J Psychiatr Res 12:189, 1975.
6. Kahn RL, Goldfarb AI, Pollack M, Peck A: Brief objective measures for the determination of mental status in the aged. Am J Psychiatry 117:326, 1960.
7. Hodkinson HM: Evaluation of a mental test score for assessment of mental impairment in the elderly. Age Ageing 1:233, 1972.

Chapter 21

# Neurologic Diseases—Stroke and Other Cerebrovascular Conditions

*Fletcher H. McDowell*

Although the variety of neurologic diseases encountered narrows with advancing age, these conditions continue to be extremely common in the geriatric group. Perhaps more importantly, they account for a large portion (if not the majority) of seriously disabling illnesses encountered in this group. Additionally, neurologic disease, when it occurs in older persons, usually causes serious disability either through impairment of normal motor and sensory function, or, perhaps even more devastating, through impairment of intellectual capacity. The most commonly encountered neurologic diseases affecting the elderly are outlined in Table 21-1. The frequency of neurological disease varies markedly with advancing age; some become more frequent causes of illness, and some do not occur at all.

*Cerebrovascular disease* is, undoubtedly, the most common neurologic problem of the elderly population, and it is usually the most devastating in terms of causing morbidity and mortality. *Degenerative diseases,* such as Parkinson's disease and amyotrophic lateral sclerosis (ALS), although they occur less often, cause significant disability. The peripheral nervous system is not immune to disease, the most common being those associated with diabetes. *Spinal cord disease,* although uncommon, still occurs, occasionally as a result of trauma; most frequently, it is the result of degenerative arthritis. *Brain tumor* declines in frequency with age, but still occurs in the geriatric age group; it is important to recognize because of the rising percentage of benign tumors encountered in elderly persons. Although *demyelinating disease* and *primary seizure disorders* occur in this age group, they occur much less frequently than at younger ages. *Primary muscle disease* is almost unknown, but occasionally disease of the muscular junction, such as *myasthenia gravis,* does occur. The frequency of *generalized brain disease* producing intellectual loss rises rapidly with advancing age. This is perhaps the most devastating of all neurologic problems affecting the geriatric group; variations of this problem include acute delirium as well as chronic progressive dementia.

This chapter presents a discussion of stroke, the most frequently occurring cerebrovascular condition, and Chapter 22 presents other common neurologic concomitants of advanced age, including Parkinson's disease, epilepsy, spinal cord disease, ALS, peripheral neuropathy, Guillain-Barré syndrome, and myasthenia gravis. The problem of dementia has been discussed in Chapter 18 and will not be addressed here.

## STROKE

### Classification, and Frequency

The nature of strokes encountered in the elderly population is identical with that encountered among younger individuals. These include (1) strokes resulting from cerebral infarction, caused by either embolic arterial occlusion or atherosclerotic or other vascular disease or (2) hemorrhagic strokes, such as subarachnoid and primary intracerebral hemorrhage. The annual incidence of stroke rises

**Table 21-1.** NEUROLOGIC DISEASES OF THE ELDERLY

**Cerebrovascular disease**
- Cerebral infarction
  - atherosclerotic
  - embolic
- Intracerebral hemorrhage
- Subarachnoid hemorrhage
- Temporal arteritis

**Degenerative diseases**
- Parkinson's disease
- Dementia—Alzheimer's disease

**Peripheral neuropathy**
- Diabetic
- Nutritional deficiency
- Toxic
- Idiopathic

**Spinal cord disease**
- Cervical spondylosis with cervical myelopathy
- Cord compression, spinal cord tumor (primary and metastatic)

**Brain tumor, primary and metastatic**
- Myasthenia gravis
- Amyotrophic lateral sclerosis

**Epilepsy, idiopathic and secondary**

**Intoxication**
- Delirium

**Cardiovascular**
- Syncope

steeply as patients enter the geriatric ages.[1,8,11,25] In the decade prior to age 65, the annual incidence in the United States is 262 per 100,000 population; for the decade age 65 to 74, it doubles to 582. For the decade age 75 to 84, it almost triples, reaching 1380; above age 85, nearly 1800 strokes per 100,000 population occur each year. It is generally believed that strokes are more common in men than in women. A national survey of stroke for 1981 indicates that this difference continues, although a number of sources indicate that the incidence for females rises rapidly after age 65 and can reach the level occurring in males by age 80.[25]

Two types of strokes are recognized by the pathologists. One involves infarction of brain tissue owing to lack of blood supply, and the other involves hemorrhage into the brain tissue owing to rupture of vessels, either over the surface (as from cerebral aneurysm) or within the substance of the brain.

## *Strokes Caused by Cerebral Infarction*

The most common cause of stroke is cerebral infarction, which occurs when an area of the brain experiences a reduction in cerebral blood flow below approximately 10 ml per 100 gm per minute. If this reduction is sustained over a period of 10 to 15 minutes and remains unrelieved by restoration of normal flow or by the development of collateral circulation from borderline areas, tissue membranes lose the ability to maintain electrolyte and other gradients between intracellular and extracellular fluid and the neural cell dies.

Cerebral infarction results from a number of causes. The most common is disturbance in the cerebral arteries, which are most commonly involved by atherosclerosis and, more rarely, with inflammatory disease e.g., cranial arteritis (see Chapter 36). Cerebral infarction can also result from cardiac disease when emboli (either from mural thrombi following myocardial infarction or from valvular lesions—such as occur with rheumatic heart disease) enter the cerebral circulation and obstruct vessels, with resulting distal ischemia and infarction. An additional cause can be disease of the blood itself. Infarction is common in polycythemia vera. Cerebral infarction in general appears to have some correlation with the hematocrit level, in that patients with an elevated hematocrit level seem to have a higher chance of stroke and reduced cerebral blood flow than those with normal or low hematocrit levels.[21-23]

*Arterial disease,* distinctly the most common cause of cerebral infarction is atherosclerotic vascular disease.[18] It is now believed that less than 4 per cent of the population who reach the age of 80 die without significant atherosclerotic vascular disease. Atherosclerotic disease becomes symptomatic only when collateral circulation in arterial beds is not available or when changes in arterial supply due to atherosclerotic diseases occur abruptly and collateral circulation does not have an opportunity to develop. Atherosclerotic disease in the cerebral arteries tends to have a preference for certain vascular sites, usually involving larger arteries rather than small ones. The most common site of origin in the cerebral arteries is the *internal carotid artery,* just above the bifurcation of the common carotid artery. Here, lesions frequently may totally obstruct the internal carotid artery or may ulcerate and become a source of emboli in the distal cerebral circulation. Other common sites in the cerebral arterial tree are along the internal carotid artery as it enters the skull and at its bifurcation. Additional sites are the beginning of the middle cerebral and anterior cerebral arteries, the vertebral and basilar arteries, and the origin of the posterior cerebral arteries. Obstruction and occlusion may occur at any of these sites, and if adequate collateral supply from other channels is not present, cerebral infarction can result. Some patients have abnormalities of the circle of Willis, with absent or attenuated posterior communicating arteries; patients who do not have posterior communicating arteries have a higher incidence of cerebral infarction than those who do have them.

In younger patients, cerebral infarction resulting from cerebral emboli of a cardiac source is more frequent than stroke occurring from progressive atherosclerotic disease of head and neck vessels. Formerly, a major cause of cerebral emboli was rheumatic heart disease, which tends to affect a much younger population. Myocardial infarction with mural thrombi provide a source of emboli in the elderly.

Stroke has a strong tendency to ensue in patients with auricular fibrillation.

## Clinical Presentation

The symptoms of cerebral infarction, from whatever the cause, are similar at any age, and the character of stroke does not seem to be influenced by age. Symptoms, however, may be influenced by the degree of atherosclerotic disease present. This tends to increase steadily as age progresses. The more pronounced the atherosclerotic disease, the more extensive the involvement of cerebral vessels, the more obstructions or occlusions, the greater the chances of stroke, and the greater the tendency for the stroke to be serious.

Cerebral infarction has three recognized presentations:[10,12,19]

1. The patient with *completed stroke* usually awakens with or experiences sudden onset of paresis and sensory loss in one portion of the body or another. This neurologic deficit stabilizes, and persistent disability remains.
2. When first seen by a physician, the patient with *progressing stroke* may show minimal evidence of paresis or sensory loss. This may progress either steadily or in a step-like fashion over a period of from 12 to 24 hours, with increasing neurologic deficit.
3. A patient with *transient cerebral ischemia*[12] experiences the sudden onset of paresis or sensory loss in the face or hand on one side, with or without speech difficulties. This gradually improves over a few minutes and leaves the patient without neurologic residua.

For each variety, the first appearance of symptoms is rather abrupt. The initial symptoms depend on the portion of the brain that is ischemic or is becoming infarcted. The area of the brain most commonly involved is the portion supplied by the *middle cerebral artery*. Ischemia or infarction in this area produces characteristic symptoms of weakness or paralysis in the face, arm, and hand on the opposite side of the body; impaired sensory perception in the same area; and in many cases, homonymous visual field defects. If the infarction is in the dominant hemisphere, there are usually speech deficits. If the infarction involves the portion of the brain anterior to the motor strip, speech difficulties will be seen largely as impairment of expression (expressive dysphasia). If infarction involves the motor strip in the inferior parietal or superior temporal region, speech impairment will be manifested by difficulty in perception and understanding speech (receptive dysphasia). Generally, following cerebral infarction, combinations of expressive and receptive dysphasia occur, with one or the other more or less predominating. When the nondominant cerebral hemisphere is infarcted, sensory difficulties may be profound. Patients may become unaware that the left side is paralyzed and may completely ignore this side.

Infarction in the portion of the brain supplied by the *anterior cerebral artery* causes paralysis and weakness of the lower extremity on the opposite side. Infarctions in this area are less common, probably because one arterior cerebral artery can supply both anterior cerebral circulations owing to the presence of adequate collateral circulation through the arterior communicating artery.

Infarction in the portion of the brain supplied by the *posterior cerebral artery* predictably causes homonymous visual field defects on the side opposite the infarction. There may also be impairment in awareness of what is seen and difficulty with reading. If more proximal portions of the brain supplied by the posterior cerebral artery are involved, infarction in the upper portion of the brainstem, the midbrain, may occur with varying degrees of paralysis, including ocular motor nerve palsy, associated with the visual field defects.

*Brainstem infarctions* are much more complicated in their presentation. The usual hallmark is evidence of a disturbance in cranial nerve function. Perhaps the most common brainstem infarction occurs in the lateral medulla, causing the *lateral medullary syndrome,* which is due to occlusion or impaired circulation in the portion of the brain supplied by the posterior inferior cerebellar artery. In this syndrome, the patient has the sudden onset of nausea, vertigo, ataxia, pain, and sensory loss in the face on the same side as the infarction and loss of sensory perception on the opposite side of the body. On examination, such patients usually have ataxia, with an intention tremor on the side of the lesion and impaired pain and temperature perception in the face on the side of the lesion and on the side opposite the lesion.

Infarctions due to *basilar artery occlusion* present a varied picture. The most profound disturbance occurs with infarction of the pons, including the basis pontis and the pontine tegmentum. This produces a quadriplegic patient, unresponsive to outside stimuli, with varying degrees of ophthalmoplegia and impaired responses to caloric stimulation. If the pontine tegmentum is preserved, the patient may be quadriplegic but can show some evidence of awareness to outside stimuli.

## Evaluation

The evaluation begins with a careful general physical examination. Cardiac disorders may be found to be the source of emboli producing cerebral occlusion. Special attention is devoted to detecting evidence of rheumatic valvular disease and cardiac dysrhythmia. Electrocardiographic (EKG) examination is always carried out, since changes may suggest the simultaneous presence of myocardial infarction. This can be the source of cerebral emboli from thrombi on the ventricle wall. Careful evaluation of peripheral arterial pulses will give information about the degree of atherosclerotic vascular disease elsewhere and the possibility of impairment to these vascular beds. Careful auscultation over the carotid arteries in the neck may reveal bruits, which may help to identify the potential source of the infarction. Careful examination of the ocular fundi should always be done, because occasionally small emboli may be present in the retinal vessels. If these are refractile and orange in color, they usually are caused by cholesterol crystals. These rarely cause vascular occlusion and impaired vision. Small white plugs or occluded vessels suggest platelet emboli. These are usually associated with some impairment in circulation to the retina and with visual symptoms in many instances.

Careful evaluation of cardiac rhythm is needed in examining any patient with stroke, because dysrhythmia, in addition to fostering emboli, may severely affect cerebral blood flow. Careful evaluation of blood pressure should be routine, since hypertension is common in patients with atherosclerotic vascular disease. Both infarcts and hemorrhages can occur with or without elevated blood pressure. It is impossible to be sure that a stroke is caused by either infarct or hemorrhage without a computed tomographic (CT) scan. It is now clear that small intracerebral hemorrhages are often the cause of what appear to be small cerebral infarcts on clinical grounds and then are discovered on CT scan to be hemorrhage.

A complete blood count, hematocrit level, and red blood cell count are important. Blood glucose should always be determined because diabetes or hypoglycemia may complicate stroke.

Whether the clinical picture is caused by hemorrhage or by infarction is easily settled by the routine performance of a computerized brain scan, which is sensitive to the presence of blood in tissues. Blood is radiodense (radiopaque) and shows up clearly in these studies. Infarcted tissue may not appear abnormal for some time after the infarction. With infarction, there may be some decrease in radiodensity of tissue as well as distortion of the normal geography of the ventricles because of the development of edema. Repeating the CT scan (if normal at onset) several days later, may show an area of decreased tissue density corresponding to the suspected area of brain infarction. The most important use of the CT scan is to distinguish between hemorrhage and infarction and to be certain that other conditions, such as brain tumor, are not causing the clinical picture.

At this point, further evaluation depends on whether or not prophylactic therapy can be considered useful in preventing further loss of brain tissue to infarction. If the patient has had a major completed stroke, little can be accomplished. If the patient rapidly recovers some function and has limited neurologic residua, consideration should be given to determine whether treatment might protect the remaining cerebral tissue at risk.

The physician must attempt to identify the source of infarction. If the patient does not have heart disease or blood disease (polycythemia vera) as a possible source, the most likely cause is atherosclerotic vascular disease. If the atherosclerotic vascular disease is located outside the head in a surgically accessible site and the patient has regained considerable neurologic function (or, in the case of transient ischemic attacks, has no residua), the physician must determine whether surgical correction of an extracranial arterial lesion might help prevent future cerebral infarction.

*Cerebral angiography* is performed by femoral catheterization, with selective opacification of the cerebral arterial tree arising from the aorta. This procedure is now used almost universally in the evaluation of cerebrovascular disease regardless of age and is safer than other methods. Complications of stroke have occurred with this method, but they are rare. Whether these are due to the breaking off of atherosclerotic plaques during catheterization is unknown. The catheter is passed to the arch of the aorta near the branching of the innominate, left carotid, and vertebral arteries. Any atherosclerotic material that is broken off between the femoral site of puncture and the arch would be swept downward, entering either the femoral arteries or possibly the renal arteries. Femoral or renal artery obstruction has not been reported as a complication. It is unlikely that releasing contrast medium by injection in the aortic arch can cause infarction. An infarction is likely to occur when a catheter is placed in the right or left common carotid artery or vertebra, slightly obstructing it, and contrast medium is injected. Pure contrast medium is highly irritating and can cause vessel damage and stroke. With *digital subtraction angiography* (DSA) now in common use, the amount of medium injected is very small (5 to 10 ml for the study of each artery) and the complication rate is minimal. *Intravenous digital subtraction cerebral angiography* has also been developed, and excellent pictures can be obtained without the hazards of arterial injection. If extracranial arterial disease is identified and can be determined as causative, consideration should always be given for surgical removal of such lesions.

### Surgical Treatment

Surgery is considered both for relieving arterial obstruction and for removing ulcerated atherosclerotic plaques. If atherosclerotic disease in other arteries distal to the surgically accessible sites is extensive, little can be done surgically. Anastomosing the temporal artery to the middle cerebral artery has been studied for bypassing obstructive disease in the intracranial portions of the carotid artery. The operation is now in widespread use but has recently been shown to be ineffective in preventing future TIA or stroke.

### Other Forms of Treatment

If surgical correction of atherosclerotic disease is not possible, other therapies may be effective.

*Anticoagulants,* first heparin and then Coumadin, have been used to prevent further transient ischemic attacks and to reduce the chances of future stroke.[3,12] The data on the effectiveness of this approach are not yet conclusive, but studies carried out over the past three decades indicate that patients receive some protection. One risk is that patients taking anticoagulants have a higher incidence of cerebral hemorrhage and subdural hematoma. In elderly frail patients who are not good surgical candidates, anticoagulants might be tried, although the problems of maintaining patients on Coumadin are considerable. Safe usage of these agents requires an intelligent patient, a cooperative family, a knowledgeable physician, and a reliable laboratory. If any one of these requirements is absent, anticoagulants should not be used.

Currently, *aspirin* with its effects as an inhibitor of platelet aggregation, has been recommended for the suppression of transient ischemic attacks and the reduction of the chance of strokes in patients identified as having atherosclerotic disease.[2,7,9] The dose varies from 300–1200 mg per day. Lower doses of aspirin have been found to effectively suppress platelet aggregation but reported studies have used 600–1200 mg per day. The rationale for this treatment is that frequently atherosclerotic plaques become ulcerated. Debris, composed primarily of platelets, is thought to collect on the surface of an ulcer; it is postulated that shedding of this debris into the cerebral circulation leads to transient obstruction, causing transient ischemic attacks and small cerebral infarctions. An ulcerated plaque is also a potential source of larger emboli, which may obstruct large vessels. Several important studies have been carried out on the effectiveness of aspirin in reducing transient ischemic attacks and in preventing future stroke.[5] Aspirin is generally believed to be an effective means of providing protection. As the result of some studies, there is concern that aspirin may be more effective if combined with other platelet antiaggregants such as dipyridamole (Persantine).[2] When surgery is not advisable and anticoagulants are contraindicated, aspirin as a prophylactic, along with other platelet aggregant inhibitors (dipyridamole), should be considered. Always, the goal of treatment of cerebral vascular accident is to protect remaining cerebral tissue from further damage by infarction and to prevent future loss of function.

## Recovery

Recovery from cerebral infarction does occur. If neurologic recovery is going to happen, it usually happens fairly promptly, often within the first 30 days after the onset. This recovery undoubtedly occurs in areas of brain tissue that have not been destroyed by infarction but whose function has been impaired by reduced (but not fatally limited) cerebral blood flow. Although a reduction in cerebral blood flow to a level of approximately 18 ml of blood flow per 100 gm of brain per minute will stop function in these tissues, if the blood flow does not drop lower than this, the tissue is apparently viable and, with restoration of blood flow, may return to normal function. Reductions to levels of 10 ml of blood per 100 gm of brain per minute for 10 minutes or more cause infarction in experimental stroke models. Cerebral blood flow reduction to profound (but not critical) levels, with restoration, followed by recovery of neurologic defects over a relatively brief period, is believed to have occurred in patients who have stroke with good recovery. Unfortunately, this is less common than the usual picture of permanent loss of voluntary motion and sensory perception in the parts of the body supplied by the infarcted nervous system.

During the recovery process, it is extremely important to identify and manage correctly all associated conditions, such as cardiac disease and blood disease, which may complicate the picture by affecting normal cerebral blood flow. Later treatment is devoted to rehabilitation of the patient with stroke.

### Rehabilitation

Although rehabilitation does not restore neurologic function,[6] it allows the patient to become adjusted to the disability, provides education about ways in which function can be carried on, and allows the patient to become as independent as possible, utilizing the intact extremities (see Chapter 14). This involves, first, protecting paralyzed extremities from deformity due to joint fixation and muscle and tendon shortening. If these deformities are allowed to develop, they can be very difficult to correct. Paralyzed or weakened extremities must be moved passively through a full range of motion once or twice daily for at least 30 to 60 days. This is the period during which neurologic recovery can be expected if it is to occur and if voluntary movement is to return. Later, without return of voluntary movement, it may be difficult, if not impossible, to avoid some joint fixation and muscle shortening, especially if the paralyzed part becomes spastic. If some voluntary movement returns, exercises are carried out daily to improve strength and to find what degree of function is possible. At the same time, exercises are also initiated in the intact extremities to increase strength and dexterity, since in severe paralysis the intact side must take over most functions. The patient will need to learn ways to dress, to eat, to get in and out of bed with minimal assistance, to walk (using support), to bathe, and to use the toilet.

Patients with cerebral infarction in the part of the brain supplied by the middle cerebral artery are generally able to ambulate, because the motor cortex of the leg may be spared and paralysis encountered in the lower extremities is less severe. Patients with nondominant hemisphere cerebral infarctions, with extensive sensory impairment and lack of awareness of their paralyzed side, are very difficult to rehabilitate because they may truly not be able to comprehend the cause and full extent of their disability. Patients who have previously shown a decline in intellectual capacity and are unable to learn, in addition to having a brain infarction, experience a great deal of trouble mastering ways to overcome disability caused by stroke. The presence of the two factors makes the outcome of stroke rehabilitation highly questionable.

Surprisingly, dysphasia, especially when it is *expressive,* does not preclude a successful outcome of stroke rehabilitation. Patients who are unable to express themselves, but are able to understand, usually can carry on quite well in rehabilitation. With proper encouragement and direction, they may achieve notable results in lessening dependency. Individuals with *receptive* dysphasia often have more trouble because of their difficulty in understanding what is being said to them and in following directions; their outlook is somewhat less positive.

The major determining factor in successful stroke rehabilitation is whether the patient has an understanding family, willing to take the patient home and help him to do what is necessary for independent living at home.[6] A supportive, warm home environment, managed by a healthy spouse, is perhaps the greatest asset for successful recovery. The possibility of a stroke victim's living at home is greatly augmented by educating the family about stroke. This includes information about what causes it, what to expect in terms of recurrence and other complications, management of personality changes, alteration of the home for easier living, need of outside help, and supportive community services. This process should involve the physician, the nursing service, social service personnel, and, if available, physical and occupational therapists. Such a coordinated team approach is mentioned in Chapter 3.

Patients most likely to achieve recovery are those with weakness rather than plegia and those with some retention of voluntary motion in the lower extremities. In general, individuals who have paralysis of the arm rarely, if ever, gain return of skillful voluntary movements. Often, only crude movements at the shoulder and elbow are possible, making a useful extremity unlikely. However, any return in voluntary motion in either the upper or lower extremity can usually be augmented by proper bracing and support.

Patients who are the least likely candidates for rehabilitation (and in whom rehabilitation probably should not be considered) are (1) those who were demented (or who were showing signs of becoming demented) before the stroke occurred, (2) those who show major declines in intellectual function following a stroke, and (3) those who have difficulties with recognizing their paretic side; this occurs most often with right hemisphere infarctions.

Age is not a major determining factor in the successful outcome of rehabilitation, but elderly patients with stroke are often very fragile, not only because of age but because of concomitant cardiac and other complicating illnesses. Depression is a significant problem among stroke patients and is a significant problem for successful rehabilitation. Although not all patients with stroke coming to a rehabilitation center are depressed, a considerable proportion are, and attention must be given to managing their depression if rapid and successful rehabilitation is to be achieved. Depression is reported to be most prevalent between 6 months and 2 years after the onset of the stroke. Also, there appear to be some anatomic correlates. Individuals with left hemisphere brain injury have been found to be more often depressed than patients with right hemisphere or brainstem infarction.[14–16] Surveys indicate that almost one third of patients are depressed at the time they are evaluated for rehabilitation after cerebral infarction.[13]

Active medical treatment programs should be considered for stroke patients who show any evidence of depression. Specialized treatment areas, specifically stroke rehabilitation, have been found to be more effective than nonspecialty units. Staff members of specialty units are frequently much more optimistic and attuned to the day-by-day problems facing a stroke patient, are more enthusiastic about rehabilitation, and generally more understanding about the problems that may be encountered; all of these factors improve outcome.

## *Strokes Caused by Hemorrhage*

### SUBARACHNOID HEMORRHAGE

Subarachnoid hemorrhage, which makes up about 6 to 9 per cent of all strokes, was once believed to be a condition largely confined to young individuals.[25] The incidence is significantly affected in the older age groups by how thoroughly patients with serious and major strokes are studied. With more accurate methods of determining the presence of subarachnoid hemorrhage and its usual cause, ruptured berry aneurysm, it is being recognized that the condition also occurs not infrequently among the elderly. Present data suggest that the peak incidence occurs between ages 45 and 55 (5.5 per 100,000 population per year) and that the incidence over age 65 is around 2 per 100,000 per year. With the advent of the CT scan, findings of subarachnoid hemorrhage as a cause of stroke in older individuals will undoubtedly increase because of the greater accuracy of detection.

The causes of subarachnoid hemorrhage at any age, are, primarily, ruptured berry aneurysm, ruptured arteriovenous anomaly, and subarachnoid hemorrhage of unknown cause. Ruptured arteriovenous anomaly with subarachnoid hemorrhage generally occurs most frequently in the younger age groups.

**Clinical Manifestations.** Symptomatology is not affected by the age of the patient. The most common symptom is the sudden abrupt onset of extremely severe headache. At first, headache may be localized to one side of the head, but usually rapidly, it becomes generalized. Often the side of the head on which the headache begins is a clue to the side of the bleeding source. Headache beginning in the frontal region, around the eyes, suggests bleeding in the anterior portion of the cerebral circulation; headache beginning in the back of the head may indicate bleeding originating in the posterior fossa. At onset of bleeding, patients may be unconscious transiently, but they quickly regain consciousness. They then complain of severe headache and show evidence of lethargy and occasionally have nausea and vomiting. Other patients may remain unconscious, and on examination, show evidence of serious neurologic deficit with hemiplegia or quadriplegia. Others, at the onset of bleeding, lapse rapidly into coma, become decerebrate, and quickly die. It is estimated that a significant percentage of sudden unexplained deaths are due to unrecognized subarachnoid hemorrhage, with dissection of blood into the ventricles, causing rapid brainstem compression and respiratory failure.

The individual with subarachnoid hemorrhage who awakens, after a period of unconsciousness, or who does not lose consciousness at all, may experience a brief period of impaired awareness, often followed by lethargy, will then complain of severe generalized headache and, after a few hours, develop a stiff neck. Stiffness of the neck is due to the chemical meningeal reaction caused by blood in the subarachnoid space.

Medical and neurologic evaluation of patients with subarachnoid hemorrhage should proceed rapidly after admission. This is done to rule out disturbances in general physical function and to assess neurologic deficits present. Frequently, EKG changes are noted after subarachnoid hemorrhage, which suggest myocardial ischemia. Careful scrutiny is needed in interpreting these changes, as they may be caused by the subarachnoid hemorrhage itself, or these changes may represent coincidental cardiac disease. Patients with subarachnoid hemorrhage who develop chemical meningitis may also be febrile. On neurologic examination, other than stiff neck, patients may show evidence of focal brain dysfunction, such as hemiparesis, sensory defects, occasionally visual field defects or, in many cases, isolated ocular motor nerve palsies resulting from specific placement of an aneurysm compressing the third nerve.

**Course and Initial Management.** A significant number (35 to 40 per cent) of patients die rapidly after the initial hemorrhage. The death rate is probably higher among elderly individuals who are fragile and who may have other complicating disorders that reduce ability to withstand a major cerebral insult. For patients who survive, initial management is directed toward providing relief of headache and taking measures to sustain respiration, blood pressure, and fluid intake. A quiet atmosphere with no physical activity is needed. If blood pressure is elevated at the time of hospital admission, it should gradually be reduced to normal levels. After the onset of the hemorrhage, patients should be kept at nearly bedrest almost all of the time. If possible, however, it generally is advisable to have patients use toilet facilities with assistance rather than put them through the difficult operation of using bedpans. Patients should not be allowed to become constipated, and they should not strain while having a bowel movement.

**Recurrence and Prevention.** Subarachnoid hemorrhage tends to recur, with each new recurrence carrying the same chance of mortality and morbidity as the initial hemorrhage. Recurrence is most likely within the first week to 10 days after the initial hemorrhage.[4,17,24]

Attempts to prevent recurrence of hemorrhage are most successful when applied as early as possible. Usually, however, this is possible only for those patients who do not lose consciousness or who experience only a brief period of coma (classified as grade 1 and grade 2). Currently, the only successful means known to prevent recurrence of hemorrhage is (1) identification of the source of hemorrhage and (2) surgical correction of it, if possible. Since surgical removal of bleeding requires identification of the type and locale of the sources,[4,17] cerebral angiography must precede any consideration for treatment. In order to achieve a complete survey of the potential sites of hemorrhage before operation is considered, angiography must demonstrate all major cerebral vessels on both sides of the brain.[4] Aneurysms are often multiple, and it may be difficult to determine exactly which aneurysm has caused bleeding. Use of CT scanning can identify the sites of bleeding within the brain and the subarachnoid hematomas that often surround an artery or an aneurysm that has ruptured. The resolution of CT scans is now almost fine enough to identify an aneurysm, but angiography is still required to outline the size and shape of the aneurysm and the character of its neck so that the surgeon can determine accurately the chances for a successful operation.

Intracranial surgery should always be approached with considerable caution because elderly patients are fragile and, with complications from other diseases, suffer a greater risk from general anesthesia and long intracranial procedures than younger individuals. Patients in good physiologic condition should certainly be considered for intracranial surgery for an aneurysm, if they are in comas of grade 1 or 2. Aneurysmal surgery is now done under microscopic visualization, and its technical quality is excellent. Operative mortality and morbidity have been reduced to around 5 per cent or less in the population as a whole.[4,17,20] Mortality and morbidity data on aneurysm surgery in the geriatric age group are not easy to obtain. In one Japanese study, in patients over 70 years old, operative mortality was 11 per cent and morbidity was 33 per cent; these figures indicate that advanced age is probably associated with greater risk for intracranial surgery.

Elderly patients in grade 3 and 4 classifications (i.e., with a more prolonged period of coma) should not be considered for surgery. These patients should be given supportive care in hope that there might be some restoration of function, with possible reconsideration later on. Because the chances of recurrent bleeding drop sharply after the second week following the initial hemorrhage, it is debatable whether the risks of surgery are lower, equal to, or higher than the chances of recurrent bleeding with its attendant mortality.

For the elderly patient who is seen 2 or 3 weeks following the initial hemorrhage and who is doing well, it is probably best to adhere to conservative treatment.

Suggested medical treatment to prevent subarachnoid hemorrhage has focused on the fact that blood in the cerebrospinal fluid (CSF) produces a fibrolytic reaction believed to be responsible for lysing clots in aneurysms, again releasing blood into the subarachnoid space.[20] Agents that prevent fibrinolysis, such as $\epsilon$-aminocaproic acid or its derivatives, have been used for this purpose. In general, these agents have not produced effective reduction of recurrent subarachnoid hemorrhage in carefully controlled treatment trials.

## INTRAPARENCHYMAL BRAIN HEMORRHAGE

**Primary Intracerebral Hemorrhage.** Primary intracerebral hemorrhage makes up about 6 per cent of all strokes. In recent studies, the highest incidence occurs in the decade age 65 through 74, (5.5 per 100,000) compared with figures a decade earlier (4 per 100,000) and a decade later (3.5 per 100,000). Since the mid-1970's, there has been a sharp decline in frequency. This is probably related to the major efforts to identify individuals with hypertension and to control high blood pressure. Primary intracerebral hemorrhage is most likely to occur in individuals with marked hypertension, yet may still occur in individuals who have never had a history of high blood pressure and, on examination, are not found to be hypertensive. With the introduction of CT scanning, the findings of small intracerebral hemorrhages have increased considerably.

Primary intracerebral hemorrhage most commonly occurs in the portion of the brain supplied by the lenticulostriate arteries. These are branches of the middle cerebral artery as it runs underneath the cerebral hemispheres laterally into the sylvian fissure. These small vessels supply most of the basal ganglia and the internal capsule. The most common site of hemorrhage is in the putamen. Other common sites are the frontal, temporal, and occipital cortices and, next in frequency, the substance of the cerebellum.

Of all types of stroke, primary intracerebral hemorrhage carries the highest mortality and morbidity. Bleeding into the brain produces a hematoma that destroys and compresses nearby neural structures and tracts. This may ultimately dissect into the ventricular system, causing a large expansion of a cerebral hemisphere on one side. The result is a shift of brain substance, herniation of the temporal lobes through the tentorium cerebelli, and brainstem compression. Smaller hemorrhages in lobes of the cerebral hemispheres are less likely to produce this sequence of events because they do not cause much shift or edema.

The classical clinical picture is the explosive onset of severe headache, nausea and vomiting, and major unilateral neurologic defect, usually with subsequent lapse into unconsciousness, coma, and relatively rapid death. Patients arriving in the emergency room with this syndrome, especially if it is accompanied by severe hypertension, should be considered as having primary intracerebral hemorrhage until proven otherwise. When other patients do not present with this classic symptomatology, the differential diagnosis between intracerebral hemorrhage and cerebral infarction may be difficult.

The most effective means of making the diagnosis is by use of CT scans. Demonstration of a large intracerebral blood clot is conclusive evidence of the condition. Lumbar puncture is not indicated because it is not necessary when CT scans are available and it carries a risk of upsetting intracranial cerebral fluid dynamics and promoting possible brain herniation.

*Management* is directed toward keeping the patient alive during the acute phase of the illness. With intracranial pressure elevations that are still life-threatening, the use of agents that dehydrate the brain, such as mannitol or urea, can be briefly helpful; however, they do not resolve the condition. Generally, intracerebral hemorrhage is self-resolving. If the patient survives the initial insult, there is usually a major morbidity with hemisensory defects that are often slow to resolve, if they ever do.

Surgery during the acute phase has been attempted. Most surgeons find that removal of a hematoma from a patient who is obtunded or in coma does not produce a desirable result and often worsens the situation. For those individuals with small hematomas who do not lose consciousness but who have neurologic deficits, self-resolution of the problem may occur. If an intracerebral hemorrhage is slow to resolve, removal of the hematoma may improve the recovery of neurologic function. Such instances are uncommon.

**Intracerebellar Hemorrhage.** In contrast to intracerebral hemorrhage, intracerebellar hemorrhage *does* require immediate consideration for surgery. This condition, if recognized at bedside, can often be dramatically helped by surgical removal of the hematoma. Patients present with a history of sudden onset of headache, nausea and vomiting, with ataxia and evidence of brainstem dysfunction, such as nystagmus, ophthalmoplegia, and disturbances in cerebellar function. Such individuals should immediately be considered as possibly having primary intracerebellar hemorrhage. If this can be demonstrated on CT scan, immediate evacuation of the hematoma may be life-saving, since further enlargement of a hematoma in this area may produce brainstem compression with impaired breathing, hypertension, and often death. The objective of surgery is to remove the hematoma prior to evidence of brainstem compression. This is the one variety of intraparenchymal hemorrhage for which surgery is indicated.

## *Other Cerebrovascular Diseases*

Several less common cerebrovascular conditions occur in the geriatric age group, but they are very infrequent and will not be presented here. Spontaneous dissection of internal carotid artery, fibromuscular dysplasia of the carotid artery, trauma to the carotid artery, and unusual inflammatory diseases (such as periarteritis) may lead to symptoms of cerebral ischemia and can produce cerebral infarction. These conditions will usually be uncovered by a careful clinical evaluation of the patient, but may require cerebral angiography for confirmation.

### References


1. Alter M, Christoferson L, Rusch J, et al: Cerebrovascular disease—frequency and population selectivity in an upper midwestern community. Stroke 1:454, 1970.
2. Canadian Cooperative Study Group: A randomized trial of aspirin and sulfinpyrazone in threatened stroke. N Engl J Med 299:53, 1978.
3. Cerebral Ischemia: The role of thrombosis and of antithrombotic therapy. Stroke 8:151, 1977.
   *An excellent review on the medical treatment of cerebral ischemia. The Joint Committee for Stroke Resources has also published a number of other reviews on subjects relating to cerebrovascular disease, including the epidemiology, stroke rehabilitation, medical and surgical management of stroke, strokes in children, transient focal cerebral ischemia, and cerebral circulation and metabolism in stroke. These are extensive review articles, excellently referenced, and should allow the reader access to most, if not all, of the important articles written on the subjects up until the time of the review. These articles have been appearing in* Stroke *since 1973.*
4. Drake CG: Management of cerebral aneurysm. Stroke 12:273, 1981.
5. Easton JD, Byer JA: Transient cerebral ischemia: medical management. *In* McDowell FH, Sonnenblick EH, Lesch M (eds.): Current Concepts in Cerebrovascular Disease. New York, Grune & Stratton, 1980.
6. Feigenson JS, Gitlow HS, Greenberg SO: The disability oriented rehabilitation unit—A major factor predicting stroke outcome. Stroke 9:5, 1979.
   *A well-referenced article on most of the previous literature relating to this topic. Dr. Feigenson summarizes the advantages of rehabilitation programs for victims of stroke.*
7. Fields WS, Lemak NA, Frankowski RF, et al: Controlled trial of aspirin on cerebral ischemia. Part II. Stroke 8:301, 1977.
8. Garraway WM, Whisnant JP, Furlan AJ, et al: The declining incidence of stroke. N Engl J Med 300:449, 1979.
9. Kurtzke JF: Controversy in neurology. The Canadian study on TIA and aspirin: A critique of the Canadian TIA study. Ann Neurol 5:597, 1979.
10. McDowell FH: Transient cerebral ischemia: Diagnostic considerations. *In* McDowell FH, Sonnenblick EH, Lesch M (eds.): Current Concepts in Cerebrovascular Disease. New York, Grune & Stratton, 1980, pp. 7–22.
11. Matsumoto N, Whisnant JP, Kurland LT, Okazaki H: Natural history of stroke in Rochester, Minn., 1955 through 1969, an extension of a previous study. Stroke 4:20, 1973.
12. Millikan CH, McDowell FH: Treatment of transient ischemic attacks: Progress in cerebrovascular disease. Stroke 9:299, 1978.
13. Reding M, Orto L, Willensky P, Fortuna I, et al: The dexamethasone suppression test. An indication of depression in stroke. Arch Neurol 42:209, 1985.
14. Robinson RG, Kubos KL, Starr LB, et al: The mood disorders in stroke patients: Importance of location of lesion. Brain 107:81, 1984.
15. Robinson RG, Starr LB, Kubos KL, Price TR: Post stroke affective disorders in cerebrovascular diseases. *In* Reivich M, Hurtig HI (eds): New York, Raven Press, 1983, pp 137–145.
16. Robinson RG, Price TR: Post-stroke depressive disorders: A follow-up study of 103 patients. Stroke 13:635, 1982.
17. Sahs AL, Perret GE, Locksley HB, Nishioka A.: Intracranial aneurysms and subarachnoid hemorrhage. Philadelphia, JB Lippincott, 1969.
   *An extensive documentation of 5000 patients who were followed in the Aneurysm Treatment Trial, which was conducted from about 1958 through 1978.*
18. Sandler M, Bourne GH: Atherosclerosis and Its Origin. New York, Academic Press, 1963.
19. Schmidley JW, Caronna JJ: Transient cerebral ischemia—pathophysiology. *In* McDowell FH, Sonnenblick EH, Lesch M (eds.): Current Concepts in Cerebrovascular Disease. New York, Grune & Stratton, 1980, pp. 23–40.
   *A well-documented, well-referenced review on the pathophysiology, diagnosis, and treatment of transient ischemic attacks and progressing stroke. It is up to date as of 1980 and contains most of the relevant reference material that might be useful to any reader. Several sections in this book have been used as references in this chapter.*

20. Suzuki J.: Cerebral Aneurysms. Tokyo, Neuron Press, 1979.
*An enormous study of the experience of the Japanese in the management of cerebral aneurysms and subarachnoid hemorrhage.*
21. Thomas DJ, Marshall J, Ross-Russel RW: Cerebral blood flow in polycythemia. Lancet 2:161, 1978.
22. Thomas DJ, Marshall J, Ross-Russel RW: Effect of hematocrit on cerebral blood flow in man. Lancet 2:941, 1978.
23. Tohgi H, Yamanoucki H, Murakami M, et al: Importance of the hematocrit as a risk factor in cerebral infarction. Stroke 9:369, 1978.
24. Walton J: Subarachnoid Hemorrhage. London, EPS Livingstone, 1956.
*A well-written book and probably the earliest complete document relating to subarachnoid hemorrhage, its cause, natural history, and treatment.*
25. Weinfeld FD: The national survey of stroke. Stroke 12:Suppl. No. 1, 1981.

Chapter 22

# Other Neurologic Diseases of the Elderly

*Fletcher H. McDowell*

## PARKINSON'S DISEASE

Since its description by James Parkinson in 1917, Parkinson's disease has become recognized as one of the most common neurologic disorders of the elderly. The disorder includes a number of subentities, including Parkinson's disease proper and several conditions with similar symptoms, usually referred to as *Parkinsonian syndromes.* Approximately one million individuals are affected by Parkinson's disease in the United States; approximately 40,000 to 50,000 new cases are identified annually.

The condition most commonly has its onset between the ages of 55 and 60. It can occur at an earlier age, however, and at later ages even into the 80s. The disease is equally common in men and women. It has been identified in all races in whom neurologic illness is carefully studied and in whom individual life spans are long enough so that the disease can show itself. A variety of types include (1) postencephalitic, (2) arteriosclerotic, (3) drug-induced, and (4) idiopathic.

**Postencephalitic Parkinson's Disease.** This type was common between the years 1920 to 1930 and usually followed a clearly identified episode of von Economo's (lethargic) encephalitis. The symptoms of Parkinson's disease usually followed the encephalitis within a few months but sometimes occurred as long as 5 to 10 years afterward. Postencephalitic Parkinson's disease affected younger individuals more often than did other forms. The occurrence of this type of Parkinson's disease is distinctly unusual now, for the most part having ceased when von Economo's encephalitis disappeared around 1930. Generally, in patients who had encephalitis, Parkinson-like symptoms were not the only neurologic abnormalities. Paralysis, ocular palsies, dystonia, episodic seizures such as oculogyric crises, and a tendency for slower progression often were evident.

**Drug-Induced Parkinson's Disease.** This form is most commonly seen after the use of medications such as reserpine and phenothiazines. Symptoms may occur within days of onset of drug use or following the drug withdrawal. Generaly, elderly patients experience bradykinesia, reduced movement, and fixed postures; younger individuals more often experience dystonia. Along with the reduced motion, patients may at times exhibit dystonic-like movements involving the head and neck and face, a sensation of restlessness and desire to be in motion, and somewhat sterotyped repetitive movements of the face and mouth. This movement disorder most often appears during the administration of the agent, and the movements may become permanent. Drug-induced Parkinsonian symptoms in elderly person tend to most closely resemble those of classic Parkinson's disease.

**"Arteriosclerotic" Parkinson's Disease.** This term is applied to individuals in whom Parkinson's symptoms first appear simultaneously with evidence of atherosclerotic changes in cerebral vessels. The connection between these two conditions has never been firm, however, and the two conditions may be simply coexisting as independent entities.

**Idiopathic Parkinson's Disease.** Most Parkinson's Disease falls into this category. Generally, there is no clear point as to when the disease begins. The most common initial symptom that patients clearly recall is the development of tremor, usually starting on one side of the body and most often in an upper extremity. The tremor often spreads to involve both sides. By the time tremor is present, most patients will recall that they have noticed a tendency to "slow down," with all of their daily activities having become a little more difficult to perform. Patients usually describe this phenomenon of slowing down as "stiffness", "rigidity", or "weakness". Frequently, patients may notice that their facial expression is less facile, a point which their families may mention. The patient may also note a change in posture, with a tendency to stoop, caused by flexion of the trunk and head and some flexion at the knees. The gait changes, and steps may be short. The patient may shuffle his feet when he walks and show a descreased swing of the upper extremities while walking. As the bradykinesia or hypokinesia increases, the patient may assume fixed postures for long periods of time without evidence of discomfort, and a mask-like expression may develop. Later, there is increased difficulty with walking, with more short, quick steps (festination) and difficulty in resuming walking after once stopping—(start hesitation). Speech may become affected, the most common disturbance being a decrease in volume; the speech may also become rapid and clipped, poorly enunciated, and extremely difficult to understand. Patients may report that they have considerable difficulty in dressing themselves and in using eating utensils to cut food. They often have trouble in getting in and out of bed, turning in bed, getting in and out of chairs, and bathing themselves. Handwriting may become small and illegible. The disease can progress to the point where initiating movement may become impossible and complete dependency occurs.

## *Physical Examination*

When examined by physicians, patients may have some or all of the major phenomena associated with the disease. When the patient walks, it is usually easy to observe that one or both arms do not swing rhythmically. The patient may not lift his feet from the floor (which results in shuffling) and may have difficulty starting to walk again if stopped.

The patient may have tremor at rest. It can usually be demonstrated when the patient performs an intentional act—the tremor briefly stops. The tremor is generally rapid and rhythmic at the rate of 4 to 8 cycles per second (H2).

When the patient is asked to perform rapid skilled movements with upper and lower extremities, there is almost invariably difficulty in doing so, especially with the hands. Patients will usually report that their skill in performing fine movements with their hands, such as buttoning and unbuttoning clothes, sewing, or using their hands for hobby work, has become limited; these functions may become impossible.

Strength may be decreased, but it usually is not grossly impaired. Passive movement of the extremities, when tremor is present, may reveal a ratchet-like sensation called "cogwheel rigidity." At times, rigidity will present evenly throughout the passive range of motion. The patient's posture, on examination, is usually obviously different from normal, with a flexion of the head, shoulders, and trunk and sometimes flexion at the knees and hips. Patients may report an awareness of poor balance and being easily pushed off balance. With severe postural instability, patients may report frequent falling. On examination, pushing the patient gently forward or backward may cause falling unless the patient is supported.

Patients may have abnormalities of ocular movement with forced eye closure. Blepharospasm at times can be demonstrated by tapping the forehead, when repeated tapping does not result in the usual decrease of blinking; at times, the eyes shut and remain shut until forceably opened.

Sialorrhea, which is common in patients with Parkinson's disease, is not associated with an increase in saliva production; it is due to a reduction in the reflex swallowing of saliva, which then collects in the mouth and runs with gravity to the nearest exit, usually the lips. As the condition progresses, patients report difficulty in swallowing, as well as choking, and aspiration. Coupled with decreased pulmonary function due to hypokinesia and rigidity in the respiratory musculature, these conditions often set the stage for aspiration pneumonia.

## *Drug Therapy Using Levodopa*

Until the discovery of dopamine deficiency and its possible correction by the administration of levodopa (L-dopa), therapy for Parkinson's disease was largely based on the use of anticholinergic agents. It was accidentally discovered during the last century that tincture of belladonna often relieved some of the symptoms of Parkinson's disease. Virtually all drug therapy until 1967 was based on atropine-like agents as the standard therapy. It was subsequently demonstrated that acetylcholine agonists increase the symptoms of Parkinson's disease and anticholinergic agents (trihexyphenidyl, benztropine, cycrimine, procyclidine) will relieve the symptoms to some degree. The efficacy of these agents had never been very great. The most commonly used anticholinergic agent is trihexyphenidyl (Artane). It is given in divided doses of 2 to 10 mg per day, starting with a low dose and gradually increasing until side effects appear or improvement stops. Common side effects are dry mouth, blurred vision, and at times urinary retention and delirium.

With the introduction of agents to reduce blood pressure (reserpine) and the discovery of drugs having a tranquilizing effect, it became common to see Parkinson-like symptoms following long-term use of these agents. It was the stimulus of drug-induced Parkinson's disease that set the stage for major discoveries as to the exact nature of the brain defect associated with the disorder. The identification of dopamine as a neurotransmitter that could reverse the effects of reserpine-induced bradykinesia or akinesia in animals immediately posed the possibility that a deficiency in this transmitter had something to do with Parkinson's disease. It was demonstrated in individuals who had died from Parkinson's disease that the dopamine content of the central nervous system (CNS) was extremely low, especially in the substantia nigra and the caudate nucleus. This led to identification of the major defect in Parkinson's disease as a decline in the number of dopamine-producing cells in the substantia nigra. This discovery was followed by the demonstration, in 1967, by Cotziàs that a precursor of dopamine (L-dopa), given in large doses, could reverse some, if not all, of the symptoms of the disorder. L-dopa has become the standard treatment since that date.

Initially, large amounts of L-dopa were required for relief of symptoms. This treatment was associated with major side effects, the most disturbing of which were nausea and vomiting. Occasionally, patients had orthostatic hypotension. If these symptoms could be tolerated and the dose increased, patients noted marked relief of hypokinesia and bradykinesia, improvement in all motor functions, and often relief of tremor. Patients treated in this way were able to perform daily activities more easily and became more independent.

It was later demonstrated that certain agents could inhibit the conversion of L-dopa to dopamine in the body and that these metabolic inhibitors did not cross the blood-brain barrier. This allowed most of the L-dopa administered to enter the brain, where the deficiency of dopamine occurred. Most L-dopa taken orally is rapidly decarboxylated into dopamine, which is then eliminated in the urine. High levels of circulating dopamine stimulate the vomiting center and can produce nausea and vomiting. With the suppression of peripheral metabolism by such agents as $\alpha$-methyldopa hydrazine, and benserazide, it has been possible to reduce the total dose of L-dopa, improve the response to the drug, and decrease markedly the incidence of side effects, e.g., nausea, vomiting, and hypotension. A limiting side effect for patients taking either regular L-dopa or L-dopa and a metabolic inhibitor is the development of abnormal involuntary movements, or *dyskinesia.* These movements most commonly involve the face, tongue, head, and upper extremities. These sometimes become so marked that they cause as much difficulty for the patient as the original Parkinson's disease. Fortunately, these symptoms are dose-related and reduction of medication dose results in their relief or cessation.

### Current Treatment

Today, it is the practice to administer L-dopa with a decarboxylase inhibitor. In the United States, the method of choice is $\alpha$-methyldopa hydrazine in combination with L-dopa (Sinemet). A relatively small dose is used initially, building up to the desired level, i.e., until maximum relief of symptoms occurs with minimal, if any, side effects. Generally, patients start with 300 mg of L-dopa/30 mg of $\alpha$-methyldopa hydrazine. Approximately 100 mg of $\alpha$-methyldopa hydrazine are needed to suppress most of the peripheral decarboxylation. In view of this fact, with small intakes of L-dopa in Sinemet combination of 10/100, not enough metabolic inhibitor is given. Therefore a new combination containing 25 mg of $\alpha$-methyldopa hydrazine and 100 mg of L-dopa has been developed. This allows patients who are taking 400 and 500 mg of L-dopa per day to have complete suppression of decarboxylation in the periphery. Currently, patients are begun on three to four tablets a day of 25/100 Sinemet with a gradually increasing dose until maximum symptom relief occurs. Dose increases can be made at 3- to 7-day intervals until two successive increments are given without evidence of improvement or until dyskinetic movements appear. With this regimen, patients who have Parkinson's disease can be expected to improve considerably. There is usually a marked decrease in bradykinesia or hypokinesia and often a marked decrease in tremor. In some instances, it has been possible to abolish all evidence of Parkinson's disease using these agents. On the average, more than half to two thirds of the patients will show 50 per cent improvement with this treatment.

### Long-Term Effects

The long-term efficacy of these agents has been investigated thoroughly since their introduction in the early 1970s. Several events may inhibit their effectiveness.

First, patients may notice that they become

aware when it is time to take another dose of medication. At the end of a previous dose period, they tend to slow down and have some evidence of return of symptoms of Parkinson's disease. They begin to cycle their symptoms around their intake of Sinemet. Initially, taking the medication may produce marked improvement, which may last many hours, followed by a decline and return of parkinsonian symptoms that are again relieved by another dose. Also, patients may notice that shortly after taking a dose considerable abnormal involuntary movement or dyskinesia may occur briefly; alternatively, these movements may occur at the end of a dose period. Generally, there is a cycling of the L-dopa blood levels in these patients.

Patients may also find that, for no reason, symptoms of Parkinson's disease return abruptly. The symptoms may last from minutes to hours, followed by complete reversal to relatively normal function. This sequence of events has been called the "on-off" phenomenon. The exact cause of this has not been demonstrated, but it does not appear to be related to the wearing off of the effect of a particular dose. Blood levels are generally high when a patient is functioning well and low when symptoms return. Possibly, the abrupt change in response to medication is due to dopamine receptor blocking, followed by hypersensitivity. The only evidence supporting either theory is that continuous intravenous administration of L-dopa, by providing a stable blood level, seems to abolish the symptom. Patients who have been treated for long periods of time are very likely to develop the "on-off" phenomenon. Unfortunately, treatment of this situation has not been terribly successful. More frequent administrations of L-dopa have been tried in order to maintain more stable blood levels. Improved absorption of L-dopa by decreasing protein intake has proved only slightly successful. Currently, the use of dopamine agonists to supplement Sinemet is being tried, with some evidence of improvement.

Another complication noted with long-term treatment by L-dopa has been the development of marked postural instability. Patients report that after several years of treatment their balance has become poor, that they frequently fall forward or backward while getting in and out of chairs or while backing up, and that occasionally they fall for no reason at all. Injuries are common. Often patients fall so frequently that they cannot safely get out of a chair. On examination, they usually show marked instability. When they are pushed forward or backward, they fall unless supported. Some patients have been found to have decreased or absent labyrinthine function. The exact cause of the development of postural instability is not clear. Loss of postural reflexes is a common phenomenon associated with Parkinson's disease, and this seems to become more marked as the disease progresses under treatment with L-dopa.

Dyskinetic movements seem to appear more readily with long-term treatment, and patients frequently notice that they occur progressively with less medication. Generally, patients report improved function along with some abnormal involuntary movements and may prefer this state to the immobility associated with return of parkinsonian symptoms. Often a compromise on dosage must be achieved to provide for minimal dyskinesia and maximum relief of symptoms.

Patients treated for long periods with L-dopa may show a high incidence of loss of intellectual capacity, and in many instances marked dementia may ensue. The dementia may become the most serious problem facing the patient and will require major changes in lifestyle. Dementia had been noted as a concomitant of Parkinson's disease long before the use of L-dopa, but it was generally not emphasized as a major phenomenon. Now that patients are able to be kept mobile and articulate for longer periods, it is clear that with the progression of the disorder, dementia is almost a constant feature. Neuropathologic CNS examination in patients with this disorder has shown changes in the brain similar to those found in patients with Alzheimer's disease. With dementia, patients frequently become quite easily confused and hallucinate readily. Often the causes of the hallucinations, changes in mentation, and delirium are the drugs given for the relief of Parkinson's disease. The most commonly offending drugs are those of the anticholinergic type, but L-dopa itself may aggravate mental confusion and cause hallucinations. If these symptoms are prominent, the agents must be decreased or discontinued.

## *Other Therapeutic Drugs*

**Antihistamines.** Antihistamines, which have a mild anticholinergic effect, have been extensively used, especially diphenhydramine (Benadryl), phenadrine, and chlorphenoxamine. These are all similar in action on the CNS and may be useful in damping a tremor and improving the response to other agents. The most commonly used of these drugs, diphenhydramine, has been found very helpful in reducing tremor when given in amounts of 50 to 100 mg per day.

**Antidepressants.** An antidepressant is sometimes extremely useful. The most commonly used agents are *imipramine* (Tofranil) or *amitriptyline.* Imipramine given in 10- or 25- mg doses, two to three times per day; amitriptyline, 25 mg, is given before bedtime, and sometimes an additional 25-mg dose is given during the day. These drugs often produce remarkable improvement for the depressed bradykinetic patient with Parkinson's disease.

**Antivirals.** It was accidentally discovered, over a decade ago, that an antiviral agent, *amantadine hydrochloride,* is effective in relieving symptoms of Parkinson's disease. When given in doses of 100 mg two to three times per day, patients may be aware of considerable relief of tremor, hypokinesia, and bradykinesia. Amantadine is often used as the initial treatment for a patient with early Parkinson's disease, especially with mild symptoms. It is useful in relieving tremor and used together with Sinemet may provide more relief than with either drug alone. It is recommended as the initial treatment for the relief of tremor when bradykinesia is not marked.

**Ergot Derivatives.** With the discovery of the effectiveness of L-dopa in relieving symptoms of Parkinson's disease, efforts were made to find agents with a similar action but not requiring the metabolic conversion of L-dopa to dopamine in the nervous system. A number of agents have been discovered and tried, but only one has come into general use. Ergot derivatives were shown to have a dopamine-like effect, and from this group of drugs, *bromocriptine* was discovered to have a distinct dopamine agonistic effect.

Bromocriptine has been used to treat patients whose response to Sinemet has been less than desirable, especially those patients with the "on-off" phenomenon. It appears to be most effective when used to supplement the dose. It has a longer period of action in the CNS and is more potent than Sinemet.

Bromocriptine is started in small doses, 2.5 mg two to three times per day, and then gradually increased in amount. As the dose is increased, the dose of Sinemet is decreased to prevent involuntary movements. Bromocriptine is increased until the symptoms of the "on-off" response are eliminated or reduced or until intolerable side effects appear. These are most commonly orthostatic hypotension and delirium. The usual dose of bromocriptine able to produce a desired effect is between 20 and 40 mg per day. Bromocriptine has been used alone as the only antiparkinsonian agent, but in general it is not as effective as when used with Sinemet. Another dopamine agonist soon to be available derived from ergot is *pergolide.* This agent so far appears to be more effective than bromocriptine.

In some respects, bromocriptine is not a very useful agent; it has the distinct disadvantage of being enormously expensive, and the number of side effects from it are so large that it is used by very few.

## *Surgical Treatment*

Over the past 25 years or so, surgical treatment of Parkinson's disease has been carried on with variable results. Thalamotomy does abolish tremor on the side opposite the lesion, but it does not halt the progression of bradykinesia and rigidity, which are usually the most debilitating symptoms of the disorder. More accurate sterotactic surgery has evolved over the past decade, and many surgeons now recommend thalamotomy to reduce tremor. Complications of the more recent forms of sterotactic surgery seem to be fewer than those previously encountered. The operation is almost exclusively reserved for young patients with Parkinson's disease who have unilateral tremor as a main manifestation.

## *Activity Level*

It is important that patients with Parkinson's disease remain as physically, socially, and intellectually active as possible.

It becomes very easy for patients to move very little and to rapidly become physically deconditioned. Exercise programs and increased activity are desirable in maintaining optimal performance. If a patient is able to do these on his own, so much the better; if not, formal physical therapy programs should be undertaken.

Patients should be encouraged to remain as independent as possible, and effort should be made to keep friends and family from making patients dependent by doing things for them. No matter how long it takes a patient to carry out daily activities, the patient should be encouraged to continue to do them unassisted when possible.

Family members may have to force social activity, since the elderly parkinsonian patient may easily become less interested in social connections and in activity outside the home. Patients often become increasingly apathetic and sometimes somnolent. Generally, it is very difficult to convince patients to take on social activities; however, once they engage in them, they generally find them interesting and enjoyable. Rarely will the patient spontaneously initiate a social activity, especially if there is some evidence of decline in intellectual capacity.

### *Prognosis and Course*

Parkinson's disease is gradually progressive. It is not possible to predict accurately how rapidly the disease will progress. The only benchmark is to determine how rapidly it has progressed between the onset of the condition and the examination by the physician; the rate of progression in the past usually signals the probable rate of progression in the future. With progression, all symptoms and signs of disorder become more marked. In addition to the motor disturbance, the patient may demonstrate a decline in intellectual capacity and may ultimately become demented.

Patients with acute increases in symptoms should be looked at extremely carefully, since the most common causes are an alteration in medication, stopping medications, the development of an intercurrent illness, or depression. The most common cause of abrupt worsening is that the patient forgets to take medication regularly, resulting in a gradually decreasing dose. Depression can markedly increase all aspects of Parkinson's disease and must be recognized and treated. Any intercurrent illness with fever may worsen the symptoms and signs of Parkinson's disease. If recent increases in symptoms cannot be explained on the basis of drug elimination or depression, the patient should be carefully examined for the possibility of other illnesses. This is especially important for the elderly patient who may be showing signs of dementia.

Generally, patients may enjoy 10 to 15 years of good function with proper treatment. Excessive use of L-dopa in the treatment of Parkinson's disease may hasten decline, but this has not been established. The marked relief of symptoms provided by L-dopa with a metabolic inhibitor is so beneficial that it should not be withheld. However, disability is what is being treated in Parkinson's disease; if patients, despite the clear clinical evidence of having the disorder, have no disability, they should not be treated until this occurs.

## EPILEPSY

Epilepsy, or seizure disorder, can occur at any age; however, it becomes distinctly less common as individuals grow older. In Turner's survey of a thousand patients who developed epilepsy from birth to age 70, only 0.4 per cent of the patients developed seizures after the age of 61. With patients achieving increased longevity since Turner's report, however, the percentage of seizures among the elderly has increased as individuals live long enough to develop conditions causing seizures.

With head trauma excluded as a possible cause, the most common reasons for seizures developing in the elderly are brain tumor, cerebrovascular disease, and drug intoxication. Seizure beginning after the age of 35 must always be considered a possible symptom of brain tumor. Abrupt onset of seizure with associated neurologic abnormalities, such as paresis or sensory loss, usually has a vascular cause. In individuals who are taking sedatives, tranquilizers, or antidepressants, the sudden development of seizures during the period when they stop such medications generally indicates a withdrawal fit.

Seizures may occur in individuals with primary and secondary CNS tumors. The frequency of seizures with tumors is not clear, but probably they occur in 30 per cent of the cases. Seizures are much more common when tumors grow slowly and involve the cerebral cortex.

The frequency of seizures in individuals with stroke is believed to be around 7 to 10 per cent. Seizures following stroke occur in two phases, one, generally short-lived, occurs immediately after the stroke. Seizures occurring later, within months or during the first year after a stroke, tend to become repetitive.

Seizures following drug intoxication usually occur during the withdrawal period. These are often one-time events, but sometimes more than one seizure is reported.

Seizures in the elderly occur about equally in both sexes. The types of seizures that occur in an elderly individual are usually no different from those occurring in younger people, except that "absence" or *petit mal* seizures are distinctly uncommon. The most frequently encountered seizures in the elderly are *generalized* or *focal,* but sometimes *psychomotor variants* or *temporal lobe seizures* are observed. The seizure usually is manifested by sudden loss of consciousness or altered awareness, accompanied by convulsive or involuntary movement. This is followed by a period of impaired mentation. The entire seizure rarely lasts more than 5 minutes.

## *Symptoms*

It is most important to determine whether an individual who is suspected of having seizures has actually had one. An aura, if present, is extremely suggestive that an episodic period of unconsciousness is due to a seizure disorder, and it must be determined whether the seizure is focal. Unilateral twitching of an arm, sensory experience, or flashes in one visual field or another are extremely helpful symptoms suggesting the site of the source of seizures. An olfactory aura may indicate that the seizure is coming from the temporal lobe, but it may not be possible to tell on which side it began.

An abrupt loss of consciousness, followed by *tonic* or *clonic seizures,* is characteristic of a generalized seizure. It is most important to look for any evidence of focal motor phenomena during such an episode. Unilateral seizures with motor disturbances limited to one arm or leg or the face clearly indicate the source of the seizure as being in the opposite hemisphere in the motor cortex. Focal seizures are extremely important because they clearly indicate a focal lesion. The most common cause of focal lesions in individuals who have epilepsy beginning past age 40 is a brain tumor. If seizures are observed by others, there is usually no dispute concerning an accurate diagnosis. If there is doubt whether episodic loss of consciousness is due to a seizure, or to syncope, the post-ictal period may provide a useful clue. Virtually always, if loss of consciousness is due to a seizure, a patient may experience a brief period of post-ictal confusion, sometimes lasting as short a time as a few seconds and sometimes lasting hours to days; this is highly suggestive of seizure rather than syncope. Phenomena such as incontinence, tongue biting, or injury during the seizure also suggest seizure disorder.

Seizures are a symptom. Elderly individuals who have seizures must be carefully evaluated. If there is no preceding history suggestive of stroke, they are then considered possible candidates for brain tumor and evaluated specifically for that. If neurologic examination shows evidence of a focal abnormality, the chances are great that a brain tumor is the source. If there is a history of *gradual onset* of focal neurologic defect plus development of seizures, brain tumor is almost certain. If there is no focal neurologic abnormality and the seizures are focal, brain tumor is still quite likely. If the seizure was generalized and neurologic examination reveals no focal abnormality, the chances of brain tumor being the cause are diminished but not absent (in the elderly) and further evaluation is always indicated.

Currently, the most effective means of evaluation is by a computerized brain scan. This will show intracranial masses, blood collections, and hypodense areas suggesting *cerebral infarction.* When there is an abrupt-onset seizure, accompanied by abrupt-onset hemiparesis or hemisensory loss, the cause of the seizure is most often vascular with cerebral infarction, although hemorrhage into a brain tumor or primary intracerebral hemorrhage cannot be excluded. It is peculiar that cerebral infarction does not produce a higher incidence of seizures, but characteristically it does not. A common seizure event occurring soon after a stroke is "partial continuous epilepsy." This involves continuous seizure activity in a part, such as part of the face or the hand, on the side opposite the stroke. There may be a continuous spiking focus on the electroencephalogram (EEG). Partial continuous seizures are often difficult to control with anticonvulsants and tend to disappear spontaneously with time. Later, patients with stroke with clear-cut evidence of hemiparesis may develop generalized or focal seizures that can usually be controlled adequately with anticonvulsants.

Seizures in the elderly are rarely, if ever, idiopathic. There is almost always a reason for their presence, and the reasons are generally serious ones that require attention. Frequently, the cause of the seizure is a treatable condition that should be dealt with before the brain is destroyed by the process causing the seizure.

For patients who develop seizures during or after the taking of medication, avoidance of medication in the future is the best course of action. For individuals addicted to or dependent on short-acting barbiturates or other tranquilizing drugs, this may be difficult. Withdrawal from medication is especially difficult for the chronic alcoholic who, after long periods of drinking and stopping, may develop seizures. The problems faced by these elderly individuals are similar to those encountered in younger age groups.

If a cause for seizures in an elderly person cannot be determined and if they recur, anticonvulsants should be given on a regular basis. The most useful anticonvulsant is diphenylhydantoin, given in doses starting at 300 mg per day. Blood levels are measured at 1 and 2 weeks to determine whether a therapeutic level has been obtained. Generally the range for a therapeutic level is from 10 to 20 $\mu$g/ml of diphenylhydantoin. This is usually all that is necessary to control seizures, but additional anticonvulsants such as phenobarbital may be needed for complete control in unusual instances.

If, during the initial evaluation of an elderly patient with seizures, a cause cannot be determined, the possibility that the patient has a brain tumor cannot be dismissed. Such patients should be followed regularly to determine whether new evidence of brain dysfunction has occurred. This is most successfully done by performing a routine neurologic examination and by asking those who know or who live with the patient to observe whether, when seizures reoccur, if there is any evidence that they are focal, and whether there is any change in personality and intellectual level.

When seizures follow an intracerebral hemorrhage or a cerebral infarction, the problem of the paresis and the disability associated with it are usually much more serious than seizures that can be controlled by anticonvulsants.

On no account should an elderly individual who develops seizures past the age of 60 be dismissed as having idiopathic epilepsy. A careful search for a cause should always be made.

## SPINAL CORD DISEASE

### *Spinal Cord Compression*

Aside from trauma, spinal cord compression in the elderly is uncommon. It can develop slowly and insidiously or with surprising rapidity. Acute spinal cord dysfunction in older persons is usually caused by compression from tumor, either primary or metastatic, or from spinal cord infarction. Metastatic tumors compressing the spinal cord tend to cause problems more acutely than primary spinal cord tumors. The symptoms are similar, usually consisting of back or neck pain, gradually progressive weakness in the legs and arms, poor balance, difficulty walking, and difficulty in climbing stairs and getting out of chairs. Symptoms may develop over a few hours and render a patient paraplegic or quadriplegic. In a patient who has a known malignancy, complaints of leg weakness or difficulties with gait are always serious and require prompt attention. If evaluation and treatment are ignored or delayed, paralysis may become complete and permanent, usually accompanied by incontinence. The examination of such patients may reveal weakness and reduced or lost reflexes, often accompanied by extensor plantar responses. Sometimes only weakness is present. Complaints of new or increasing leg, back, or arm weakness should never be ignored in the elderly, especially if there is a history of malignancy.

Further evaluation should be carried out immediately, including x-ray films of the spine and computed tomography (CT scanning).

If there is a clear-cut decrease in motor and sensory level, treatment can be directed at the appropriate spinal cord level. Usually, however, myelography is needed for accurate localizing of the site of the lesion. When it is likely that metastatic tumor is the cause of cord compression, decamethazone therapy and irradiation of the area of compression are initiated. These procedures must be carried out on an emergency basis, because if compression is not relieved rapidly, the prognosis for recovery is very poor. When there is no history or evidence of malignancy elsewhere, an exploratory laminectomy is recommended.

### *Spinal Cord Infarction*

Spinal cord stroke is uncommon at any age, but it occasionally occurs in the elderly. The thoracic portion is the most vulnerable area of the spinal cord because the limited segmental arterial input to the anterior spinal artery reduces the chance that collateral circulation might prevent infarction. A patient with spinal cord infarction usually reports the abrupt onset of back pain, which may radiate around the trunk, and the sudden onset of leg weakness or paralysis, with few complaints of sensory disturbance other than pain. On examination, there is loss of voluntary movement below the level of infarction. Initially, although reflexes are lost, there may be no signs of corticospinal tract disease or major sensory loss, thus giving rise to the diagnosis of hysteria. Urinary retention is the rule and patients may eventually develop distended bladders.

The infarction generally involves the center of the spinal cord, which is dependent on the anterior spinal artery for its blood supply. This area contains the corticospinal tracts and anterior horns. The sensory tracts are more peripheral in the cord, and there is a better chance of blood supply coming from the posterior spinal arteries and surface branches.

With time, pain subsides and evidence of corticospinal tract dysfunction becomes clear on neurologic examination, with hyperreflexia, spasticity, and extensor plantar responses. Bladder and bowel incontinence are the rule and require special care if any degree of automatic and predictable bladder and bowel function is to restored.

## *Chronic Spinal Cord Disease*

The most common cause of chronic spinal cord disease is *cervical spondylosis* with cervical myelopathy. This is almost exclusively a geriatric condition. The cause of the condition is degenerative arthritis, common in the cervical spinal column of most individuals 60 years of age or over. Hypertrophic arthritic changes that occur around the intervertebral spaces in the cervical spine often become sizable enough to compress the spinal cord and interfere with blood supply of the spinal cord on its ventral surface. Blood supply to the spinal cord primarily comes from the anterior spinal artery and its sulcal and coronal arteries. These enter the center of the cord and supply the corticospinal tracts, the anterior horns, and the crossing sensory fibers. It is believed that with overgrowth of bone around the vertebral spaces, there is compromise of the usual space for the spinal cord, and with repeated flexion and extension of the neck, there is intermittent compression of the arterial supply to the spinal cord. When this occurs over a long period of time, it produces a gradual ischemic cell loss and the onset of rather specific symptoms of myelopathy associated with cervical spondylosis.

Characteristically, patients report that they begin having difficulty walking. They may complain of leg weakness and stiffness, and when observed, they may have developed a slightly spastic gait. They also may be aware that hand function has deteriorated, with loss of strength in some of the intrinsic muscles. At times patients may report loss of muscle substance in the hands and forearms. Also they may be aware of some loss of sensory perception, usually for pain and temperature, in the fingers of one or both hands. These symptoms progress until the patient is unable to walk. Associated urgency and frequency of urination and at times urinary incontinence develop. Patients often report limitation of motion in the neck and pain in the neck on flexion, extension, and rotation.

### Physical Examination

On neurologic examination, there is a highly characteristic picture. There is no evidence of involvement of head function and no evidence of atrophy or change in muscles supplied by the cranial nerves or upper two or three cervical roots. Examination of the hands usually reveals specific weaknesses in intrinsic hand muscles and at times fasciculations with biceps weakness and preservation of triceps strength. Examination may reveal atrophy of these muscles, reduced biceps tendon reflexes, and hyperactive triceps reflex. Examination of sensory perception may reveal impaired perception of pain and temperature in the hands. In the lower extremities, the patient exhibits descreased voluntary motion, difficulty with rapid skilled movement, hyperactivity of knee and ankle reflexes, extensor plantar responses, and an increase in resistance to passive motion. These findings indicate corticospinal tract dysfunction. On sensory examination, in the lower extremities there may be some impairment of vibration and position perception. The combination of upper motor neuron disturbances in the arms and hands and corticospinal tract disturbances in the lower extremities, with a degree of spinal cord dysfunction in the cervical region, is characteristic of the condition. X-ray films of the neck generally show evidence of marked osteoarthritic disease at the level of C-4, C-5, C-6, and C-7. The most common site is C-5/C-6.

When this combination of symptoms and signs is evident and there is x-ray evidence of cervical osteoarthritic changes with limitation of motion in the head and neck, a lumbar myelogram should be done. If there is marked encroachment on the dye column in the cervical spinal region, and especially if there is a block in this region, decompressive laminectomy should be considered. This can be done posteriorly with removal of a lamina over several sections to allow the spinal cord more space or by anterior removal of the osteoarthritic lipping between the cervical vertebrae. This relieves the encroachment by the bony changes in the cervical spine. Surgery helps the condition and may stop further progression of the disorder.

### Differential Diagnosis

The differential diagnosis needs to be carefully evaluated, since a similar combination of symptoms and signs can be noted in patients with amyotrophic lateral sclerosis (ALS). If electromyography (EMG) shows fasciculations in any muscles other than those of the upper extremities, the diagnosis of amyotrophic lateral sclerosis should be seriously considered. Careful examination of the thigh and muscles of the head and neck should routinely be done, especially if there is any suggestion of fasciculation seen on examination.

## AMYOTROPHIC LATERAL SCLEROSIS

Amyotrophic lateral sclerosis (ALS) is a progressive disorder of unknown cause, characterized by muscle weakness and wasting and by motor neuron degeneration in the spinal cord and brain. Rarely found in the elderly, its most common period of onset is between the ages of 40 and 60. It occurs more often among men than women. Geographically, the areas of highest frequency are the island of Guam and some parts of Japan. In a small percentage of cases, ALS is familial.

### *Clinical Features*

Weakness, usually symmetric, most often starts in the peripheral muscles of the arms and legs and, occasionally, in the muscles of the head and neck. Ultimately, the muscles supplied by the cranial nerves (resulting in disordered speech, difficulty swallowing, and facial weakness) and the muscles of the arms and legs are almost always involved; occasionally, the muscles of the head and neck are affected. Along with the progressive weakness, the muscles atrophy and weight loss occurs. Fasciculations, usually observed by the physician on examination, are occasionally noted by the patient. Patients often report discomfort from muscle cramps.

### *Physical Examination and Diagnosis*

On examination, the involved muscles are weak and wasted. Fasciculations of these muscles can usually be seen easily, and fibrillations may be found on EMG. Patients often have impaired tongue movement, weakness of palate, difficulties in swallowing, and facial and jaw weakness. Deep tendon reflexes may be hyperactive, and there may be abnormal reflex responses such as an extensor plantar response. These indicate some degree of corticospinal tract involvement. At times reflexes may be absent or depressed. No sensory disturbances are found.

Confirmation of the disorder can be obtained by EMG examination of weak muscles, which will almost invariably show fibrillations and fasciculations.

### *Prognosis and Course*

The course of ALS is progressive, the mean survival time being approximately 3 years after diagnosis. If the disorder predominantly affects musculature of the head and neck, demise may be hastened by impaired respiration and aspiration. The course of the illness is not altered by the age of the patient, but older individuals are less likely to withstand the rigors of respiratory and other forms of supportive treatment that may be necessary.

### *Differential Diagnosis*

It is most important to make certain that the patient's disorder is not due to a treatable condition common in the elderly. The most frequently encountered differential is with spinal cord compression caused by cervical osteoarthritis. In this condition, muscle atrophy and weakness are largely confined to muscles supplied by cervical spinal cord segments. Weakness and wasting predominantly involve the hand and arm muscles with signs of corticospinal tract involvement in the legs. In ALS, weakness, wasting, and fasciculations are found in both the upper and lower extremities and in muscles of the head and neck.

### *Treatment*

There is no treatment; supportive measures are all that can be offered as the disease relentlessly takes its course. A realistic problem facing those who who care for ALS patients is whether supportive care should be given and, if so, how long it should be carried out. There is little to be gained for the elderly in supportive treatment with artificial respiration when there is a hopeless outlook.

## PERIPHERAL NEUROPATHY

Peripheral neuropathy is a common neurologic disorder in the elderly. It is frequently overlooked as the cause of abnormal gait, poor balance, and leg weakness. When a patient complains of increasing difficulty in walking in the dark, bumping into objects or falling, unexplained difficulties with gait, or recent onset of concern about balance and a fear of falling, a careful examination should be conducted for peripheral neuropathy. Patients also may complain of paresthesia (abnormal sensations) and numbness.

Evidence of peripheral neuropathy appears in the lower extremities first, in those peripheral nerves which have the largest axons. The disorder generally begins gradually, and patients usually have a great difficulty in determining exactly when their symptoms began. It is usually symmetric in presentation, although some presentations may be asymmetric. In the absence of trauma, asymmetric neuropathy is suggestive of diabetes mellitus. Frequently, the disorder is completely asymptomatic; this is characteristic of diabetic peripheral neuropathy in most cases.

As neuropathy progresses, the sensory motor levels move up the lower extremities and, later, the patient may experience paresthesia and loss of sensory perception and strength in the upper extremity as well.

### *Physical Examination*

On examination, weakness and atrophy of the more peripheral muscles will be noted. Tendon reflexes are usually absent or reduced, or they are obtainable only by reinforcement. There is no impairment of rapid skilled movements if strength remains to move a particular part. Evidence of fatigability can generally be found, and the usual resistance to passive motion of a limb is somewhat reduced. On examination for sensory perception, the physician may note decreased vibratory perception and position sense, reduced perception of pain and touch and, frequently, hyperalgesia to pressure. Peripheral neuropathy may predominantly affect sensory systems, or its effect may be predominantly motor; generally, it is a mixture of both.

Most instances of peripheral neuropathy in the elderly are due to metabolic causes, principally diabetes and nutritional deficiency. Occasionally, one encounters toxic neuropathies in which ingestion of a medication or heavy metal interferes with neural metabolism. Chronic alcoholism is often associated with peripheral neuropathy, usually resulting from nutritional deficiency. Rarely, no explainable cause can be found.

### *Diabetic Peripheral Neuropathy*

The most common cause of peripheral neuropathy in the elderly is diabetic neurovascular disease. This tends to be asymptomatic and is usually discovered when examination of an elderly diabetic patient reveals absent ankle jerks, some weakness of dorsiflexion of the toes and feet, reduced vibratory sense at the ankles, and some impairment in position sense in the toes. Occasionally, patients report difficulty with gait and balance, pain, paresthesia, and weakness in legs and feet.

There is usually an easily detectable increase in sensory level of pain and touch perception at the ankles or the midportion of the lower extremity. These changes in neurologic function may be the first evidence that an individual has diabetes, and an elderly patient who has these findings should be checked for this disorder. In addition, older individuals who are known to be diabetic should be screened carefully for symptoms of peripheral neuropathy.

#### COURSE

Diabetic peripheral neuropathy can be progressive to the point where it becomes disabling. It may produce difficulties with balance and walking, especially when vision cannot be used to correct for inadequate position sense in the legs and feet. It may also be associated with autonomic dysfunction, with orthostatic hypotension, impotence, and urinary and fecal incontinence. Advanced disturbances of the autonomic system may also produce changes in intestinal activity with gastric atony. Peripheral sensory impairment may become marked enough that unnoticed joint destruction may result from minor injury and a Charcot's joint develops, especially in the ankle joints.

At times diabetic neuropathy may cause pain. This occurs when there is evidence of local involvement of a peripheral nerve, with muscle weakness, atrophy, pain and tenderness in the same area, usually the thigh *(diabetic amyotrophy)*. This presentation, usually asymmetric, is not uncommon in the elderly and is believed to be due to involvement of the small vessels of peripheral nerves, causing infarction of a nerve branch. This cause has not been firmly established, however.

Diabetic neuropathy may involve the oculomotor nerves, especially the third nerve. Patients will note the sudden onset of diplopia and ptosis and on examination are found to have weakness or paralysis of abduction, upward, and downward gaze. The pupil is often spared. This neuropathy has been related to occlusion of small vessels supplying the nerve. Individuals with peripheral neuropathy due to diabetes may have nutritional deficiency associated with major loss of weight. However, this is extremely uncommon because most diabetics now receive adequate treatment before this situation occurs.

#### Treatment

Treatment is rarely satisfactory. More careful regulation of diabetes has been recommended. This is believed to halt progression of the neuropathy, but it does not improve lost function. Patients with orthostatic hypotension can sometimes obtain relief of symptoms by leg binding or tight stockings or by the use of fluorinated steroids to increase blood volume. The condition tends to be progressive, and even these measures at some point will not be effective. Treatment of incontinence in such patients is extremely difficult, and external catheter or absorptive clothes are used to prevent wet and macerated skin. Intestinal stasis that is due to diabetic neuropathy can sometimes be alleviated by the use of dopamine antagonists (metaclopramide, domperidone).

### *Nutritional Neuropathy*

Elderly individuals who live alone and cook for themelves often become negligent about the character of their diet, frequently existing on meals that are totally inadequate in vitamins. After a period of time on such a diet, evidence of peripheral neuropathy may develop. Chronic alcoholics are also susceptible in this regard. Alcoholism is associated with a high carbohydrate intake and a low intake of thiamine and other vitamins, eventually leading to impaired neural metabolism and failure of peripheral nerve function. Patients with nutritional deficiency/peripheral neuropathy should be carefully screened for the possibility of chronic alcoholism.

Nutritional deficiency neuropathy tends to be symmetric, producing both motor and sensory deficiencies simultaneously. The most striking disturbances are found early in the feet, with footdrop as evidence of weakness in the lower extremities. Usually, the patient complains of a "pins and needles" sensation in the feet and often pain in the soles on standing or walking. Examination reveals muscle atrophy and weakness in the anterior tibial muscles and, to a lesser extent, in the posterior leg muscles. Tendon reflexes may be absent, and resistance to passive motion may be reduced.

Decreases in vibratory perception and position sense will usually be detectable. There is almost always hyperalgesia to pressure in the involved parts, especially the toes and soles of the feet. Decreased perception of pain and touch can usually be found. The degree of the involvement of the peripheral nerves is evidenced by the height of the level. In most cases when peripheral neuropathy causes a decreased sensory level at the knees, patients will have major difficulty in function, thus calling the physician's attention to this disturbance if it has not been noted already.

A number of specific vitamin deficiencies that can occur in the elderly have been associated with peripheral neuropathy. Thiamine (vitamin $B_1$) deficiency produces a beriberi-like syndrome with and without peripheral edema. Thiamine deficiency is usually manifested by peripheral neuropathy without edema, or dry beriberi. True beriberi with peripheral edema and cardiac failure is extremely unlikely in Western societies. Pellagra, a result of niacin (vitamin $B_3$) deficiency, can be associated with peripheral neuropathy; almost invariably it is accompanied by some evidence of dementia, dermatitis, and diarrhea.

### *Other Forms of Neuropathy*

*Pernicious anemia* may also be associated with peripheral neuropathy. Usually this is accompanied by evidence of damage to the posterior and lateral spinal cord columns and anemia. At times, however, symptoms of peripheral neuropathy may be the initial evidence of pernicious anemia.

A variety of peripheral neuropathies have been reported to occur with *carcinoma.* A primary sensory neuropathy has been described in patients who have bronchogenic carcinoma, and mixed motor and sensory neuropathies have been described in individuals with gastrointestinal, ovarian, thyroid, and bronchial carcinoma. A motor and sensory neuropathy has been observed in patients with lymphoma. Although these occurrences are rare, these causes should be considered when unexplained peripheral neuropathy is detected.

*Toxic neuropathy* may perhaps be less frequent in elderly individuals than in the young and middle aged, because elderly individuals are generally retired and no longer active at work where they might be exposed to a variety of toxins. Lead neuropathy, occasionally seen in elderly individuals, may be associated with a peripheral neuropathy in which pain, parasthesias and wristdrop predominate.

Certain medications may cause peripheral neuropathy. These include isonizid, stilbamadine, and emetine. Occasionally, peripheral neuropathy occurs with corticosteroid administration and with nonsteroidal anti-inflammatory agents such as phenylbutazone.

### *Treatment*

When the cause of the peripheral neuropathy is identified, treatment can usually be outlined for that particular condition. For patients who have a nutritional deficiency, a wholesome diet with adequate vitamin intake is essential. For those with inability to absorb vitamin $B_{12}$, injections of vitamin $B_{12}$ are critical to interrupting the process and restoring some function. In both situations, the progress toward recovery may be quite slow, occurring over a period of many months. Usually, the acute symptoms of parasthesias and pain resolve fairly rapidly when adequate nutrition is established. For those patients who have had exposure to toxic substances that can cause neuropathy, removal of patient from contact with these substances is essential. In specific conditions (e.g., arsenic poisoning), heavy metal chelating agents such as dimercaprol (BAL) may be useful. When peripheral neuropathy is associated with carcinoma, treatment should be primarily directed toward the removal of the primary tumor with hope that some of the peripheral nerve damage will be reversed.

At times, patients with chronic progressive peripheral neuropathy will exhibit no evidence of nutritional deficiency, diabetes, deficiency in absorption of vitamin $B_{12}$ or exposure to heavy metals or drugs that could have produced impaired peripheral nerve function. There is very little that can be done in these cases, although treatment with nutritional support and high vitamin intake has been recommended.

## ACUTE ONSET PERIPHERAL NEUROPATHY (GUILLAIN-BARRÉ) SYNDROME

Peripheral neuropathy may have an acute onset with rapid development of ascending weakness and, at times, loss of sensation. This condition usually begins in the lower extremities, spreading to the upper extremities, but the symptoms may begin in the upper extremities. Guillain-Barré syndrome is frequent in the elderly, and its incidence rises with increasing age.

Frequently, the patient will give a history of a gastrointestinal or respiratory illness preceding the onset of weakness. Weakness beginning in the legs can rapidly spread to involve the entire body and can seriously impair respiration. Often there is facial weakness, with unilateral or bilateral and ophthalmoplegia being noted in some cases.

On examination, motor signs are more common than sensory. There is flaccid limb paralysis with absent reflexes. Sensory impairment is usually slight and can be completely absent. The neurologic changes are caused by swelling of nerve roots which may produce axonal degeneration.

Recovery from paralysis is the rule, but patients may be left with permanent motor loss in the peripheral hand and leg muscles. For the elderly, recovery is less certain, and the hazards and difficulties of caring for patients who are completely paralyzed and require artificial ventilation decrease the chances of a hopeful outcome. Although most motor recovery occurs within 4 to 6 months, complete recovery may require 12 to 36 months. There is no specific treatment, and survival depends on good medical management of respiratory failure and severe weakness and especially on skilled nursing care.

## MYASTHENIA GRAVIS

Myasthenia gravis is an autoimmune disease that interferes with neural muscular transmission as a result of immunologic destruction of acetylcholine receptors. The cause is yet undetermined. The disease can have its onset in any age group, including the elderly. In young adults it is more common in women, but it is equally common in men and women past the age of 40.

Classically, the most frequently encountered symptoms are disturbances of eye movement. The patient usually complains of double vision (diplopia) or is noted to have ptosis. Occasionally, patients will also be observed to have dysarthria or show some evidence of facial weakness or weakness in the muscles of the neck. They will occasionally report difficulty getting out of chairs or difficulty walking up and down stairs. They may also be aware that symptoms of weakness are more intense at some times of the day than others. Frequently patients find that they feel better earlier in the day. As the day passes on, they become increasingly weak.

When patients expressing these complaints are examined, there is usually objective evidence of weakness in muscles. Most often there is some evidence of ptosis, usually asymmetric, and weakness in eye muscles supplied by both the oculomotor nerve and the abducent nerve. It is striking that almost invariably the disturbance in eye movements is asymmetric. Proximal muscles are generally weaker than distal muscles, and the pattern is generally asymmetric. Skilled movements are usually normal unless weakness is pronounced. Sensory perception is normal. Evidence of easy fatigability can be confirmed by repeated tapping of the biceps or patellar reflex; the response will decline with repeated stimulation. At times there will be some loss of muscle substance. Electromyography shows disturbance in neuromuscular transmission with declining responses to electrical stimulation.

Occasionally myasthenia gravis is associated with a thymoma. Although this most often is evident in younger patients, every patient with myasthenia gravis should have a chest film taken to determine whether a thymoma is present. Myasthenia gravis can also occur with hyperthyroidism.

## Treatment

Treatment involves using drugs that block the destruction of acetylcholine by acetylcholinesterase. When the diagnosis is in question, the use of an intravenous anticholinesterase agent such as endrophonium (10 mg) can be helpful. In the presence of this disease, administration of this drug usually produces dramatic relief of the symptoms for up to 1 hour. For maintenance therapy, neostigmine is generally the drug of choice. It is given on a regular basis orally, starting at doses of 15 mg three times a day and building up with time to achieve maximum relief of symptoms. This may require doses reaching more than 150 mg per day. Other anticholinesterase agents with a longer period of action are pyridostigmine and ambenonium. At times, patients benefit by epinephrine or ephedrine or, occasionally, adrenocorticotropic hormone (ACTH) or adrenal corticosteriods. Recently, plasmapheresis has been effective in reducing the levels of immune complexes directed against acetylcholine receptors and has in some cases dramatically relieved the symptoms.

In older patients, myasthenia gravis may be limited to the extraocular muscles, and there may be complaints of diplopia and ptosis. Oral medication rarely successfully corrects these abnormalities; the problems may be relieved in part by alternating eye patches to avoid diplopia and eyelid lifts attached to eyeglasses to overcome ptosis.

## Adverse Drug Reactions

Symptoms of myasthenia gravis can be made worse by a variety of other medications, especially some antibiotics. These include polymyxin (such as colistin, polymyxin B), and aminoglycoside (streptomycin, kanamycin, gentamicin, tobramycin). The unnecessary use of any of these antibiotics should be avoided, especially in patients with generalized myasthenia. Patients with myasthenia are hyper-reactive to agents that produce a degree of neuromuscular block (procainamide, propanolol, phenytoin, chlorpromazine) and to CNS depressants (barbiturates, narcotics).

Myasthenia gravis can occasionally remit spontaneously. In other instances, the course is not strikingly progressive. In some patients, symptoms may worsen abruptly as a result of a "myasthenic crisis." In such a crisis, for unexplained reasons, increased amount of anticholinesterase drugs are required; alternatively, sudden worsening of symptoms may be due to an overdose of these drugs, causing depolarization of the motor end plate and block. The symptoms in these two states are similar.

Treatment is first directed toward support of respiration. Testing the patient with a short-acting anticholinesterase preparation (endrophonium) may help determine which mechanism is involved. This should be attempted only if the patient is being cared for in an intensive care unit that is equipped to give assisted ventilation. If the symptom worsening is due to cholinergic intoxication, anticholinesterase medication should be stopped and supportive therapy given; after a few days, anticholinesterase agents can be restarted. The mortality associated with these crises is high unless proper supportive care is available and applied.

### References

**_Parkinson's Disease_**

Birkmayer W, Hornikiewicz, O: Advances in Parkinsonism Basel, Roche, 1976.

Dorros S: Parkinson's: A Patient's View. Cabin John, Md., Seven Locks Press, 1981.
*A patient's experience with Parkinson's disease.*

Javey-Agid F, et al: Biochemical neuropathy of Parkinson's disease. Neurol 40:189, 1984.

*An up-to-date discussion of the basis for understanding Parkinson's disease.*

Marsden CD, Falk S: Disorders of Movement. Boston, Buttersworth Scientific, 1982.

*A good review and discussion of all movement disorders.*

McDowell FH, Barbeau A: Second Canadian-American Conference on Parkinson's Disease. New York, Raven Press, 1974.

*Good background for pathology and usefulness of L-dopa up to that date.*

Poirier LJ, Sourkes TL, Bedard PJ: The Extrapyramidal System and Its Disorders. Advances in Neurology Series, No. 6, New York, Raven Press, 1979.

Quinn NP: Anti-parkinson drugs today. Drugs 28:236, 1984.

*An excellent review of treatment of Parkinson's disease, up to date and beautifully referenced.*

### Epilepsy

Penfield WG, Rasmussen TB: Epileptic Seizure Patterns. Springfield, Ill, Thomas, 1951.

Scholf C, Yarnell PR, Ernest MD: Origin of seizures in elderly patients. JAMA 238:1177, 1977.

Schmidt RP, Wilder BJ: Epilepsy. Philadelphia, F.A. Davis, 1968.

Turner WA: The Morrison lectures on epilepsy. Br Med J 1:733, 1910.

Woodbury DM, Penvy JK, Schmidt RP: Antiepileptic Drugs. New York, Raven Press, 1972.

### Spinal Cord Disease

Brain WR, Northfield D, Wiltinson M: The neurological manifestations of cervical spondylosis. Brain 75:187, 1952.

Nugent GR: Clinicopathologic correlations in cervical spondylosis. Neurology 9:273, 1959.

*These references, while old, are excellent.*

### Amyotrophic Lateral Sclerosis

Mulder DW. The Diagnosis and Treatment of amyotrophic Lateral Sclerosis. Boston, Houghton-Mifflin, 1980.

### Peripheral Neuropathy

Dyck PJ, Thomas, RK, Lambert EH, Bunge R: Peripheral Neuropathy, 2nd ed. Philadelphia, W.B. Saunders Co., 1984.

*This four-volume text provides an up-to-date summary of the extensive information available on this subject.*

Sumner AJ: The Physiology of Peripheral Nerve Disease. Philadelphia, W.B. Saunders Co., 1980.

### Guillain-Barré Syndrome

Dowling PC, Cook SD, Prineas JW: Guillaine-Barré syndrome. Ann Neurol (Suppl) 9:1, 1981.

*This symposium reviews recent information on etiology, diagnosis and treatment of this syndrome.*

### Myasthenia Gravis

Lisak, RP, Barchi RL: Myasthenia Gravis. Philadelphia, W.B. Saunders Co., 1982.

Oosterhuis H. JGH: Myasthenia Gravis, New York: Churchill Livingstone, 1984.

Walton J: Disorders of Voluntary Muscle. New York, Churchill Livingstone, 1981.

## Chapter 23

# Sleep and Aging

*Sonia Ancoli-Israel*
*Daniel F. Kripke*

As we get older, many of us become aware of changes in our sleep. Older people sleep less deeply, wake up more frequently during the night, and awaken earlier in the morning. In the past, it was thought that older people need less sleep because they are less active. However, research has shown that healthy sleep durations are about the same in older and younger adults. This chapter will examine the sleep of elderly people — how sleep changes, why sleep changes, and the consequences of these changes.

## NATURAL HISTORY AND COURSE OF SLEEP: OBJECTIVE SLEEP PARAMETERS

Sleep is divided into two types: rapid eye movement (REM) sleep and non-rapid eye movement (NREM) sleep. NREM is further subdivided into four stages: stage 1, 2, 3, and 4. Stage 1 is the very lightest level of sleep. Stages 2, 3, and 4 get progressively deeper. To study sleep, one needs to record, at minimum, brain waves using electroencephalography (EEG); eye movement; and muscle tension of the chin.

During NREM, eye movements are slow and there is a normal degree of muscle tension (Fig. 23–1). During REM, which is the dream stage, eye movements are rapid (thus the name — rapid eye movement sleep) and there is almost no muscle tension (Fig. 23–2). In fact, during REM we are paralyzed except for the eyes and the respiratory system. This is a protective mechanism that keeps us from acting out our dreams. When people wake up from their dreams, they sometimes experience a feeling of paralysis. This sleep paralysis usually lasts only a few moments and is normal.

During the night we cycle through the different stages of sleep. As we get older, the pattern of cycles begins to change (Fig. 23–3). Although there have been many studies examining sleep patterns in humans, relatively few have dealt with the aged. Feinberg and colleagues have done some of the most extensive research in this area. The general conclusion that can be drawn is that the sleep of the older person is more disturbed. When comparing young adults (19 to 36 years) with normal aged adults (64 to 92 years), Feinberg and associates[1,2] reported that total sleep time and stage 4 (EEG slow-wave) sleep were less for normal aged adults than for younger adults. Sleep latency, (i.e., the time from when the person goes to bed until first sleep occurs) was greater for normal aged adults than for young adults. In addition, normal aged adults had more arousals during the night than did young adults. These results have been supported by many other researchers including Prinz,[3] Prinz and Raskind,[4] and Spiegel.[5]

## EPIDEMIOLOGY OF SLEEP COMPLAINTS: SUBJECTIVE REPORTS

Sleep complaints are a major health problem in the United States. Ten per cent to 45 per cent of individuals of all ages responding to a series of surveys done from 1959 to 1979 complained of "insomnia" or trouble sleeping.[6,7] In each study, the prevalence of subjective sleep complaints increased with age and was highest among people over 65 years of age. Subjective self-reported sleep patterns are not always consistent with the objective findings. There is general agreement that increases in age are associated with reported increases in subjective total sleep time (TST);

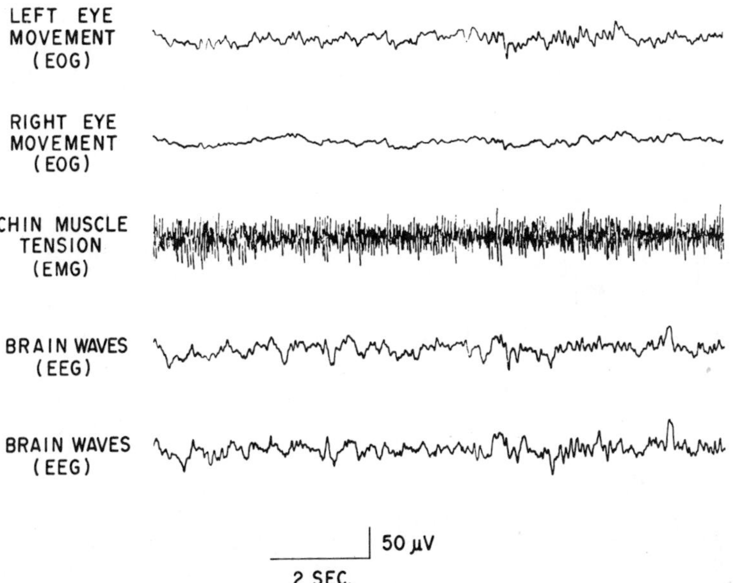


**Figure 23–1.** Non-rapid eye movement (NREM) sleep. Chin muscle tension is high, and brain waves are slow in frequency and high in amplitude. EOG = electro-oculogram; EMG = electromyogram; EEG = electroencephalogram.

sleep latency (SL), i.e., the time it takes to fall asleep; wake time after sleep onset (WASO); number of awakenings during the night; number of daytime naps; and use of sleeping pills.[8] Thus, self-reported subjective sleep increases with age, whereas objectively recorded sleep decreases.

Epidemiologic studies suggest that people with sleep complaints are at greater risk for excess mortality. From 1959 to 1960, the American Cancer Society distributed health questionnaires to 1,000,000 Americans, and after 6 years, 98.4 per cent follow-up was obtained. Kripke and associates[8a] found that in these data, about 6.5 per cent of all deaths were statistically associated with short sleep (under 7 hours) or long sleep (over 8 hours), that is, those that reported short or long sleep had a higher mortality

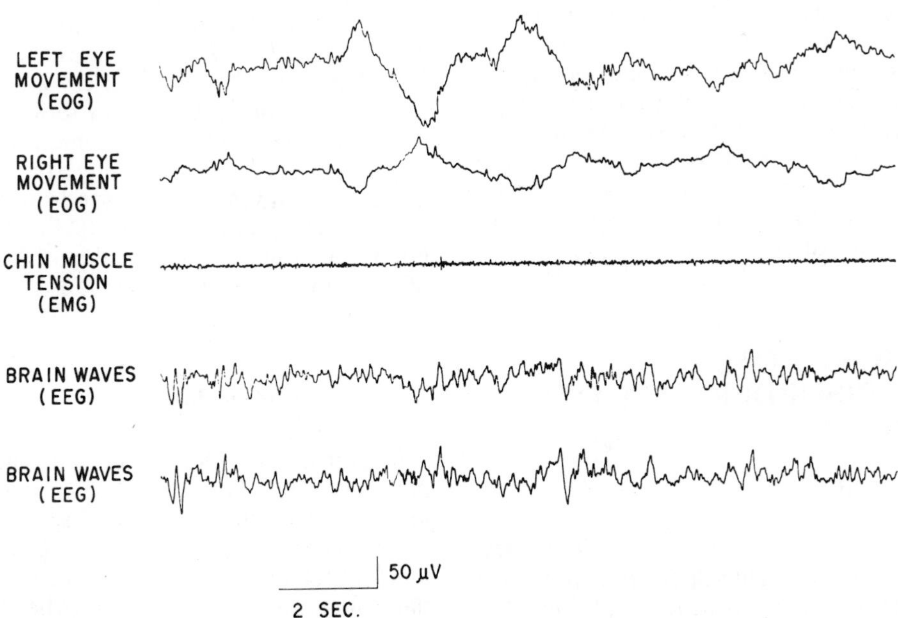


**Figure 23–2.** Rapid eye movement (REM) sleep. Chin muscle tension is very low and brain waves are faster in frequency and lower in amplitude than during NREM. EOG, electro-oculogram; EMG = electromyogram; EEG = electroencephalogram.

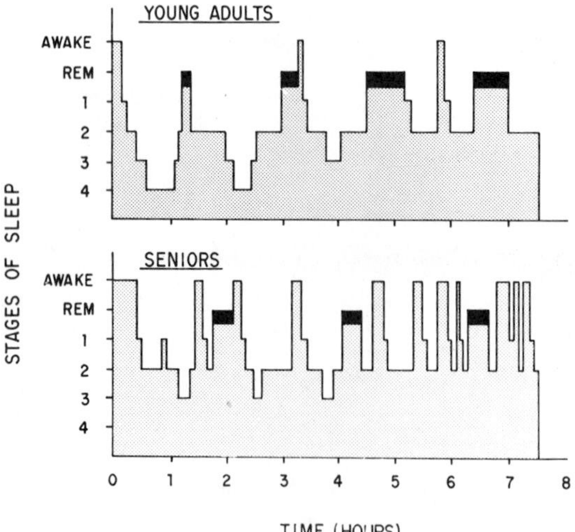


**Figure 23-3.** Normal sleep cycles. As we get older, it takes us longer to fall asleep and we have less deep sleep, more awakenings, and less REM.

rate at six-year follow-up. More deaths were associated with reported long sleep than with reported short sleep. Eighty-six per cent of deaths associated with reported long and short sleep occurred among those over 60 years of age. Similar results have been reported by Belloc.[9]

Since both the objective and subjective works indicate a higher rate of disturbances of sleep among the elderly, especially midsleep awakenings, it becomes necessary to re-evaluate the question of sleep disturbances in this population. The main question to be answered is whether these changes in sleep reflect normal maturation or pathologic processes. Our belief is that many of these changes are caused by one of two specific pathophysiologic processes, namely sleep apnea and nocturnal myoclonus. We will review these sleep disorders in detail because they are especially prevalent in the aged. We will then review the more general procedure for making diagnoses and some of the other sleep disorders.

# THE MOST COMMON SLEEP DISORDERS AMONG THE AGED

## *Sleep Apnea*

Sleep apnea is one of the most serious sleep disorders and can be a life-threatening problem. Sleep apnea is a repetitive process of respiratory cessation during sleep. The sleep apnea syndromes encompass three disorders: (1) Obstructive sleep apnea involves the collapse of the pharyngeal airway, with partial or complete blockage of airflow. (2) Central sleep apnea results from failure of the respiratory neurons to activate the phrenic and intercostal motor neurons that mediate respiratory movements. (3) Mixed sleep apnea is a combination of obstructive and central sleep apneas.[10,11] Sleep apnea is diagnosed when there is a cessation of breathing for at least 10 seconds, 30 times a night (or at least five episodes per hour of sleep). Most apnea episodes are terminated by transient arousals. In addition, episodes of hypoventilation may produce anoxia or arousal even when complete sleep apnea does not occur.

Recent reviews have suggested a variety of mechanisms, sometimes working in combination, that can cause sleep apnea, such as obesity; micrognathia; jaw or nasal deformities; thyroid, pituitary, or neurologic impairments; and alterations of respiratory reflexes during sleep.[10-13] Cardiac catheterization studies and studies done before and after tracheostomy[14] have shown that one of the consequences of sleep apnea is hypertension, both transient and persistent. Lugaresi and associates[12] have shown that the partial obstruction of snoring may also cause nocturnal hypertension. Carskadon and Dement[15] demonstrated that sleep apnea is associated with increased daytime sleepiness even among those elderly subjects who offer no sleep complaints. Other consequences of sleep apnea include anoxia, impairments of mental function, disorders of sleep maintenance, excessive daytime sleepiness, cardiac arrhythmias, cardiorespiratory failure, and ultimately, death during sleep.[16,17] Estimates from the Stanford Sleep Disorders Clinic case series[18] and from our own Sleep Disorders Clinic case series[19] indicate that when severe obstructive apnea is identified, 20 per cent of patients who refuse treatment die within the first year after the syndrome is recognized; most die of what is called "heart failure," but it is unclear if the heart failure was a sequela of sleep apnea or some other cause.

## *Nocturnal Myoclonus*

Nocturnal myoclonus (or periodic movements in sleep) is a syndrome of periodic leg jerks, which occur every 20 to 40 seconds during episodes lasting from minutes to hours. The leg jerks repeatedly arouse the patient.[20,21] Nocturnal myoclonus can be diagnosed when the number of periodic leg movements per hour of sleep is equal to or greater than five.[20] In this disorder, periodic episodes of leg jerk alternate with normal sleep. Since the patients are repeatedly disturbed, they often complain both of insomnia and excessive daytime sleepiness. Although some patients with this syndrome suffer partial disability, the long-term risk is unknown.

There is evidence[20,22] that nocturnal myoclonus is often associated with sleep apnea. Thus, this syndrome may have some pathophysiologic relationship with sleep apnea in addition to being an independent syndrome.[21]

### *Prevalence of Sleep Apnea and Nocturnal Myoclonus*

The true prevalence of sleep apnea or nocturnal myoclonus has not yet been established in any population. Dement and co-workers[23] have stated that the ultimate prevalence of sleep apnea may mirror the prevalence of loud snoring. Snoring increases markedly with age, and about 45 per cent of males and 32 per cent of females over age 65 are estimated to snore.[12] In a population sample from San Marino, Italy, Lugaresi[24] found that hypertension was twice as common among persons who snore, even after controlling for age, sex, and obesity. This suggests either that a large proportion of all those people who snore have sleep apnea or that the partial obstruction of snoring causes a similar form of cardiorespiratory compromise.

Several studies have suggested that sleep apnea is especially prevalent among the aged.[15,22,25-28] Carskadon and Dement[15] studied 24 asymptomatic elderly people in good general health and found that 37.5 per cent had sleep apnea. We studied 24 seniors with sleep complaints[22] and found that in this sample as well, 37.5 per cent had at least 30 episodes of apnea per night. (In addition, another 37.5 per cent had nocturnal myoclonus.)

We are currently studying the prevalence of sleep apnea in a randomly-selected sample of the elderly population in San Diego. In the first 100 subjects (65 years and over) who had their sleep recorded, 28 per cent had at least 30 episodes of sleep apnea on the recorded night. Of those with episodes of apnea, 21 per cent had sleep complaints, whereas 79 per cent had *no* sleep complaints. Of these same 100 subjects, 38 per cent had at least five leg jerks per hour of sleep. It is thus clear that mild sleep apnea and mild nocturnal myoclonus are very prevalent among older people, and more severe sleep apnea and nocturnal myoclonus are common.

## EVALUATION OF SLEEP COMPLAINTS

A scientific, medical approach to sleep disorders (both insomnia and excessive sleep) has been developed. With a carefully planned sequence of history-taking and all-night polygraphic recordings (polysomnograms), it has been possible to provide specific etiologic diagnoses and treatment recommendations for the majority of patients with sleep complaints.

### *Evaluation*

Evaluation begins with a complete sleep history. Whenever possible, it is important to interview the bed partner, because the bed partner often notices problems in the patient's sleep of which the patient is unaware.

A sleep history includes questions about a typical night's sleep, daytime functioning, and details of drug and alcohol use as well as the medical history. Key data include the following:

1. Time to bed (is it the same every night?)
2. Sleep latency (how long does it take to fall asleep?)
3. Number of arousals during the night
4. Final awakening time
5. Is the schedule the same on weekdays and weekends? (are times of waking up irregular?)
6. Estimated time spent actually sleeping at night

These data help determine the person's sleep pattern. It is often advisable to have the patient keep a sleep diary for several weeks prior to the interview to help provide a reliable perspective. Patients often learn more about their own patterns by keeping a diary.

Other questions attempt to differentiate between sleep apnea and nocturnal myoclonus. Does the patient snore, gasp for breath, stop breathing, or wake up confused (sleep apnea)? When the patient awakens, is there morning headache (sleep apnea)? Does the patient kick repetitively or have restless legs (nocturnal myoclonus)? However, it is important to remember that some patients will not be aware of any of these symptoms.

Questions on daytime functioning include the following:

1. How do you feel when you get up in the morning?
2. Do you nap deliberately during the day?
3. Do you find yourself falling asleep while

reading, watching television, at a play or movie, while talking with friends, during sex, or while driving?

These questions try to establish if the patient is falling asleep at inappropriate times, which would suggest disturbed sleep at night.

Drug, alcohol, food (caffeine), and medical histories are all important for determining interactions as well as the cause and effect of the sleep disturbance (see Incompatible Clinical Syndromes, page 245).

After the history is complete, it is sometimes necessary to refer the patient to a sleep disorders center for evaluation. A full-night recording can then be done. The traditional clinical polysomnogram records a minimum of seven channels: brain waves, using EEG; eye movement, using electro-oculography (EOG); chin muscle tension, using electromyography (EMG); leg movements using EMG, heart rate, using electrocardiography (EKG); and two respiration channels. The patient is recorded for at least one full night and sometimes for two nights.

A new portable recording device is now also available as a screening tool.[29] This portable recorder is placed on the patient in the afternoon, and the patient can be sent home to sleep in his or her own bed. (For hospital inpatients, the equipment can be used at the patient's bedside.) Respiration, wrist activity (for determining wake from sleep), and leg muscle tension are recorded. This system is more convenient and comfortable for the patient and less expensive than a laboratory polysomnogram.

It is only with a complete full-night recording that one can absolutely rule out sleep apnea. If a polysomnogram cannot be obtained, the clinician must proceed with extreme caution.

### *Differential Diagnosis*

The Association of Sleep Disorders Centers (ASDC)[30] has established a diagnostic classification system for sleep and arousal disorders. The two major categories of classification are Disorders of Initiating and Maintaining Sleep (DIMS) and Disorders of Excessive Somnolence (DOES). Other categories include Disorders of the Sleep-Wake Schedule and Dysfunctions Associated with Sleep, Sleep Stages, or Partial Arousals (Parasomnias).

The types of sleep disorders most commonly seen among the elderly are psychophysiologic insomnia, sleep apnea, nocturnal myoclonus, insomnia or hypersomnia associated with the use of drugs or alcohol, or insomnia secondary to a psychiatric or medical disorder (e.g., depression).

Psychophysiologic insomnia can be classified as either DIMS or DOES. When transient, this disorder is generally associated with acute emotional conflicts associated with anxiety or depression. Persistent psychophysiologic insomnia may be due to poor sleep habits, causing the process of going to sleep to become associated with frustration and arousal.[8]

As already mentioned, sleep apnea generally presents with complaints of excessive sleepiness (DOES) but may also present with complaints of insomnia (DIMS). The type of apnea associated with DIMS is usually central sleep apnea. Sleep apnea associated with DOES is usually obstructive or mixed. Patients with sleep apnea complain of snoring and difficulty breathing at night. These people often sleep in separate bedrooms because of their loud snoring. They have short sleep latencies but experience multiple arousals during the night. Often an interview with the spouse provides the best information.

People with nocturnal myoclonus most often complain of insomnia (DIMS) because of the multiple arousals caused by the repetitive leg kicks. Bed partners often sleep in separate beds because of the constant kicking. Once again, a certain proportion will complain of excessive daytime somnolence due to the disturbance of their sleep at night. In this case also, an interview with the bed partner is useful.

## MANAGEMENT

The geriatric population is the largest group of hypnotic drug users. Basen[31] indicated that people over 60 years of age, although composing only 14 per cent of the population, receive 33 per cent of all hypnotic prescriptions. There have been no long-term clinical studies of hypnotics in any age group, and certainly not among the aged. When considering prescription of a hypnotic drug for an older patient, one must first recognize that the risks may well outweigh the benefits. There is no substantial scientific evidence that any hypnotic drug is useful for treatment of any long-term condition, particularly among the aged.[32] It is our impression that hypnotics usually do more harm than good. A number of very significant risks of all hypnotics have been identified, including oversedation and hangover, hypotension, restlessness, aggression, confusion, personality impairment, weakness and falling, addiction, induction of liver enzymes, exacerbation of sleep apnea, and overdose deaths.

Most hypnotics are more likely to produce side effects in older patients. The major advantage of the benzodiazepines (drugs such as flurazepam, diazepam, or temazepam), are their relative safety in overdose, lower addiction risk, and weak interactions with other drugs. However, flurazepam and diazepam have very long half-lives in older subjects, i.e., 2 to 8 days. They tend to accumulate over several days or weeks. Adverse drug effects should always be considered when mental deterioration occurs in a patient being treated with long-acting benzodiazepines, and unfortunately, the intoxication syndrome is slow to resolve. Shorter-acting benzodiazepines, such as temazepam and oxazepam, are slowly absorbed and consequently, they are of little use in hastening sleep onset. Chloral hydrate has the advantages of rapid onset and rapid metabolism, but it is unclear whether it is otherwise safe and well-tolerated. The barbiturates appear to have above-average risk for overdose, addiction, and drug interaction, and they have no demonstrated advantages. In fact, in a review of the psychopharmacology of the aged, Raskind and Eisdorfer[33] argued that barbiturates are totally contraindicated in the elderly. Hypnotics are only indicated for treatment of transient situational conditions or for occasional use.

For the depressed elderly patient, a sedating tricyclic, such as doxepin in low doses (10 to 50 mg), is often the best choice for combined hypnotic and antidepressant effects.

For many sleep complaints, physicians should look to alternative treatments. Some alternative treatments for the management of sleep complaints include behavior modification techniques, relaxation training, and biofeedback. Most important, a patient with difficulty sleeping should keep very regular bedtimes and wake-up times to stabilize habits and circadian rhythms. Even if the patient did not fall asleep until 4:00 A.M., he should get up at his scheduled time. A patient with difficulty sleeping should never stay in bed when he is not sleepy. This keeps the patient from having negative associations and frustrations in the bedroom. Avoiding daytime naps is also useful in some cases because naps, like sleeping late in the morning, can disturb rhythms and reduce the amount of sleep a person gets at night.

For the patient with sleep apnea, the treatment depends on the severity of the disorder. In the mild case with very few complications (e.g., little or no daytime sleepiness, no cardiac arrhythmias during the episodes), no treatment is currently indicated. Obese patients will often benefit from weight loss. In moderate to severe cases, imipramine or progesterone (for obstructive or central sleep apnea) and acetazolamide (for central sleep apnea) can be tried. In life-threatening obstructive apnea, a tracheostomy or pharyngoplasty can be considered.

A few words must be said about the interaction of hypnotics with sleep apnea. It is known that hypnotics depress the respiratory drive in the waking state. Some evidence suggests that hypnotics also make sleep apnea worse.[34,35] As already discussed, there is a high prevalence of sleep apnea among both symptomatic and asymptomatic elderly people. Hypnotics prescribed to these patients could exacerbate their oxygen desaturation and create serious medical risks. Sleep apnea cannot be diagnosed by history alone. Therefore, we do not believe that even a careful history can assure a clinician that a patient in this age range can receive hypnotics safely.

For the patient with nocturnal myoclonus, clonazepam or diazepam at bedtime often provide symptomatic relief. This is the only situation in which we consider prescribing a hypnotic for long-term use, knowing that the long-term effects of these treatments have not been studied.

If the insomnia is secondary to some medical problem, then the primary problem should be treated rather than the sleep problem. Treatments for problems that affect sleep include analgesics for pain, antacids for dyspepsia, aminophylline for nocturnal asthma, cardiac medications for nocturnal angina, and chemotherapy and psychotherapy for depression and other psychiatric disorders.[8] The time of day that medication is administered should also be considered. For example, tricyclic antidepressants are usually best given at bedtime.

For the patient with no objective sleep disorders, education on good sleep habits and on what to expect (e.g., it is reasonable to sleep less if you are not tired during the day; you may expect to wake up several times at night) may resolve the problems.

For a more complete discussion of management of sleep disorders in the elderly, the reader is referred to works by Miles and Dement[8] and by Mendelson.[32]

## INCOMPATIBLE CLINICAL SYNDROMES

There are several drugs and medical conditions that adversely affect sleep. Tolerance and withdrawal from sedative-hypnotics can produce insomnia. Drugs such as theophylline, isoproterenol, phenytoin, and L-Dopa, all frequently used in the elderly, may produce insomnia as a side effect.[32] Tricyclic antidepressants may exacerbate nocturnal myoclonus, although they may relieve depression and sleep apnea. Benzodiazepines can exacerbate sleep apnea, although they help nocturnal myoclonus. Diuretics that produce alkalosis can also exacerbate central sleep apnea.[36] Diuretics likewise increase nocturia and thus disrupt sleep. Alcohol, although often used to induce sleep, will actually cause insomnia with excessive use. The alcohol withdrawal that occurs several hours after bedtime ingestion can disrupt sleep.[37]

Central nervous system stimulants and depressants can be associated with excessive daytime somnolence. Drug metabolism is slower in the elderly; therefore there may be a daytime carry-over of drowsiness caused by a hypnotic taken at night.[32] Antihistamines, major and minor tranquilizers, methyldopa, and amitryptyline may all produce excessive daytime somnolence.

Medical conditions that are highly prevalent and affect the sleep of the elderly include chronic pain, arthritis, nocturia, chronic brain syndrome, and nocturnal dyspnea.[8] As already mentioned, careful treatment of these conditions should help alleviate the associated sleep problems.

## CONCLUSION

Elderly patients with either short or long sleep need careful evaluation. We should not prescribe sedative-hypnotics to this population. There is evidence that most people overestimate their sleep latency time and underestimate their total sleep time.[38] Without objective documentation, the clinician cannot be sure of the true problem. The majority of elderly people have sleep apnea, nocturnal myoclonus, or both. We must become more aware and more sensitive to the older patient's daily, and nightly, routine in the hopes of being able to establish a diagnosis. In summary, we must re-evaluate our approach to treating the widespread sleep complaints of the elderly population.

### References

1. Feinberg I: Changes in sleep cycle patterns with age. J Psychiatr Res 10:283, 1974.
2. Feinberg I, Koresko RL, Heller N: EEG sleep patterns as a function of normal and pathological aging in man. J Psychiatr Res 5:107, 1967.
*One of the first studies done on sleep in the aged.*
3. Prinz PN: Sleep Changes with Aging: Psychopharmacology of Aging. New York, Spectrum Publications, 1980.
4. Prinz PN, Raskind M: Aging and sleep disorders. *In* Williams R, Karacan I (eds.): Sleep Disorders: Diagnosis and Treatment. New York, John Wiley and Sons, 1978, pp. 303–321.
5. Spiegel R: Sleep and Sleeplessness in Advanced Age. New York, Spectrum Press, 1981.
6. Kripke DF, Simons RN, Garfinkel L, Hammond EC: Short and long sleep and sleeping pills: Is increased mortality associated? Arch Gen Psychiatry 36:103, 1979.
7. McGhee A, Russel SM: The subjective assessment of normal sleep patterns. J Ment Sci 108:642, 1962.
8. Miles LE, Dement WC: Sleep and aging. Sleep 3:119, 1980.
*A special issue of Sleep devoted to "Sleep and the Aged." This is an excellent review of the literature.*
8a. Kripke DF, Ancoli-Israel S, Mason W, Messin S: Sleep-related mortality and morbidity in the aged. *In* Chase MH (ed.): Sleep Disorders: Basic and Clinical Research. New York, Spectrum Publications, 1983, pp. 415–429.
9.. Belloc NB: Relationship of health practices and mortality. Prev Med 2:67, 1973.
10. Guilleminault C, Dement WC: Sleep Apnea Syndromes. New York, Alan R. Liss, 1978.
*This book is a most comprehensive collection of papers on sleep apnea.*
11. Phillipson EA: Control of breathing during sleep. Am Rev Respir Dis 118:909, 1978.
*This paper reviews respiratory physiology during sleep.*
12. Lugaresi E, Coccagna G, Cirignotta F: Snoring and its clinical implications. *In* Guilleminault C, Dement WC (eds.): Sleep Apnea Syndromes. New York, Alan R. Liss, 1978, pp. 13–22.
13. Lugaresi E, Coccagna G, Mantovani M: Hypersomnia with Periodic Apneas. New York, SP Medical and Scientific Books, Spectrum Publications, 1978.
*A physiologically oriented presentation.*
14. Tilkian A, Guilleminault C, Schroeder J, et al: Sleep-induced apnea syndrome: Prevalence of cardiac arrhythmias and their reversal after tracheostomy. Am J Med 63:348, 1977.
15. Carskadon MA, Dement WC: Respiration during sleep in the aged human. J Gerontol 36:420, 1981.
*A study of elderly people who had no sleep complaints.*
16. Tilkian A, Guilleminault C, Schroeder J, et al: Hemodynamics in sleep-induced apnea. Studies during wakefulness and sleep. Ann Intern Med 85:714, 1976.
17. Tolle F: Understanding the sleep apnea syndromes. J Indiana State Med Assoc 73:21, 1980.
18. Guilleminault C: Primary and Secondary Sleep Apnea Syndromes. Paper presented at the annual meeting of the Association for the Psychophysiological Study of Sleep, 1980.
19. Ancoli-Israel S, Kripke DF, Menn SJ, Messin S: Benefits of a sleep disorders clinic in a Veterans Administration Medical Center. West J Med 135:14, 1981.
20. Coleman RM: Periodic movements in sleep (nocturnal myoclonus) and restless legs syndrome. *In* Guilleminault C (ed.): Sleeping and Waking Disorders: Indications and Techniques. Menlo Park, Addison-Wesley Publishing Co, 1982, pp. 265–296.
*This chapter presents the history and current understanding of nocturnal myoclonus.*
21. Guilleminault C, Tilkian A, Dement WC: The sleep apnea syndromes. Annu Rev Med 27:465, 1976.
22. Ancoli-Israel S, Kripke DF, Mason W, Messin S: Sleep

apnea and nocturnal myoclonus in a senior population. Sleep 4:349, 1981.
*A study of elderly people with sleep complaints.*

23. Dement WC, Carskadon MA, Richardson G: Excessive daytime sleepiness in the sleep apnea syndrome. *In* Guilleminault C, Dement WC (eds.): Sleep Apnea Syndromes. New York, Alan R. Liss, 1978, pp. 23–46.
24. Lugaresi E, Cirignotta F, Coccagna G, Piana C: Some epidemiological data on snoring and cardiocirculatory disturbances. Sleep 3:221, 1980.
*This entire issue of Sleep is devoted to "Control of Breathing During Sleep," making this issue a comprehensive up-to-date reference.*
25. Block AJ, Boysen PG, James WW, Hunt LA: Sleep apnea, hypopnea, and oxygen desaturation in normal subjects. N Engl J Med 300:513, 1979.
26. Block AJ, Wynne JW, Boysen PG: Sleep-disordered breathing and nocturnal oxygen desaturation in postmenopausal women. Am J Med 69:75, 1980.
27. Reynolds CF, Coble PA, Block RS, et al: Sleep disturbances in a series of elderly patients: Polysomnographic findings. J Am Geriatr Soc 28:164, 1980.
28. Webb P: Periodic breathing during sleep. J Appl Psychol 37:899, 1974.
29. Ancoli-Israel S, Kripke DF, Mason W, Messin S: Comparisons of home sleep recordings and polysomnograms in older adults with sleep disorders. Sleep 4:283, 1981.
30. Association of Sleep Disorders Centers: Diagnostic classification of sleep and arousal disorders. 1st ed. (Prepared by the Sleep Disorders Classification Committee, HP Roffwarg, Chairman.) Sleep 2:1, 1979.
*This special issue of Sleep presents the currently accepted criteria for diagnosing sleep disorders.*
31. Basen MM: The elderly and drugs—Problems, overview and program strategy. Public Health Rep 92:34, 1977.
32. Mendelson WB: The Use and Misuse of Sleeping Pills. New York, Plenum Medical Book Co., 1980.
*A comprehensive book on the advantages and disadvantages of sleeping pills in all age groups. There is a chapter on hypnotics in the elderly.*
33. Raskind M, Eisdorfer C: Psychopharmacology of the aged. *In* Simpson (ed.): Drug Treatment of Mental Disorders. New York, Raven Press, 1976, pp. 237–266.
34. Dolly FR, Block AJ: The effect of flurazepam on sleep-disordered breathing and nocturnal oxygen desaturation in asymptomatic subjects. Am Rev Respir Dis 125:107, 1982.
35. Mendelson WB, Garnett D, Gillin JC: Single case study: Flurazepam-induced sleep apnea syndrome in a patient with insomnia and mild sleep-related respiratory changes. J Nerv Ment Dis 169:261, 1981.
36. Findley L, Ancoli-Israel S, Kripke DF, et al: Sleep Apnea in Congestive Heart Failure. Am Rev Resp Dis 125:253, 1982.
37. Taasan WC, Block AJ, Boysen PG, et al: Alcohol increases sleep apnea and oxygen desaturation in asymptomatic men. Am J Med 71:240, 1981.
38. Carskadon MA, Dement WC, Mitler MM, et al: Self-reports versus sleep laboratory findings in 122 drug-free subjects with complaints of insomnia. Am J Psychiatry 133:1382, 1976.
*This article compared subjective reports with objective sleep recordings.*

## *Additional Reading*

1. Guilleminault C, Eldridge FL, Simmons FB, Dement WC: Sleep apnea syndrome—Can it induce hemodynamic changes? West J Med 123:7, 1975.

## Chapter 24

# The Aging Eye

Carol R. Kollarits

Blindness is the disability feared most by elderly Americans. This fear is rational, since 3 per cent of the patients studied in the mobile population of the Framingham Study cohort were found to be legally blind.[1] In a recent study of geriatric patients confined to nursing homes, more than 25 per cent were legally blind.[2]

This chapter acquaints the physician caring for geriatric patients with his or her responsibilities in the early diagnosis of potentially blinding eye diseases. In addition, emergency management of ocular trauma and management of common ocular complaints of the elderly are outlined. A brief description is given of common surgical techniques and medications used by ophthalmologists, since the geriatric physician will often be called upon to advise patients concerning interaction of medications or need for certain types of eye surgery.

## ANATOMIC REVIEW

Figure 24–1 represents a vertical cross section through a human eye and orbit. The upper lid is elevated by the action of the levator muscle (innervated by cranial nerve III). The lids are closed by contraction of the subcutaneous orbicularis muscles (cranial nerve VII) in both the upper and lower lids. The inner surfaces of the lids are lined with conjunctiva. The conjunctiva forms a continuous lining from the inner surfaces of the lids over the sclera up to the junction of the sclera with the cornea. The tear film is a mixture of conjunctival mucus, aqueous tears secreted by the lacrimal gland, and oil from glands opening at the lid margin. The tear film lubricates the movement of the lids over the cornea.

The anterior chamber is filled with aqueous humor produced by the ciliary body behind the clear lens. The lens is suspended by collagen fibers called *zonules* from the ciliary body. The ciliary body contains several muscles that, when contracted, cause the lens to increase its anteroposterior diameter and bring the eye into focus on near objects. The central portion of the eye is filled with vitreous humor, a matrix of collagen fibrils containing a hyaluronic acid gel. The retina is a tissue that is ten cell layers thick and extends from the optic nerve to the edge of the ciliary body. The choroid is a vascular layer underlying the retina. The tough, white outer coat of the eye is the sclera. The optic nerve consists of axons from the nerve fiber layer of the retina. These axons synapse in the lateral geniculate body, which gives rise to second order neurons that proceed to the occipital cortex.

The six extraocular muscles insert into the sclera to move the eye. The lateral rectus muscle is innervated by cranial nerve VI. The superior oblique muscle is innervated by cranial nerve IV. The medial rectus, inferior rectus, inferior oblique, and superior rectus, as well as the previously mentioned levator muscle, are innervated by cranial nerve III. The sphincter muscle of the iris is innervated by parasympathetic fibers carried in cranial nerve III. The dilator muscle of the pupil is innervated by sympathetic fibers. The anatomic origins and pathways by which these fibers reach the pupil dilator muscles have been reviewed elsewhere.[3]

## EYE EXAMINATION

The screening area of every physician's office should be equipped with a well-illuminated Snellen chart for estimating visual acuity at a distance of 20 feet. The examiner should obtain the best corrected visual acuity of each eye separately with the patient's current spectacles. Pupil light responses should be checked with a flashlight, including the "swinging flashlight test" for every patient. (Fig. 24–2). Next, the intraocular pressure of each eye should be esti-

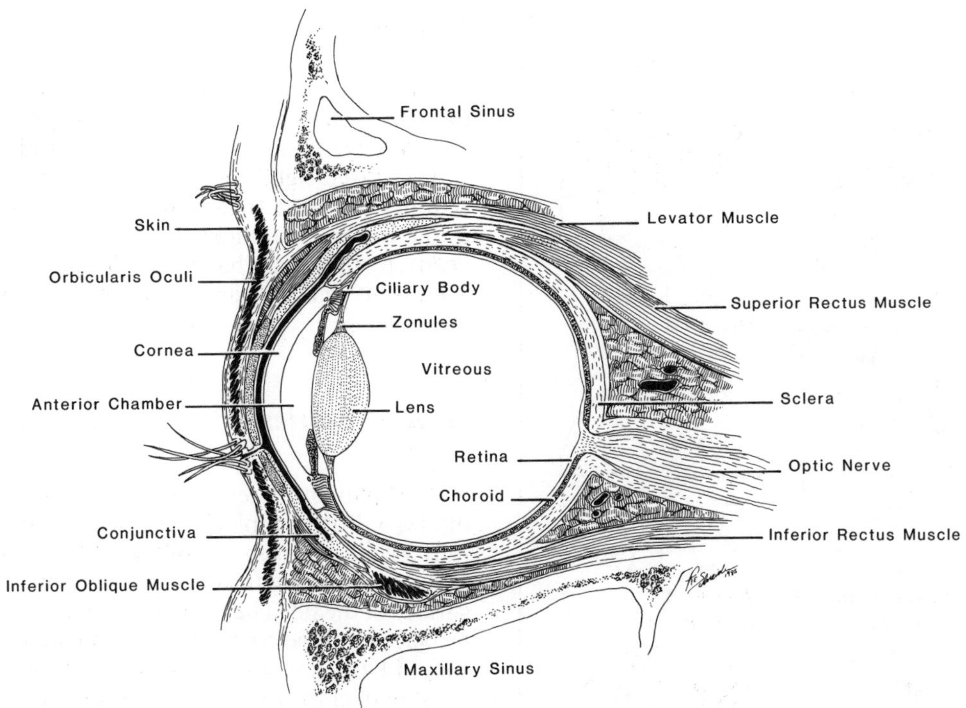


**Figure 24-1.** Artist's representation of a cross-section of the eye.

mated by one of the four methods illustrated in Figure 24–3. Of these, the least expensive is palpation of the eye. This is of practical value only in acute angle-closure glaucoma, in which one eye will be rock hard whereas the other eye, usually with normal pressure, will feel like a grape when palpated through the eyelid. The Schiotz tonometer, although not as accurate as the air puff tonometer or the Goldmann applanation tonometer, is much less expensive than either of these. The use of the Schiotz tonometer is readily learned. The patient should be asked to lie down or recline in a chair with a comfortable head and neck rest. The physician or nurse applies a drop of topical anesthetic solution to each eye. After about 30 seconds, the Schiotz tonometer can be rested gently on the patient's cornea and a reading obtained from each eye in turn. Annual intraocular pressure estimation should be performed as a screening test for chronic simple glaucoma. In addition, ophthalmoscopic examination of the optic disc and retina of both eyes should be performed at yearly intervals.

Ophthalmoscopy is accomplished more easily if the patient's pupils are dilated. One drop of 10 per cent phenylephrine hydrochloride (Neo-Synephrine) in each eye will dilate the pupils of most eyes with blue irises within 15 to 20 minutes. More darkly pigmented eyes require two or three sets of drops, given at 5-minute intervals. Blood pressure measurements should be done prior to instilling the drops, since 10 per cent Neo-Synephrine will raise systemic blood pressure in a significant percentage of patients. In hypertensive patients, $2\frac{1}{2}$ per cent Neo-Synephrine may be used to avoid further blood pressure elevation. The only contraindications to pupillary dilation are recent head injury, a history of angle-closure glaucoma, or previous admonition by an ophthalmologist that the patient's pupils should not be dilated (because of the possibility of dislocating an iris-fixated intraocular lens).

## COMMON OCULAR PROBLEMS

### *Presbyopia*

The most common ocular complaint of Americans over 40 years is diminished ability to focus clearly at normal (less than arm's length) reading distances. This is presbyopia. It is caused by thickening (increased anteroposterior diameter) of the lens within the eye as a result of continued growth of the lens fibers. In the young eye, focusing on a near object is accomplished by contraction of the muscles in the ciliary body, with subsequent reduction in the tension of the zonules and elastic capsule of the lens.

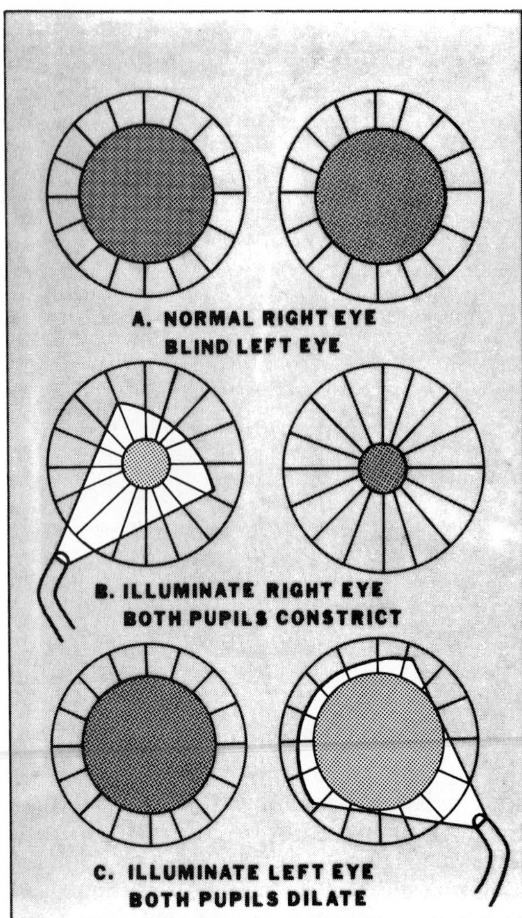


**Figure 24–2.** Swinging flashlight test for a Marcus Gunn afferent pupillary defect. In dim illumination, the blind left eye has the same size pupil as its normal fellow eye *(A)*. Illumination of the normal eye causes both pupils to constrict equally (direct and consensual pupillary miosis) as in *(B)*. Swinging the flashlight over to illuminate the blind eye results in an apparent dilation of the pupil because the blind eye has dilated consensually in response to loss of illumination of the normal eye *(C)*. (*From* Mehelas and Kollants: Pupillary clues to neuro-ophthalmic diagnosis. Postgrad Med 71:199, 1982. Reproduced with permission.)

The resultant increase in anteroposterior lens thickness is allowed to continue until the desired distance of focus is reached. In the older eye, the already thickened lens responds more slowly to change in tension of the elastic capsule. Some individuals notice that they can, with some effort, focus clearly for reading but then find that when they look up, their distance vision is blurred and remains blurred for several seconds to a few minutes as the lens very slowly resumes its previous anteroposterior diameter. These symptoms are relieved by the use of reading glasses or the addition of bifocal segments to the patient's distance spectacle correction.

## *Second Sight*

After being presbyopic for many years, some individuals find that they can once again focus clearly for reading without using their bifocals. This "second sight" phenomenon is caused by acquired myopia (nearsightedness) secondary to increasing lens thickness. The protein composition of the lens changes at this time, usually leading to lens opacification (cataract formation).

## *Ocular Injuries*

If the patient presents with *pain* following an injury, a drop of topical anesthetic can be carefully instilled by gently pulling down the lower eyelid and placing the drop on the conjunctival surface of the lid. The examiner's fingers should be placed well below the lash margin and the lid should be pulled away from the eye by rolling the skin over the inferior orbital rim rather than pushing the lid downward. Pushing the lid may transmit pressure to an injured eye, causing pain and prolapse of vitreous and retina through a corneoscleral laceration. Once the anesthetic drop is instilled, patients with superficial injuries feel nearly complete relief from pain. Deeper injuries are usually still painful, in spite of the topical anesthetic drop.

If a *corneal abrasion* is suspected, it can often be more readily identified by placing a fluorescein strip in the tear film just long enough to color the tears yellow. After the patient blinks, the abraded area of the cornea will stain bright yellow, making it more readily distinguished from the normal, nonstaining corneal surface. Corneal abrasions can be treated with instillation of an antibiotic ointment and firm patching. The lids should be patched sufficiently tightly so that they cannot open under the patch and allow the patch to further abrade the cornea. Use of a patch for 24 hours will permit most corneal abrasions to heal.

If a *penetrating ocular injury* is suspected on the basis of an irregular pupil, or if an obvious *laceration* is evident upon inspection, the eye should not be patched; rather, a metal shield should be taped over the eye to prevent further damage while the patient is being transported to an ophthalmologist for definitive surgical management.

Evaluation and treatment of eye injuries are aided by having a fully equipped eye emergency tray. Suggested contents of such a tray are listed in Table 24–1.

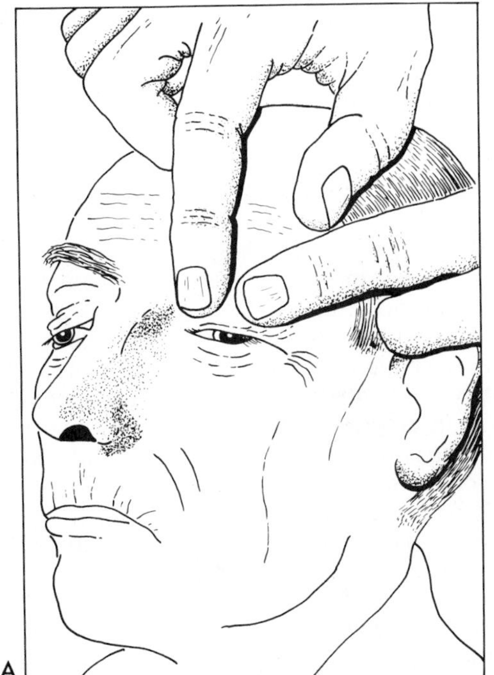


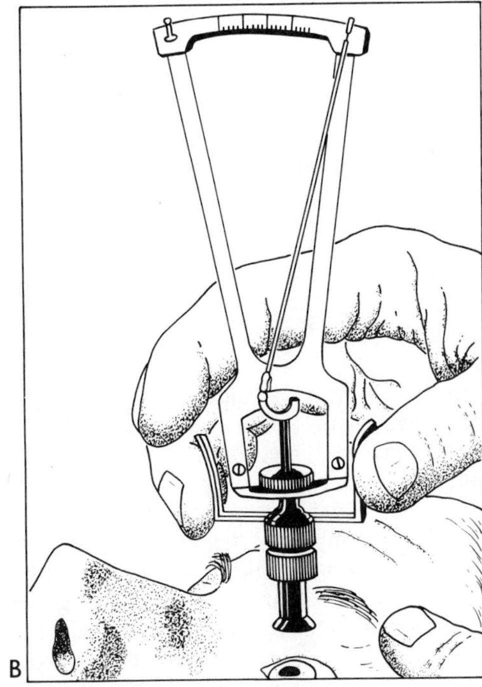


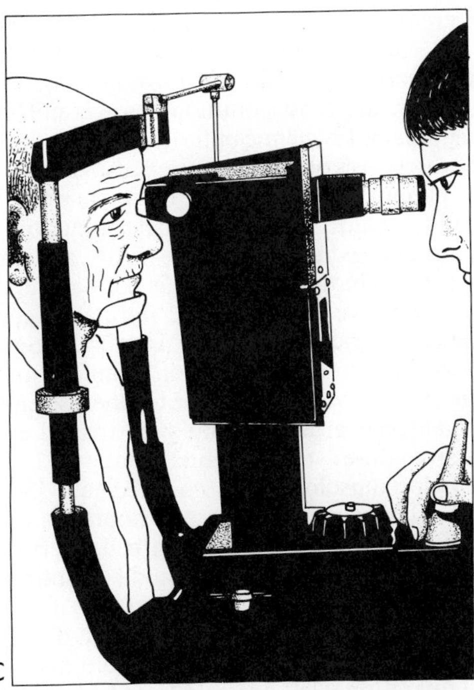


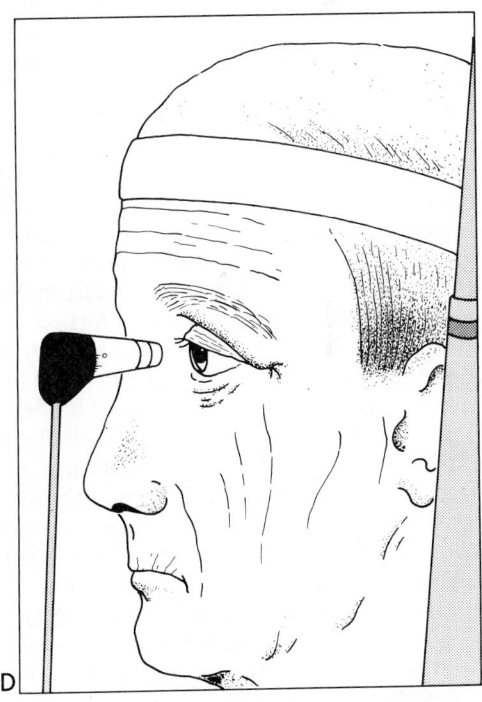


**Figure 24–3.** Methods of intraocular pressure estimation.

(A). Finger palpation is useful only when a large difference exists between the intraocular pressure of the two eyes, as in unilateral angle-closure glaucoma.

(B). Schiotz tonometry can be learned readily, and because the tonometer is relatively inexpensive, it can be used in every physician's office to screen for chronic simple glaucoma.

(C). The air-puff tonometer can be used for screening large numbers of patients, but it is far more expensive than Schiotz's tonometer.

(D). Goldmann's applanation tonometer, used with a slit lamp, is the standard instrument for glaucoma diagnosis and management by most ophthalmologists. It is expensive and requires considerable skill.

**Table 24–1.** CONTENTS OF EYE TRAY

| |
|---|
| Oval eye pads |
| Paper tape (1 in.) |
| Sterile gauze (4 in. × 4 in.) |
| Sterile fluorescein strips |
| Topical ocular anesthetic |
| Antibiotic ointment |
| Sterile irrigating solution |

## *Sudden Visual Loss*

Patients reporting a sudden loss of vision should have visual acuity checked with the Snellen chart and recorded. Pupil responses should be examined carefully. In a patient with acute severe visual loss in one eye, a Marcus Gunn afferent pupillary defect will be present when the swinging flashlight test is performed (Fig. 24–2). If the Marcus Gunn pupil is not present in the affected eye, then visual loss is due to an opacity of the media (cataract or vitreous hemorrhage) or there is *no* visual loss (patient is hysterical or malingering). If the pupils are normal, confrontation visual field testing should be done to rule out a homonymous hemianopia due to a stroke, because many patients will interpret the loss of the right half of the visual field of each eye as blindness of the right eye.

The most common causes of *monocular painless visual loss* in the elderly are (1) subretinal hemorrhage (macular degeneration), (2) central retinal artery or vein occlusion, (3) ischemic optic neuropathy (caused by atherosclerosis or giant cell arteritis), (4) retinal detachment, and (5) vitreous hemorrhage resulting from diabetic retinopathy or retinal hole formation. Central retinal artery occlusion can seldom be reversed in time to allow recovery of vision, but the patient requires work-up for sources of emboli. The most common origin of emboli blocking the central retinal artery is atheromatous plaques at the carotid bifurcation and the mitral valve.[4] Patients with central retinal vein occlusion also have a poor prognosis for visual recovery. Patients with a branch retinal vein occlusion have a much better chance of recovery of useful vision, but many of them will require laser treatment.[5] Patients with venous occlusive disease need to be evaluated for systemic hypertension, chronic simple glaucoma, and any disease that increases blood viscosity. These include polycythemia, leukemia, the coagulopathies, and macroglobulinemia.

Patients with sudden visual loss in one eye should be examined by an ophthalmologist on an emergency basis. *Binocular sudden visual loss* is most commonly caused by bilateral occipital lobe infarcts. The pupil responses are normal if the visual loss is a result of occipital infarction.

## *Gradual Visual Loss*

Progressive, unrelenting visual blurring occurring over months or years is most often due to cataracts. Visual loss from macular degeneration often has a intermittent downhill course that the patient may not be able to report accurately. Untreated chronic simple glaucoma results in progressive peripheral visual field loss that the patient may not notice until the central vision is threatened. Gradual visual loss may also be caused by optic nerve atrophy.

Every patient with optic atrophy (pallor of the optic disc) and gradual visual loss should be evaluated for tertiary syphilis, diabetes mellitus, pernicious anemia and other anemias, brain tumor, and poor nutrition (possibly associated with chronic alcoholism and cigarette smoking —"tobacco-ethanol amblyopia").

Patients with ischemic optic neuropathy may present with optic atrophy in one eye and an apparently edematous disc in the other eye. This is the classical "Foster Kennedy syndrome," often ascribed to sphenoid ridge meningioma. However, the most common cause is not meningioma but ischemic optic neuropathy due to atherosclerosis or giant cell arteritis. Work-up of the patient with ischemic optic neuropathy should include skull films, determination of erythrocyte sedimentation rate (ESR), and temporal artery biopsy. If the ESR is normal and the skull films are interpreted as normal, a computed tomography (CT) scan of the brain should be obtained to rule out an intracranial tumor. Acute visual loss, whether due to atherosclerosis or giant cell arteritis, should be treated with massive doses of systemic steroids (1 gm methylprednisolone sodium succinate [Solu-Medrol] intravenously every 12 hours for 3 to 5 days). If the diagnosis of giant cell arteritis is made, oral corticosteroids should be continued until the ESR is reduced to normal even if vision is not corrected, since patients with this disorder have an increased mortality rate from myocardial infarction if left untreated (see Chapter 36). In desperate situations, when steroid therapy has failed to restore vision in the patient's only remaining eye, transient blood pressure elevation with intravenous l-norepinephrine may be considered.[6]

The hereditary causes of progressive optic nerve or retinal degeneration usually present themselves prior to age 50 years and will have been diagnosed previously.

In the absence of observed ocular abnormalities, unexplained visual loss should be considered to be caused by brain tumor until proved otherwise by appropriate studies.

## *Tearing and Irritation*

Many older people are troubled by irritation, the sensation of a foreign body, and excessive tearing. All these can be symptoms of a "dry eye syndrome." If no foreign body or trichiasis (ingrown lashes rubbing on the cornea) is found after inspection of the eye with fluorescein staining of the tear film, a presumptive diagnosis of dry eye syndrome can be made. Treatment consists of an artificial tear preparation containing a long-chain polymer that mimics the action of the mucus that is often deficient in the tears of the elderly. Tears Naturale or a similar preparation should be used regularly four times daily and especially before reading or other activities that require frequent eye movements. If the artificial tear preparation does not relieve the excessive tearing, the ophthalmologist should evaluate the patient for dysfunction of the nasolacrimal duct or abnormal lid position.

## *Drooping Lids*

Irritation may be caused by malpositions of the lower lid. Entropion (turning in) and ectropion (turning out) are both caused by laxity of the orbicularis muscle and require surgical procedures that tighten this muscle. Laxity of the orbicularis muscle over the upper lid results in *blepharochalasis*—the development of an extra lid fold, often containing herniated orbital fat. This lid fold may hang down onto the upper lashes and make it difficult for the patient to elevate the lids sufficiently to see. In true ptosis of the upper lid, the entire lid droops downward over the cornea and the lid fold disappears. This is usually caused by dehiscence of the levator muscle, but *myasthenia gravis* and *Horner's syndrome* should be ruled out.

Horner's syndrome may cause minor ptosis of both upper and lower lid, making the affected eye appear smaller because of the narrowed lid fissure. The pupil will be smaller in the affected eye than in the other eye, and the skin on the same side of the face will produce less sweat. If the patient has no other neurologic signs, a chest film with apical lordotic views should be obtained to rule out the presence of a Pancoast tumor or tuberculosis of the apex of the lung affecting the sympathetic pathway to the pupil.[3] If the x-ray results are negative and the patient develops no other neurologic symptoms, no further work-up is necessary.

## *Light Flashes, Floaters, and Visual Hallucinations*

Flashing lights that the patient localizes to one eye (rather than one half of the visual field in both eyes) are usually due to a *vitreous detachment.*

When the vitreous detaches from the optic nerve, a circular condensation of *collagen fibers* may float free just in front of the macula and is seen as a nearly transparent "doughnut" by the patient. Other "wiggly lines," "worms," or "threads" that move when the eye moves and continue to move across the patient's visual field for a short time after the eye stops moving are also examples of collagen fibers floating in the vitreous in front of the retina. These floaters are usually no cause for alarm, but if the patient describes floaters appearing as a "swarm of gnats" in the field of one eye, this usually represents red blood cells from a retinal tear. Since retinal tears may cause retinal detachment, a patient with this complaint should definitely be examined by an ophthalmologist.

*Brain tumor* or *cortical ischemia* may cause visual hallucinations. With the lesion affecting the temporal lobe, the patient may have the sensation that he is seeing a movie of some past episode in his life. A lesion of the occipital cortex causes unformed hallucinations, such as flashing light or zigzag lines. The most common example is the visual aura of migraine, which is not necessarily accompanied or followed by a migraine headache.

## *Diplopia*

Paralysis of the third, fourth, or sixth cranial nerves may cause diplopia (double vision) that is rather troublesome to the patient in the field of gaze of the affected extraocular muscle(s). Patching the affected eye may be necessary to allow the patient to recover from a cerebral vascular accident or head trauma without the added distraction of diplopia. Corrective muscle surgery is usually not done for 6 months following head injury or stroke because spontaneous recovery is possible in that time. The young patient who complains of diplopia with one eye covered is usually hysterical, but the elderly individual who describes monocular diplopia often is suffering from a "double focus" cataract. Visual acuity may be quite good with such a cataract, but the diplopia may be sufficiently annoying to justify cataract extraction. Intermittent vertical diplopia is a common sign of basivertebral artery insufficiency in the elderly. Double vision or ptosis that occurs only in the evening is most likely due to myasthenia gravis.[7] If symptoms are not present during a morning examination, another examination should be carried out as late in the day as possible and if double vision or ptosis can be documented, an edrophonium chloride (Tensilon) test may alleviate the symptoms and confirm the suspected diagnosis of myasthenia gravis.[7]

## *Purulent Discharge and Lid Crusting*

*Bacterial conjunctivitis* is characterized by a purulent discharge that often mats the lids shut when the patient wakes up in the morning. This is not accompanied by pain and should be relieved within 3 to 4 days by frequent use of antibiotic drops.[8]

Infection of the lid margins *(marginal blepharitis)* is manifested by greasy crusts around the bases of the lashes and swelling and redness of the underlying skin. Warm, moist compresses should be applied to the affected lids four times daily, followed by gentle scrubbing of the lid margins with cotton-tipped applicators dipped in baby shampoo. After the lids have been gently dried, a drop of antibiotic solution (such as Neosporin) should be applied into the inferior cul-de-sac. At night, the bedtime lid scrub should be followed by instillation of an antibiotic ointment, with gentle massage into the skin of the lid margins. Ointment is used at bedtime because it keeps the antibiotic in contact with the infected areas for a longer period of time. Drops are used during the day because they do not blur the patient's vision. Use of an antidandruff shampoo on the hair of the scalp often aids in the cure of chronic blepharitis having a seborrheic component.

## *Painless Red Eye*

Painless, watery discharge, accompanied by conjunctival hyperemia and symptoms of fullness of the lids, is most likely due to a viral or chlamydial conjunctivitis. Topical antibiotics should be used as for the treatment of bacterial conjunctivitis, to prevent a bacterial superinfection in these conditions. Sulfonamide eye drops may be used in suspected viral or chlamydial conjunctivitis, but they are not effective in the average case of bacterial conjunctivitis because of the large amount of para-aminobenzoic acid present in purulent discharge. If the symptoms continue beyond 1 week or if the patient complains of pain, an ophthalmologist should be consulted.

Redness, watery discharge, and itching are most commonly caused by allergy. A decongestant preparation (such as Naphcon-A) should be prescribed, one drop four times daily. If the patient obtains some relief with the decongestant drops but still is symptomatic, oral antihistamines should be used. *Under no circumstances should topical steroid drops be used by any physician other than an ophthalmologist because of the dangers of potentiating viral infections and inducing glaucoma.*[9]

Subconjunctival hemorrhage presents as a dramatic bright red infiltration over the sclera. No treatment other than reassurance should be given, and no work-up is required if the patient has no cutaneous petechial hemorrhages and no history of recent easy bruising or bleeding.

## *Painful Red Eye*

A patient with a red, painful eye, with an apparent corneal ulcer (white spot on cornea), should be referred to an ophthalmologist *as an emergency. No antibiotic drops or ointment should be instilled prior to referral,* since this may suppress growth of organisms cultured from corneal scrapings. Bacterial corneal ulcers are usually painful, whereas ulcers caused by herpes simplex may not be very painful.

In addition to bacterial or viral corneal ulcers, a red, painful eye may be caused by angle-closure glaucoma or iritis. In angle-closure glaucoma, the pupil of the affected eye is dilated, compared with the pupil of the normal eye, and has a significantly increased intraocular pressure that can easily be detected by finger palpation[3] or tonometry. In iritis, the pupil of the affected eye is smaller than that of the normal eye and the pressure can be quite low. For either condition, the patient should be referred to an ophthalmologist for definitive management.

## *Glaucoma*

Chronic simple glaucoma affects at least 2 per cent of the population over the age of 40. It is an asymptomatic disease that, unlike the much rarer acute angle-closure glaucoma, causes no pain. The gradual loss of vision from prolonged elevation of intraocular pressure is often unnoticed by the patient until a significant amount of visual field is gone. The normal range of intraocular pressure is 9 to 23 mm Hg. Patients having intraocular pressure higher than the normal range or documentation of progressive increase in the cup-disc ratio over a period of years should be referred to an ophthalmologist for evaluation of possible chronic simple glaucoma.

## *Periocular Pain*

The most common cause of periocular pain is *sinus disease.* Because of the proximity of the sinuses to the orbit (Fig. 24–1) and common innervation (cranial nerve V), sinus pain is often referred to the eye. In the absence of decreased vision, elevated intraocular pressure, or redness, most complaints of ocular pain deserve a trial of decongestant therapy and sinus x-ray examination.

The lancinating pain of *tic douloureux* and the throbbing pain of *migraine* may also involve the eye. Tic douloureux responds well to carbamazepine (Tegretol), whereas migraine may be reduced in frequency by use of propranolol hydrochloride (Inderal). For patients with frequent, debilitating migraine, Inderal should be started at a dosage of 10 mg per day and gradually increased to a dosage of 40 mg per day. The dose may need to be reduced if orthostatic hypotension is produced. Some patients who have a definite warning aura occurring 15 to 30 minutes prior to the onset of the headache can abort the headache by taking one 10-mg tablet of Inderal and one 5-grain tablet of aspirin as soon as they notice the warning migraine aura.

Pain in the distribution of the ophthalmic division of the trigeminal nerve may be caused by *herpes zoster.* Often the patient complains of pain when combing the hair for up to 10 days prior to the appearance of the vesicles. No specific ocular therapy is indicated unless vesicles develop on the tip of the nose on the same side as the "shingles." When this occurs, the eye usually has severe inflammation, often resulting in chronic pain and accelerated cataract formation. As in any elderly person with herpes zoster, systemic evaluation should be done for leukemia, lymphoma, and other diseases affecting the immune system. Post-herpetic pain may be severe and prolonged over several months. Tegretol is often useful in the management of this pain. There is some evidence that systemic steroids given during the acute attack may reduce the severity and duration of the post-herpetic pain.

Throbbing pain accompanied by an ipsilateral paralysis of cranial nerve III (upper lid ptosis, dilated pupil, eye displaced down and laterally) should be considered to be caused by an *intracranial aneurysm* until a normal arteriogram has been obtained. Painful ophthalmoplegia caused by the Tolosa-Hunt syndrome may be treated with steroids after aneurysm and diabetes mellitus have been ruled out. Paralysis of the third cranial nerve caused by diabetes mellitus does not involve the pupil and usually is not accompanied by the severe pain seen in patients with aneurysm or Tolosa-Hunt syndrome. If caused by diabetes, the paralysis will disappear spontaneously within 90 days.

## *Cataract*

Any decrease in transparency or alteration of optical homogeneity of the lens is called a cataract.[10] Cataract formation begins in everyone over 30 years of age but progresses at varying rates in different individuals. Total opacification of the lens, resulting in a white, "mature" or "ripe" cataract, actually occurs in very few people. This is especially true now with the improvement of modern surgical techniques, and decreased visual acuity (usually 20/50 or worse) has become the major indication for cataract surgery.

Compared with a normal lens, a mature cataract has excess water, $Na^+$ ions, $Ca^{++}$ ions, and insoluble proteins. The mature cataract has abnormally low levels of $K^+$ ions, free amino acids, glutathione, inositol, and soluble lens proteins.[10] Some of these changes in lens chemistry may result from exposure to ultraviolet light or other (unknown) toxic environmental influences. Cataract formation is more common in diabetics because of increased hydration resulting from the presence of excessive sorbitol and fructose in the diabetic lens. Inhibition of the enzyme aldose reductase reduces sorbitol accumulation in the lens and may retard the development of cataracts in diabetics.[10] Use of topical aldose reductase inhibitors by diabetics is now being investigated in clinical trials. Unfortunately, no other eye drops or external therapy has been shown to reverse cataract changes that may already be present. For most patients with cataracts, surgical extraction is the only alternative to progressive visual loss.

## SIDE EFFECTS OF OCULAR MEDICATIONS

*Instillation of a drop of medication in the conjunctival cul-de-sac is equivalent to giving the same amount of medication intravenously.*[9] It should be apparent that systemic anaphylactic reactions can occur just as easily as local allergic responses to the active pharmaceutical agent, its vehicle, or the preservative added to the drug and its vehicle. Redness and itching of the lid skin are allergic reactions often seen in patients taking atropine. Some patients may complain of dryness of the mouth and flushing of the skin while taking atropine. This is a true pharmacologic side effect rather than an allergic reaction. Any of the topical antibiotic drops can cause a local allergic reaction and are capable of causing anaphylaxis in patients with histories of prior exposure to the drug. Chloramphenicol eye drops have (rarely) been associated with aplastic anemia. Topical corticosteroid-containing eye drops cause elevation of intraocular pressure in one third of the normal population. Corticosteroid drops may potentiate a herpes simplex or fungal keratitis. In addition, patients with tissue antigen HLA A1 are likely to develop corticosteroid-induced cataracts, whether the steroid is given topically or systemically.[11]

Of the medications used to treat glaucoma, *pilocarpine* has the lowest reported incidence of systemic side effects. It does produce blurring of vision because of induced spasm of accommodation in young patients, and decreased vision because of the decreased pupil size, which in turn reduces the amount of light entering the eye. This may severely reduce vision in an eye with a cataract. *Timolol maleate* drops have been known to precipitate status asthmaticus and congestive heart failure. *Epinephrine* drops can cause cardiac arrythymias, as well as deposition of pigment in the conjunctiva. The carbonic anhydrase inhibitors *acetazolamide* (Diamox) and *methazolamine* (Neptazane) are prescribed for the management of severe glaucoma when combinations of eye drops have failed to control the intraocular pressure sufficient to prevent continued visual loss. Diamox is chemically similar in structure to the sulfonamides and may cause blurred vision, decreased appetite, a metallic taste in the mouth, dizziness, and renal stones. These side effects are less frequent with Neptazane but are not entirely absent.[9]

## OCULAR SURGERY

### *Cataract Extraction*

Cataract extraction is the most commonly performed operation in the United States today, with close to half a million being performed each year. The ophthalmologist has a choice of several types of cataract surgery: intracapsular extraction, extracapsular extraction, and phakoemulsification.[12] The success rate for each of these procedures is at least 95 per cent. Thus, the risk of visual loss as a result of the operation is 5 per cent or less.

Complications may be slightly higher in patients choosing to have an intraocular lens implanted at the time of surgery. Nevertheless, most patients accept this increased risk because the quality of postoperative vision with an intraocular lens implant is remarkably better than vision with thick spectacles. The aphakic (without lens) eye requires thick, powerful spectacles to focus light on the retina following loss of the dioptric power of the natural lens. Such a powerful lens causes magnification of images, "pincushion" distortion, image jump, and other annoying or dangerous optical phenomena. These optical problems can be eliminated if the patient can wear a contact lens correction on the aphakic eye. Unfortunately, most elderly individuals are unable or unwilling to handle standard hard contact lenses and not all patients are able to use the "continuous or permanent wear" soft lenses.

The ophthalmologist and patient together should select the type of surgery to be performed. The geriatric physician should refer patients to the ophthalmologist, who selects patients appropriately for surgery (those having visual acuity of 20/50 or less); most operated patients obtain good visual results. Patients often ask whether a laser can be used to remove a cataract. The new neodymium-YAG laser can be used to cut the anterior capsule of the cataract prior to surgery or to remove opacities in the posterior capsule following extracapsular cataract surgery. Complete removal of the cataract cannot be done with the laser; rather, it requires one of the surgical techniques mentioned previously.

If the patient has been advised to have cataract surgery but does not believe that vision is significantly compromised to justify surgery, near vision should be checked with the patient wearing current bifocals. If the patient can read newsprint with the affected eye, surgery can usually be deferred. Sometimes the patient is eager to have cataract surgery, but the ophthalmologist may recommend that no surgery be done. This is often because macular degeneration or chronic simple glaucoma has reduced the patient's vision to the point where the cataract is less responsible than the optic nerve or retinal damage for the decreased vision. When other intraocular diseases coexist with a cataract, the time when cataract surgery should be performed becomes a matter of careful judgment by the ophthalmologist.

## Retinal Surgery

The argon laser is most commonly used in the treatment of diabetic retinopathy and macular degeneration.[13,14] Diabetic patients with decreased vision resulting from macular edema or exudates may show improvement following focal laser therapy of the leaking blood vessels responsible for the edema or exudates. Diabetics with normal vision may receive laser panretinal ablation to prevent future loss of vision if they have neovascularization of the disc, neovascularization elsewhere, or vitreous hemorrhage.[13] Patients with macular degeneration should undergo fluorescein angiography, a procedure performed to detect abnormal blood vessels entering the subretinal space from the underlying choroid. If these vessels are not directly under the foveal avascular zone or under the nerve fiber bundle connecting the macula and the optic disc, they sometimes can be ablated with laser therapy. This may result in stabilization of vision and prevention of future visual loss; however, it is relatively rare for a patient to regain normal vision.[14] Retinal pigment epithelial detachments can sometimes be sealed with resulting improvement in visual acuity.

The argon laser may be used to seal retinal holes; however, it is often not useful in the treatment of *retinal detachment* because the detached retina is nearly transparent. Most retinal detachments (85 to 90 per cent) can be repaired by applying cryotherapy to the causative retinal hole(s) and indenting (buckling) the sclera overlying the hole with an external silicone band or explant. The scleral buckle places the detached retina closer to its original position against the choroid. If the cryoretinopexy has created sufficient inflammation, the retinal hole will seal shut on the buckle, and the subretinal fluid will be reabsorbed.

## Glaucoma Surgery

Recently, the argon laser has been used to treat the trabecular meshwork in eyes of patients with *chronic simple glaucoma* on maximum medical therapy. The indication for laser trabeculopexy is continued visual loss and consideration of regular surgical intervention. If the laser trabeculopexy is not successful in lowering the intraocular pressure, a routine surgical trabeculectomy or another filtering procedure can be performed on the eye.

*Angle-closure glaucoma* is much less common than chronic simple glaucoma, but it is less likely to be neglected because its most common symptom is severe pain. The pain results from abrupt elevation of intraocular pressure from blockage of the trabecular meshwork by the peripheral iris. In addition to pain, the elevated pressure causes corneal edema, creating colored halos around lights observed with the affected eye. The angle closure can be relieved by creating an iridotomy (hole in the iris) either with the argon laser or by regular surgical iridectomy.

## Corneal Surgery

Corneal transplants may be performed for corneal decompensation following cataract surgery. Corneal decompensation may be painful and may also be debilitating to the patient's vision. Corneal transplant for this indication has at least an 85 per cent success rate. Corneal surgery for the correction of refractive errors (to eliminate the need for wearing spectacles) is still highly experimental.

## Enucleation

If total blindness affects an eye (i.e., the patient experiences no perception of light when exposed to the brightest illumination available) and the eye is free of pain and cosmetically acceptable, it should be left alone. If the eye becomes painful because of corneal degeneration, neovascular glaucoma, or other ongoing intraocular pathologic processes, it should be enucleated. In about 6 weeks, the patient's conjunctiva is usually healed sufficiently to permit fitting of a cosmetically acceptable prothesis. Most elderly patients are extremely reluctant to part with an eye, even when it is causing sufficient pain to induce continuous nausea and vomiting. The relief of pain obtained after an enucleation is gratifying.

Enucleation of an eye with a malignant melanoma has become a subject of controversy recently. Eyes with small, asymptomatic melanomas discovered on routine examination should probably be observed, without enucleation. Eyes with larger melanomas that are causing visual symptoms are probably in a rapid growth phase and may already have metastasized prior to the manipulation involved in enucleation. Enucleation is definitely not indicated for metastatic carcinoma within the eye, since this condition ordinarily responds well to radiation therapy.

### *Orbital Surgery*

Primary orbital tumors often respond well to surgical excision. If at all possible, suspected metastatic cancer in the orbit should be treated without biopsy, since biopsy is often followed by bleeding, pain, proptosis, and other complications. Primary tumors of the lid (usually basal cell carcinoma on the lower lid and squamous cell carcinoma on the upper lid) should be excised aggressively, with frozen section control and oculoplastic repair, if necessary, since these tumors have a high cure rate if entirely resected.

## BLINDNESS AND LOW VISION

In most states, *legal blindness* is defined as a visual acuity of 20/200 or worse in the better eye with the best possible spectacle or contact lens correction. A person may be legally blind, also, with visual acuity better than 20/200, if the visual field is constricted to less than 20 degrees in the eye with the larger visual field. "Low vision," "legal blindness," and "total blindness" are not synonymous. A legally blind patient may be able to read with proper low vision aids,[15] and a patient with low vision (20/50 to 20/200) may benefit immensely from low vision aids. Any patient with a visual handicap that cannot be improved by regular spectacles or surgery should be referred to a low vision service, after complete examination by an ophthalmologist. In referring a patient for a low vision evaluation, the physician must be careful not to raise the patient's expectations too high.[16] Patients with expectations of receiving a "bionic eye" or a "pair of glasses that will make me see again" will be disappointed when they are asked to learn to work with magnification devices. Yet, low vision aids and training may enable the patient to continue a meaningful, productive life in spite of a visual handicap.[17,18]

### References

1. Leibowitz HM, Krueger DE, Maunder LR, et al: The Framingham eye study monograph. An ophthalmological and epidemiological study of cataract, glaucoma, diabetic retinopathy, macular degeneration, and visual acuity in a general population of 2631 adults, 1973–1975. Surv Ophthalmol 24:335, 1980.
2. Mehelas, TJ, Kiess RD, Kollarits CR, et al: Visual loss in geriatric residents of northwestern Ohio nursing homes. Ohio State Med Assoc J Mar: 235, 1984.
3. Mehelas TJ, Kollarits CR: Pupillary clues to neuro-ophthalmic diagnoses. Postgrad Med 71:199, 1982.
4. Kollarits CR, Lubow M, Hissong S: Retinal strokes: Incidence of carotid atheromata. JAMA 222:1273, 1972.
5. Archer DB, Ernest JT, Newell FW: Classification of branch retinal vein obstruction. Trans Am Acad Ophthalmol Otolaryngol 78:148, 1974.
6. Kollarits CR, McCarthy RW, et al: Norepinephrine therapy of ischemic optic neuropathy. J Clin Neuro Ophthalmol 1:283, 1981.
7. Bajandas FJ: Neuro-ophthalmology Board Review Manual. Thorofare, NJ, Charles B. Slack, 1980.
8. Fedukowicz HB: External Infections of the Eye. 2nd ed. New York, Appleton-Century-Crofts, 1978.
9. Havener WH: Ocular Pharmacology. 4th ed. St. Louis, C.V. Mosby Co., 1978.
10. Cotlier E: The lens. *In* Moses RA (ed.): Adler's Physiology of the Eye. St. Louis, C.V. Mosby Co., 1981.
11. Kollarits CR, Swann ER, Shapiro RS, et al: HLA A1 and steroid-induced cataracts in renal transplant patients. Ann Ophthalmol 14:1116, 1982.
12. McIsaac M: Ophthalmic surgery in the elderly. Primary Care 9:173, 1982.
13. The Diabetic Retinopathy Study Research Group: Photocoagulation treatment of proliferative diabetic retinopathy. The second report of diabetic retinopathy study findings. Ophth AAOO 85:82, 1978.
14. Gass JDM: Stereoscopic Atlas of Macular Diseases: Diagnosis and Treatment. 2nd ed. St. Louis, C.V. Mosby Co., 1977, pp. 40–74.
15. Wise JB, Witter SL: Argon laser therapy for open-angle glaucoma: A pilot study. Arch Ophthalmol 97:319, 1979.
16. Adams GL, Pearlman JT, Sloan SH: Guidelines for psychiatric referral of visually handicapped patients. *In* Pearlman JT, Adams GL, Sloan SH (eds.): Psychiatric Problems in Ophthalmology. Springfield, Ill, Charles C. Thomas, 1977, pp. 142–151.
17. Fay EE: Clinical Low Vision. Boston, Little, Brown and Co., 1976.
18. Stetten D: Coping with blindness. N Engl J Med 305:458, 1981.

## Chapter 25

# Otologic Disorders

*Robert G. Anderson*
*William L. Meyerhoff*

Aging is a lifelong process that begins at birth and affects the entire body. This chapter reviews the normal physiologic manifestations of aging in the external auditory canal, middle ear, and vestibular and auditory portions of the inner ear. Rehabilitation of the elderly individual with impaired hearing is also discussed.

## EXTERNAL AUDITORY CANAL

### *Normal Anatomy*

Changes of the auditory canal associated with aging are better understood with knowledge of the normal anatomy of this structure. The external canal extends from the conchal cartilage and tragus laterally to the tympanic membrane medially (Fig. 25–1). The skin of the outer one half to one third of the canal is 0.5 mm to 1 mm thick, contains numerous hair follicles and sebaceous and cerumen glands, and has well-developed dermal and subcutaneous layers (Fig. 25–2).[1] The skin of the medial one half to two thirds of the canal, in contrast, is thin (0.2 mm), firmly attached to the underlying periosteum, and has no subcutaneous layer and only infrequent small hair follicles and glands.

### *Age-Related Changes*

#### Hair and Cerumen

Two kinds of hair grow in the external auditory canal. Minute vellus hairs, although more plentiful laterally, cover almost all of the ear canal. Tragi, the larger, laterally situated hairs, are found only in adult males. These tragi are a secondary sex characteristic and tend to become coarser, longer, and more noticeable beginning in the third or fourth decades of life.[2] In addition to the lateral external auditory canal, these large tragi are also present on the tragus, antitragus, and helix.

Cerumen glands are actually modified apocrine sweat glands. Apocrine sweat glands are most abundant in the axillae, nipples of the breast, and the external auditory canals. In the ear canals and axillae they are believed to be responsible for the distinctive odors of cerumen and sweat, respectively. Cerumen glands open onto the skin or more frequently into the hair follicle just external to the opening of the sebaceous gland ducts. In the hair follicle (apopilosebaceous duct), sebum, apocrine secretions, and desquamated epithelial cells combine to form either wet or dry cerumen, the two genetically controlled phenotypes.[3,4] It is well known that with aging the axillary apocrine sweat glands atrophy and undergo a physiologic decrease in activity. Biopsy studies have also shown a corresponding decrease in the number of cerumen glands in the ear canals of older subjects. The reduction in number and activity of cerumen glands is consistent with the *tendency* for cerumen to become drier in older individuals. However, there is no strict correlation between age and the amount or color of ear wax.[2]

Cerumen impactions tend to occur more frequently in older males than in women or young men because the large tragi in the aging male ear canal become entangled in the drier, accumulated wax, preventing the natural dislodgment of cerumen. Subsequent impactions may be removed in several ways. If the wax is relatively soft, irrigation of the ear canal with water at body temperature may be attempted. Firmly impacted cerumen often resists removal even

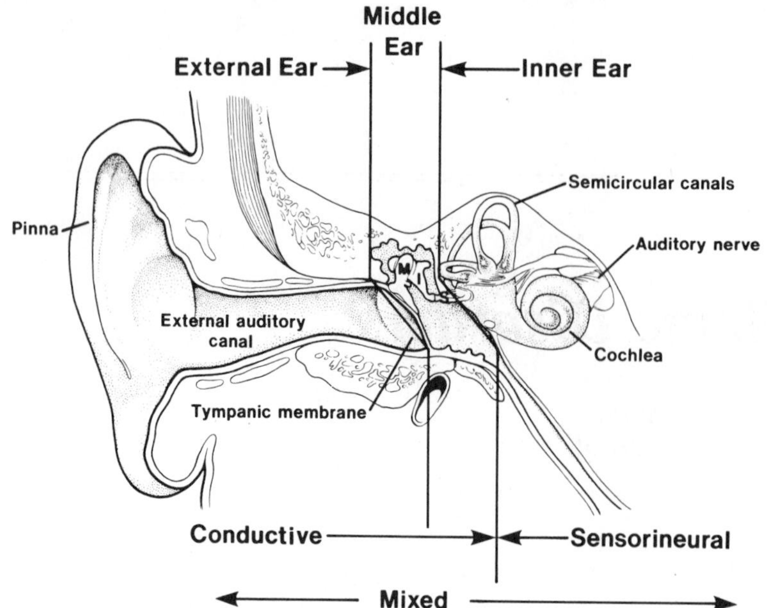


**Figure 25-1.** Types of hearing loss. This cross section demonstrates the external, middle, and inner regions of the ear. The type of hearing loss is also classified according to the region of the ear involved. M = malleus; I = incus; S = stapes.

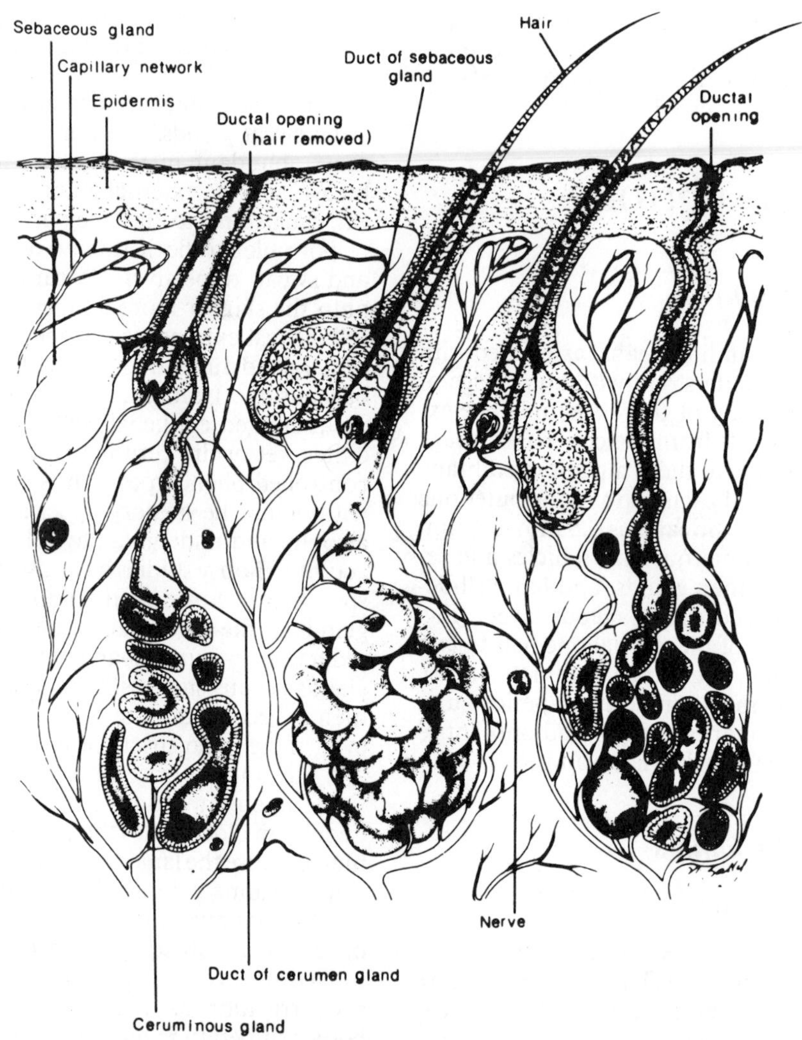


**Figure 25-2.** Drawing of skin of lateral portion of external auditory canal. (From Main T, Lim D: The human external auditory canal secretory system: An ultrastructural study. Laryngoscope 86:1164, 1976. Reproduced with permission.)

with vigorous irrigation and must therefore be manually extracted using a cerumen curette and otoscope. Care must be taken to avoid trauma to the ear canal, especially the medial portion of the canal, which is covered by thin, easily traumatized skin. Ceruminolytic agents are available and may be used to soften dry, firmly impacted cerumen. Generally, ceruminolytics are used for no more than 48 hours, following which the softened wax may be irrigated from the ear canal. Irrigation and ceruminolytics should not be used in the presence of tympanic membrane perforations.

## Pruritus

Anatomic and biochemical changes related to aging leave the skin atrophic and often inadequate to cope with the environment. In elderly individuals, itching of the skin, in general, can be attributed to dryness, but it is sometimes a major complaint even when no apparent clinically significant abnormality is present. This itching is a frequent but unwelcome symptom associated with senile skin and may be present in the external auditory canal. The problem may be exacerbated by vigorous efforts to remove accumulated dry cerumen with cotton-tipped applicators and other foreign instruments.

Dry skin results from atrophy of the epithelium and epidermal sebaceous glands. Secondarily, this causes a decrease in hydration and oiliness of the skin, which results in pruritus.[5] Strong soaps and shampoos may pool in the external auditory canal and irritate the skin. Bathing with hot water, especially in the winter when the ambient air is dry, removes moisture from the skin. Drying the external canal with rubbing alcohol or an alcohol-vinegar (acetic acid) mixture may help prevent external otitis, but also removes fat and increases dryness, leading to further irritation and itching. Frequently, chronic pruritus of the external auditory canal is not a sign of chronic otitis externa or serious dermatologic problems but merely an itch-scratch-itch cyle initiated by the dry skin associated with aging. Efforts must be directed toward breaking this cycle by avoiding moisture, trauma, and defatting agents in the external canal and occasionally by using emollients, which act as an epidermal seal, slowing the loss of moisture from the skin. Several drops of glycerine instilled in the ear canal daily will decrease the dryness and frequently preclude the need for alcohol douches after bathing and swimming. If alcohol douches are used in the elderly, they should be followed by the instillation of glycerine or another emollient.

## Infections

The aging process does *not* cause a higher incidence of infections of the external canal. However, otitis externa, when it does occur, is manifested by otalgia and tenderness of the ear canal. Progression of the disease results in serous or purulent discharge, conductive hearing loss, increasing tenderness, fever, and periauricular erythema and swelling. Initially the ear canal should be thoroughly cleaned, following which the patient is instructed to avoid getting water in the infected ear. Antibiotic-steroid otic drops are used three times daily for 7 to 10 days, and if periauricular erythema and auricular tenderness are marked, oral antibiotics may be prescribed. In individuals prone to recurrent otitis externa, efforts should be directed toward preventing water from entering the ears, avoiding all trauma (cotton-tipped applicators, fingers), and moisturizing the canal skin with glycerine. If water cannot be avoided, drying agent ear douches, such as Domeboro otic (aluminum acetate) or alcohol (alcohol-vinegar), may be used. These should be followed by an emollient to prevent excessive drying of the canal skin.

The well-described entity of malignant (necrotizing) otitis externa is a Pseudomonas osteitis and osteomyelitis of the temporal bone, and although it is most common in elderly diabetics, it has also been documented in children.[6–9] It is more likely related to a compromised vasculature and immunologic system than to the age of the patient.

## Tumors

The vast majority of tumors of the external auditory canal are squamous cell carcinomas, basal cell carcinomas, and ceruminomas. Ceruminomas include (1) adenomas, (2) pleomorphic adenomas, (3) adenoid cystic carcinoma, and (4) adenocarcinoma. Although the *median* ages at which all these tumor types occur range from 50 to 61 years, numerous cases have been reported in the third decade of life and a few cases in the teenage years.[10–13] Thus, tumors of the external auditory canal, although more prevalent in older individuals, cannot be considered manifestations of the aging process. Nonetheless, they should be considered in all patients who complain of chronic otalgia (with or without otorrhea), hearing loss, vertigo, or facial nerve paralysis. Any tissue removed from the external auditory canal should undergo histologic examination.

## MIDDLE EAR

### *Normal Anatomy*

The middle ear includes the tympanic cavity and auditory ossicles (malleus, incus, and stapes). The joints between the ossicles (incudomalleal and incudostapedial joints) are true synovial diarthrodial joints.

### *Age-Related Changes*

#### MIDDLE EAR JOINTS

The non-diseased middle ear undergoes age-related changes that are most obvious in the middle ear joints. The earliest changes in the joints consist of fraying, fibrillation, and vacuolation of the articular cartilages. Subsequent changes include hyalinization of the joint capsule, thinning and calcification of the articular cartilages, hyaline deposition in the articular disc, and, occasionally, narrowing of the joint space. The most severe arthritic changes include calcification of the joint capsule, diffuse calcification of the articular cartilages and disc, and fusion or obliteration of portions or all of the joint space. Two thirds of people 30 to 70 years of age have mild to severe arthritic changes in middle ear joints; all individuals over 70 years of age show moderate to severe arthritic changes in the middle ear joints. There is no sex predilection for these arthritic changes, which are symmetric in both ears and usually more severe in the incudomalleal joint.[14]

Arthritic changes have been evaluated audiometrically, and even complete obliteration of the joint space has no identifiable effect on sound transmission through the middle ear.[15] It is now accepted that aging alone does not result in conductive hearing loss (middle ear presbycusis).[16–18]

#### TUMORS

Middle ear and mastoid tumors occur in individuals in the same age range as do tumors of the external auditory canal, and therefore they cannot be considered manifestations of aging. These diagnoses should be considered in patients of all ages with the symptoms previously described for tumors of the external auditory canal.

## INNER EAR

### *Normal Anatomy*

The inner ear is encased in a dense bony capsule and consists of the vestibule, three semicircular canals (balance), and the cochlea (hearing). In the vestibular system, the semicircular canals sense head rotation (angular acceleration) and the utricle senses head position (linear acceleration).

### *Age-Related Changes in Vestibular Dysfunction*

Dizziness, which in this discussion includes the sensations of unsteadiness, dysequilibrium, and vertigo, is a common complaint of older individuals. Several studies have shown that almost 60 per cent of elderly people living in their homes and over 80 per cent of patients in general outpatient geriatric clinics complain of dizziness.[19,20]

Balance, or the sensation of equilibrium, is maintained by inner ear vestibular function, vision, and appropriate kinesthetic signals from the body. In evaluating the contribution of vestibular dysfunction in dizziness of the aged, it is necessary to eliminate other possible etiologic factors. Thus, visual disturbances and musculoskeletal and neurologic disorders, in addition to the well-known metabolic causes of dizziness, must be considered in the elderly patient complaining of a balance disturbance (Table 25–1). The effects of aging on (1) the histologic changes of the vestibular end-organ, (2) routine vestibular function tests (electronystagmography), and (3) performance on quantitative ataxia tests will be discussed. (See also Chapter 6, page 26).

The vestibular portion of the inner ear has not been studied as extensively as the cochlea; however, several investigators have documented the age-related loss of sensory epithelia and other components of the labyrinth. There is almost a 40 per cent decrease in the number of myelinated vestibular nerve fibers in individuals over 74 years of age compared with those less than 35 years of age.[21] This correlates very well with Rosenhall's findings of a 20 to 40 per cent decrease in the number of hair cells in the cristae and maculae in the inner ears of older age groups.[22]

A number of researchers have evaluated the effects of aging on vestibular function tests, with various findings and conclusions.[23–26] Although these tests (electronystagmography) are relatively insensitive and are used primarily to iden-

Table 25-1. DISORDERS ASSOCIATED WITH DIZZINESS

| Peripheral Vestibular System | Central Nervous System |
|---|---|
| Meniere's disease | Demyelinating diseases (multiple sclerosis, diffuse sclerosis, acute disseminated encephalitis) |
| Chronic otitis media | Localized encephalitis |
| Vestibular neuronitis | Metastatic tumors of the brain stem |
| Luetic (neurosyphilis) | Posterior fossa tumors |
| Iatrogenic (otologic surgery) | Seizures (temporal lobe epilepsy) |
| Head trauma | Orthostatic hypotension |
| Cupulolithiasis | Vascular lesions or disease (thrombotic and embolic) |
| Ototoxic drugs | **Systemic and Metabolic** |
| Otosclerotic inner ear syndrome | Hypoglycemia |
| Alternobaric vertigo | Hypothyroidism |
| Primary tumors of temporal bone (congenital cholesteatoma, glomus tumor, facial nerve neuroma, squamous cell carcinoma) | Anemia |
| Metastatic tumors of temporal bone (prostate, breast, kidney, lung) | Drug intoxication |
| Cerebellopontine angle tumors (acoustic neuroma, cholesteatoma, meningioma) | Allergic inner ear syndrome |
| | **Cervical** |
| | Cervical vertigo |

tify an imbalance between the two vestibular end-organs, it is generally accepted that certain parameters of vestibular function indicate that the aging vestibular end-organ is less sensitive to caloric stimulation than it is in younger age groups.

In addition to studies directed specifically to the peripheral vestibular system, tests have been developed to evaluate and compare balance function in general. Graybiel and Fregly,[27] in 1966, developed a new quantitative ataxia test battery. This battery included the following: walking heel to toe on a 0.75-in. rail with eyes open, standing heel to toe on a 0.75-in. rail with eyes open, standing on a 2.75-in. rail with eyes closed, standing on alternate legs with eyes closed, and the sharpened Romberg test. Examining 1055 *healthy* subjects from 16 to 60 years of age, Fregly and associates[28] found a statistically significant deterioration of balance function in the 31-to 40-year-old group compared with individuals 16 to 31 years of age.[28] There appeared to be a marked, almost linear, decrease in performance with increasing age. Although previously discussed factors may play a role, this decrease in balance-maintaining function has a high degree of correlation with the histologic age-related changes in the vestibular end-organ.

## Conditions of Dysequilibrium

In addition to a general decrease in vestibular sensitivity, at least four age-related conditions of dysequilibrium have been described:

1. Cupulolithiasis.
2. Ampullary dysequilibrium.
3. Macular dysequilibrium.
4. Vestibular ataxia of aging.[27]

**Cupulolithiasis.** Known as postural vertigo, benign positional vertigo, or benign paroxysmal vertigo, cupulolithiasis is characterized by sudden severe episodes of vertigo precipitated by a particular head position. This disorder is believed to be caused by dense deposits of insoluble breakdown products from the utricle and semicircular canals, which settle in the ampulla of the posterior semicircular canal. These deposits fix to the cupula and cause cupular deflections when the head is repositioned. Cupulolithiasis may result from head injury, ear surgery, possibly otitis media, or inner ear vascular occlusion or may occur spontaneously in individuals beyond the fourth decade of life. When cupulolithiasis occurs in older subjects, it not infrequently persists indefinitely. If incapacitating, surgical section of the responsible vestibular nerve may alleviate the problem. More often, however, patients learn to live with this disease and avoid the head positions that initiate the dizziness.

**Ampullary Dysequilibrium.** Vertigo of ampullary dysequilibrium occurs with angular head movements, such as turning the head quickly to the right or left or on extension or flexion of the head. A sense of rotation may persist for several seconds after the movement has been completed, or the sensation of downward movement may continue for several seconds after a stooping movement has been made. Pathologic documentation of this problem is lacking, and treatment is directed toward eliminating the precipitating movement.

**Macular Dysequilibrium.** Macular dysequilibrium of aging is characterized by vertigo precipitated by a change of head position relative to the direction of gravitational force after the head has been maintained in a given position for some time. For example, upon attempting to rise from bed, the patient may have such a pronounced sensation of dysequilibrium that sitting up may have to be accomplished in stages. Orthostatic hypotension may cause similar symptoms but is usually accompanied by other signs of intracranial ischemia. As with ampullary dysequilibrium, an explanation of the problem to the patient and the suggestion that the patient carefully avoid movements that elicit these symptoms are all that is indicated.

**Vestibular Ataxia.** Vestibular ataxia of aging is characterized by a constant sensation of dysequilibrium with ambulation. Walking is hesitant, with frequent side steps and a fixed head position to gain optimum advantage of visual points of reference. Although there is no pathologic documentation, the symptoms are suggestive of a loss of vestibular control over the lower limbs. This condition is most common in the seventh and eighth decades and often persists for the remainder of the patient's life.

#### Rehabilitation

It is apparent that the vestibular system is not spared the effects of aging. Older individuals do suffer from dizziness and have more difficulty maintaining equilibrium than younger individuals. Efforts should be directed toward diagnosing and treating known otologic and systemic causes of dysequilibrium and improving patients' visual and proprioceptive contact with the environment. The use of thin-soled shoes, canes, or walkers and removal of area rugs or carpets may be suggested. Visual contact with the environment may be enhanced by using night lights, wearing eyeglasses (either newly prescribed or a stronger prescription) or undergoing corneal or cataract surgery.

## AUDITORY DYSFUNCTION

### *Types of Hearing Loss*

Hearing impairment is classified as conductive, sensorineural, or mixed. *Conductive* hearing loss may be caused by anything that precludes the normal transmission of sound through the external auditory canal, tympanic membrane, or middle ear. Various conditions that frequently result in conductive hearing loss include impacted cerumen, tympanic membrane perforation, otitis media, and discontinuity or fixation of the middle ear ossicles (e.g., otosclerosis). *Sensorineural* hearing loss occurs when the inner ear, auditory nerve (cranial nerve VIII), brainstem, or cortical auditory pathways are not functioning properly. A *mixed* hearing loss is a conductive loss superimposed on a sensorineural loss (Fig. 25-1).

### *Audiometric Evaluation*

Hearing sensitivity is measured in units of sound that are known as decibels (dB). A decibel is not a fixed value of sound but represents a logarithmic ratio based on a standard reference level of acoustic pressure. In standardized hearing tests, discrete frequencies of sound from 250 cycles per second [hertz (Hz)] to 8000 Hz are presented in a prescribed manner until the listener responds to the stimulus being presented, thus establishing the threshold of hearing sensitivity. A hearing threshold of 15 dB or less at any given frequency is considered normal, and the more decibels of sound that are required for a person to hear, the poorer the hearing. Although an average hearing threshold of 30 dB or less in the speech frequencies (500 to 3000 Hz) is usually satisfactory for routine listening needs, amplification may be indicated if psychosocial needs or work-related requirements demand better hearing.

Hearing for pure tones is measured in two ways for each ear. Air conduction (AC) is the measured level of sound transmitted through the ear canal and middle ear ossicles to the inner ear. Bone conduction (BC), on the other hand, involves placing a vibrator on the mastoid bone behind the ear and directly stimulating the inner ear, thus bypassing the external and middle ears. If measurements of hearing sensitivity by AC and BC are equal and less than 15 dB, no significant impediment to hearing exists. If they are equal and greater than 15 dB, a sensorineural or nerve-type hearing loss is present. In a conductive hearing loss, the threshold for AC is greater than for BC. A threshold greater for BC than for AC implies faulty testing, patient confusion, or malingering.

Although pure tone hearing tests provide significant information regarding auditory function, another important consideration involves the ability to understand speech. *Speech discrimination* or understanding is determined by using a standardized list of specific single syllable (monosyllabic) words, which are presented to the patient at a comfortably loud listening level. Results are computed in percentages based on the number of words the patient correctly repeats, with 100 per cent being a perfect speech discrimination score. Thus, the higher the speech discrimination score, the better the ability to understand speech. In general, individuals with scores lower than 70 to 80 per cent will have noticeable problems understanding speech.

### *Presbycusis*

In the United States, hearing loss constitutes one of the most common physical disabilities. For older adults, the major auditory dysfunction is the result of presbycusis. Several studies have indicated that approximately 25 per cent of people between 65 to 74 years of age and almost 50 per cent of people 75 years of age or older experience hearing difficulties.[30,31] There are currently more than 25 million people in the United States over the age of 65 years.[32] This represents a significant number of people with presbycusis or noise-induced hearing loss or a combination of the two.

Since Zwaardemaker[33] first described the clinical manifestations of high tone hearing loss in the aged, numerous contributions have been made to our knowledge of presbycusis. Researchers have attempted to determine the effect on hearing of diet, metabolism, arteriosclerosis, noise, stress, and heredity.[34-36] Elegant histopathologic studies have elucidated end-organ and central nervous system pathologic processes, and correlated these changes with various audiometric patterns.[29,37,38]

Clinical studies have demonstrated that hearing in populations not exposed to noise is better than in individuals from noisy industrialized areas. Also, better hearing is maintained in the higher frequencies in populations with lower serum cholesterol than in those with high serum cholesterol and higher rates of coronary artery disease. Black males in industrial areas have been shown to have better hearing than age-matched White males with no history of exposure to industrial noise. This finding indicates a possible genetic factor in hearing loss. Most likely, arteriosclerotic vascular disease, industrial or occupational noise exposure, and heredity all play major roles in hearing loss of the elderly.[39-41]

Identification of potentially treatable causes of hearing loss is of utmost importance, and the diagnosis of presbycusis should be a "diagnosis of exclusion" (Table 25-2). Not infrequently the patient will reveal a history of ototoxic drug treatment, significant noise-exposure, or a familial predisposition to sensorineural hearing loss occurring earlier than would normally be expected for presbycusis. In cases of familial predisposition, medical or surgical treatment is of no benefit. If the audiogram and history are typical of noise-induced hearing loss (maximum hearing loss at 4 KHz), protective ear devices may help to prevent further hearing loss.

## Classification

Initial reports by Crowe[42] and Saxen[43] described two pathologic types of deafness. One mainly involved the organ of Corti (sensory presbycusis), whereas the other primarily involved the cochlear neurons (neural presbycusis). In 1964, Schuknecht[37] suggested two additional categories, one involving the stria vascularis and termed metabolic presbycusis and the other thought to be due to an alteration of the complex motion mechanics of the inner ear caused by stiffening of the basilar membrane (inner ear conductive deafness) (Fig. 25-3).

Since there is usually more than one area of degeneration present in a given ear, the diagnosis of one of the four types is not frequently made. The general term, presbycusis, therefore describes a slowly progressive, *otherwise unexplained,* symmetric, sensorineural hearing loss, which begins in middle to older age and is usually worse in the frequencies above 2000 Hz (Fig. 25-4).

## Characteristics

Certain characteristics of presbycusis have been established. It appears that in the majority of subjects, the pattern of the pure tone hearing loss is consistent over the years. This suggests that the site of the pathology remains unchanged with aging. Only about 8 per cent of the patients with presbycusis will have a change in the pure tone *pattern* (flat or descending), although almost all patients will experience a progressive increase in pure tone thresholds.[44]

A well-documented auditory handicap in older people is their decrease in speech discrimination. Many elderly people report that they can hear people talking but cannot understand what is being said. Regardless of how loudly speech is presented to the patient with decreased discrimination, a large percentage of the words will remain unintelligible. In presbycusis, particularly the pure neural type, the discrimination loss for speech is greater than would be predicted from the pure tone audiogram. Another significant characteristic of presbycusis is the finding that speech discrimination for a given pure tone hearing level is worse in older patients than in younger patients.[45] This effect is minimal with a pure tone average of less than 10 dB but increases considerably with greater pure tone losses (Fig. 25-5). Other parameters of speech discrimination tests, e.g., word rate per minute and overlapping or interruption of words, confirm that older patients have poorer speech discrimination than young patients with the same pure tone averages. This raises the question of whether the decreased performance of older individuals on speech discrimination tests is due to peripheral end-organ disease or central auditory pathway disease, possibly starting as far peripherally as the first order cochlear neurons and extending proximally to the auditory cortex of the temporal lobe. Many researchers believe

**Table 25–2.** CAUSES OF BILATERALLY SYMMETRIC SENSORINEURAL HEARING LOSS*

| Disorder | Characteristics | Diagnosis | Treatment |
|---|---|---|---|
| Meniere's disease | Episodic attacks of fluctuant SNHL, vertigo, tinnitus, aural fullness or pressure; bilateral in 20–30% of cases | History of typical attacks with symptom-free intervals; hearing loss involves low tones initially and later all frequencies; rule out neurosyphilis | Medical: Diuretics and low-salt diet<br>Surgical: Decompression or shunt of endolymphatic sac; section of vestibular nerve |
| Luetic hearing loss (late acquired syphilis) | Frequently bilateral SNHL with no characteristic audiometric pattern; speech discrimination score often worse than would be predicted on basis of pure tone thresholds; often associated with vestibular symptoms; may mimic Meniere's disease | Positive FTA-ABS test, with or without clinical history of syphilis | Penicillin and oral steroids |
| Paget's disease | Slowly progressive SNHL and CHL; SNHL worse in high frequencies; maximum CHL of 20–30 dB at 500 Hz | Skeletal deformities of skull and long bones of extremities, elevated serum alkaline phosphatase and urinary hydroxyproline | Calcitonin |
| Hypothyroidism | Slowly progressive SNHL affecting all frequencies equally | Usual clinical stigmata of hypothyroidism; decreased serum $T_4$ | Desiccated thyroid or synthetic mixture of $T_4$ and $T_3$ |
| Ototoxic drugs | Hearing loss with or without vestibular dysfunction following treatment with known ototoxic drug | History | None |
| Hereditary Progressive SNHL | Progressive SNHL beginning at earlier age than expected for presbycusis; possible positive family history | Family history | None |
| Noise-induced hearing loss | History of prolonged exposure to loud continuous noise or brief exposure to loud impulse noise | History; characteristic audiogram with maximum hearing loss at 4000 Hz; may not be distinguishable from presbycusis | None; use of ear protectors may prevent further loss from noise exposure |
| Head trauma | Severe head injury often resulting in loss of consciousness and bilateral temporal bone fractures | History | None |
| Cochlear otosclerosis and far-advanced clinical otosclerosis | Far-advanced clinical otosclerosis (stapedial fixation) and cochlear otosclerosis (SNHL) may appear on audiogram as severe to profound SNHL; patient will have good speech modulation (unlike in profound SNHL) and will be wearing or will have worn a bone conduction hearing aid; possibly a family history for otosclerosis | History is suggestive but surgical exploration of stapes footplate is diagnostic and therapeutic; post-stapedectomy patient may be able to wear ear-level hearing aid with good results | Stapedectomy, sodium fluoride |

* The hearing loss from any of these diseases may be improved with hearing aids unless it is of such a degree that hearing aids will be inadequate or unsatisfactory. Individuals with bilateral profound SNHL may be candidates for a cochlear implant and should be evaluated by an otologist to determine their suitability for such a device.

*Abbreviations:* SNHL-sensorineural hearing loss; FTA-ABS test- fluorescent treponemal antibody test; CHL-conductive hearing loss; Hz-hertz (cycles per second); dB-decibel (arbitrary unit of sound intensity).

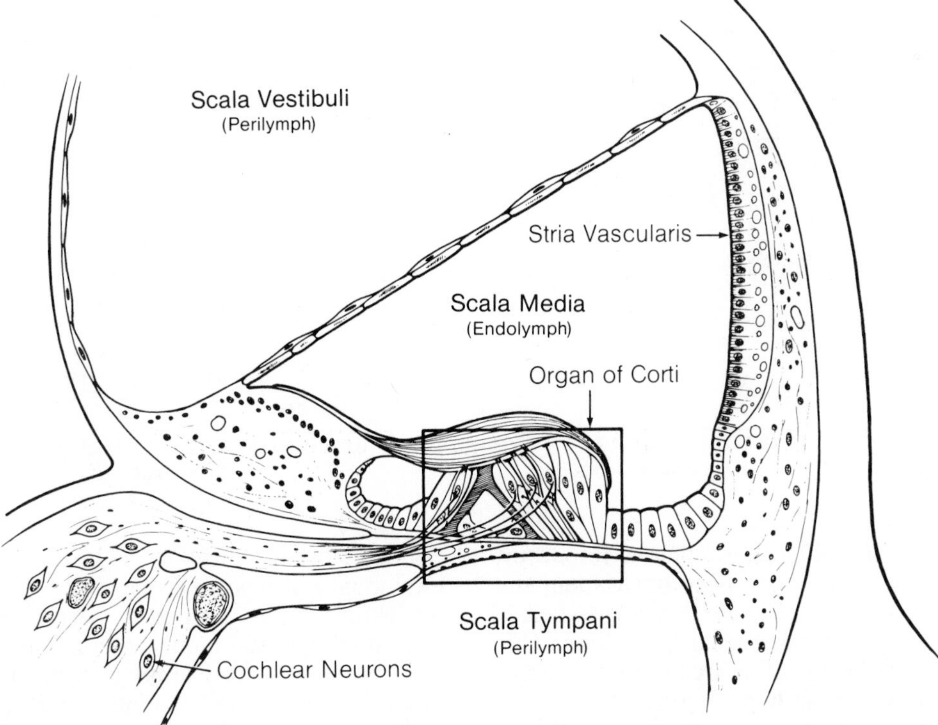


**Figure 25–3.** Cross section of the cochlea showing the cochlear neurons, organ of Corti, and stria vascularis.

that central factors (such as decreased cell counts in the temporal lobes, increased time for information processing in the brain, and possibly increased synaptic delays in the central auditory pathways) are responsible for the decreased speech discrimination abilities of the elderly.[46,47]

Further limitations in hearing concern a decrease in directional hearing. Many older people experience difficulty in identifying very small

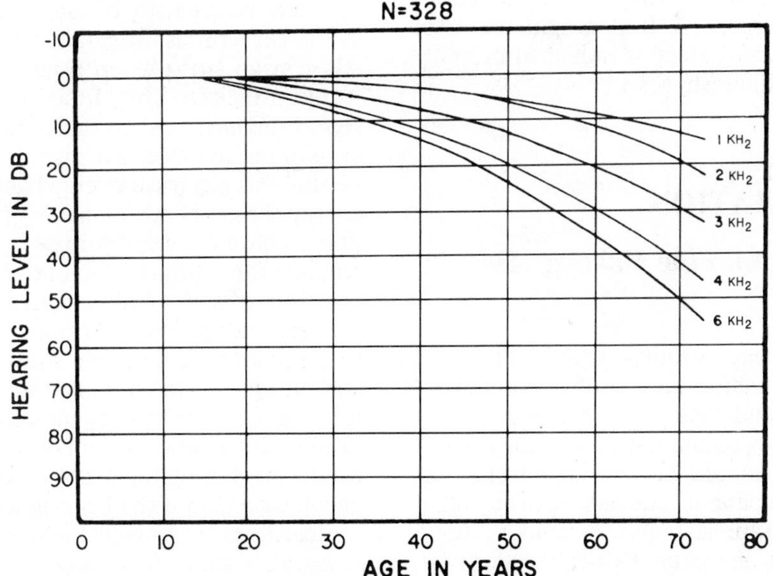


**Figure 25–4.** Hearing level as a function of age (non-noise occupation). Hearing threshold shifts from 1 to 6 KC. Note that the pure tone hearing levels *(thresholds)* increase with age, especially in the higher frequencies. (From Glorig A, Davis H: Age, noise and hearing loss. Ann Otol 70:556, 1961. Reproduced with permission.)

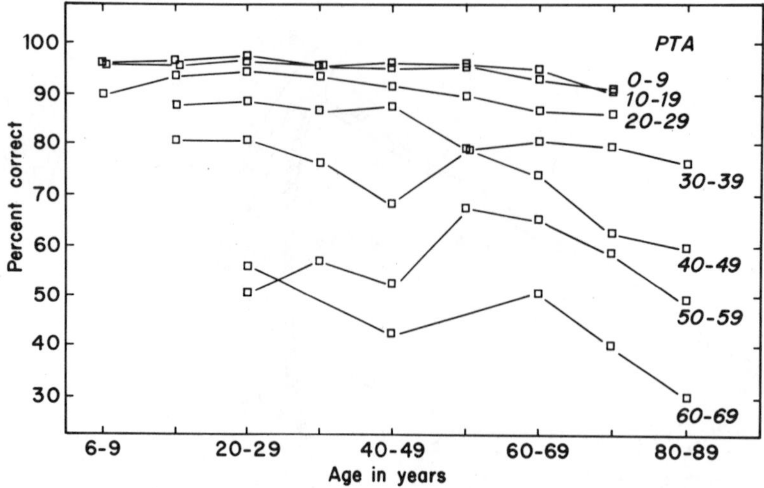


**Figure 25–5.** For a given pure tone hearing loss, the percentage of correct responses for speech discrimination decreases with increasing age. PTA = pure tone average. (From Jerger J: Audiological findings in aging. Adv Otorhinolaryngol 20:115, 1973. Reproduced with permission.)

interaural time differences. This is important when several people are positioned about the listener or when the listener is trying to hear a speaker when there is background noise. This loss of directional hearing creates further problems with understanding of speech.[48]

It is obvious that presbycusis is more than a *simple* loss of hearing. It is a complex disorder involving loss of speech processing and discrimination as well as perception of pure tones. Understanding the emotional distress that accompanies this deteriorating sensory function in older individuals will help in suggesting rehabilitative measures. Careful explanations of the problem, reassurance that the patient is not "going deaf," and encouragement and motivation to continue participating in social functions are very important. A trial amplification of sound with hearing aid(s) is indicated in many individuals with presbycusis.

# AUDITORY REHABILITATION

## *Factors Determining Hearing Aid Candidacy*

Once a thorough otologic examination and audiologic evaluation have confirmed bilateral sensorineural and medically untreatable hearing loss, auditory rehabilitation and the use of a hearing aid(s) should be considered and discussed with the patient. The success of any rehabilitative program is highly dependent upon such factors as the patient's health, alertness, and motivation. For many elderly people, the support and assistance of family members, nursing home staff, and interested friends are critical to the successful use of hearing aids. An individual with hearing impairment who thrives on senior citizen activities, participation in church groups, and family interaction may derive great benefit from amplification. However, one who is debilitated, confined to bed, or generally not motivated may have only limited use for such a device, regardless of the degree of hearing loss.

## *Physical Aspects of Hearing Aids*

A hearing aid is a miniature amplifier of acoustic energy, designed specifically to improve human hearing. Its primary function is to increase the intensity of sound and to deliver it to the ear with as little distortion as possible.[49] All hearing aids use essentially the same electronic principle. They function by converting sound (acoustic energy) into electrical energy, amplifying the electrical signal, and then converting this electrical energy back into acoustic energy. They operate on battery power and contain a volume control for use by the patient to regulate the amount of sound that is received. Selection of a given aid is based on how much the hearing needs to be improved, the various frequencies that need the most amplification, and the upper limit of sound that the patient can tolerate. Current hearing aids can often be adjusted to fit a patient's individual and changing needs, precluding the necessity of purchasing a new hearing aid if the hearing loss changes.

Hearing aids are available in several different styles, all of which function in basically the same fashion. The selection of a particular style of hearing aid will depend upon the patient's type and degree of hearing loss, cosmetic desires, personal preference, and manual dexterity for inserting the aid and adjusting the controls (Fig. 25-6). The postauricular (behind-the-ear) aid is currently the most commonly recommended device because of its small, neat appearance, wide application, and versatility of fitting. The body aid is capable of delivering greater power for more severe hearing losses and is also appropriate for patients who may have difficulty manipulating the smaller hearing aid controls on the ear level models. Patients with a variety of hearing losses are now able to use the cosmetically appealing all-in-the-ear aid successfully, although this is somewhat less adaptable for fitting purposes than the other styles.

### *Determining the Appropriate Hearing Aid*

When a patient is believed to be a candidate for a hearing aid, a hearing aid evaluation by a qualified audiologist will allow selection of the best aid, proper ear mold, and style of the aid and will determine whether one or both ears should be aided. Although actual procedures vary among audiologists, the intent of a hearing aid evaluation is always to determine whether amplification is needed and which features will be most effective in improving communication for a particular patient.[50]

It is particularly important, especially for the elderly patient, that he or she actually experiences hearing aid use prior to procuring his or her own aid. Elderly individuals are usually the most difficult to fit because of acquired poor listening habits, unwillingness to make changes in their lives, poor discrimination ability, and often decreased tolerance to loud sounds. On the basis of a formal hearing aid evaluation, it is usually possible to predict whether a patient will reject or be able successfully to incorporate hearing aid use into his or her daily life. The final decision is whether to aid one ear (monaural fitting) or both ears (binaural fitting). Although there is currently no standard clinical test procedure available to prove the advantages of binaural amplification, the literature suggests that binaural aids assist in localization of sound and provide increased sound intensity.[51,52] There are also several studies showing improved speech discrimination ability through the use of binaural hearing aids.[53,54] In the geriatric population, the additional cost of two aids must be weighed in light of actual communication needs. Binaural aids may be considered if the pure tone hearing loss is bilaterally symmetric (thresholds for each ear within 15 dB of each other) and speech discrimination scores for each ear are within 16 per cent to 20 per cent of each other. Initial use of *binaural* aids must be strictly on a trial basis to allow the patient the opportunity to experience the potential benefits to be gained in everyday listening before a financial commitment is made.

Family members frequently expect the new aid to return the long-impaired hearing to normal. This is not a realistic expectation. It is often necessary to counsel the family regarding the limitations of the elderly patient's newly aided auditory ability.

## OTHER REHABILITATIVE PROGRAMS

In some instances, the use of amplification alone may be insufficient to compensate satis-

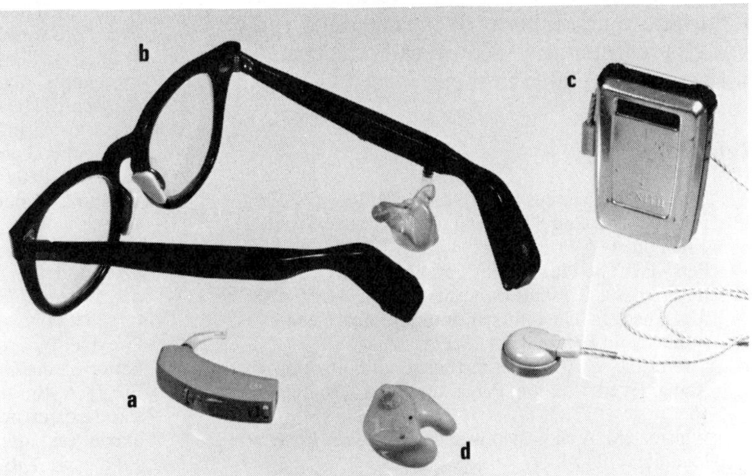


**Figure 25-6.** Commonly used hearing aids. *(a)* Postauricular (behind-the-ear) aid. *(b)* Eyeglass hearing aid. *(c)* Body aid. *(d)* All-in-the-ear hearing aid.

factorily for communication deficits caused by a hearing loss. For the elderly patient who wishes to remain an actively involved member of the community, supplementary auditory rehabilitation programs may be appropriate. Programs for communication counseling are generally conducted by a certified audiologist and consist of a regular series of sessions designed to teach seemingly obvious strategies, such as watching the face of the speaker for supplementary communicative cues. Many other more subtle strategies are available to allow the patient more enjoyment from communicative encounters.

Lip-reading instruction may also be available to the elderly hearing-impaired patient. Lip-reading skills are more often slowly acquired rather than learned in a short course, and it is unrealistic to have high expectations that lip reading alone, as a rehabilitative alternative, will make up for limitations in communication as a result of hearing loss. The benefit of lip-reading services for the hearing impaired elderly may be in helping them to develop a greater awareness of the visual aspects of communication (e.g., facial expression, gestures, environmental clues), which can often successfully supplement aided hearing. These lessons, when offered in group sessions, can be rewarding psychologically to the hearing impaired elderly.

## CONCLUSION

Some of the most significant age-related changes experienced by the elderly are found in the auditory and vestibular regions of the inner ear. Hearing loss, both for pure tones and speech discrimination, and vestibular dysfunction resulting in a decreased ability to maintain equilibrium, are problems affecting a significant segment of society. Thorough evaluation, treatment, and rehabilitation of these elderly individuals are imperative if they are to receive the full benefits available to them.

### References


1. Senturia BH, Marcus MD, Lucente FE: Diseases of the External Ear. 2nd ed. New York, Grune & Stratton, 1980, pp. 4–6.
2. Perry ET: The Human Ear Canal. 1st ed. Springfield, Ill, Charles C Thomas Publishers, 1957, pp. 57–70.
3. Matsunaga E: The dimorphism in human normal cerumen. Ann Hum Genet 25:273, 1962.
4. Montagna W: Advances in Biology of Skin. Vol. VI. Aging. 1st ed. London, Pergamon Press, 1964, pp. 1–16.
5. Waisman M: A clinical look at the aging skin. Postgrad Med 66:87, 1979.
6. Chandler J: Malignant external otitis. Laryngoscope 78:1257, 1968.
   *This is the original article describing "malignant" otitis externa and defining its characteristics, morbidity, and mortality.*
7. Chandler J: Malignant external otitis: Further considerations. Ann Otol 86:417, 1977.
   *Dr. Chandler, who first described this disorder, adds further clinical information on the diagnosis and treatment of this serious disease. This is an excellent article, well worth reading.*
8. Horn KL, Gherini S: Malignant external otitis of childhood. Am J Otol 2:402, 1981.
9. Joachims HZ: Malignant external otitis in children. Arch Otolaryngol 102:236, 1976.
10. Crabtree JA, Britton BH, Pierce MK: Carcinoma of the external auditory canal. Laryngoscope 86:405, 1976.
11. Dehna LP, Chen KTK: Primary tumors of the external and middle ear. Arch Otolaryngol 106:13, 1980.
12. Johns ME, Headington HT: Squamous cell carcinoma of the external auditory canal. Arch Otolaryngol 100:45, 1974.
13. Lewis JS; Cancer of the ear. Laryngoscope 70:551, 1960.
14. Etholm B, Belal A: Senile changes in the middle ear joints. Ann Otol 83:49, 1974.
15. Elpern BS, Greisen O, Anderson HC: Experimental studies on sound transmission in the human ear. Acta Otolaryngol 60:223, 1965.
16. Klotz RE, Kilbane M: Hearing in an aging population. Preliminary report. N Engl J Med 266:277, 1962.
17. Melrose J, Welsh OL, Luterman DM: Auditory responses in selected elderly men. J Gerontol 18:267, 1963.
18. Sataloff J, Vassallo L, Menduke H: Presbycusis: Air and bone conduction thresholds. Laryngoscope 75:889, 1965.
19. Droller H, Pembarton J: Vertigo in a random sample of elderly people living in their homes. J Laryngol Otol 67:689, 1953.
    *This article documents the suspicions of many geriatricians about the prevalence of imbalance in the nonhospitalized and otherwise functional elderly.*
20. Orma E, Koskenoja M: Postural dizziness in the aged. Geriatrics 12:49, 1957.
21. Bergstrom B: Morphology of the vestibular nerve. II. The number of myelinated vestibular nerve fibers in man at various ages. Acta Otolaryngol 76:173, 1973.
22. Rosenhall U: Degenerative patterns in the aging human vestibular neuro-epithelia. Acta Otolaryngol 76:208, 1973.
23. Arslan M: The senescence of the vestibular apparatus. Pract Otorhinolaryngol 19:475–483, 1957.
24. Bruner A, Norris T: Age related changes in caloric nystagmus. Acta Otolaryngol Suppl 282:1, 1979.
25. Karlsen E, Hassanein R, Goetzinger C: The effects of age, sex, hearing loss and water temperature on caloric nystagmus. Laryngoscope 91:620, 1981.
26. Mulch G, Petermann W: Influence of age on results of vestibular function tests. Ann Otol Suppl 56, 88:1, 1979.
    *This is a review of previous studies on vestibular function test results in the elderly. Reasonable explanations are presented for conflicting findings and conclusions by the various researchers.*
27. Graybiel A, Fregly A: A new quantitative ataxia test battery. Acta Otolaryngol 61:292, 166.
28. Fregly A, Smith M, Graybiel A: Revised normative standards of performance of men on a quantitative ataxia test battery. Acta Otolaryngol 75:10, 1973.
    *Fregly presents objective evidence documenting the loss of balance-maintaining ability beginning in the fourth decade and increasing with advancing age. It is*

*a well-written clearly stated article with rather impressive findings.*

29. Schuknecht HF: Pathology of the Ear. 1st ed. Cambridge, Mass, Harvard University Press, 1974, pp. 388–409.
30. U.S. Department of Health, Education, and Welfare: Prevalence of selected impairments, United States, 1971. DHEW Publication No. (HRA) 75–1527. Rockville, MD, 1975.
31. U.S. Public Health Service: Hearing status and ear examination: Findings among adults, United States 1960–1962. Health Services and Mental Health Administration. PHS Publication No. 1000, Series 11, No. 32. Public Health Service, Washington, D.C., U.S. Govt. Printing Office, 1968.
32. U.S. Dept. of Commerce: 1980 Census of Population, Bureau of the Census. Pub. No. PC80-S1-1, Washington, D.C., U.S. Government Printing Office, 1981.
33. Zwaardemaker H: Der Verlust an hoehen Toenen mit zunehmendem Alter: Ein neues Gesetz. Arch Ohr Nas-Kehlk-Heilk 32:53, 1891.
34. Johnsson L, Hawkins J: Vascular changes in the human inner ear associated with aging. Ann Otol 81:364, 1972.
35. Naritomi H, Meyer J, Sakai F, et al.: Effects of advancing age on regional cerebral blood flow. Arch Neurol 36:410, 1979.
36. Rosen S, Olin P: Hearing loss and coronary heart disease. Arch Otolaryngol 82:236, 1965.
37. Schuknecht HF: Further observations on the pathology of presbycusis. Arch Otolaryngol 80:369, 1964.
38. Suga F, Lindsay J: Histopathological observations of presbycusis. Ann Otol 85:169, 1976.
39. Rosen S: Presbycusis study of a relatively noise-free population in Sudan. Ann Otol 71:727, 1962.
    *This article presents a strong case against the inevitability of presbycusis as a disease of "aging." The author reasonably suggests that diet, cigarette smoking, exercise, noise pollution, and stress play major roles in the hearing loss common beyond middle age in industrialized societies.*
40. Royster LH, Thomas WG: Age effected hearing levels for a white nonindustrial noise exposed population (NINEP) and their use in evaluating industrial hearing conservation programs. Ann Ind Hyg Ass J 40:504, 1979.
    *Possible genetic factors in hearing loss of the elderly are explored by Royster and Thomas, who compared the hearing of Blacks and Whites. They found that noise-exposed Black males had better hearing than White males not exposed to high levels of noise.*
41. Rosen S, Plester D, El-Mofty A, Rosen HV: Relation of hearing loss to cardiovascular disease. Trans Am Acad Ophthalmol Otol 68:433–444, 1964.
42. Crowe SJ, Guild SR, Polvogt LM: Observations on the pathology of hightone deafness. Johns Hopkins Hosp Bull 54:315, 1934.
43. Saxen A: Pathologie und Klinik der Altersschwerhoerigkeit. Acta Otolaryngol. Suppl 23, 1937.
44. Dayal VS, Nussbaum MA: Patterns of puretone loss in presbycusis. Acta Otolaryngol 71:382, 1971.
45. Jerger J: Audiological findings in aging. Adv Otorhinolaryngol 20:115, 1973.
46. Calearo D, Lazzaroni A: Speech intelligibility in relation to the speech of the message. Laryngoscope 67:410, 1957.
47. Hinchcliff R: The anatomical locus of presbycusis. J Speech Hear Disord 27:301, 1962.
48. Matzker J, Springborn E: Richtungshoeren und Lebensalter. Z Laryngol Rhinol 37:739, 1958.
49. Pollack MD: Electroacoustic characteristics. *In* Pollack MD (ed.): Amplification of Hearing Impaired. 1st ed. New York, Grune and Stratton, 1975.
50. Burney PA: A survey of hearing aid evaluation procedures. ASHA 14:439, 1972.
51. Tillman T, Kasten R, Horner J: The Effect of the Head Shadow on the Reception of Speech. Convention of the American Speech and Hearing Association, 1963.
52. Wright HN: Binaural hearing and the hearing impaired. Arch Otolaryngol 70:485, 1959.
53. Harris JD: Monaural and binaural speech intelligibility and the stereophonic effect based upon temporal cues. Laryngoscope 75:428, 1965.
54. Heffler HA, Schultz MD: Some implications of binaural signal selection for hearing aid evaluation. J Speech Hear Res 7:279, 1964.

## Chapter 26

# Falls

*Henry M. Wieman*
*Evan Calkins*

Falls are one of the most important problems in geriatrics. Their importance relates in part to the increased susceptibility of older people to the serious consequences of falling, such as hip fractures or subdural hematomas. It has been estimated that accidents, two thirds of which are falls, are the fifth most common cause of death among the elderly[1] and contribute to an unknown number of additional deaths. Even when not accompanied by physical injury, falls limit freedom for many elders through subsequent fear of falling again. Falls may be important indicators of a serious or potentially serious underlying medical disorder which, if not identified or reversed, has a high likelihood of leading to death.[2] Thus, falls constitute a serious threat to life, health, and quality of life of elderly people (Fig. 26–1).

Most studies indicate that women suffer more falls and higher mortality and morbidity from falls than men.[1,3] Osteoporosis contributes to this difference.[4] Other factors include the fact that women are more likely to live alone and to experience a longer period of disability and dependency.[5]

Elderly persons are very apt to conceal from their physician the occurrence or frequency of falls.[2] This may be the result of forgetfulness, denial, fear, or unwillingness to communicate fully with the physician. In the minds of many people falling is associated with a degree of incapacity that is almost infantile, which people who have led independent and useful lives are apt to suppress or conceal. Therefore, it is very important that the physician specifically ask any new patient about the occurrence of falls and review this possibility with patient or family or both at repeated intervals.

These statements primarily concern the elderly person living in the community, who comes to a physician for periodic visits. Falls are also an important problem for many elderly people in hospitals and nursing homes.[6] It is our view that the etiology and management of falls occurring in the nursing home setting are significantly different from those of falls occurring in community dwelling elderly. In considering the range of conditions that may be associated with falls, it is helpful to differentiate those factors that are relevant for the community dwelling elderly from those that are relevant for patients in an institutional setting.

## ETIOLOGY OF FALLS

Table 26–1 lists the causes of falls in the elderly. In any individual, several mechanisms predisposing one to falls are probably at work. Some authors have drawn a dichotomy between environmental and person-centered falls,[3] but most agree that, in most cases, the fall results from an interaction between the person and environmental defects.[7]

Table 26–2 lists the clinical presentations likely to ensue from different types of falls. Frequently patients will be unable to recollect or reconstruct the precise sequence of symptoms or events that preceded the fall. This is especially true for patients who have a cognitive deficiency. Nevertheless, a careful history from patient and family will often provide important clues to the type of fall and the correct diagnosis.[8]

### *Falls Caused by Environmental Factors*

Factors in the physical environment are important and usually obvious.[9,10] These include

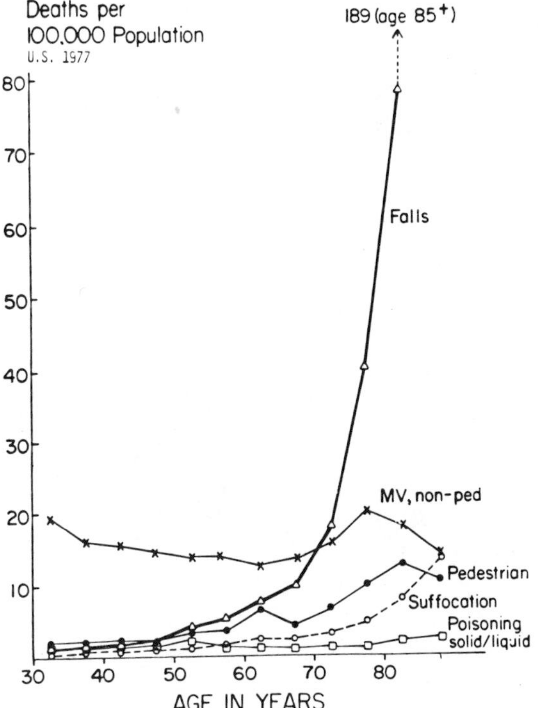


**Figure 26-1.** The frequency of deaths from accidents of various kinds in people from infancy to 80 years of age. Above age 70, falls become the most frequent cause of accidental death. (From Baker SP, Harvey AH: Fall injuries in the elderly. Clin Geriatr Med 1(3):502, 1985.)

**Table 26-1.** CAUSES OF FALLS IN THE ELDERLY

1. Environmental factors
   - Physical environment
     - Slippery floors
       - Smooth surface
       - Urine or other fluid on floor
     - Throw rugs
     - Obstructions (including grandchildren)
     - Door steps or uneven steps
     - Bathroom hazards: lack of handles, slippery bathtub
     - Poorly designed stairs or walkways
       - Absence of railings
   - Visual environment
     - Inadequate light
     - Poor marking of steps and other hazards
2. Central nervous system
   - Dementia, depression, somnolence
   - Cerebrovascular insufficiency (strokes and TIAs), carotid and vertebral artery insufficiency
   - Anemia
   - Normal pressure hydrocephalus
3. Neurosensory deficit
   - Vestibular dysfunction
   - Visual abnormality
4. Cardiovascular disease
   - Arrhythmia, including Stokes-Adams
   - Postural hypotension
5. Metabolic derangements
   - Hyponatremia or hypovolemia
   - Hypoglycemia
6. Loss of proprioception (cord or peripheral nerves)
   - Cervical spondylosis
   - Peripheral neuropathy
7. Musculoskeletal deficit, including abnormalities in gait
8. Inappropriate patterns of care
   - Restraints
   - Drugs

such hazards as throw rugs, slippery floors, inappropriately placed furniture, toys, and even grandchildren. They also include poorly designed stairs and walkways and absence of railings and handles (Fig. 26-2). Once the hazard has been pointed out, the problem is apt to be remedied. Therefore, physical hazards are a more common cause of falls in the person who comes to the hospital with a fractured hip than in an individual who complains of repeated falls, in whom a variety of causes or predisposing factors may be at work (Table 26-2).

## *Central Nervous System*

Demented patients fall frequently.[8,12] Whether this is because of inattention, somnolence, poor judgment, or specific psychomotor deficits associated with degenerative processes of the brain has not yet been elucidated clearly. Many falls that occur in nursing homes characterized by patients sliding off furniture are related to somnolence rather than to musculoskeletal deficiency or syncope. Both depression and dementia have been implicated in falls.[13]

Falls are frequently associated with small cerebral infarcts or more commonly, transient is-

**Table 26-2.** TYPES OF FALLS

1. Slips and trips: The patient may falsely attribute the fall to these causes when in reality it is due to a physical deficit.
2. Falls while attempting a difficult maneuver (such as climbing over a bed rail).
3. Syncope: The loss of consciousness immediately precedes the fall, and may, itself, be preceded by a brief interval of giddiness or unsteadiness.
4. Seizure: The loss of consciousness accompanies the fall. It may be preceded by an aura. It may or may not be accompanied by clonic movements and incontinence.
5. Drop attack: Sudden loss of muscular tone without loss of consciousness.
6. Vertigo: The patient experiences true dizziness (the room seems to spin) and falls to one side or the other.
7. Sliding off furniture: due to weakness or somnolence.

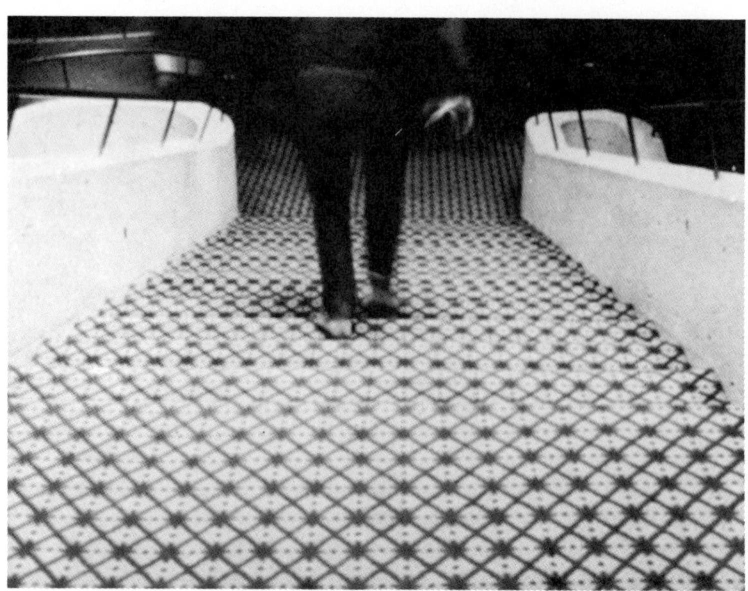

**Figure 26–2.** An illustration of the importance of environmental design in the prevention of falls. Vivid patterns, on floor or steps, can obscure essential visual information about the position of each tread. (From Archea JC: Environmental factors in stair accidents by the elderly. Clin Geriatr Med 1(3):561, 1985).

chemic attacks. The patient may not remember or may dismiss as unimportant the symptoms of cerebral ischemia and may incorrectly attribute the fall to a trip or slip. In a number of cases, the cerebrovascular insufficiency reflects loss of patency of carotid or vertebral vessels. The significance of a bruit over the carotid artery as a clue to the presence of obstruction to the artery is currently under active debate.[14,15]

Additional information on cerebral ischemia is presented in Chapter 21.

Insufficiency of the vertebral artery is a fairly common cause of intermittent syncope and falls. Upon careful questioning, the patient with this syndrome will often state that the symptoms occur when he or she is looking up and to one side, as when reaching for a high object. The condition is especially apt to occur in patients with moderately severe cervical spondylosis.

Epilepsy is not a frequent cause of falls in the elderly but is often overlooked. Since it is one of the more readily reversible causes, it is important to be alert to this possibility. The patient need not present with the classic history, since epilepsy may be present merely as a recurrent confusion. A CT scan and an electroencephalogram taken subsequent to the fall may be negative; both may also show "abnormalities" in normal elderly.[16]

Normal pressure hydrocephalus results in ataxia early in its course and for this reason may predispose to falls. However, the frequency and treatability of that condition remain controversial.[17]

## *Neurosensory Deficit*

The special senses, especially vision and vestibular function, are important for normal equilibrium.[11] The visual contribution to equilibrium becomes more important to older people as proprioception declines. Illusions and ambiguous visual information may induce falls, for example on escalators or ramps.[9] These problems arise from the faulty processing of information from the peripheral visual field; visual acuity does not predict sensitivity to illusions of disequilibrium. Although distorted vision contributes to falls, blindness itself does not necessarily lead to increased falls.[18]

Although vertigo is common in the elderly, it is not a frequent cause of falls. Its presence or occurrence can easily be identified in cognitively alert patients through careful questioning. From the point of view of etiology, vertigo can be divided into two types.

Peripheral vertigo refers to auditory or vestibular disease. The more common diseases are positional vertigo, labyrinthritis, and Meniere's disease. Positional vertigo can be avoided by carefully watching one's position. Labyrinthitis, accompanied by low-pitched tinnitus and hearing loss, is self-limited but may require meclizine or antihistamine therapy. Meniere's disease is a severe, unrelenting disease that warrants otolaryngologic consultation.

Central vertigo relates to disease of the brain. Although it is not common, if vertigo cannot be readily attributed to peripheral causes, exploration of central possibilities beginning with a CT scan is mandatory.

## *Cardiovascular Disease*

The relationship between syncope and falls is an important one and is receiving considerable attention at present.[19-21] One of the problems faced by physicians and investigators is that the association between syncope and falls may not be clearly identified by the patient. Patients will frequently inappropriately attribute their fall to environmental causes or "bad luck."[22] Thus, syncope may be a more important antecedent to falls than is generally appreciated.

The most common causes of syncope are cardiac in origin. Two syndromes predominate: cardiac arrhythmias, including Stokes-Adams attack, and postural hypotension. Conduction abnormalities and premature ventricular contractions become more frequent in the elderly. As with a number of other age changes, differentiating harmless concomitant problems of age from actual disease is fraught with difficulty and controversy. Nevertheless, Gordon and others[20] found treatable cardiac arrhythmias in 12 of 37 elderly patients subject to falls. Lipsitz and coworkers[19] found an increase in the frequency of falls in patients with multifocal paired premature ventricular contractions (PVCs) but did not find this relationship in those with single PVCs. In addition, in his study the frequency of brady-tachycardia syndrome was the same in people who had experienced syncope as in the control group who had not.

Orthostatic blood pressure instability is common among the elderly[23] and has been studied extensively. Postural hypotension should be suspected in persons who become faint or experience "dizziness" (by which they usually mean giddiness) following a sudden change in position, such as rising from bed or a chair. In addition, postprandial syncope, associated with transient hypotension, commonly occurs in elderly persons following eating or defecation.[21] (The latter association contributes to the frequency of falls in the bathroom.) The frequency of orthostasis as a cause of syncope or falls or both in enhanced by the use of many drugs (see further on).

## *Metabolic Derangements*

The most frequently encountered metabolic problem leading to falls is that of dehydration, whether due to diarrhea, fever and inadequate fluid intake, or excessive use of diuretics. The clinical expression of this problem is most apt to be syncope or postural hypotension, although drop attacks and even vertigo may ensue. Other metabolic derangements that may predispose to falls include hypokalemia, hypercalcemia, hypomagnesemia, hypoglycemia, and azotemia.

## *Loss of Proprioception and Abnormal Gaits*

Most older people experience, to some degree, a mild loss of proprioception, thus contributing to the importance of the environmental factors cited earlier.[24] More severe loss of proprioception is frequently seen in persons with pernicious anemia, diabetic neuropathy, or other diseases of the spinal cord such as cervical spondylosis. Abnormalities of gait also contribute to the risk of falling.[25] Investigators have begun to define gait characteristics of the elderly.[26] A variety of abnormal gaits have been described,[27] but it is not clearly understood which gaits predispose to falls. Why some patients with normal gaits fall while others with very disordered gaits ambulate safely remains obscure. Postural sway can be measured by a force platform.[25] Postural response to threats to equilibrium are difficult to study but crucial to the issue of falls.[29]

## *Musculoskeletal Deficits, Including Abnormalities of Gait*

Musculoskeletal disease should not be overlooked as a common cause of falls. Gross deformities, such as flexion deformity of the hip or knee, obviously predispose to falls.

While "drop attacks" may be due to a variety of causes, including postural hypotension, they are frequently caused by weakness of the muscular support to the lower extremity, most commonly the quadriceps muscle. Studies of muscle function in normal elderly have confirmed the presence of age-related changes in length-tension relationships for the quadriceps muscle which, if severe, will interfere with an elderly individual's ability to stand erect.[30] The muscles become progressively fatigued during standing and may "give out," resulting in a fall. A simple assessment of strength of the quadriceps muscles by a physician or physical therapist will provide support for this diagnosis.

### *Adverse Effects of Therapy*

The problems we have cited, with the exception of environmental factors, may be operative in any elderly person, whether he or she is living independently or in an institutional environment. The frequency of occurrence of the problems, however, will be different, depending upon the patient's situation. For example, in acute care hospitals, elderly persons are apt to be kept in bed for inordinate periods of time due, at least in part, to concern by ward staff that if a patient is walking around he or she may fall. In point of fact, this policy is a major contributing factor to the incidence of falls in acute care hospitals, because of the muscular weakness that inevitably occurs, especially in the elderly, following even a few days in bed.[31] Balance and muscle strength are trainable. Lack of practice of the ambulatory skill is one of the costs of immobility.[28]

By far the most common cause of falls in the institutionalized patient is confusion or an effort to combat confusion or inappropriate behavior as a result of the use of restraints, either pharmacologic or physical.

For elderly persons, the first night in the hospital is a period of exceptional hazard. The unfamiliar environment, coupled with the presence of underlying illness, leads, almost inexorably, to some degree of confusion. Use of bed rails and absence of illumination contribute to the problem. Innumerable patients sustain hip fractures during this first night in the hospital while attempting to climb over bed rails in the darkness.[32]

An even more common cause of falls in the institutionalized elderly is often an integral part of the situation of long-term care. Motivated by the high frequency of falls as a result of many of the factors noted above, in an institutional setting the nursing staff is apt to resort to the use of restraints by Poseys. The patient whose urinary control is frequently diminished faces the problem of attracting the nurse's attention, getting released from the Posey, and walking to the toilet, with a high frequency of falls en route.[33]

One of the most frequent antecedents to falls is the inappropriate use of drugs.[34] This is true both for independent elderly and for the institutionalized person. Drugs that are especially apt to predispose to falls include those that induce somnolence (hypnotics), postural hypotension (diuretics, nitrates, antihypertensive agents, and tricyclic antidepressants), and confusion (cimetidine and digitalis).

For a more detailed presentation of the various problems leading to falls, please consult the index.

## APPROACH TO DIAGNOSIS AND MANAGEMENT OF FALLS

The context of a fall demands primary consideration. An active, independent elderly patient who falls deserves close attention for clues to specific causes, such as cardiac or neurologic disease or inappropriate use of drugs, including alcohol. A chronically debilitated nursing home resident is more likely to fall because of an accumulation of multiple dysfunctions. The evaluation of a very frail patient who falls should be viewed as a search for opportunities for improvement rather than for a single diagnosis.

All patients who fall deserve a careful history and physical examination. In the history, one should attempt to differentiate the type of fall, as illustrated in Table 26–2, and define the time sequence, including potential predisposing factors. The history may be difficult to elicit or interpret. A patient with a hip fracture may have fallen as a result of a slip or from syncope and sustained the fracture as a result; alternatively, she may have fractured the hip after an apparently minor twist of the ankle which occasioned a fall. Occasionally patients will describe hearing a snap or crack, experiencing sudden pain in the groin, and then falling.[4]

Preventive and therapeutic efforts should be directed toward the specific etiologic or predisposing factors believed to be present and are described in appropriate sections of this book. A few general principles will be presented here.

### *Syncope*

As mentioned earlier, patients will frequently ascribe to a slip or trip an episode which was, in fact, initiated by syncope. An example is the occurrence of a fall following getting up from the toilet. The frequent association of defecation with postural hypotension may be overlooked and the fall ascribed to a slippery floor or lack of handrails.

Patients whose falls appear to be related to syncope should be studied carefully for central nervous system, cardiovascular, or metabolic disease. In addition to a complete physical examination, including a neurologic assessment, the laboratory studies should include serum electrolyte levels, hematologic studies, serum magnesium and calcium values, blood glucose, serum creatinine concentrations, and an electrocardiogram. Patients suspected of having cardiac arrhythmias should be studied with a Holter monitor and the arrhythmia, if present, should be treated appropriately. Evaluation and treatment of patients with symptoms suggestive of a transient ischemic attack (TIA) or stroke are controversial[14,15] and are described more fully in Chapter 21. In elderly patients, carotid endarterectomy is seldom attempted; patients with TIAs or recurrent strokes not accompanied by a reversible contributing factor such as anemia should be treated with small doses of aspirin if no history of ulcer is found.

The presence of epilepsy as a cause of syncope or falls may be very difficult to detect in elderly patients. In one patient whom we recently followed, the chance observation that her episodic syncope was followed by a rise in serum thyroid-stimulating hormone level provided the only clue to the presence of epilepsy. Dilantin therapy has completely ablated her attacks. Electroencephalograms and CT scans should be obtained in patients suspected of having intracerebral disease, although these studies seldom provide important clues to the etiology of falls and may show nonspecific abnormalities.[16]

## *Vertigo*

Vertigo, or the false sensation of motion, especially rotation, does not appear frequently as an antecedent to falls.[8] When vertigo does occur, nystagmus can be observed if the examiner is present during the appearance of this symptom.[35] Before the clinician undertakes an extensive investigation, he should check the ear canal for impacted cerumen, which occasionally causes vertigo. In any case, a more accurate history should be obtained.

## *Hypotension*

Most people, as they age, exhibit some degree of postural hypotension. It is important to examine all elderly patients, including those who complain of falls and those who do not, for this condition. In a busy office practice with patients who do not complain specifically of falls, comparison of pressures in the sitting and standing positions is adequate. A difference of 20 mm systolic or the occurrence of giddiness following standing is grounds for concern.[36] For a patient in whom one suspects the occurrence of falls, the physician should record the blood pressure while the patient is recumbent and then immediately after standing, watching for a difference of 20 mm systolic or the presence of giddiness or unsteadiness. In patients who fall early in the morning, following breakfast, or after going to the bathroom, one should consider the possibility that eating or defecating has led to the appearance or exacerbation of postural hypotension.

When postural hypotension has been identified, the search for contributing factors starts with a blood hemoglobin reading and an electrolyte determination; more intensive studies such as Holter monitoring may be indicated.[21] Therapy includes appropriate preventive action, such as reduced doses of diuretics, smaller meals, or avoidance of walking after eating or immediately after arising from bed or chair. The use of support stockings may prove helpful. If the hypotension is severe, treatment with low doses of fludrocortisone (Florinef) or supplemental sodium chloride may be indicated.

## *Musculoskeletal Deficits*

Although the classic explanation for drop attacks is the presence of posterior cerebral ischemia secondary to vertebral artery disease, similar manifestations may be due to quadriceps weakness, especially in persons with underlying orthopedic or rheumatic disease. Careful assessment of quadriceps strength by an experienced physician or physical therapist will assist in evaluating the potential importance of this factor. A systematic program of quadriceps strengthening exercises, with the knee at full extension, undertaken three times weekly will often lead to significant improvement over the course of two or three months.

## *Drugs*

A careful evaluation of the patient's intake of drugs, including prescription drugs, over-the-counter preparations, and alcohol, is an essential component of the evaluation of falls. Drugs that are apt to lead to falls include diuretics, anticholinergic agents (such as tricyclic antidepressants), nitrates, and hypnotics.[34]

## Prevention

For many patients who fall, both independent and institutionalized, prevention becomes the most important aspect of therapy. In developing a plan of care for community dwelling elderly, especially those who for any reason are prone to falls, a careful inspection of the home environment is an important preventive measure. This should preferably be done by someone who is skilled in detecting hazards and knowledgeable about appliances, such as an occupational therapist. The inspection should include careful examination of floor coverings, stairs, and bathrooms. In view of the increased need for illumination and altered color perception of most elderly persons, such inspection should address visual as well as physical aspects of environment[11] (see Chapters 4 and 24). The nature and sources of available assistive devices are presented in Chapter 15.

The patient who experiences confusion is always at risk for falls, and a carefully planned program of prevention is equally important. If possible, recently hospitalized elderly patients should be placed in a room near the nurse's desk where they can be observed. Bed rails should be avoided if possible. Instead, a comfortable chair should be placed close to the bed, and the layout of the furniture should be pointed out clearly to the patient before saying goodnight. The patient should be visited and, in many instances, toileted frequently during the night. Should delirium ensue, the therapeutic methods outlined in Chapter 20 are recommended.

The necessity for use of physical restraints, such as Poseys, should be evaluated with care. While the threat of fractures represents an understandable concern on the part of nurses and other caregivers, the adverse effects of immobility and functional restriction on quality of life and general health must also be taken into consideration.[31]

When the ischemic episodes are believed to be caused by carotid atherosclerosis, carotid endarterectomy is seldom undertaken in persons of very advanced age, and therapy with aspirin is usually indicated.

When falls are believed to be due to vertebral artery insufficiency and triggered by neck motion (as when looking for a high object), preventive therapy consists of either instruction to the patient to avoid this particular position or use of a protective neck collar.

## Summary

Finally, we conclude with a reminder concerning the *multiplicity* of factors that may lead to falls. Some of these will be summative. For example, environmental factors, which are important to all elderly persons, are especially important to people with orthopedic, visual, or proprioceptive problems. In other instances, patients will experience several simultaneous causes of falls, or fall-inducing symptoms, each acting independently. An example is the patient with frequent attacks of vertigo caused by vestibular disease who also has infrequent but severe Stokes-Adams attacks. Identifying the presence of one precipitating factor does not preclude a search for others.

There is a great need for additional research in this field. While this summary reflects our present state of knowledge, a recent initiative on the part of the National Institute of Aging to accelerate research on this important topic will undoubtedly lead to important new information in the near future.

Of all the syndromes characteristic of the elderly population, none deserves more careful attention than falls.

### References


1. Rubenstien LZ: Falls in the elderly: A clinical approach. West J Med 136:273, 1983.
   *A good review of the epidemiology, causes of, and approaches to falls; risk factors such as recent admission to an institution, sedation, and environmental hazards are emphasized.*
2. Gryfe CI, Amies A, Ashley MJ: A longitudinal study of falls in an elderly population: I. Incidence and morbidity. Age Ageing 6 (1977 supplement): 201 1977.
   *This longitudinal study from the Jewish Home in Toronto is the largest and most rigorous original epidemiologic study of falls available. Fracture, injury, and gross fall rates in this intermediate care setting are well documented. They had more fractures of ribs and upper limbs than other authors report.*
3. Riffle KL: Falls: Kinds, causes and prevention. Geriatr Nursing (NY) 3:165, 1982.
4. Melton JL, Riggs BL: Risk factors for injury after a fall. Clin Geriatr Med 1(3):525, 1985.
   *The entire issue of this series is devoted to falls and merits the attention of anyone interested in the subject. This article highlights the role of osteoporosis and lack of soft-tissue padding due to malnutrition as risk factors for fractures after a fall.*
5. Katz S, Branch LG, Brannon MH, et al: Active life expectancy. N Engl J Med, 309:1218, 1983.
   *This study highlights the fact that recent prolongation*

*of life expectency has prolonged the period of dependence. Women live through a markedly longer period of debility than men.*

6. Berry G, Fisher RH, Land S: Detrimental incidents including falls in an elderly institutional population. J Am Geriatr Soc 29:322, 1981.
7. Amerman P: The ecology of falls. Presented at the scientific session of the Gerontologic Society of America, 1985, New Orleans, LA.
8. Isaacs B: Are falls a manifestation of brain failure? Age Ageing 7(1977 supplement):97, 1977.
*This study reviews historical features antecedent to falls: trips, dizziness, rapid head movement, etc. The role of lack of attentiveness and somnolence is emphasized and cardiac arrhythmias and drop attacks are downplayed.*
9. Owen DH: Maintaining posture and avoiding tripping: Optical information for detecting and controlling orientation and locomotion. Clin Geriatr Med 1(3):581, 1985.
*The role of vision in maintaining postural equilibrium is explored here to complement reference 27. The role of environmental hazards interacting with gait abnormalities and visual debility is well described.*
10. Duthie EG, Gambert SR: Accident and fall prevention in the elderly. Wisconsin Med J 82:22, 1983.
*Review of epidemiology and causes of falls. Good discussion of adaptive equipment and architectural precautions.*
11. Leibowitz HW, Shippert CL: Spatial orientation mechanisms and their implication for falls. Clin Geriatr Med 1:571, 1985.
*Visual cues from the environment determine sense of verticality and equilibrium; this information takes on great value when proprioception is threatened.*
12. Mossey JM: Social and psychologic factors related to falls among the elderly. Clin Geriatr Med 1:541, 1985.
*This very complete review of research in this area emphasizes the lack of convincing social or psychological documentation.*
13. Billig NA, Ahmed SW: An assessment of depression and dementia associated with hip fracture. Presented at the 1985 Gerontological Society of America, New Orleans, LA.
14. Barnes RW, Archie JP, Batson RC: Advocates in vascular controversies. Surgery 95:739, 1984.
15. Hertzer NR, Beven EG, Young JR, et al: Incidental asymptomatic carotid bruits in patients scheduled for peripheral vascular reconstruction: Results of cerebral and coronary angiography. Surgery 96:535, 1984.
16. Obrist WD: Cerebral blood flow and EEG changes associated with aging and dementia. *In* Blazer DG (ed): Handbook of Geriatric Psychiatry. New York, Van Nostrand Reinhold, 1983.
*Authoritative account of the EEG in aging patients.*
17. Adams RD: Altered cerebrospinal fluid dynamics in relation to dementia and aging. *In* Amaducci L, Davison AN, Antuono P (eds): Aging of the Brain and Dementia (Aging V. 13). New York, Raven Press, 1980.
18. Margulic I, Librach G, Schadel M: Epidemiological study of accidents among residents of homes for the aged. J Gerontol 25:342, 1979.
*This review of falls in homes for the aged in Israel demonstrates a lower rate of falls among blind residents compared with the sighted. Whether this change was due to immobility or greater caution should be studied.*
19. Lipsitz LA, Galvagno EC, Wei JY, Rowe JW: Risk factors for syncope in the elderly. Presented at the scientific session of the Gerontological Society of America, November 1985, New Orleans, LA.
20. Gordon, M. Huang M. Gryfe CI: An evaluation of falls, syncope, and dizziness by prolonged ambulatory cardiographic monitoring in a geriatric institutional setting. J Am Geriatr Soc 30:6, 1982.
*Twenty-four hour EKG monitoring showed a high yield of treatable cardiac arrhythmias among fainting and falling patients. More recent studies (references 10, 16) are less sanguine.*
21. Lipsitz LA: Abnormalities in blood pressure homeostasis that contribute to falls in the elderly. Clin Geriatr Med 1:637, 1985.
*In documenting the antecedents to syncope, situations such as eating and defecating were found as commonly as abnormal heart rhythms. Syncope was not found to be a common cause of falls in this well-staffed nursing home.*
22. Hurd PD, Bluestein M, Hazlett AJ: Falls, medication and the attribution of responsibility. Presented at the scientific session, Gerontologic Society of America, November 1985, New Orleans, LA.
23. Caird FL, Andrew CB, Kennedy RD: Effect of posture on blood pressure in the elderly. Br Heart J 35:527, 1973.
*This classic report from Scotland documents the high rate of serious orthostatic changes in normal elderly people.*
24. Sabin TD: Biologic aspects of falls and mobility in the elderly. J Geriatr Soc 30:51, 1982.
*This scholarly work argues for the role of peripheral neuropathy and loss of proprioception as the cause of the common problems of gait and mobility among the aged.*
25. Overstall PW, Johnson AL, Exton-Smith AN: Instability and falls in the elderly. Age Ageing 7(1977 supplement):92, 1977.
*This study recorded postural sway measured on a pressure platform. Correlation with falls was weak. Those who fell due to tripping had less sway than those who did not fall.*
26. Koller WC, Glatt SL, Fox JH: Senile gait: A distinct neurologic entity. Clin Geriatr Med 1:661, 1985.
27. Rodstein M: Falls in the aged. *In* Cape RDT, Coe RM, Rossman I (eds): Fundamentals of Geriatric Medicine. New York, Raven Press, 109–116, 1983.
*A general overview of falls and research on causes. In contrast to references 10 and 13, drop attacks are emphasized. Gait disturbances are well reviewed.*
28. Overstall PW: Prevention of falls in the elderly. J Geriatr Soc 20:481, 1982.
29. Larish D, Penna D, Leo K: Control of static and dynamic posture in the aged. Presented at the scientific session of the Gerontologic Society of America, November 1985, New Orleans, LA.
30. Pendergast DW: Personal communication. 1985.
31. Cape RDT, Dodd S, Shorrock C, et al: Immobilization in the aged: Medical and psychological effects. Proceedings of the Ontario Psychogeriatric Society (Toronto, 1977), 29–36.
*This article emphasizes the medical and human costs of restraints.*
32. Editorial: Cotsides—Protecting whom from what? Lancet Aug 18:383, 1984.
*Cotsides is the British word for bed siderails. This editorial convincingly argues against their routine use and pleads for humane and compassionate respect for our patients' freedom and dignity.*
33. Ashley MJ, Gryfe CI, Amies A: A longitudinal study of falls in an elderly population: II Some circumstances

of falling. Age Ageing 6(1977 supplement):211, 1977. *This article describes the circumstances of the falls enumerated in the Gryfe study (reference 2). The high frequency of falls related to toileting (over 50% among the very old and even higher in men than in women) and high risk of falls from the sitting position are the most unexpected features of the study.*

34. MacDonald JB: The role of drugs in falls in the elderly. Clin Geriatr Med 1:621, 1985. *The best review of articles on the subject of falls and drugs by the author who first proved that barbiturates cause hip fractures (reference 25).*

35. Goodhill V: Tinnitis and dizziness in the aged. *In* Rossman I (ed): Clinical Geriatrics. Philadelphia, Lippincott, 393–409, 1979.

36. Caird FI, Kennedy RD, Williams BO: Practical Rehabilitation of the Elderly. London, Pitman, 1983. pp. 48 ff.

## Chapter 27

# Sexuality and the Elderly

*William B. Applegate*

Although sexual activity tends to decline in frequency and vigor with age, many older people continue to have an interest in sex and an active sex life.[1] Unfortunately, many in our society, physicians included, have a rather limited definition of human sexuality. Many still view sexuality as primarily procreational or place excessive emphasis on coitus and achieving an orgasm, as opposed to taking the broader view that sexuality may involve a variety of activities and has recreational, emotional and life-enhancing aspects. Continued sexuality may be important to the emotional health and identity of many elderly people. In a recent survey of elderly people reporting sexual dysfunction, 22 of 31 responders reported negative personal effects from their dysfunction, and in 18, the negative effects involved a poorer self-image.[2]

## PREVALENCE OF SEXUAL ACTIVITY

### *Males*

It is apparent, from several studies, that male sexuality declines with age.[3-5] Figure 27–1 depicts Kinsey's data on number of orgasms per week from all activities and from intercourse.[6] Kinsey stated that "the rate at which males slow up in these last decades does not exceed the rate . . . in the previous age groups."[3] Kinsey and associates[3] and Pfeiffer[1] reported that 70 to 75 per cent of healthy males are still sexually active at ages 60 to 65, but by age 80, this declines 20 to 25 per cent.[1,3] It appears that the *degree* of sexual interest shows a significant inverse correlation with age; the incidence of some interest is much less affected by age.[4] Single and postmarital males have a frequency of sexual activity only slightly less than that of married males.[3] Factors associated with continued sexual activity in the elderly male include frequency and enjoyment of sexual activity in the younger years, age, health, social class, and physical function.[7] Kinsey and associates[3] and Verwoerdt and co-workers[4] reported that total sexual activity is higher for men than women at all ages.

### *Females*

Kinsey and associates[8] reported that frequency of coitus for married women follows a gradual declining course similar to that of men but that solitary sexual activities such as masturbation and nocturnal dreams to orgasm gradually increase until the fourth decade, remain constant until the sixth decade, and then decline gradually. The prevalence of continued coitus in married women at age 65 is about 50 per cent.[9] Frequency of intercourse for unmarried and postmarital women is much less than that for married women, although rates of masturbation are higher.[9] Factors predictive of continued sexual activity in married females include marital status, health, age, and past sexual enjoyment.[7]

The waning of sexual activity is more in terms of frequency and vigor than of kind. For both sexes, declines in the rate of coitus are more related to aging changes in the male.[7-9] Finally, for a substantial number of men and women, sexual relations end only with death.

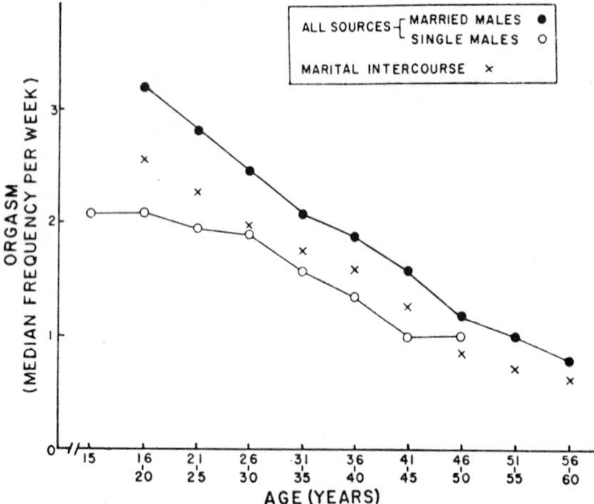


**Figure 27–1.** Frequency of total sexuality as measured by frequency of orgasms (From Botwinick J: Drives, expectations, and emotions. *In* Birren JE (ed.): Handbook of Aging and the Individual. Chicago, University of Chicago Press, 1959.)

## ALTERNATIVE SEXUAL ACTIVITY

Unmarried women over 65 years outnumber single men by four to one; therefore, it is important to consider alternative sexual outlets. Masturbation and bisexuality are very sensitive topics with elderly people. The physician should probe gently about alternative sexual activity when necessary, always being mindful to honor the individual patient's value system. At age 50, about 50 per cent of single men and women and 10 to 30 per cent of married men and women masturbate at least occasionally.[3,8,9] At times, the physician may be asked about technique or complications, such as irritation of the clitoris, urethra, or vagina.

Older people tend to hold more conservative views on sexuality, with 85 to 90 per cent disapproving of homosexuality.[10] Some of these views may be a cohort effect and subject to future change. One recent study of 100 randomly selected female gynecology patients, average age 31, reported that almost one third had seriously considered bisexuality.[11]

## PHYSIOLOGY OF THE HUMAN SEXUAL RESPONSE

Before exploring changes in the sexual response with age, it is appropriate first to summarize the basic physiology of human sexuality. Sexual arousal or libido is a cerebral process that, for instance, can still occur despite a spinal cord transection and may involve the limbic system.[12] Spinal centers in the thoracolumbar cord stimulate erections in the male owing to psychologic input and higher nervous system activity, whereas sacral centers mediate erections in the male in response to direct genital stimulation.[13] The afferent portion of the local reflex arc involves the fibers of the pudendal nerve to the sacral cord, whereas parasympathetic fibers of the nervi erigentes (pelvic nerves) make up the efferent portion (Fig. 27–2). Although erection is under parasympathetic control, the smooth muscle contractions necessary for ejaculation are under sympathetic control. Also, the internal sphincter of the bladder is contracted by sympathetic impulses by way of the hypogastric plexus to prevent retrograde ejaculation.[12]

In the female, the local genital response consists of vasocongestion mediated again by the parasympathetic nervous system. Once again, psychologic and higher nervous input is probably mediated through the thoracolumbar spinal cord, whereas the local reflex arc is mediated through the sacral spinal cord. Female orgasm, in part, consists of a series of contractions of the perineal muscles, which are analogous to those involved in ejaculation.[12] For both the male and the female, the orgasmic experience consists, at least in part, of an emotional experience located in the higher central nervous system.

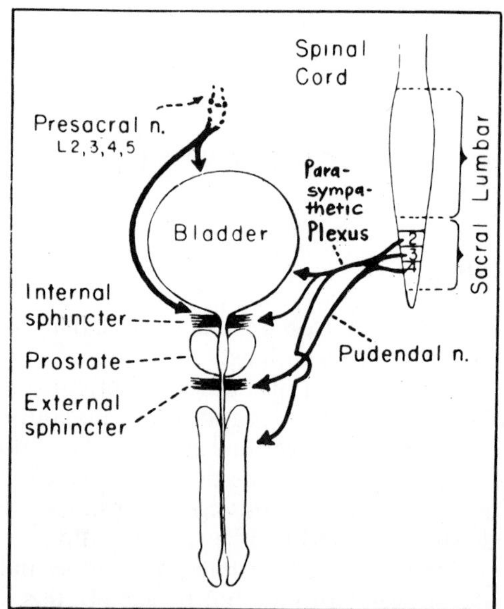


**Figure 27–2.** Schematic anatomy of the bladder and penis. (From Ellenberg M: Sex and diabetes. Diabetes Care 2:5, 1979. Reproduced with permission from the American Diabetes Association, Inc.)

## AGING SEXUAL RESPONSE

### Males

Masters and Johnson have reported the most extensive study of aging sexual physiology.[14-16] The sexual response in the aging male is generally slower and of diminished intensity. There are changes in each of the four stages of the sexual response, which include excitement, plateau, orgasm, and resolution. During the excitement phase, the elderly male is slower to achieve erection. Achieving an erection often takes minutes, rather than seconds, and is less spontaneous, often requiring direct stimulation from the sexual partner. The older man develops less intense physiologic reactions to stimulation, including a decrease in sexual blush and less muscle tension. The plateau phase usually lasts longer in the older male, but this often gives the older man a greater control and greater ability to stimulate his partner. Once he has reached the plateau phase, his erection is fairly secure.

Ejaculation is less forceful and shorter in duration, lasting only 1 to 2 seconds versus 2 to 4 seconds in youth. The volume of semen is less, usually only 1 to 2 ml versus 3 to 5 ml in youth. In addition, there is often a decrease in ejaculation demand, so that at regularly recurring intervals, the male may simply not develop the pressure to ejaculate.[16] During the resolution phase, erection is rapidly lost, and the refractory period is usually longer, often extending for 12 to 24 hours. Despite these changes, the male's subjective level of pleasure derived from sexual activity does not change at all with age.

### Females

Just as with the aging male, sexual responsiveness in the aging female is slower and reduced in intensity.[14-16] With the loss of ovarian functions, the vaginal barrel becomes constricted and the vaginal walls become thin and atrophic. These changes, which may be ameliorated by continued sexual activity or exogenous estrogens, may lead to fissures and pain on intercourse. During the excitement phase, there is delayed onset of vaginal lubrication, which may take several minutes and necessitate direct stimulation. Increased use of artificial (water-soluble) lubricants may be needed. During excitement, the labia do not become as engorged and may still hang in limp folds. The clitoris and surrounding structures may atrophy, but sensation from stimulation is not thought to be decreased. With atrophy of the mons pubis and labia, irritation or pain may be induced with stimulation of the clitoris. As with the male, the plateau phase may be prolonged and onset of orgasm delayed. Often, the duration and intensity of the orgasm is diminished. As with the aging male, the resolution phase is quite rapid. Despite these physiologic changes, the subjective level of pleasure obtained from sexual activity does not change with age.

## APPROACH TO SEXUAL DYSFUNCTION IN THE ELDERLY PATIENT

### Initial Approach

As data cited previously indicate, although there is a decline in total sexual activity with age, many older people continue to have both an interest in sex and an active sex life.[3,4] It is difficult for the clinician to know the best approach to intervention when a patient reports a decline in sexual activity. Elderly people are, at times, reluctant to discuss sexual matters, even when they feel the need.[17] It is known that older males troubled primarily with sexual concerns may present to the clinician's office with repetitive somatic complaints such as back pain.[17] The older woman with sexual problems may present with genitourinary complaints. As part of the routine evaluation of new patients, the physician should inquire gently about the older person's sex life and invite discussion. At times, the older person may initially refuse to discuss such matters, only to open up to discussion after a few pertinent questions about his or her sex life are asked during the review of systems. In addition, physicians themselves may experience difficulties when they attempt to take a sexual history of older people. They must accept the fact, stated previously, that sexuality may be very important and appropriate for the elderly. Also, some physicians may, at times, feel inhibited when discussing sexuality because of their own cultural or ethical backgrounds or because of personal sexual difficulties. Such inhibitions must be overcome if the physician is to effectively manage these problems in elderly people.

If an older person reports that sexual activity is declining or has ceased, the physician should actively pursue further counseling or treatment only if one or the other partner is troubled by the change or indicates a willingness to proceed. However, in either event, the physician should try to acquaint the patient, at least briefly, with information regarding the age-related physiologic changes mentioned in the previous section. These changes are often misinterpreted by elderly people. A man who experiences a delay in achieving erection may not know that this is a normal physiologic change with age, which responds to direct stimulation. Instead, he may develop a fear of failure, develop performance anxiety, and fail to perform or begin to avoid sexual contact.[16] The woman who sees these changes in her husband and who has developed aging changes herself, along with fears of diminished attractiveness, may interpret his delayed response as an expression of his loss of interest, and she, too, may begin to avoid sex.[16] Often both males and females place great importance on an orgasm. If the male experiences occasional loss of ejaculatory demand, either he or his wife may again have reactions similar to those just described. Also, if the woman is slow to lubricate or reach orgasm, the elderly male may begin to be anxious about his sexual capabilities.

The widow's syndrome and the widower's syndrome, identified by Masters and Johnson, are two aging-related syndromes of sexual dysfunction that the physician may encounter fairly frequently.[16] These syndromes are found in elderly people who have undergone a year or more of sexual continence, often because of illness or death of a spouse. In the case of the male, when a sexual opportunity ultimately presents again, erectile failure may result. This usually promotes great fear and anxiety and may lead to continuing impotence. However, if the male is fortunate enough to have a knowledgeable and patient partner, the problem is usually reversible in days to weeks. In the case of the female, during the period of sexual continence, the vaginal barrel constricts and lubrication is retarded. With a patient and knowledgeable partner, the syndrome is reversible in 6 weeks to 3 months. In either case, the couple in question should focus on intimacy and closeness and allow sexual stimulation to proceed gradually.[18]

## *Evaluation*

When a male or female patient complains of sexual dysfunction of a more established nature and is willing to pursue the matter beyond receiving information on aging, the following general approach should be used: Sexual dysfunction in the elderly male usually presents as erectile failure or loss of libido.[15] Even in the elderly, psychogenic problems are a frequent cause. Psychogenic impotence may be sudden in onset or cyclical in nature; libido is usually diminished.[12] It may be associated with specific life events and is often selective in that there may be no erectile failure during masturbation and firm morning erections are still, at least periodically, present (but decline in frequency with age).[13] Clinical depression is a very common cause of diminished libido and erectile problems.[18] Many experts advise a referral to a psychologist for evaluation of psychogenic impotence and suggest that the Minnesota Multiphasic Personality Inventory, or test for depression, be administered.[19]

Organic impotence tends to have a more gradual onset—decrease or total absence of morning or nocturnal erections and gradual decrease in the quality or firmness of erections.[13] Classically, libido is not affected; however, emotional and organic problems often overlap, making these distinctions less than absolute.[12] Prior to further diagnostic evaluation, the patient's medication regimen should be reviewed, since a wide variety of medications, including alcohol and over-the-counter medications, impair sexual function (Table 27–1).[19,20] Antihypertensive medications are particularly likely to affect sexual function, and this may, in turn, affect compliance. If any question exists regarding a medication, it should be discontinued or a replacement found. Alcohol consumption should be discontinued or decreased markedly. If problems persist, a complete medical work up, including history, physical examination, and laboratory studies, is indicated (Table 27–2). Special attention should be paid to signs of diabetes mellitus or its complications (e.g., funduscopic changes, signs of peripheral or autonomic neuropathy), or generalized vascular disease (e.g., bruits), since both these conditions predispose to impotence in males (see later discussion).[19] In general, any older person who is significantly compromised by a chronic disease or metabolic abnormality can develop loss of

**Table 27–1.** DRUGS THAT DEPRESS SEXUAL FUNCTION

| | |
|---|---|
| Alcohol | Estrogens (in men) |
| Alpha-methyldopa | Guanethidine |
| Anticholinergic agents (often nonprescription) | Monoamine oxidase inhibitors |
| Antineoplastic agents | Narcotics |
| Barbiturates | Phenothiazines |
| Benzodiazepines | Propranolol |
| Butyrophenones | Reserpine |
| Cannabis | Spironolactone |
| Cimetidine | Thiazide diuretics |
| Clofibrate | Thioxanthenes |
| Clonidine | Tricyclic antidepressants |

**Table 27–2.** ORGANIC CAUSES OF SEXUAL DYSFUNCTION

| |
|---|
| Arteriosclerosis, generalized |
| Cardiorespiratory embarrassment |
| Diabetes, other endocrine diseases |
| Drugs, alcohol |
| Genitourinary disorders (prostatitis, perineal prostate surgery) |
| Hematologic disorders (pernicious anemia, leukemia, anemia) |
| Infections, febrile reactions |
| Inflammation, active |
| Metabolic disorders (electrolytes) |
| Miscellaneous disorders (renal failure, cirrhosis) |
| Neurologic disorders (parkinsonism, peripheral neuropathy, spinal cord lesions, organic brain syndromes) |

libido or impotence; hence, laboratory studies are indicated including tests to determine a blood count, fasting blood sugar, sedimentation rate, electrolytes, urea nitrogen values, liver function, calcium levels, and thyroid function. A chest x-ray is also indicated. The role of serum testosterone levels are controversial in the elderly, since there is no clear correlation between lower testosterone levels and sexual function.[21]

However, since Spark and associates[22] have shown that a higher proportion of impotence in elderly males may be attributable to endocrine problems than was formerly thought, the serum testosterone level should be determined. Levels of follicle-stimulating hormone, luteinizing hormone, and prolactin should be checked to see if they are low.[22]

At present, the most effective test for differentiating psychogenic from organic impotence is the recording of nocturnal penile tumescence (NPT), which many advocates employ as a screening test prior to a medical evaluation.[23,24] Such tracings during sleep monitor nocturnal erections, which usually occur during rapid eye movement (REM) sleep. Since this test alone does not measure the quality of an erection, if the screening is done at home, some patients who have early organic impotence may be misclassified as false-negatives, since they may still have erections that are not firm. If the study is done in a sleep laboratory, the quality of the erection can be checked and the presence or absence of REM sleep can be ascertained, since if REM sleep is suppressed, erections may not occur. Correction does have to be made for the patient's age, since penile tumescence does decline somewhat with age.[23] Further, useful evaluation would include measurement of penile blood pressure.[25] Penile systolic pressure should not be more than 40 mm Hg below brachial systolic pressure. If penile systolic pressure is more than 60 mm Hg below brachial systolic pressure or the penile index (penile systolic pressure divided by brachial systolic pressure) is less than 0.6, then arterial insufficiency is possible and phalloarteriography may be indicated[25] (see later discussion, page 287).

Sexual dysfunction in the elderly female frequently presents as dyspareunia, vaginismus, or loss of libido.[15,16] In general, the same observations about psychogenic dysfunction and loss of libido discussed in relation to the male also apply to the female. Psychologic evaluation, review of the medication regimen, and general medical work up may be indicated. Instead of erectile failure, atrophic changes in the vaginal wall tend to lead to vaginal constriction and irritation with intercourse (see Chapter 35).[15,16] Administration of exogenous estrogen can help reverse some of these changes and, hence, help maintain sexual function.[26] In addition to dyspareunia associated with the estrogen-deficient state, pain with intercourse may set up vaginismus, an involuntary spasm or constriction of the muscle around the vaginal outlet or outer third of the vagina.[16,20] Most women with vaginismus will have severe pain on physical examination if a finger or small speculum is introduced into the vagina. Atrophic changes may reverse after a period of weeks to months of gradual sexual stimulation. Use of lubricants is often necessary. For some women, pelvic exercises and use of dilators of gradually increasing diameter are helpful. Once progress is made, resumption of intercourse in the female astride position may give the woman a greater sense of control.

## *Counseling and Therapy*

If sexual dysfunction exists and is not clearly organic, some form of sex therapy may be indicated. Although most elderly couples are unlikely to pursue sophisticated sex therapy, Masters and Johnson[15] have demonstrated 50 per cent improvement rates with elderly couples willing to undergo therapy. Counseling regarding techniques for reducing "spectatoring" (constantly monitoring one's own sexual performance) or performance anxiety by focusing on sensate pleasure may be helpful. Communication with sexual partners should be stressed. The patient and partner should be advised to focus on warmth, intimacy, and physical closeness rather than being preoccupied with orgasms or vaginal penetration. Alternative techniques, such as masturbation, can be explored; and couples can be advised that certain positions may circumvent physical disability. Both partners should be advised that the sexual response is a natural reflex that may paradoxically be inhibited by attempts to force it to occur.[15]

## THE DIABETIC PATIENT

### *Males*

The prevalence of erectile impotence increased with age in diabetic males (Fig. 27–3).[13] Although it has been frequently stated that the presence of impotence is related to the duration of disease, recent work has called this theory into question.[12] Impotence may be the presenting complaint in a diabetic. Diabetic men with erectile difficulties have greater frequency of peripheral and autonomic neuropathies than diabetic males without problems with erection.[13]

Problems with erection in diabetic patients may present with a relatively acute onset (days to weeks) and, in such cases, are usually related to acute metabolic decompensation and are reversible.[13] In the compensated elderly diabetic, the onset of impotence is often more gradual and progressive (see decription of organic impotence) and is usually related to neuropathy of the pelvic nerves. Classically, it is stated that diabetic males with impotence do not have a loss of libido, but the combination of emotional reaction to the loss of function and diminution of sex drive that may occur with age may result in diminished libido.[12] Orgasmic and ejaculatory capacity are usually not lost in diabetic men. However, a minority of males will have retrograde ejaculation due to inadequate closure of the internal sphincter of the bladder.

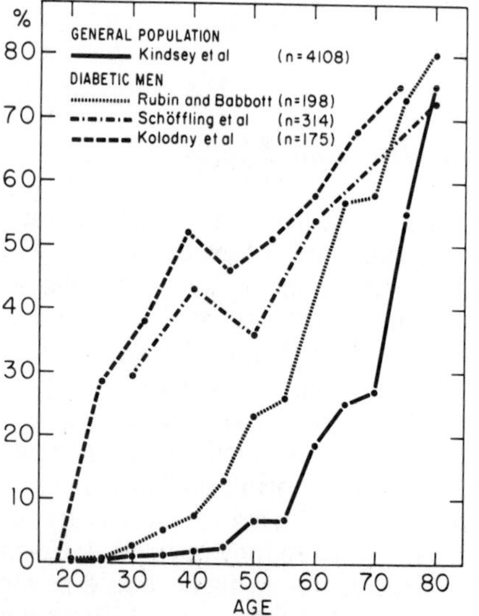


**Figure 27–3.** Frequency of impotence in the general population and in diabetic males. (From Schiavi RC, Hogan B: Sexual problems in diabetes mellitus: Psychological aspects. Diabetes Care 2:10, 1979. Reproduced with permission from the American Diabetes Association, Inc.)

### *Females*

Much less is known about sexual function in female diabetics. Two recent reports are conflicting. Kolodny[27] compared 125 diabetic women, ranging in age from 18 to 42 years, with hospitalized women who had been ill for at least 3 months. Thirty-five per cent of the diabetic women, as opposed to six per cent of the controls, reported an absence of the orgasmic response. On the other hand, Ellenberg[28] studied 100 diabetic women, aged 24 to 73 years, 54 of whom had distinct neuropathies. No clear impairment of sexual desire was seen, and 82 per cent reported continued orgasmic ability. Theoretically, the analog of erectile ability in the male would be vasocongestion and lubrication in the female. It is possible that these facilities could be impaired, but orgasmic ability retained, as in the male; but this has yet to be documented.

To date, it appears that sexual function in the elderly, stable diabetic male is more likely to be compromised than in the elderly stable diabetic female. Therapy involves, of course, close control of the diabetes and counseling, as described in the section on sexual dysfunction.

## CARDIOVASCULAR DISEASE AND SEXUALITY

When cardiovascular disease develops in an elderly man or woman, sexual activity frequently diminishes. The clinician should involve himself or herself with the sexual concerns of the cardiac patient.

In general, elderly people who can tolerate mild physical exertion, such as walking up two flights of stairs, can tolerate most forms of sexual activity.[20] On the average, sexual intercourse is estimated to consume about 150 calories.[17] The average heart rate is higher during treadmill testing of cardiac patients, and the death rate from this test is only about one in 10,000 tests.[17] Deaths reported during sexual intercourse are rare. Hellerstein and Friedman[29] compared marital sexual activity in 48 males after myocardial infarction with that of 43 middle-aged males who were at high risk for coronary artery disease but without evidence of such. They found that the mean number of orgasms per week declined significantly within 6 months after myocardial infarction. In a subsample of patients who underwent physiologic monitoring during sexual activity, the mean peak heart rate during orgasm was 117 beats per minutes (range 90 to 144 beats per minute). The average maximal heart rate during daily work activity (mostly sedentary jobs) was somewhat higher at 120 beats per minute. Evidence of cardiac ischemia on the electrocardiogram was no more frequent with sexual activity than with normal work.

Thus, the patient who has had a recent myocardial infarction or has stable angina pectoris can perform routine sexual activity safely if he or she can tolerate minimal exertion. Physical conditioning improves both the frequency and quality of sexual activity.[29]

It should be noted that these data were obtained from middle-aged married couples and may not apply to extramarital or nonroutine sexual experiences. There is some evidence to suggest that extramarital sexual activity or sexual activity conducted after a meal or heavy ethanol intake may be more physiologically stressful.[30]

Literature on physiologic changes in female cardiac patients who undertake sexual activity is virtually nonexistent.

At times fear of precipitating an attack of angina or a heart attack can inhibit sexual activity. For instance, both a decrease in libido and an increase in impotence are frequently encountered after a myocardial infarction. Recent studies indicate that impotence develops in 20 to 30 per cent of patients after a heart attack, and 40 to 66 per cent of patients report a decrease in libido.[30] This problem is multifactorial, including anxiety, effect of medications, and change in self-image. Counseling should be undertaken to alleviate fears and when appropriate, to advise continued function. Whenever possible, the sexual partner should be involved in a joint counseling session, since it is known that the partner may, at times, not believe the reported advice. Unfortunately, recent surveys indicate that few coronary patients receive adequate sex counseling.[30]

Most stable postcoronary patients are capable of resuming sexual activity within 2 to 4 weeks after discharge.[20,29] If questions persist, an exercise tolerance test is helpful to document tolerance to stress. If the patient is capable of sustaining a maximum heart rate of 120 to 130 beats per minute for a short time, then resumption of sexual activity can be advised, especially if this activity is with the patient's regular sexual partner. Patients should be advised at first to use comfortable positions and avoid vigorous exertion or extremely lengthy sessions. Patients should be counseled to avoid cigarettes, and those with more severe disease should be advised to avoid sexual activity after a heavy meal or the intake of alcohol.

The same basic principles apply to the patient with stable angina pectoris.[20] Prophylactic use of nitroglycerin or long-acting nitrates prior to sexual activity may relieve psychologic stress as well as decrease physiologic stress on the heart. Regular use of beta-blockers may also be helpful, but propranolol has been reported to cause impotence in some people. A progressive exercise program will often improve tolerance to physical stress and decrease the likelihood of chest pain. Use of standing or sitting positions during intercourse may reduce attacks of angina, possibly by reducing the left ventricular end-diastolic volume. The prohibitions mentioned previously about smoking and diet apply here as well.

Generalized atherosclerosis, even in the absence of coronary insufficiency may be associated with erectile dysfunction.

Researchers, using phalloarteriography to study impotent males estimated that 25 per cent of cases of erectile dysfunction were caused by vascular disease.[31] Wagner and Metz[31] reported that 40 to 50 per cent of males referred to a vascular service for peripheral vascular disease had erectile dysfunction. Atherosclerotic changes that may affect erection can be located in the distal part of the aorta, the common or internal iliac arteries, the internal pudendal artery, or one or more of the penile arteries. If vascular changes exist in the larger arteries, intermittent claudication or symptoms of peripheral vascular disease are often, but not always, present. Usually there is a history compatible with organic impotence, as described previously. Most commonly, some degree of erection can be achieved but cannot be maintained for a sufficient length of time. Michal and associates[32] have reported an interesting variant called the "external iliac steal syndrome," which is frequently confused with psychogenic impotence. In this variant, an erection is achieved while the patient is lying still, but when activity commences with greater gluteal and leg muscle activity, the erection may be lost because blood flow through the internal iliac artery may reverse, the lower extremity being supplied by collaterals from the pelvic area. The diagnostic evaluation includes an examination of the lower vascular system, nocturnal penile tumescence studies, and possibly arteriography.

### *Sexual Function and Prostate Surgery**

The proportion of males requiring surgery for benign prostatic hypertrophy or prostatic cancer increases with age. Many elderly men greatly fear these procedures, and there is widespread belief that any form of prostate surgery will impair potency. When questioned about sexual function, some elderly males respond that their sexual activity ceased after prostate surgery. The clinician caring for an elderly patient facing prostate surgery should always address the issue of sexual function if the patient indicates he is still sexually active or has sexual interest.

Few men subjected to a transurethral resection of the prostate experience any difficulties with potency. Finkle and Prior[33] reported on potency in elderly men (aged 50 to 81 years) who underwent various types of prostate surgery (Table 27–3). Potency after all operations was present in 65 per cent of patients aged 55 to 69 years and 34 per cent of patients aged 70 years and over. Age-related data were not available for the different types of surgery, but overall, 95 per cent of men were potent after transurethral surgery. The transurethral resection of prostatic tissue does not affect either the pelvic nerves that control erection and ejaculation or the blood flow to the penis. Most of the impotence that occurs after this type of surgery is probably due to psychogenic causes. Up to 90 per cent of men will develop retrograde ejaculation into the bladder after transurethral surgery because the internal sphincter of the bladder is usually cut.[20] Since semen is directed retrograde into the bladder, these men lose the sensation of semen spurting through the urethra with ejaculation, and this may be a cause for concern in some patients. However, erectile capability and the potential for orgasm are not impaired. Finding spermatozoa in a centrifuged urine specimen obtained immediately after orgasm is diagnostic of retrograde ejaculation.[20] Preoperative counseling regarding this problem is strongly recommended.

The percentage of men potent after suprapubic prostatectomy is a little lower (see Table 27–3). Since this approach involves an incision in the anterior wall of the bladder and dissection around the bladder neck, most patients experience retrograde ejaculation. The percentage of men potent after retropubic prostatectomy (unless radical surgery is performed) is essentially the same. Potency after perineal prostatectomy is related to the extent of surgical dissection. Finkle and Taylor[34] have reported that 71 per cent of men with perineal prostatectomy retain potency and that 43 per cent of men after radical dissection are still potent. However, the latter data are presented from a retrospective study in which most patient charts contained inadequate information; therefore, the percentages could be spuriously high. Most observers continue to report that 90 to 98 per cent of patients who have undergone a radical perineal prostatectomy with extensive dissection (usually for prostate cancer) are impotent postoperatively.[20] On the other hand, other studies indicate that the use of less extensive surgery, combined with radiation implants, will result in significantly less loss of sexual function.[35]

Counseling has recently been shown to influence sexual capabilities after prostate surgery. Zohar and associates[36] reported that men who were given counseling prior to surgery were significantly less likely to develop impotence.

**Table 27–3.** POTENCY STATUS FOLLOWING PROSTATECTOMY*

| | Type of Operation | | | |
|---|---|---|---|---|
| | ***Peri-neal*** | ***Trans-urethral*** | ***Supra-pubic*** | ***Total*** |
| No. of patients | 35 | 32 | 35 | 102 |
| Potent preop | 24 | 22 | 22 | 68 |
| Potent postop | 17 | 23 | 20 | 60 |
| % retaining potency | 71 | 95 | 87 | 84 |

* Reproduced with permission from Finkle AL and Prior DV: Sexual potency in elderly men before and after prostatectomy. JAMA 196:125, 1966.

## SEXUAL COUNSELING FOR THE CANCER PATIENT

It is beyond the scope of this chapter to discuss in detail the problems with sexuality that occur with a variety of types of cancer and their respective treatment. For an excellent in-depth review of this area, the reader is referred to the chapter on the oncology patient in Kolodny's textbook on sexual medicine.[20] Several issues should be considered here. First, receiving the diagnosis of any of the more serious forms of malignant disease is a severe threat to the individual, frequently resulting in depression, altered body image, guilt, despair, and marital difficulties. Such emotional problems may well impair libido. Cancer patients of either sex are likely to experience an increased desire for physical closeness, while, at the same time, displaying a diminished interest in coitus.[20]

* See Chapter 37.

For the purposes of this discussion, problems associated with sexuality after a woman has undergone mastectomy will be reviewed. A recent study by the Masters and Johnson Institute of 60 women who had undergone mastectomy indicated that only four of the women reported prior counseling sessions with either physicians or nurses, but almost one half wished such discussions had been available.[37] After mastectomy, there was a definite change in sexual activity levels. Fifty-two per cent of these women had reported a frequency of intercourse of once a week prior to surgery, whereas only 35 per cent reported continuing this rate after surgery. The proportion of women who reported they never or rarely had coital orgasm rose from 17 per cent prior to surgery to 40 per cent in the first 3 months after surgery. Also, the frequency of breast stimulation during sexual activity declined significantly. Thirty-eight per cent of husbands had not viewed the incision site within the first 3 months after the mastectomy.[37]

When a woman is facing a mastectomy, the clinician should begin counseling well in advance of the surgery. It is helpful to inquire about the patient's sexual status to determine the importance of sexual activity in her life. Even if sexual activity is low, the clinician should remember that self-image and female sexuality are inexorably linked. The woman, and possibly her husband, should be involved in discussions about the various types of surgery available, and, if medically indicated, consideration should be given to less disfiguring surgery. The husband should be encouraged to visit his wife frequently in the hospital and, if feasible, view his wife's body soon after surgery.[20] If a mastectomy is performed, fitting of a breast prosthesis should be considered as well as the possibility of reconstructive surgery in those people or couples to whom such issues are very important. The woman should be counseled by a lay group such as Reach for Recovery to deal with her emotional response to the surgery and to sexual activity as soon as possible if chemotherapy or other medical issues do not supervene.

## SEXUAL COUNSELING FOR THE ARTHRITIS PATIENT

Although the types of chronic arthritis are diverse, they all can limit sexuality. In general, sexual activity may be limited because of the constitutional symptoms associated with arthritis, because of pain associated with active disease, or because contractures and limitation of motion may impede active movement or certain positions.[20] Curry[38] and Todd and associates[39] studied sexual behavior in adult patients with degenerative arthritis of the hip and have found some disruption in sexual activities in 67 per cent and 52 per cent of persons studied, respectively.

Counseling should first focus on issues of self-image in the arthritis victim and the establishment of effective communication between the sexual partners. The clinician should gently explore the possibility of alternative methods of sexual expression if one partner is severely limited. The Arthritis Foundation publishes a useful book that counsels patients on a variety of topics related to sexuality, including use of a variety of positions.[40] The lateral position is useful if either partner has back involvement. If the woman has hip involvement, a modification of the male superior position, with the male supporting most of his own weight, or the rear entry position is useful. If the man has hip or knee involvement, the female astride position may be most comfortable. In addition, patients should be counseled to plan sexual activity for the time of day when they feel the best and plan their medication schedule to provide relief during intercourse. At times, a warm shower or bath before sex will be relaxing and relieve stiffness.

## SEXUALITY IN THE NURSING HOME SETTING

The nursing home is frequently a sexually restrictive environment, with inadequate facilities for individuals or couples to have privacy for sexual activity.[41] Although few data are available, current studies appear to indicate that most nursing home residents approve of sexual activity for residents but indicate little or no personal activity.[41,42] Also, many elderly people have conservative or negative feelings about masturbation, but such activity does continue into old age and may be the only form of sexual activity available. Also, at times, families of nursing home residents raise serious objections to elderly parents or relatives engaging in sexual activity. Such objections may derive from family taboos with regard to sexuality or from concern about a possible inheritance. The nursing home staff may not have strong negative feelings about resident sexual activity but may do little to change the nursing home environment to facilitate sexual privacy.[42] The physician should promote change in the nursing home to facilitate privacy and freedom for alternative sexual expression for those residents who have such needs.

## References


1. Pfeiffer E: Sexual behavior in old age. *In* Busse E (ed.): Behavior and Adaptation in Late Life. Boston, Little, Brown and Co., 1969.
2. Kofoed L, Bloom JD: Geriatric sexual dysfunction: A case survey. J Am Geriatr Soc 30:437, 1982.
3. Kinsey AC, Pomeroy WB, Martin CE: Sexual Behavior in the Human Male. Philadelphia, W.B. Saunders Co., 1948, pp. 218–262.
4. Verwoerdt A, Pfeiffer E, Wang HS: Sexual behavior in senescence. II. Patterns of sexual activity and interest. Geriatrics 24:137, 1969.
5. Pfeiffer E, Verwoerdt A, Wang HS: Sexual behavior in aged men and women. Arch Gen Psychiatry 19:753, 1968.
6. Botwinick J: Drives, expectations, and emotions. *In* Birren JE (ed.): Handbook of Aging and the Individual. Chicago, University of Chicago Press, 1959.
7. Pfeiffer E, Davis GC: Determinants of sexual behavior in middle and old age. J Am Geriatr Soc 20:151, 1972.
8. Kinsey AC, Pomeroy WB, Martin CR, Deghard PH: Sexual Behavior in the Human Female. Philadelphia, W.B. Saunders Co., 1953.
9. Christenson CV, Gagnon JH: Sexual behavior in a group of older women. J Gerontol 20:351, 1965.
10. Snyder GE, Spreitzer E: Attitudes of the aged toward nontraditional sexual behavior. Arch Sex Behav 5:249, 1976.
11. Wall S, Kaltreider N: Changing social-sexual patterns in gynecologic practice. JAMA 237:565, 1977.
12. Schiavi RC, Hogan B: Sexual problems in diabetes mellitus: Psychological aspects. Diabetes Care 2:9, 1979.
    *Excellent review of both psychologic and physical aspects of sexual function in diabetic males and females. Provides information on diagnostic evaluation and treatment.*
13. Ellenberg M: Sex and diabetes: A comparison between men and women. Diabetes Care 2:4, 1979.
    *Review of differentiation of psychogenic from organic impotence. Provides data on sexual dysfunction in male and female diabetics.*
14. Masters WH, Johnson VE: Human Sexual Response. Boston, Little, Brown and Co., 1966.
    *Still the definitive work on the physiology of the human sexual response.*
15. Master WH, Johnson VE: Human Sexual Inadequacy. Boston, Little, Brown and Co., pp. 316–350, 1970.
    *Although based on a relatively small sample of elderly persons, the chapters on the aging male and female and related sexual problems are still definitive.*
16. Masters WH, Johnson VE: Sex and the aging process. J Am Geriatr Soc 29:385, 1981.
    *Concise, informative summary of aging changes, with mention of syndromes of particular importance in the elderly.*
17. Glover BH: Sex counseling of the elderly. Hosp Pract 12:101, 1977.
    *Broad overview of sex counseling in the elderly.*
18. Shearer MR, Shearer ML: Sexuality and sexual counseling in the elderly. Clin Obstet Gynecol 20:197, 1977.
    *Excellent general review of physiologic and counseling issues. Good discussion of loss of libido and organic problems.*
19. Furlow WL: Diagnosis and treatment of male erectile failure. Diabetes Care 2:18, 1979.
    *Although focused on the diabetic, presents a clear, concise approach to the evaluation of the impotent male.*
20. Kolodny RC, Masters WH, Johnson VE: Textbook of Sexual Medicine. Boston, Little, Brown and Co., 1979.
    *Outstanding textbook on sexual problems that pertain to clinical medicine. Good review of aging sexual physiology and excellent chapters on sexual problems related to certain disease states.*
21. Tsitouras PP, Martin CE, Harman SM: Relationship of serum testosterone to sexual activity in healthy elderly men. J Gerontol 37:288, 1982.
22. Spark RF, White RA, Connolly PB: Impotence is not always psychogenic. JAMA 243:750, 1980.
23. Karcan I, Williams RL, Thornby JI, Salis PJ: Sleep-related penile tumescence as a function of age. Am J Psychiatry 132:932, 1975.
24. Beutler LE, Gleason DM: Integrating the advances in the diagnosis and treatment of male potency disturbance. J Urol 126:338, 1981.
25. Kempczinski RF: Role of the vascular diagnostic laboratory in the evaluation of male impotence. Am J Surg 138:278, 1979.
26. Semmens JP, Wagner G: Estrogen deprivation and vaginal function in postmenopausal women. JAMA 248:445, 1982.
27. Kolodny RC: Sexual dysfunction in diabetic females. Diabetes 20:557, 1971.
28. Ellenberg M: Sexual aspects of the female diabetic. Mt Sinai J Med 44:495, 1977.
29. Hellerstein HK, Friedman EH: Sexual activity and the postcoronary patient. Arch Intern Med 125:987, 1970.
30. Masur FT: Resumption of sexual activity following myocardial infarction. Sexuality and Disability 2:98, 1979.
31. Wagner G, Metz P: Impotence (erectile dysfunction) due to vascular disorders. J Sex Marital Ther 6:223, 1980.
32. Michal V, Kranor R, Pospichal J: External iliac "steal syndrome." J Cardiovasc Surg 19:255, 1978.
33. Finkle AL, Prior DV: Sexual potency in elderly men before and after prostatectomy. JAMA 196:125, 1966.
34. Finkle AL, Taylor SP: Sexual potency after radical prostatectomy. J Urol 125:350, 1981.
35. Herr HW: Preservation of sexual potency in prostate cancer patients after prostatectomy. J Urol 116:332, 1976.
36. Zohar J, Meiray D, May B, Duist N: Factors influencing sexual activity after prostatectomy. J Urol 116:332, 1976.
37. Frank D, Danbash RL, Webster SK, Kolodny RC: Mastectomy and sexual behavior. Sexuality and Disability 1:16, 1978.
38. Curry HL: Osteoarthritis of the hip joint and sexual activity. Ann Rheum Dis 29:488, 1970.
39. Todd RC, Lightowler CDR, Harris J: Low function arthroplasty of the hip joint and sexual activity. Acta Orthop Scand 44:690, 1973.
40. Boggs J: Arthritis, living and loving. Atlanta, GA, Arthritis Foundation, 1982.
41. Koss MJ: Sexual expression of the elderly in nursing homes. Gerontologist 18:372, 1978.
42. Wasow M, Loeb MB: Sexuality in nursing homes. J Am Geriatr Soc 28:73, 1979.


## *Additional Reading*


1. Kolodny RC, Kahn CB, Goldstein HH, et al: Sexual dysfunction in diabetic men. Diabetes 23:306, 1973.
2. Rubin A, Babbott D: Impotence and diabetes mellitus. JAMA 168:498, 1958.
3. Schöffling K, Federlin K, Ditschurneit H, et al: Disorders in sexual function in male diabetics. Diabetes 12:519, 1963.

## Chapter 28

# Hypothermia

*Rudolph M. Navari*
*Thomas W. Sheehy*

Hypothermia is defined as a condition in which central or core body temperature is equal to or less than 35° C (95° F).[1-3] *Accidental hypothermia* is a term frequently used to distinguish environmentally induced hypothermia from hypothermia that develops secondary to medical conditions or surgical treatment.[2-7]

## CLASSIFICATION

Several classifications for hypothermia have been developed. These are based either on etiology or on the severity of hypothermia as determined by body temperature measurements. Exposure is a prerequisite to all types of hypothermia, but contrary to popular belief, it need not be prolonged.[3]

Etiologically, there are three common types of hypothermia.[8] *Immersion hypothermia* occurs when cold stress exceeds maximum body heat production. Mountain climbers inadequately clothed in cold weather and long distance swimmers exposed to hot and cold waters are prone to this type of hypothermia. *Exhaustion hypothermia* results from depletion of the body's readily available energy sources. It occurs in long distance runners; miners, steel workers, and other manual laborers; and so on. *Subclinical hypothermia* is usually found in the elderly, resulting from an impairment to their central temperature-regulating center. Often older patients are unable to adjust their body temperatures readily to extremes. They may have consistently low core body temperatures due at least in part to impaired ambient temperature perception, impaired capacity to shiver, decreased total body water, and inability to conserve heat by vasoconstriction.

Clinically, hypothermia is classified according to the degree of core body temperature:[9,10] (1) *mild* hypothermia refers to a core body temperature of 32 to 35° C (90 to 95° F); (2) *moderate* hypothermia, to a core body temperature of 30 to 32° C (86 to 89° F); (3) *severe* hypothermia, to a core body temperature below 30° C (86° F). This classification system is useful both for assessment of clinical severity and for treatment of the condition.

## PATHOPHYSIOLOGY

Figure 28–1 outlines the general physiologic responses to cold.[2] When cold is perceived by peripheral afferent thermoreceptors, stimuli are sent, via the spinal thalmic tracts, to that portion of the anterior hypothalmus that coordinates and controls central body temperature. In turn, the hypothalmic temperature-regulating center stimulates the sympathetic nervous system, the extrapyramidal tract, and the anterior pituitary gland. Stimulation of the autonomic nervous system increases the heart rate, vasoconstricts the dermal blood vessels, and vasodilates muscle blood vessels. Extrapyramidal tract stimulation induces shivering, which tends to increase vasodilation in muscles. Stimulation of the anterior pituitary gland leads indirectly to increased thyroxine and corticosteroid release. Together, these events are designed to prevent heat loss and to increase body heat production.

In the elderly, these physiologic responses may be blunted or lost. Table 28–1 outlines altered physiologic responses and changes in the elderly that increase their risk for hypothermia. Progressive thermoregulatory impairment occurs in many elderly individuals as they age.[11] In a progressive 5-year study, Collins and associates[11] found that in the elderly peripheral

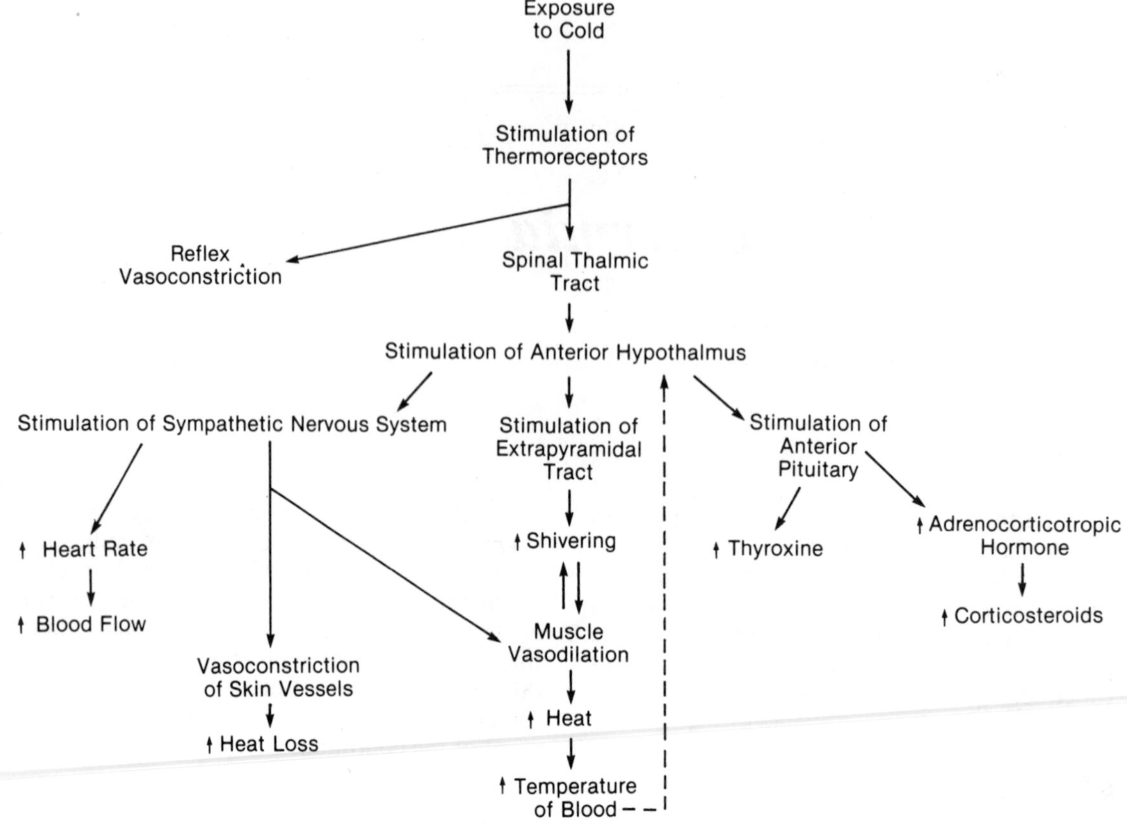


**Figure 28-1.** General physiologic responses to cold.

blood flow decreased at rest, reflex vasoconstrictor response showed impairment, and the incidence of orthostatic hypotension increased. Together, these findings suggested impairment of the autonomic nervous system. A subsequent study of the same patients suggested that they had impaired thermal discrimination.[12] Although they preferred the same environmental temperature as younger individuals (22 to 23° C) [71.6 to 73.4° F]), they were unable to adjust to ambient temperatures as readily.

**Table 28-1.** ABNORMAL PHYSIOLOGIC MECHANISMS IN THE ELDERLY IN RELATION TO HYPOTHERMIA

1. Impaired recognition of decreased temperature (decreased)
2. Decreased resting peripheral blood flow
3. Decreased activity of autonomic nervous system
4. Decreased mobility
5. Decreased muscle mass
6. Decreased vasoconstriction
7. Decreased ability to alter respiratory response to changes in environmental temperatures
8. Decreased shivering

Thermal perception is commonly impaired among the aged. Many elderly patients are unable to discern temperature differences at 5° C (9° F) with their fingers.[13] In contrast, younger individuals can detect differences of as little as 0.5° C (0.9° F). Comparative studies have also revealed that elderly individuals, immobilized in cabinets and subjected to temperature changes from 5 to 15° C (41 to 59° F) have more rapid falls in body temperature, impaired ability to maintain body temperature, less perception of cold, and increased oxygen consumption. Those with chronic low body temperatures were more susceptible to hypothermia, for they have less body heat to lose than normothermic individuals.[13]

## ETIOLOGY

Predisposing causes of hypothermia are numerous as shown in Table 28-2.[11,13,14] Historically, hypothermia has been regarded as a province of the infant and the elderly. This concept arose from earlier studies in Great Britain, which revealed that 0.68 to 3 per cent of hospital

**Table 28–2.** PREDISPOSING CONDITIONS OF HYPOTHERMIA IN THE ELDERLY

| |
|---|
| **Accidental** |
| Environment |
| Poor living conditions |
| **Central Nervous System Dysfunction** |
| Cerebrovascular disease |
| Wernicke's encephalopathy |
| Head trauma |
| Neoplasms |
| Mental illness |
| **Drug-Induced** |
| Phenothiazines |
| Ethanol |
| Barbiturates |
| Anesthetics |
| Phenformin |
| Antidepressants |
| **Nutrition** |
| Protein-calorie deficiency |
| Cirrhosis |
| **Infections** |
| Sepsis |
| Pneumonia |
| **Renal Dysfunction** |
| Uremia |
| **Endocrine Dysfunction** |
| Hypothyroidism |
| Hypoadrenalism |
| Hypopituitarism |
| Hypoglycemia |
| Diabetes mellitus |
| **Cardiovascular Dysfunction** |
| Myocardial infarction |
| Peripheral vascular disease |
| Congestive heart failure |
| Pulmonary embolus |

admissions during the winter months were as a result of hypothermia. Most of these patients were either elderly (42 per cent) or infants.[3,15] More recent experience, however, shows that accidental hypothermia occurs at all ages and does not necessarily require prolonged exposure to cold temperatures.[1,9,16] In the young adult, hypothermia is usually secondary to stressful athletic events, to boating or automobile accidents, to infection, or to metabolic derangements, e.g., diabetic ketoacidosis, uremia, hypothyroidism.[16,17] In community hospitals, combinations of alcohol, hypoglycemia, infection, and certain drugs are now recognized as major predisposing causes of hypothermia, along with age.[9]

### *Age*

Age alone is a prominent cause of hypothermia. Mild hypothermia, that is, a body temperature below 34° C (93.2° F), occurs in a substantial number of the aged.[13,18–21] In England, 11 to 15 per cent of the elderly living at home or alone were found to be hypothermic.[21,22] This high incidence was attributed to a variety of environmental factors, including poor heating facilities, living alone, being housebound, and even a lack of indoor plumbing. Yet, Fox and associates[20] were unable to correlate any of these factors with low body temperatures in the elderly. Central heating is not the answer to prevention of hypothermia in the elderly.[6]

### *Acute Illness*

Hypothermia secondary to acute illness is also more common in the elderly.[3,23] It may accompany or follow pneumonia, congestive heart failure, hypoglycemia, renal failure, and so on. Cerebrovascular accidents, head trauma, metabolic encephalopathies, and progressive mental deterioration may further reduce the elderly patient's awareness of cold and lessen his or her physical activity, further predisposing to hypothermia.

### *Cardiovascular Collapse*

Conditions causing cardiovascular collapse, such as congestive heart failure, myocardial infarction, septicemia, pulmonary embolism, and so forth, can readily give rise to hypothermia. These conditions too are more likely to occur in the aged patient.[24]

### *Endocrine Dysfunction*

Classically, myxedema and hypoglycemia are considered the most common endocrine causes of hypothermia.[25–27] However, diabetic ketoacidosis is an even more common cause, particularly in the elderly.[17,28,29] Conversely, pituitary and adrenal failure are rarely responsible for hypothermia.

## CLINICAL FINDINGS

Diagnosis requires a high index of suspicion for hypothermia. All primary care and geriatric facilities as well as emergency departments should have rectal thermometers capable of recording body temperatures as low as 24° C (75.2° F). The presenting signs of hypothermia are listed in Table 28–3, along with associated complications.

Table 28–3. CLINICAL ASPECTS OF ELDERLY HYPOTHERMIA

| Presenting Signs | Complications |
|---|---|
| ***Cardiovascular*** | |
| Hypotension | Shock |
| Arrhythmias | Cardiac arrest |
| Myocardial infarction | Congestive heart failure |
| ***Pulmonary*** | |
| Aspiration | Bronchopneumonia |
| Dyspnea, apnea | Respiratory arrest |
| ***Central Nervous System*** | |
| Depressed mental status | |
| Hyporeflexia | |
| Depressed pupillary response | |
| ***Gastrointestinal*** | |
| Pancreatitis | |
| Upper gastrointestinal bleeding | |
| ***Renal*** | |
| Oliguria, anuria | Acute renal failure |
| Metabolic acidosis | |
| Polyuria | |
| ***Sepsis*** | |
| ***Hematologic*** | |
| Disseminated intravascular coagulation | |
| Thrombocytopenia | |
| Leukopenia | |

MacLean and associates[25] categorized hypothermia into three clinical stages based on body temperature.

## Stage 1 — Responsive Phase

These patients have mild hypothermia and body temperatures of 32.2 to 35° C (90 to 95° F). If they are otherwise normal, patients in this stage are usually capable of adjusting physiologically to their hypothermia. They tend to generate and retain body heat, hence the term "responsive" phase. In this phase, the body's metabolic rate increases, as does blood pressure, cardiac rate, cardiac output, and respiratory rate. The patient shivers unless this response is lost owing to aging. Cutaneous vasoconstriction occurs and renders the skin pale and cold to the touch. Diuresis ensues as vasoconstriction increases the volume of the central circulation.

## Stage 2 — Slowing Phase

With temperatures below 32.2° C (90° F), the ability to generate heat is seriously impaired. Now, the respiratory rate, the heart rate, and the cardiac output begin to decline. Muscles tend to stiffen and shivering decreases perceptively. Central nervous system symptoms become evident, due presumably to central tissue hypoxia and to increased blood viscosity. Disorientation, hallucinations, and coma may develop. Cerebellar signs, dysarthria, hyporeflexia, cranial nerve deficits, and decreased pupillary responses may be observed.[30,31]

Arrhythmias and hypotension are the main manifestations of cardiovascular involvement. Experimental studies have shown bradycardia to occur almost regularly as the temperature drops below 90° F (32.5° C). Myocardial irritability becomes evident as the temperature approaches 30° C (86° F). Atrial fibrillation with slow ventricular response develops at 80 to 85° F (27 to 30° C).[32–34] Ventricular fibrillation is likely to occur at lower temperatures. Electrocardiographically, there may be an increase in the P-R interval, Q-T prolongation, and T wave inversion.[32–37] Osborn's sign (camel-hump sign) or the "J" wave is a common but nonspecific sign of hypothermia. It is found on the electrocardiogram in about one fourth of hypothermic individuals. The J wave simply refers to the extra upward deflection at the junction of the QRS complex and S-T segment. Sometimes, cardiac creatinine phosphokinase (CPK) and lactase dehydrogenase levels are elevated. Whether these elevations result from a cellular "leak" due to impaired cell membrane integrity or to microinfarction is not clear at present.[37]

Hypotension is common, with the blood pressure falling progressively as the temperature falls.[32–34] At one time or another, cold-induced bradycardia, decreased tissue oxygen requirements, hypovolemia, and vasoconstriction have all been blamed for hypotension. Most likely, a combination of these events is responsible. Together, or alone, depressed cardiac output, hypotension, and arrhythmias may lead to florid congestive heart failure, shock, and cardiac arrest.

Hypoventilation may result from decreased respiratory rate and reduced minute ventilatory volume. A shift to the left in the oxyhemoglobin dissociation curve decreases the amount of dissolved oxygen in blood. Hence, blood gas levels must be corrected for the body temperature. The laboratory should always be notified of the patient's temperature, so that correction can be made and a more accurate blood gas analysis rendered.[33] Less oxygen is available for cellular metabolism in hypothermic patients, but fortunately, cold tends to decrease tissue oxygen requirement.[33]

The impaired cough reflex associated with both age and hypothermia, along with diminished consciousness and dehydration, makes the hypothermic patient more susceptible to pulmonary infections, notably, bronchopneumonia. Respiratory arrest, too, may occur at temperatures below 24° C (75° F).

Bowel sounds in this stage of the disease are usually difficult to discern because of hypomotility. Muscle stiffness may make the abdominal muscles sufficiently rigid to make abdominal palpation difficult. Occasionally hemorrhagic pancreatitis ensues, presumably as a result of hypothermia-induced microvascular sludging. Drug metabolism can be altered as the result of hypothermia-induced reduction in hepatic conjugating and detoxifying activity. Hepatic failure, however, is rare in nonalcoholic patients.[33]

### *Stage 3 — Poikilothermic Phase*

Extreme temperatures are evident in this stage, sometimes below 24° C (75° F). At this temperature, a rigor-mortislike appearance is evident, and patients in this phase have been mistaken for corpses. They are cold and stiff to touch and feel frozen. As Fitzgerald and Jessop and others state,[33,38] the differential diagnosis is death. Elderly patients with complete loss of thermoregulation can become poikilothermic, i.e., their body temperature assumes the prevailing ambient temperature.

## TREATMENT AND GENERAL CARE

### *General*

Hypothermia is a medical emergency, and when possible, the patient should be managed in an intensive care setting.[39–41] On initial contact, any wet clothing should be removed and the patient wrapped in blankets or other insulating materials. Once the patient is admitted for care or treatment, careful and continuous monitoring of the pulse, arterial blood pressure, and respiration is essential. Initially, and throughout the critical period, accurate and continuous core temperature measurements by rectal core thermometer are prescribed. Adequate intravenous access and a patent airway must be established early. Supplemental oxygen is given after blood has been obtained for measurement of arterial blood gases. Initial orders should include assays of serum electrolytes, glucose, creatinine, and amylase; complete blood count including platelets; urinalysis; hepatic function studies; blood cultures; and tests of stool for occult blood. Blood cultures are performed immediately, since sepsis is a common cause of hypothermia. In addition, an electrocardiogram and chest x-ray should be requested.

The physical examination must be thorough, and the examiner should make a diligent search for signs indicative of the precipitating causes of hypothermia, as listed in Table 28–2. The elderly, in particular, are prone to a number of illnesses that may be directly responsible for their hypothermia.

Certain findings commonly encountered in hypothermia can be treated rapidly. Hypoglycemia is extremely common in hypothermic patients admitted to a community hospital. Forty-one per cent of Fitzgerald and Jessop's patients had initial serum glucose levels below 50 mg per dl.[33] Thus, use of 5 per cent glucose in normal saline should be part of the initial solute therapy. Hypothermia also predisposes to hypovolemia. Initial fluid repletion with 100 to 200 ml of 5 per cent glucose in normal saline per hour is customary. Since sepsis is another important cause of hypothermia, some but not all authorities recommend that following performance of appropriate cultures, broad spectrum antibiotics should be given empirically.[3,9,18] Bradycardia, if severe, may require the use of atropine and/or isoproterenol. If these drugs fail, cardiac pacing is necessary until rewarming methods have stabilized the cardiovascular system. The use of pressor agents for hypotension has to be assessed individually. Hypothermic patients often fail to respond normally to these and other drugs.

A central venous line is established. This is extremely helpful in monitoring elderly hypothermic patients, in whom the risk for hypervolemia secondary to fluid overload or to the rapid shifts of extravascular and intravascular fluids is greatest during rewarming.[40] Previously, intravenous corticosteroids were recommended as part of initial treatment.[3] Now, most believe that they are not necessary unless there is a history of adrenal suppression or insufficiency or evident pulmonary aspiration.[8,39–44] Fluid intake and output and electrolytes and platelets must be assessed. If oliguria or anuria ensues, treatment with furosemide or mannitol may be necessary. Potassium chloride or sodium bicarbonate may be required if the degree of hypokalemia and acidosis becomes intense.

Finally, an adequate airway must be maintained. Aspiration is common, especially among elderly individuals or comatose patients. Some physicians recommend administration of 1 to 3 L of oxygen per minute by nasal cannula for all patients. For those patients whose airways cannot be kept clear of secretions, an endotracheal tube may be required. In these patients aspiration should be done only after insertion of the endotracheal tube.

## *Specific Measures*

The most controversial aspect of hypothermia is the method of rewarming. Therapeutic recommendations are usually based on the degree of hypothermia, i.e., mild, moderate, or severe. Table 28–4 shows the various methods of rewarming that have been previously employed.

Passive external rewarming (PER) has been the traditional method. The patient is placed in a warm room (>25° C [77° F]), covered with blankets or other coverings, and given warm intravenous fluids (37.5° C [98° F]). The patient warms at his own pace, using heat generated by his own body. If the procedure is successful, rewarming is gradual (0.5° C [33° F] per hour). This method has been recommended for use in the elderly and for patients with mild hypothermia.[3] Some have criticized this method as being too slow to prevent some of the complications and metabolic consequences of hypothermia.[45]

Active external rewarming (AER) involves immersion of the trunk in hot water (40 to 45° C [104 to 113° F]) or, alternately, the use of electric blankets or hot water bottles.[19] This method is controversial. Critics claim that rapid external rewarming produces rapid cutaneous vasodilation. It is argued that this, in turn, results in a decrease in peripheral vascular resistance, hypotension, decreased coronary perfusion, and a shunting of cool blood to the myocardium, where it may further reduce the temperature and lead to cardiac arrhythmias.[26,30,40–50] This technique has been used successfully in younger adults who are alcoholics or who have accidental hypothermia,[19,53] and there are isolated reports of its effectiveness in the aged.[40,51,52] Most authorities, however, consider this method too dangerous for elderly patients, particularly those with fragile cardiovascular systems.

Active core rewarming (ACR) has been used in treating patients with hypothermia ranging from moderate to severe.[39,45,48,49,51,53,54] The techniques are numerous and include inhalation of heated oxygen;[44,45] peritoneal dialysis;[41,55–60] hemodialysis;[61] irrigation of the mediastinum,[62] stomach,[59] and colon[13] with warm fluids; use of warming parenteral fluids; and extracorpuscular blood rewarming.[48] Proponents suggest that this method has distinct advantages over other methods, claiming that it leads to a preferential warming of the myocardium, with an increase in cardiac output, a decrease in cardiac irritability, and a rapid return to a near normal core temperature.[45,48,49]

ACR may be necessary in individuals with severe hypothermia and/or cardiac instability or insufficiency that fails to respond to conventional methods of resuscitation. Elderly patients with severe hypothermia may respond to PER if their cardiovascular status is stable.[42,44,63,64] Inhalation of heated oxygen or extracorpuscular blood rewarming may be necessary if serious cardiac arrhythmias ensue or diabetic coma evolves.[44] In two studies, AER was used successfully with low mortality in patients of advanced age.[51,52]

**Table 28–4.** REWARMING METHODS

| |
|---|
| **Passive External (PE)** |
| Warm environment (> 25° C [77° F]) |
| Insulating material |
| **Active External (AE)** |
| Immersion in hot water |
| Electric blankets |
| **Active Core (AC)** |
| Inhalation of heated steam |
| Face mask |
| Endotracheal tube |
| Dialysis |
| Hemodialysis |
| Peritoneal |
| Irrigation |
| Mediastinal via thoracotomy |
| Colonic |
| Intragastric balloon |
| Extracorporeal blood rewarming |

## *Comparative Treatment Studies*

There has been controversy over the most effective rewarming methods because there were not enough studies involving sufficient numbers of hypothermic patients to permit prospective comparisons of treatment efficacy. Recently, such studies have become available (Table 28–5).[1,19,44,64–66]

Weyman and associates[19] studied 39 patients with accidental hypothermia. Contributing factors were present in most. Twenty-eight were intoxicated with ethanol, two overdosed with heroin, and eight had serious underlying medical disorders. Thirty-three were treated by AER and six by PER. The major complications attributed to AER, namely hypotension and cardiac irritability, did not occur. Only five of these patients were 65 years of age or older. Mortality was 6.25 per cent among the 31 patients with hypothermia alone. It was 75 per cent among the eight patients whose hypothermia accompa-

Table 28–5. COMPARISON OF HYPOTHERMIC STUDIES—TREATMENT AND MORTALITY

| | Weyman et al[19] | Davidson and Grant[9] | Hudson and Conn[65] | O'Keefe[64] | Frank and Robson[53] | Ledingham and Mone[51] | Fitzgerald and Jessop[33] | Miller et al[44] |
|---|---|---|---|---|---|---|---|---|
| **Patients (number)** | 39 | 60 | 16 | 62 | 10 | 44 | 22 | 114 |
| **Age (years)** | 52 | 53 | 53 | 58 | — | 60 | 63 | 59 |
| **Mean Age (years)** | 22–83 | 17–99 | 21–81 | 14–87 | 24–68 | 40–70 | 30–80 | — |
| **Core temperature °C** | | | | | | | | |
| **Range** | 22.6–34.4 | 26.9–35 | 20–33.3 | — | 26.5–33 | 20.0–34.3 | 23.8–35 | —<br>30.8 |
| **Precipitating Factors (patients)** | | | | | | | | |
| ***Alcohol*** | 28 | 14 | — | 39 | — | 4 | 20 | — |
| ***Drugs (other)*** | 2 | — | — | — | — | 18 | — | — |
| ***Medical Illness*** | 8 | 18 | 8 | 10 | 7 | 19 | 18 | 23 |
| **Treatment** | | | | | | | | |
| ***AER**** | 33 | 11 | — | — | — | 42 | — | 14 |
| ***PER†*** | 6 | 40 | 8 | 56 | 10 | — | 22 | 68 |
| ***Other*** | — | 9 | 8 | — | — | 2 | — | 53 |
| **Mortality with Hypothermia Only (%)** | 6 | 3.3 | 0 | 11 | 0 | 6 | — | 12 |
| **Mortality with Medical Illness (%)** | 75 | — | 88 | 67 | 0 | 53 | 36 | 48 |

* AER = active external rewarming.
† PER = passive external rewarming.

nied significant medical conditions. Several of these patients were refractory to both rewarming methods.

Miller and co-workers[44] reviewed 114 hypothermic patients with 135 presentations, treated in an urban emergency department by various methods of rewarming. The mean age of these patients was 59.4 years (± 17.6 years). The rates of rewarming were 0.71° C (33.27° F) per hour with PER, 0.74° C (33.33° F) per hour with heated aerosol via mask, 1.22° C (34.19° F) per hour with heated aerosol via endotrachial tube, 0.90° C (33.62° F) per hour with AER using heated whirlpool or electric blankets. Overall, mortality was 11.9 per cent, but it was 47.9 per cent for those with serious underlying disease. Mortality according to rewarming methods was 64 per cent with AER (9/14), 7.7 per cent with heated aerosol with a mask (1/13), 5.8 per cent with PER (4/68), and 5.0 per cent with heated aerosol via endotrachial tube (2/40). Usually patients with severe hypothermia were treated with the heated aerosol endotrachial tube method. In this study, the survivors had a higher mean arrival temperature than nonsurvivors.

Davidson and Grant[9] studied 60 patients with hypothermia over a 2-year period in a surburban hospital. Over one half of the patients were 60 years of age or older. Neither the severity nor the incidence of hypothermia was related to the ambient air temperatures or season of the year. Diabetes mellitus and alcohol abuse were found to be risk factors. Again morbidity was related to the presence of underlying disease.

Hudson and Conn[65] reported on 16 patients with hypothermia. Seven of eight patients (two over 65 years of age) with significant cardiovascular disease died. None of the remaining eight had cardiovascular disease and all survived. The degree of hypothermia was similar in both groups. PER was adequate for most patients.

O'Keefe[64] studied 62 hypothermic patients, with a median age of 58 years (range 14 to 87 years). Fifty-six or 90 per cent were treated with PER only. Overall mortality was 11 per cent. All but one death occurred in patients with serious associated medical conditions. Mortality in this subset of patients was 67 per cent. Sixty-three per cent of the patients were alcoholics, 24 per cent had mental disorders, and 14 per cent had severe medical problems (e.g., pneumonia, edema, and liver disorders). O'Keefe concluded that for both young and old, PER is adequate for all degrees (mild, moderate, severe) of hypothermia, provided that the patient's cardiovascular status is stable.

Frank and Robson[53] used rapid immersion rewarming, aggressive fluid resuscitation, and intensive care in ten hypothermic patients, ages 24 to 68 years, without a single death. They strongly believe that this technique reduces mortality in patients with severe hypothermia.

Recently, Ledingham and Mone[51] had considerable success with AER. Their series consisted of 44 hypothermic patients with a mean age of 60 years (range 40 to 70 years). Forty-two were rewarmed with a radiant heat cradle at a rate of 1° C (33.8° F) per hour. Overall mortality was 27 per cent. Only two patients died during treatment. Again, mortality was attributed to underlying disease and not to hypothermia. The authors concluded that AER was safe, even for the elderly hypothermic patient. The mortality reported was less and the morbidity was comparable with those found in other trials employing AER. Nonetheless, severe hypotension was a problem among their patients during rewarming.[44]

Fitzgerald and Jessop[33] studied 22 hypothermic patients with a mean age of 63 years (range 30 to 80 years). All had serious concomitant disease. In the majority, hypothermia was attributed to alcohol (91 per cent) hypoglycemia (41 per cent), and infection (41 per cent). Age and hypothyroidism were clinically significant in three patients. All patients were treated with PER. Mortality was 35 per cent. None of the patients with alcoholic hypothermia died. Again, most deaths were attributable to associated medical conditions, namely, infection, renal failure, and cardiovascular disease.

## PROGNOSIS

The mortality among hospitalized elderly patients with hypothermia varies from 20 to 85 per cent.[1,9,13,19,44,45,64–67] Using PER, Mills[68] reported a mortality of 12.5 per cent within 24 hours and 50 per cent within 30 hours in elderly patients admitted with rectal temperatures of less than 32.3° C (90° F). Goldman and associates[19] reported a mortality of 38.5 per cent in elderly patients with primary hypothermia and a rectal temperature of less than 35° C (95° F). Elderly hypothermic patients with temperatures of less than 32.3° C (90° F) should survive if properly treated and if they have no serious underlying medical problems.[3,64]

Mortality has been related to several factors, namely, (1) the degree of hypotension on admission;[44] (2) the duration of hypothermia prior to treatment;[70] (3) the temperature on arrival; (4) associated underlying conditions, particularly cardiovascular disease;[9,16,44,64,65] and (5) the development of complications.[19,50]

It is important to remember that patients should not be pronounced dead until their core body temperatures reach normal with rewarming. There have been numerous cases recorded of full recovery, even after hours of persistent asystole requiring prolonged cardiopulmonary resuscitation.[13,42,71]

Mills[72] recently summarized the management approach to hypothermic patients. Although the rewarming technique is important, he places more emphasis on careful and detailed supportive care of the patient. Variance in supportive care rather than the rewarming techniques may be responsible for the large differences in mortality found among the reported series.

## AFTEREFFECTS IN THE AGED

The aftereffects of hypothermia are also more significant in the aged. Many develop a tendency for recurrent hypothermia. Survivors of hypothermic attacks have been found to have lower than normal resting body temperatures, along with impaired shivering and vasoconstriction. This residual hypothalmic dysfunction places them at an increased risk for subsequent attacks of hypothermia, even in the presence of moderately cold temperatures.[55]

## PREVENTION

Prevention of hypothermia in the elderly centers on two main aspects of care: adequate living conditions and preventive health care.[73,74] Physicians and paramedical personnel should question elderly patients about their living conditions. Whenever possible, a diet should be prescribed that is adequate and provides sufficient calories during the cold temperature months. Activity, when possible, should be encouraged. Drugs with hypothermic action, such as sedatives, phenothiazines, ethanol, and depressants, should be avoided. The elderly should be encouraged to wear sufficient clothing in the winter and to use bedding designed to prevent heat loss. If they live alone, the suitability of their quarters, i.e., insulation, heating, and so on, should be ascertained.[75]

Elderly patients should be seen more frequently during winter months in order to keep tighter control on conditions predisposing to hypothermia, such as diabetes mellitus, malnutrition, peripheral vascular disease, congestive heart failure, and infection.

## CONCLUSION

Hypothermia is a serious problem among the elderly due to their increased susceptibility to cold and to their altered physiologic responses to low temperatures. The aged are also subject to certain diseases and drugs that further predispose them to hypothermia and heighten the mortality associated with hypothermia. In any elderly individual, careful evaluation for cardiovascular, renal, and endocrine diseases as well as nutritional deficiency and sepsis must be undertaken when hypothermia is encountered. These entities tend to increase mortality associated with hypothermia in both young and old. Supportive care and appropriate rewarming must be accompanied by aggressive treatment of these concomitant conditions.

### References


1. Stine RJ: Accidental hypothermia. JACEP 6:413, 1977.
2. Reuler JB: Hypothermia: Pathophysiology, clinical settings, and management. Ann Intern Med 89:519, 1978.
3. Wollner L, Spalding JMK: Accidental hypothermia in the elderly. *In* Brocklehurst JC (ed.): Textbook of Geriatric Medicine and Gerontology. 2nd ed. Edinburgh, Churchill Livingstone, 1978, pp. 246–253.
4. Petersdorf RG: Hypothermia. Arch Intern Med 139:399, 1979.
5. Edwards RJ Jr: Accidental hypothermia. JACEP 6:426, 1977.
6. Besdine RW: Accidental hypothermia: The body's energy crisis. Geriatrics 34:51, 1979.
7. Thompson MK: The care of the older patient in winter. Practitioner 223:787, 1979.
8. Lloyd EL: Treatment of accidental hypothermia. Br Med J 1:413, 1979.
9. Davidson M, Grant E: Accidental hypothermia. A community hospital perspective. Postgrad Med 70:42, 1981.
10. Johnson LA: Accidental hypothermia: Peritoneal dialysis. JACEP 6:556, 1977.
11. Collins KJ, Dore C, Exton-Smith AN, et al: Accidental hypothermia and impaired temperature homeostasis in the elderly. Br Med J 1:353, 1977.
12. Collins KJ, Exton-Smith AN, Dore C: Urban hypothermia: Preferred temperature and thermal perception in old age. Br Med J 282:175, 1981.
13. Bristow G, Smith R, Lee J, et al: Resuscitation from cardiopulmonary arrest during accidental hypothermia due to exhaustion and exposure. Can Med J 117:247, 1977.
14. Horvath SM, Radcliff CE, Hutt BK, Spurr GB: Metabolic responses of old people to a cold environment. J Appl Physiol 8:145, 1955.
15. Goldman A, Exton-Smith AN, Francis G, O'Brien A: Report on a pilot study of low temperatures in old people admitted to hospitals. J R Coll Physicians Lond 11:291, 1977.
16. Williams RG, Schocken DD, Morey M, Koisch FP:

Medical aspects of competitive distance running. Postgrad Med 70:41, 1981.
17. Gale EAM, Tattersall RB: Hypothermia: A complication of diabetic ketoacidosis. Br Med J 2:1387, 1978.
18. Andrew PJ, Parker RS: Treating accidental hypothermia. Br Med J 2:1641, 1978.
19. Weyman AE, Greenbaum DM, Grace WI: Accidental hypothermia in an alcoholic population. Am J Med 56:13, 1974.
20. Fox RH, Woodward PM, Exton-Smith AN, et al: Body temperatures in the elderly: A national study of physiological, social, and environmental conditions. Br Med J 1:200, 1973.
21. Salvosa CB, Payne PR, Wheeler BF: Environmental conditions and body temperatures of elderly women living alone or in local authority homes. Br Med J 4:656, 1971.
22. Society and Medical Officers of Health. A pilot survey into the occurrence of hypothermia in elderly people living at home. Public Health 82:223, 1968.
23. Whittle JL, Bates JH: Thermoregulatory failure secondary to acute illness: Complications and treatment. Arch Intern Med 139:418, 1979.
24. Vaughan MS, Vaughan RW, Cork RC: Postoperative hypothermia in adults: Relationship of age, anesthesia, and shivering to rewarming. Anesth Analg 60:746, 1981.
25. MacLean D, Griffiths PD, Browning MC: Metabolic aspects of spontaneous rewarming in accidental hypothermia and hypothermic myxedema. Quart J Med 43:371, 1974.
26. Coni KK: Deep posterior tibial compartmental syndrome after accidental hypothermia in an elderly hypothyroid patient. A Am Geriatr Soc 29:77, 1981.
27. Lovel TWI: Myxedema coma. Lancet 1:823, 1962.
28. Stoner HB, Frayn KN, Little RA, et al: Metabolic aspects of hypothermia in the elderly. Clin Sci 59:19, 1980.
29. MacLean D, Murison J, Griffiths PD: Acute pancreatitis and diabetic ketoacidosis in accidental hypothermia and hypothermic myxedema. Br Med J 4:757–761, 1973.
30. Milner JC: Hypothermia. Ann Intern Med 89:565, 1978.
31. Harvey GR: Physiologic changes encountered in hypothermia. Proc R Soc Lond 66:1053, 1973.
32. Brewin EG: Physiology of hypothermia. Int Anesthesiol Clin 2:803, 1964.
33. Fitzgerald FT, Jessop C: Accidental hypothermia: A report of 22 cases and review of the literature. Adv Intern Med 27:128, 1982.
34. Black PR, Van Devanter S, Cohn LH: Effects of hypothermia on systemic and organ system metabolism and function. J Surg Res 20:49, 1976.
35. Schwab RH, Lewis DW, Killough JH, Templeton JY: Electrocardiographic changes in rapidly induced deep hypothermia. Am J Med 248:290, 1964.
36. Wollner L: Accidental hypothermia and temperature regulation in the elderly. Gerontol Clin 9:347, 1967.
37. Thompson R, Rich J, Chmelik F: Evolutionary changes in the electrocardiogram of severe progressive hypothermia. J Electrocardiol 10:67, 1977.
38. Sereda WM: Treatment of hypothermia. Can Med Assoc J 112:931, 1975.
39. Welton DE, Mattox KL, Miller RR, Petmecky FF: Treatment of profound hypothermia. JAMA 240: 2291, 1978.
40. Ledingham IM, Mone JG: Accidental hypothermia. Lancet 1:391, 1978.
41. Reuler JB, Parker RA: Peritoneal dialysis in the management of hypothermia. JAMA 240:2289, 1978.
42. Editorial: Treating accidental hypothermia. Br Med J 2:1383, 1978.
43. Levy LA: Severe hypophosphatemia as a complication of the treatment of hypothermia. Arch Intern Med 40:128, 1980.
44. Miller JW, Danzl DF, Thomas DM: Urban accidental hypothermia: 135 cases. Ann Emerg Med 9:456, 1980.
45. Lloyd EL: Accidental hypothermia treated by central rewarming through the airway. Br J Anaesth 45:41, 1973.
46. Brown CG: Accidental hypothermia. Postgrad Med 71:39, 1982.
47. Editorial: Treating accidental hypothermia. Lancet 1:701, 1978.
48. Wickstrom P, Ruiz B, Lilja GP, et al: Accidental hypothermia. Core rewarming with partial bypass. Am J Surg 131: 622, 1976.
49. Truscott DG, Witmer BF, Clein LJ: Accidental profound hypothermia. Successful resuscitation by core rewarming and assisted circulation. Arch Surg 106:216, 1973.
50. Tolman KG, Cohen A: Accidental hypothermia. Can Med Assoc J 103:1357, 1970.
51. Ledingham IM, Mone JG: Treatment of accidental hypothermia: A prospective study. Br Med J 1:1102, 1980.
52. Meriwether WD, Goodman RM: Severe accidental hypothermia with survival after rapid rewarming. Am J Med 52:505, 1972.
53. Frank DH, Robson MC: Accidental hypothermia treated without mortality. Surg Gynecol Obstet 151:379, 1980.
54. Gregory RT, Doolittle WH: Accidental hypothermia. Alaska Med 15:48, 1973.
55. MacMillan AL, Corbett JL, Johnson RH, et al: Temperature regulation in survivors of accidental hypothermia of the eldery. Lancet 2:165, 1967.
56. Hayward JS, Steinman AM: Accidental hypothermia: An experimental study of inhalation rewarming. Aviat Space Environ Med 46:1236, 1975.
57. Grossheim RL: Hypothermia and frostbite treated with peritoneal dialysis. Alaska Med 15:53, 1973.
58. Soung LS, Swank L, Ing TS, et al: Treatment of accidental hypothermia with peritoneal dialysis. Can Med Assoc J 117:1415, 1977.
59. Johnson LA: Accidental hypothermia. Peritoneal dialysis. JACEP 6:556, 1977.
60. Davis FM, Judson JA: Warm peritoneal dialysis in the management of accidental hypothermia. New Zealand Med J 94:207, 1981.
61. Lee HA, Ames AC: Hemodialysis in severe barbiturate poisoning. Br Med J 1:1217, 1965.
62. Linton AL, Ledingham IM: Severe hypothermia with barbiturate intoxication. Lancet 1:24, 1966.
63. Editorial: Rewarming for accidental hypothermia. Lancet 1:251, 1978.
64. O'Keefe KM: Accidental hypothermia: A review of 62 cases. JACEP 6:491, 1977.
65. Hudson LD, Conn RD: Accidental hypothermia. Associated diagnoses and prognosis in a common problem. JAMA 227:37, 1974.
66. Altus P, Hickman JW, Pina I, Barry PP: Hypothermia in the sunny south. South Med J 73:1491, 1980.
67. Vaisrub S: Accidental hypothermia in the elderly. JAMA 239:1888, 1978.
68. Mills GL: Accidental hypothermia in the elderly. Br J Hosp Med 10:691, 1973.

69. Goldman A, Exton-Smith AN, Francis G, O'Brien A: Report on a pilot study of low temperatures in old people admitted to hospital. J R Coll Phys Lond 11:291, 1977.
70. Exton-Smith AN: Accidental hypothermia. Br Med J 4:727, 1973.
71. Southwick FS, Dalgish PH Jr: Recovery after prolonged asystolic cardiac arrest in profound hypothermia. JAMA 243:1250, 1980.
72. Mills WJ Jr: Accidental hypothermia: Management approach. Alaska Med 22:9, 1980.
73. Cardon TC Jr: Saving the hypothermic patient. JAMA 240:2761, 1978.
74. Rango N: Old and cold: Hypothermia in the elderly. Geriatrics 35: 93, 1980.
75. Allen WH: Accidental hypothermia in Hertfordshire during the winters of 1966–67. Public Health 83:229, 1969.

# MEDICAL-SURGICAL DISORDERS

Chapter 29

# Cardiac Disease in the Elderly

Arthur J. Moss

Cardiac disease is the major cause of morbidity and mortality in the elderly. The older individual, in contrast with his or her younger brethren, has to contend with marked acceleration of the aging process as well as an increased probability of cardiac disease that is likely to significantly impair already compromised cardiac function. Nearly half of the population over 65 years of age has existing evidence of cardiac disease as manifest by a prior myocardial infarction, active angina, symptoms or signs of congestive heart failure, or electrocardiographic abnormalities.[1] The clinician caring for elderly patients is continuously challenged because it is important for him or her to differentiate between the decline that normally occurs with age and problems resulting from specific cardiac disease.

In the first portion of this chapter, background information will be provided concerning the biochemical, physiologic, and anatomic changes that occur in the heart with age. Specific cardiac diseases in the elderly will be highlighted, and the differential diagnosis of the common clinical syndromes associated with cardiac dysfunction will be emphasized. The past decade has seen the extensive application of noninvasive testing in the outpatient evaluation of patients with cardiac disorders, and the usefulness of these new techniques, as they apply to the geriatric cardiac patient, are presented. Finally, the rapid advances in and the current status of cardiac therapeutics in terms of drugs, pacemakers, surgery, and angioplasty will be described, since these modalities of treatment have contributed significantly to the improved well-being of the geriatric cardiac patient.

## CHANGES IN THE HEART WITH AGE

An understanding of the alterations that occur in the anatomy, biochemistry, and physiology of the aging heart is clinically important if one is to develop a rational schema for the diagnosis and management of cardiac disease in the elderly. Investigations of intact hearts from senescent animals and findings of age-associated changes in cardiac performance provide useful information for understanding the setting of geriatric heart disease. A comprehensive review of this subject is provided in a monograph by Weisfeldt.[2] Recent evidence summarized by Lakatta and coworkers[37,51] suggests caution in interpreting these putatively age-associated decreases in cardiac performance, since they may reflect age-related diseases rather than the aging process per se (Editor's Note).

### Anatomic Changes

Progressive changes occur in the fibrous skeleton and the valves of the heart with age.[3] In both of these structures, the collagen tissue becomes more sclerotic and there is a progressive deposition of calcium in the so-called wear-and-tear areas of the heart. Nodular thickenings occur on the closure lines of the valves, predominantly in the mitral and aortic leaflets, and degenerative changes develop at the sites of maximum cusp movement, leading to increased valvular stiffness. These changes in the aortic valve, commonly referred to as aortic valve sclerosis, explain the systolic ejection murmur frequently heard in the elderly. In both the aortic and the mitral valves, minor degrees of mucoid degeneration occur with age, and these changes may be associated with insufficiency murmurs.

Calcification of the cardiac skeleton, especially the mitral annulus, may be associated with mitral insufficiency and atrioventricular conduction abnormalities. The latter results from compromise of the bundle of His and related structures. Histologic changes are also evident in the sinoatrial and atrioventricular nodes, with an age-associated reduction in the number of pacemaker cells and an increase in the amount of fibrous tissue and fat.[4] There is a loss of Purkinje fibers in the bundle of His and in the major left and right bundles, with a lesser degree of loss in the distal branches.

The myocardium also undergoes age-related changes, and a yellow-brown pigment called lipofuscin accumulates in the aging myocardial fibers. The functional significance of this pigment deposition is unclear. Current speculation suggests that lipofuscin deposition may be related to quantitative changes in oxidative enzyme activity.

These anatomic and histologic changes with age explain the increased propensity of the elderly to degenerative valvular and myocardial diseases, varying degrees of heart block, and sinus node dysfunction. In some elderly individuals, the degenerative changes may progress rapidly over the course of a few years, resulting in functionally significant disease.

## *Biochemical and Biophysical Changes*

The heart is dependent on oxidative metabolism, and it is unlikely that any major disturbance in these energy production pathways can be tolerated by the organism. Several investigators using in vitro techniques have documented modest decreases in cardiocellular mitochondrial enzyme activities involving fatty acid oxidation, the tricarboxylate cycle, and oxidative phosphorylation in the aging heart.[5] This diminution is explained in part by a reduction in the number of mitochondria per unit volume as well as a shift of specific activity away from active fatty acid oxidation. Reduction in these energy related pathways may well contribute to diminished functional performance in the aging heart.

Calcium ion uptake and release by the sarcoplasmic reticulum within the myocardial cell is central to the cardiac contractile process. When the myocardial cell is excited, calcium enters the cell through voltage-dependent channels in the myocellular membrane and is simultaneously released from the sarcoplasmic reticulum, thereby increasing the concentration of intracellular free calcium ions to a critical level. This calcium binds with the troponin C molecule on the actin filament, permitting actin-myosin cross-bridging, with subsequent sarcomere shortening. Re-uptake of calcium by the sarcoplasmic reticulum and efflux of calcium from the cell terminates contraction and promotes sarcomere relaxation. The aged heart contracts and relaxes more slowly than the younger heart. Recent studies from the National Institute of Aging indicate that the reduction in the rate of these time-related phenomena is associated with a decrease in the rate of calcium release and removal by the sarcoplasmic reticulum.[6] In any event, it is clear that older patients could be quite susceptible to the cardiodepressant effects of the newer calcium antagonists such as verapamil and diltiazem.

Various electrophysiologic characteristics of the myocellular action potential, including the level of the resting membrane potential, the rate of rise of the action potential (dV/dt), the plateau duration, the repolarization time, and the effective refractory period, are similar in hearts from adult and senescent animals.[6] In contrast, the rate of spontaneous automatic firing of pacemaker cells in the sinus node and in the Purkinje network of the ventricles declines with age.[7] This decreased automaticity results primarily from a reduction in the rate of phase 4 depolarization in pacemaker cells—an active energy-requiring process. Reduced pacemaker automaticity in the senescent heart would explain the increased occurrence of sinus node dysfunction in the elderly and the enhanced susceptibility of these patients to the bradycardic effects of antiarrhythmic agents. In addition, conduction is slowed through nodal tissue, such as the atrioventricular node, possibly from altered phase 4 depolarization in pacemaker cells located in the junctional regions of nodal tissue. Also, the conduction velocity of the electric impulse is diminished in Purkinje fibers of senescent hearts.[8]

One of the most striking changes that occur in the heart with advancing age is a reduction in the response to stress. Lakatta[9] investigated adrenergic-mediated stress in the aged heart of animals and man and found an age-related decline in the postsynaptic response to beta-adrenergic stimulation. The findings suggested a reduction in either the number or the function of myocardial adrenergic receptors in older hearts. Other investigators have shown that isolated muscle from older animals has fewer adrenergic receptors than muscle from younger animals. In this regard, recent studies have suggested a decline in the number of digitalis-associated myocardial receptors with age, a finding that may explain the reduced inotropic effect of digitalis in the aged. The reduction in the number or function of adrenergic and digitalis receptors with age may be part of a universal characteristic of the aging process and probably applies to a wide spectrum of physiologic and pharmacologic receptors located throughout the body. The net result would be a diminished effectiveness of agonists such as catecholamines and an enhanced sensitivity to antagonists such as beta-blockers and calcium channel blockers in the elderly individual.

### *Physiologic Changes*

There is a slight but definite decline in the average resting heart rate with age.[4] At age 30, the resting heart rate averages 76 beats per minute, with a reduction of about 4 beats per decade over the course of the subsequent 50 years. The "intrinsic heart rate" (the heart rate after pharmacologic denervation by simultaneous cholinergic and adrenergic blockade) also diminishes with age but to a lesser degree than the resting heart rate. These observations suggest an age-associated reduction in vagal innervation to the heart. The maximum heart rate during exercise diminishes markedly with age.[4] The decline in maximum heart rate is not due to reduced sympathetic activity, since plasma norepinephrine increases with age, particularly with exercise.[10] Rather, the findings suggest either a reduction in receptors, or sinus node pacemaker cells, or both.

Atrial and ventricular ectopic beats occur more frequently in those in the older than the younger age group, even in the absence of demonstrable organic heart disease. Several investigators have carried out cross-sectional studies using 24-hour Holter electrocardiogram (ECG) recordings in the evaluation of the frequency and complexity of cardiac arrhythmias in different age groups. Fleg and Kennedy[11] reported the 24-hour Holter ECG findings in 98 elderly (aged 60 to 85 years) healthy subjects. Although the sample size was small, the study indicated that a healthy population of elderly subjects has a substantial prevalence of atrial and ventricular ectopic beats. These findings argue for restraint in the treatment of asymptomatic ectopic beats in older patients.

Cardiac output progressively declines with age, especially at rest in the recumbent position. Furthermore, longitudinal studies of aging and studies comparing cardiovascular function in younger and older healthy subjects have demonstrated decreases in *maximum* stroke volume, cardiac output, and oxygen uptake in older individuals in response to exercise. A recent study by Port and associates[12] evaluated the effects of age on radionuclide left ventricular ejection fraction at rest and during upright bicycle exercise. Age did not influence left ventricular function at rest, but the ejection fraction was significantly reduced during exercise in subjects over age 60. Wall motion abnormalities during exercise were seen with increasing frequency in older subjects, and these changes were not associated with abnormalities in end-diastolic volume or blood pressure.

The reduction in activity-related left ventricular function with age may be due to one of four mechanisms: (1) a depression of the Frank-Starling relationship between stroke work and end-diastolic fiber length (heterometric autoregulation); (2) increased afterload in terms augmented peripheral vascular resistance; (3) decreased contractility due to disease; and (4) decreased contractility due to aging. As pointed out earlier, the impaired release and uptake of calcium by sarcoplasmic reticulum and the diminished number of adrenergic cardiac receptors in the senescent heart provide a reasonable explanation for the observed reduction in myocardial contractility with age.

## HEART DISEASE

Heart disease in the aged patient includes the usual spectrum of cardiac lesions observed in the younger patient as well as less commonly recognized disorders somewhat specific to the elderly. This categorization is clinically useful, and the various cardiac disease entities are presented in this format (Table 29 – 1). It should be emphasized that the principal manifestations of cardiac disease include alterations in the level of consciousness; disorders of cardiac rhythm; low cardiac output states, with or without overt congestive heart failure (CHF); and ischemic-type cardiac pain. These clinical syndromes are highlighted in the subsequent section.

### *Cardiac Disease Commonly Occurring in the Elderly*

#### Coronary Heart Disease

Cardiovascular disease is the most common cause of death in the elderly, and the vast majority of these deaths are due to coronary artery

**Table 29-1.** CLASSIFICATION OF CARDIAC DISEASE IN THE ELDERLY

| **Commonly Occurring Cardiac Diseases** |
|---|
| Coronary heart disease |
| Hypertensive heart disease |
| Valvular heart disease |
| Rheumatic valve disease |
| Congenital bicuspid aortic stenosis |
| Nonrheumatic aortic insufficiency |
| Cardiomyopathy |
| Miscellaneous cardiac disease |
| Atrial septal defect |
| Pulmonary heart disease |
| Pericarditis |
| Infective endocarditis |
| **Cardiac Diseases Somewhat Specific to the Elderly** |
| Calcific degenerative disorders |
| Mitral annular disease |
| Aortic valvular sclerosis |
| Sclerodegenerative disease of the conducting system |
| Mucoid degeneration of the cardiac valves |
| Senile cardiac amyloidosis |

disease from arrhythmias or myocardial failure. Although the pathology of ischemic heart disease is similar in those over and under age 65, certain features are particularly associated with older patients. Pomerance[13] has pointed out that large fibrous infarcts in patients with no history even suggestive of past coronary events are rarely seen except in the elderly. With an acute myocardial infarction elderly patients have a fourfold increased mortality when compared with younger patients. Advanced age is associated with a disproportionately high in-hospital mortality rate, even in the so called "good-risk" myocardial infarction patient. Latting and Silverman[14] reported that the major causes of death in hospitalized patients aged 70 years and older with acute myocardial infarction were shock and cardiac rupture.[14] This high incidence of myocardial rupture in the elderly may be due to chronic pathologic changes that affect the myocardium.

The symptom presentation of coronary heart disease in the elderly may be quite atypical. Classic anginal chest pain is the exception rather than the rule. Exertional angina may present with dyspnea, acute fatigue, or atypical discomfort. The symptoms resulting from myocardial ischemia may mimic other common problems in the elderly. Discomfort located in the back, shoulders, elbows, or hands may suggest arthritis. Epigastric discomfort and burning, particularly if they come on at night, are often misdiagnosed as peptic ulcer disease. Postprandial discomfort is frequently ascribed to a coexisting hiatus hernia. From my own clinical experience, a hiatus hernia rarely causes troublesome postprandial symptoms, and this condition is vastly overdiagnosed. The resulting error has significantly compromised the clinical identification and management of patients with serious ischemic heart disease.

Although the diagnosis of angina is more difficult in the elderly, the clinical significance of nocturnal, decubitus, postprandial, or crescendo angina is similar to that in younger patients. These patterns of angina are frequently associated with severe three vessel coronary disease and a high likelihood for life-threatening complications.

Even in the presence of acute myocardial infarction, the symptom presentation in the elderly is more frequently atypical than classic (Table 29-2). Chest pain is rarely perceived as being severe, and the older patient is more likely to complain of dyspnea than chest discomfort. Pulmonary edema in the absence of chest pain is a rather common presentation of myocardial infarction in patients over age 70 years. Pathy[15] has pointed out that syncope, cerebral vascular accidents, and peripheral vascular occlusions are reasonably common presentations of acute coronary disease in the elderly. These complications are usually secondary to an arrhythmia, hypotension, or an embolus complicating the myocardial infarction.

## Hypertensive Heart Disease

As pointed out in the Framingham study,[16] hypertension is the leading cause of CHF in all

**Table 29-2.** SYMPTOM PRESENTATION OF ACUTE MYOCARDIAL INFARCTION IN THE ELDERLY*

| **Frequent Presenting Clinical Features** |
|---|
| Sudden dyspnea |
| Exacerbation of heart failure |
| Typical substernal chest discomfort |
| Indigestion |
| Acute confusion |
| **Less Frequent But More Misleading Presenting Features** |
| Stroke |
| Syncope |
| Vertigo, lightheadedness, or faintness |
| Peripheral vascular occlusion |
| Palpitations |
| Renal failure |
| Pulmonary embolus |

* Adapted from Pathy MS: Clinical presentation of myocardial infarction in the elderly. Br Heart J 29:190, 1967.

age groups, but especially in the elderly. Hypertensive heart disease represents one of the end-organ effects of chronic sustained blood pressure elevation. The patient with hypertension may remain asymptomatic for many years, and the ravages of the disorder in terms of cerebral, retinal, renal, vascular, and cardiac abnormalities may not become evident until the individual passes retirement age. In the early stages, concentric left ventricular hypertrophy develops, with a progressive decrease in left ventricular diastolic compliance. The left ventricular end-diastolic pressure may be minimally increased at rest, but elevates significantly with exercise, resulting in exertional dyspnea. At this phase, the heart may be of normal size with only slight chamber dilation, the radionuclide ejection fraction is probably within the normal range, and the ECG is likely to show early voltage changes of left ventricular hypertrophy. The rate of subsequent progression of hypertensive heart disease is extremely variable from one individual to another. A multiplicity of factors, including the degree of hypertension, the chronicity of the blood pressure elevation, the size and patency of the nutritive coronary vessels, the intrinsic sensitivity of the myocardium to circulating catecholamines, and other yet to be identified factors, determines the subsequent clinical course. Frequently, progressive myocardial damage ensues with secondary cardiomegaly, chamber dilation, congestive heart failure, and an ischemic strain pattern on ECG. The blood pressure normalizes during this later congestive phase in association with a falling cardiac output. Left bundle branch block, bifascicular and trifascicular heart block, ventricular irritability, and sinus node dysfunction may develop and further compound an already tenuous cardiac state. The older members of the population with a long-standing history of chronic hypertension are at high risk for developing this compromised cardiac state, especially when other compensatory mechanisms are also deteriorating.

## Valvular Heart Disease

The common valvular heart disorders in the aged include acquired rheumatic valve disease, congenital bicuspid aortic stenosis, and nonrheumatic aortic insufficiency. Rheumatic heart disease is generally acquired during childhood and adolescence, and severe multivalvular disease usually results from multiple episodes of rheumatic fever. The mitral valve is more frequently involved than the aortic, and survival to old age with a single valve lesion is not unusual. As emphasized by Selzer and Pasternak,[17] the basic lesion of rheumatic heart disease is mitral stenosis. Mitral stenosis in the aged is frequently associated with atrial fibrillation, moderate degrees of secondary pulmonary hypertension, heavy valve calcification, and a tendency to systemic emboli. The classic physical findings of a rumbling diastolic murmur, an opening snap, accentuated first heart sound ($S_1$), and a palpable right ventricular impulse may be difficult to identify in the elderly due to alterations in the thoracic cage from emphysema, kyphosis, and similar degenerative structural conditions. Since rheumatic mitral stenosis is a relatively uncommon disorder in older patients, one should be alert to certain clues that provide a high index of suspicion. Dyspnea and fatigue in association with CHF, atrial fibrillation, and relative right ventricular preponderance on the ECG are such findings, and the physician should request a chest x-ray and an echocardiogram. The echocardiogram is an extremely sensitive and specific test not only for ascertaining the diagnosis of mitral stenosis but also for providing a crude estimation of the severity of the lesion and the degree of left atrial and right ventricular enlargement. On rare occasions, the echocardiogram may reveal an unanticipated atrial myxoma, which can mimic the clinical picture of mitral stenosis.

Aortic stenosis has only a few causes, and the clinical picture of this disorder in the elderly is remarkably similar regardless of the specific etiology. The orifice area of the aortic valve is reduced, the valve is calcified, and the cusp commissures are fused. *Congenital* aortic stenosis is associated with a bicuspid valve, whereas *rheumatic* aortic stenosis is engrafted on a normal tricuspid valve. As in younger patients with aortic stenosis, the occurrence of anginal chest pain, effort dyspnea, or exertional syncope has ominous implications because these symptoms develop only in the setting of a critical reduction in the aortic valve area. The development of CHF is a late manifestation of the disease, and it reflects the secondary development of severe myocardial dysfunction. The diagnosis of aortic stenosis is usually suggested by a harsh systolic ejection murmur that is loudest in the primary aortic area, with radiation to the neck. The intensity of the heart murmur bears a poor relationship to the severity of the stenosis. Rather, the severity of the lesion can be evaluated better by the quality of the carotid pulse, the intensity of the aortic second sound ($S_{2A}$), and the prominence of the left ventricular impulse.

In patients with critically significant aortic stenosis, the carotid pulse is slow rising, $S_{2A}$ is diminished to absent, and the left ventricular impulse has a sustained quality when the patient is examined in the left lateral decubitus position. Some of these signs may be absent in the elderly patient with severe aortic stenosis as a result of arteriosclerosis of the large vessels, accentuation of the pulmonary second sound ($S_{2P}$), and emphysematous enlargement of the thoracic cage. The ECG invariably shows left ventricular hypertrophy, with a "strain" pattern of ST and T wave changes. The chest x-ray usually reveals significant aortic valve calcification, often in association with dilatation of the ascending aorta and a convex hypertrophic configuration to the left heart border. The echocardiogram is very useful in evaluating the presence and severity of the aortic valve lesion as well as the degree of secondary left ventricular hypertrophy. The clinical course of patients with aortic stenosis is usually stable for extended periods of time. The decline is rapid once symptoms develop, and this is when cardiac catheterization is indicated. The decision-making process is primarily concerned with the timing of the operation. Surgical intervention is indicated when cardiac symptoms develop and hemodynamic studies confirm critical aortic stenosis with a valvular gradient of more than 50 mm Hg or a calculated valve area of less than 0.8 $cm^2$.

In contrast to aortic stenosis, aortic insufficiency may be due to any one of several causes, and the disorder occurs in either a chronic or acute form. The chronic type of aortic insufficiency is usually caused by deformity of the leaflets, usually as a result of rheumatic scarring, but congenital and postendocarditic conditions may produce a similar hemodynamic abnormality. Less commonly, aortic insufficiency may result from dilation of the aortic annulus, such as might occur with syphilitic aortitis, Marfan's syndrome, or rheumatoid spondylitis. Chronic aortic insufficiency, if not punctuated by episodes of bacterial endocarditis, is surprisingly well tolerated, and many patients with this disorder survive into old age. However, the clinical course is inexorably progressive, with the rate of decline determined by the magnitude of the volume overload on the left ventricle and the degree of myocardial impairment. Dyspnea and fatigue are the early symptoms, and the full-blown picture of CHF develops late in the clinical course, usually in association with the occurrence of atrial fibrillation. Atypical chest pain is common, and anginal pain may be due to relative coronary insufficiency from the low aortic diastolic pressure or from coexisting intrinsic coronary artery disease.

The clinical diagnosis of aortic insufficiency is not difficult because several prominent physical findings almost always coexist, and these findings also provide valuable information about the severity of the hemodynamic burden on the left ventricle. The major findings include a high-pitched diastolic murmur, which is best heard along the left sternal border with the patient in the sitting position; a prominent precordial rocking motion; bounding peripheral pulses of the water-hammer type; and a wide pulse pressure, with diastolic pressure below 70 mm Hg. Chest x-ray reveals enormous cardiomegaly, much greater than is seen with aortic stenosis, and significant left ventricular hypertrophy is invariably present on the ECG. The echocardiogram provides useful information about left ventricular chamber size, myocardial wall motion, the configuration of the aortic root, and qualitative data on the severity of the insufficiency. As in aortic stenosis, the timing for cardiac catheterization and surgical intervention is a matter of clinical judgment. Patients with these disorders should have concomitant follow-up with a cardiovascular specialist to assist in the decision-making process.

Acute aortic insufficiency is usually due to either bacterial endocarditis with valve perforation or acute aortic root dilation from aortic dissection. In both cases there is an abrupt volume overload on the left ventricle without the development of prior compensating mechanisms, and the underlying conditions require aggressive in-hospital management, generally culminating in high-risk surgical intervention.

### Cardiomyopathy

Disorders of cardiac muscle frequently develop in the older population, and a useful categorization of cardiomyopathy includes both the etiology and the type of functional abnormality. Alcoholic cardiomyopathy and hemochromatosis with cardiomyopathy are both treatable disorders and should be considered in every patient regardless of age who has unexplained cardiac muscle disease. The diagnosis of alcoholic cardiomyopathy is suggested from the history and is otherwise a diagnosis by exclusion. In contrast, the diagnosis of hemochromatosis is suggested by an unusual color to the skin, and the disorder is easily confirmed by serum iron and iron-binding capacity. In the vast majority of elderly patients with cardiomyopathy, the etiology is not uncovered and the patient is categorized as having an idiopathic cardiomyopathy. Goodwin[18] has functionally subdivided cardiomyopathy into congestive, restrictive, hypertrophic, and obliterative types. Most patients with cardiomyopathy present with a congestive picture characterized by dyspnea, fluid retention, cardiomegaly, and arrhythmias. The hypertrophic type is of special interest because there may be obstruction and the clinical presentation can be similar to that of valvular aortic stenosis. The condition is more common in the elderly than is generally appreciated.[19] In brief, hypertrophic obstructive cardiomyopathy (HOCM) is characterized by septal thickening out of proportion to that of the left ventricular free wall (asymmetric septal hypertrophy) and secondary narrowing of the left ventricular outflow tract. Patients with hypertrophic obstructive cardiomyopathy frequently present with angina, syncope, or palpitations. Clinical signs may include a very brisk upstroke to the carotid pulse, a prominent fourth heart sound, a reduplicated apical impulse, and a parasternal systolic ejection murmur that is accentuated by the Valsalva maneuver. The ECG may have deep Q waves in the inferior and apical leads from the septal hypertrophy as well as a left ventricular hypertrophy pattern. The echocardiogram is essential in the clinical confirmation of this disorder because it provides precise information about the magnitude of the asymmetric septal hypertrophy, the degree of outflow tract obstruction, and the presence of any abnormalities in the mitral valve support apparatus. Therapy with beta-blockers, which is diametrically opposite to that given for most other cardiomyopathies and aortic stenosis, may be associated with dramatic symptomatic improvement. Surgical resection of the muscular septum is rarely required in the elderly patient.

## Miscellaneous Cardiac Disease

Many patients with atrial septal defect who do not develop pulmonary hypertension survive into the retirement years. The clinical findings result from chronic volume overload of the right ventricle, with right ventricular hypertrophy and engorgement of the pulmonary vasculature. The flow rate through the pulmonary circulation is usually two to four times that of the systemic circulation, and the pulmonary pressure remains near normal levels unless pulmonary hypertension develops. The elderly survivors of this congenital condition have usually been spared the development of significant pulmonary hypertension. Patients with atrial septal defect may present with exertional dyspnea, fatigue, palpitations, or right-sided failure. The latter is often precipitated by the development of atrial fibrillation. Patients often have a history of repeated respiratory tract infections. On cardiac examination, one may find cardiomegaly, a hyperdynamic right ventricular impulse, a widely split and fixed second heart sound, and a moderately intense systolic ejection murmur, which is best heard in the pulmonic area. The ECG reveals complete or incomplete right bundle branch block and prominent atrial P waves if the patient is still in sinus rhythm; first-degree heart block is a common but not an invariable finding. The chest x-ray usually reveals the diagnosis, showing marked enlargement of the right heart chambers, the main pulmonary artery, and the peripheral arterial branches. The echocardiogram shows right ventricular enlargement and a loss of continuity of the atrial septum and thus further confirms the diagnosis. Patients with atrial septal defect frequently have concomitant mitral valve prolapse, which can also be identified by echocardiography. The differential diagnosis for the outpatient physician performing the examination includes rheumatic mitral valve disease with pulmonary hypertension, cardiomyopathy, and cor pulmonale complicating chronic lung disease. The definitive diagnosis requires confirmation by cardiac catheterization. In the absence of severe pulmonary hypertension, most 60- to 70-year-old patients with atrial septal defect would benefit from surgery. However, these older individuals are often reluctant to consider surgical intervention, and appropriate medical management can provide considerable stability and symptomatic improvement.

Pulmonary hypertension secondary to hypoxic chronic lung disease with right ventricular hypertrophy and congestive heart failure, i.e., cor pulmonale, is a difficult problem in all age groups, but especially in the elderly. Chronic hypoxia accentuates the pulmonary hypertension and causes secondary polycythemia. Complicating atrial tacharrhythmias are common and further compound the heart failure. The cause of chronic cor pulmonale is usually chronic bronchitis-emphysema, with obstructive airway disease. Other considerations in the older age group include the late secondary effects of thoracic deformities, such as kyphoscoliosis and hypoxic diffusion syndromes associated with diffuse pulmonary parenchymal disease, as seen with idiopathic pulmonary fibrosis or chronic sarcoidosis. Patients with cor pulmonale benefit dramatically from nearly continuous low flow oxygen because it lowers hypoxic-induced pulmonary hypertension. Oxygen therapy is the mainstay of treatment in this population, but caution must be exercised in relation to the flow rate of oxygen utilized if the patient is dependent on an hypoxic drive for ventilation. Decongestive measures and bronchodilator therapy must be tailored to the individual because these patients are extremely sensitive to the adverse side effects of most cardiac and pulmonary medications.

Acute pericarditis rarely occurs in the elderly, but effusive pericarditis is a more common disorder in the older population than is generally appreciated. Causes of significant effusions include metastatic cancer to the pericardium (usually from squamous carcinoma of the lung), tuberculosis, uremic pericarditis, bacterial infections in the compromised host, and viruses. The primary concern is the development of life-threatening pericardial tamponade. The diagnosis should be considered in the presence of the classic triad of pulsus paradoxus; Kussmaul's sign, with inspiratory ascent of the neck veins; and pulsatile neck veins. The last-named sign is due to the combination of a high venous filling pressure and a transient torrential inflow of blood across the open tricuspid valve, followed by an abrupt reduction of inflow from diminished right ventricular diastolic compliance resulting from the tense pericardial effusion. Echocardiography provides information about the presence and magnitude of the pericardial fluid, but not about the danger of impending tamponade. Tamponade may occur in association with either benign or malignant conditions, and prompt, aggressive intervention (needle aspiration and/or surgical drainage) is required. The decision-making process to intervene is dependent on a high index of suspicion, which results from the appearance of the triad of the aforementioned clinical findings.

### Infective Endocarditis

The clinical aspects of infective endocarditis have changed considerably over the past 20 years as a result of alterations in the susceptible population, earlier diagnosis and treatment, and an expanding armamentarium of antibiotics. Durack[20] has highlighted the following recent trends in infective endocarditis: (1) The median age of patients has increased; (2) there is an increased male to female ratio; (3) the proportion of acute cases has increased; (4) fewer patients develop the signs of advanced subacute bacterial endocarditis, such as Osler's nodes, Janeway lesions, or Roth's spots; (5) the proportion of cases due to streptococci has decreased; and (6) the number of cases caused by gram-negative organisms, fungi, and miscellaneous unusual microbes has increased. Endocarditis in the elderly has become more common, even though degenerative valvular disease seems to present a relatively low risk for infection. Since many of the elderly patients are edentulous, *Streptococcus viridans* is less frequently the offending organism in this age group than in younger patients. In contrast, elderly patients are more likely to have urologic problems, and enterococcal infection of the valves has become more prevalent. The prosthetic valves are particularly vulnerable to infection, especially with organisms of low virulence such as *Staphylococcus epidermidis.* Pre-existing mitral or aortic valve disease is no longer a prerequisite for endocarditis. As in the past, the triad of fever, anemia, and a heart murmur are the findings that should raise the clinical suspicion of endocarditis. Elderly patients may be afebrile, and if a patient with recent clinical deterioration has unexplained anemia and a heart murmur, endocarditis should be considered. Because of the protean manifestations of this disorder, there are a wide range of possibilities in the differential diagnosis. Echocardiography has been used to detect valvular vegetations, and when findings are positive, this method is helpful. It should be emphasized that a negative finding does not exclude endocarditis as the diagnosis. Isolation of an organism from blood cultures is an essential step in establishing the diagnosis, and blood should be drawn for both aerobic and anerobic cultures. The choice of antibiotic should be dictated by the sensitivity of the cultured organism.

Within the context of endocarditis, the clinician providing outpatient care for the elderly has two responsibilities: (1) to prevent endocarditis through appropriate prophylaxis; and (2) to diagnose infective endocarditis early so that complications can be avoided by prompt treatment. Prophylaxis begins with identification of the patient at risk, requires appropriate patient education, and culminates in patient compliance with an up-to-date preventive regimen. As pointed out by Durack,[20] common errors in endocarditic prophylaxis for dental or genitourinary procedures include starting antibiotics too early (they should be started one hour before the procedure), continuing antibiotics too long (therapy needs to be rendered only for 2 days), using inappropriately low antibiotic doses, failing to cover minor procedures, not appreciating the increased risk posed by prosthetic valves (more vigorous therapy is required), and confusing prevention of rheumatic fever (long-term, low dose of antibiotics) with prevention of endocarditis (short-term, high dose of antibiotics). For specific antibiotic guidelines for prophylaxis of endocarditis, the clinician is referred to recommendations published in the *Medical Letter*[21] and by the American Heart Association.[22]

## *Cardiac Disorders Somewhat Specific to the Elderly*

Pomerance[23] categorized the pathologic cardiac findings in the aged and was the first to emphasize a spectrum of findings that was unique to the elderly. In addition, she pointed out that heart failure in the geriatric patient is often associated with two or more pathologic processes, e.g., coronary heart disease and calcific degenerative disease.

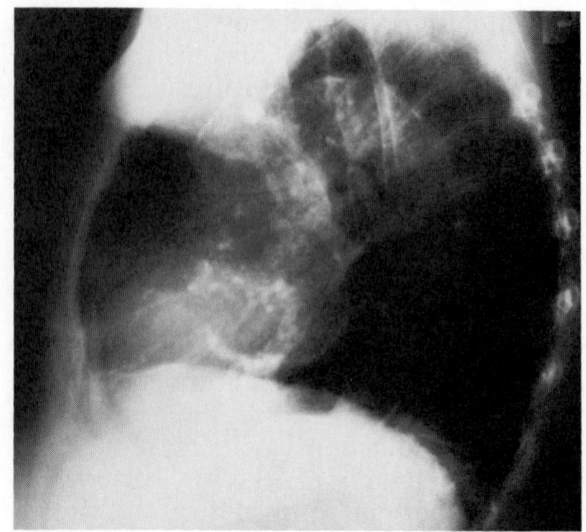

**Figure 29-1.** Lateral chest x-ray that reveals the characteristic J-shaped calcification involving the mitral anulus. This calcific degeneration of the fibrous skeleton of the heart occurs only in the elderly and can produce mitral insufficiency and atrioventricular conduction defects.

### Calcific Degenerative Disease

Calcific degenerative changes involving various cardiac structures frequently occur in the aged. The two most common anatomic sites in which these changes develop are the fibrous skeleton of the heart and the fibrous portion of the aortic cusps. In their milder forms, these degenerative conditions produce minimal functional abnormality, but when the degenerative process is extensive, hemodynamic and electrical dysfunction may dominate the clinical picture.

The mitral annulus and the supporting structures of the cardiac skeleton become progressively involved in a degenerative process that is limited to the elderly population. Calcium deposition reduces normal annular movement during systole, thereby contributing to various degrees of mitral insufficiency. In its full-blown picture, the development of massive calcification of the mitral annulus is associated with severe mitral regurgitation; involvement of the atrioventricular conduction system occurs with the development of heart block (Lev's disease).[24] This degenerative condition is more frequently observed in females than in males and is especially common in patients with diabetes mellitus and a history of hypertension. The diagnosis is suggested by a somewhat harsh systolic murmur at the apex in association with some degree of heart block. The disorder is substantiated either by the presence of a J-shaped calcification on lateral chest x-ray (Fig. 29-1) or prominent reflectivity in the mitral annular region on echocardiogram. These patients are at increased risk for developing complete heart block, and they frequently present with a history of syncope. Pacemaker therapy is the treatment of choice for this type of heart block.

The other degenerative condition frequently encountered in the elderly is sclerosis and calcification of the fibrous portion of the aortic cusp, with variable reduction in cusp morbidity. In most cases the degree of distortion resulting from cusp calcification is mild, and the predominant effect is a moderately intense, aortic systolic ejection murmur. Aortic valve sclerosis generally remains an innocuous condition without adverse hemodynamic effects. Occasionally, the valvular calcification becomes quite intensive, with immobilization of the cusps and functionally significant aortic stenosis similar to that seen with rheumatic aortic stenosis or congenital biscuspid aortic valve disease. In such cases, the clinical and hemodynamic findings are similar to those described previously in the section on valvular aortic stenosis.

### Sclerodegenerative Disease of the Conducting System

Lenegre's disease is a sclerodegenerative disorder of obscure origin that involves the His-Purkinje conducting system of the heart.[25] This disorder is one of the most common causes of right bundle branch block and left anterior hemiblock (bifascicular block) in older patients. The natural history of this disease is a slow progression to complete heart block over several years. Patients with this condition frequently have a history of transient syncope, but when examined after an episode, the only abnormality is the electrocardiographic finding of bifascicular block. Several syncopal episodes may occur before sustained complete heart block ensues. Early appreciation of the likelihood of Lenegre's disease following the first syncopal episode permits initiation of pacemaker therapy to prevent subsequent episodes, and it is hoped, to avoid syncope-induced injury, such as a fractured hip. Lenegre's disease is a "first cousin" to Lev's disease. As pointed out in the prior section, Lev's disease is caused by a calcific degenerative process of the fibrous skeleton, with invasion of the major conducting fascicles from without, whereas Lenegre's disease involves intrinsic degeneration of the His-Purkinje network. The clinical courses of Lenegre's and Lev's disease are remarkably similar.

### Mucoid Degeneration of the Cardiac Valves

Primary mucoid degeneration of the cardiac valves, but principally the mitral and aortic valves, varies greatly in severity. This disorder may occur at any age, but it is more severely manifest in the elderly. The pathologic process involves the central fibrous portion of either the mitral or aortic valve, or rarely both valves. Mucoid degeneration with myxomatous change in the ground substance of the valves produces leaflet enlargement, with redundancy and eventual prolapse. In all probability, the process evolves slowly over a long period of time. The cause of this condition is not known, but the normal aging process is probably a contributing factor. Some investigators believe that this disorder in the elderly simply represents an exaggeration and progression of the common mitral valve prolapse (floppy mitral valve) condition seen in healthy young adults. In the elderly, the mucoid degeneration may produce significant mitral or aortic insufficiency. In addition, disruption of the mitral valve support apparatus secondary to chordal rupture and dilation of the aortic root may occur with their associated compounding problems.

With mitral valve prolapse, the physical findings consist of an apical mid-to-late systolic murmur and a non-ejection click caused by systolic prolapse of the valve. If aortic insufficiency develops with involvement of the aortic valve, the volume of regurgitation is often quite massive, with rapid clinical deterioration. In such cases, the murmur of aortic insufficiency is usually full-length throughout diastole, with an Austin Flint presystolic rumble at the apex if the regurgitant jet impacts on the anterior leaflet of the mitral valve. The echocardiogram provides definitive evaluation of the valvular prolapse.

The physician caring for elderly patients with valvular prolapse should be alert to disease progression with resulting massive valvular insufficiency, infective endocarditis, cerebral emboli from valvular thrombi, and complex arrhythmias. Such complications may develop suddenly, with rapid clinical deterioration in a previously stable patient.

### Senile Cardiac Amyloidosis

The deposition of amyloid within the myocardium and its associated vessels is a distinctive process in individuals over age 65. The pathologic distribution and the immunologic characteristics of senile cardiac amyloidosis are different from those of primary systemic amyloidosis and secondary amyloidosis. Pomerance[26] found fine atrial deposits of amyloid in 50 per cent of elderly patients at autopsy, with ventricular involvement in 16.5 per cent. The occurrence of this disorder increases sharply with age. Macroscopically, there is often nothing to suggest cardiac amyloidosis. The large, firm, waxy hearts resulting from primary amyloidosis do not occur in the senile form. Rather, nodular deposits of amyloid first appear in the atrial endocardium and later in the ventricular subendocardium. In advanced cases, small deposits of amyloid may be found in the valves, and rarely within the conducting system.

The clinical significance of senile cardiac amyloidosis is related to the extent and severity of myocardial involvement. Small deposits limited to atria are probably insignificant, but more extensive cardiac involvement may be associated with atrial fibrillation or cardiac failure. This disorder frequently complicates other coexisting conditions such as coronary heart disease and mitral annular calcification, thus adding insult to injury. Patients with senile cardiac amyloidosis may have an increased sensitivity to digitalis, but a well-documented series has not been reported. There is no distinctive ECG pattern in patients with senile cardiac amyloidosis, but atrial fibrillation and nonspecific ST and T wave changes are frequently observed findings. The unique echocardiographic findings of primary systemic amyloidosis along with generalized increased reflectivity from the entire myocardium do not occur in the senile form. In brief, senile cardiac amyloid, a frequent concomitant of senescence, appears to produce hemodynamic and arrhythmic problems only in the rare situation when cardiac involvement is extensive.

## CLINICAL SYNDROMES

### *Syncope*

Syncope (transient loss of consciousness) may be due to a serious, life-threatening cardiac problem, and this symptom should always be treated with clinical respect. If the cause of the syncope is not promptly diagnosed and appropriate treatment is not initiated early, recurrent syncope may be associated with secondary injuries from falls, especially in the elderly. It is not unusual for older patients to ignore their first episode of syncope, especially if it is of short duration and not associated with any sequelae. The primary care physician may be the first one to uncover an interim history of syncope during a routine office visit, and this physician should initiate the necessary medical work-up. At this point, the general physician may function in a triage capacity by trying to determine the organ system responsible for the prior, unobserved syncopal episode. For example, the physician may refer the patient to a cardiologist if a cardiac arrhythmia is suspected, to a vascular surgeon if carotid bruits are detected and extracranial vascular disease is considered, or to a neurologist if a seizure disorder or a brain tumor is a likely possibility. In any event, appropriate clinical evaluation in the office should permit an accurate diagnosis of the cause of the problem in the vast majority of patients.

#### CLINICAL CLASSIFICATION OF SYNCOPE

A clinically useful classification of syncope in terms of the temporal aspects of the onset and offset of the event is presented in Table 29–3. When the syncopal episode begins slowly with gradual loss of consciousness followed by a similar slow recovery phase, hyperventilation or hypoglycemia is frequently the cause. If the patient is observed during such an episode, the pulse remains full with an adequate rate, and the return of full consciousness is not prompt even though the patient is supine.

When the syncope begins abruptly but the recovery is slow, suggesting a postictal state, a seizure disorder or its equivalent is usually the cause. This diagnosis is further substantiated if there was urinary incontinence or tongue biting during the spell.

**Table 29–3.** CLINICAL CLASSIFICATION OF SYNCOPE IN TERMS OF THE TEMPORAL ASPECTS OF ONSET AND OFFSET

| **Gradual Onset and Offset** |
|---|
| Hyperventilation |
| Hypoglycemia |
| **Abrupt Onset and Gradual Offset** |
| Seizure disorder |
| Head trauma |
| **Abrupt Onset and Abrupt Offset** |
| Vascular or autonomic disorders |
| Orthostatic hypotension |
| Vasovagal syncope |
| Extracranial vascular disease |
| Cardiac disorders |
| Aortic outflow tract obstruction |
| Obstruction of venous return |
| Transient cardiac arrhythmias |

In general, cardiovascular syncope is abrupt in onset and offset. The patient may have no forewarning of the episode; he or she collapses to the ground, often sustaining some personal injury in the fall and quickly regains full consciousness without postictal sequelae. The entire episode is very brief, lasting from 15 seconds up to 2 to 3 minutes. The patient is usually lucid within a few minutes of the episode.

**Cardiovascular Syncope.** Abrupt onset-offset syncope can be etiologically grouped into peripheral vascular, extracranial cerebral vascular, or cardiac causes. Orthostatic hypotension is common in elderly patients and may be caused by sympathetic autonomopathy, venous varicosities, or drugs. Vasovagal syncope from abrupt parasympathetic discharge, usually precipitated by emotions, emesis, or pain, can cause generalized vasodilatation with hypotensive loss of consciousness and compounding bradycardia. Syncope from extracranial vascular disease is very infrequent. Carotid disease usually presents with unilateral weakness, and orthostatic syncope rarely occurs unless there is high-grade, bilateral, severe carotid stenosis. The subclavian steal syndrome is associated with transient dizziness resulting from compromise to the posterior circulation, and similar symptoms of vertigo occur with vertebrobasilar disease. Vertebrobasilar "drop attacks" are distinctly uncommon.

Nonarrhythmic cardiac conditions in which syncope occurs include aortic outflow disease, with either aortic valvular stenosis or hypertrophic obstructive cardiomyopathy, and obstruction to venous return from conditions such as superior vena caval obstruction or atrial myxoma. The physician usually becomes suspicious of these disorders on cardiac examination.

Cardiac arrhythmic syncope is the most common cause of transient loss of consciousness in the elderly, yet it is often the most difficult to diagnose. Bradyarrhythmic syncope may result from transient parasympathetic overactivity or spontaneous slow heart rhythm, with a brief episode of sinus arrest or atrioventricular block in the susceptible individual. Such patients generally have intrinsic carotid sinus hypersensitivity, underlying sinus node dysfunction, or atrioventricular conduction disturbance from Lenegre's or Lev's disease. The atrial brady-tachycardiac syndrome is the most common arrhythmic cause of syncope in the elderly, and it represents a common manifestation of sinus node dysfunction.[27]

In elderly patients with acute myocardial infarction, arrhythmic syncope may overshadow any associated symptoms of chest pain. Ischemic rhythm disorders such as heart block or complex ventricular tachyarrhythmias, including even transient ventricular fibrillation, can occur. An ECG taken after a syncopal episode may uncover changes of an unanticipated acute myocardial infarction.

Older individuals tolerate rapid heart action poorly, and syncope may occur with heart rates of supraventricular and ventricular tachycardia that might cause only minor symptoms in younger patients. Recurrent paroxysmal supraventricular tachycardia is a common disorder, and extremely rapid heart rates can be achieved if preexcitation pathways exist such as might occur in the Wolff-Parkinson-White syndrome. Transient ventricular tachycardia is usually seen in association with significant underlying heart disease or may be secondary to cardioactive drugs. Elderly patients are very sensitive to medication, and tachyarrhythmic syncope can easily be produced from inadvertent toxicity or the adverse effects of digitalis, as well as quinidine, disopyramide, or the tricyclic antidepressants.[28]

### Clinical Evaluation of Patients with Syncope

A precise history of the chronologic aspects of the syncopal episode is the most important part of the evaluation. Any individual who witnessed the patient's prior syncopal episode should be interviewed. On examination, the blood pressure should be taken with the patient supine and upright and in both arms. Careful auscultation for carotid and subclavian bruits should be performed. Evaluation of the change in systolic heart murmurs with hand grip and the Valsalva maneuver can provide valuable information regarding the differential diagnosis between aortic valve disease and hypertrophic obstructive cardiomyopathy. The systolic murmur of the latter is diminished with hand grip–induced hypertension and is accentuated during the strain phase of the Valsalva maneuver. An apical systolic murmur of mitral insufficiency may be the only finding to indicate possible underlying mitral annular disease, with its potential for producing intermittent heart block (Lev's disease).

The carotid sinus maneuver and forced hyperventilation have proved invaluable in the evaluation of patients with syncope. In the absence of carotid bruits, transient unilateral carotid sinus massage with the patient supine during electrocardiographic monitoring is safe, and it often uncovers sinus or atrioventricular nodal dysfunction (Fig. 29–2). The development of transient sinus arrest or heart block, along with symptoms such as lightheadedness, similar to those accompanying syncopal episodes, pinpoints the problem. Forced hyperventilation with frequent and deep respirations for 1 to 2 minutes may produce symptoms of lightheadedness, dizziness, or near syncope that mimic spontaneous episodes. These two office procedures may provide a quick, precise diagnosis and avoid a costly, usually unproductive, workup using invasive studies.

The resting 12-lead electrocardiogram is frequently normal in patients with syncope, but it may reveal evidence of electrical abnormality, which suggests an arrhythmic cause of the syncope. Findings such as first-degree heart block, right bundle branch block with left axis deviation, sinus bradycardia, or complex ventricular rhythm should alert the physician to the possibility of an arrhythmic etiology. If a cardiac arrhythmia is suspected, multiple 24-hour Holter recordings should be obtained. A chest x-ray may reveal significant mitral annular calcification (see Fig. 29–1), which frequently occurs in association with conduction defects.

## *Palpitations*

Cardiac arrhythmias are common in the elderly. In the absence of major symptoms such as syncope, and when there is no significant coexisting heart disease, subjective palpitations are for the most part benign. Patients describe palpitations using a variety of terms to indicate a

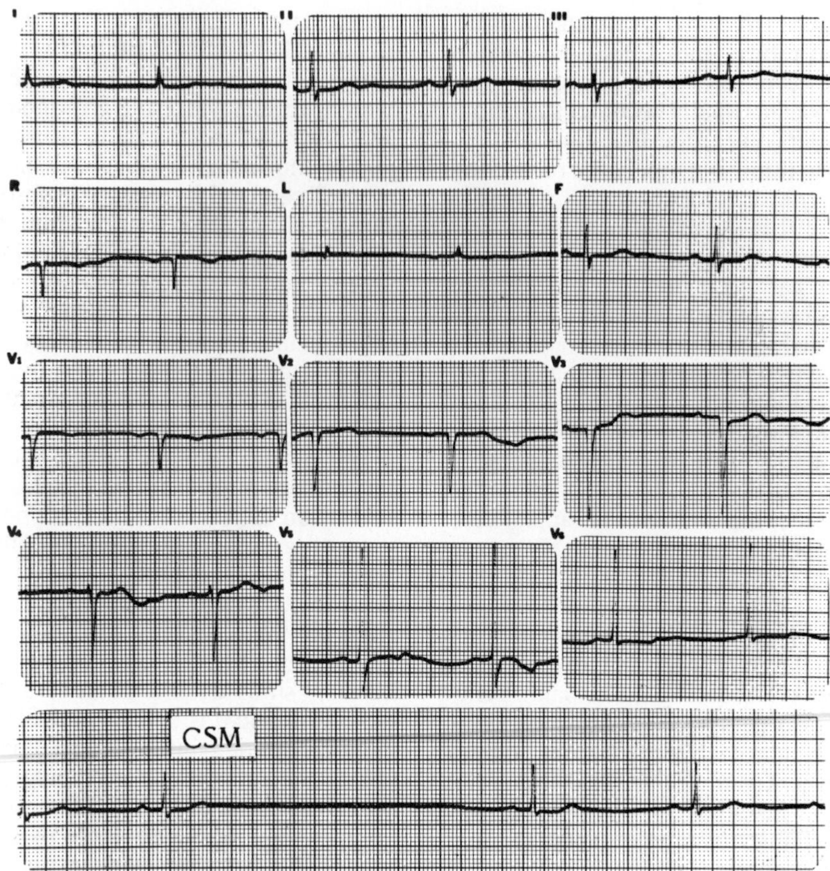


**Figure 29–2.** Electrocardiogram of a 70-year-old patient with episodes of severe lightheadedness and near syncope. The patient was not receiving any medication. Sinus bradycardia, borderline first-degree heart block, and an old anterior myocardial infarction are evident. With the patient supine, right carotid sinus massage (CSM) produced a transient 2.5 second sinus arrest, with lightheadedness similar to spontaneous episodes.

disagreeable awareness of the heart beat. Frequently applied terms include fluttering, racing, jumping, skipping, flip-flops, or simply a strong beating. Some patients are more descriptive and report the feeling as a "bird in the chest," a "fish out of water," or a "jackhammer in the neck."

The rhythm responsible for the palpitation may not be present when the patient is seen, and the patient should be requested to tap out with a finger the subjective palpitation that he or she has experienced. This maneuver is useful in differentiating between isolated premature beats, the irregular rhythm of atrial fibrillation, and regular tachycardias. If the pulse rate or rhythm were taken during an episode, it would be important to know because it would provide valuable diagnostic data.

The patient should be queried about any coexisting symptoms during the palpitations. Diaphoresis suggests hemodynamic compromise, anginal pain may be primary or secondary, and dyspnea indicates left ventricular dysfunction. Polyuria and polydipsia frequently occur in association with paroxysmal supraventricular tachycardia or episodic atrial flutter-fibrillation.[29]

Common intermittent arrhythmias in the older outpatient include benign atrial premature beats, the spectrum of episodic supraventricular tachyarrhythmias; the atrial brady-tachy syndrome, with alternating slow and rapid heart rhythms; and ventricular premature beats (VPBs). Unless the patient is observed during an episode, the specific arrhythmia responsible for the palpitations may be difficult to interpret from the history, examination, and resting electrocardiogram. An auscultatory nonejection click in association with an apical mid-to-late systolic murmur raises the question of mitral valve prolapse with associated arrhythmias. The diagnosis of latent thyrotoxicosis, the so-called apathetic thyrotoxicosis of the elderly, is overrated as a cause of unexplained palpitations. Alcohol, caffeinated beverages, cardioactive drugs, and anxiety are common factors precipitating and exacerbating troublesome palpitations.

In addition to a routine electrocardiogram, 24-hour Holter recordings with a diary of any symptoms, exercise stress testing, and an echocardiogram are important noninvasive laboratory studies for clarifying the type and even the cause of the palpitations. Not infrequently, anxious patients complain of subjective racing of the heart that is nothing more than mild acceleration of the sinus rate, with sinus tachycardia in the range of 120 beats per minute.

As a general rule, the aged individual with "benign" palpitations should be reassured and not treated with antiarrhythmic medication. The drugs are generally ineffective in controlling the palpitations and have a high frequency of significant adverse side effects, and their cost and compliance requirements add an additional burden to an already troubled individual. Reassurance and withdrawal of all possible offending therapy is the treatment of choice if the palpitations appear benign and if there is no significant, life-threatening, coexisting cardiac disease.

## *Congestive Heart Failure*

Congestive heart failure (CHF) is a major complication of cardiac disease in the elderly, and the prevalence of this disorder increases progressively with age. CHF may be due to many diverse causes, but chronic hypertension, silent or overt coronary heart disease, and valvular disease account for most cases. The cardiac aging process, with progressive deterioration in ventricular function unrelated to specific disease entities, probably plays an exacerbating role. Certainly, the circulatory reserve of the elderly, especially in response to stress, is reduced.[9] In the presence of cardiac disease, the severity of the CHF is largely dependent on the extent of myocardial damage, and the degree of global cardiac dysfunction is closely correlated with the amount of myofiber loss.[30] Significant compromise of renal and hepatic functions often produces an added burden.

Numerous factors can contribute to exacerbation of CHF in an individual with existing cardiac disease. Silent myocardial infarction, increased hypertension, subclinical pulmonary emboli, and the development of new atrial fibrillation are common problems in the elderly that precipitate overt CHF. In addition, fever, infection, and anemia are poorly tolerated by elderly patients with borderline compensated CHF, and the development of these coexisting medical problems will aggravate the situation.

The physical demands of everyday life on ambulatory elderly individuals require a greater percentage of total circulatory reserve than is needed for younger people, thus making the older individual more vulnerable to CHF. Regardless of the cause of the underlying cardiac problem, a common decompensating factor in the elderly is dietary sodium excess. Attempts to limit dietary salt intake are difficult for the older person living alone. Low-salt foods are expensive and not readily available. Episodic dietary indiscretion is a frequent cause of unexplained exacerbation of CHF necessitating an urgent office visit.

### Extracardiac Factors in CHF

Complex adjustment mechanisms are set into motion by the low cardiac output state of CHF. Initially these compensatory mechanisms are beneficial, but overcompensation may become dysfunctional. An understanding of these factors is essential for rational therapeutic intervention.

Patients with chronic CHF have diminished concentrations of myocardial norepinephrine due to reduced cardiac synthesis of this compound. In contrast, arterial norepinephrine concentrations are increased as a result of generalized activation of the sympathetic nervous system. The effect of the latter is to initially maintain the systemic pressure, but in chronic CHF, the compensatory increase in arteriolar resistance creates an augmented afterload, which makes it more difficult for the failing heart to eject blood. An important cornerstone of modern therapy for CHF is the reduction in peripheral resistance by vasodilator therapy.

The renin-angiotensin-aldosterone system is also activated in CHF, resulting in renal salt and water retention, systemic and renal arteriolar vasoconstriction, and secondary increase in afterload resistance.[31] There is a reduction in total renal blood flow, and in the more severe forms of CHF, the glomerular filtration rate is decreased, resulting in prerenal azotemia.

CHF is also associated with an increased secretion of antidiuretic hormone. It certainly contributes to excess fluid retention and to the hyponatremia, which frequently accompany heart failure.

### Clinical Findings

The classic clinical findings of CHF are well described in most medical textbooks. However, the symptoms and signs of early CHF in the elderly individual may be obscure and difficult to interpret. Exertional dyspnea, fatigue, bibasilar rales, and mild ankle edema are usually the earliest findings of CHF, but each of these symptoms and signs may have other explanations. The coexistence of emphysema, musculoskeletal abnormalities, and chronic venous disease of the lower extremities compounds the problem. Generally, the early diagnosis of CHF requires the presence of a combination of these findings buttressed by recent weight gain, physician awareness of an underlying heart problem, and knowledge of physical, social, or environmental factors that can stress the circulatory system. The integration of this clinical information into a total picture, a so-called gestalt, which is based on clinical experience with the elderly, permits earlier and more precise diagnosis by the seasoned physician.

More overt types of CHF are easy to diagnose, but some of the presenting findings may mimic other diseases. Left ventricular failure with cardiac asthma may be mistaken for chronic obstructive lung disease or asthmatic bronchitis, and frequently the auscultatory findings are indistinguishable. Pulsations of the deep jugular veins and distention of the external jugular system when the patient is sitting in a 90-degree position are important signs of heart failure. Many physicians only look at the external jugular veins, which can be misleading. Distention of these veins may be due to local factors in the musculoskeletal structures of the neck and thus provide false information to the uninitiated. Elevated pulsations of the deep jugular system are a reliable sign of elevated central venous pressure. However, the deep jugular veins can be distended to such a degree that pulsations are only evident at the angle of the jaw with the patient in the 90-degree upright position. Right upper quadrant discomfort, hepatomegaly, and ascites are found in advanced CHF, but these findings may resemble fatty nutritional cirrhosis or metastatic liver disease. Once again, it is the associated findings that provide valuable information in the differential diagnosis.

Cardiac examination in elderly patients with CHF is generally less precise than in younger individuals. Emphysema, resulting in an increase in the anteroposterior dimension of the thoracic cage, increases the distance between the chest wall and the heart and attenuates transmission of sounds. A displaced apical impulse of cardiomegaly may not be felt, the heart size may be indeterminate, and auscultatory heart sounds may be distant. Thus, third heart sound ($S_3$) and fourth heart sound ($S_4$) gallops may not be heard even in the presence of flagrant heart failure, and heart murmurs may be reduced by one or two grades in intensity due to the low output state.

## *Anginal Discomfort*

The diagnosis of angina pectoris is made largely from the patient history, and the elderly frequently have atypical presentations. Age-related neurologic and cognitive deficits often make elucidation of the history difficult. The pattern of the discomfort that is precipitated by physical or emotional factors or that awakens the patient at night is more important in establishing the diagnosis than the character or location of the pain. Classic substernal discomfort, with radiation to the neck, jaw, or inner aspects of the arms, that lasts 5 to 10 minutes does not tax the diagnostic ability of the physician for patients of any age group. The geriatric patient with anginal discomfort may present with episodic weakness or dyspnea, unexplained diaphoresis, indigestion, interscapular ache, or arthritic-type shoulder-elbow discomfort. These symptoms have been categorized as anginal equivalents. Frequently there is a consistency to the repeated episodes, with recurrence that is predictable.

A therapeutic trial with sublingual nitroglycerin often provides sensitive and specific diagnostic information about the cause of atypical symptoms. Prompt and consistent relief of the aforementioned episodes with nitroglycerin establishes the diagnosis. The resting ECG may reveal nonspecific ST and T wave changes, a left bundle branch block pattern, or Q waves of an old myocardial infarction, findings that are not sufficiently specific to establish the diagnosis of angina. In fact, the ECG may be entirely normal in the presence of unequivocal angina.

Confirmation of the diagnosis of angina may require a treadmill exercise test. Supervised low to moderate level activity testing may establish the diagnosis of angina and determine the relative severity of the underlying coronary disease process. Occurrence of the patient's characteristic discomfort/sensation within the first few minutes of activity testing, with significant ST and T wave changes that regress during recovery, usually indicates major two or three vessel coronary disease or left main coronary disease. Many elderly patients cannot perform an exercise test owing to associated musculoskeletal abnormalities. In such situations, coronary angiography may be required for more precise diagnosis, depending on the intractability of the angina and the physician's judgment regarding the potential for intervention with coronary artery bypass graft surgery.

Although anginal pains are usually due to coronary disease, patients with aortic valvular stenosis or hypertrophic obstructive cardiomyopathy may present with angina despite normal coronary vessels. The heart murmurs in the latter condition may be unimpressive, but the ECG in both conditions generally reveals significant ischemic ST and T wave abnormalities. The echocardiogram should be used to diagnose or rule out these obstructive outflow tract conditions.

Decubitus angina, nocturnal angina, and postprandial angina have the same prognostic clinical implications in the elderly as they do in younger patients. Extensive trivessel coronary disease or left main coronary stenosis is the underlying pathologic state in these types of angina, and the 1-year mortality is high.[32]

Nonspecific management involves normalization of blood pressure, decongestive therapy, correction of dysfunctional rhythm disturbances, and correction of coexisting medical conditions, such as anemia and thyroid abnormalities. Specific therapy with nitrates, beta-blockers, and calcium antagonists and the indications for coronary bypass graft surgery in the elderly will be presented in a later section.

## DIAGNOSTIC LABORATORY STUDIES

When indicated, diagnostic tests should be used to complement the routine history and physical examination. Standard laboratory tests, including a blood count, blood chemistries, ECG, and chest x-ray will not be covered in this chapter. Rather, the focus will be on four specialized noninvasive cardiac diagnostic procedures that provide important information about structural and functional abnormalities of the heart. These noninvasive tests are particularly useful in the evaluation of elderly patients in whom more involved invasive procedures may carry a significant risk. However, in certain situations, invasive hemodynamic cardiac catheterization or coronary and left ventricular angiography are required, and the indications for these special in-hospital studies will also be discussed.

### *Holter ECG Recording*

The 24-hour Holter ECG has become an important noninvasive diagnostic technique in the evaluation of patients with cardiac rhythm disturbances or symptoms of angina. The Holter recording provides data on the spectrum of heart rates (mean, zeniths, nadirs) during daily activities; the occurrence and complexity of extra heart beats and arrhythmias; the development of conduction disturbance, such as bundle branch block or atrioventricular heart block; and changes of active myocardial ischemia in terms of ST and T wave alterations.

A Holter recording is obtained for the following reasons: (1) to evaluate patient's symptoms, such as syncope, palpitations, and angina; (2) to assess pharmacologic antiarrhythmic or anti-ischemic therapy; (3) to determine sensing and pacing function of implanted pacemakers; (4) to evaluate rhythm stability or instability prior to hospital discharge after myocardial infarction or open heart surgery; and (5) to monitor a patient's response to physical and nonphysical stress. Monitoring a patient using the 24-hour Holter ECG may uncover a potentially life-threatening arrhythmia in any one of the preceding situations. It has also been used in the assessment of prognosis after myocardial infarction, since the probability of 1-year cardiac mortality is directly related to the frequency of ventricular premature beats, expressed as the average number of beats per hour.[33]

In the evaluation of patients with infrequent episodic events in which an arrhythmia is suspect, multiple 24-hour Holter recordings are indicated. Holter monitoring frequently complements a formal treadmill exercise tolerance test (ETT) in the evaluation of cardiac patients. The Holter is more sensitive in detecting arrhythmias, but the exercise tolerance test provides more accurate assessment of the adequacy of coronary perfusion and global cardiovascular performance.[34]

### *Exercise Tolerance Test*

Several exercise protocols exist that permit adjustment of the workload to the capability of the patient. The treadmill is the most widely used technique for exercise testing, although bicycle stress testing is also available in some institutions. An important advantage of the treadmill is the ease of adjustment of the grade and the speed of walking to the agility of the patient. This is especially important in the elderly because of limitations imposed by musculoskeletal problems.

During exercise testing, the ECG is monitored continuously, the blood pressure is recorded intermittently, and the patient is asked to relate any symptoms of chest discomfort, dyspnea, or extreme fatigue. The test can be safely carried out in the elderly, and the procedure will provide valuable diagnostic and functional information during dynamic performance.[35]

The specific treadmill exercise protocol to be used depends on the indications for the test. The test can be used to provide functional information about tolerance for a specific level of activity, for diagnostic assessment of patients with suspected angina, to determine the severity of known underlying coronary disease, or to provoke arrhythmias. The referring physician should realize that exercise testing in the elderly carries some risk, albeit small, and good clinical judgment and knowledge of the indications as well as the absolute and relative contraindications are of paramount importance when deciding to perform such a test.

The most standard exercise test is the submaximal Bruce protocol, which is targeted to 75 per cent to 90 per cent of the age-predicted heart rate. The initial walking rate begins at 1.7 miles per hour at a 10 per cent grade, and the speed and grade are progressively increased at 3-minute intervals. This protocol is overly stringent for elderly patients, and frequently the exercise test is terminated prematurely because of leg and joint problems rather than because of cardiac symptoms or signs. Elderly patients seem to perform better when the speed is kept constant and the grade gradually increased. The modified Balke-Ware protocol[36] has many advantages over the Bruce test because the walking is constant at 2.0 to 3.3 miles per hour, with a 2 to 5 per cent increase in grade every 2 to 3 minutes. For low-level exercise testing, the protocol is terminated after 6 minutes, with a peak oxygen consumption that is only three times baseline (3 METS)—a level equivalent to the metabolic needs of limited home activity. For higher level testing, the protocol can be continued for additional time at steeper grades.

The diagnostic and performance criteria for the accurate interpretation of exercise testing in the elderly is less than clear-cut. Most of the standards have been established on younger individuals. Elderly patients, especially elderly women, have a relatively high rate of false-positive ischemic ST-segment changes during exercise testing. In younger patients, submaximal exercise testing has a 60 per cent to 70 per cent sensitivity and a 90 per cent specificity in identifying the presence and absence of significant underlying coronary disease. The sensitivity and specificity percentages are considerably less in the older age group.

## *Echocardiogram*

Echocardiography has been an important addition to the diagnostic armamentarium of the physician, and this noninvasive procedure is particularly well suited for use in elderly patients. This technique provides dynamic visualization of the cardiac structures and is very useful in evaluating the pericardium and pericardial space, the ventricular walls, the ventricular septum, the valves, the dimensional size of the atrial and ventricular chambers as well as the outflow tracts, and the presence of mass lesions such as thrombi or myxoma. One can use the older, single dimensional motion (M)-mode approach, which provides an "ice-pick" view of the heart or the newer two-dimensional cross-sectional scanner, which provides images in a plane through the heart. By directing the two-dimensional echo transducer through multiple axes, a three-dimensional spatial image can be reconstructed in the mind's eye.

The echocardiogram provides useful information about ventricular function. Systolic wall motion abnormalities, including global hypokinesia as well as regional areas of akinesia and dyskinesia (aneurysm), can be detected, and it is possible to visualize intramural thrombi. Recent echo studies suggest that abnormalities in ventricular diastolic compliance can also be identified, and this is particularly important, since ventricular compliance is known to decrease with advancing age.[37]

Alterations in mitral valve function (stenosis, insufficiency, and prolapse) are easily detected by echocardiography. In addition, calcification of the mitral annulus can be visualized as a dense band of hyper-reflective echoes at the base of the mitral valve. Calcific aortic valvular stenosis is easily differentiated from hypertrophic obstructive cardiomyopathy. Moreover, the degree of stenosis or outflow tract obstruction can now be accurately estimated from pulsed Doppler echocardiography, which qualitatively evaluates blood flow velocity. Valvular vegetations, when large, can also be visualized. Both M-mode and cross-sectional echocardiography are extremely accurate in determining the presence or absence of pericardial effusion, and thus these techniques are useful in evaluating the cause of cardiomegaly in the elderly.

Every technique has its limitations, and this is especially true of echocardiography. Many elderly patients have chest cage deformities and coexisting emphysema, which contribute to technical difficulties in the ultrasonic examination of the heart. The success rate for technically satisfactory echocardiograms declines progressively with age, and the echo window is narrower in older than in younger subjects.

## *Radionuclide Imaging*

Radionuclides are widely employed in the assessment of cardiac performance, myocardial perfusion defects (cold spot imaging), and acute myocardial necrosis (hot spot imaging). The tests are relatively noninvasive and require only the intravenous injection of short-lived radionuclides. The studies can be repeated without excessive radiation. Cardiac imaging requires a scintillation camera (single or multicrystal) and a computer-based processing unit for organizing and analyzing the scintillation data. Performance and perfusion studies can be done at rest and during or after exercise. These tests are especially useful in the elderly, since they can be done on an outpatient basis; they provide accurate and quantitatively precise information about cardiac function; and they are clinically efficacious in improving accuracy of diagnosis and patient management.

The radionuclide ejection fraction test is utilized in the evaluation of global and regional cardiac performances. The radionuclide commonly used is technetium 99m. The tests are performed either by the first transit through the central circulation (first-pass technique) or by analysis of the radioactively labeled blood pool during multiple cardiac systolic and diastolic cycles (*mu*ltiple *ga*ted method, which is referred to by the acronym MUGA). The global ejection fraction is the fraction of the diastolic volume ejected during systole, i.e., the stroke volume divided by the end-diastolic volume. In normal subjects, the resting ejection fraction is greater than 0.60 and usually increases during exertional activity.

Recent studies involving healthy volunteers found that the resting radionuclide ejection fraction does not decline with age. Port and associates[12] reported that the resting radionuclide ejection fraction was above the normal value of 0.60 in most healthy subjects over age 60. However, in contrast to the exercise radionuclide ejection fractions in younger subjects, those in the elderly declined abnormally—a finding suggesting underlying subclinical myocardial dysfunction and a reduction in reserve capacity.

Radionuclide ejection fraction tests provide valuable information on cardiac performance in patients with coronary disease, CHF ventricular aneurysm, hypertensive heart disease, and obstructive as well as nonobstructive cardiomyopathy. Recent studies in coronary disease indicate that the 1-year cardiac mortality increases progressively as the quantitated radionuclide ejection fraction declines. A radionuclide ejection fraction greater than 0.50 is associated with a very favorable outcome, an ejection fraction less than 0.35 reflects significant underlying heart disease, and an ejection fraction under 0.20 is associated with an ominous prognosis with a 1-year mortality of 35 per cent. Regional wall motion abnormalities, especially those developing during exercise, identify the effects of localized coronary disease. Elevated ejection fractions are consistently found in patients with hypertrophic obstructive cardiomyopathy. Serial measurements of the radionuclide ejection fraction can be used to evaluate the efficacy of therapeutic interventions, such as decongestive measures, coronary angioplasty, or corrective cardiac surgery, as well as the rate of progression of cardiac disease over time in a given patient. Also, separate right and left ventricular performances can be assessed, and this is useful in the evaluation of patients with cor pulmonale and coronary heart disease.

Myocardial perfusion imaging with the radionuclide thallium-201 is best performed during exercise, with a follow-up resting study a few hours later. Such a sequence of testing permits evaluation of the presence or absence of a perfusion deficit during exercise and during redistribution at rest. Exercise perfusion deficits that disappear during reperfusion at rest permit identification of reversible hypoperfused areas associated with significant localized coronary stenosis. A perfusion deficit that persists during both exercise and rest is most consistent with previous infarction and scar without reversible ischemia. When properly performed on the elderly patient, myocardial perfusion imaging may provide sufficient information to obviate the need for coronary angiography.

Myocardial imaging with the infarct-avid radionuclide technetium-99m pyrophosphate permits identification of an area of acute myocardial necrosis. Images are obtained in multiple positions in order to more accurately identify an involved region. This test is usually performed in the hospital in patients with equivocal clinical findings of acute myocardial infarction. The test is most valuble in patients who present several days after an acute event and in those with a left bundle branch block pattern that precludes a specific ECG confirmation of infarction.

## *Cardiac Catheterization and Coronary Angiography*

Cardiac catheterization and coronary angiography are utilized to enhance diagnostic accuracy in patients with significant coronary, valvular, or congenital heart disease. In elderly patients, these procedures should be performed when there is a reasonable possibility that surgical intervention may be required for treatment of life-threatening problems or disabling symptoms. In experienced hands, these diagnostic studies are associated with only a minimally increased morbidity and mortality risk in patients over age 70. In this age group, severe trivessel coronary stenosis and/or left main stenosis, significant aortic stenosis, and atrial septal defect with greater than a two-to-one shunt are eminently correctable if the clinical situation so dictates. Precise evaluation of the extent and severity of the coronary disease process, the functional state of the left and right ventricles, the severity of the valvular lesions, and the magnitude of any existing shunt is essential in the decision-making process regarding medical or surgical management.

## CARDIAC THERAPEUTICS

During the past decade there has been a significant expansion in the therapy for cardiovascular disease for all age groups. In conjunction with the addition of many new therapeutic agents, there has ensued a better understanding of drug pharmacokinetics and pharmacodynamics in the elderly, thereby improving the science of drug therapy in this patient population. Emphasis will be placed on the more troublesome adverse effects that frequently occur with cardioactive agents in the older population. Pacemakers have been available for over 20 years, and their use has resulted in major inroads into the treatment of symptomatic and life-threatening bradycardias. However, because problems with pacemakers are sufficiently common, every physician caring for the elderly must stay abreast of the ongoing developments in the field. Cardiac surgery is showing efficacious results in the elderly, with an acceptably low operative mortality and morbidity. Age is no longer a contraindication for open heart surgery in appropriately selected cases. Finally a new technique, angioplasty, is available for dilating stenotic vessels, including the coronary arteries, with considerably less morbidity than occurs with surgical intervention. This section will focus on recent developments in cardiac therapeutics involving the application of drugs, pacemakers, open heart surgery, and angioplasty in elderly patients.

### *Drugs*

#### Digitalis

Some of the traditional uses of digitalis therapy are being re-examined because of the high rate of adverse side effects and the questionable efficacy with chronic administration.[38,39] In addition, newer approaches to the treatment of CHF may be superseding the use of digitalis. Digitalis remains the most effective agent for the control of the ventricular response to atrial fibrillation.

Digoxin is the most frequently prescribed digitalis preparation. Digoxin is widely distributed, and it is excreted primarily by the kidney. Older patients have a reduction in lean body mass and a decrease in renal function—two factors that contribute to the high incidence of digoxin toxicity in the elderly. Dose reduction should be predicated on the size of the patient and the estimated or quantitated creatinine clearance. It should be remembered that the creatinine clearance is frequently reduced to 50 per cent of normal in older patients, even when the blood urea nitrogen is within normal limits.

Two recent studies suggest that digitalis use in the early posthospital phase of myocardial infarction is associated with an increased cardiac mortality.[39,40] The adverse effect of digitalis was significant even after adjustment for differences in the severity of the underlying cardiac disease between those patients treated with digitalis and those not treated with digitalis.

Several recent studies have substantiated an important interaction between digoxin and quinidine, with serum digoxin concentrations approximately doubling during coadministration of these two agents.[41] The clinical significance of this interaction is under active investigation. At the present time, one should exercise prudence when concomitantly administering digoxin and quinidine in the elderly patient.

#### Antiarrhythmic Agents

The efficacy of the existing oral antiarrhythmic agents (quinidine, procainamide, and disopyramide) is probably overestimated, whereas their potential for producing serious adverse side effects in older patients is underestimated. Most indications for antiarrhythmic therapy occur in-hospital, with complex cardiac rhythms complicating acute cardiac disease. Frequently, the antiarrhythmic therapy is inappropriately maintained long after the indication or need. The primary indication for chronic antiarrhythmic treatment in the elderly is in the small subset of patients with recurrent life-threatening ventricular arrhythmias or troublesome paroxysmal atrial tachyarrhythmias. To date, no definitive study demonstrating beneficial results with routine antiarrhythmic therapy in postinfarction patients has been published.

If antiarrhythmic therapy is initiated, assuming a valid indication, the dose should be adjusted on the basis of arrhythmia control, the desired therapeutic blood level, and the avoidance of adverse side effects. All the available antiarrhythmic agents can initiate life-threatening cardiac problems, and each has unique side effects. Overall, older patients are considerably more vulnerable to these adverse effects than are younger individuals. Quinidine, and to a lesser extent disopyramide, can induce prefibrillatory tachyarrhythmia, (torsades de pointes), which usually produces syncope and may culminate in death. Disopyramide has significant negative inotropic effects, and it can precipitate CHF and hypotension in patients with pre-existing heart disease.[42] In addition, several investigators have described life-threatening electromechanical dissociation following disopyramide therapy in older patients with depressed ventricular function. Disopyramide should probably not be prescribed to elderly patients, not only because of these cardiotoxic effects but also because its use results in an almost universal occurrence of urinary retention in men, constipation, severe drying of the mouth, and worsening of glaucoma. Procainamide is usually well tolerated initially, but troublesome side effects such as fever or a lupus-like arthritis are common with chronic therapy. The elderly are particularly vulnerable to the toxic build-up of the procainamide metabolite, *N*-acetyl procainamide (NAPA). This metabolite is almost exclusively excreted by the kidney, and with chronic therapy in patients with compromised renal function, *N*-acetyl procainamide toxicity can develop very subtly.

## Diuretics

The available diuretics can be classified into three groups depending on their site and mechanism of action: (1) loop diuretics (furosemide, ethacrynic acid, and bumetanide); (2) distal convoluted tubule diuretics (thiazides); and (3) potassium-sparing diuretics (spironolactone, triamterene, and amiloride). The loop diuretics are the most potent agents available, with an excellent dose-response relationship over a wide range of doses. In patients with low cardiac output or CHF, even large oral doses of the loop diuretics may be ineffective owing to reduced gastrointestinal absorption. However, small intravenous doses of these agents may produce significant diuresis. Thiazide diuretics are moderately potent agents. These drugs are of limited efficacy in patients with reduced glomerular filtration rates and in older patients with diminished cardiac output.

The thiazide and the loop diuretics may produce significant hypokalemia, especially when these agents are used in combination. The long-acting thiazide diuretic, chlorthalidone, is especially likely to induce hypokalemia with chronic therapy. Supplemental oral potassium may prevent hypokalemia, but the available potassium salts are not very palatable and compliance is frequently a problem. The potent diuretics can cause dehydration and may precipitate prerenal insufficiency in older patients with borderline renal function. Potassium supplements in such situations may precipitate dangerous hyperkalemia.

The potassium-sparing diuretics are the least potent of the available agents. The antikaluretic action of these diuretics may produce unexpected hyperkalemia; consequently these drugs should be used with extreme caution in older patients. I have personally seen several cases in which the potassium-sparing diuretics precipitated hyperkalemic heart block; the conduction disturbance disappeared with drug withdrawal and a permanent pacemaker was not required.

## Vasodilator Therapy

The concept of vasodilator therapy for the treatment of CHF was introduced in the mid 1970s. Initially, the standard antihypertensive agents that were available were utilized primarily to reduce peripheral systemic resistance (afterload reduction). Subsequently, the additional importance of reducing filling pressure through venous vasodilation (preload reduction) was appreciated. Currently, the most effective vasodilator regimens involve individual agents or combinations of agents that reduce both afterload and preload.

Several oral vasodilating drugs are very useful in the management of CHF on an outpatient basis. The use of hydralazine in a gradually increasing dosage (up to 50 mg every 6 hours) in combination with full-dose nitrates (either oral isosorbide dinitrate or topical nitroglycerin ointment) is an effective regimen. Prazosin has balanced vasodilator effects on arterioles and veins and may be used in place of the hydralazine-nitrate combination. However, prazosin is frequently associated with orthostatic hypotension with initial dosing, and tachyphylaxis is common during chronic administration. These effects limit the usefulness of this agent as a primary vasodilator in the older age group. Captopril, a recently introduced angiotensin-converting enzyme inhibitor that reduces the concentration of angiotensin II, is an important addition to vasodilator treatment of CHF. Angiotensin II is a potent vasoconstrictor and stimulator of aldosterone secretion, two dysfunctional effects of the activated renin-angiotensin system that develop in CHF. Captopril has been useful in the treatment of CHF that is refractory to direct-acting vasodilators.

### NITRATES

Nitrates are the mainstay of treatment for angina. They are dilators of arterial and venous smooth muscle and have a potent effect on large coronary vessels. Sublingual and chewable preparations have a very short duration of action and are useful primarily in the treatment or prophylaxis of a typical episode of angina pectoris. The oral preparations, isosorbide dinitrate or erythrityl tetranitrate, are efficacious in controlling angina if large doses of these agents are used at frequent 4-hour dosing. For example, the effective oral antianginal dosage of isosorbide dinitrate is generally in the range of 30 mg every 4 hours while awake. However, there is considerable individual variation. Topical nitroglycerin, either nitroglycerin ointment or the newly introduced slow-release transdermal patches, permits continuous cutaneous absorption over sustained periods of time. The transdermal patches require application only once a day and are as effective as other more frequently administered nitrates. These topical preparations are especially useful in patients with decubitus, nocturnal, and postprandial angina.

Most elderly patients tolerate nitrates well, but some are troubled with profound orthostatic hypotension and intolerable headaches,which preclude the use of these agents. When nitrates are initially introduced, it is wise to evaluate the patient's response to an individual tablet of sublingual nitroglycerin in the office. Since nitrates come in a variety of doses, minor side effects can usually be managed by dose reduction. Topical nitrates may irritate the sensitive skin of the elderly; however, rotation of the application sites usually resolves this problem.

### BETA-ADRENERGIC BLOCKING AGENTS

Several beta-adrenergic blocking drugs are currently available for treating angina, the postinfarction state, and hypertension. The current list of agents includes propranolol, metoprolol, nadolol, timolol, and atenolol. The primary action of all these drugs is competitive blockade of the beta-adrenergic receptors, but considerable variation exists among the agents in the duration of action (half-life), lipid solubility, relative selectivity (heart versus other adrenergic receptors), metabolism and excretion, and side effects. Furthermore, the blood concentrations of a given dose of some of these agents can vary 20-fold between individuals. Recent studies indicate that plasma concentrations are higher after oral administration to elderly patients than is the case in younger individuals,[43] and this may account for the increased frequency of adverse side reactions that have been noted with propranolol with advancing age. If beta-blockers are prescribed for patients over 70 years, the initial dose should be low, with a gradual increase upwards, as indicated by the clinical response and the patient's tolerance to the medication.

In most of the reported postinfarction trials with beta-blockers, the cut-off age for eligibility was 70 to 75 years.[44-46] However, the Danish investigators attempted to enroll all postinfarction patients, irrespective of age, in a study of alprenolol.[47] Mortality reduction was demonstrated for patients 65 years of age or younger. Patients 66 years of age or older had an increased 1-year mortality with alprenolol in comparison with placebo treatment (49 per cent versus 35 per cent, $p < 0.08$). These findings suggest caution in the routine use of beta-blockers in older age postinfarction patients.

The standard contraindications to the use of beta-blockers apply to all age groups: left ventricular dysfunction, CHF, history of bronchial asthma, sinus node dysfunction, and vasospastic (Prinzmetal's) angina. The elderly are particularly susceptible to the bradycardiac effects of these agents. A subtle yet troublesome side effect of propranolol in older patients is its ability to induce subclinical depression or alterations in memory and cognitive function. Many elderly patients who have been on chronic propranolol therapy are not aware of these changes or else they and their family have come to accept a decline in mental function as part of the cerebral aging process. It is only when propranolol is discontinued or switched to a less lipid-soluble beta-blocker, such as atenolol, that the full impact of the adverse effects of the agent is appreciated.

### CALCIUM CHANNEL BLOCKERS

Three recently introduced calcium channel blocking agents (nifedipine, verapamil, and diltiazem) are efficacious in the management of exertional, vasotonic, and vasospastic angina. This class of agents represents a significant addition to the therapeutic armamentarium for the management of ischemic heart disease. These agents have a multiplicity of membrane and intracellular activities that can affect myocellular function as well as the contractile state of smooth muscle.

Nifedipine appears to be a safe agent but has annoying side effects such as dizziness, headaches, hypotension, and gastrointestinal upset in approximately 10 per cent of treated patients. Nifedipine is indicated primarily for the treatment of angina, but it is also being used as a complementary vasodilator for blood pressure control and afterload reduction. Verapamil, in contrast with nifedipine, depresses myocardial contractility and slows atrioventricular nodal conduction. The physiologic properties of verapamil can produce serious adverse side effects, including CHF and high-grade atrioventricular block. Patients receiving beta-blockers, digitalis, or antiarrhythmic agents are especially vulnerable to the dysfunctional physiologic properties of verapamil. Only sparse data are available on the use of verapamil in the elderly, but physiologic reasoning suggests a high likelihood of potentially life-threatening problems with the use of this drug in vulnerable patients. Presently, advanced age should serve as a relative contraindication to the routine use of this agent.

## *Pacemakers*

More pacemakers are implanted in the elderly than in any other segment of the population. Indications for pacemaker implantation have broadened since the device was originally introduced for the treatment of episodic syncope due to high-grade heart block. Pacemakers are now being utilized in the treatment of symptomatic patients with bradycardic sinus node disease, atrial-tachycardia syndrome, and refractory re-entrant tachycardias.

With the advent of microelectronics, an explosion in pacemaker technology has ensued resulting in the introduction of multiprogrammable generators, dual chamber pacemakers, and the so-called intelligent pacemaker. Briefly, the current generation of pacemakers can be programmed after implantation for rate, output voltage, sensitivity, pulse width, mode (demand or fixed-rate), and a variety of other parameters, depending on the needs of the patient. The pacing site may be located in the atrium or ventricle or in both chambers for special types of synchronous or sequential pacing. Pacing has become so complex that a special pacemaker code has been developed for uniformity in categorizing the chamber(s) paced, the chamber(s) sensed, and the mode(s) of response (Table 29–4). Thus, a ventricular-inhibited pacemaker would be coded VVI, indicating the *V*entricular chamber is paced, the *V*entricular chamber is sensed, and the pacer generator is *I*nhibited by sensed ventricular activity.

Unipolar and bipolar systems are available, with no real advantage of one over the other. Most electrodes are positioned pervenously to stimulate the endocardium, but the subxyphoid or transthoracic surgical approach is occasionally required when the pervenous method is not technically feasible. Presently, 85 per cent of the pacemakers implanted in the United States are of the ventricular-demand type (VVI), 10 per cent are atrial-demand units (AAI), and the remaining 5 per cent are specialized devices.

Pacemakers may be associated with a variety of problems. The most common ones include battery pocket erosion due to chronic low-grade infection with *Staphylococcus epidermidis,* electrode dislodgement from improper place-

**Table 29–4.** THREE-POSITION PACEMAKER CLASSIFICATION CODE

| | Letter Position<br>*First* | <br>*Second* | <br>*Third* |
|---|---|---|---|
| ***Category*** | Chamber(s) Paced | Chamber(s) Sensed | Mode of Response |
| ***Letters Used*** | V—Ventricle<br>A—Atrium<br>D—Double | V—Ventricle<br>A—Atrium<br>D—Double<br>0—None | I—Inhibited<br>T—Triggered<br>D—Double<br>0—None |
| *Examples* | VVI = *V*entricular paced, *V*entricular sensed, and *I*nhibited by sensed ventricular activity; this is the code for the typical ventricular demand pacemaker.<br>DVI = *D*ual chambers paced, *V*entricular sensed, and *I*nhibited by sensed ventricular activity; this is the code for the sequential atrioventricular pacemaker. | | |

ment, electrode perforation of the thin-walled right ventricle, and high threshold with inconstant pacing. The geriatric patient is especially prone to the "pacemaker syndrome" when a ventricular-demand pacemaker is implanted to maintain an adequate heart rate in patients with bradycardic sinus node disease. This syndrome is characterized by a low cardiac output state and orthostatic hypotension despite an adequate heart rate. In elderly patients with impaired myocardial function, the normal sequence of atrial then ventricular contraction is an important factor in optimizing global cardiac performance. Direct pacing of the ventricle eliminates sequential atrioventricular contraction and can cause significant cardiac dysfunction despite an adequate pacing rate. This problem can be avoided or corrected in patients with sinus node disease by using either an atrial pacemaker, if atrioventricular conduction is intact, or a dual chamber sequential pacer if heart block exists.

Regular follow-up of patients with these implanted units is essential for the optimal care. The general physician who cares for such patients is not in a position to do this, but he or she must insist that monthly transtelephone monitoring be carried out either by a cardiologist, by the pacemaker manufacturer, or by a commercial monitoring service. This periodic monitoring is an important safety measure for the identification of early sensing and pacing problems, such as premature battery depletion, random electronic component failures, and electrode dislodgement.

## *Cardiac Surgery*

With the improvement in the techniques of cardiac surgery, including hypothermic cardiopulmonary bypass, there has been a dramatic reduction in operative mortality and perioperative morbidity. As the safety of cardiac surgery has increased, there has been a gradual and progressive extension of surgical intervention to patients in the older age group. The three most common surgical heart operations in the elderly are coronary artery bypass graft (CABG) surgery, valve replacement, and atrial septal defect repair. Frequently the last two operations are combined with CABG surgery. There is no good reason to delay or deny surgical intervention when critical disease exists that is amenable to corrective surgery at an acceptably low operative risk.

The specific indications for cardiac surgery have already been presented in the section on cardiac diseases. It is important for the general physician to realize that the best operative results are found in surgical units in which the volume of operations is large and older patients make up a significant percentage of the surgical experience. The success rate is significantly influenced by the quality of the preoperative preparation, the anesthesia, and the postoperative care as well as the technical competence of the surgical team. Although this is a truism for all surgery, it is especially pertinent to the elderly undergoing cardiac surgery because their compensatory reserve is stretched to the very limit and minor errors in management are not tolerated.

The surgical mortality for CABG, aortic valve replacement, and atrial septal defect repair is approximately two- to threefold higher in patients 70 years of age and older than in younger patients.[48] The surgical risk increases proportionately with age, but many dramatically successful results have been achieved in patients in the eighth decade of life. It should be realized that overtly healthy individuals in their mid-80s have an additional life expectancy of approximately 5 years. The decision regarding surgical intervention in this age group requires exquisite clinical judgment, and the primary care physician should work in close harmony with the cardiologist and the cardiac surgeon to determine if it is appropriate to procede with cardiac surgery. The generalist should not be intimidated by the specialist. As the late President John F. Kennedy said, one should not rely entirely on the judgment of experts.

## *Coronary Angioplasty*

Percutaneous transluminal coronary angioplasty (PTCA) was introduced for the treatment of localized proximal coronary stenosis in 1977 by Gruntzig and co-workers.[49] Initially the procedure was limited to single vessel coronary disease in younger patients. However, with increasing experience and generally favorable results comparable to that of CABG surgery, multivessel disease in all age groups is being subjected to balloon dilation. The procedure does not take much longer than a diagnostic coronary angiogram, but it does require surgical standby backup for emergency bypass if complications develop. When successful, the patient need only stay in the hospital for 2 days after the dilation procedure. The markedly reduced morbidity of PTCA is especially appealing for older patients.

The guidelines for patient selection are rapidly changing. Presently, symptomatic anginal patients of all age groups with localized proximal stenosis involving one or two major coronary vessels should be considered for this procedure. The success rate in experienced hands is in the range of 70 to 80 per cent. Older patients are more likely to have calcified lesions, resulting in a reduced probability of effective dilation. In addition, the elderly have more tortuous angulated coronary vessels. As a result there is increased difficulty reaching the site of stenosis with the dilating catheter in these vessels. The current patency rates 1 year after effective dilation are in the range of 75 per cent.[50] With further improvements in this technique, PTCA is likely to become safer and more effective in the elderly, and it should have more widespread application. It holds great promise for simplifying the management of older patients with obstructive coronary disease.

## CONCLUSION

The accurate diagnosis and optimal management of cardiac disease in the geriatric patient is a challenge to the medical profession. The proportion of elderly patients is increasing, and cardiac disease remains the most prevalent disorder in this age group. However, new and more effective therapies continue to be released. When one looks back and observes the dramatic progress that has been made in this field during the past 20 years, one experiences an optimistic sense of excitement about advances that will be available to the next generation of physicians at the turn of the century.

### References


1. Kennedy RD, Andrews GR, Caird FI: Ischaemic heart disease in the elderly. Br Heart J 39:1121, 1977.
2. Weisfeldt ML: The Aging Heart, Its Function and Response to Stress. New York, Raven Press, 1980. *This book is the twelfth volume of a series of edited monographs on aging by Raven Press. The authors provide valuable pathophysiologic data on the aging cardiovascular system and place the available data into a useful clinical perspective.*
3. Pomerance A: Pathology of the myocardium and valves. *In* Caird FI, Dall JLC, Kennedy RD (eds.): Cardiology in Old Age. New York and London, Plenum Press, 1976, p. 11.
4. Kennedy RD, Caird FI: Physiology of aging of the heart. *In* Noble RJ, Rothbaum DA (eds.): Geriatric Cardiology. Philadelphia, F. A. Davis Co., 1981, p. 1.
5. Hansford RG: Metabolism and energy production. *In* Weisfeldt ML (ed.): The Aging Heart. New York, Raven Press, 1980, p. 25.
6. Cavoto FV, Kelliher GJ, Roberts J: Electrophysiological changes in the rat atrium with age. Am J Physiol 226:1293, 1974.
7. Roberts J, Goldberg PB: Changes in cardiac membranes as a function of age with particular emphasis on reactivity to drugs. *In* Cristofalo VJ, Roberts J, Adelman RD (eds.): Advances in Experimental Medicine and Biology. Vol. 61. Explorations in Aging. New York, Plenum Press, 1975, p. 119.
8. Rosen MR, Reder RF, Hordof AJ, et al: Age-related changes in Purkinje fiber action potential of adult dogs. Circ Res 43:931, 1978.
9. Lakatta EG: Age-related alterations in the cardiovascular response to adrenergic mediated stress. Fed Proc 39:3173, 1980.
10. Zeigler MG, Lake CR, Kobin LJ: Plasma noradrenaline increases with age. Nature 261:333, 1976.
11. Fleg JL, Kennedy HL: Cardiac arrhythmias in healthy elderly population. Chest 81:3, 1982.
12. Port S, Cobb FR, Coleman RD, Jones RH: Effect of age on the response of the left ventricular ejection fraction to exercise. N Engl Med 303:1133, 1980.
13. Pomerance A: Cardiac pathology in the elderly. *In* Noble RJ, Rothbaum DA (eds.): Geriatric Cardiology. Philadelphia, F. A. Davis Co., 1981, p. 9.
14. Latting CA, Silverman ME: Acute myocardial infarction in hospitalized patients over age 70. Am Heart J 100:311, 1980.
15. Pathy MS: Clinical presentation of myocardial infarction in the elderly. Br Heart J 29:190, 1967.
16. Kannel WB, Castelli WP, McNarmara PM, et al: Role of blood pressure in the development of congestive heart failure. The Framingham Study. N Engl Med 287:781, 1972.
17. Selzer A, Pasternak RD: Congenital and valvular heart disease. *In* Noble RJ, Rothbaum DA (eds.): Geriatric Cardiology. Philadelphia, F. A. Davis Co., 1981, p. 169.
18. Goodwin JF: The frontier of cardiomyopathy. Br Heart J 48:1, 1982.
19. Whiting RB, Powell WJ, Dinsmore RE, Sanders CA: Idiopathic hypertrophic subaortic stenosis in the elderly. N Engl J Med 285:196, 1971.
20. Durack DT: Infective and non-infective endocarditis. *In* Hurst JW (ed.): The Heart. New York, McGraw Hill, 1982, p. 1250.
21. Antimicrobial prophylaxis: Prevention of bacterial endocarditis. T Med Lett 19:40, 1977.
22. Kaplan EL, Anthony BF, Bisno A, et al: Prevention of bacterial endocarditis. Circulation 56:139A, 1977.
23. Pomerance A: Pathology of the heart with and without cardiac failure in the aged. Br Heart J 27:697, 1965.
24. Lev M: Anatomic basis for atrioventricular block. Am J Med 37:742, 1964.
25. Lenegre J: The pathology of complete atrioventricular block. Prog Cardiovasc Dis 6:317, 1964.
26. Pomerance A: Senile cardiac amyloidosis. Br Heart J 27:711, 1965.
27. Moss AJ, Davis RJ: Brady-tachy syndrome. Prog Cardiovasc Dis 16:439, 1974.
28. Moss AJ, Schwartz PJ: Delayed repolarization (QT or QTU prolongation) and malignant ventricular arrhythmias. Mod Concepts Cardiovasc Dis 51:85, 1982.
29. Wood P: Polyuria in paroxysmal tachycardiac and paroxysmal atrial flutter and fibrillation. Br Heart J 25:273, 1963.
30. Dash H, Johnson RA, Dinsmore RE, Harthorne JW: Cardiomyopathic syndrome due to coronary artery disease. I. Relation to angiographic extent of coronary disease and to remote myocardial infarction. Br Heart J 39:733, 1977.
31. Cannon PJ: The kidney in heart failure. N Engl J Med 296:26, 1977.

32. Bruschke AVG, Proudfit WL, Sones FM: Progress study of 590 consecutive non-surgical cases of coronary disease followed 5 – 9 years. I. Arteriographic correlations. Circulation 47:1147, 1973.
33. Bigger JT, Weld FM: Analysis of prognostic significance of ventricular arrhythmias after myocardial infarction. Shortcomings of Lown grading system. Br Heart J 45:717, 1981.
34. Kennedy HL: Comparison of ambulatory electrocardiography and exercise testing. Am J Cardiol 47:1359, 1981.
35. Laslett LJ, Amsterdam EA, Mason DT: Exercise testing in the geriatric patient. Internal Medicine. Sept. 1980, p. 53.
36. Wolthuis R, Groelicher V, Fischer J: A new practical clinical treadmill protocol. Am J Cardiol 39:697, 1977.
37. Gerstenblith G, Frederikson J, Yin F, et al: Echocardiographic assessment of a normal aging population. Circulation 56:273, 1979.
38. Johnston GD, McDevitt DG: Is maintenance digoxin necessary in patients with sinus rhythm? Lancet 1:567, 1979.
39. Moss AJ, Davis HT, Conard DL, et al: Digitalis-association cardiac mortality after myocardial infarction. Circulation 64:1150, 1981.
40. Bigger JT, Weld FM, Rolnitzky LM, Ferrick KJ: Is digitalis treatment harmful in the year after acute myocardial infarction? Circulation 64:83, 1981.
41. Hager WD, Genster P, Mayersohn M, et al: Digoxin-quinidine interraction. N Engl J Med 300:1238, 1979.
42. Podrid PJ, Schoeneberger A, Lown B: Medical intelligence. Congestive heart failure caused by oral disopyramide. N Engl J Med 302:614, 1980.
43. Castleden CM, Kaye CM, Parsons RL: The effect of age on plasma levels of propranolol and practolol in man. Br J Clin Pharmacol 2:303, 1975.
44. The Beta-Blocker Heart Attack Study Group: The B-blocker heart attack trial. JAMA 246:2073, 1981.
45. The Norwegian Multicenter Study Group: Timolol-induced reduction in mortality and reinfarction in patients surviving acute myocardial infarction. N Engl J Med 304:801, 1981.
46. Hjalmarson A, Elmfeldt D, Herlitz J, et al: Effect on mortality of metoprolol in acute myocardial infarction. A double-blind randomised trial. Lancet 2:823, 1981.
47. Andersen MP, et al: Effect of alprenolol on mortality among patients with definite or suspected acute myocardial infarction. Lancet 2:866, 1979.
48. Jolly WW, Isch JH, Shumacker HB: Cardiac surgery in the elderly. *In* Noble RJ, Rothbaum DA (eds.): Geriatric Cardiology. Philadelphia, F.A. Davis Co., 1981, p. 195.
49. Gruntzig A: Transluminal dilatation of coronary artery stenosis. Lancet 1:263, 1978.
50. Holmes DR, Vlietstra RE, Smith HC, et al: Restenosis following percutaneous transluminal coronary angioplasty (PTCA): A report from the NHLBI PTCA registry. Am J Cardiol 49:905, 1982.
51. Lakatta EG, Yin FCP: Myocardial aging: Functional alterations and related cellular mechanisms. Am J Physiol 242:H927, 1982.

## *Additional Reading*

1. Caird FI, Dall JLC, Kennedy RD (eds.): Cardiology in Old Age. New York and London, Plenum Press, 1976.
*An excellent compendium of articles on the physiologic, pathologic, and clinical aspects of cardiology in the elderly.*
2. Noble RJ, Rothbaum DA (eds.): Geriatric Cardiology. Philadelphia, F. A. Davis Co., 1981.
*An overview of geriatric cardiology, which focuses not only on population studies but also on the individual elderly patient with documented or potential cardiac disease. It is a clinically oriented book, with chapters contributed by outstanding experts in the field.*

## Chapter 30

# Pulmonary Disease

*Roy L. Donnerberg*
*Gerald F. Dixon*

Many parameters of lung function decline with aging. Although accumulative injury from environmental pollution and remote disease processes play some role, it is apparent that age-dependent alterations in the lung's mechanical functions and the lung's defense mechanisms compromise the respiratory system in the aged. These modifications of function contribute to the disabilities and limitations resulting from breathlessness in the elderly. Lung infection, including bronchitis and pneumonia, increases in incidence with aging, and pulmonary infections rank as the fourth leading cause of death in the elderly.[1,2] An understanding of the senescent-related declines in lung function and the unique aspects of pulmonary diseases in the aged is valuable in the care of the geriatric patient.

## AGE-ASSOCIATED ALTERATIONS IN MORPHOLOGY AND FUNCTION OF THE LUNG

Structural changes and the resultant physiologic consequences contribute greatly to the mechanical alterations that occur in the respiratory system with aging. Since lung size and form result from the interplay of retractile (elastic) forces of the lung and the expansive forces of the thoracic cage, alterations in the morphology and function of the aged lung can be attributed to the senescent changes in the thoracic cage as well as in the pulmonary parenchymal ultrastructure. The older lung has a decrease in base-to-apex diameter and an increase in the anterior and posterior diameter. Macroscopic mounts of lungs from older people show reductions in alveolar surface and enlargement of bronchioles and alveolar ducts.[3] Following age 30, there is approximately a 4 per cent loss of lung surface for each decade of life.[4] Ultrastructurally, lung collagen and elastin, which are largely responsible for the retractile properties of the lung, are quantitatively unchanged with age. However, the elastic forces of the lung are clearly reduced, rendering the lung more distensible and compliant. (The term compliance refers to changes in volume per given change in pressure.) These changes in elastic forces may be attributable to qualitative changes in elastin fibers, which do not show fragmentation but do exhibit an increase in cross linkages between the polypeptide chains with aging.[5-10]

In contrast to the lung itself, the thoracic cage becomes more elastic and less compliant with aging, and to a greater degree than the reverse is true in the lung. Thus, the compliance of the total system, i.e., lung and chest wall, is decreased with aging.

Another important component of lung function is surfactant. Surface-acting materials contribute significantly to the mechanical fòrces of the lung. At this time there is no study to show that the physiology of surfactant differs in the old lung compared with the young lung.[11-13] In addition, the importance of respiratory muscle performance in physiologic measurements and in the pathophysiology of lung diseases has been recently recognized.[14-16] The maximum power (static force) of respiratory muscles can be recorded as pressure change at the mouth with a given lung volume. Studies have revealed reduced inspiratory and expiratory forces with aging.[17] Endurance and coordination are other parameters of muscle function, and since respiratory muscles and skeletal muscles have physiologic similarities, declines in respiratory muscle performance in the elderly would be expected.[18]

It is evident that age-associated changes in the lung's form and function in the elderly are complex. However, in spite of individual variations, changes in pulmonary function occurring with aging can be summarized as listed in Table 30-1 and as diagrammed in Figures 30-1 and 30-2.

## *Lung Volumes and Airflows*

After maturity the compliance of the lung increases.[19] Since there is an interdependence of all structures in the lung, form and function of the small airways and alveolar spaces are significantly influenced by this alteration in lung recoil. Age-associated changes in the elastic recoil of the lung may play a dominant role in alterations in lung volumes, expiratory flows, and gas exchange. With advancing age, the total lung capacity (TLC) changes little or reduces slightly when corrections are made for reduced height of the older individual.[20] Residual volume (RV) and functional residual capacity (FRC) increase substantially, however. This occurs as a result of alterations in opposing compliance of the lung and chest wall as well as alterations in function of the small airways. It is of interest that the vital capacity (VC) has been found to have a direct relationship with longevity in older patients, and there is a strong association between mortality and reduced vital capacity, with and without the presence of cardiovascular diseases and emphysema.[21]

A number of studies have shown declines with old age in the forced expiratory volumes in one second ($FEV_1$), the maximum forced midexpiratory flow (FEF 25 to 75 per cent) and the maximal expiratory flow at 50 per cent of the vital capacity.[22-24] The driving pressure of the alveolar gas during expiration is a sum of the recoil pressure of the lung and the pressure applied around the lungs. As a result, decreased elastic recoil of the lung plays an important role in these age-associated declines in expiratory flows. Especially at low lung volumes, the decrease in lung elastic recoil necessary for the support of the small airways may also allow narrowing of airways, resulting in increased airway resistance, which contributes in turn to reduced expiratory flows.[25] In addition, respiratory muscle weakness and lack of muscle coordination can add to the reduced expiratory flow found in the aged.

## *Gas Exchange*

With reduced recoil, the lung settles within the chest in older people to a greater degree than in young adults, progressively reducing the caliber of the dependent airways and alveolar spaces. The small airways thus open at a larger lung volume and close earlier at a larger lung volume (closing volume) during tidal ventilation, resulting in reduced ventilation to the dependent alveolar spaces, where perfusion of capillary blood remains normal. This decrease in ventilation of alveolar spaces disturbs the important delicate matching of ventilation ($\dot{V}_A$) and perfusion ($\dot{Q}$) and results in a low ventilation to perfusion ratio ($\dot{V}_A/\dot{Q}$). With less ventilation, less oxygen is delivered to the alveolar gas and the capillary blood.[26] Pulmonary capillary blood flowing from these regions is oxygen deficient, and overall low arterial oxygen tension

**Table 30-1.** AGE-ASSOCIATED CHANGES IN STUDIES OF PULMONARY FUNCTION AND ARTERIAL BLOOD GASES

| | |
|---|---|
| **Spirometry** | |
| $FEV_1$* | Decreased |
| Maximum expiratory flow at 50% VC † | Decreased |
| Maximum midexpiratory flow | Decreased |
| **Lung Volumes** | |
| Total lung capacity | Decreased (slightly) |
| Residual volume | Increased |
| Closing volume | Increased |
| **Diffusing Capacity** | Decreased |
| **Alveolar-Arterial Oxygen Gradient** | Increased |
| **Arterial Blood Gases** | |
| pH | Unchanged |
| $Pa_{CO_2}$ | Unchanged |
| $Pa_{O_2}$ | Decreased |

* $FEV_1$ = forced expiratory volumes in one second.
† VC = vital capacity.

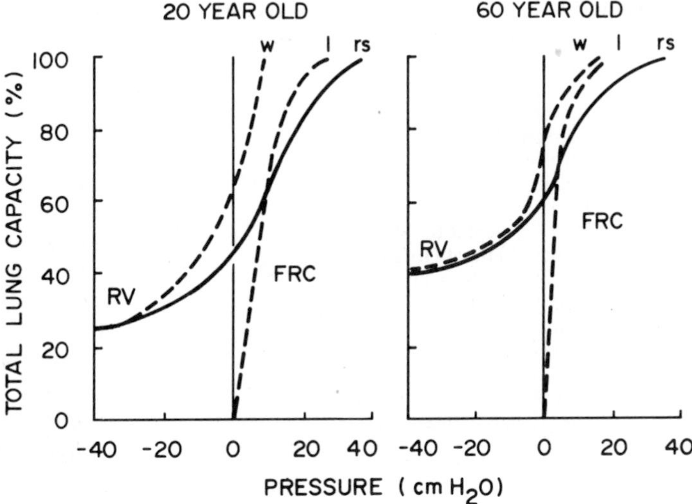


**Figure 30–1.** This figure diagrams the relationships between lung volumes as noted and the respective pressures in the young and old. The lung (l) of older people expands to a larger volume per given pressure change than that of young adults. The chest wall (w) requires greater pressure change per given volume change in the elderly. The total system (rs) in the elderly is less compliant. (From Murray L (ed.): The Normal Lung. Philadelphia, W.B. Saunders Company, 1976. Reproduced with permission.)

(hypoxemia) results.[27] Although mild hypoxemia is common with aging, the carbon dioxide excretion remains adequate and the arterial carbon dioxide tensions remain normal.

With aging, there is a reduction in the diffusing capacity of the lung ($DL_{CO}$) associated with a decline in alveolar surface area and capillary bed.[4,28] Aging also affects the control of ventilation. Elderly men have decreased ventilatory responses to both hypoxia and hypercapnia.[29] Exercise capacity, defined as maximum oxygen consumption, also decreases with age.[20] This decrease in exercise capability is a reflection of changes in the combined cardiopulmonary systems.[30] In spite of this decreasing capability, training and conditioning can result in high levels of fitness in older men.[31]

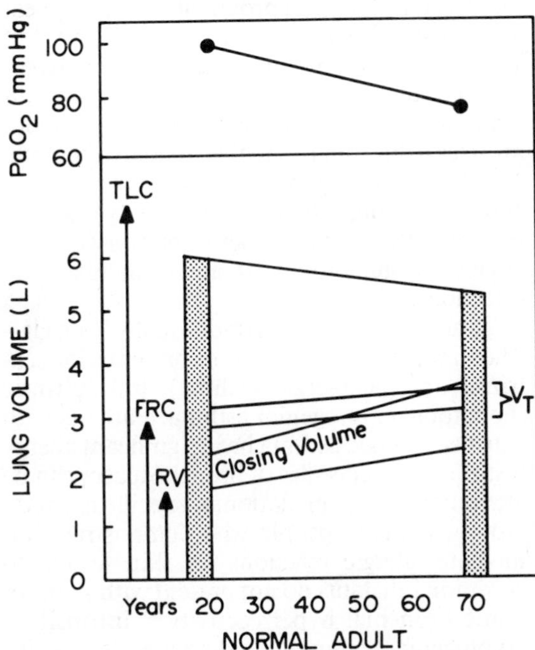


**Figure 30–2.** This figure shows relative changes in different lung volumes with age. Note the dramatic alterations in residual volume (RV) and closing volumes. The functional residual capacity (FRC) may increase slightly and the tidal volume ($V_T$) remains about the same. The total lung capacity (TLC) decreases slightly. Together with these changes there is a decrease in the $Pa_{O_2}$ (resting—room air) with age. (From Pontoppidan H: Acute respiratory failure in the adult. N Engl J Med 287:692, 1972. Reproduced by permission of the New England Journal of Medicine.)

## AGE-ASSOCIATED ALTERATIONS IN LUNG DEFENSE SYSTEMS

The lung has a close interface with pollutants of the ambient air and is repeatedly exposed to aspiration of foreign material. Multiple systems of defense against both intrinsic and extrinsic insults have developed. The major respiratory tract defense system against extrinsic induced injury are listed in Table 30–2. It is readily apparent that the elderly are frequently predisposed to impairments in these delicate systems. Mucous transport by the mucociliary system, which is responsible for the cleaning action in proximal airways, is reduced in elderly people with chronic lung disease.[32] Dehydration, commonly found in the debilitated geriatric patient, further compromises this function. Transfer of IgA across the nasal epithelium is reduced in the aged; this may also occur in the lower respiratory tract.[33] T-cell mediated defense mechanisms have been found to be defective in certain older individuals. This was found to be associated with increased mortality from lung infec-

**Table 30-2.** LUNG DEFENSE SYSTEMS

| |
|---|
| **Anatomy** |
| Turbulence |
| Aerosol impaction |
| Gas scrubbing |
| **Mechanics** |
| Cough |
| Expiratory flow |
| Irritant receptor threshold |
| **Normal Flora of Oropharynx** |
| **Mucociliary System** |
| Ciliary action |
| Mucous viscosity |
| **Alveolar and Airway Cells** |
| Macrophages—phagocytosis |
| Lymphocytes—antibody production |
| Neutrophils—phagocytosis |

tions.[34] Normal flora of the oropharynx change with aging and debilitation. In persons of advanced age, especially those in dependent-living life-styles, gram-negative bacilli can colonize the oropharynx.[35] Correlated with this is the observed higher incidence of and mortality from gram-negative bacillary pneumonias in the aged.[36,37] Bentley[38] has drawn attention to the possible influence of age-associated lung hypoxia and the function of the alveolar macrophages in the aged, since these cells are deleteriously affected by hypoxia.[38] The clinical applications of these aspects of lung function are obvious. Since nutrition and hydration influence immunity, muscular strength, and mucous membrane function, the nutritional state of the elderly should be evaluated regularly and corrected when indicated. Maneuvers such as elevation of the head of the bed, purêed diets, adequate hydration, and proper oral hygiene are all simple preventive measures to reduce pulmonary infections. Specific aspects of pulmonary infections are covered in Chapters 44 and 45.

## ASTHMA, CHRONIC BRONCHITIS, AND EMPHYSEMA IN THE ELDERLY

Although asthma, chronic bronchitis, and pulmonary emphysema vary in etiology, these diseases present with similar manifestations of small airway obstruction. Increased expiratory airflow resistance resulting from narrowing of the airway lumen can be associated with spasm of the smooth muscle within the walls of the airways, mucosal inflammation with edema and secretions, or loss of centrifugal support of the peripheral airways. In these diseases, one or more of these mechanisms of airway obstruction may exist. Chronic obstructive lung diseases are of greater importance as causes of disability than as causes of death. As a result of improved medical care and increased survival, obstructive lung diseases are increasingly common in geriatric patients. The prevalence of these diseases in the population segment over 60 years is approximately 30 per 1000 persons for asthma, 40 per 1000 persons for chronic bronchitis, and 60 per 1000 men for emphysema.[39] The mortality from these diseases increases with age from approximately 200 per 100,000 for people between 65 and 70 years to 450 per 100,000 for those over age 75.[40]

### *Asthma*

Although chronic bronchitis and emphysema are three times more common than asthma in the elderly, the pathophysiology of asthma serves as an example of the reversible mechanisms of airway obstruction in these diseases. Asthma is characterized by hyperreactivity of the airways. Receptors within the upper respiratory tract, larynx, and proximal bronchi appear to initiate reflexes of bronchoconstriction.[41-44] The basic pathophysiology in asthma is hyperactivity and hyperresponsiveness of various structures of the bronchi, including smooth muscles, cilia, and bronchial glands. In asthma, this degree of hyperactivity may vary greatly and rapidly. Bronchial hyperreactivity is seen in patients with asthma, upper respiratory tract allergies, chronic bronchitis, and bronchial, viral infections.

Clinically, asthma has traditionally been classified according to patterns of presentation: extrinsic (atopic-allergic asthma) and intrinsic (nonatopic-cryptogenic) asthma. Patients with extrinsic allergic asthma have significant allergy histories, and episodes of bronchospasm can be attributed to the inhalation of specific agents.[45] However, many people who demonstrate immediate allergic reactions on skin testing to common inhalants do not present with symptomatic bronchial hyperreactivity.[46] Intrinsic or cryptogenic asthma characteristically begins suddenly, usually in adult life, and is not associated with skin test reactivity to inhaled antigens. With provocative aerosol challenges, nonspecific agents (methacholine-histamine-citric acid, etc.) cause minimal bronchial reactivity in normal patients, but a more pronounced hyperresponsiveness and bronchospasm in all asthmatics. Specific inhaled agents (antigenic inhalants) cause hyperresponsiveness only in persons with extrinsic allergic asthma.[47-49]

Elderly patients with asthma frequently complain of uncomfortable and distressing breathlessness. Characteristically, this occurs episodically. Dyspnea in asthma may develop very quickly as a result of exposure to a number of noxious stimuli, including ambient air thermal differences, aerosols, and fumes. Wheezing and dyspnea while the patients is at rest are the clinical hallmarks of this disorder. Cough and mucoid sputum production are frequently prominent symptoms in asthma; not uncommonly, chronic cough may be the only presenting symptom.

The physical findings in asthmatics include an increased respiratory rate, prolongation of expiration, use of accessory respiratory muscles, and wheezing. With marked airway narrowing, as seen in severe asthma attacks, total air movement may be reduced, and the lung may be greatly expanded because of trapped air. These two phenomena result in less sound production and reduced transmission of sounds to the chest wall. Thus, wheezing by auscultation may be markedly reduced or totally absent in advanced states of bronchospasm. Other causes of airway obstruction and pulmonary edema may also cause wheezing. More reliable methods of grading the degree of bronchospasm in asthma include evaluation of the degree of work of accessory respiratory muscles, increased pulsus paradoxus, and decreased peak expiratory flows.[50] Pulmonary function studies in asthmatics show reduced expiratory flows, which may improve markedly after use of bronchodilator drugs. During acute attacks the residual volume (RV) and total lung capacity (TLC) are increased while the diffusing capacity ($DL_{CO}$) remains normal. Chest radiographs usually show hyperinflation of the lungs.

Long-term therapy should begin with avoidance of inhalation of noxious agents, especially antigenic dust for those patients with extrinsic allergic asthma. Immunotherapy, with the injection of minute quantities of antigens, may be helpful in patients with allergic asthma.[51,52] However, therapy for asthma is largely pharmacologic. The majority of elderly patients with asthma are treated with oral or inhaled bronchodilator drug therapy. Cromolyn sodium may have a role in the treatment of some patients, and steroids are also effective. Therapy should be staged according to the patient's symptomatic requirements and responses. The overall goal is to give the patient sufficient reduction of bronchial spasm and cough to allow an acceptable life-style.

For bronchodilator drug therapy, $beta_2$-adrenergic drug agonists may be used initially and are well tolerated in the elderly.[53,54] Metaproterenol, terbutaline, and albuterol in the recommended dosages are the most commonly used oral compounds because of their airway selectivity and prolonged action. Administration of these drugs by aerosol allows for few symptomatic side effects.[55] However, the elderly patient may have problems coordinating inspiration with the inhaler. Reservoir devices are now marketed to help in the administration of these drugs. Theophylline is a bronchodilator that is available in many forms, some producing sustained blood levels, and thus allowing a convenient once-or twice-a-day dose. Theophylline is metabolized in the liver. Old age, liver congestion, and use of cimetidine and erythromycin are some of the many factors that decrease metabolism of the theophyllines. Toxic levels are considered to be above the range 18 to 20 $\mu$ per milliliter. All patients should be informed to reduce oral dosages if toxic symptoms of headache, nausea, and vomiting occur, and serum level monitoring is recommended in older patients, especially during acute illnesses. For intravenous therapy, aminophylline is the most frequently used preparation. In the elderly, because of reduced aqueous body compartments and reduced metabolism, 3 mg per kilogram of theophylline (based on ideal body weight) over 20 to 30 minutes is a recommended loading dose, with 0.45 mg per kilogram or less per hour as a maintenance dose for acute attacks.[56-59] During intravenous administration, frequent monitoring of blood drug levels is recommended. Theophylline may have other advantages in addition to its bronchodilatory action. These include increased strength and endurance of the diaphragm and central neurogenic respiratory stimulation.[60] Combinations of terbutaline and aminophylline orally provide for synergistic activity, thus allowing for fewer side reactions.[61]

Corticosteroids are indicated in patients with refractory bronchospasm. For outpatient therapy, prednisone in doses of 10 to 20 mg daily in the morning or on alternate mornings may be effective in relieving bronchospasm in patients who respond inadequately to theophylline and beta-agonist preparations. Steroids have been found to reduce bronchial inflammation and to upgrade adrenergic receptor activity.[62] After prolonged administration, steroids should be reduced gradually, to prevent the complications of adrenal insufficiency. Corticosteroids may also be given via the inhaled route as beclomethasone. The usual dosage is two inhalations three or four times daily. The obvious advantage of this form of therapy is the relative lack of systemic side effects.[63] Problems with pharyngeal colonization with *Candida* have been encountered, but the incidence of pharyngitis may be reduced by having the patient gargle with water after each use of the inhaler.

Cromolyn sodium blocks release of vasobronchoactive materials from lung cells.[64] It has been used to help prevent attacks of bronchial reactivity rather than reverse established bronchospasm.[65] This drug may be added to the regimen of asthmatics not responding to other drug therapy. It may block certain mechanisms of hyperreactivity more effectively than other drugs.[66] The recommended dosage is 20 mg delivered to the bronchi by the inhalation of either an aerosolized solution or a dry powder.

Asthmatics are subject to acute exacerbations of their condition, manifested by severe, and at times life-threatening, airway obstruction. These acute episodes may be related to infections or exposure to irritating fumes and aerosols. Patients present with increasing severity of airway obstruction and the $FEV_1$ becomes progressively reduced.[67] When the $FEV_1$ approaches 1.5 L or less, severe impairment of lung ventilation/perfusion ratios and serious hypoventilation may occur, resulting in $CO_2$ retention and respiratory acidosis. This condition of status asthmaticus is associated with decreasing responsiveness and/or decreasing numbers of adrenergic receptors. Large doses of corticosteroids can be helpful and lifesaving. Prednisone may be given orally in doses of 60 mg or more daily during these acute episodes. In more severe states, intravenous administration of hydrocortisone, 100 mg every 2 to 4 hours, or methylprednisolone, 20 mg per kilogram every 6 hours, can be carried out.[68] Ventilatory assistance may be necessary when severe $CO_2$ retention with respiratory acidosis develops as a result of severe bronchial obstruction and/or respiratory muscle fatigue.

## *Chronic Bronchitis*

Current criteria for the diagnosis of chronic bronchitis include the presence of excess bronchial mucus and/or a chronic productive cough, not due to other diseases, of 3 months duration for more than 2 successive years.[4] There is an increasing incidence of chronic bronchitis with age.[69] This may result from accumulative effects of inhaled air pollution and cigarette smoke but also may reflect age-associated changes in the mucous and bronchial defense mechanisms.

Patients with chronic bronchitis present with symptoms of chronic cough, frequently productive of sputum which, during acute exacerbations, may be colored and purulent. Auscultation of the chest in bronchitis may reveal basilar inspiratory crackles (rales) and sonorous rhonchi. Cor pulmonale with congestive heart failure is frequent and recurrent.

Patients with chronic bronchitis experience early and severe hypercapnia and hypoxemia. It has been postulated that these individuals lack the neurogenic drive to increase minute ventilation necessary to compensate for the increase in dead space ventilation and ventilation/perfusion mismatching. However, the pathophysiology of respiratory failure in chronic bronchitis is probably much more complex.[70,71] The alveolar spaces remain intact and are well perfused in this condition. Airway obstruction due to mucosal edema and secretions, bronchospasm, and/or increases in dead space ventilation results in pronounced reduction of gas transport. Therefore, hypoxemia can be severe and can give rise to polycythemia and increase pulmonary artery hypertension, resulting in cor pulmonale. In this condition, lung volumes change little, although some increase in residual volume (RV) may occur. Expiratory flows are reduced and may improve slightly with bronchodilatation. The diffusing capacity ($DL_{CO}$) remains near normal. Pulmonary function tests may help in identifying the predominant disease processes in patients (Table 30–3). The chest radiograph may show a prominent heart with increased vascular markings.

Therapy of chronic bronchitis is directed toward reducing inhaled irritants. An important first step is to encourage patients to stop smoking. Although reversibility of bronchial constriction is not as great as in asthmatics, bronchodilator drug therapy may improve symptoms. Long-term steroid therapy as described previously may be beneficial in some patients. Medications should be used in a stepwise manner and given clinical trials. Especially in patients who have symptoms of cough and sputum production, full dose antibiotic therapy directed toward the predominant bacterial organism may be helpful. This therapy may be directed initially empirically toward the most common sputum isolates of *Hemophilus influenzae* and *Streptococcus pneumoniae.* With acute exacerbations, sputum cultures and specific antimicrobial therapy are indicated.

## *Emphysema*

Pulmonary emphysema is defined as a condition characterized by tissue destruction and air

**Table 30-3.** PULMONARY FUNCTION STUDIES IN CHRONIC OBSTRUCTIVE PULMONARY DISEASES

| | Asthma | Chronic Bronchitis | Emphysema |
|---|---|---|---|
| TLC* | large | normal | large |
| $FEV_1$† | reduced | reduced | reduced |
| Reversibility of Obstruction | marked | moderate | minimal |
| $DL_{CO}$‡ | normal | normal | reduced |

* TLC = total lung capacity.
† $FEV_1$ = forced expiratory volumes in one second.
‡ $DL_{CO}$ = diffusing capacity of the lung.

space enlargement distal to terminal bronchioles.[4] Although cellular and subcellular mechanisms for this tissue destruction can only be theorized at this time, present evidence suggests a delicate balance between the tissue defense mechanisms, which lead in turn to destructive processes, and body mechanisms developed to limit tissue destruction. Cigarette smoke and perhaps other toxic materials induce macrophages and other cells to release proteolytic enzymes that deleteriously alter lung tissue. These enzymatic activities are modified by a protective $alpha_1$-globulin present in body tissues. The effectiveness of this protective system undoubtedly varies greatly among individuals, especially in certain persons in whom a genetically linked deficiency of $alpha_1$ is found. Clinically, emphysema presents most frequently in middle-aged or older patients with a normal $alpha_1$-globulin serum level who have been heavy cigarette smokers.

It is of interest that there are similarities in the alterations of lung functions with the normal aging processes and the pathologic processes of emphysema. An increased incidence with age of significant emphysema in the lungs of nonbronchitics has been reported.[4] Whether this is entirely age-dependent or is a result of accumulative environmental insults to pulmonary tissue is not clear. At this time, emphysema is considered to result from disease processes and not normal aging.

Patients with significant pulmonary emphysema present with breathlessness and undue dyspnea. Initially this is noticed with physical exertion. The escalation of symptoms is usually more rapid in patients who continue to smoke and may be slowed considerably in individuals who stop smoking.[72] Physical findings include increased respiratory rates, prolonged expiration, use of accessory respiratory muscles with inspiration, and use of abdominal muscles during expiration. Patients with severe emphysema are usually thin and have reduced muscle mass. The chest and lungs are enlarged. Breath sounds are generally reduced. The chest radiograph shows hyperinflated lungs and a narrow cardiac silhouette.

The basic pathologic picture is unevenly distributed areas of tissue destruction in the lung. This loss of both the alveolar air space and capillary bed does not disturb ventilation/perfusion matching significantly unless advanced disease is present. These tissue alterations result in lack of support of small airways, particularly during expiration. It is important to remember that some degree of bronchial wall inflammation with spasm may be present.[73] Patients with predominant emphysema and minimal bronchitis may have only slightly reduced arterial oxygen and slightly reduced $CO_2$ gas tension during the early stages of these diseases. This does not result in cyanosis or alveolar hypoxia and pulmonary hypertension. Thus cor pulmonale is a late complication, associated with severe emphysematous change resulting from irreversible reduction of capillary bed as well as vasoconstriction related to alveolar hypoxia. Polycythemia is not common. Pulmonary function studies in emphysema patients show reduced expiratory flows ($FEV_1$ and peak flows), with little change following administration of bronchodilators. The TLC, RV, and FRC are grossly increased because of abnormal function of small airways and loss of lung recoil. The early and usually severe reduction of the ($DL_{CO}$) in the face of an enlarging lung is particularly characteristic of emphysema.

## THERAPEUTIC PROGRAM FOR ELDERLY PATIENTS WITH CHRONIC OBSTRUCTIVE PULMONARY DISEASE

The management of chronic obstruction airways disease in the elderly needs to be individualized according to symptomatology, physiologic impairment, and other concomitant disorders. Cigarettes and other environmental pollutants must be avoided. Influenza and pneumococcal prophylaxis immunizations are important. Theophylline therapy may reduce airway resistance, serve as a ventilatory stimulant, and improve respiratory muscle performance. Other bronchodilator therapy, including use of albuterol, terbutaline, or metaproterenol, can be carried out depending upon the patient's symptomatic response. In advanced or severe cases of chronic airways obstruction, oral or inhaled steroids may give symptomatic improvement in some patients. A trial of prednisone (10 to 60 mg per day in the morning daily or on alternate days) in those patients who are refractory to other forms of therapy may be initiated. Some patients show significant symptomatic and physiologic improvement, and steroid therapy may be considered.[74,75] Steroid therapy is given preferably every other day in the morning for long-term therapy, and the dosage should be low, 10 mg or less, either daily or every other day. Antibiotics (ampicillin, sulfamethoxazole-trimethoprim, or tetracycline) should be used, especially during exacerbations of bronchial infections. Patient or family education regarding timing of medication and possible side effects is essential for optimal therapeutic benefits.

Acute exacerbations of respiratory failure in patients with chronic airways obstruction may require hospitalization. Bronchopulmonary infection or congestive heart failure are responsible for the majority of these exacerbations and should be treated appropriately. Intravenous medications (bronchodilators, diuretics, antibiotics, steroids) generally result in a more rapid and predictable response than oral therapy. Supplemental oxygen enrichment of inspired gas optimizes oxygenation, may reduce the work of breathing, and may serve as a bronchodilator. Oxygen therapy may reduce the neurogenic respiratory drive, especially in patients with $CO_2$ retention. With severe hypoxemia, hypercapnia, or respiratory acidosis, endotracheal intubation and ventilatory support may be necessary. The decision to intubate a patient should be based upon the expected reversibility of the acute episode, the patient's quality of life, and the prognosis of any underlying conditions. Since acute disease may result in irreversible pulmonary damage, some patients after intubation may be committed to continuous mechanical ventilation following this therapy. The medical, psychological, social, and financial ramifications of permanent ventilatory assistance add considerable complexities to the clinical management of acute respiratory failure in patients with advanced emphysema.

In chronic respiratory failure, in addition to pharmacologic therapy, supplemental oxygen is of proven benefit. In patients with cor pulmonale with a $Pa_{O_2}$ of less than 55 mm or 60 mm Hg (resting—room air), supplemental oxygen (1 to 4 L per minute via nasal cannula) 24 hours a day significantly improves function and survival.[76] Patients with $CO_2$ retention may be dependent upon hypoxemia for their ventilatory drive, and in those persons, long-term low flow supplemental oxygen is indicated for correction of hypoxemia but must be cautiously prescribed and monitored by measurement of arterial blood gases.

The psychologic effects of continuous supplemental oxygen must not be underestimated. Unlike other forms of medication, which only slightly alter a patient's life-style, supplemental oxygen can be physically cumbersome, resulting in restricted mobility. Additionally, the attention generated by family, friends, and acquaintances may be socially embarrassing and anxiety provoking. Thorough patient and family education regarding the reasons and benefits of supplemental oxygen is helpful. Fortunately, great advances have been made in the size and appearance of respiratory equipment, which helps in the acceptance of oxygen therapy. However, the physician needs to be mindful of mental depression or rejection when oxygen is prescribed.

The rehabilitation of the patient with chronic obstructive pulmonary disease (COPD) is very involved.[77,78] The approach should be multidisciplinary, including the physician, respiratory technologist, clinical nurse specialist, nutritionist, and physical therapist. Understanding the underlying pathophysiology helps the patient and his or her family anticipate and cope with associated problems. The diet should insure adequate calories to prevent loss of muscle protein and strength. In some patients with significant sputum production, percussion and postural drainage of the chest may be helpful to mobilize secretions. Physical conditioning programs utilizing treadmills or walking are beneficial in keeping patients motivated and physically active. Patients who are receiving supplemental oxygen should increase their flow rates by 1 to 3 L per minute while exercising to prevent oxygen desaturation. Respiratory muscle exercises utilizing the diaphragm and abdominal and accessory muscles result in improved exercise capacity in some patients.[79] There are few indications for mucolytics, expectorants, and intermittent positive pressure breathing.

## PULMONARY EMBOLI IN THE ELDERLY

Sudden death occurs more commonly among the elderly than any other age group. One frequent cause of sudden death in this age group is pulmonary embolism.[80] Pulmonary embolism is somewhat unique in that it is a complication rather than a primary disease. The vast majority of emboli originate as thrombi in the lower extremities, although fat, tumor, or air can also embolize to the lung.

Factors that predispose to pulmonary emboli are especially prevalent in older people. These include prolonged bed rest, congestive heart failure, fractures or other injuries to the lower extremities, chronic deep venous insufficiency of the legs, and carcinoma (Table 30-4). Symptoms of pulmonary emboli vary from indolent to explosive in the elderly. In the acute syndrome, patients classically present with the sudden onset of dyspnea, chest pain, and hemoptysis. However, more common presentations in the elderly include apparent progression of underlying cardiac and/or pulmonary disease, transient dyspnea or chest discomfort, syncope, atypical pleural effusions, and atypical bronchopneumonia (Table 30-5). Ante mortem, the diagnosis of pulmonary embolism is accurately made in only approximately 50 per cent of cases when compared with autopsy findings.[81]

Blood gases may be misleading as arterial oxygenation decreases with age. Impedance plethysmography of the leg is helpful in detecting deep vein thrombosis of the thighs and is also noninvasive and well tolerated by the elderly. Venography is usually well tolerated but is associated with the risk of thrombophlebitis.[82] Ventilation/perfusion isotopic lung scanning is helpful in the evaluation of suspected pulmonary emboli, provided that there is no underlying lung disease. This may be diagnostic if multiple, nonmatched areas are present.[83] The ventilation portion of this study is often difficult for the older patient because of the cooperation that is required.

**Table 30-4.** CONDITIONS THAT PREDISPOSE TO VENOUS STASIS/ THROMBOSIS IN THE ELDERLY

| |
|---|
| Prolonged bed rest |
| Congestive heart failure |
| Trauma to the lower extremities |
| Chronic venous insufficiency of the lower extremities |
| Varicosity of veins |
| Carcinoma (especially pancreatic and bronchogenic) |

**Table 30-5.** UNCOMMON PRESENTATIONS OF PULMONARY EMBOLI IN THE ELDERLY

| |
|---|
| Progression of underlying cardiac disease |
| Progression of underlying pulmonary disease |
| Transient dyspnea |
| Transient chest pain |
| Palpitations |
| Syncope |
| Change in mental status |
| Congestive heart failure refractory to therapy |
| Atypical pleural effusions |
| Atypical pneumonias |

Pulmonary angiography is the best means of establishing the diagnosis of pulmonary embolism. In the elderly, the risk of complications, such as arrhythmias, congestive heart failure, and cardiac perforation, is increased.[84] High pulmonary artery pressure, which is commonly found in patients with chronic obstructive pulmonary disease, many prevent the performance of this procedure. An additional risk is radiocontrast-induced renal failure, which occurs more frequently in patients with renal insufficiency, dehydration, and diabetes mellitus, all of which are commonly encountered in the elderly.

Chronic pulmonary embolization may be difficult to diagnose in the geriatric patient. Presentations include further worsening of heart failure, progression of COPD, arrhythmias, hyperventilation, signs of pulmonary hypertension, and renal deterioration. These facts should be kept in mind in the evaluation of an elderly individual with lung disease.

Initial therapy of pulmonary embolism is heparin. Contraindications for this therapy, including recent cerebrovascular accidents, bleeding diathesis, and peptic ulcer, are occasionally found in the elderly and necessitate placement of an inferior vena cava (IVC) umbrella or IVC plication/ligation.[85] Both of these procedures may not be curative, and each has attendant complications or side effects.

Heparin therapy should be given by constant infusion at a relatively high concentration to avoid fluid overload (10,000 units heparin per 250 ml of IV solution). The partial thromboplastin time (PTT) should be maintained at approximately one and a half to two times normal. The patient should be kept at bed rest for approximately 1 week and then allowed to walk with assistance. The platelet count should be monitored for heparin-induced thrombocytopenia. Since most elderly patients will continue to be predisposed to the recurrence of emboli, long-term anticoagulation therapy should be considered. Sodium warfarin (Coumadin) is the drug of choice because it can be taken orally. However, in the elderly, this drug is often difficult to regulate because of dietary indiscretions and other medications that interfere with Coumadin activity. In addition, patients over age 60 with significant medical-surgical disorders are at increased risk of bleeding. The prothrombin time (PT) should be maintained at one and a half to two times normal, with frequent determinations to avoid excessive anticoagulation. Thrombolytic therapy (streptokinase or urokinase) can also be cautiously considered in the treatment of pulmonary embolism in the elderly, although there have been no studies that have shown that this mode of treatment results in improved mortality compared with conventional heparin therapy.[86]

Prophylaxis for pulmonary emboli can be of significant benefit to an older person. Elderly patients with fractures of the lower extremities who will be immbolized for 10 or more days, people with severe congestive heart failure, acute myocardial infarct patients, or major surgical candidates (especially abdominal, thoracic or gynecologic surgery) should be given 5000 units of heparin subcutaneously every 12 hours during the period of immobilization.[87]

## INTERSTITIAL LUNG DISEASE

The interstitial lung diseases are a heterogenous group of disorders that involve both the alveoli and lung parenchyma. There are over 130 disorders that are associated with the presence of fibrosis in the lung interstitium.[88,89] Among the known causes are occupational or environmental inhalants including silica, asbestos, and coal dust. Several chemotherapeutic agents including bleomycin, cyclophosphamide, methotrexate, and busulfan and certain antimicrobials such as nitrofurantoin can cause interstitial lung disorders. Congestive heart failure, infectious disorders, collagen diseases, and neoplastic diseases can also affect the interstitium of the lung. Patients over 65 years may also be at special risk for the development of pulmonary fibrosis because of repeated nocturnal aspiration.[90,91] The largest group of interstitial lung diseases are not associated with any known predisposing cause and are called idiopathic.

Presenting symptoms in the elderly commonly include severe dyspnea, cough, and systemic complaints referable to the underlying disorder. Physical examination may be nondiagnostic, but respiratory distress and inspiratory crackles (rales) are common. Chest radiographs of geriatric patients with interstitial lung disease are usually abnormal, showing evidence of nodular and/or reticular infiltrates. A lung biopsy not uncommonly demonstrates nonspecific alveolar and interstitial inflammation and fibrosis. If an offending agent can be identified, it should be avoided. A trial of corticosteroids (prednisone 40 to 60 mg per day) may relieve the dyspnea and cough. Oxygen therapy is indicated for those patients who demonstrate hypoxemia and/or severe respiratory distress. For a discussion of tuberculosis, pneumonia, and pulmonary carcinoma in the elderly, see Chapters 42, 44, and 45.

### References


1. Foy HM, Cooney MK, Allan I, Kenny GE: Rates of pneumonia during influenza epidemics in Seattle, 1964 to 1975. JAMA 241:253, 1979.
2. Bureau of the Census: A Monthly Chartbook of Social and Economic Trends. Washington, DC: Department of Commerce, September 1976.
3. Weibel ER: Morphometry of the Human Lung. New York, Academic Press, 1963, pp. 54–55.
4. Thurlbeck WM: Chronic Airflow Obstruction in Lung Disease. Philadelphia, W.B. Saunders Company, 1976, pp. 190–197, 12–95, 96–230.
5. Pierce JA, Ebert RV: Fibrous network of the lung and its changes with age. Thorax 20:469, 1965.
6. Adamson JS: An electron microscopic comparison of the connective tissue from the lungs of young and elderly subjects. Rev Resp Dis 98:399, 1968.
7. Sanberg LB, Soskel NT, Leslie JG: Elastin structure biosynthesis and relation to disease states. N Engl J Med 304:566, 1981.
8. Kohn RR: Changes in connective tissue. *In* Cander L, Moyer JH (eds.): Aging of the Lung. New York, Grune and Stratton, 1964, pp. 13–20.
9. Blumenthal HT, Yu Sy, Ridley AM: Comparison of aging changes in elastin tissue of the lungs and arteries. *In* Cander L, Meyer JH (eds.): Aging of the Lung. New York, Grune and Stratton, 1964, pp. 21–40.
10. Pierce JA: Biochemistry of aging in the lung. *In* Cander L, Meyer JH (eds.): Aging of the Lung. New York, Grune and Stratton, 1964, pp. 61–69.
11. Morgan TE: Pulmonary surfactant. N Engl J Med 284:1185, 1971.
12. Clements JA: Pulmonary surfactant. Am Rev Resp Dis 101:984, 1970.
13. King RJ: The surfactant systems of the lung. Fed Proc 33:2238, 1974.
14. Macklem PT, Roussos CS: Respiratory muscle fatigue: A cause of respiratory failure? Clin Sci 53:419, 1977.
15. Roussos CH, Macklem PT: The respiratory muscles. N Engl J Med 307:786, 1982.
16. Macklem PT: Respiratory muscles: The vital pump. Chest 78:753, 1980.
17. Black LE, Hyatt RE: Maximal respiratory pressure: Normal values and relationship to age and sex. Am Rev Resp Dis 99:696, 1969.

18. Shock NW, Norris AH: Neuromuscular coordination as a factor in age changes in muscular exercise. *In* Jokl E, Brunner D (eds.): Physical Activity and Aging. Munich, Karger, 1970, pp. 92–99.
19. Turner JM, Mead J, Wohl ME: Elasticity of human lungs in relation to age. J Appl Physiol 33:711, 1972.
20. Murray JF: The Normal Lung. Philadelphia, W.B. Saunders Company, 1976, pp. 307–324.
21. Kannel WB, Hubert H: Vital capacity as a biomarker of aging. Biological Markers of Aging, NIH Publication No. 82-2221, Washington, DC, Government Printing Office, 1982, pp. 145–160.
22. Knudson RJ, Lebowitz MD, Holberg CJ, et al: Changes in normal maximal expiratory flow volume curve with growth and aging. Am Rev Resp Dis 127:725, 1983.
23. Knudson RJ, Slatin RC, Lebowitz MD, et al: The maximal expiratory flow-volume curve. Am Rev Resp Dis 113:587, 1976.
24. Milne JS, Williamson J: Respiratory function tests in older people. Clin Sci 42:371, 1972.
25. Gelb AF, Zamel N: Effect of aging on lung mechanics in healthy non-smokers. Chest 68:538, 1975.
26. Hozland J, Milic-Emili J, Macklem PT, et al: Regional distribution of pulmonary ventilation and perfusion in elderly subjects. J Clin Invest 47:81, 1968.
27. Kanber GJ, King FW, Eshchar YR, et al: The alveolar-arterial oxygen gradient in young and elderly men during air and oxygen breathing. Am Rev Resp Dis 97:376, 1968.
28. Georges R, Saumon G, Loiseau: The relationship of age to pulmonary membrane conductance and capillary blood volume. Am Rev Resp Dis 117:1069, 1978.
29. Peterson DA, Pack AI, Silage DA, et al: Effects of aging on ventilatory and occlusion pressure responses to hypoxia and hypercapnia. Am Rev Resp Dis 124:387, 1981.
30. Horvath SM, Borgia JF: Cardiopulmonary gas transport and aging. Am Rev Resp Dis 129 (Suppl):S68, 1984.
31. Cantwell JD, Watt EW: Extreme cardiopulmonary fitness in old age. Chest 65:357, 1974.
32. Santa Cruz R, Landa J, Hirsch J, et al: Tracheal mucous velocity in normal men and patients with obstructive lung disease: Effects of terbutaline. Am Rev Resp Dis 109:458, 1974.
33. Alford RH: Effects of chronic bronchopulmonary disease and aging on human nasal secretion IgA concentrations. J Immunology 10:984, 1968.
34. Roberts-Thomson IC, Whittingham S, Youngchaiyud U, et al: Ageing immune response and mortality. Lancet 368, 1974.
35. Valenti WM, Trudell RH, Bentley DW: Factors predisposing to oropharyngeal colonization with gram negative bacilli in the aged. N Engl J Med 298:1108, 1978.
36. Oswald NC, Simon G, Shooter RA: Pneumonia in hospital practice. Br J Dis Chest 55:109, 1961.
37. Garb JL, Brown RB, Garb JR, et al: Differences in etiology of pneumonias in nursing home and community patients. JAMA 240:2169, 1978.
38. Bentley DW: Pathogenesis of bacterial pneumonia in the elderly: The effect of normal aging processes. *In* Stul, K (ed): Geriatric Education: Lexington, MA, Collamore Press, 1981.
39. U.S. Department of Health, Education and Welfare: Prevalence of Selected Chronic Respiratory Conditions. Vital Health Statistics No. 84, Washington, DC, Government Printing Office, 1970.
40. U.S. Veterans Study. Am Med News, June 8, 1984.
41. Boushey HA, Holtzman MJ, Sheller JR, et al: Bronchial hyperreactivity. Am Rev Resp Dis 121:389, 1980.
42. Leff A: Pathophysiology of asthmatic bronchoconstriction. Chest 82 (Suppl):S13, 1982.
43. Deal EC, McFadden ER, Ingram RH, et al: Airway responsiveness to cold air and hyperpnea in normal subjects and in those with hay fever and asthma. Am Rev Resp Dis 121:621, 1980.
44. Menkes HA: Airway reactivity and the need for a simple test. Am Rev Resp Dis 121:619, 1980.
45. Mathews KP: Respiratory atopic disease. JAMA 248:2587, 1982.
46. Burrows B, Lebowitz MD, Barbee RA: Respiratory disorders and allergy skin-test reactions. Ann Intern Med 84:134, 1976.
47. Salome CM, Schoeffel RE, Woolcock AJ: Effect of aerosol fenoterol on histamine and methacholine challenge in asthmatic subjects. Thorax 36:580, 1981.
48. Myers JR, Corrao WM, Braman SS: Clinical applicability of a methacholine inhalational challenge. JAMA 246:225, 1981.
49. Chatham M, Bleeker ER, Norman P, et al: A screening test for airways reactivity. Chest 82:15, 1982.
50. Fischl MA, Pitchenik A, Gardner LB: An index predicting relapse and need for hospitalization in patients with acute bronchial asthma. N Engl J Med 305:783, 1981.
51. Patterson R, Norman P, Van Metre T: Immunotherapy—immunomodulations. JAMA 248:2759, 1982.
52. Lichtenstein LM: An evaluation of the role of immunotherapy in asthma. Am Rev Resp Dis 117:191, 1978.
53. Webb-Johnson DC, Andrews JL: Bronchodilator therapy. N Engl J Med 297:476, 1977.
54. Paterson JW, Woolcock AJ, Shenfield GM: Bronchodilator drugs—state of the art. Am Rev Resp Dis 120:1149, 1979.
55. Larsson S, Svedymyr N: Bronchodilating effect and side effects of $beta_2$-adrenoceptor stimulants by different modes of administration. Am Rev Resp Dis 116:861, 1977.
56. Krivoy M, Alroy G: Maintenance oral theophylline therapy: suggested schedule in elderly patients. Respiration 40:233, 1980.
57. Jusko WJ, Koup JR, Vance JW, et al: Intravenous theophylline therapy: Nomogram guidelines. Ann Intern Med 86:400, 1977.
58. Weinberger M, Hendeles L, Bighley L: The relation of product formulation to absorption of oral theophylline. N Engl J Med 299:852, 1978.
59. Ziment I: Respiratory Pharmacology and Therapeutics. Philadephia, W.B. Saunders Company, 1978, pp. 190–218.
60. Aubier M, Detroyer A, Sampson M, et al: Aminophylline improves diaphragmatic contractility. N Engl J Med 305:249, 1981.
61. Wolfe JD, Tashkin DP, Calvarese B, et al: Bronchodilator effects of terbutaline and aminophylline alone and in combination in asthmatic patients. N Engl J Med 298:363, 1978.
62. Motulsky HJ, Insel PA: Adrenergic receptors in man. N Engl J Med 307:18, 1982.
63. Hodson ME, Batten JC, Clarke SW, et al: Beclomethasone dipropionate aerosol in asthma. Am Rev Resp Dis 110:403, 1974.
64. Burgher LW, Elliott MR, Kass I: A perspective on the role of cromolyn sodium as an antiasthmatic agent. Chest 60:210, 1971.
65. Breslin FJ, McFadden ER, Ingram RH: The effects of cromolyn sodium on the airway response to hyper-

pnea and cold air in asthma. Am Rev Resp Dis 122:11, 1980.

66. Pepys J: Basic mechanisms in acute and chronic allergic lung disease. Immunol Allergy Pract 3:13, 1981.
67. Weiss EB: Status Asthmaticus. Baltimore, University Park Press, 1978.
68. Tanaka RM, Santiago SM, Kuhn GJ, et al: Intravenous methylprednisolone in adults in status asthmaticus. Chest 82:438, 1982.
69. Freeman E: The Respiratory System. *In* Brocklehurst JC: Textbook of Geriatric Medicine and Gerontology. Edinburgh, Churchill Livingstone, 1978, pp. 433–449.
70. Murciano D, Aubier M, Milic-Emili J, et al: Central respiratory drive in acute respiratory failure of patients with chronic obstructive lung disease. Am Rev Resp Dis 122:191, 1980.
71. Aubier M, Murciano D, Milic-Emili J, et al: Effect of $O_2$ administration on ventilation and blood gases in acute respiratory failure of patients with chronic obstructive lung disease. Am Rev Resp Dis 122:747, 1980.
72. Fletcher C, Peto R, Tinker C, et al: The Natural History of Chronic Bronchitis and Emphysema. New York, Oxford University Press, 1976.
73. Thurlbeck WM: Smoking, airflow limitations, and the pulmonary circulation. Am Rev Resp Dis 122:183, 1980.
74. Mendella LA, Manfreda J, Warren CPW, et al: Steroid response in stable chronic obstructive pulmonary disease. Ann Intern Med 96:17, 1982.
75. Albert RK, Martin TR, Lewis SW: Controlled clinical trial of methylprednisolone in patients with chronic bronchitis and acute respiratory insufficiency. Ann Intern Med 92:753, 1980.
76. Trial Group: Continuous or nocturnal oxygen therapy in hypoxemic chronic obstructive lung disease. Ann Intern Med 93:391, 1980.
77. Lertzman MM, Cherniac RM: Rehabilitation of patients with chronic obstructive pulmonary disease. Am Rev Resp Dis 114:1145, 1976.
78. Hodgkin JE: Chronic obstructive pulmonary disease. Park Ridge, IL, American College of Chest Physicians, 1979, pp. 1–102.
79. Belman MJ, Mittman C: Ventilatory muscle training improves exercise capacity in chronic obstructive pulmonary patients. Am Rev Resp Dis 121:273, 1980.
80. Morrell MT: The incidence of pulmonary emboli in the elderly. J Geriatrics 25:138, 1970.
81. Morrell MT, Dunnill MS: Postmortem incidence of pulmonary emboli in a hospital population. Br J Surg 55:347, 1968.
82. Rosenow EC III, Osmundson PJ, Brown ML: Pulmonary embolism. Mayo Clin Proc 56:161, 1981.
83. Neumann RD, Sostman HD, Gottschalk A: Current status of ventilation/perfusion imaging. Semin Nucl Med 10:198, 1980.
84. Moser KM: Diagnosis and management of pulmonary emboli. Hosp Pract 15:57, 1980.
85. Abramson DI: Medical and surgical management of deep venous thrombosis in pulmonary embolism. Pract Cardiol 7:111, 1981.
86. Sasahara AA, Sharma GV, Tow DV, et al: Clinical use of thrombolytic agents in venous thromboembolism. Arch Intern Med 142:684, 1982.
87. Stein PD: Low dose heparin for prevention of pulmonary embolism and significance of normal lung scan. Results of a survey of three ACCP scientific sections. Cardiopul Med 21:12–14, 1982.
88. Crystal RG, Fulmer JD, Roberts WC, et al: Idiopathic pulmonary fibrosis. Ann Intern Med 85:769, 1976.
89. Fulmer JD: The interstitial lung diseases. Chest 82:172, 1982.
90. Chernow B, Johnson LF, Janowitz WR, et al: Pulmonary aspiration as a consequence of gastroesophageal reflux. Dig Dis Sci 24:839, 1979.
91. Orringer MB: Respiratory symptoms and esophogeal reflux. Chest 76:618, 1979.

Chapter 31

# Renal and Lower Urinary Tract Diseases in the Elderly

John W. Rowe

In a normal young adult, renal capacity far exceeds the ordinary demands for solute and water conservation and excretion. Although renal function is substantially diminished in old age, under ordinary circumstances the aged kidney still provides for adequate regulation of the volume and composition of extracellular fluid. However, the reduced function of the aged kidney has important clinical implications for diagnosis and treatment of many disorders. Although normal aging has no influence on urinalysis, it does strongly influence the interpretation of most other standard clinical tests of renal function, including serum creatinine, blood urea nitrogen (BUN), and radiologic studies.

## NORMAL RENAL CHANGES WITH AGE

Advancing age is associated with progressive loss of renal mass in man, with renal weight decreasing from 250 to 270 gm in young adulthood to 180 to 200 gm by the eighth decade.[1] The loss of renal mass is primarily cortical, with relative sparing of the renal medulla. The number of hyalinized or sclerotic glomeruli identified on light microscopy increases from 1 to 2 per cent during the third to fifth decade, and to 12 per cent after age 70.[2-4]

Several age-related changes have been documented in the renal tubule, including thickening of the tubular basement membrane. Of particular interest is the observation that diverticula of the distal nephron, which are essentially absent in kidneys from young individuals, become increasingly prevalent with advancing age, reaching a frequency of three diverticula per tubule at age 90.[5] It has been suggested that these diverticula represent the origin of the simple retention cysts commonly seen in the elderly.[6]

Changes in the intrarenal vasculature with age, independent of hypertension or other renal disease, are probably responsible for most clinically relevant changes in renal function with age. Normal aging is associated with variable sclerotic changes in the walls of the larger renal vessels. These sclerotic changes do not encroach on the lumen and are augmented in the presence of hypertension.[1,5-7] Smaller vessels appear to be spared, with fewer than 20 per cent of senescent kidneys from nonhypertensive individuals displaying arteriolar changes.[8]

A progressive reduction in renal plasma flow of approximately 10 per cent per decade, from 6 dl per minute in young adulthood to 3 dl per minute by 80 years of age is well-established.[9] Detailed studies indicate selective loss of cortical vasculature, with preservation of medullary flow. These cortical vascular changes probably account for the patchy cortical defects commonly seen on renal scans in healthy elderly adults.

The major clinically relevant renal functional defect arising from these histologic and physiologic changes is a progressive decline, after maturity, in the glomerular filtration rate (GFR), estimated by the clearance of insulin or creatinine. Age-adjusted normative standards for creatinine clearance have been established.[10,11] Creatinine clearance is stable until the middle of the fourth decade, when a linear decrease of about 8.0 ml per minute per 1.73 $m^2$ per decade begins.

Absence of a reciprocal elevation in serum creatinine associated with the decrease of GFR with age is of major clinical importance.[10] Since muscle mass, from which creatinine is derived, falls with age at roughly the same rate as GFR, the rather drastic age-related loss of renal function is not reflected in an elevation of serum creatinine. Thus serum creatinine values result in the overestimation of GFR in the elderly. Depressions of GFR that are so severe as to result in elevations of serum creatinine above 1.5 mg per dl are rarely due solely to normal aging and indicate the presence of an additional disease state.[11]

Brenner and colleagues[12] have recently presented an innovative, unitary hypothesis to explain the progressive nature of the reduction in renal function that accompanies normal aging as well as a number of disease states. They suggest that the high protein content of most human diets and the resultant chronic high-solute load delivered to the kidneys is associated with chronic renal vasodilatation. The resultant persistent high glomerular capillary pressure and flow may lead to extravasation of macromolecules into the glomerular mesangium, thus inducing a reaction that leads to progressive glomerular sclerosis. As glomeruli stop functioning, the solute load per nephron is increased and the deteriorative process accelerates.

## ADJUSTMENT OF MEDICATIONS IN HEALTHY ELDERLY PEOPLE

In clinical practice, the doses of many drugs excreted primarily by the kidneys are routinely adjusted to compensate for age-related alterations in renal function. Dose adjustments are required in medications excreted by way of glomerular filtration, such as digoxin, aminoglycoside antibiotics, and cimetidine, as well as agents dependent on tubular function for their elimination, such as penicillins and procainamide. Unfortunately, these adjustments are nearly always based on serum creatinine values, resulting in overdose in elderly patients, in whom serum creatinine level exaggerates renal function. Often the BUN determination provides a better estimate of renal function in the elderly. Ideally, dose adjustments should be based on creatinine clearances; when only serum creatinine is available, the influence of age must be considered if an appropriate drug regimen is to be constructed.

## RENAL DISEASES

There is a marked influence of age on the prevalence of diseases affecting the urinary tract. In addition, the substantial age-related reductions in renal function noted previously influence the presentation and response to treatment of renal disease and make the elderly especially vulnerable to the development of renal, fluid, and electrolyte complications of extra-renal diseases.

### *Acute Glomerulonephritis*

Acute glomerulonephritis is receiving increasing attention as a disease in which presentation and prognosis are clearly age-related. In children and young adults, acute glomerulonephritis is often associated with recent streptococcal infection, and the presentation is fairly uniform, with hematuria, heavy proteinuria, edema, and hypertension. In young patients, the prognosis is generally good when glomerulonephritis is associated with post-streptococcal disease; the outcome is variable when the disease is found in patients who have not had a recent streptococcal infection.

In elderly patients, acute glomerulonephritis is manifestly different.[13,14] The presentation is nonspecific, with nausea, malaise, arthralgias, and a rather striking predeliction for pulmonary infiltrates initially. Commonly, the clinical syndrome is believed to represent worsening of a pre-existing illness, especially congestive heart failure (CHF). Proteinuria is generally moderate. Hypertension or edema may indicate a post-streptococcal etiology, which is unusual in the elderly and results in a favorable prognosis. Otherwise, the prognosis is poor, with the most frequent histologic finding being crescentic glomerulonephritis, with focal, segmental necrotizing and fibrosing glomerulitis.[14] Although management is presently controversial, some patients respond to a combination of corticosteroids and immunosuppressive agents, including azothioprine or cyclophosphamide.

### *Nephrotic Syndrome*

Nephrologists have traditionally taught that age plays an important role in the etiology of nephrotic syndrome, with the likelihood of lipoid nephrosis decreasing and amyloidosis increasing with advancing age. In 1971, Fawcett and coworkers[15] reviewed one hundred consecutive cases of biopsied adults with nephrotic syndrome, 25 of whom were over 60 years of age. They found no impact of age on the frequency of any specific histologic type of glomerular change. In particular, minimal-change disease and amyloidosis were seen with equal frequency in young and old patients, and additionally, there was no impact of age on the generally excellent response of patients with the former entity to corticosteroids. Thus, age has no specific impact on the diagnosis or management of nephrotic syndrome.

## *Renal Vascular Disorders*

### Renal Arterial Thromboemboli

Occlusive arterial disease is an important cause of both acute and chronic renal failure in the elderly. Renal arterial thromboemboli occur in any setting associated with peripheral embolization, such as acute myocardial infarction, chronic atrial fibrillation, and subacute bacterial endocarditis. The manifestations of a renal embolus in the elderly may vary from an essentially clinically silent event to a full-blown syndrome, including severe flank pain and tenderness, hematuria, hypertension, spiking fevers, marked reduction in renal function, and elevations of serum lactate dehydrogenase. Small emboli are very difficult to detect, since renal scans may show focal perfusion defects in many apparently normal elderly patients. Major emboli may be suggested by findings of differential contrast excretion on pyelography and confirmed by renal scanning and aortography. Surgery is often not useful in treating severe acute thromboembolism, but anticoagulant therapy may be of major benefit.[16,17] In cases in which renal function is discernibly impaired, improvement may occur over a period of several days to weeks.

### Renal Arterial Atheroemboli

Patients with severe atherosclerosis may suffer embolization of material from atheromatous plaques into the renal circulation, either spontaneously or following aortic surgery or aortography. Renal failure may be acute in onset, associated with massive bilateral embolization, or more chronic, progressing gradually over several weeks. Evidence of embolization to other organs, including the gut, pancreas, skin, and lower extremities, is common. Renal pathologic findings characteristically include the presence of amorphous material, with elongated, biconvex, needle-shaped cholesterol crystals in small- to medium-sized arteries. The prognosis is poor, with no treatments resulting in predictable improvement. Despite hemodialysis, many patients die, presumably owing to the effects of severe atherosclerosis on other organs.[18,19]

### Renal Arterial Thrombosis

Thrombotic occlusive renal arterial disease frequently complicates severe aortic and renal arterial atherosclerosis, especially in the setting of decreased renal blood flow caused by CHF or volume depletion. Symptoms may be remarkably absent. In cases in which renal function was previously good, the only manifestation of unilateral thrombosis may be a doubling of serum BUN, creatinine, and perhaps a modest increase in blood pressure. In patients with pre-existing renal impairment and azotemia, renal arterial occlusion may precipitate CHF, marked hypertension, and the emergence of the uremic syndrome. Intravenous pyelography is generally of less diagnostic benefit than renal scanning, and definite diagnosis is made angiographically. There should be a careful evaluation for coexisting abdominal aortic aneurysm, which may lead to renal arterial occlusion by extension of atheromata or dissection. Angiography should involve the least amount of contrast material possible in order to minimize the likelihood of a nephrotoxic reaction, which although generally limited to several days of oliguria and mild azotemia, may take the form of severe acute oliguric renal failure. When technically feasible, surgical revascularization should be carefully considered. Substantial return of renal function can be obtained after prompt revascularization, and in some cases, recovery occurs even if surgery is delayed until several months after the vascular occlusion.

## *Acute Renal Failure*

Age influences renal disease by either altering the prevalence of specific diseases or by affecting the presentation, course, and response to treatment of conditions seen in both early and late adult life. Acute renal failure is seen more frequently in old patients simply because the common inciting events, including hypotension associated with marked volume depletion, bleeding, major surgery, sepsis, and the injudicious use of antibiotics, are more common in multiply impaired elderly people, who are often at increased risk because of pre-existing moderate renal insufficiency.

One common cause of acute renal failure in the elderly deserving of special mention is renal failure induced by the administration of radiographic contrast agents, whether for intravenous pyelography or for angiography. Reductions in renal function after use of these agents seem to be particularly common in patients who are volume depleted or have pre-existing reductions in GFR, both conditions of high prevalence in the elderly. In addition, patients with diabetes and myeloma appear to be especially vulnerable to contrast agent–induced nephrotoxicity.[20,21] It has recently been shown that nonsteroidal anti-inflammatory agents that inhibit prostaglandin synthesis may also induce impairments in renal function in patients with decreased renal blood flow or certain renal diseases, especially lupus nephritis.

The management of acute renal failure in the elderly is a complex and demanding task worthy of the effort. The aged kidney retains the capacity to recover from acute ischemic or toxic insults over the course of several weeks. Although the usual "acute tubular necrosis" (with 2 to 10 days of oliguria followed by a diuretic phase and, in turn, recovery of function) may be seen in the elderly, "nonoliguric" acute renal failure is being recognized with increasing frequency.[22,23] In these cases, renal function, as reflected in serum BUN and creatinine levels, is impaired for several days after a brief hypotensive episode associated with surgery, sepsis, overmedication, or volume depletion or after the administration of nephrotoxic radiographic contrast agents. After this brief period of azotemia, renal function gradually returns to its previous level. Despite this transient and reversible loss of renal function, oliguria is not a prominent component of the clinical picture. Since the clinical hallmark of renal failure is generally thought to be a dramatic reduction in urine output, cases of nonoliguric acute renal failure may go unrecognized. This may result in the inadvertent overdose of patients during the period of impaired renal function with medications excreted predominantly by way of renal mechanisms, including digitalis preparations and aminoglycoside antibiotics, such as gentamicin. Whether these patients may later develop permanent loss of renal function is currently under study.

The principles employed in the management of younger patients with full-blown acute renal failure complicated by oliguria are used in the management of elderly patients with this condition. The most important principle is the careful exclusion of urinary obstruction as a cause of the renal failure. This is particularly true in men with prostatic hypertrophy or prostatic carcinoma or in women with gynecologic malignancy.[24]

The major causes of death during acute renal failure are associated with diseases, volume overload precipitating acute pulmonary edema, hypertensive crisis, hyperkalemia, gastrointestinal bleeding, and infection. Dialysis, whether it be hemodialysis or peritoneal dialysis, is effective in the elderly, and the complication rate seems to be dictated more by coincident cardiovascular disease than by the patient's age. Dialysis often substantially simplifies management. One should not wait until an emergency situation is present before initiating dialysis in cases in which it is very likely that renal function will not return before the dialysis will be needed. The immediate indications for emergency dialysis include pulmonary edema unresponsive to diuretics, hyperkalemia, uremic pericarditis, and seizures or uncontrolled bleeding on a uremic basis. The use of intravenous catheters placed in the femoral vein for dialysis has been a major advance in the management of elderly patients with acute renal failure.[25] These catheters are easily placed and circumvent the need for implantation of arteriovenous shunts for access for dialysis in acute renal failure.

Aside from the initiation of dialysis, careful attention to several other factors is necessary. Water and salt balance must be monitored carefully. Due to catabolism, the usual patient with acute renal failure will lose about $\frac{1}{2}$ kg of body mass per day.[24] Attempts to keep body weight constant will result in the gradual expansion of the extracellular fluid and consequent increase in blood pressure and risk of precipitation of cardiac failure. Similarly, overzealous fluid restriction will impair the patient's general condition and central nervous system function and may delay the recovery of renal function. In general, the administration of approximately 6 dl of fluid a day provides adequate fluid balance.

Potassium balance is crucial; hyperkalemia must be avoided if possible and treated promptly if present.[26] Acidosis progresses with the length and degree of renal failure, and sodium bicarbonate should be administered in an effort to maintain circulating bicarbonate levels in the range of 15 to 19 mEq per L. Administration of sodium bicarbonate may expand extracellular fluid volume, and thus patients should be watched carefully for the development of congestive failure.

Infection is a common and lethal complication of acute renal failure. Urine infection secondary to unnecessary urinary catheterization is particularly common. Little is gained from placing a urinary catheter in an oliguric patient, in whom volume status and serum levels of BUN, creatinine, and potassium are better guides of progress and to treatment than urinary output. Infection of intravenous lines is also common, and these lines should be scrupulously monitored and discontinued when possible.

Additional routine measures in the treatment of acute renal failure include the administration of oral phosphate-binding agents in an effort to minimize the elevation of serum phosphorous associated with acute renal failure and the administration of a diet limited in protein content in order to blunt the rise in BUN. Of major importance is careful attention to the alteration in the dose interval of medications excreted by way of the kidney and recognition of the enhanced sensitivity of elderly uremic patients to psychotropic medication, such as hypnotics and major tranquilizers.

## *Chronic Renal Failure*

Many forms of chronic renal failure are more commonly seen late in life because the renal disease is secondary to other age-dependent disease. Examples include hydronephrosis secondary to prostatic hypertrophy or cancer, renovascular hypertension or renal failure secondary to atherosclerosis, multiple myeloma, drug-related causes of renal insufficiency, and, perhaps most common, prerenal azotemia from CHF or volume depletion.

Although the general principles of management of renal failure are similar in young and old adults, the geriatric patient with chronic renal insufficiency presents with several special characteristics. As noted previously with regard to diagnosis, serum creatinine in the elderly generally fails to increase to as high levels as in the young, despite equivalent levels of residual renal function.[10] Since serum creatinine does not reflect the degree of renal failure, many debilitated uremic elderly patients with creatinine levels less than 10 mg per dl will not be recognized as uremic, whereas substantially higher levels are common in younger uremic patients.

Another factor often delaying recognition of chronic renal failure in the elderly is the presentation of renal failure as decompensation of a previously impaired organ systems before the emergence of specific symptoms of uremia. Examples include worsening of pre-existing heart failure, hypertension due to inability to excrete salt and water, gastrointestinal bleeding in the presence of gastrointestinal malignancy or ulcer, or mental confusion in a borderline demented patient who becomes increasingly azotemic.

Once the presence of chronic renal failure is established, the definitive cause should be identified. Most renal failure in the elderly is due to chronic glomerulonephritis, hypertensive and atherosclerotic vascular disease, diabetes, or, in some cases, late-presenting polycystic kidney disease. The most important diagnostic consideration is strict exclusion of potentially reversible causes, such as urinary tract obstruction (particularly in men with symptoms of prostatism), renal arterial occlusion (which may be repairable), hypercalcemia, or the use of nephrotoxic agents.

If no reversible component is identified, the patient should be followed closely so that the rate of loss of renal function can accurately be judged. Appropriate adjustments to account for the renal failure should be made in the dose schedules of all medications, especially digoxin. Hypertension should be controlled carefully. As serum phosphate rises, phosphate-binding antacids should be given with meals in order to suppress hyperphosphatemia, hypocalcemia, and the resultant adverse effects on bone.[27] As serum phosphate falls in response to treatment, serum calcium will generally rise toward the normal range. If hypocalcemia persists after normalization of phosphate, it should be treated with preparations of Vitamin D or its congeners (i.e., Vitamin D—50,000-unit tablets, twice daily to three times daily; dihydrotachysterol, 0.2 to 0.4 mg twice daily or 1,25-dihydroxyvitamin $D_3$, 0.25 to 0.5 uq twice daily), in order to increase intestinal calcium absorption.[28]

Anemia associated with chronic renal failure often requires more aggressive management in elderly patients because of coexisting cardiac disease. Red cell indices are not a reliable estimate of iron deficiency in uremia. Iron deficiency should be excluded by evaluation of serum iron and ferritin, and oral or parenteral iron supplements should be administered if indicated. In the absence of iron deficiency, anemia of chronic renal failure will respond to monthly injections of androgens (e.g., nandrolone decanoate, 200 mg IM).[29] If symptomatic anemia persists, which it often does, regular transfusions of red cells are indicated.

Dietary management of elderly patients with chronic renal failure is often overdone, thus compounding the nutritional impact of the disease. Protein and salt restriction is often needed in young individuals to suppress the volume expansion and BUN elevations. Under normal conditions many elderly patients ingest 60 to 70 gm of protein and 4 to 5 gm of salt daily, and strict limitations of these dietary constituents is often unnecessary. Similarly, although hyperkalemia should be avoided and dietary potassium controlled, the reductions required in the elderly are often moderate. Acidosis should be controlled with the addition of oral sodium bicarbonate tablets, with the aim of keeping serum bicarbonate levels near 18 to 20 mEq per L. The best approach to these modifications is careful alteration of the diet to suit the proven needs of the individual patient.

Pruritus is a major problem in elderly uremic patients, especially in the presence of coexisting xerosis. In addition to skin moisteners, ultraviolet treatments have been found effective and safe for elderly uremic patients.[30,31] Administration of so-called "antipruritic" agents such as antihistamines and ataractics are rarely helpful, since they act primarily by causing sedation and may have adverse effects on the nervous system in the elderly.

### Dialysis in the Elderly

Chronic maintenance dialysis, generally hemodialysis but occasionally chronic ambulatory peritoneal dialysis, remains the mainstay of treatment of elderly uremic patients. Elderly patients often do very well on dialysis, with the frequency of complications seemingly more related to coexisting extrarenal disease than age itself. Psychologically, elderly patients often are more able to adapt to chronic dialysis than their younger counterparts. Once it is clear that a patient will need chronic maintenance dialysis at some time in the near future, early creation of an arteriovenous fistula for access to hemodialysis is important. This is particularly true in the elderly, since such fistulas often mature rather slowly. At present, renal transplantation is generally not considered in individuals over age 60 years.

## DISORDERS OF FLUID AND ELECTROLYTE BALANCE

Under normal circumstances, age has no effect on plasma sodium or potassium concentrations, plasma pH, or the ability to maintain normal extracellular fluid volume. However, adaptive mechanisms responsible for maintaining constancy of the volume and composition of the extracellular fluid are impaired in the elderly. Because of these physiologic changes, acute nonrenal illness in geriatric patients is often complicated by development of derangements in fluid and electrolyte balance, which delay recovery and prolong hospitalization.

### Extracellular Volume Depletion

Normal aging is associated with a blunting of the renal response to salt restriction. Thus, although the aged kidney is eventually able to decrease urinary salt to very low levels when salt intake is minimal, it may take several days for this adaptive response to develop fully.[32] This may account for the common observation that elderly patients seem to develop volume depletion rapidly during acute illnesses such as pneumonia.

This tendency of the senescent kidney to lose salt is due to both nephron loss (with increased osmotic load per nephron and resultant mild osmotic diuresis) and also to important age-related reductions in renin and aldosterone. Basal and post-stimulation levels of renin are diminished by 30 to 50 per cent in the elderly.[33] The lowered renin levels are associated with 30 to 50 per cent reductions in plasma concentrations of aldosterone, as well as with significant reductions in the secretion and clearance rates of aldosterone.[34,35]

Management of extracellular volume depletion and of its effects on cardiac, central nervous system, and renal functions includes the prompt administration of sodium chloride. If extracellular depletion is mild, oral administration of foods with high sodium content over several days is often sufficient. When volume depletion is severe, as reflected by decreased blood pressure or orthostatic hypotension, the intravenous administration of isotonic saline is indicated. Decreased tissue turgor, a useful sign of volume depletion in young adults, may be a less reliable sign in frail, nutritionally impaired elderly patients. The administration of hypotonic fluids, such as 5 per cent glucose in water, is to be avoided, since it leads to hyponatremia while failing to correct the salt depletion and may aggravate the patient's overall condition.

### Extracellular Volume Expansion

Just as old patients are more likely to develop volume depletion when deprived of salt and water, volume expansion is also a commonly encountered problem. Primarily because of its lower GFR the senescent kidney is less able to excrete an acute salt load than the younger kidney. Geriatric patients, especially those with existing cardiac disease, are thus at risk for expansion of the extracellular fluid volume when faced with an acute salt load (from inappropriate intravenous fluids, dietary indiscretion, or, as commonly occurs, after the administration of sodium-rich radiographic contrast agents, such as those used in intravenous pyelography).

In the absence of pre-existing cardiomegaly, administration of excess fluid generally does not result in the precipitation of acute CHF but rather in modest weight gain and the appearance of mild peripheral edema. Over the course of several days, this excess salt is generally excreted. The administration of oral diuretics is indicated if the volume expansion aggravates pre-existing heart failure or hypertension. The mainstay of management of acute volume expansion with pulmonary congestion remains the intravenous administration of potent diuretics such as furosemide or ethacrynic acid.

### Hyperkalemia

Age-related decreases in GFR, renin, and aldosterone, mentioned previously, contribute to the elderly patient's increased risk of developing hyperkalemia in a variety of clinical settings, especially when the patient has gastrointestinal bleeding (a major source of potassium) or is given potassium salts intravenously. This tendency toward hyperkalemia is further aggravated in any clinical setting associated with acidosis, since the senescent kidney is sluggish in its response to acid loading, resulting in prolonged depression of pH and concomitant potassium elevation. Similarly, diuretics such as spironolactone or triamterene, which impair renal potassium excretion, should be administered with caution to the elderly, especially those with coincident renal disease. The concomitant administration of these agents and potassium should be avoided.

The initial management of hyperkalemia includes discontinuation of sources of additional potassium in diet, discontinuation of potassium-sparing diuretics, and the prompt maximization of renal function in patients with volume depletion or heart failure. Severe hyperkalemia requires prompt treatment with intravenous calcium salts (calcium chloride or calcium gluconate), which directly antagonize the effect of hyperkalemia on the myocardium. Also indicated are sodium bicarbonate, glucose, and insulin. Such emergency treatment is of only temporary benefit in controlling serum potassium and has no effect on total body potassium. Therefore, while these emergency efforts are taking place, efforts toward total body potassium depletion should be initiated. These include the oral or rectal administration of sodium-potassium exchange resin (Kayexalate) and potent intravenous diuretics such as furosemide or ethacrynic acid.

An important hyperkalemic syndrome that is not infrequently seen in elderly patients, especially diabetics, is hyporeninemic-hypoaldosteronism.[36] Patients with this syndrome present with hyperkalemia in the presence of moderate degrees of renal impairment, especially interstitial renal disease. Physiologic investigations reveal very low circulatory levels of aldosterone, generally low levels of renin, and normal levels of basal and post-stimulation cortisol.[37] These physiologic alterations result in blunted urinary potassium excretion and mild metabolic acidosis, which is easily reversed by the administration of fludrocortisone.[38]

### Hypernatremia

The clinical impact of the aged kidney's inability to properly regulate salt balance under stress is compounded by similar abnormalities in water metabolism. The capacity of elderly individuals to conserve water and elaborate a concentrated urine under conditions of either water deprivation or infusion of antidiuretic hormone (ADH) is impaired.[39,40] The cause of the decreased concentrating capacity of the aged kidney probably relates to the concomitant decline in GFR and an age-related decrease in renal response to ADH.

Although the decline in water-conserving capacity with age is not so severe as to have clinical significance under conditions of free access to water, it may become important when fluid intake is limited in the presence of exaggerated insensible losses, such as with fever. Under such conditions, elevations of the serum sodium concentration to levels that impair mental function (greater than 160 mEq per L) are commonly seen in the geriatric age group. Both the salt- and water-losing tendencies of the senescent kidney contribute to the common clinical presentation of acutely or subacutely ill elderly patients with hypertonic volume depletion.

In the initial management of the patient with severe hypertonic volume depletion, it is important to focus on volume repletion as potentially life-saving and to treat such patients with rapid intravenous infusion of isotonic saline until cardiovascular stability is attained. In the presence of marked hypernatremia, these isotonic fluids are actually "hypotonic" relative to the patient's plasma, and serum sodium will begin to fall as volume is expanded. Once blood pressure and intravascular volume are corrected, hypotonic fluids should be administered until the serum sodium is below 150 mEq per L.

Severe hypertonic dehydration in the elderly is uniformly associated with marked alterations in consciousness. Although the volume and the composition of the extracellular fluid may be normalized within 72 hours of admission, alterations in mental state commonly persist for some time, and slow recovery over 2 weeks is not infrequent. Thus persisting confusion, despite normal electrolytes, should not necessarily precipitate invasive clinical evaluation. Patience is often rewarded in such cases, and the complications and cost of lumbar punctures and invasive radiologic procedures are avoided.

### Hyponatremia

Perhaps the most serious and least recognized electrolyte problem in geriatric patients is their tendency to develop water intoxication. The clinical presentation of hyponatremia is nonspecific, with depression, confusion, lethargy, anorexia, agitation, and weakness the most common findings. When hyponatremia is severe (serum sodium concentrations below 110 mEq per L), seizures and stupor may be seen and central nervous system damage may be irreversible. It is not unusual for geriatric patients to become hyponatremic in the setting of any stress, including surgery, fever, or acute viral illness.

Clinical evaluation of the elderly hyponatremic patient usually reveals that one of three general conditions is causing the disorder. One general cause is decreased renal capacity to excrete water as a consequence of acute or chronic reductions in renal blood flow. This is seen in patients with extracellular volume depletion, CHF, hypoalbuminemia associated with cirrhosis or nephrosis, or drug-induced hypotension. In addition to evidence from history and physical examination of the possible presence of any of these disorders, laboratory examination often reveals prerenal azotemia, with BUN elevations out of proportion to the elevations in serum creatinine. A second group of patients have hypernatremia secondary to the salt wasting induced by diuretics or, less commonly, by adrenal insufficiency.

A third group of patients display a constellation of findings consistent with oversecretion of ADH as a cause of the water retention. These findings include low serum sodium, evidence of good renal function (low BUN), mild extracellular fluid expansion (normal to slightly full neck veins, trace edema), and evidence of inappropriate renal water retention (urine osmolality greater than maximally dilute and, in many cases, more concentrated than serum). In addition, because of the slight extracellular fluid expansion and subsequent reduction in aldosterone secretion and elevation of GFR, excess ADH secretion is associated with the presence of modest to large amounts of sodium in the urine.

Excess ADH secretion is commonly associated with pneumonia, tuberculosis, stroke, meningitis, subdural hematoma, and a variety of other pulmonary and central nervous system disorders. Although patients in all age groups may develop hyponatremia in these settings, the elderly seem particularly prone to this complication. The elderly are more prone to develop drug-induced ADH excess. In one study, elderly patients accounted for most cases of hyponatremia developing from use of chlorpropamide.[41] Although the hyponatremic patient is unable to excrete a water load, after resolution of the acute illness, water metabolism is normal. In many cases, the same patient returns several weeks or months later with another acute illness and again develops hyponatremia.

One must maintain a high degree of suspicion for hyponatremia in geriatric patients, particularly in view of the slow, insidious nature of the development of water intoxication and its nonspecific clinical presentation. Physicians caring for the elderly should be cautious in the prescription of medications known to increase ADH secretion, such as chlorpropamide, and barbituates and in the administration of hypotonic fluids in the setting of recent surgery or any acute illness.

Management of water intoxication is dictated by the level and rate of fall of the serum sodium and by the clinical manifestations and cause of the disorder. In all cases, strict water restriction is appropriate. Medications possibly associated with water intoxication, such as diuretics or agents that increase ADH, should be withheld. In cases in which hyponatremia is associated with reduced renal blood flow, therapy should be aimed at maximizing renal function by correction of CHF, volume repletion of patients with extracellular fluid depletion, or restoration of blood pressure to normal in hypotensive patients.

In cases of excess ADH secretion, fluid restriction alone generally results in a slow return of plasma osmolality toward normal levels. In resistant cases or when fluid restriction is impractical, the water-retaining effects of ADH can be inhibited by oral administration of demethylchlortetracycline in doses of 300 mg twice to three times daily. This nephrotoxic agent induces a state of partial nephrogenic diabetes insipidus and predictably results in correction of hyponatremia over the course of several days. Since it is a nephrotoxic agent, the serum creatinine and BUN levels should be followed carefully.

In patients with severe hyponatremia (serum sodium concentrations less than 110 mEq per L), the most effective approach is the administration of hypertonic saline; 500 ml of 3 per cent sodium chloride can be administered safely, intravenously, to most patients over a 12-hour period and will generally increase the serum sodium 8 to 10 mEq per L, thus placing the patient out of immediate danger while other therapeutic modalities are initiated. Simultaneous administration of high doses of intravenous furosemide to promote brisk diuresis and hypertonic saline has been found to be effective in patients with severe hyponatremia and appears to be associated with less risk of volume expansion.[42]

## URINARY TRACT INFECTIONS

### *Asymptomatic Bacteriuria*

Physicians taking care of elderly patients are frequently faced with a decision regarding the most appropriate managment of a patient, often a resident of a long-term care facility, who is found on routine screening to have pyuria and bacteriuria with greater than 100,000 organisms per ml of carefully collected urine. If there are no symptoms referrable to urinary tract infection and if repeat culture confirms the original finding, the patient can be said to have asymptomatic bacteriuria (ASB). Increasingly prevalent in people of advanced age, this condition is found in as many as one fifth of community-dwelling elderly and in approximately one third of nursing home residents.[43,44] Although the pathophysiology of ASB is unknown, it is found with increasing prevalence in individuals with significant central nervous system disease (e.g., dementia, cerebral vascular disease, or Parkinson's disease), in diabetics, and in patients who are immobilized. Adequate long-term studies of the risk associated with asymptomatic bacteriuria have not been reported, but present experience indicates that ASB is not associated with appreciable risk and therefore it is probably best left untreated, with careful follow-up of the patients for any evidence of decreasing renal function or for the evolution of symptoms that may be associated with urinary tract infections.

A common clinical situation is the admission of an old person to an acute care facility with fever and other signs of systemic infection. Initial evaluation will often disclose bacteriuria and pyuria, which may or may not have been present on previous examinations. In such patients, culture and Gram stain of the urine should be performed, along with blood cultures and routine evaluation for other sources of infection. If a urine Gram stain is not available, these patients are generally best treated with broad spectrum antibiotics until the results of blood cultures have been returned. It is dangerous to assume that the systemic infection originated in the urinary tract, and many patients will have another source of infection coincident with asymptomatic bacteriuria that can mislead the clinician. Thus the findings of bacteriuria and pyuria in such patients should not be interpreted as a definitive localization of the source of infection. A thorough evaluation of other potential sources is important. As with any potential urinary tract infection, if the patient had been previously treated with sulfamethoxazole-trimethoprim for a substantial period of time, one must be aware that enterococcal urinary infection is more likely and can frequently lead to sepsis. In such cases, organism-specific antibiotics effective against enterococci, such as ampicillin, are frequently indicated.

### *Bacterial Cystitis*

The guidelines for the diagnosis and management of acute bacterial cystitis in elderly individuals generally follow those for their younger counterparts.[45] Findings of significant bacteria and pyuria, accompanied by symptoms of lower urinary tract infection, should be treated with organism-specific antibiotics for 10 to 14 days. Repeat urine cultures should be obtained at the end of antibiotic treatment. If symptoms recur, it is likely that reinfection is present with a new organism rather than a relapse of the previously treated infection. Nonetheless, repeat culture is mandatory and, if reinfection is present, a second course of organism-specific antibiotics for 10 to 14 days is indicated. In cases of relapse, a 6-week treatment with antibiotics may be effective in eradicating the infection. In individuals who develop chronic recurrent urinary tract infection, whether as a result of relapse or reinfection, a thorough evaluation of the urinary tract for obstruction, stones, diverticula, or other possible sources of infection is indicated. This evaluation generally begins with an intravenous pyelogram. However, the physician should be aware that this procedure may be associated with nephrotoxicity in the elderly. Patients at greatest risk for contrast agent–mediated losses of renal function as a result of intravenous pyelography appear to be individuals who are volume depleted, are diabetic, or have multiple myeloma. In such patients, pyelography should only be performed in situations in which the patient is not volume-depleted; nephrotomography often provides a useful alternative method of evaluation and can be used to avoid the necessity of a repeat pyelogram in cases in which standard pyelography fails to discern suspected abnormalities. In patients who have chronic recurrent urinary tract infection in which no anatomic cause is identified, chronic suppressant therapy is effective. Present evidence suggests that a single nightly dose of sulfamethoxazole-trimethoprim or nitrofurantoin is very effective. However, in patients with impaired renal function, nitrofurantoin is best avoided, since it is not found in appreciable quantities in the urine in these patients, and it may accumulate in the blood, resulting in chronic neuropathy.

A special consideration relevant to large numbers of elderly patients is the management of bacteriuria and pyuria in the presence of a chronic in-dwelling bladder catheter.[46] In general, bacteriuria in this setting does not require treatment if there is no evidence of symptoms of urinary tract or systemic infection. These patients occasionally develop such purulent urine that catheter drainage is impaired; this can be managed easily with irrigation of the urinary catheter with dilute acetic acid solutions. A policy of surveillance cultures at regular intervals in catheterized patients is of substantial value in providing guidance for acute antibiotic treatment in cases in which urosepsis develops.

## *Pyelonephritis*

As with other life-threatening infections, the symptoms of pyelonephritis may be vague in frail elderly individuals when compared with those in younger adults, who will almost uniformly present with fever and flank pain. Acute pyelonephritis should be treated as a medical emergency, with prompt institution of organism-specific antiobotics.[47] However, many elderly patients with pyelonephritis will respond very slowly to treatment despite prompt appropriate administration of antibiotics and will continue to evidence confusion, flank pain, tenderness, and fever for several days. Persistence of these symptoms often triggers an unnecessary evaluation of the urinary tract, including intravenous pyelography and cystoscopy, with retrograde catheterization, in order to exclude obstruction as a causative factor. However, if cultures indicate that appropriate antibiotics had been administered, the physician should be patient and withhold intravenous pyelography and other studies for at least a week, as long as there are no clinical signs of deterioration. Unnecessary intravenous pyelography, especially in volume-depleted, acutely ill patients, may be associated with impairments of renal function.

## *Perinephric Abscess*

Perinephric abscess deserves special consideration in any discussion of urinary infection in the elderly. Chronic renal parenchymal infection, often extending beyond the borders of the renal capsule, may be very insidious in the elderly and present in a nonspecific fashion, with weight loss and weakness. This disorder generally develops in the presence of renal stag horn calculi and is generally resistant to antibiotic therapy. Surgical intervention often results in dramatic improvement in the patient's general functional status. In such cases, a renal mass can often be palpated, and a flat plate of the abdomen will disclose a stag horn calculus.

### References

1. Tauchi H, Yoshioka T, Kobayashi H: Age changes in the human kidney of the different races. Gerontologia 17:87, 1971.
2. McLachlan MS, Guthrie JC, Anderson CK, et al: Vascular and glomerular changes in the aging kidney. J Pathol 121:65, 1977.
3. Sworn MJ, Fox M: Donor kidney selection for transplantation. Br J Urol 44:377, 1972.
4. Kaplan C, Pasternack B, Shah H, et al: Age-related incidence of sclerotic glomeruli in human kidneys. Am J Pathol 80:227, 1975.
5. Darmady EM, Offer J, Woodhouse MA: The parameters of the aging kidney. J Pathol 109:195, 1973.
6. McLachlan MSF: The aging kidney. Lancet 2:143, 1978.
7. Yamaguchi T, Omae T, Katsuki S: Quantitative determination of renal vascular changes related to age and hypertension. Jap Heart J 10:248, 1969.
8. Moritz AR, Oldt MR: Arteriolar sclerosis in hypertensive and non-hypertensive individuals. Am J Pathol 12:679, 1973.
9. Wesson LG: Physiology of the Human Kidney. New York, Grune & Stratton, 1969, p. 98.
10. Rowe JW, Andres R, Tobin JD, et al: The effect of age

on creatinine clearance in man: A cross-sectional and longitudinal study. J Gerontol 31:155, 1976.

11. Rowe JW, Andres R, Tobin JD: Letter: Age-adjusted normal standards for creatinine clearance in man. Ann Intern Med 84:567, 1976.
12. Brenner BM, Meyer TW, Hostetter TH: Dietary protein intake and the progressive nature of kidney disease. N Engl J Med 307:652, 1982.
13. Arieff A, Anderson RJ, Massay SG: Acute glomerulonephritis in the elderly. Mod Geriatr 3:77, 1973.
14. Potvliege PR, DeRoy G, Dupuis F: Necropsy study on glomerulonephritis in the elderly. J Clin Pathol 28:891, 1975.
15. Fawcett IW, Hilton PJ, Jones NF, et al: Nephrotic syndrome in the elderly. Br Med J 2:387, 1971.
16. Parker JM, Lord JO: Renal artery embolism: A case report with return of complete function of the involved kidney following anticoagulant therapy. J Urol 106:339, 1971.
17. Moyer JD, Rao CN, Widrich WC, et al: Conservative management of renal artery embolus. J Urol 109:138, 1973.
18. Thurlbeck WM, Castleman B: Atheromatous emboli to the kidneys after aortic surgery. N Engl J Med 257:442, 1957.
19. Kassirer JP: Atheroembolic renal disease. N Engl J Med 280:812, 1969.
20. Kamdar A, Weidmann P, Makoff DL, et al: Acute renal failure following intravenous use of radiographic contrast dyes in patients with diabetes mellitus. Diabetes 26:643, 1977.
21. Alexander RD, Berkes SL, Abvelo G: Contrast media-induced oliguric renal failure. Arch Intern Med 86:56, 1978.
22. Anderson RJ, Linas SL, Berns AS, et al: Nonoliguric acute renal failure. N Engl J Med 296:1134, 1977.
23. Bhat JG, Gluck MC, Lowenstein J, et al: Renal failure after open heart surgery. Ann Intern Med 84:677, 1976.
24. Levinsky NG, et al: Acute Renal Failure in the Kidney. *In* Brenner BM, Rector F (eds.): The Kidney. 2nd edition, Philadelphia, W. B. Saunders Co., 1981, p. 1181.
25. Matalon R, Nidus BD, Cantacuzino D, et al: Intermittent hemodialysis with repeated femoral vein puncture. JAMA 214:1883, 1970.
26. Cohen JJ, et al: Disorders of Potassium Balance in the Kidney. *In* Brenner BM, Rector F (eds.): The Kidney. 2nd edition, Philadelphia, W. B. Saunders, 1981, p. 908.
27. Slatopolsky E, Bucker NS: The role of phosphorus restrictions in the prevention of secondary hyperparathyroidism. Kidney Int 4:141, 1973.
28. Massey SG, Goldstein DA: Role of parathyroid function in uremic toxicity. Kidney Int 13:839, 1978.
29. Hendler ED, Goffinet JA, Ross S, et al: Controlled study of androgen therapy in anemia of patients on maintenance hemodialysis. N Engl J Med 291:1046, 1974.
30. Gilchrest BA, Rowe JW, Brown RS, et al: Ultraviolet phototherapy of uremic pruritus. Ann Intern Med 91:17, 1979.
31. Shultz BC, Roenigk WH Jr: Uremic pruritus treated with ultraviolet light. JAMA 243:1836, 1980.
32. Epstein M, Hollenberg NK: Age as a determinant of renal sodium conservation in normal men. J Lab Clin Med 87:411, 1976.
33. Crane MG, Harris JJ: Effect of aging on renin activity and aldosterone excretion. J Lab Clin Med 87:947, 1976.
34. Flood C, Gherondache C, Pincus G, et al: The metabolism and secretion of aldosterone in elderly subjects. J Clin Invest 46:960, 1967.
35. Weidmann P, De Myttenaere-Bursztein S, Maxwell MH, et al: Effect of aging on plasma serum and aldosterone in normal man. Kidney Int 8:325, 1975.
36. Schambelan M, Stockigt JR, Biglieri EG: Isolated hypoaldosteronism in adults. A renin deficiency syndrome. N Engl J Med 287:573, 1972.
37. Oh MS, Carroll HJ, Clemmons JE, et al: A mechanism for hyporeninemic hypoaldosteronism in chronic renal disease. Metabolism 23:1157, 1974.
38. Sebastian A, Schambelan M, Lindenfeld S, et al: Amelioration of metabolic acidosis with fludrocortisone therapy in hyporeninemic-hypoaldosteronism. N Engl J Med 297:576, 1977.
39. Rowe JW, Shock NW, DeFronzo R: The influence of age on urine concentrating ability in man, Nephron 17:279, 1976.
40. Lindeman RD, Lee TD Jr, Yiengst MJ, et al: Influence of age, renal disease, hypertension, diuretics, and calcium on the anti-diuretic response to suboptimal infusion of vasopressin. J Lab Clin Med 68:206, 1966.
41. Weissman PN, Shenkman L, Gregerman RI: Chlorpropamide hyponatremia. N Engl J Med 284:65, 1971.
42. Hantman D, Rossier B, Zohlman R, and Schuer R: Rapid correction of hyponatremia in the syndrome of inappropriate secretion of antidiuretic hormone. Ann Intern Med 78:870, 1973.
43. Akhtar AJ, Andrews GR, Caird FL, Fallon RJ: Urinary tract infection in the elderly: A population study. Age Ageing 1:48, 1972.
44. Brocklehurst JC, Bee P, Jones D, Palmer MK: Bacteriuira in geriatric hospital patients. Age Ageing 6:240, 1977.

## Chapter 32

# Hypertension in the Elderly

*Robert C. Tarazi*

Both arterial pressure and age are continuous variables. Hence the notion of "hypertension in the elderly" can at best constitute only a relative entity, not a condition qualitatively different from increased blood pressure in the adult population.

Hypertension is the result of the interaction of different pressor mechanisms; these are relatively limited in number, and the various types of hypertension differ from each other, not so much by the presence of any single pressor factor but rather by the way in which these factors are integrated.[1] Age affects many of these physiologic mechanisms in a graded way. There is therefore no arbitrary limit at which hypertension suddenly becomes a qualitatively different disease. Nevertheless, some characteristics begin gradually to assume a greater importance with advancing years, influencing both the clinical picture and response to treatment. One outstanding example is the gradual reduction in compliance of the aorta and large vessels with age; this reduction is more frequent among older patients, but it certainly can occur in younger subjects[2,3] and will have the same consequences regardless of the patient's chronologic age. Its occurrence does not negate the importance of other pressor factors but will modulate their expression.

Although the reduced arterial distensibility with its secondary exaggeration of systolic hypertension and diminished effectiveness of baroceptor reflexes[4] is perhaps the better known of the vascular changes that develop with age, there are others, possibly more subtle in their expression but no less important in their therapeutic consequences. These include a gradual reduction in beta-adrenergic receptors in the heart and blood vessels[5-7] and changes in liver and kidney function that can alter the excretion rate of antihypertensive agents.[8] The reduction in vascular beta-receptors enhances the vasoconstrictor effect of alpha-adrenergic stimuli and may alter response to alpha-blocking agents; fewer cardiac beta-receptors may entail a reduction in cardiac contractile reserve.[7,9,10] A diminished excretion rate of drugs can enhance their hypotensive potential or risk from adverse side effects.

Most age-dependent changes can be accelerated by hypertension, whether these changes are reduced aortic distensibility,[11] diminution in beta-adrenergic receptors,[12] or impaired renal function. Chronologic age becomes, therefore, less important than the medical history of the patient; safe and effective treatment will depend more on careful assessment of the individual than on dogmatic decisions based on arbitrary values of blood pressure and age.

## SYSTOLIC HYPERTENSION IN THE ELDERLY

Traditionally, physicians have been more familiar with decisions based on diastolic blood pressure (DBP) levels, both for diagnosis and treatment of hypertension. Stepped-care therapy is based entirely on the degree of diastolic pressure elevation.[13] There are many reasons for this bias, such as the assumed greater lability of systolic blood pressure (SBP) and its purported dependence on cardiac action in contrast to the closer relation of diastolic pressure to peripheral arteriolar vasoconstriction.[14] Although both of these impressions have repeatedly been shown to be mistaken,[15,16] they remain, nevertheless, influential.

Conversely, the discussion of hypertension in elderly patients is much too often dominated by questions about isolated systolic hypertension.

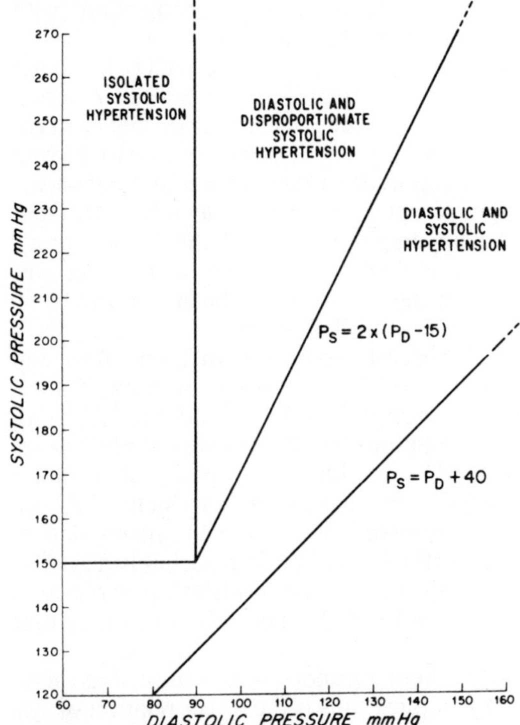


**Figure 32–1.** The relationship between diastolic ($P_D$) and systolic ($P_S$) blood pressures would have been given by the first line ($P_S = P_D + 40$) if aortic distensibility remained the same whatever the $P_D$ level. However, since distensibility is reduced as diastolic blood pressure increases, the systolic pressure rises relatively more than the diastolic, as shown by the equation of the second line. Inappropriate systolic elevations for the level of diastolic pressure can cover the whole spectrum from $P_S > 2 \times (P_D - 15)$ to isolated systolic elevations. (From Koch-Weser J: Correlation of pathophysiology in primary hypertension. Am J Cardiol 32:499, 1973.)

Although legitimate, these questions address only part of the problem and, thus, sometimes distort the approach to one of the important and frequent diseases of the elderly.[8] Hypertension in patients over 60 years of age is *not* limited to isolated elevations of systolic pressure; it is just as liable to be diastolic as well as systolic or more frequently both. The risk of cardiovascular disease increases with elevations in either the diastolic or systolic level, often more steeply with the latter.[17,18] The epidemiologic characteristics of hypertension and its risks in patients over 60 years of age have been defined in several excellent reviews.[19–21] The efficacy of treatment of diastolic hypertension in that age group was convincingly demonstrated by the Hypertension Detection and Follow-up Program and other studies.[8] The problems of pure systolic hypertension are, in my opinion, only partly due to the absence of definite proof of efficacy for its treatment; the clear relation between systolic pressure levels and risk from cardiovascular disease[17,18,22,23] would have tipped the decision toward treatment were it not for the difficulties and side effects of treatment. In fact, the question raised today as regards hypertension in the elderly does not challenge its risks or the advisability of treatment as much as the safety of therapy or its practicality in that high-risk population.[24]

Wiggers[25] long ago defined the relation between the diastolic pressure and distensibility of the aorta and large vessels; because this distensibility is reduced as DBP increases, pulse pressure (everything else being equal) increases as hypertension develops (Fig. 32–1). The implication is that added loss of elasticity of these large vessels (windkessel) will lead to an even steeper slope of the relation between SBP and DBP, which attains its maximum in isolated systolic hypertension due to aortic sclerosis. The practical results are that a larger drop of SBP must be expected for an equal reduction of DBP during treatment of these patients (Fig. 32–2), with a greater risk of transient but alarming side effects and hence, the need for reduced dosage of drugs and a much more gradual approach to blood pressure control.

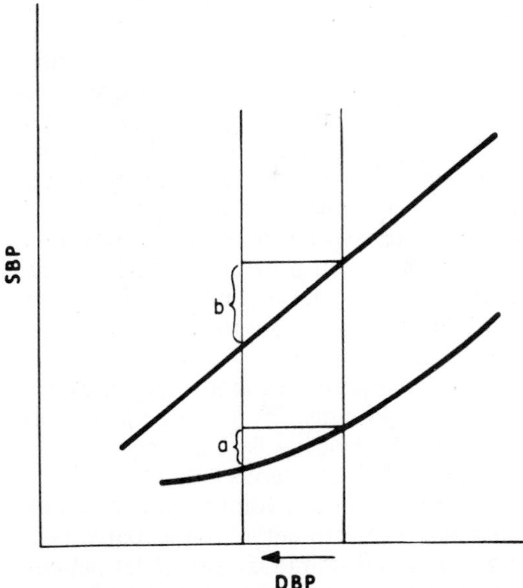


**Figure 32–2.** The steeper slope of the relation between systolic blood pressure (SBP) and diastolic blood pressure (DBP) (see Fig. 37–1) signifies that one should expect a greater drop of SBP in patients with inappropriate systolic hypertension (b > a) for the same reduction in diastolic pressure. (From Tarazi, RC, Lagaini F, and Dustan HP: The role of aortic distensibility in hypertension. *In* Milliez P and Safar M, eds: Recent Advances in HT. Vol. 2. Reims, France, Laboratoires Boehlinger Ingelheim, 1975, pp. 133–142.)

Thus, it is important to view the relationship of systolic to diastolic pressure levels as a continuum and *not* to subdivide patients with hypertension into two groups only, i.e., those with diastolic hypertension and those with isolated systolic hypertension. Between these two groups are a large number of patients who have, along with an elevated diastolic pressure, a greater than expected increase in systolic pressure. This "inappropriate systolic hypertension" can be of different degrees but its implications are the same, that is, therapeutic problems in those patients are similar to the problems encountered in isolated systolic hypertension; common to both are the marked variations in systolic pressure, the brittleness of blood pressure control, and the borderline baroceptor adequacy.

## PATHOPHYSIOLOGIC ASPECTS

### *Cardiac Function and Hemodynamic Patterns*

An increase in total peripheral resistance remains the hemodynamic hallmark of established hypertension in both young and older subjects.[26] Cardiac output can be normal for the patient's age but is more frequently reduced;[3,27,28] the combination of a small stroke volume and high pulse pressure suggests reduced aortic distensibility (see below). There are, however, some exceptions, such as patients who present with an evident hyperkinetic circulation despite a long-standing hypertension;[29] this combination seems rare in patients over the age of 65, but when present, the high cardiac output and signs of sympathetic stimulation suggest the need for sympatholytics in therapeutic planning.

Plasma volume is frequently low in elderly hypertensive patients,[27,28] which helps explain to some degree their low cardiac output. When associated with poor venous tone and static dependent edema, the low volume may contribute to the poor adjustment of these patients to upright posture.[30] Paradoxically, older patients often have a low plasma renin activity despite their low plasma volume, possibly because of reduced autonomic reflexes or blunted end-organ responsiveness.[31] Whatever the basic mechanism (blunted baroceptors, low plasma renin activity, or contracted intravascular volume), its important practical consequences are the marked sensitivity of most elderly hypertensives to diuretics and the need in these patients to begin antihypertensive medication with about half the adult dose.

*Cardiac performance* is at special risk in older hypertensive patients because of a combination of factors, including the greater incidence of coincidental coronary or arrhythmic heart disease, the reduction of cardiac output and beta-adrenergic receptors with age and left ventricular (LV) hypertrophy,[6,7,10] and the inappropriate increase in SBP.[32] The reduction of cardiac output with age has recently been confirmed by carefully controlled studies;[7] the result is a higher systemic resistance to blood flow and greater impedance to cardiac ejection. The reduced responsiveness to beta-adrenergic stimulation will blunt the effectiveness of cardioadrenergic drive, robbing the heart of a major supportive mechanism and reducing its contractile reserve.[9] The result is greater dependence on the Frank-Starling mechanism to meet extraloads and a predisposition to ventricular dilation and further encroachment on cardiac reserve.

Of particular importance because of its therapeutic implications is the direct relation of systolic pressure levels to the cardiac load; it is the systolic not the diastolic pressure that is the variable used to define ventricular afterload[32] and hence the oxygen-expensive types of cardiac work. This relationship is therefore particularly important in patients with reduced cardiac function or potential heart disease. Indications for antihypertensive therapy based exclusively on diastolic pressure levels miss the evident importance of systolic pressure for patients with inappropriate systolic hypertension or those with cardiac problems. Many studies have directly demonstrated the marked reduction in stroke volume and increase in LV end-diastolic pressure associated with even modest increases in SBP (Table 32–1). More accurate appreciation of the impact of systolic hypertension on the heart will improve the physician's understanding of the cardiac hypertrophy and diminished performance that is seen in older patients, and often ascribed to some unspecified degenerative effect of age, and offer a possibility for treatment.

When a physician is confronted with a multiplicity of causes for cardiac dysfunction, as is often the case in older patients, the more important causes are those for which something can be done. Careful reduction of SPB may help improve cardiac performance. To a purely quantitative definition of hypertension it is appropriate to add in some cases a biologic dimension; a SBP that depresses cardiac function is too high for that particular patient and should indicate

**Table 32–1.** HEMODYNAMIC EFFECTS OF INCREASED SYSTOLIC BLOOD PRESSURE (SBP)*

| | Control | ↑SBP† |
|---|---|---|
| Systolic pressure (mm Hg) | 122 ± 6 | 133 ± 8† |
| Diastolic pressure (mm Hg) | 87 ± 4 | 85 ± 4 |
| LVEDP‡ (mm Hg) | 5.1 ± 0.5 | 6.0 ± 0.6† |
| Cardiac index L/m² | 1.71 ± 0.16 | 1.58 ± 0.17† |
| SV/EDV§ | 0.42 ± 0.04 | 0.35 ± 0.04† |

Urschel CW, Covell JW, Sonnenblick EH, Ross J Jr, and Braunwald E: Effects of decreased aortic compliance on performance of the left ventricle. Am J Physiol 214:298, 1968.

* Increase obtained by inserting a rigid bypass along the aorta.

† = $p < 0.01$.

‡ LVEDP = left ventricular end-diastolic pressure.

§ SV/EDV = ejection fraction.

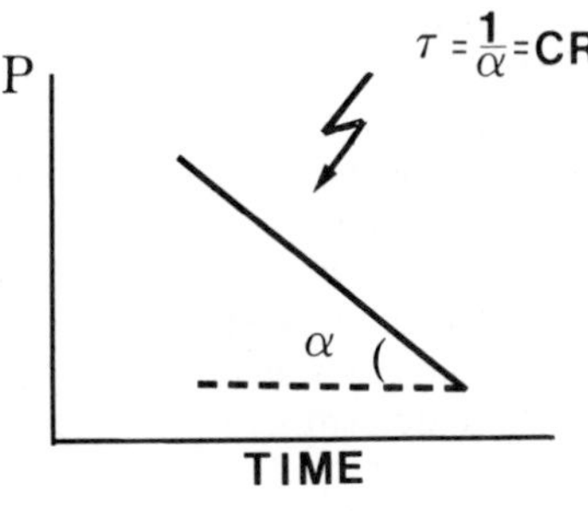


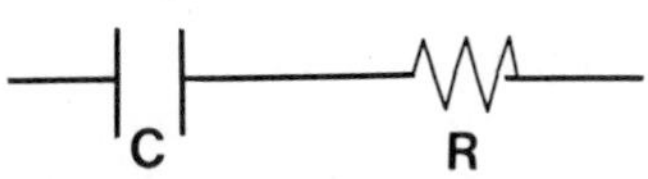


**Figure 32–3.** The fall in arterial pressure from the dicrotic notch until the beginning of the next cardiac cycle is exponential and can be likened to a simple model linking in series a capacitance (C) with a resistive element (R). Arterial compliance can therefore be calculated from the slope of the diastolic part of the pulse and from simultaneously determined total peripheral resistance. This method has been validated in man by Simon and associates.[34]

careful consideration of antihypertensive measures.

## *Aortic Compliance and Arterial Dynamics*

Arterial compliance reflects the viscoelastic properties of the walls of the large arteries and determines the effectiveness of their role in buffering the wide fluctuations in pressure generated by the heart (windkessel effect).[25] Although there is a general tendency for arterial compliance to diminish with age and for hypertension in the elderly to be associated with aortic rigidity, there are enough exceptions to suggest that investigations are sometimes needed in problem cases.[2,3]

Many indices have been proposed to determine aortic compliance in humans;[3,33–35] some such as the ratio of pulse pressure to stroke volume (PP/SV, mm Hg rise in pressure per ml blood ejected) can be useful as easy approximations of systemic arterial compliance (SAC).[3] Others are more precise mathematic derivations from the slope of fall in intra-arterial pressure during diastole (Fig. 32–3).[34,35] In our experience and that of others, there has been a close correlation in most older patients between PP/SV ratio and the index derived from pulse pressure tracings; many exceptions, however, were found among young subjects. The paradox is explained by the dependence of SBP on more than one factor; it depends in part on aortic distensibility but also in part on the velocity of ventricular ejection of blood. In case the inappropriate elevation of SBP is related to a reduction in aortic compliance, the two indices agree, but if ventricular ejection is abnormally rapid, then SBP may be high even though arterial compliance is normal or only slightly reduced.[36]

The compliance of the arterial system is not a fixed characteristic dependent only on the biochemical and structural characteristics of its walls. The "tone" of large arteries is influenced by different neurohumoral factors, particularly sympathetic activity,[37,38] and reacts differently to various vasodilators. The work of Safar and associates[39–41] has brought to light the frequent divergence between the effect of vasodilators on the small resistance vessels and their effects on the large arteries. Some like hydralazine lower peripheral resistance by peripheral vasodilation but reduce the diameter of the larger vessels, whereas converting-enzyme inhibitors and particularly calcium entry blockers dilate both the small peripheral vessels and the large arteries.[42] As these differences are confirmed and better appreciated, they will add a new dimension to our therapeutic choice of vasodilators. Those that produce arterial as well as arteriolar dilation may prove more suitable for patients with peripheral arterial disease. This subject will be discussed further under Therapeutic Considerations.

## *Baroceptor Function in Older Patients*

One of the more significant features in circulatory homeostasis is the gradual reduction in baroceptor sensitivity that develops with age, both in normotensive and in hypertensive subjects.[4] The early clinical observations of blunted arterial pressure responses to a Valsalva maneuver in older patients were further extended and quantified by studies of the heart rate response to induced variations in systolic blood pressure; baroceptor sensitivity was defined by the slope of the relation determined between the SBP levels and RR intervals.[43] This sensitivity was gradually reduced with advancing age, and within each decade was significantly lower in hypertensive than in normotensive subjects.[4]

The blunting of baroceptor reflexes in older hypertensives suggests that complaints of hypotension and dizziness on standing or straining will be frequent when antihypertensive therapy is initiated in patients over 60 years old. The combined effects of age and hypertension have the elderly living at the edge, as it were, of baroceptor compensation. The balance can be easily tipped to inadequate postural adjustment and even fainting by everyday events such as the toning down of sympathetic activity by supine rest or by the use of simple sedatives, which can depress baroceptor sensitivity further.[30] The practical implications are that elderly patients should be warned against sudden standing-up, jumping out of bed, straining, and so on, and especially that physicians should avoid prescribing drugs that interfere with the effectiveness of baroceptor reflexes.

## EVALUATION OF ELDERLY HYPERTENSIVES

Evaluation of a patient's condition can never be limited to one system alone or to investigation of a single abnormal finding; we are concerned with the patient as a whole, not with a blood pressure value, whether it is measured in the office, at home, or over 24 hours. This is particularly true of the patient over 60 years in whom hypertension is apt to be associated with other problems that will influence the whole therapeutic approach. Atherosclerosis, with signs and symptoms of vascular insufficiency in various organs; diabetes mellitus; depression, osteoarthritis; and obstructive pulmonary disease are all common in elderly patients, and each will impose its restriction on the choice of antihypertensive drug. Analgesics given over the counter may interfere with the antihypertensive effects of furosemide or of captopril; sedatives and antidepressants may impair baroceptor reflexes and exaggerate postural hypotension. Adequate evaluation begins therefore with a careful medical history to assess the patient's personality, memory, and understanding of his or her disease as well as of *all* the medications being used.

The duration of hypertension is particularly important; in the majority of patients, hypertension dates back to their middle years and represents classic essential hypertension.[23] Evaluation is then mostly directed to assessment of target organ damage and of concomitant atherosclerosis and other diseases, with particular attention to the heart, to the possibility of carotid or peripheral vascular disease, and to the level of renal excretory function.[23] In other patients, the increase in pressure will have developed de novo above the age of 55 or there has been an acute exacerbation of a stable hypertension. Under these conditions, a search for atherosclerotic renal artery stenosis is warranted.[8,44] Investigations may also be warranted for either primary or secondary aldosteronism if hypokalemia develops easily and limits therapy.[8]

### *Blood Pressure Recording*

Careful, repeated measurements of blood pressure are needed in all hypertensives, young and old, in order to avoid overdiagnosis, needless anxiety, and side effects of unnecessary treatment. Extremely wide variations in SBP readings are common in the elderly. Multiple blood pressure measurements should therefore be obtained before deciding on treatment (at least three measurements on each of at least three office visits over a period of weeks). An alternative is to have the patients measure their own blood pressures regularly at home for a couple of weeks.

In addition, two questions must be carefully answered: (1) What is the response of arterial pressure to upright posture? (2) What is the effect of arterial stiffness on auscultatory blood pressure measurements? Caird and associates[45] reported a drop of 20 mm Hg or more in systolic pressure on standing in 24 per cent of 494 subjects above age 64. The poor cardiovascular adjustment to posture implies the potential for more side effects during treatment and the need to use small doses and avoid drugs that impair baroceptor reflexes. As regards the second question, older patients frequently have a greater discrepancy between auscultatory and intra-arterial blood pressure levels than do younger subjects; some with apparent severe hypertension were shown to be almost normotensive by direct intra-arterial records.[46] This "pseudohypertension" is probably related to the difficulty of compressing a stiff and possibly calcified brachial artery.

## THERAPEUTIC CONSIDERATIONS

Controversies still surround the advisability and modalities of antihypertensive therapy in elderly patients.[47] The controversy will not be solved by statistics and epidemiologic studies alone; in my opinion its persistence really reflects more a fear of complications and a reluctance to meddle with patients who have reached a great age unmolested by vascular disease. An editorial in the Lancet expressed the situation in a most precise, elegant and practical way. Three questions summarize the physician's dilemma: (1) Is there an increased risk associated with hypertension in the elderly? (2) Is this risk reversible by therapy? (3) At what cost in iatrogenic disease might some increase in survival be purchased and can the labor and expense of detecting and treating symptomless hypertension in this age group be justified in social and economic terms?[47]

The answers today are quite clear for some points, still doubtful for others, and, as regards the last point, involve a value judgment rather than a scientific decision. It is a demonstrated fact that hypertension, whether diastolic or systolic, is associated with increased cardiovascular risk. The favorable effect of therapy in treating diastolic hypertension in patients over 60 or 65 years has been proved in many trials both in the United States[19] and abroad.[20,48] Table 32-2 is one of many that can be found in the many excellent reviews of the subject. There is no definite evidence that antihypertensive therapy is beneficial in elderly patients with isolated systolic hypertension, but there is also no evidence that adequate and cautious treatment is harmful.

I do not think the questions raised can be solved only by more statistical evidence. The problem is clinical, the objects stem from bedside observations, and the answer will come from a better understanding of pathophysiology applied with common sense. The Lancet editorial expressed this very well indeed.

> Therapeutic misadventures are more likely in the elderly because of inappropriate dosage, impaired cardiovascular homoeostasis, erratic pill-taking, and polypharmacy for multiple diseases. Few would urge the conversion of a happy independent hypertensive into a depressed invalid, chair-bound or bed-bound for fear of postural hypotension, in pursuit of a theoretical prolongation of life, but such instances are grounds not so much for neglecting hypertension as for avoiding a casual approach.[47]

This is the reason for the long discussion of pathophysiology in this chapter; its reasoned application should make antihypertensive treatment safer and therefore more acceptable. There are many published discussions of antihypertensive drugs for older patients such as the excellent summary by Kirkendall and Hammond,[8] the personal opinion of Gifford,[23] and the recommendations of the National High Blood Pressure Education Committee.[44] Two basic principles are stressed by all:

1. The initial doses and subsequent increments of any antihypertensive agents selected should be quite small (half the usual adult dose) because of the many factors that enhance their hypotensive effect in older patients. These include low plasma volume, impaired mechanisms of cardiovascular homeostasis, reduced excretion rate of some drugs, and greater sensitivity to sympatholytics and alpha-blockers because of enhanced sympathetic vasoconstrictor tone.
2. Drugs that interfere with baroceptor reflexes should be avoided if at all possible because of the borderline "baroceptor compensation" of older patients.

**Table 32-2.** INCIDENCE OF MORBID EVENTS IN PATIENTS AGED 60 AND OLDER AT RANDOMIZATION*

| Blood Pressure Prior to Randomization (mm Hg) | Control Group *Rand†* | Control Group *Events* | % | Treated Group *Rand†* | Treated Group *Events* | % |
|---|---|---|---|---|---|---|
| 90-104 | 21 | 13 | 61.9 | 19 | 8 | 42.1 |
| 150-114 | 22 | 14 | 63.9 | 19 | 3 | 15.8 |
| Total | 43 | 27 | 62.8 | 38 | 11 | 28.9 |

From Kirkendall WM, Hammond JJ: Hypertension in the elderly. Arch Intern Med 140:1155, 1980.
* Veterans Administration Cooperative Study on Morbidity in Hypertension
† Rand = number of patients randomized.

To the extent that general rules can really be summarized in a few sentences and still be helpful, one might suggest from the preceeding discussion that antihypertensive therapy in older patients could begin, if indicated, with small doses of a diuretic to which small doses of an adequate vasodilator could be added later. Hydralazine has been suggested because it does not interfere with baroceptor reflexes and can be well tolerated; however, it could induce or worsen angina pectoris.[8] The hemodynamic pattern produced by converting-enzyme inhibitors and most calcium entry blockers appears favorable; the latter can serve more than one purpose if the hypertensive patient also suffers from some form of arterial insufficiency, peripheral or coronary.

Of potentially great importance is the *better understanding of vasodilators* that has been developing in the past few years. To the early concept of peripheral vasodilators as drugs that lower total peripheral resistance (TPR) by relaxing the resistance vessels, two aspects have been added; their effect on veins and their action on the large arteries. Drugs classified as vasodilators because their first hemodynamic effect is to lower TPR can be subdivided according to the following:

1. Mode of action, whether it is neural or humoral or a direct effect on the vascular smooth muscle.
2. Venodilating effect. At one end of the spectrum are those drugs that produce marked venodilation and lower cardiac output; at the other end are those with little if any venodilating effect, which lead to marked tachycardia and increased output. Those with balanced venoarteriolar effect will lower TPR without altering cardiac output significantly.[49]
3. Effect on large arteries. It has been pointed out in a series of impressive studies[39-42] that the effects of different vasodilators on the large (brachial) arteries differ in time course, intensity, and, more importantly, in direction from their effects on small arterioles. Thus hydralazine dilates the resistance vessels but actually decreases the diameter of the large arteries. Converting-enzyme inhibitors and calcium entry blockers dilate both the large arteries and the small resistance vessels. Nitroglycerine can dilate the brachial artery without reducing TPR.

Another approach to the choice of a vasodilator has been developed based on the patient's level of plasma renin activity. Converting-enzyme inhibitors are more potent in high renin hypertension, at least acutely.[50] More relevant to our discussion is the reported marked effectiveness of calcium entry blockers in patients with low-renin conditions;[51,52] they are also particularly effective in older patients. It is not completely settled whether the enhanced effectiveness of calcium entry blockers is related to the prevalence of low renin in patients above 60 years or to the blunting of baroceptor reflexes, which may interfere with blood pressure response to vasodilators. Nevertheless, the fact remains that treatment with calcium entry blockers might prove effective for more than one reason in older patients. It is important, however, to avoid (1) those drugs that depress heart rate in patients with poor cardiac function or abnormal cardiac conduction and (2) those that may overstimulate the heart in patients with angina pectoris.

## References

1. Tarazi RC, Gifford RW Jr: Systemic arterial pressure. *In* Sodeman WA Jr, Sodeman TM (eds.): Pathophysiology. 6th ed. Philadelphia, W.B. Saunders Company, 1979, pp. 198–229.
2. Ho JK, Lin CY, Galysh FT, et al: Aortic compliance: Studies on its relationship to aortic constituents in man. Arch Pathol 94:537, 1972.
3. Tarazi RC, Lagaini F, Dustan HP: The role of aortic distensibility in hypertension. *In* Milliez P, Safar M (eds.): Recent Advances in Hypertension. Vol. 2, Reims-France, Laboratoires Boehlinger Ingelheim, 1975, pp. 133–142.
4. Gribbin B, Pickering TG, Sleight P, Peto R: Effect of age and high blood pressure on baroreflex sensitivity in man. Circ Res 29:424, 1971.
5. Amer SM, Gomoll AW, Perhuch JL Jr, et al: Aberrations of cyclic nucleotide metabolism in the hearts and vessels of hypertensive rats. Proc Nat Acad Sci 71:4930, 1974.
6. Baker SP, Potter LT: Cardiac $\beta$-adrenoceptors during normal growth of male and female rats. Br J Pharmacol 68:65, 1980.
7. Rodeheffer RJ, Gerstenblith G, Becker LC, et al: Exercise cardiac output is maintained with advancing age in healthy human subjects: Cardiac dilatation and increased stroke volume compensate for a diminished heart rate. Circulation 69:203, 1984.
8. Kirkendall WM, Hammond JJ: Hypertension in the elderly. Arch Intern Med 140:1155, 1980.
9. Saragoca M, Tarazi RC: Left ventricular hypertrophy in rats with renovascular hypertension. Alterations in cardiac function and adrenergic responses. Hypertension 3:II-171, 1981.
10. Tarazi RC: The progression from hypertrophy to heart failure. Hosp Pract 18:101, 1983.
11. Wolinsky H: Effects of hypertension and its reversal on the thoracic aorta of male and female rats. Circ Res 28:622, 1971.
12. Ayobe MH, Tarazi RC: Beta-receptors and contractile reserve in left ventricular hypertrophy. Hypertension 5 (Suppl I):I-192, 1983.

13. Joint National Committee: The 1984 Report of the Joint National Committee on Detection, Evaluation and Treatment of High Blood Pressure. Arch Intern Med 144:1045, 1984.
14. Fishberg AM: Hypertension and Nephritis. Philadelphia, Lea and Febiger, 1939.
15. Ayman D: Essential hypertension: The diastolic blood pressure; its variability. Arch Intern Med 48:89, 1931.
16. Berne RM, Levy MN: Cardiovascular Physiology. St Louis, C.V. Mosby Company, 1981, pp. 94–108.
17. Kannel WB: Role of blood pressure in cardiovascular morbidity and mortality. Prog Cardiovasc Dis 17:5, 1974.
18. Kannel WB, Wolf PA, McGee DL, et al: Systolic blood pressure, arterial rigidity and risk of stroke. JAMA 245:1225, 1981.
19. Hypertension Detection and Follow-up Program Cooperative Group: Five year findings of the Hypertension Detection and Follow-up Program: Part I: Reduction in mortality. Part II: Mortality by race, sex and Age. JAMA 242:2562, 1979.
20. National Heart Foundation of Australia Study: Treatment of mild hypertension in the elderly: Report by the Management Committee. Med J Aust 2:398, 1981.
21. Dyer AR, Stamler J, Shekelle RB, et al: Hypertension in the elderly. Med Clin North Am 61:513, 1977.
22. Colandrea MA, Friedman GD, Nichaman MZ, et al: Systolic hypertension in the elderly: An epidemiologic assessment. Circulation 41:239, 1970.
23. Gifford RW Jr: Isolated systolic hypertension in the elderly. JAMA 247:781, 1982.
24. Jackson G, Pierscianowski TA, Mahon W, Condon JR: Inappropriate antihypertensive therapy in the elderly. Lancet 2:1317, 1976.
25. Wiggers CJ: Circulatory dynamics. *In* Physiologic Studies. Modern Medical Monograph. New York, Grune and Stratton, 1952.
26. Tarazi RC: The hemodynamics of hypertension. *In* Genest J, Kuchel O, Hamet P, Cantin M (eds.): Hypertension. 2nd ed. New York, McGraw-Hill Book Company, 1983, pp. 15–42.
27. Adamapoulos PN, Chrysanthalkopoulis SG, Frohlich ED: Systolic hypertension: Non-homogenous disease. Am J Cardiol 36:697, 1975.
28. Messerli FH, Sundgaard-Riise K, Ventura HO, et al: Essential hypertension in the elderly: Haemodynamics, intravascular volume, plasma renin activity, and circulating catecholamine levels. Lancet 2:983, 1983.
29. Ibrahim MM, Tarazi RC, Dustan HP, et al: Hyperkinetic heart in severe hypertension: A separate clinical hemodynamic entity. Am J Cardiol 35:667, 1975.
30. Tarazi, RC, Fouad FM: Circulatory dynamics in progressive autonomic failure. *In* Bannister R (ed.): Autonomic Failure: A Textbook of Clinical Disorders of the Autonomic Nervous System. Oxford, England, Oxford University Press, 1983, pp. 96–113.
31. Niarchos AP, Laragh JH: Hypertension in elderly. Mod Con Cardiovasc Dis 49:43, 1980.
32. Tarazi RC, Levy MN: Cardiac responses to increased afterload. Hypertension 4 (Suppl II):II-8, 1982.
33. Abboud FM, Houston JH: The effects of aging and degenerative vascular diseases on the measurement of arterial rigidity in man. J Clin Invest 40:933, 1981.
34. Simon AC, Safar ME, Levenson JA, et al: An evaluation of large arteries compliance in man. Am J Physiol 237:H550, 1979.
35. Randall OS, Esler MD, Bulloch GF, et al: Relationship of age and blood pressure to baroreflex sensitivity and arterial compliance in man. Clin Sci Mol Med 51 (Suppl 3):357s, 1976.
36. Tarazi RC: Hypertension in the elderly: *In* Robinson RR, Dennis VW, Ferris TF, et al (eds): Nephrology, vol. 2. New York, Springer-Verlag, 1984, pp. 1154–1162.
37. Freis ED: Hemodynamics of hypertension. Physiol Rev 40:27, 1960.
38. Alicandri CL, Fariello R, Agabiti-Rosei E, et al: Influence of the sympathetic nervous system on aortic compliance. Clin Sci Mol Med 59 (Suppl 6):279s, 1980.
39. Simon AC, Safar MA, Levenson GA, Kehder AM, Levy BI: Systolic hypertension. Hemodynamic mechanism and choice of antihypertensive therapy. Am J Cardiol 44:505, 1979.
40. Simon AC, Safar ME, Levenson JA, et al: Action of vasodilating drugs on small and large arteries of hypertensive patients. J Cardiovasc Pharmacol 5:626, 1983.
41. Safar ME, Simon AC, Levenson JA, Cazor JL: Hemodynamic effects of diltiazem in hypertension. Circ Res 52 (Suppl I):169, 1983.
42. Simon AC, Levenson JA, Bouthier J, et al: Effects of acute and chronic angiotensin-converting enzyme inhibition on the human hypertensive large arteries. J Cardiovasc Pharmacol 7:S45, 1985.
43. Bristow JD, Honour AJ, Pickering GW, et al: Diminished baroreflex sensitivity in high blood pressure. Circulation 39:48, 1969.
44. National High Blood Pressure Education Program: Statement on Hypertension in the Elderly. Revised on 1980, Bethesda, Maryland, pp. 1–7.
45. Caird FI, Andrews GR, Kennedy RD: Effect of posture on blood pressure in the elderly. Br Heart J 35:527, 1973.
46. Taguchi JT, Suwangool P: "Pipe-stem" brachial arteries. A cause of pseudohypertension. JAMA 228:733, 1974.
47. Editorial: Hypertension in the elderly. Lancet 1:684, 1977.
48. Kuramoto K, Matsushita S, Kuwajima I: The pathogenetic role and treatment of elderly hypertension. Jap Circ J 45:833, 1981.
49. Tarazi RC, Dustan HP, Bravo EL, Niarchos AP: Vasodilating drugs: Contrasting haemodynamic effects. Clin Sci Mol Med 51:575s, 1976.
50. Tarazi RC, Bravo EL, Fouad FM, et al: Hemodynamic and volume changes associated with captopril. Hypertension 2:576, 1980.
51. Buhler FR, Hulthen L, Kiowski W, et al: The place of the calcium antagonist verapamil in antihypertensive therapy. J Cardiovasc Pharmacol 4:S350, 1982.
52. Fouad FM, Pedrinelli R, Bravo EL: Clinical and systemic hemodynamic effects of nitrendipine. Clin Pharmacol Ther 35:768, 1984.

## Chapter 33

# Urinary Incontinence in the Elderly

*Ananias C. Diokno*

Micturitional disorders are common among the elderly.[1] Unfortunately, they have not received as much attention as other more acute, life-threatening medical disorders. In addition, there is a prevalent misconception among the elderly and their families that most micturitional disorders are a natural result of aging and that there is nothing that can be done about such problems. Compounding the problem is the lack of knowledge of many care providers about major aspects of urologic disorders affecting the elderly. As a consequence, many urologic ailments are not revealed by the patient, are not diagnosed, and, if identified, are treated by benign neglect.

Urinary incontinence or involuntary loss of urine is one such micturitional disturbance that affects the elderly to a major extent.[2,3] Although the prevalence of urinary incontinence in the elderly living in a community in the United States is not known, several European studies have reported that prevalence rates vary from 1.6 to 49 per cent.[1,4,5] However, the present consensus is that the true prevalence rate is in the 15 to 30 per cent range. The major discrepancy in the results is in most part due to differences in the definition of urinary incontinence.

The clinician caring for the elderly does not have to be convinced that urinary incontinence is much more prevalent among the institutionalized elderly than among those living in a community. European hospital surveys of older people revealed that as many as 48 per cent of institutionalized elderly may be incontinent.[6] Willington estimated that 30 per cent of unselected elderly admissions are incontinent.[7] Furthermore, a survey sponsored by the Department of Health, Education and Welfare in 1975 on long-term care facilities reported that 55 per cent of patients surveyed had some problem with urinary control and an additional 5 per cent were using a catheter or other collecting device.[8]

The impact of urinary incontinence goes beyond the individual himself to the family members as well as to the society as a whole. For the individual, chronic loss of urine can lead to skin irritation, infections, and ulcerations. Psychologically, it has led elderly into isolation and depression.[9] There are immeasurable economic losses from soiled linens, carpeting, and other household furnishings. The lack of knowledge about incontinence on the part of many family members coupled with the lack of knowledge about therapeutic options on the part of some care providers, has resulted in unnecessary institutionalization of the affected individual.

## ANATOMY AND NEUROPHYSIOLOGY OF THE LOWER URINARY TRACT

Urinary incontinence is a complex disorder whose causes, mechanisms, and treatments are diverse. A major mistake is to consider urinary incontinence one entity and to treat it as such. In reality, there are several types, depending upon the mechanism of urine loss. In order to understand the pathophysiology of incontinence, a brief review of the anatomy and neurophysiology of the lower urinary tract is in order.

The body of the urinary bladder, or bladder fundus, and the proximal urethra should be considered as one unit both anatomically and functionally.[10] Both segments originate from the vesicourethral sac of the urogenital sinus, and both possess smooth muscle and elastic tissue in their walls. The smooth muscle of the bladder extends down into the urethra and contributes to the bulk of the wall of the proximal urethra.

There are three important components that play a major role in the maintenance of continence: the detrusor muscle, the proximal urethra or internal sphincter, and the periurethral striated muscle or external sphincter (Fig. 33–1). The smooth muscle of the bladder and urethra has certain intrinsic properties that are completely independent of any nervous control from the central nervous system. The viscoelastic properties of the smooth muscle and elastic tissue allow the bladder to accommodate a large volume of fluid within its cavity under low intravesical pressure.

Fluid present within the urinary bladder cavity is prevented from leaking out through the urethra by the resistance exerted by the internal sphincter or proximal urethra. The resistance is the sum total of the forces originating from the mucosa, smooth muscle, and elastic tissue, constituting the internal sphincter. This segment of the urethra includes the proximal urethra, which is the proximal three fourths of the female urethra and the prostatic and membranous urethra in the males. Under low intravesical pressures, the internal sphincter is sufficient to contain the urine within the cavity.[11]

When high bladder pressures occur as a result of increased intra-abdominal pressure, as in coughing, straining, or laughing, the action of the internal sphincter is enhanced by the periurethral striated muscle or external urinary sphincter. This striated muscle originates from the urogenital diaphragm and the levator ani and encircles the internal sphincter. The greatest concentration of this muscle is at the midurethra in females and the membranous urethra in males.[12]

Although the storage function of the urinary bladder can be accomplished without the aid of the nervous system, evacuation is dependent upon impulses emanating from the cerebrospinal axis.[13] The micturitional center in the brain is located in the frontal lobe. The corticoregulatory tract from this center controls the micturition center located in the midbrain. From the pontine mesencephalic center, fibers descend and synapse at the spinal cord center located at S2, S3, and S4. At this level, two important motor neurons are identified. The ventral, or anterior, horn cells provide the pudendal nerves, whereas the lateral horn cells produce the pelvic nerve. From the low thoracic and high lumbar segments of the spinal cord emanate the presacral or hypogastric nerves, which innervate the bladder and urethra (Fig. 33–2).

The pelvic nerve is a parasympathetic mixed nerve. The efferent fibers carry the motor impulses that effect micturition to the detrusor muscle. The afferent fibers carry the pain, temperature, and distention perception from the bladder. The pudendal nerve is a somatic nerve that innervates the external sphincter. It also supplies the sensory perception to the perineum and genitalia. (see Fig. 33–2).

The presacral nerve is a sympathetic nerve that innervates the bladder and urethra. There are two distinct sympathetic receptors in the lower urinary tract. The alpha-adrenergic re-

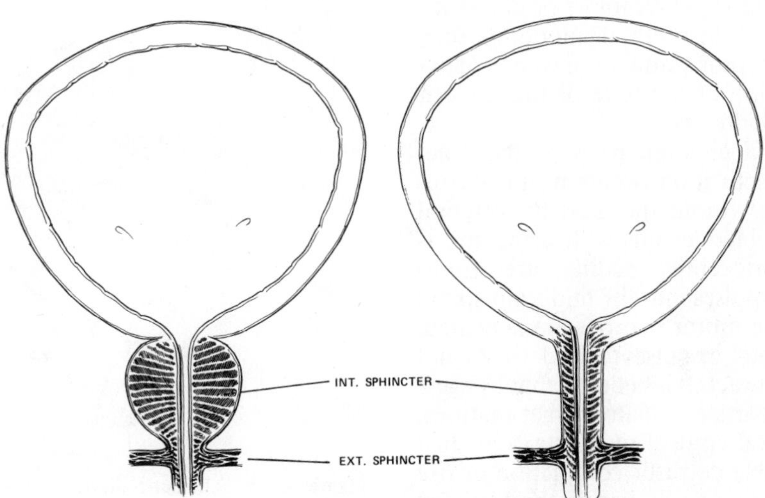


**Figure 33–1.** Schematic diagram demonstrating the two urethral sphincters.

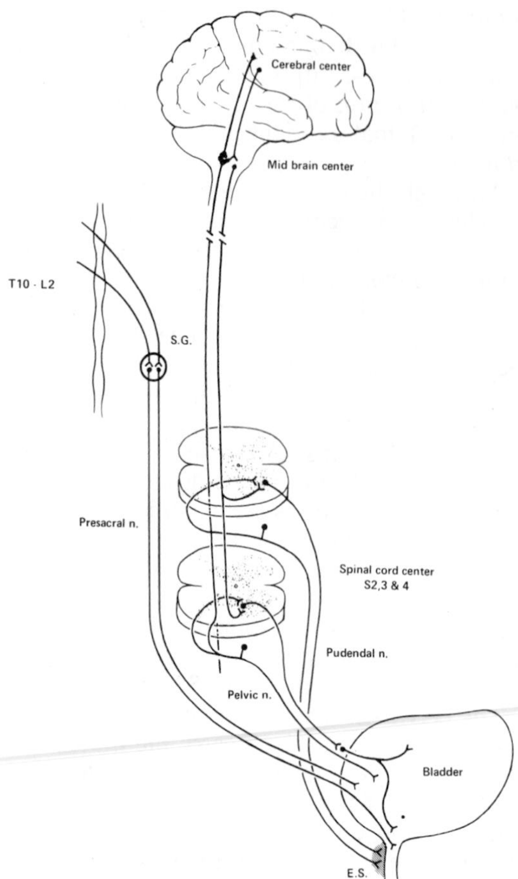


**Figure 33–2.** Cerebrospinal control of micturition. Note the cerebropontine and pontine-spinal axis and the pelvic, pudendal, and presacral nerves.

ceptors are highly concentrated in the trigone and proximal urethra, whereas the beta receptors are concentrated in the body or fundus of the urinary bladder (see Fig. 33–2).[14] Stimulation of alpha-adrenergic receptors produces increased tonicity of the urethral smooth muscle, whereas beta receptor stimulation causes relaxation or reduction of the tone of the smooth muscle of the bladder wall.

In infants and children prior to the toilet training age, micturition occurs in an uncontrolled fashion, without the need for cerebral control. As the bladder fills with urine and is stretched, proprioceptive endings are stimulated to send impulses into the midbrain-spinal cord center. The motor neurons are activated, transmitting motor impulses to the detrusor and causing it to contract. It is believed that by age 2 to 4 years, the corticoregulatory tract matures, providing cortical control to micturition. Just before measurable detrusor contraction or rise in intravesical pressure, the periurethral striated muscle relaxes completely. As the detrusor contracts, the bladder neck opens. A sustained detrusor contraction ensues, producing a strong continuous urinary stream. (Figs. 33–3 and 33–4).

## PATHOPHYSIOLOGY OF URINARY INCONTINENCE

Involuntary loss of urine can occur in any age group, although it appears to be more prevalent at both extremes of age. The mechanisms of incontinence are the same regardless of age; however, the prevalence of the various types varies in these age groups.

The basic determinant of urine loss is the pressure differential between the bladder and the urethra. Urinary incontinence will develop whenever the intravesical pressure equals or overcomes the maximum intraurethral pressure. This can occur in a variety of ways: an increase in intravesical pressure, a fall in intraurethral pressure, or a combination of the preceding, such that the detrusor pressure equals or exceeds the maximum urethral pressure. In addition, anatomic lesions such as vesicovaginal fistula and ectopic ureter will lead to urinary incontinence.

Detrusor dysfunction leading to urinary incontinence can be categorized as detrusor hyperreflexia, hypertonia, and hypotonia. Detru-

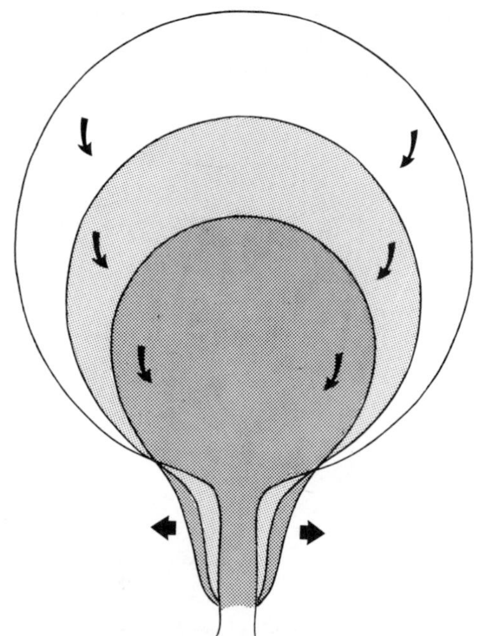

**Figure 33–3.** Schematic diagram of the contraction of the detrusor and the opening of the bladder outlet during voiding.

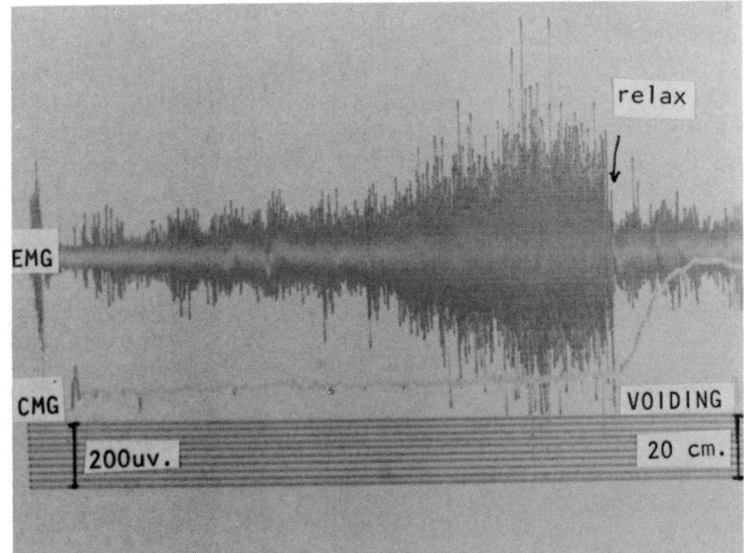


**Figure 33-4.** Combined cystometrograph (CMG) and external sphincter electromyograph (EMG) showing normal bladder and sphincter activity. Note the external sphincter relaxation just prior to and throughout the period of detrusor contraction, or voiding.

sor hyperreflexia and hypertonia can produce abnormally high intravesical pressure exceeding that of the intraurethral pressure. Detrusor hyperreflexia is neurogenic in origin, whereas hypertonia is myogenic in etiology. Detrusor hypotonia leads to chronic urinary retention, which in time produces pressure equal to or exceeding that of the intraurethral pressure. Hypotonia may be of neurogenic or non-neurogenic origin.

Sphincter dysfunction causing urinary incontinence can occur as a result of internal or external sphincter problems or both. The most common cause of stress incontinence is pelvic musculofascial relaxation and reduction of urethral resistance. In addition, injury to the membranous urethra during prostatectomy or following pelvic trauma can also produce urinary incontinence on the basis of reduced urethral sphincter competence. External sphincter paralysis or injury can lead to urinary incontinence owing to reduction of the total urethral resistance. Outlet obstruction as in prostatism can lead to urinary retention and produce incontinence with a mechanism similar to that occurring with detrusor hypotonia.

## GENERAL EVALUATION OF URINARY INCONTINENCE

Whenever one is confronted with an elderly person with urinary incontinence, a thorough history should be obtained from the patient, caretaker, or significant other. The recent and past history related to urine loss; urologic, gynecologic, neurologic and related medical and psychologic illnesses; and use of medications should be obtained.

Physical examination should include pelvic, rectal, and neurologic examinations. Sensory testing of the perineum should be accomplished as well as testing of the tone of the anal sphincter. On rectal examination, one should ascertain the possible presence of fecal impaction and palpate the prostate gland.

An evaluation of incontinence is incomplete without the analysis of the urine. A clean-catch urine sample is acceptable if the urine is normal. If urinalysis reveals pyuria or bacteriuria, an attempt should be made to ensure that this finding is not a result of contamination. In males, the prepuce should be retracted away from the meatus and the glans penis rinsed adequately before collecting the midstream urine sample. We have observed tremendous difficulty in getting elderly females to carry out strict aseptic midstream collection of the urine sample. In this situation, whenever the initial "clean-catch" urine is abnormal, we always resort to sterile catheterization, which we believe is the best and easiest way to confirm the presence of urinary infection rather than contamination. Iatrogenic infection following single sterile catheterization is an extremely rare phenomenon in our experience. On the contrary, we have seen many elderly women treated for multiple recurrent urinary infections on the basis of urinary frequency and a clean-catch urine showing infection. On many occasions we have confirmed the presence of contaminated clean-catch urine following examination of a catheterized sample. In addition, whenever there is a question of residual urine, a single sterile catheterization should be performed to measure the post-void residual.

In many of our patients with incontinence, history, physical examination, urinalysis, and simple office testing are all that we need to establish a fairly adequate diagnosis and provide the basis for specific therapeutic trial as long as the therapy is reversible and of low risk to the patient. Extensive or complex urodynamic testing should be reserved for complicated cases, whenever a surgical procedure is contemplated, or whenever a trial of treatment fails. Complicated cases include individuals with complex symptomatology, a previous anti-incontinence surgical procedure, and/or postsurgical incontinence. All patients who are to undergo a surgical procedure for incontinence should have an adequate preoperative evaluation. Whenever a trial of pharmacologic manipulation fails in a case of apparently simple or uncomplicated incontinence, further studies are needed to elucidate the real nature of the incontinence.

Urodynamic examination can be divided into basic and complex tests. The basic tests include uroflowmetry,[13] cystometry,[15] sphincter electromyography,[18] urethral pressure profilometry,[19] and cystourethroscopy. More complex and dynamic tests include simultaneous pressure measurements of the bladder, urethra, and rectum at rest and with exertion.[20] In conjunction with these pressure measurements, urinary flow rates, sphincter electromyograms, and radiographs of the bladder and urethra can be obtained.[21] It should be emphasized that not all tests enumerated are necessary to make an accurate diagnosis. The simplest test that will diagnose the problem should be used, and the more complex tests should be reserved for the complicated or unexplained incontinence.

## TYPES AND TREATMENTS OF URINARY INCONTINENCE

Urinary incontinence can be considered either transient or established.

### *Transient Urinary Incontinence*

The transient nature of urinary incontinence is frequently observed in conjunction with acute medical illness, medications, urinary tract infection, constipation, diarrhea, and vaginitis. Transient incontinence should be suspected in any situation that can cloud one's sensorium, such as in metabolic derangement, electrolyte imbalance, use of medications, and episodes of cardiovascular crisis. In addition, conditions that can directly stimulate or inhibit bladder function can also lead to acute-onset urinary incontinence.

The major objective in the management of transient incontinence is to recognize the cause and to treat it aggressively. Constipation should be relieved. When incontinence is associated with urinary tract infection, the infection should be treated effectively. Atrophic vaginitis should be treated with the use of an estrogen preparation. The usual choice is conjugated estrogen (Premarin) cream. The cream is applied with an applicator, so that a gram or two of the cream is delivered once or twice per week for 6 weeks. A maintenance dose may be necessary. Obviously, metabolic derangement and other acute medical problems should be attended immediately.

### *Established Incontinence*

Established incontinence is characterized by being chronic, persistent, or recurrent. On the basis of the mechanism of incontinence, loss of urine control can be divided into four categories: urge, stress, overflow, and functional types.

#### Urge Urinary Incontinence

Urge urinary incontinence is characterized by an uncontrolled loss of urine preceded by an urge to void. The problem is usually described as failure to hold urine long enough to reach a toilet. In certain people who have a reduced perception of bladder distention, incontinence is described as sudden loss of urine in any position without any warning and with no associated stress. The volume of urine loss can be a few drops to several hundred milliliters with complete bladder emptying. The incontinence can occur day or night. In addition to incontinence, these patients are bothered by urinary frequency, nocturia, and even suprapubic discomfort.

Urge incontinence is caused by sudden increases in intravesical pressure due to detrusor hyperreflexia or detrusor hypertonia. Detrusor hyperreflexia is seen in patients with neurologic lesions above S2, S3, and S4. The lesion produces loss of inhibition of the detrusor reflex arc, causing the detrusor to contract when the stretch receptors are stimulated by the distending bladder. The patient's mechanism for controlling the detrusor hyperreflexia is to contract the external sphincter. However, the intravesical pressure generally overcomes, partially or completely, the sphincter resistance, producing loss of urine by means of the urethra.

In patients with detrusor hypertonicity, the bladder has lost the ability to accommodate urine. As a result, high pressure develops under small volume. This high intravesical pressure overcomes the resistance at the urethral level, causing the involuntary loss of urine.

Detrusor hyperreflexia is seen in patients with cerebrovascular accident, brain tumor, incomplete spinal cord injury, parkinsonism, multiple sclerosis, and other lesions affecting the spinal cord above the sacral cord center. Detrusor hypertonia is seen in patients with interstitial cystitis, radiation cystitis, cyclophosphamide cystitis, chronic cystitis, prostatomegaly, and, rarely, carcinoma in situ of the bladder.

Diagnosis can be made by obtaining a detailed history of the nature of the incontinence and by carrying out physical and cystometric examinations.[15] Cystourethroscopy may be necessary in certain cases. In the history, the symptoms of urge, urinary frequency, nocturia, and loss of urine day and night are typical of this condition. Past history of radiation or previous recurring infection will help in the evaluation. On physical examination one should look specifically for evidence of neurologic disorders, such as hemiplegia, paraparesis, or lower extremity spasticity. Cystometric examination will confirm the diagnosis. In patients with detrusor hyperreflexia, uninhibited contractions can be documented on cystometry (Fig. 33–5). In detrusor hypertonia, small-capacity bladder and poor compliance will be documented (Fig. 33–6). There will be no residual urine, and bladder perception will be normal. Hyperreflexia can be distinguished from hypertonia by observing the effect of an anticholinergic agent on intravesical pressure. In the cystometrogram of a hypertonic patient, the curve will remain unchanged. In the patient with hyperreflexia, the uninhibited contraction will be suppressed or reduced. Cystourethroscopy will reveal a normal bladder and outlet, or it may confirm the presence of various types of cystitis or prostatomegaly encroaching into the trigone.

**Treatment.** Urge incontinence is treated primarily with the use of anticholinergic or anticholinergic-antispasmodic preparations. These preparations inhibit uncontrolled bladder contractions or enlarge the functional bladder capacity. These agents are especially appropriate for long-term maintenance use; they are not intended to cure the problem. However, they have been found to be effective in 80 to 85 per cent of patients with uninhibited bladder contractions and symptoms of urinary frequency, urgency, and incontinence.[22] The two most commonly used drugs are oxybutynin chloride and propantheline bromide. The usual dosage of oxybutynin for the elderly is 5 mg orally twice or three times a day. Propantheline is usually given as a 15 mg dose three or four times a day. Another drug in the same spectrum is dicyclomine (20 mg orally three times a day). Imipramine, because of its indirect alpha-adrenergic effect and mild anticholinergic effect, has also been used effectively at a dosage of 25 mg twice or three times a day. Caution should be exercised when using these drugs with the elderly because they are sensitive to these medications. Toxic effects include dry mouth, blurred vision, nervousness, and constipation. The initial dose

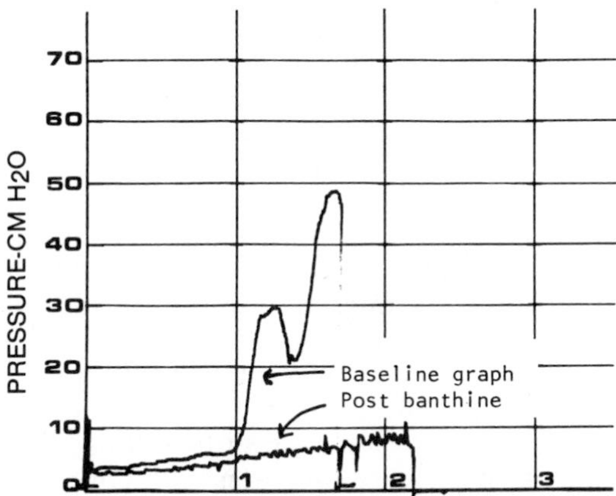


**Figure 33–5.** A cystometrograph showing uninhibited contractions in the baseline graph that were totally abolished by intravenous methantheline bromide.

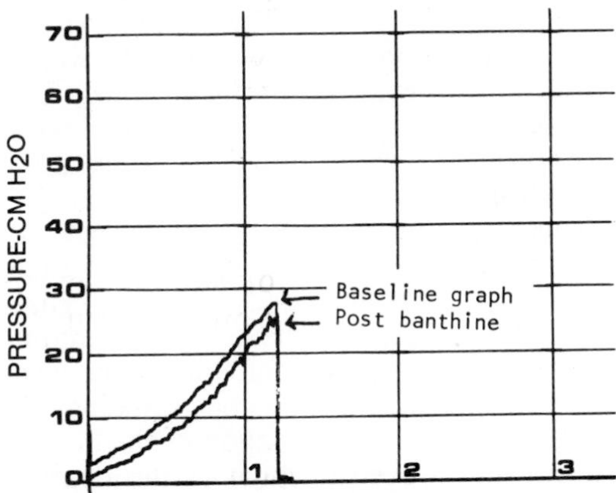


**Figure 33–6.** A cystometrograph demonstrating the ineffectiveness of methantheline bromide (Banthine) on the hypertonic detrusor.

may need to be reduced to half the recommended dose. With the reduced dose, control of urge incontinence can still be achieved without causing significant side effects.

Recent reports have suggested that behavioral management, such as bladder training techniques to improve the perception of bladder fullness and delay voiding, has been effective in improving the symptoms of patients with urge incontinence.[23] These modes of therapy may be combined with drug therapy to effect control. However, the effectiveness of behavioral therapy for the elderly has not been established. Preliminary experience with this technique suggests that memory, physical condition, will power, and long-term commitment are prerequisites for its success; these factors may be difficult to obtain in some elderly people.

The group of patients who fail to respond to the pharmacologic as well as the behavioral treatments can be considered for other treatment modalities, including selective sacral rhizolysis, bladder denervation procedures, and bladder augmentation procedures. Selective sacral rhizolysis is a percutaneous procedure done by a neurosurgeon to deactivate one or two of the nerve roots to the bladder. The augmentation procedure is a surgical procedure and as such may be indicated only for the surgically fit. It should also be recognized that this more aggressive therapy should be reserved for the few patients with severe symptoms and is seldom applicable to the elderly.

## Overflow Urinary Incontinence

Overflow urinary incontinence is characterized by periodic or continuous dripping of urine. The patient usually describes his or her problem as always being wet, owing to small volume urinary leakage day and night. These patients will also describe hesitancy and straining to void. Urinary stream, if present, will be described as very weak and interrupted. This type of incontinence is also called paradoxical incontinence because of the overflow nature of this disturbance.

This type of urinary leakage is associated with conditions leading to chronic retention of urine, such as prostatism and paralytic type of neurogenic bladder; or, in patients with hypotonic bladder, it is secondary to infrequent voiding or chronic obstruction. The long-standing obstruction and/or overdistention of the bladder walls leads to overstretching of the detrusor muscle, which in time leads to loss of muscle tone. On occasion, patients who chronically use tranquilizers have been reported to present with this condition. The overdistended bladder produces a chronically elevated bladder pressure; this, in turn, overcomes the intraurethral pressure whenever pressure is applied to the bladder or whenever a quantity of urine is pushed into the bladder by ureteral peristalsis.

Besides obtaining a history of prostatism, infrequent voiding, excessive fluid intake, and use of diuretics, the physician will usually find on physical examination evidence of a large distended bladder. Rectal examination may identify a hard nodular prostate gland, suggestive of prostatic adenocarcinoma. It should be emphasized that rectal examination alone is not useful in making a diagnosis of obstructive benign prostatic hyperplasia. There are many instances in which the hypertrophied prostate gland encroaches into the lumen, causing obstructive symptoms, and yet the prostate gland on rectal examination is relatively small. There are also instances of a markedly enlarged prostate on rectal examination due to outward growth of the prostate, which produces no outlet obstruction. Diagnosis of overflow can be confirmed by measuring the residual urine post void. Cystometry will reveal a large-capacity bladder with no or weak voluntary detrusor contraction.

In patients with suspected paralytic bladder, the Urecholine supersensitivity test of Lapides will confirm the presence of significant bladder denervation.[10] This test is done by performing the standard cystometrography, usually utilizing water or carbon dioxide as the infusing agent. The intravesical pressure is measured at 1 dl of volume. The patient is administered 2.5 mg of bethanechol chloride subcutaneously, and the cystometrogram is obtained again 15 to 20 minutes later. A positive response is characterized by an increase in bladder pressure of 20 cm over the control intravesical pressure at 1 dl of volume. False-positive response is observed in patients with azotemia; false-negatives are seen in patients with very early denervation or limited denervation to the bladder.

Urethrocystoscopy is mandatory in patients with paradoxical incontinence to rule out anatomic obstruction. The urethra should be carefully studied for strictures. Use of bougie à boule to calibrate the entire urethra in females and the anterior urethra in males will establish the presence of stricture. Cystourethroscopy findings, although very subjective, will usually identify those patients with obvious anatomic outlet obstruction. In complicated cases, more extensive urodynamic tests may be necessary to evaluate the actual cause of chronic retention.

**Treatment.** Treatment for overflow incontinence should be directed to the cause of inadequate bladder emptying. Prostatism and urethral strictures are often the cause of obstructive uropathy among men. Anatomic obstruction is extremely rare in women. Attempts should be made to relieve the obstruction by prostatectomy or release of stricture if at all possible. The transurethral approach is now the most popular and the least invasive procedure for the elderly. Age alone should not be a contraindication for surgery to relieve obstruction.

In those in whom surgical therapy is not feasible and for those with nonobstructive hypotonic bladder, the use of either clean intermittent catheterization or an indwelling Foley catheter is the next treatment of choice. Clean intermittent catheterization, introduced by Lapides in 1972, has been proved to be a safe and effective long-term treatment for patients with bladder-emptying dysfunction.[24] This is obviously preferable to long-term use of an indwelling Foley catheter and should be seriously considered for the alert, competent, ambulatory elderly. Patients can be taught clean intermittent self-catheterization by an experienced teacher (nurse, enterostomal therapist, or physician's assistant). Our experience with the use of this technique in the elderly has been gratifying.

On occasion, bladder rehabilitation can be accomplished not only by intermittent catheterization but also with the use of a cholinergic agent and an alpha-adrenergic blocker.[25] The principle in this treatment is to stimulate the bladder with bethanechol chloride, a cholinergic agent, and relax the urethral internal sphincter with the use of phenoxybenzamine, an alpha-adrenergic blocker. The usual dosage of bethanechol is 25 to 50 mg orally every 6 to 8 hours, whereas the dosage for phenoxybenzamine is 10 mg orally every 8 to 12 hours. As in other drug therapy, caution should be exercised in using these drugs in the elderly. The lowest dose with longest interval should be used initially and the dose gradually increased if necessary. These drugs should not be used for patients with cardiovascular disease, peptic ulcer disease, or labile vital signs.

For patients with overflow incontinence who are not candidates for, or do not respond to, surgery, intermittent catheterization, drug therapy, or urethral or suprapubic catheter drainage is the last recourse. Although bacteriuria is highly prevalent in patients with long-standing indwelling catheters, no attempt should be made to eradicate these bacteria, since resistant strains will result. Catheter bacteriuria should be treated only prior to instrumentation or if the patient is symptomatic. The catheter should be replaced every 4 weeks, and the usual catheter care should be instituted to avoid complications.

### Stress Urinary Incontinence

Stress urinary incontinence is characterized by sudden loss of urine associated with increased physical activity or exertion, such as coughing, laughing, and lifting. The volume of urine loss varies tremendously from a few drops to massive loss of urine. In general, the incontinence is observed with physical activity and is seldom observed at night unless coughing and other strenuous movements, such as sexual intercourse, are performed while in bed. Patients with this disorder usually have no other voiding complaints.

Stress incontinence is mainly a manifestation of abnormally reduced urethral resistance. In women, the most common cause is relaxation of the musculofascial attachments of the bladder to the pelvis. This leads to hypermobility of the proximal urethra, which leads to shortening of the functional urethra or the internal sphincter. Lapides[16] believes that the urethral shortening causes reduced urethral resistance. Enhorning[17] proposes that the loss of urethral resistance is due to the prolapse of the proximal urethra below the urogenital diaphragm during stress, so that the increased intra-abdominal pressure applied to the bladder is not equally applied to the proximal urethra.[17] Other causes of stress incontinence in women include trauma to the proximal urethra following resections or incisions, devascularized urethra, atrophic urethritis, and paralytic external sphincter.

In men, the most common cause of stress incontinence is injury to the membranous urethra following pelvic trauma or as a complication of transurethral surgery. Another cause is paralytic sphincter.

An accurately taken patient history will enable the investigator to discover the probable cause of stress incontinence. In women, a history of pregnancy is generally essential in the development of pelvic relaxation. Prior gynecologic or urologic surgery may be associated with the stress incontinence. Incontinence is usually reduced or absent at night while in bed in contrast to the frequent wetting occurring during the day while active. A careful history will permit one to distinguish stress incontinence from pure urge incontinence. Incontinence of the stress type will occur simultaneously with exertional activity, such as coughing and lifting. In urge incontinence, leakage usually occurs several seconds after exertion or stress movement has taken place. This is due to the fact that urge incontinence is the result of micturitional reflex activity stimulated by the sudden increase in intravesical pressure.

Physical examination is crucial and many times is the key to making the diagnosis. In performing the pelvic examination the physician should note the presence of perineal excoriation, atrophic vaginitis, bacterial vaginitis, uterine prolapse, urethral caruncle, and hemorrhoids. Saddle sensation should be tested to identify possible pudendal nerve injury or disease. The finding of unilateral or bilateral saddle anesthesia or hypesthesia may be the only physical sign of a neurogenic cause of incontinence. The anal tone should be tested at the time of the rectal examination. Weak or flaccid anal tone may also be suggestive of a neurologic defect.

In the performance of the pelvic examination, the physician should note the degree of pelvic relaxation. The degree of cystocele, urethrocele, and rectocele should be carefully assessed by observing the specific structure while having the patient strain. The occurrence of incontinence should be noted during this maneuver. However, it should be emphasized that the presence of a cystocele or urethrocele is a sign of pelvic relaxation but has no direct relationship to the occurrence of stress incontinence. In fact, a cystocele may have a protective effect because of its ability to absorb increases in intravesical pressures. This is also the reason why cystocele repair alone may cause postoperative manifestation of stress incontinence not previously present. Ascertaining the severity of a cystocele in patients with stress incontinence is important in determining the approach and technique for surgical repair. The presence of a severe, symptomatic cystocele in the presence of stress incontinence is an indication for a vaginal approach. However, if the cystocele is asymptomatic and nonprolapsing, the bladder-suspension procedure can be approached in a number of ways.

Anterior vaginal wall palpation has several objectives. First, urethral diverticula should be searched for. Diverticula of the urethra appear as cystic, sometimes tender masses located in the anterior vaginal wall at the mid-urethra. When these masses are milked towards the meatus, a milky, purulent discharge may be observed at the meatus. These findings are diagnostic of urethral diverticula. Secondly, the pliability of the anterior vaginal wall should be tested. The anterior vaginal wall is lifted superiorly, using the forefinger and middle finger at each side of the bladder neck. This maneuver not only determines whether the bladder can be lifted and therefore suspended but also determines the elasticity of the anterior vaginal wall. In certain cases the anterior vaginal wall is very rigid and inelastic and when lifted provokes significant pelvic and vaginal pain. In these cases, the bladder suspension procedure is probably contraindicated.

Before the physician makes a diagnosis of stress incontinence, the involuntary loss of urine should be documented. In 1961, Lapides[16] described a simple office test to document objectively, urethral shortening and incontinence. He recommends the use of a measuring 18-Fr. catheter, which is inserted into the bladder, with the catheter balloon inflated with 5 ml of sterile water. The bladder is then filled through the catheter with approximately 3 dl of sterile water or normal saline solution. The urethral length from the vesicourethral junction to the meatus is measured visually with the aid of a calibrated Foley catheter while the patient is in the lithotomy position. The patient is asked to stand, and again the urethral length is measured, followed by the removal of the catheter. As soon as the catheter is removed, the patient is asked to strain by coughing. The degree of incontinence, if any, is noted. In patients with stress incontinence, the urethral length will be observed to shorten as the position is changed from supine to standing. No change or even lengthening is generally observed in the continent female.

As mentioned earlier, stress incontinence is only a manifestation of several processes that should be distinguished if one is to consider an invasive or irreversible form of therapy such as surgical procedure. This is necessary because each type of stress incontinence has a different method of surgical therapy. However, if one is contemplating a reversible or noninvasive therapy, then a good history, physical examination, and documentation of stress incontinence will be sufficient to start such therapy.

Stress incontinence may be mimicked by, or combined with, urge incontinence. Because the approaches to therapy for stress incontinence are so different from those for urge incontinence, the exact type of incontinence should be distinguished before aggressive and invasive therapy is undertaken.

A systematic examination should distinguish the urge from the stress type of incontinence. In patients with pure stress incontinence, a cystometrogram will demonstrate a flat curve without any sign of uninhibited or uncontrolled contractions. In contrast to patients with overflow incontinence, voiding should be efficient and residual urine should be nil. To identify neurogenic bladder and sphincter as the cause of incontinence, a Urecholine supersensitivity test and needle sphincter electromyography are performed.[18] These are highly specific tests that are performed as part of the complex urodynamic assessment.

Cystourethroscopy is mandatory in patients with post-prostatectomy incontinence as well as in all patients in whom urethral trauma or disease is suspected. The presence of scar tissue at the region of the membranous urethra usually suggests trauma or devascularization, which may lead to an ineffective posterior urethra. In patients with primary stress incontinence, the incompetent proximal urethra can be visualized with the endoscope. The orifices of urethral diverticula can also be seen with the endoscope.

In complicated cases in which the simple approach does not clarify the diagnosis, complex urodynamic tests can be used and are available in many medical centers. These tests include simultaneous measurements of bladder, urethral, and rectal pressures; radiographic monitoring of the bladder and urethra at rest; bladder filling; straining; and voiding (Fig. 33–7).[13] These tests help clarify the pathophysiologic mechanism of many complicated incontinence cases.

**Treatment.** Treatment for stress urinary incontinence can be divided into nonsurgical and surgical approaches. The nonsurgical procedures consist of physical therapy and pharmacologic intervention. The physical therapy consists of urethral-sphincter, or Kegel, exercises.[26] This mode of therapy has been advocated for a long time. However, its real benefits and long-term effects in elderly people with stress incontinence are still untested. The basic mechanism for the approach is daily exercise of pelvic musculature, specifically the urogenital diaphragm, to increase its tone and to effect increased urethral resistance. The patient should be cautioned of the probability of developing pelvic pain and having sexual stimulation while doing the exercise.

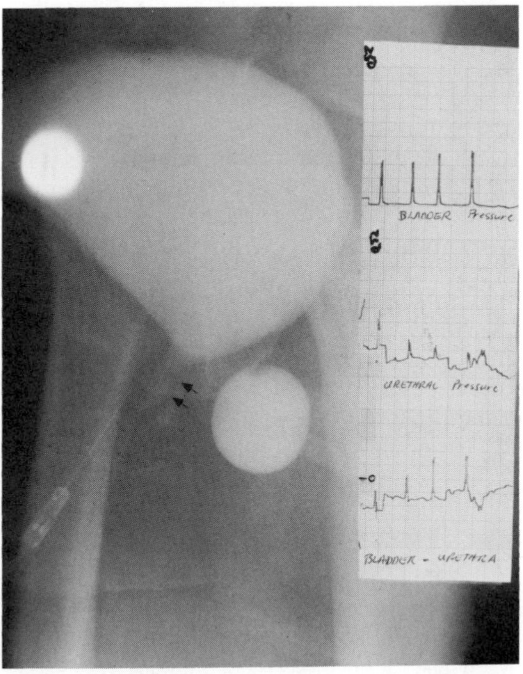


**Figure 33–7.** Simultaneous cystography and bladder and urethral pressure measurements while the patient is straining. Note the presence of contrast material in the urethra, associated with measurements of higher bladder pressure than urethral pressure. This is classic for stress urinary incontinence due to sphincter incompetency.

Pharmacologic therapy is directed to the stimulation of the alpha-adrenergic receptors located at the trigone and internal sphincter. The alpha-adrenergic agents are indicated for stress incontinence of mild to moderate degree. When used in these cases, a 75 per cent success rate can be expected. The alpha-adrenergic agents recommended for stress incontinence are phenylpropanolamine and ephedrine.[27,28] The dosage for the phenylpropanolamine is 50 to 100 mg orally twice daily. Ephedrine can be given at a dosage of 25 mg orally three to four times daily. These drugs are contraindicated in patients with hypertension and thyroid disease.

Surgical therapy for stress incontinence can be divided into bladder suspension procedures and prosthetic implantation procedures. The standard treatment for stress urinary incontinence due to pelvic relaxation is a bladder suspension procedure. This operation can be accomplished through either a suprapubic, vaginal, or combined suprapubic and vaginal approach. Regardless of the approach, the procedure has a success rate of 85 to 90 per cent. With the numerous simplified techniques to suspend the bladder, this procedure should not be denied elderly patients with simple stress urinary incontinence as long as they are good surgical and anesthesia risks.

The artificial urinary sphincter is a device that can be implanted in patients with severe urinary incontinence due to a paralytic sphincter, a fibrous or traumatized urethra, or post-prostatectomy incontinence. This device is made of silicone rubber and is composed of three parts: the pressurized balloon, the deflate bulb, and the cuff. These parts are interconnected by an assembly unit that controls the flow of fluid within the system. The entire device is surgically implanted: the cuff around the bulbous urethra or bladder neck, the deflate bulb in the labia or hemiscrotum, and the pressurized balloon in the prevesical space. It is a semi-automatic device that automatically pressurizes the cuff and occludes the urethra. The cuff is opened by squeezing the deflate bulb, causing a transfer of fluid from the cuff to the balloon. The overall success rate of this device is approximately 70 to 80 per cent. The operation is contraindicated in patients who are unable to empty their bladders completely and in patients who have memory problems.

### Functional Incontinence

Functional incontinence is the term used to describe urinary incontinence observed in patients with normal bladder and urethral function. This problem appears to be due to inability to comprehend the need to void in appropriate places or inability to communicate the sense of urgency or the imminence of voiding. As a consequence, voiding of large amounts with total emptying of the bladder occurs in inappropriate situations and environments. The patient may be either totally unaware of the event or aware of and sensitive to the urinary accident.

Functional incontinence is classically seen in patients with severe dementia and closed head injuries. It should be emphasized that this diagnosis is made only after the usual evaluation process has been done and the pathologic process has been eliminated.

**Treatment.** The treatment for functional incontinence and other forms that fail to respond to all standard treatment modalities is directed to containing the urinary leakage with the use of pads, external devices, and catheters. Males are better suited than females for the use of external catheters. Numerous devices are now available. This is fortunate because there is not one external catheter that fits everyone. In most instances the device is held in place by a double adhesive strip wrapped around the penis. The condom portion is rolled over the strip and connected to a urinary drainage bag. It should be emphasized that initial fitting and application of the device should be performed by personnel who are familiar with the device and should not be relegated to the novice.

For men who cannot use the condom catheter and for women who are incontinent, superabsorbent pads can be used to contain the urine. Exciting new developments in the field of absorbent pads have occurred within the last few years. The ideal situation is to use the most absorbent yet least bulky pad placed inside the undergarment. Nurse gerontologists and enterostomal therapists have been extremely helpful in fitting these patients with the appropriate device or the best material to contain the involuntary urine loss (see Chapter 4).

### Complex Urinary Incontinence

Complex urinary incontinence is a term used for incontinence secondary to combined urge and stress incontinence. Our experience at the continence clinic at The University of Michigan suggests that this problem is prevalent among the elderly. The presenting complaint may be purely that of stress incontinence or urge incontinence, but generally both symptoms can be obtained in the history. It appears that these patients have a long-standing mild or moderate stress incontinence and that the urge incontinence is of more recent onset.

Although the diagnosis can be suspected from the history and physical examination, the techniques used to diagnose the individual types of incontinence may be used to make an accurate diagnosis.

**Treatment.** The treatment for this problem should be directed to the most predominant symptom. In general, urge incontinence is the predominant component and should be tackled in a manner similar to that used in patients with urge incontinence. If incontinence persists and the leakage is primarily stress-related, then it should be treated also. A combination of anticholinergic and alpha-adrenergic drugs has been used with success. Care should be taken to avoid the usual side effects of these medications by reducing the initial dose. If stress incontinence persists, the bladder suspension procedure can be performed, realizing that urge incontinence should be controlled pharmacologically in the postoperative period.

The ultimate recourse in some patients is the use of an indwelling Foley catheter. In women, the urethral indwelling catheter is adequate and acceptable. However, in men, because of the high incidence of epididymitis and urethritis, suprapubic cystostomy should be seriously considered whenever permanent drainage is contemplated. With these available treatment modalities, every elderly person suffering from urinary incontinence should have an opportunity to control, if not correct, this problem.

## References

1. Brocklehurst JC, Griffiths L, Fry J: The prevalence and symptomatology of urinary infection in an aged population. Gerontol Clin 10:242, 1962.
2. Willington FL: Introduction. *In* Willington FL (ed.): Incontinence in the Elderly. New York, Academic Press, 1976, pp. 3–21.
   *This book is a must for the gerontologist taking care of urinary incontinence.*
3. Vetter NS, Jones DA, Victor CR: Urinary incontinence in the elderly at home. Lancet 2(8254):1275, 1981.

4. Akhtar AJ, Brow GA, Crombie A, et al: Disability and dependence in the elderly at home. Age Ageing 2:102, 1973.
5. Yarnell JWG, Boyle GJ: The prevalence and severity of urinary incontinence in women. J Epidemiol Community Health 35:71, 1981.
6. Wells T, Brink C: Urinary incontinence: Assessment and management. *In* Burnside I (ed.): Nursing and the Aged. New York, McGraw-Hill, 1981, pp. 519–548.
*A very informative chapter with many practical recommendations.*
7. Willington FL: Significance of incompetence of personal sanitary habits. Nurs Times 71:340, 1975.
8. U.S. Department of Health, Education, and Welfare: Long-term Care Facility Improvement Study. Washington, DC, U.S. Government Printing Office, 1975.
9. Sutherland SS: The psychology of incontinence. *In* Willington FL (ed.): Incontinence in the Elderly. New York, Academic Press, 1976, pp. 52–69.
10. Lapides J, Diokno AC: Urine transport, storage and micturition. *In* Lapides J (ed.): Fundamentals of Urology. Philadelphia, W. B. Saunders Co., 1976, pp. 190–241.
*An excellent chapter to read to understand the physiology of micturition and the types of neuropathic bladder dysfunction.*
11. Lapides J: Structure and function of the internal vesical sphincter. J Urol 80:34, 1958.
12. Lapides J, Sweer RB, Lewis LW: Role of striated muscle in urination. J Urol 77:247, 1957.
13. Raz S, Bradley WS: Neuromuscular dysfunction of the lower urinary tract. *In* Harrison JH, Gittes RF, Perlmutter AD, et al (eds.): Campbell's Urology. 4th ed. Philadelphia, W. B. Saunders Co., 1979, pp. 1215–1270.
14. Awad SA, Bruce AW, Carro-Ciampi G, et al: Distribution of alpha and beta adrenoceptors in human urinary bladder. Br J Pharmacol 50:525, 1974.
15. Lapides J: Cystometry. JAMA 201:618, 1967.
*Quick reading material to learn all about cystometry.*
16. Lapides J: Stress incontinence. J Urol 85:291, 1961.
17. Enhorning G: Simultaneous recording of intravesical and intraurethral pressure. Acta Chir Scand (Suppl) 276:1, 1961.
18. Diokno AC, Koff SA, Bender LF: Periurethral striated muscle activity in neurogenic bladder dysfunction. J Urol 112:743, 1974.
19. Gershon CR, Diokno AC: Urodynamic evaluation of female stress urinary incontinence. J Urol 119:787, 1978.
20. Bruskewitz R, Raz S: Urethral pressure profile using microtip catheter in females. Urology 14:303, 1979.
21. McGuire EJ: Radiographic evaluation. *In* McGuire EJ (ed.): Urinary Incontinence. New York, Grune & Stratton, 1981, pp. 75–85.
22. Vinson RK, Diokno AC: Uninhibited neurogenic bladder in adults. Urology 4:376, 1976.
*A review of uninhibited bladder in adults, a common problem in the elderly.*
23. Frewen WK: Role of bladder training in the treatment of the unstable bladder in the female. Urol Clin North Am 6:273, 1979.
*Dr. Frewen's experience in bladder training of the unstable bladder is presented in this manuscript.*
24. Lapides J, Diokno AC, Gould FR, Lowe BS: Further observations on self-catheterization. J Urol 116:169, 1976.
25. Sonda LP, Gershon C, Diokno AC, Lapides J: Further observations on the cystometric and uroflowmetric effects of bethanechol chloride on the human bladder. J Urol 122:775, 1979.
26. Kegel A, Powell T. The physiologic treatment of urinary stress incontinence. J Urol 63:808, 1950.
*The original Kegel technique for treatment of bladder control problems is discussed in this paper.*
27. Diokno AC, Taub M: Ephedrine in treatment of urinary incontinence. Urology 5:624, 1975.
28. Stewart BJ, Banowsky LHW, Montague DK: Stress incontinence: Conservative therapy with sympathomimetic drugs. J Urol 115:558, 1976.

Chapter 34

# Prostate Gland Disease

Ananias C. Diokno
Robert J. MacGregor

The prostate gland is a specialized glandular organ investing the male posterior urethra. Its major function appears to be the production of enzyme buffers important in sperm transportation and in the fertilization process. The prostate is of major clinical importance in the elderly because of its tendency for hyperplastic changes, generally manifesting as an obstruction to urinary flow, and carcinomatous changes in the gland, which can present in a variety of ways.

## BENIGN PROSTATIC HYPERPLASIA

### Incidence

Benign prostatic hyperplasia (BPH) is one of the most common problems encountered by clinical urologists. Patients under the age of 40 years with BPH are rare. The incidence increases after this age. Autopsy data indicate a prevalence of 95 per cent in persons dying at age 80 and over. The autopsy data do not necessarily reflect the true incidence of *clinically significant* BPH; however, the mean age for detection of BPH is 60 to 65 years.[1] It has been estimated that 10 per cent of males will probably require an operation for BPH if they live to 80 years.[2]

### Pathology

Hyperplastic change characteristically occurs in the periurethral glands of the prostate. Increase in the number and size of these glands produces a nodule that compresses "true" prostate tissue. This produces a "surgical capsule," which is an important landmark in enucleation surgery. The fibromuscular stroma also undergoes hypertrophy and hyperplasia. The ratio of adenomatous hyperplasia to fibrous hyperplasia is variable. Predominance of adenomatous hyperplasia often leads to the prostate becoming very large and requiring open removal. When the hyperplasia is predominantly fibromuscular, obstructive symptoms may not be associated with prostatic enlargement on rectal examination.

### Biogenesis

The etiology of BPH is not known at present. There is undoubtedly a hormonal basis for BPH, evidenced by the absence of BPH in men castrated before puberty, increased levels of dihydrotestosterone in BPH glands,[3] and a variable response to estrogen administration and castration. However, it would seem that the hormonal milieu affects mainly the ductal epithelium.[4] This may explain the variable success of hormonal manipulation in treating obstructive symptoms. There is to date no convincing evidence that medication is able to alter the pathogenetic factors influencing the course of BPH, including clinical obstruction.

### Pathophysiology of Obstruction

BPH causes obstruction to urine flow in several ways. Adenomatous BPH causes lobular encroachment into the lumen of the posterior urethra, impeding urine flow. Fibromuscular BPH produces rigidity of the proximal vesical neck area, preventing the normal funneling and shortening mechanism essential to normal voiding. Both mechanisms increase urethral resistance, and the bladder responds by increasing the strength of voiding contractions. Vesical muscular hypertrophy occurs. When this is prolonged, trabeculae, cellule, and saccule formation occurs. Mucosal outpouching between hypertrophied smooth muscle develops, and this is called bladder diverticulum. As urethral resistance increases, a pressure is reached above which the bladder is no longer able to respond. Bladder decompensation then occurs. Muscles become stretched, and later, muscle atrophy and fibrosis occur. Residual urine will increase gradually until the bladder is always at or near capacity; overflow, or paradoxical, incontinence then occurs. Increased pressures in the bladder have to be overcome by ureteral peristalsis, and ureteral response, including dilation and elongation, occurs. Prolonged raised intravesical pressure will cause progressive hydronephrosis, loss of tubular function, and progressive renal insufficiency and failure.

## *Presentation*

The slow and gradual progression of BPH causes symptoms to change very gradually, and it is not unusual for patients to present to a physician after the onset of symptoms or to seek advice only after the acute sequelae of obstruction sets in.

### Irritable Bladder Symptoms

Prostatic enlargement encroaches on the trigone area, producing symptoms of frequency and urgency. Nocturia is also common. Urgency and urge incontinence may also be due to detrusor hyperreflexia, a condition unrelated to BPH.

### Obstructive Symptoms

The classic obstructive symptoms include hesitancy and decrease in the caliber and force of the urinary stream. In addition, the urinary stream may be interrupted and associated with straining. In the advanced stage, the patient may complain of incomplete bladder emptying as well as suprapubic discomfort.

### Urinary Incontinence

Involuntary loss of urine may be due to detrusor hyperreflexia, detrusor irritability, or chronic retention with overflow. It is not unusual to encounter elderly patients with mixed causes of incontinence.

### Urinary Retention

Urinary retention is often the presenting complaint of patients with BPH, and it may be precipitated by a sudden increase in urinary output, e.g., recent onset of diuretic therapy, a drinking binge, or onset of diabetes. It is also commonly seen following surgical procedures or illness requiring hospitalization. Besides diuresis, drugs such as anticholinergic and alpha-adrenergic agents can precipitate urinary retention.

### Urinary Tract Infection or Epididymitis

Urinary tract infection in the elderly may be noted incidentally, but generally an increase in irritative symptoms is described. There may be fever and low abdominal discomfort. Epididymitis presents as a painful, scrotal swelling, usually with fever and leucocytosis.

These conditions in the elderly usually indicate a failure of the normal voiding mechanisms. Although other conditions such as neurogenic bladder or urethral stricture are often implicated, BPH remains a major cause of urinary tract infections in the elderly.

### Hematuria

Blood in the urine may be microscopic or gross. In cases of gross hematuria, it may be initial, terminal, or total and is usually painless. Gross hematuria is termed initial if it is observed at the beginning of voiding, terminal if it is at the end, and total if it is throughout urination. Hematuria in BPH is presumably due to rupture of prostatic veins at the surface of the prostatic urethra.

### "Silent" Presentation

Occasionally patients with BPH present with constituent symptoms of renal insufficiency and deny any urinary symptoms. The renal insufficiency is caused by prolonged obstructive uropathy leading to hydroureteronephrosis.

## *Patient Evaluation*

### History

Elderly patients may be unable or unwilling to give an accurate description of their voiding complaints. Answers to questions related to the urinary tract are often best obtained from patients' relatives. The history should include information on progression of symptoms, inciting events such as illness or operation, presence or absence of hematuria, symptoms of urinary tract infection, medications, other medical illness, and prognosis of the patient in relation to ambulation or future nursing care requirements. History of previous pelvic or genital operations or history of neurologic disorders may help in the differential diagnosis of voiding dysfunction.

### Physical Examination

Patients being examined for BPH should also be checked for concurrent cardiac and pulmonary conditions. Specific examination of the genitourinary system includes examination of the costovertebral angle for tenderness or renal mass, presence or absence of distended bladder with or without tenderness, and presence of epididymal swelling indicating epididymitis; inspection of the prepuce and urethral meatus; and palpation of the urethra to exclude stricture disease. Rectal examination is performed to exclude neoplasm or acute prostatic abscess. The size of the prostate relates little to the severity of symptoms in BPH. If possible, the patient's voiding stream should be observed.

### Urinalysis and Residual Urine Measurement

When the patient has acute urinary retention or when increased residual urine cannot be eliminated on physical examination, catheterization is performed under careful aseptic conditions after the patient has attempted to void in private surroundings. Urinalysis is mandatory. Urine culture should be carried out if there is evidence of infection. Residual urine volumes greater than 100 ml are considered abnormal and indicate bladder decompensation.

### Renal Function Evaluation

Measurements of blood urea nitrogen, serum creatinine concentration, and serum sodium and potassium concentrations should be obtained, especially if the patient is to undergo prostatic surgery.

### Excretory Urography (EU)

There have been recent studies suggesting that EU is not cost-effective prior to prostatectomy.[5] It is our belief that this procedure is still warranted to evaluate the anatomy of the urinary tract, to observe any unsuspected pathologic condition, and to provide an anatomic baseline prior to operative intervention. It is certainly indicated when hematuria or urinary tract infection is present. The study should be conducted with caution in elderly patients, especially those with azotemia, diabetes, dehydration, or multiple myeloma because renal failure can develop. Avoidance of dehydration appears to reduce the risk of such a complication.

### Uroflowmetry

Uroflowmetry, a noninvasive test to measure urinary flow characteristics, was introduced into clinical practice in recent years. The patient with a full bladder is asked to void directly into a flowmeter. The flowmeter automatically records the flow in the form of a graph. The voided volume is automatically recorded. From the graph, the duration of voiding can be measured, allowing the examiner to determine the average flow rate. In addition, the maximum or peak flow rate can also be studied.

This study provides a good objective means of documenting a poor stream. However it should not be relied on heavily, since in the early compensated stage of prostatism, the flow may be totally normal. Because the urinary flow rate depends upon the volume voided, variations will occur in the same subject. Siroky and associates[6] have devised a nomogram relating maximum and average flow rate to voided volume.

### Endoscopic Evaluation

Cystourethroscopy should be performed whenever obstructive symptoms are severe. It is also indicated in the work-up for urinary tract infection and hematuria. The endoscopic appearance of the posterior urethra does not correlate well with patient symptoms. The size of the prostate is assessed during endoscopy to determine which operative approach is to be used.

## *Treatment*

Indications for surgery are urinary retention, significant obstructive symptoms, and recurrent urinary tract infections. These symptoms, when combined with endoscopic evidence of outlet obstruction, are sufficient indications for intervention. Early surgical intervention before significant residual urine develops is advised to avoid serious complications such as urinary tract infection, azotemia, or irreversible bladder decompensation. If at all possible, surgical intervention is preferred for all ambulatory elderly patients with prostatism, since the alternative is lifelong use of a catheter. However, in poor-risk and totally bedridden patients, the inconvenience of voiding and the necessity of using internal or external catheters dictate the need for the most conservative therapy.

## *Conservative Management*

Many patients with acute retention caused by hospitalization, operation, or change in therapy will respond to several days of catheterization followed by a trial of voiding. The patients should have antibiotic coverage during this voiding trial and should be followed closely for progression of symptoms. A conservative approach is indicated if there is a history of no or minimal prior obstructive symptoms, a successful voiding trial with minimal or no residual urine, and an absence of subsequent urinary tract infection.

Intermittent clean catheterization is an alternative to prolonged use of an indwelling urethral catheter.[7] It is useful in those patients whose prostatectomy should be delayed, e.g., following myocardial infarction or recovery from a major operation. Poor-risk patients or those who cannot master intermittent catheterization may be treated with Foley catheterization for long periods, with adequate catheter care. On occasion, suprapubic cystostomy drainage may ultimately be required.

### Prostatectomy

The advent of transurethral prostatectomy has markedly reduced the mortality and morbidity from surgical relief of prostatic obstruction. Preoperative preparation includes the stabilization of renal function and the correction of fluid and electrolyte imbalance. Cardiovascular and pulmonary status should be optimized. Preoperative dehydration is prevented during the fasting period by an intravenous fluid supplement. Any urinary tract infection is rigorously treated in the perioperative period. Transurethral prostatectomy is best performed with the patient under spinal anesthesia. The size of the gland and the experience of the resectionist are two major factors that will influence the endoscopic approach. Experience has shown that prolonged resection predisposes the patient to significant blood loss, infection, fluid overloading, and electrolyte imbalance. If the gland cannot be removed in approximately 1 hour, the prostate is usually removed by open enucleation techniques. The commonly used techniques include (1) a transvesical suprapubic prostatectomy, in which the bladder is opened, and (2) a retropubic prostatectomy, in which the adenoma is enucleated through an incision in the prostatic capsule. Both techniques are applicable to large gland removal. The major drawback of an open procedure is that hospitalization is generally longer because of the suprapubic wound care, which is not required following removal by the transurethral route.

Following endoscopic removal of the prostate, the catheter is generally removed on the second postoperative day. The patient is discharged on oral antibiotics and should strictly avoid activities increasing intra-abdominal pressure for the first 6 weeks until the prostatic fossa is fully healed; otherwise, delayed bleeding may occur.

**Complications of Prostatectomy.** The early complications of hemorrhage, infection, hyponatremia, and epididymitis are uncommon with careful patient selection for endoscopic prostatectomy and good endoscopic technique.

Postprostatectomy incontinence often will resolve with continued healing. Persistent incontinence of a mild to moderate degree usually responds to alpha-adrenergic agents such as ephedrine sulfate (25 mg four times a day) or phenylpropanolamine (one spansule twice a day). Careful urodynamic evaluation is required with prolonged incontinence. True stress incontinence can be managed in a variety of ways. Kegel exercises can be used for mild to moderate incontinence. The usefulness of this therapeutic approach has not, however, been documented satisfactorily. In severe cases, use of collecting devices and perineal superabsorbent pads may be acceptable to the patient. Surgical management can be accomplished with the use of an artificial urinary sphincter.

**Recurrence of Obstructive Symptoms.** Recurring symptoms occur in a small proportion of patients and usually indicate a regrowth of prostatic tissue not completely removed at the time of prostatectomy. Careful evaluation is necessary to exclude a bladder or prostatic neoplasm or neurogenic bladder dysfunction. Urethral strictures and postoperative vesical neck contracture can be identified at the time of endoscopy. Absence of obstruction may be an indication of a decompensated bladder. This may respond to bethanechol chloride therapy (50 mg every 6 hours) or may require intermittent clean catheterization.

### Suprapubic Tube Placement

The placement of a permanent suprapubic tube is a useful alternative treatment of BPH for debilitated or poor-risk male patients. It is also indicated for patients with decompensation or in situations in which the patient is incapable of normal bathroom habits. The presence of a prostatic and long, pendulous urethra makes male patients very susceptible to urethritis, prostatitis, and epididymitis when using an indwelling urethral catheter. These problems, except urethritis, are not encountered in females, in whom an inlying urethral catheter is a practical and acceptable form of urinary drainage. In males, an inlying urethral catheter may not be tolerated, and these patients should be switched to suprapubic drainage at the earliest sign of urethral complications. Long-term care of the tube includes changing it every 4 to 6 weeks, daily irrigations with one fourth per cent acetic acid to prevent catheter encrustations, and careful management to prevent catheter obstruction. Long-term antibiotics should not be used, and only symptomatic urinary infections treated.

## CANCER OF THE PROSTATE

Neoplastic transformation in the prostate gland is a common event. Sarcomatous change is largely confined to the pediatric age group. Carcinomatous change involving the prostatic ducts is usually transitional cell in origin and exhibits a course and prognosis similar to that of transitional cell carcinoma of the bladder invasive to the prostate gland. Adenocarcinoma of the prostate is extremely common in the elderly. The response of these tumors to hormonal manipulation was initially believed to provide a promise of a curative approach to this neoplasm. However, 40 years of experience have failed to support this impression. Early diagnosis of the disease presents the best opportunity for curative therapy. The careful examination of the prostate gland in the elderly patient remains the hallmark of early detection.

### *Incidence*

Adenocarcinoma of the prostate accounts for 17 per cent of tumors in men and is the third most common cause of cancer death in men over 55 years, following lung and colorectal tumors. Death rates for White American males are estimated at 14 per 100,000.[8]

There is evidence that there is an increasing incidence of prostate cancer with age.[9] The clinical significance of this fact has to be weighed against the observation that prostate tumors presenting at a younger age are more lethal tumors.[10] Conversely, tumors presenting in patients of great age often display a more protracted natural history and may not be a major component of patient morbidity or mortality. These tumors may become more of a risk factor as medical advances increase male life expectancy.

### *Etiology*

The etiology of malignant transformation in the prostate remains unclear. Its increasing incidence with age may suggest a progressive failure of immune mechanisms. Racial factors are implicated by the increased incidence in Black Americans, with a 21.9 per 100,000 death rate, and a decreased propensity in Japanese men, with a 1.85 per 100,000 death rate. Environmental factors are suggested by an increased incidence in Japanese males in America and an increased incidence noted in workers exposed to cadmium. There seems little doubt that an altered response to hormonal stimulation is involved in the malignant transformation, and this theory is supported by the decreased incidence in eunuchoid patients[11] and by tumoral response to hormonal manipulation and antiestrogen therapy. The relationship of tumor incidence to the presence of benign prostatic hyperplasia (BPH) remains unclear.

### *Pathology*

Adenocarcinoma constitutes 95 per cent of the prostatic tumors, with transitional cell carcinoma, squamous cell carcinoma, sarcomata, and secondary neoplasms being extremely rare.

Malignant transformation appears to commonly involve the peripheral glands or true glands of the prostate. Although multifocal transformation is the rule,[12] peripheral involvement is of major clinical importance because the tumor is easily felt rectally. Conversely, endoscopic resections of the prostate that do not extend close to the prostatic capsule may miss areas of neoplasm.

Tumors are generally graded pathologically in terms of differentiation and also cellular anaplasia. The presence of perineural infiltration may aid in the diagnosis of a neoplasm but has little prognostic significance.[13] The grading classification of Gleason,[14] based on the overall architectural appearance of the tumor, appears to offer excellent correlation with the clinical course and may replace more traditional cellular classifications.

A common staging classification is seen in

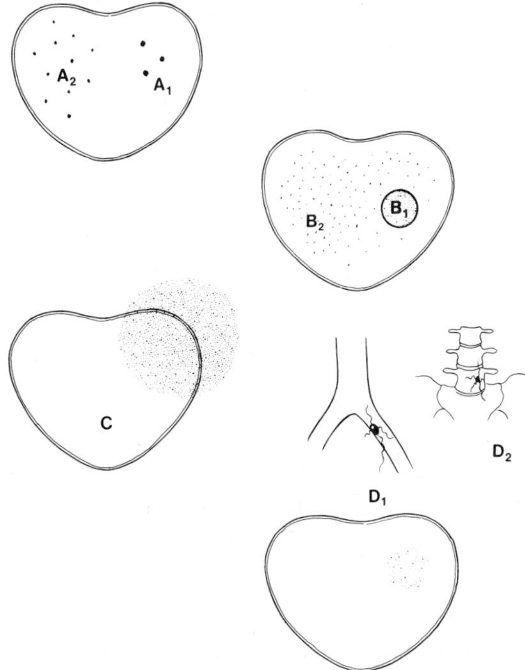


**Figure 34–1.** Stages of prostatic carcinoma. Stage A—confined to the prostate, undetected clinically; Stage B—confined to the prostate, clinically evident on rectal examination; Stage C—extends to the prostatic capsule but has not metastasized; Stage D—metastatic.

Figure 34–1. Clinical staging markedly understages the disease. Fully 35 to 40 per cent of patients have widespread disease at presentation.[15] It is also evident that progression of disease through stages A to D may proceed in an orderly sequence. A2 lesions behave in a manner similar to C lesions and have a poorer prognosis than B lesions. Spread of this tumor is by direct invasion. Denonvilliers' fascia provides a rather effective barrier to spread into the rectum except in the most anaplastic of lesions. Lymphatic spread by permeation and embolization affects the obturator nodes. These nodes are not well visualized by routine pedal lymphangiography. Hematogenous spread is said to involve the sacral plexus of Batson, possibly explaining the high percentage of pelvic and lumbar bony metastatic deposits. Distant spread occurs to the lung, liver, and adrenal gland. Prostatic neoplastic cells elaborate prostatic acid phosphatase, whose activity is detectable in serum in two thirds of patients with spread outside the prostate gland.[16]

## Clinical Presentation

The presentation of this tumor, especially in those patients (35 to 40 per cent) who present with distant metastases, is extremely varied. Therefore, detection requires constant vigilance and awareness on the part of the clinician. It is hoped that more thorough screening of patients will result in detection of the disease at earlier stages.

**Incidental Findings on Rectal Examination.** A nodule of hard consistency with or without induration and asymmetry is a common presentation. The nodule may be small and occupy only a portion of one lobe, or it may extend to involve the entire prostate gland. A hard prostate gland, with or without a nodule, should alert the physician. Such findings should be considered to indicate malignancy until proved otherwise. Other conditions that mimic prostatic carcinoma include benign focal adenomatous hyperplasia, prostatic calculi, granulomatous prostatitis, and prostatic infarction.

**Obstructive Symptoms.** Symptoms of obstruction such as slow or intermittent stream and dribbling with or without nocturia are common. A high index of suspicion should be aroused when these symptoms occur with fairly rapid onset or in relatively young patients. Acute or chronic retention is not as common a symptom of prostatic cancer as it is of benign prostatic hyperplasia.

**Irritative Symptoms.** Urgency, frequency, and a feeling of incomplete emptying may be the only manifestation of prostatic cancer. As in benign disease, several conditions can produce such symptoms.

**Hematuria.** Hematuria is rare as a presenting feature and usually indicates advanced disease.

**Presentations of Metastasis.** The presentations of metastasis are many and varied and include bone pain, paraplegia from crush fractures, cachexia, anemia, and pleural effusion. In almost all cases of prostate cancer, the findings in rectal examination will be highly suggestive of malignancy.

## Diagnosis

The diagnosis of prostatic carcinoma is generally made either as an incidental finding following transurethral prostatic surgery (stage A disease) or by prostatic biopsy. Also, the presence of elevated serum acid phosphatase should make one suspect the presence of a disseminated prostatic carcinoma. In patients with elevated acid phosphatase levels, the diagnosis should be confirmed histologically by needle biopsy prior to any definitive treatment. Prostatic biopsy may be carried out via the transperineal or transrectal route with the patient under local or general anesthesia.[17] Rarely is an open biopsy indicated. Needle aspiration of prostatic lesions is gaining acceptance in centers where cytologists have the expertise and experience to make diagnoses based on small amounts of aspirated tissue.[18]

### Staging

Clinical staging starts with the rectal examination. As soon as the neoplasm is confirmed histologically, other tests are necessary to assess the extent of the malignancy.

1. *Serum acid phosphatase assay.* This assay, which uses various substrates, differs from center to center and, as previously noted, is usually positive when the tumor has spread outside the gland. Radioimmunoassay has assisted in the standardization of the test but appears to be ineffective in detecting localized intraprostatic tumors and has been shown to be unsuccessful in mass screening of patients. The measurement of serum acid phosphatase continues to be useful in assessing early response to hormonal treatment. The levels may be falsely elevated in cases of osteosarcoma, Gaucher's disease, and thrombocytopenia.[19]

2. *Renal function test and intravenous urogram.* These tests are obtained to identify evidence of trigonal involvement and ureteric obstruction.

3. *Bone scan and radiography.* Technetium 99m polyphosphate injection followed by scanning at 3 to 4 hours is a very sensitive test for detection of metastatic involvement. It is less specific than radiographic evaluation, so that hot spots should be x-rayed to exclude Paget's disease, osteomyelitis, arthritis, and incompletely healed fracture sites. When in doubt, the physician should use tomography to evaluate the hot spot. When the metastatic lesion is far advanced, osteoblastic lesions, the most common radiographic finding, will be observed. The pelvis and the lumbosacral vertebra are the most common sites of bony metastasis.

4. *Pelvic lymphadenectomy.* This procedure is considered diagnostic rather than therapeutic, since there is little evidence that pelvic lymphadenectomy in any way influences the natural history of the disease. However, it may be an important guide to therapy. Pelvic lymphadenectomy should be offered to those patients, usually younger, in whom radical extirpation is planned, in order to rule out extensive disease. In addition, it may be of assistance in designing radiation therapy in those centers that modify their therapy in accordance with staging procedures. Complications of pelvic lymphadenectomy include pulmonary embolism, lymphocele formation, and peripheral edema. The last-named complication especially is seen when lymphadenectomy is followed by radiation therapy. Simplified staging pelvic lymphadenectomy is preferred to the more radical approach in order to avoid such complications.

## *Treatment**

The treatment options for prostatic carcinoma depend upon two major factors. These factors include the stage of the disease and the general health of the patient. In general, when the disease is localized within the prostate, the objective is to ensure eradication of the malignancy. The therapeutic options include transurethral resection of the prostate gland, radical prostatectomy, or radiation therapy. When the disease is disseminated, the major goal is palliative in nature, either with no therapy in asymptomatic cases, localized radiation therapy to the metastatic lesion, or hormonal manipulation using either estrogen or bilateral orchiectomy.

In stage A1 disease, in which the disease is diagnosed following a simple prostatectomy, no further treatment is indicated, especially in elderly patients. Occasionally, a repeat transurethral resection of any residual tissue may be recommended to ensure that no residual neoplasm is left in the prostatic fossa.

Stage A2 disease, because of its high malignant potential and behavior, is grouped with stage B1 and stage B2 disease in terms of therapy. The current consensus is that patients in these groups should undergo pelvic lymphadenectomy to rule out extensive disease. Once it is confirmed that the disease is localized, the options are radiation therapy using the internal or external mode or radical prostatectomy via the perineal or retropubic approach.

Deep radiation therapy is generally given over a 6-week course and requires daily attendance at the radiation therapy unit. Side effects include initial nausea and diarrhea. The late side effects of radiation cystitis and proctitis occur in about 15 per cent of patients. The rate of impotence approaches 50 per cent (see Chapter 27).

Interstitial implantation of $^{125}$I seeds is performed through a suprapubic incision. The radiation seeds are implanted into the prostate gland after the total required radiation dosage is carefully measured. Side effects with this technique are much less than with the external radiation technique.

Radical prostatoseminal vesiculectomy can be performed either through a retropubic supra-

---

* For information on treatment of prostatic cancer and sexual function, see Chapter 27.

pubic approach or through a perineal approach. These approaches lead to 90 per cent or more incidence of impotency and 10 to 40 per cent incidence of urinary incontinence.

Presently, there is controversy as to which is the best approach for this group of patients with localized disease. Whether anything at all should be done is also influenced by the general health of the patient. Obviously a good physical and mental state of health and a life expectancy of at least 5 years are prerequisites to surgery. Physiologic differences among elderly patients make it impossible to limit or recommend a cutoff age beyond which invasive intervention cannot be performed. Presently we favor the most conservative approach in patients discovered to have prostatic carcinoma at age 75 years and beyond. For stage C disease, deep external radiation therapy is the preferred treatment. Patients with stage D disease should be divided into two categories: asymptomatic and symptomatic patients. For the symptomatic group the treatment should be directed to the relief of symptoms. The principal form of therapy is either bilateral orchiectomy or estrogen administration. Bilateral orchiectomy is preferred for patients with cardiovascular disease or patients in whom compliance with drug therapy is expected to be a problem. Estrogen can be used in patients who refuse orchiectomy or in whom surgical intervention is contraindicated. The dose of estrogen should be 3 mg daily. Higher doses are associated with increased mortality secondary to myocardial infarctions and cerebrovascular accidents, believed to be due to increased thromboembolic phenomena.

Localized bone pain can be treated with a short course of local radiation therapy. This should be instituted following relapse from hormonal therapy. Systemic therapy, with, for example, cyclophosphamide or extramustive phosphate, is not generally recommended for the elderly because of intolerable side effects. Analgesics are used to control intractable pain. Brompton's mixture given round the clock is an alternative to intermittent analgesic regimens.

Urinary diversion may be indicated in patients with uremia due to bilateral ureteral obstruction or in patients with impassable outlet obstruction. Percutaneous nephrostomy can be used to drain the kidney. This is less invasive and can be done with the patient under local anesthesia. Suprapubic cystostomy is the procedure of choice for those with incorrectable bladder outlet obstruction.

Prostatic cancer will become more of a problem as the life expectancy of the male population increases. Early diagnosis and a flexible approach to treatment will allow optimal treatment with the least discomfort and infringement on the dignity of the patient.

## References


1. Harbitz TB, Haugen OA: Histology of the prostate in elderly men. Acta Pathol Microbiol Scand 80:756, 1972.
2. Lytton B, Emery JM, Harvard BM: The incidence of benign prostatic hyperplasia. J Urol 99:639, 1968.
3. Gloyna RE, Wilson JD: A comparative study of the conversion of testosterone to 17-beta-hydroxy-5-alpha-androstan-3-one (Dihydrotestosterone) by prostate and epididymis. J Clin Endocr 29:970, 1969.
4. Huggins C, Stevens R: The effect of castration on benign hypertrophy of the prostate in man. J Urol 43:705, 1940.
5. Bauer DL, Garrison RW, McRoberts JW: The health and cost implications of routine excretory urography before transurethral prostatectomy. J Urol 123:386, 1980.
6. Siroky MB, Olsson CA, Krane RJ: The flow rate nomogram: I. Development. J Urol 122: 665, 1970.
7. Lapides J, Diokno AC, Silber SJ, Lowe BS: Clean intermittent self-catheterization in the treatment of urinary tract disease. Trans Am Assoc Genitourin Surg 63:92, 1971.
   *A good primer on the basis of unsterile urethral catheterization as a treatment for bladder emptying dysfunction.*
8. Segi M, Kurihara M, Matsuyama T: Some aspects of cancer of the prostate gland (quoted by Gyorkey F). *In* Busch H (ed.): Methods in Cancer Research. Volume X. New York, Academic Press, 1973, p. 280.
9. Hirst AE Jr, Bergman RT: Carcinoma of the prostate in men 80 or more years old. Cancer 7:136, 1954.
10. Tjadan HB, Culp DA, Flocks RH: Clinical adenocarcinoma of the prostate in patients under 50 years of age. J Urol 93:618, 1965.
11. Moore RA: Endocrinology of Neoplastic Disease. New York, Oxford University Press, 1947, p. 194.
12. Byar DP, Mostofi FK: Carcinoma of the prostate. Prognostic evaluation of certain pathologic features in 208 radical prostatectomies examined by the step section technique. Cancer 30:5, 1972.
13. Larson DL, Rodin AE, Roberts DK, et al: Perineal lymphatics: Myth or fact. Am J Surg 112:488, 1966.
14. Gleason DF, Mellinger GT: Prediction of prognosis for prostatic adenocarcinoma by combined histological grading and clinical staging. J Urol 111:58, 1974.
    *This aids the clinician in the prognosis and management of prostatic carcinoma.*
15. Byar DP: The Veterans Administration cooperative urological research group studies of cancer of the prostate. Cancer 32:1126, 1973.
    *A recommended article for all students of prostate carcinoma. The basis for the choice of specific hormonal therapy is documented in this study.*
16. Mobley TL, Frank IN: Influence of tumor grade on survival and serum acid phosphatase levels in metastatic carcinoma of the prostate. J Urol 99:321, 1968.
17. Emmett JL, Barber KW Jr, Jackman RJ: Transrectal biopsy to detect prostatic carcinoma: A review and report of 203 cases. J Urol 87:460, 1962.
18. Linsk JA, Axilrod HD, Solyn R, DeLaurdac C: Transrectal cytologic aspiration in the diagnosis of prostatic carcinoma. J Urol 108:455, 1972.
19. Prout GR: Chemical tests in the diagnosis of prostatic carcinoma. JAMA 209:1699, 1969.
    *An excellent presentation on the value of serum acid phosphatase in the diagnosis of prostatic carcinoma.*

## Chapter 35

# Gynecologic Problems

*Jay S. Schinfeld*
*Bertram H. Buxton*
*George Ryan, Jr.*

The template of superior geriatric gynecologic health care is forged during the early reproductive years prior to menopause. Enlightened women, encouraged and guided by their physicians, assume responsible health habits regarding their diet, physical activity, weight control, and use of tobacco, alcohol, and other drugs. Appropriate behavior modification may decrease the complications of hypertension, diabetes, osteoporosis, and cardiopulmonary disease. Identification and treatment of young women at high risk for osteoporosis may prevent severe and irreversible bone loss.[1,2]

Despite this widely accepted blueprint for ensuring good health in the latter years, there are a number of gynecologic problems that become manifest after the menopause in spite of good health habits. The preventive aspects of geriatric gynecologic health care in the older, postmenopausal woman include periodic health examinations, which strengthen the patient/doctor relationship and provide an opportunity for patient health education. These examinations also give the physician an opportunity to evaluate the mental and social functions of the patient.

Annual screening of gynecologic interest in the older postmenopausal patient should include a blood pressure check and breast, pelvic, and rectal examinations. A Hemoccult test of obtained stool, along with a complete blood count and urinalysis, and a Papanicolaou cervical smear are strongly recommended. Mammography, a cholesterol screen (perhaps every 5 years), a complete SMA (Sequential Multiple Analyses), chest x-ray, and an electrocardiogram (EKG) are usually recommended.[3-6]

Cancer of the breast is either the second or third most prevalent malignancy of the female in her latter years, and its incidence increases with age.[7,8] A careful breast examination, therefore, is warranted at least on an annual basis, and more frequently in women with a positive family history[9] or previous history of breast disease. Second primaries have been reported in 8 to 20 per cent of patients who have had a previous intraductal or lobular cancer of the breast.[10] Other high-risk factors are nulliparity and a history of endometrial cancer.[10,11] In the older woman, especially if not obese, the breasts are easier to examine and have less confusing findings than those of the menstruating woman, whose breast tissues still reflect cyclic hormonal changes. Since the American Cancer Society has recommended an annual mammogram in women past the age of 50 as a means for discovering small breast lesions before they can be palpated by a physician, it is prudent to communicate this fact to patients.[8] However, the practice of our group is to order mammography (1) if indicated by physical findings, (2) in the high-risk patient, or (3) to allay anxiety in overly cancer-conscious patients. Self-examination, if acceptable to the patient, should be encouraged. Any patient with suspicious findings should be checked by low-dose xero-mammography or sent to a consultant for further evaluation. Skin lesions of the breast should be re-evaluated after local therapy to determine response to therapy. Bilateral pruritic areolar skin lesions should arouse suspicion of mammary Paget's disease. The severity and incidence of "fibrocystic" disease of the breast are lessened in the older postmenopausal female, but occasionally needle aspiration with cytologic examination may be required to evaluate the rare cystic mass in the postmenopausal breast. Any noncystic mass or one persisting after aspiration should be evaluated by biopsy.

The ovary, although it becomes hormonally senescent, may develop cancer at any age, and any palpable ovary in a postmenopausal woman demands further investigation.[12]

Annual Pap smears have usually been advocated for women over the age of 60. These are mandatory for women who have had abnormal smears in the past (i.e., patients who have had cervical or vaginal dysplasia).[13] About 36 per cent of women will have undergone a hysterectomy by the age of 60, and it is reasonable for these women to have Pap smears on a 3-year interval basis if they are not at high risk from previous genital dysplasia or cancer. Symptomatic women over 70 years of age are similarly evaluated. Although the Pap smear is highly effective in identifying cervical cancer, it is only 50 to 65 per cent accurate in screening for endometrial malignancy and, thus, cannot be utilized to rule out endometrial cancer. A comprehensive technique of cervical scraping, endocervical aspiration, and submission for laboratory evaluation of material aspirated from the endometrial cavity has, in our experience, increased the ability to discover a nonsymptomatic endometrial cancer. About 20 per cent of patients who eventually develop cancer of the vulva will give a history of either malignant or premalignant lesions of the upper genital tract.[14]

## ESTROGEN REPLACEMENT THERAPY

In the United States in the 1960s, estrogen replacement therapy (ERT) was prescribed to most postmenopausal patients. However, starting in 1975, a series of studies demonstrated an association between ERT and endometrial hyperplasia and cancer.[15-18] Patients and physicians refused to consider replacement therapy, and as a result, many women suffered from estrogen deficiency symptoms. Since 1978, better-controlled research of both a retrospective and prospective nature has been carried out that assists in understanding the risks and benefits of ERT in postmenopausal women.[19-21]

Women reach menopause, the final menstrual event, around 51.6 years of age, with the prospect of continuous estrogen use for more than 30 years. However, menopause may begin at a younger age naturally or artificially.[22] There remain no easy answers to questions concerning who shall receive ERT and for how long. However, many women both require and desire estrogen for protection of their bodies and quality of life.

ERT is used to treat or prevent vasomotor instability symptoms known as flushes and flashes. These are probably mediated through catecholamine interaction at the level of the hypothalamus. Current research has shown a relationship between luteinizing hormone (LH) surges and the onset of skin temperature changes and flushes and flashes.[23] These symptoms can be totally debilitating, affecting marital and social behavior. Only 25 to 35 per cent of women who are postmenopausal come to the physician requesting therapeutic intervention, either because they are reticent to discuss their problems or because they are only mildly affected.

A more important reason to consider ERT is the proven association of the climacteric and osteoporosis (see Chapter 39).[24] Estrogen inhibits osteoclasts, which are responsible for bone degradation. A change in diet and exercise or an increase in weight may predispose older women to an increased risk of hip and wrist fractures. Hip fractures are the twelfth leading cause of death in women; survivors may be significantly limited in their activities.

Many women will benefit from ERT to maintain vaginal and bladder health, and ERT can help prevent aseptic urethritis and vaginal synechiae. There is also convincing new evidence suggesting improvement in cardiovascular status, lessened skin aging, decreased depression, and less memory loss.[25,26] There is no proof that pulmonary embolism, cerebral vascular accidents, or myocardial infarctions are associated with the generally accepted dosages of estrogen used today.

The evidence for an association between endometrial hyperplasia and the subsequent development of endometrial cancer with ERT was first presented in the early 1970s.[15-18] Some reports showed an increased relative risk of developing endometrial cancer of 2- to 12-fold, but many of these early studies were criticized because of their designs and pathologic interpretations.[19,20]

Currently, there have been several well-documented reports that suggest that there is indeed an association between estrogen use and endometrial cancer, related to dose and duration of exposure.[13,14] Many patients, aware of these findings through the media and earlier discussions with their physicians, will not consider estrogen use with the uterus in situ.

However, it is important to look at this association in terms of actual percentages and the risks of developing carcinoma of the uterus. The expected incidence of endometrial cancer in nonusers of estrogen is approximately one per thousand women at risk.[32] Prolonged use of estrogen alone would increase this risk to approximately three to eight women per thousand. However, studies have shown that the women with endometrial carcinoma that is associated with ERT have as high as a 95 per cent 5-year survival rate.[21] This is due, in part, to the earlier diagnosis and treatment of the carefully, frequently monitored patients who have sufficient medical care associated with the prescription of ERT.

In an excellent study, Schiff and associates,[28] at the Boston Hospital for Women, followed 25 symptomatic postmenopausal women with an intact uterus who were randomly assigned in this double-blind study to either a cyclic (3 weeks on, 1 week of placebo) or continous (daily) regimen with conjugated estrogens. The incidence of endometrial hyperplasia was 3.7 per hundred women months in the continuous groups and 4.5 per hundred women months in the cyclic group (not statistically significant). Patients with endometrial hyperplasia tended to spot or bleed at abnormal intervals. The opinion of the study was that these rates of hyperplasia were unacceptably high.

However, the administration of a progestin for at least 10 days can reduce to zero the incidence of hyperplasia in patients who have had no prior hyperplasia or carcinoma.[27,29] It has been shown that progestins have a definite and pronounced antiproliferative effect on the endometrium[30] and are useful in reversing hyperplasia in 93 per cent of patients. In addition, progestins are effective in decreasing both the incidence and severity of vasomotor symptoms and, theoretically, may be weakly protective for osteoporosis. In two long-term studies by Nachtigal and associates[31] and Hammand and associates,[27] respectively, there was no development of carcinoma when cyclic progestin therapy was employed, regardless of the dose of estrogen replacement. Vaginal bleeding at an unexpected time required an endometrial biopsy or dilatation and curettage to rule out significant disease. The report by Judd and co-workers,[32] representing the opinion of the American College of Obstetricians and Gynecologists, and that by Gambrell[29] found that an initial screening biopsy was not cost-effective. However, in our menopause unit we believe that a baseline biopsy allows us to tailor our management and reassure our patients, especially the patients who refuse to accept the use of cyclic progestin therapy, with its associated bloating, breast fullness, and withdrawal bleeding.

Therefore, if there is no pre-existing hyperplasia or carcinoma, as demonstrated by endometrial biopsy, we believe that ERT for 21 to 25 days, combined with a progestin for approximately 10 to 14 days a month, can decrease the risk of development of significant endometrial disease to acceptable ranges for both the physician and the patient. Any endometrial carcinomas that may develop tend to be detected and treated early, with an excellent cure rate for the patients in this group.

There is little good evidence of an association between breast cancer and ERT. Studies have suggested that oral contraceptives are protective against the development of benign tumors in the breast and that these doses do not significantly increase the risk of breast carcinoma.[33] No protective association of ERT has been shown for either benign or malignant breast neoplasia.[34] Epidemiologically, age-adjusted incidence and death rates for breast carcinoma have remained stable in the last several years, despite increased estrogen use in postmenopausal patients. Most case control studies have shown no significant association between estrogen use and breast cancer.[27,31,34] One study showed a risk if there was "high exposure to estrogen in patients with intact ovaries," but patients on conjugated estrogen doses of 0.625 mg were at no increased risk. Factors that may protect against breast cancer include pregnancy, lactation, late menarche, and early bilateral oophorectomy.[34,35] In general, there is little evidence that women on ERT, without a personal or family history of breast carcinoma or pre-existing fibrocystic or other disease of the breast, have an increased risk of development of breast carcinoma.[36]

Recently, there has been some theoretic evidence that even women without an intact uterus may benefit from the addition of progestins to counteract the unopposed estrogen effect on the breast tissue. Gambrell and Vasquez,[37] in a prospective study, have obtained some evidence that estrogen therapy may provide protection against the development of breast carcinoma when it is combined with progestin.

Contraindications to ERT include undiagnosed vaginal bleeding, acute liver disease, chronic impaired liver function, acute vascular thrombosis, neuro-ophthamalogic disease, and breast or endometrial carcinoma. Relative risk may be increased in patients with pre-existing hypertension, uterine leiomyomata, fibrocystic disease of the breast, familial hyperlipidemias, migraine headaches, chronic thrombophlebitis, endometriosis, and gallbladder disease.

In our menopause unit at the University of Tennessee College of Medicine, patients undergo an initial interview during which the risks and benefits of ERT are assessed and presented with specific reference to the patient and her past medical history. Proper nutrition and exercise, avoidance of excessive use of nicotine and alcohol, and proper diet are emphasized. The patient is then presented a series of options: estrogen replacement therapy, estrogen and progestin replacement therapy, progestin only therapy, or nutritional/behavioral/activity modification. We currently suggest using low doses of conjugated estrogens, 0.625 mg for 21 to 25 days. This dose has been shown to be protective for osteoporosis. Ten mg of medroxyprogesterone acetate are given during the 12th through twenty-first cycle day or seventeenth through thirtieth, when no estrogens are taken, as many women require some therapy continuously to prevent vasomotor symptoms.

## COMMON GYNECOLOGIC PROBLEMS

Eighty per cent of gynecologic problems in women over 60 years of age relate to postmenopausal bleeding, vulvovaginal inflammations or infections, genital prolapse, or alterations in bladder function.[38] Often symptoms must be tactfully elicited from the patient.

Tissue changes resulting merely from the aging process are difficult to differentiate from those induced by the estrogen-deficient state. The aging process is associated with decreased cell division and growth and a decrease in the repair capacity of tissue, with fatty infiltration, cellular atrophy, and increased cell pigmentation. Degenerative changes leading to a loss in elastic tissue have also been ascribed to aging, as have a decreased vascularity and a decrease in smooth muscle tone.[45] Estrogen target tissues show decreased cellularity, a thinning of the epithelium with a decrease in elastic tissue, and an increased vaginal alkalinity with increased propensity for infection. Atrophy of the vaginal canal results in foreshortening, with the urethral meatus receding posteriorly along the roof of the vagina.[48] These changes are to some extent reversible or improved by the use of estrogen replacement. Changes due to aging that occur in estrogen-dependent tissues are aggravated and perhaps accelerated by the estrogen-deficient state.

### *Postmenopausal Bleeding (PMB)*

The occurrence of genital bleeding one or more years past the last menstrual period requires investigation. Although the source of bleeding may be benign or originate from sites other than the genital tract, one third of the cases reveal evidence of a premalignant or malignant endometrial or cervical lesion.[39] Malignancy of the cervix is far less frequent in the postmenopausal age group, but malignancy of hyperplasia of the endometrium occurs more often. A negative Pap smear will not rule out the possibility of endometrial disease. Another third of the patients show a benign endometrium or endometrial polyps, whereas another third have atrophic endometrium.[40] Bleeding from an atrophic friable vaginal epithelium may coexist in any or all of these categories.

A discussion of various means of cytologic tissue sampling of the endometrial cavity goes beyond the scope of this chapter, but patients should be referred for such investigation if postmenopausal bleeding is present. Dilatation and curettage remain the standard means for investigating postmenstrual bleeding. Gambrell's data[29] indicate that endometrial sampling *prior* to the indications of ERT is not cost-effective and that biopsy is indicated only in patients with unscheduled or heavy bleeding rather than the expected light withdrawal bleeding at the end of cyclic estrogen/synthetic progesterone administration. He indicates that cyclic progesterone may be discontinued in women in whom estrogen replacement is terminated when, over a 3-month period, they no longer bleed after finishing progesterone therapy.

### *Infections and Inflammations*

Bacterial vaginitis is more common in the older postmenopausal female than in her younger counterpart. Since the atrophic vaginal epithelium is thinner and more friable, subepithelial entry of bacteria occurs more easily.[41,42] Topical estrogen treatment usually establishes a healthier vaginal epithelium, which is more resistant to bacterial invasion. Estrogen can be used alone or with topical antibacterial creams or a 10 per cent Betadine (povidone-iodine) douche. Trichomoniasis is not common in postmenopausal patients, but Candidiasis causing vulvovaginitis, especially in those patients with glucose intolerance, is more frequent. Antifungal drugs (miconazole nitrate 2 per cent or clotrimazole 1 per cent cream), with appropriate glucose control, will quickly bring these fungal problems under control. Use of a 1 per cent solution of gentian violet remains an effective antifungal therapy.[43] It can be applied by the physician; applications can be repeated every 10 to 14 days. More frequent use may cause irritation. A sanitary pad may be used for protection of the patient's underclothing.

Pelvic infections and abscess formation are rare in the older, postmenopausal patient but may result in increased mortality and morbidity if not suspected.[41] Abscesses in these patients may be secondary to diverticulitis or may follow endometrial biopsy. The symptoms can be quite variable, but usually fever, abnormal bleeding, pelvic pain, tenderness, and mass are present. Antibiotic treatment must be guided by renal function.

Inflammatory and acute vulvar lesions may be treated with a cool, half-strengthened 5 per cent Burow's solution (aluminum acetate).[44] Vulvar lesions are, of course, myriad and may represent dermatologic conditions occurring elsewhere, such as psoriasis and seborrheic and contact dermatitis.[42] Vulvar dystrophies include atrophic and dysplastic types as well as the combined atrophic and hyperplastic lesions. The main symptom of dystrophic lesions is pruritis. The atrophic lesion lichen sclerosus is best treated by local application of 2 per cent testosterone propionate in sesame oil or white petrolatum.[44] Estrogen is not effective in treating vulvar atrophy and, if used, leads to increased atrophy of this tissue. Corticosteroid creams are successfully used for treatment of hypertrophic dystrophy. Lichen sclerosus improves more slowly than vulvar hyperplasia. Therefore, mixed atrophic and hypertrophic lesions should be treated first with corticosteroid creams, with the addition of testosterone later to control the atrophic component.[44] The application of testosterone may gradually be reduced to once or twice a week, but the condition invariably will become symptomatic again if therapy is discontinued completely. Infrequently, with testosterone propionate, the side effects of clitoral hypertrophy and increased libido may occur but only rarely are hirsutism and voice changes noted.

Crotamiton (Eurax), a potent antipruritic, mixed with corticosteroids (seven parts of corticosteroids to three parts of Eurax), may occasionally be used.[42]

When vulvar lesions are seen, the only accurate basis for diagnosis and establishment of an initially appropriate treatment is biopsy. All erosions; raised, ulcerated and pigmented lesions; or lesions that persist despite treatment necessitate biopsy. It is difficult to differentiate with exactness the nature of lesions by clinical inspection. Therefore, biopsy is reassuring to both patient and physician and directs the appropriate therapeutic approach. The Keys' punch biopsy is an easily performed office procedure,[42] but the primary physician may want to refer a patient requiring this procedure to a gynecologist. Staining the vulva with toluidine blue and then washing it with 1 per cent acetic acid may be helpful in identifying suspicious areas for biopsy. Suspicious areas retain the toluidine blue stain.

Bartholinitis in the older, postmenopausal female should always arouse suspicion of the uncommon malignancy of Bartholin's glands, and cytologic or histologic evaluation by needle aspiration or biopsy is indicated.

## *Genital Prolapse*

In the United States, the incidence of genital prolapse in the older, postmenopausal female has been decreasing, probably owing to the decreased parity of American women and earlier operative intervention, when tissues are less attentuated and the patient's general health is better.[45]

The symptoms caused by genital prolapse include a "bearing down" sensation, fullness and pressure in the vaginal and pelvic areas, backache, and, occasionally, urinary incontinence. The clinical presentation of genital prolapse includes cystocele, urethrocele, rectocele, enterocele, and descent of the uterus and/or cervix. The degree of relaxation is usually determined by the amount of descent of the involved segment when the patient is at rest and/or when she is straining. When the cervix protrudes beyond the introitus when the patient is at rest, the prolapse is judged to be severe. Total eversion of the vagina is called procidentia. If, with straining, the cervix protrudes beyond the introitus, the prolapse is labeled moderate. If, with straining, the cervix descends close to but not through the introitus, the prolapse is mild.

Stress incontinence is not a symptom of cystocele but may be associated with it if there is also an anatomic defect in the support to the urethrovesical junction or urethral incompetence.

A latent enterocele may be difficult to demonstrate in a reclining patient, and examination of the patient in a semi-sitting or even a standing position may be necessary. Since more than one third of American women at age 60 years have had a hysterectomy,[46] postoperative prolapse of the vaginal vault may pose a perplexing problem, especially in those women who wish to preserve a functional vagina. The expectation of sexual function must be communicated clearly by the referring physician to the gynecologic surgeon, who may then plan his or her surgery accordingly. ERT or biweekly introvaginal estrogen cream applications cannot reverse pelvic relaxation that has already occurred but may reverse symptoms resulting from associated atrophic epithelium. It may be used preoperatively for 2 to 3 weeks to improve the vaginal tissues for better postoperative healing.

Since correction of pelvic relaxation is rarely an emergency or a lifesaving procedure, surgical intervention can often be tailored to the patient's schedule and convenience so that her hospital stay and postoperative convalescence can be free of anxiety and allow protection from overactivity for optimal tissue healing.

The use of pessaries for support and management of pelvic relaxation is generally a temporizing measure until surgery can be planned. Occasionally, an elderly patient with medical complications that contraindicate surgery requires permanent use of a pessary, usually a Gellhorn or inflatable device, which can be removed and cleaned every 4 to 6 weeks. The use of estrogen cream, one-half applicator full weekly, helps the vaginal epithelium to tolerate the pessary, lessening the likelihood of abrasion or ulceration of the atrophic thin and friable vaginal tissue. The Gellhorn pessary has a stem that keeps the device in the axis of the vagina and a central port along the stem for drainage. Intercourse is not recommended for patients with this type of pessary but may be possible with a Smith-Hodge pessary.

## *Alteration in Bladder Function*

Urinary complaints may be elicited by careful history taking. Brockelhurst[46] studied a female population ages 45 to 64 and found that 57 per cent had some degree of incontinence. In the over 65-year age group, 23 per cent of the older women admitted to some form of incontinence. Pure stress urinary incontinence was present in 12 per cent.[47] Many older women appear to accept some incontinence as an expected manifestation of aging (see Chapter 33).

The spectrum of urinary symptoms in older postmenopausal women also includes burning, urgency, frequency (both diurnal and nocturnal), inability to stop the urinary stream, and, more rarely, difficulty in urination. Pain, burning, and frequency, both day and night, usually indicate infection. Urgency with incontinence may also reflect the presence of infection. There is a sixfold increase in urinary tract infections in older postmenopausal women compared with perimenopausal females, ages 45 to 55.[47] This is due to the increased vulnerability of the atrophic tissues to bacterial invasion and to an increased incidence of residual urine after voiding. Treatment includes increased fluid intake during the daytime and specific antibiotic therapy, as determined by urine culture and sensitivity testing.

Occasionally, patients will present with nonspecific chronic recurrent urethritis for which no dominant causative organism is found. Empiric therapy with urinary antibiotics or analgesics, urethral dilatations, and tranquilizers may be used individually or in combination. Local estrogen therapy may be helpful in incontinent women with estrogen deficiency demonstrated by vaginal smear or with obvious clinical evidence of vaginal atrophy. Cytologic and histologic evidence obtained pre- and post-treatment will confirm urethroepithelial response to estrogen, favoring enhanced urethral competence. Local estrogen therapy will also be accompanied by an increase in periurethral vascularity, which contributes to urethral support and function.[48] Estrogen receptors have been found in the urethra, the bladder trigone area, and the periurethral tissues.[49] If urge incontinence or other urinary symptoms persist after anti-infection treatment and local estrogen therapy, as described previously, further evaluation is required. When there is no discernible anatomic dislocation or abnormality of the bladder neck, urge incontinence may be treated by various medications, including anticholinergic agents, such as propantheline bromide (Pro-Banthine) or emepronium bromide. Antispasmodics such as flavoxate hydrochloride (100 to 200 mg four times daily) may also be tried.

For patients suspected of having adult enuresis, imipramine may be utilized. This drug acts as an anticholinergic agent centrally as well as locally. Ornade spansules are another popular anticholinergic medication that may be tried in patients with urgency incontinence due to a hyperactive detrusor muscle. Kegel exercises, although effective in younger women, rarely contribute to improving pure stress incontinence in older postmenopausal women.[46]

The use of bladder drills along with psychotherapy (biofeedback technique) may be helpful in women with pure urge incontinence. In these women, there is associated detrusor hyperactivity, nocturnal and diurnal frequency, and no overt bladder pathologic condition. Complete relief has been reported in 90 per cent of these women, with objective cystometric improvement of detrusor control in 77 per cent.[47] Sensory or motor deficit involving the perineum or sphincteric response to clitoral stimulation or any historical evidence of neurologic problems requires that urologic evaluation with cystometry be obtained. Historical evidence of diabetes and multiple sclerosis implies a neurologic component as the etiology of urinary problems, particularly incontinence.

In pure stress incontinence there is loss of the posterior urethrovesicle angle or a downward displacement of this angle; this requires surgical intervention for cure. If urgency is present and infection has been ruled out, there may still be a mixed etiologic basis for incontinence (e.g., detrusor instability). In these cases, surgery may improve the incontinence but not completely cure it. Often, therefore, clearing up infection, trials of medical therapy, and estrogen therapy may precede the overt decision to refer patients with urinary incontinence for surgical correction.

Although the disorder to be corrected is rarely life threatening, surgery may increase the quality of the patient's life, adding to her comfort and happiness. Surgery may be possible, even in women with cardiac, pulmonary, and renal problems, if it is carefully planned and timed (see Chapter 47).

## CONCLUSION

It is possible to maintain a woman's physical and mental health during the decades after menopause with careful and complete examinations, counseling, and establishment of a good doctor-patient relationship. Although there may be an increased risk of carcinoma in patients undergoing ERT, current literature shows that this risk may be modified and minimized in the vast majority of cases, with benefits far outweighing risks in selected individuals.

### References*


1. Christiansen C, Christiansen MS, Transbol I: Bone mass in postmenopausal women after withdrawal of estrogen/progesterone replacement therapy. Lancet 1:459, 1981.
2. Nachtigall LE, Nachtigall RH, Nachtigall RD, et al: Estrogen replacement therapy. I: A ten year prospective study in the relationship to osteoporosis. Obstet Gynecol 53:277, 1979.
3. American Cancer Society: Guidelines for the cancer-related checkup. Recommendations and rationale. CA 30:194, 1980.
4. Medical Practice Committee, American College of Physicians: Periodic health examination: A guide for designing individualized preventive health care in the asymptomatic patient. Ann Intern Med 95:729, 1981.
5. Spitzer WO: Report of the task force on the periodic health examination. Canad Med Assoc J 121:1193, 1979.
6. Standards for Obstetrics-Gynecological Services. 5th ed. Washington, The American College of Obstetricians and Gynecologists, 1982, p. 45.
7. American Cancer Society Cancer Statistics, 1982. CA 32:17, 1982.
8. American Cancer Society: Breast cancer detection demonstration project: A five year summary report. CA 32:209, 1982.
9. Lilienfield AM: The epidemiology of breast cancer. Cancer Res 23:1503, 1963.
10. Schottenfeld D, Berg J: Incidence of multiple primary cancers. IV. Cancers of the female breast and genital organs. JNCI 46:161, 1971.
11. Lowe CR, MacMahon D: Breast cancer and reproductive history of women in South Wales. Lancet 1:153, 1970.
12. Barber HRK, Graber EA: The postmenopausal palpable ovary syndrome. Obstet Gynecol 38:921, 1971.
13. Moertel CG, Dockerty MB, Baggenstoss AH: Multiple primary malignant neoplasms. Cancer 14:238, 1961.
14. Walker AM, Jick H: Declining rates of endometrial cancer. Obstet Gynecol 56:733, 1980.
15. Ziel HK, Finkle WD: Increased risk of endometrial carcinoma among users of conjugated estrogens. N Engl J Med 293:1167, 1975.
16. Weiss NS, Szekely DR, Austin DF: Increasing incidence of endometrial cancer in the United States. N Engl J Med 294:1259, 1976.
17. Smith DC, Prentice R, Thompson DJ, et al: Association of exogenous estrogen and endometrial cancer. N Engl J Med 293:1164, 1975.
18. Mack TM, Pike MC, Henderson BE, et al: Estrogens and endometrial cancer in a retirement community. N Engl J Med 294:1262, 1976.
19. Cramer DW, Knapp RC: Review of epidemiologic studies of endometrial cancer and exogenous estrogen. Obstet Gynecol 54:521, 1979.
20. Horwitz RI, Feinstein AR: Alternative analytic methods for case-control studies of estrogens in endometrial cancer. N Engl J Med 299:1089, 1978.
21. Robboy SJ, Bradley R: Changing trends and prognostic features in endometrial cancer associated with exogenous estrogen therapy. Obstet Gynecol 54:269, 1979.
22. Stillman RJ, Schinfeld JS, Schiff I, et al: Ovarian failure in long-term survivors of childhood malignancy. Am J Obstet Gynecol 139:62, 1961.
23. Tataryn IV, Meldrum DR, Frumar AN, et al: LH, FSH, and skin temperature during the menopausal hot flash. J Clin Endocrinol Metab 49:125, 1979.
24. Lindsay R, Hart C, Aitken JM, et al: Long-term prevention of post-menopausal osteoporosis by estrogen. Lancet 1:1038, 1976.
25. Ross RK, Pagini-Hill A, Mac TM, et al: Menopausal oestrogen therapy and protection from ischaemic heart disease. Lancet 1:858, 1981.
26. Bush TL, Cowan LD, Barrell-Connor E, et al: Estrogen use and all cause mortality. JAMA 249:903, 1983. *An important but somewhat controversial study of osteoporosis prevention.*
27. Hammond CB, Jelovseck FR, Lee KL, et al: Effects of long term estrogen replacement. II. Neoplasia. Am J Obstet Gynecol 133:537, 1979.
28. Schiff I, Sela HK, Cramer D, et al: Endometrial hyper-


* References 1 through 20 are the commonly discussed references concerning ERT and endometrial cancer.

plasia in women on cyclic or continuous estrogen regimens. Fertil Steril 37:79, 1982.
29. Gambrell RD Jr: Preventing endometrial cancer with progestin. Contemp Ob/Gyn 17:133, 1981.
30. Whitehead MI, Townsend PT, Pryse-Davies J, et al: Effects of estrogens and progestins on the biochemistry and morphology of the postmenopausal endometrium. N Engl J Med 305:1599, 1981.
31. Nachtigall FLE, Nachtigall RH, Nachtigall RD, et al: Estrogen replacement therapy. II. Prospective study in a relationship of carcinoma and cardiovascular and metabolic problems. Obstet Gynecol 54:75, 1979.
32. Judd HL, Cleary RE, Creaseman WT, et al: Estrogen replacement therapy. Obstet Gynecol 58:267, 1981. *A must paper to read from the American College of Obstetricians and Gynecologists.*
33. Sartwell PE, Arthes FG, Tonascia JA: Epidemiology of benign breast lesions: Lack of association with oral contraceptive use. N Engl J Med 288:551, 1973.
34. Ross RK, Paganini-Hill A, Gerkins V, et al: A case control study of menopausal estrogen therapy and breast cancer. JAMA 243:1635, 1980.
35. Hoover K, Gary LA, Cole EP, McMahon B: Menopausal estrogens and breast cancer. N Engl J Med 295:401, 1976.
36. Gambrell RD, Massey FM, Castaneda TA, Boddie AW: Estrogen therapy and breast cancer in postmenopausal women. J Am Geriatr Soc 38:251, 1980.
37. Gambrell RD Jr, Vasquez JM: Estrogen therapy and breast cancer—is the verdict in? Contemp Ob/Gyn 19:38, 1982.
38. Parsons L, Summers SC: Gynecology. Volume II. 2nd ed. Philadelphia, W.B. Saunders Co. 1978, p. 1646.
39. Gambrell RD Jr: Clinical use of progestins in the menopausal patient: Dosage and duration. J Reprod Med 27:531, 1982.
40. Mack HC: The glycogen index in the menopause: A study of certain estrogen functions based on a new method of staining vaginal smears. Am J Obstet Gynecol 45:402, 1943.
41. Ledger WJ: Infections in elderly women. Clin Obstet Gynecol 20:1, 1977.
42. Friedrich EG Jr: Therapeutic principles and techniques: Evaluation and management of diseases of the vulva. Clin Obstet Gynecol 21:983, 1978.
43. Tovell HNM, Young AW Jr: Classification of vulval diseases. Clin Obstet Gynecol 21:955, 1978.
44. Kaufman RH, Gardner HL: Vulva dystrophies. Clin Obstet Gynecol 21:1081, 1978.
45. Semmens JP, Wagner G: Estrogen deprivation in vaginal function. JAMA 248:445, 1982.
46. Brockelhurst JC: Textbook of Geriatric Medicine in Gerontology. Edinburgh and London, Churchill and Livingstone, 1973.
47. Soloman S, Panagotopolocus P, Oppenheim A: Urinary psychology studies as an aid to diagnosis. Obstet Gynecol 76:57, 1958.
48. Smith P: Age changes in the female urethra. Br J Urol 44:667, 1972.
49. Iosif CS, Batra S, Canders EK, Astebt B: Estrogen receptors in the human female lower urinary tract. Obstet Gynecol 141:817, 1981.

## Chapter 36

# Musculoskeletal Diseases in the Elderly

*Evan Calkins*
*Theodore Papademetriou*
*Hanimi R. Challa*

Aches and pains in the musculoskeletal system constitute the most frequent complaints of the elderly.[1-5] This is true for several reasons. First, a number of the diseases that underlie these symptoms, such as osteoarthritis, osteoporosis, pseudogout, and polymyalgia rheumatica, occur with increasing frequency in advanced age. Second, most of these musculoskeletal disorders are not fatal but linger, causing pain and discomfort for many years. These diseases also accumulate, one musculoskeletal disorder frequently predisposing to others. As a result, many older people suffer from several musculoskeletal conditions simultaneously.

Musculoskeletal diseases are often difficult to diagnose. This stems, in part, from the wide diversity of conditions that may underlie the complaints. These include not only disorders commonly classified as "rheumatic" in nature but also a wide range of diseases whose origins lie in other organ systems. In contrast to the long list of possible etiologies, musculoskeletal symptoms are limited to a short list of specific complaints: pain, tenderness, swelling, stiffness, and limitation of motion. Correct diagnosis often requires careful attention to what may appear to be small details in history, physical examination, and, to a lesser extent, laboratory procedures.

This chapter is intended to provide a guide to the correct diagnosis and treatment of musculoskeletal symptoms in the elderly. It is divided into three segments: (1) general considerations in diagnosis (history, physical examination, and laboratory procedures); (2) age-specific aspects of the presentation, course, and treatment of common musculoskeletal disorders; and (3) a "problem-oriented" approach to diagnosis and management of several important specific syndromes.

## GENERAL CONSIDERATIONS IN DIAGNOSIS

### *History*

The history should be complete. The physician should determine when the symptoms began, even though their onset may have been decades ago (presuming, of course, an adequate memory on the part of the patient or family). Careful attention should be given to the course of the disease. Did certain factors such as trauma, acute medical illness, or severe psychological stress precede the initial manifestations? Was the subsequent course steady or intermittent? What, if any, factors preceded or "triggered" the exacerbations of the condition? Careful attention should also be given to the presence or absence of constitutional symptoms, such as anorexia, weight loss, night sweats, and vasomotor instability. These symptoms are helpful in differentiating one of the inflammatory diseases, such as rheumatoid arthritis, from a degenerative or metabolic disorder.

The important symptom *morning stiffness* provides a good example of the importance of a careful history. Many patients experience muscular and joint stiffness when they arise from bed. The duration of stiffness provides an important diagnostic clue. If this symptom lasts for several minutes only (up to 20), it is much more consistent with a degenerative process, such as osteoarthritis, rather than an inflammatory disease, such as rheumatoid arthritis or polymyalgia rheumatica. In patients with active rheumatoid arthritis, the stiffness characteristically lasts for at least 1 hour and may last the entire day, the duration of morning stiffness paralleling the extent of disease activity.

## *Physical Examination*

The physician should observe, carefully, the patient's ability to ambulate, transfer, and use, effectively, a wheelchair, a walker, or other assistive devices. The physician should avoid the temptation to try to help the patient accomplish these maneuvers; this assistance often results in greater discomfort on the patient's part. In addition, such efforts deprive the physician of an excellent opportunity to observe how the patient makes use of his or her musculoskeletal system to accomplish these tasks.

The skin should be scrutinized for tophi, rheumatoid or other nodules, rash/ecchymosis, lymphadenopathy, and so on. All peripheral joints should be examined for thickening of the synovium, tenderness, increased joint fluid, ligamentous laxity and instability, deformity, and limitation of range of motion. These observations should be recorded. The physician should learn how much pressure on one of the small joints of the hand can be tolerated by a normal person, without eliciting pain. Muscle groups and, when indicated, individual muscles and tendons are examined. In patients with rheumatoid arthritis, one should be particularly mindful of the presence of ruptured tendons, especially extensors and flexors of the fingers and thumb, because these complications, if identified early, are often susceptible to surgical repair. With practice, the physician should be able to perform a good examination of all joints in a cooperative patient in about 10 to 12 minutes. In a confused elderly person with limited mobility owing to musculoskeletal involvement this examination will take at least twice as long.

The neurologic examination should include assessment of tendon reflexes, Babinski's reflex, Hoffmann's sign, and sensitivity to pinprick. In patients with back symptoms suggesting the possibility of cord compression, one should assess the degree of bladder distention and check for the possibility of loss of pin prick sensation in the perianal area. Cord compression is a medical emergency and may lead to irreversible paraplegia unless corrected promptly.

## *The Problem of Multiple Diseases*

Merely because a patient has clear-cut stigmata of one disease, such as rheumatoid arthritis, does not mean that the symptoms at hand need necessarily be due to that disorder. They may instead be due to a coincidental disease, the clinical manifestations of which are more obscure.

Occasionally one will encounter patients with rheumatoid arthritis who also suffer from hyperthyroidism or myxedema. The former can mimic, or reinforce, the constitutional symptoms accompanying the rheumatic disease. Myxedema may also closely mimic rheumatoid arthritis, both conditions resulting in the appearance of "slowing down." A deepening tone of voice, characteristic of patients with myxedema, may also be encountered in those with rheumatoid arthritis, owing to involvement of the larynx. Myxedema frequently causes a form of plastic rigidity that, superficially, resembles the stiffness of rheumatoid arthritis. If a patient with rheumatoid arthritis also has one of these thyroid disorders, appropriate treatment of the endocrine disease almost invariably results in striking amelioration of the symptoms of the rheumatoid arthritis.

Patients with osteoarthritis will not infrequently develop acute articular symptoms due to concomitant acute gout or pseudogout. Both of these conditions are especially apt to become manifest following surgery or other stress. Failure to recognize that the acute symptoms are due to a condition other than the osteoarthritis itself will result in the loss of an opportunity for appropriate treatment.

Even more serious is the possibility that the physician may fail to recognize the presence of septic arthritis in a patient with chronic joint involvement due to rheumatoid arthritis or osteoarthritis. Patients with joint damage due to chronic arthritis are at increased risk for the development of pyogenic arthritis, both via the hematogenous route and secondary to aspiration or local injection of medication into the joint. Patients with long-standing arthritis of any sort should be suspected of having superimposed joint infection if any joint exhibits greater than usual pain, tenderness, or swelling.

Patients with rheumatic diseases frequently exhibit progressive and disabling hand symptoms. Although these symptoms may be due to the rheumatoid process per se, the physician should be alert to the possibility that the symptoms may reflect, at least in part, compression neuropathy involving the median nerve at the carpal tunnel or neuropathy secondary to cervical spine involvement. Careful history and physical examination and, when appropriate, electromyogram (EMG) studies will lead to the correct diagnosis.

## *Laboratory and Diagnostic Procedures*

The laboratory work-up is guided by the history and physical findings. If the patient presents evidence of a *generalized* rheumatic disease, there is a cluster of laboratory studies that, in our view, should be obtained in virtually all cases (Table 36 – 1). In interpreting the erythrocyte sedimentation rate, it is important to remember that normal values for the sedimentation rate are higher in the elderly than in the young. Values of 40 to 50 mm/1hr. are frequently encountered in elderly persons who appear in all respects perfectly healthy (Fig. 36 – 1).[5a] Serum acid phosphatase activity should be measured in male patients, especially those with back pain. Estimations of serum calcium and phosphorus levels and alkaline phosphatase activity are indicated because symptoms of hyperparathyroidism may closely mimic generalized forms of arthritis. Use of serum protein electrophoresis is important to explore the possibility of multiple myeloma. Determination of the concentration of serum albumin is helpful for several reasons; for example, it can indicate the presence of protein calorie malnutrition. The presence of diffuse hyperglobulinemia will provide additional evidence of a chronic inflammatory disorder. As noted elsewhere in this chapter, serum thyroid function tests should be obtained if there is the suspicion of a thyroid disorder. An antinuclear antibody study should be obtained in patients with generalized inflammatory arthritis, especially if it involves the small joints and is accompanied by rash, hematologic or renal manifestations, or severe constitutional manifestations. However, the physician should be mindful of the fact that the frequency of positive antinuclear antibody reactions increases significantly in the elderly population.[4,6–10] Whether this reflects immunologic changes associated with normal aging per se or whether it reflects age or time-related increases in autoimmune disease is still not entirely clear.[10]

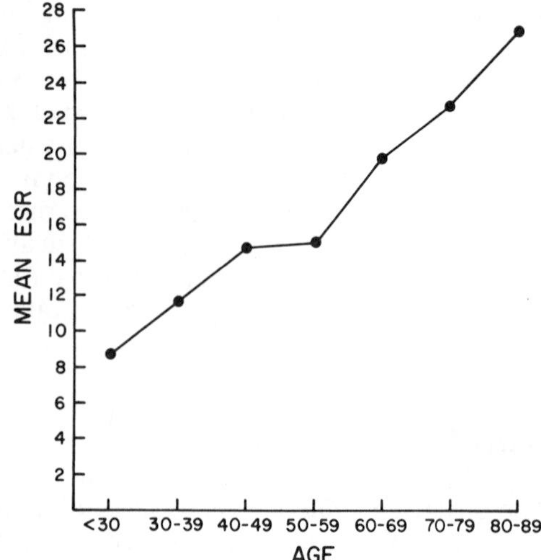


**Figure 36 – 1.** Increase in the mean erythrocyte sedimentation rate (ESR) with advancing age, Wintrobe method, measured in millimeters per hour. (From Hayes CS, Stinson IN: Erythrocyte sedimentation rate and age. Arch Ophthalmol 94:939, 1976. Copyright © 1976, American Medical Association. Reproduced with permission.)

**Table 36 – 1.** IMPORTANT LABORATORY STUDIES IN THE DIAGNOSIS OF MUSCULOSKELETAL DISEASES

| |
|---|
| **Obtain Always or Almost Always** |
| Complete blood cell count and differential |
| Erythrocyte sedimentation rate |
| Serum calcium, phosphorus, and alkaline phosphatase levels |
| Serum urate and creatinine concentration |
| Total serum protein; serum protein electrophoresis (most instances) |
| X-ray of hands and other joints, as indicated clinically |
| **Obtain if Appropriate (see text)** |
| Rheumatoid factor assay |
| Antinuclear antibody test |
| Triiodothyronine ($T_3$) and thyroxine ($T_4$) measurements |
| Synovial fluid examination for crystals, bacteria (culture), and cell count |
| Other diagnostic studies, such as arthrogram |

It is customary to obtain a rheumatoid factor assay in all patients suspected of having rheumatoid arthritis. Although this procedure has become so routine that its omission will undoubtedly lead to censure, its diagnostic value is relatively low in patients of any age. This is especially true in the elderly, in whom, as with the antinuclear antibody study, there is an increase in positive reactions in the population as a whole.[4,6–10] Connotations of adverse prognosis, given to younger patients who exhibit high titer rheumatoid factor assays, do not appear to hold in persons of advanced age.

X-rays will be helpful in diagnosing both systemic and localized disease of the musculoskeletal system. To avoid obtaining unnecessary or inappropriate films, the primary physician should either become familiar with the optimal views required to assess specific problems or should seek consultation from a rheumatologist, orthopedist, or radiologist before requesting x-rays. For example, when history and physical examination suggest instability of a C1 to C2 area, due to rheumatoid arthritis, views should be obtained with the neck in both the flexed and extended position, being cautious to avoid extremes of motion of the neck. In cases in which sacroileitis is suspected, a posteroanterior or "angled" view of the sacroiliac joints should be obtained. X-rays of the knees should always be obtained with the patient in the standing position, to demonstrate varus-valgus deformities or narrowing of one or both of the joint compartments of the knee. In patients with shoulder pain, one should request an anteroposterior projection to show joint space narrowing and joint cysts. In addition, it is important to obtain internal and external rotation views and axillary views to assess the possible presence of calcific deposits.

*Polytomography* can provide more information than plain radiography in some types of rheumatic involvement, e.g., in avascular necrosis of the head of the femur or humerus.

*Computed tomography* (CT) scan is used with increasing frequency for the study of the musculoskeletal system. It is highly accurate in the detailed assessment of spinal fractures and instability and in the diagnosis of pathologic conditions of the spine, such as disc disease, facet joint arthropathy, spinal stenosis, involvement of the sacroiliac joints,[11] and paravertebral abscess.

A *bone scan,* using a technetium compound, can provide important information about the extent of bone involvement and also its metabolic state. This procedure is helpful in the evaluation of primary and metastatic bone tumors, metabolic bone disease, and infections of bones and joints. Early inflammatory joint disease may be detected by increased uptake by inflamed synovium. Scans of the sacroiliac joints are useful in assessing ankylosing spondylitis. The bone scan is also used in assessing pain in patients with total joint replacements, in whom it will identify possible areas of osteomyelitis or component loosening. A bone scan will provide evidence of "stress fractures" at an early stage when the plain radiograph may not show any changes. Fractures of the spine in patients with osteoporosis will show increased uptake or remain "hot" for a considerable period of time (e.g., up to a year); this can be helpful in differentiating recent from older compression fractures.

*Arthrography* is a useful procedure in the evaluation of joints. In the knee, the first joint to be studied by this procedure, arthrography is helpful in demonstrating menisceal tears, synovial nodules (as in villonodular synovitis), and popliteal cysts. In the shoulder, arthrography is of importance mainly in the diagnosis of rotator cuff tears.

*Arthroscopy* has been used for evaluation of intra-articular disease, particularly of the knee. Biopsy of the synovial tissue can be carried out by this procedure. Arthroscopy is beginning to be used for the treatment of certain joint conditions; the scope of its use as a means of treatment is enlarging as more experience is accumulating.

*Synovial fluid examination* should always be examined in persons with recent onset of synovial effusion. It should also be examined in persons with established arthritis, either osteoarthritis or rheumatoid arthritis, and long-standing joint effusions if the joint in question becomes tender or exhibits other inflammatory symptoms, such as pain or warmth, to a disproportionate degree as compared with other joints.

The various studies of the synovial fluid may be classified as having (1) great, (2) marginal, or (3) questionable diagnostic significance.

1. The first group includes Gram's stain of thin smear of aspirate, bacteriologic cultures of fluid, and examination of fluid for crystals. These are the determinations upon which the definitive diagnosis of infection, gout, and pseudogout depends, and without them, these diagnoses cannot be made properly.
2. The second group includes total and differential cell count. These are indicative of the degree of inflammation and can be helpful, but are not diagnostic for a specific disease entity.
3. The third group includes other determinations, such as estimation of fluid viscosity, mucin clot test, measurement of glucose concentration, rheumatoid factor assay, and assays for immune complexes. These determinations are interesting but only occasionally useful, and they are much less important in the differential diagnosis than are the preceding studies.

*Biopsy of the synovium,* done either through the arthroscope or as an open procedure, will identify the presence of tumor or tumorous conditions of the synovium (villonodular synovitis). Biopsy will also permit confirmation of the diagnosis of tuberculosis or fungus infection.

*Bone biopsy* can be helpful in early stages of metabolic bone disease when the biochemical and radiographic findings are not diagnostic. In elderly patients with generalized bone pain and/or compression fractures of the spine, a bone biopsy will permit differentiation between osteoporosis and osteomalacia or hyperparathyroidism. This procedure can be carried out with little patient discomfort by means of a specially designed needle.

Tissue fixation of materials obtained at biopsy is often a source of confusion. When biopsying the synovium, tophi, or other tissue for identification of urate crystals, the specimen should be fixed in alcohol because the urate crystals are soluble in aqueous fixatives. All other tissues should be fixed in formalin, with the exception of specimens for electron microscopy or for special histologic or immunohistologic studies. Since these procedures are important in the diagnosis of muscle disease (if appropriate laboratories are available), specimens of muscle should, ideally, be fixed for routine histologic studies (in formalin), for immunohistologic studies (in liquid nitrogen), and for electron microscopy.

## *Design of the Work-up*

In an elderly person with musculoskeletal complaints, the entire battery of indicated diagnostic studies should rarely, if ever, be performed in a "crash program" over the course of a few days. Although there are certain determinations that should be initiated at the time of first visit or admission, such as synovial fluid examination in patients suspected of having septic arthritis or acute gout, other examinations and laboratory procedures and a complete history, should be spread out over the course of several "sittings" to avoid patient fatigue. It is often advisable to establish a *preliminary* diagnosis based on the initial examinations and to initiate simple symptomatic therapy, even at the outset. This might include use of salicylates and heat and periodic rest. More sophisticated and specific therapy can be instituted later when the precise diagnosis has been established.

It is important, however, that one works steadily toward the establishment of the correct diagnosis. Merely to conclude that a patient has a "collagen vascular disease" does not provide grounds for appropriate management. Instead, one must ask, which collagen vascular disease is it? If the manifestations and laboratory findings do not clearly fit one of the well-defined entities, one should suspect that the patient has two diseases or that the entire symptoms complex is due to an entity not usually included within the spectrum of rheumatic diseases, such as metastatic carcinoma, sarcoidosis, tuberculosis, and hyperparathyroidism.

# AGE-SPECIFIC ASPECTS OF SYSTEMIC RHEUMATIC DISEASES

The frequency of different rheumatic and musculoskeletal diseases varies markedly with advancing age. This fact alone provides initial guidance in the differential diagnosis of musculoskeletal symptoms in the elderly (Table 36–2). The likelihood that these symptoms may be due to an entity other than the rheumatic or "connective tissue" diseases increases with advancing age.

## *Osteoarthritis*

Osteoarthritis is one of the most common disorders to affect older people. Kellgren and Lawrence[12] found radiologic changes indicative of this disorder in 87 per cent of females and 83 per cent of males aged 55 to 64 years. Twenty-two per cent of females and 15 per cent of males in this age group complained of symptoms referable to this condition.

### PATHOPHYSIOLOGY

There is some uncertainty as to the extent to which the underlying process and pathologic changes reflect biologic changes of aging per se or events of a traumatic, a metabolic, or an immunologic nature. These events are more frequently encountered in persons of advanced years, and their effects accumulate with the passage of time.[13]

The process of aging itself is accompanied by important biochemical and structural changes both in the fibrous component of cartilage (collagen) and in the matrix.[14-20] In addition, aging is accompanied by changes in subchondral bone with the result that this tissue, which in younger people shares the stress-absorbing function of cartilage, becomes increasingly prone to microfractures.[19] As these heal, the remodeled trabeculae are more rigid than normal bone and less effective as shock absorbers. Thus, the everyday trauma of walking, jumping, etc. is transmitted to the articular cartilage which itself has become

**Table 36-2.** FREQUENCY OF MUSCULOSKELETAL DISEASES IN YOUTH AND OLD AGE

| | Youth (2-25 years) | Midlife (30-50 years) | Old Age (65+) |
|---|---|---|---|
| Still's disease | + | ± | − |
| Ankylosing spondylitis | ++ | + | − |
| Reiter's disease | ++ | + | − |
| Rheumatic fever | ++ | + | − |
| Arthritis accompanying ulcerative colitis | + | ++ | ± |
| Septic arthritis | | | |
| Gonococcal | ++ | + | ± |
| Staphylococcal and other infections | + | ++ | +++ |
| Gout | ± | ++ | ++ |
| Idiopathic systemic lupus erythematosus (SLE) | +++ | ++ | + |
| Rheumatoid arthritis | ++ | ++ | ++ |
| Polymyositis | + | ++ | ++ |
| Scleroderma | + | ++ | ++ |
| Drug-induced SLE | + | + | +++ |
| Paget's disease | − | + | ++ |
| Osteoarthritis | − | + | +++ |
| Polymyalgia rheumatica and temporal arteritis | − | − | ++ |
| Calcium pyrophosphate deposition disease | − | + | +++ |
| Osteopenia | + | ± | +++ |
| Metastatic carcinoma and multiple myeloma | − | + | +++ |

*Key:* − = Rare or not occurring; ± = very infrequently; + = infrequently; ++ = commonly occurring; +++ = very frequently.

less flexible with age, resulting in degenerative changes.

Certain inherited disorders,[21] such as ochronosis, Wilson's disease, hemochromatosis, and calcium pyrophosphate deposition disease (pseudogout), result in the deposition, in cartilage, of abnormal substances that weaken the fabric of the cartilage itself. Other inherited disorders also enhance the rate of progression of degenerative changes by leading to laxity of the ligaments essential to the support of a given joint.

Inherited postural abnormalities, such as scoliosis, place added strain on the entire skeletal system. Structural abnormalities caused by the presence of other articular diseases, such as rheumatoid arthritis and gout, also predispose to secondary degenerative changes. Histologic changes resulting from these processes include circumscribed zones of granularity that progress to ulceration, fissuring, thinning, and, eventually, complete loss of cartilage. The degenerative processes just described are accompanied by the proliferation of bone and cartilage at the periphery of the joint, thus accounting for osteophytic spurs and Heberden's nodes.[22] These are the bony "knobs" frequently occurring adjacent to the distal interphalangeal joints. Heberden's nodes may occasionally be inflamed, tender, and cystic. (They may result in limitation of motion but do not cause serious crippling.) Bouchard's nodes, a less severe form of these nodes, sometimes occur adjacent to the proximal interphalangeal joints. They should be differentiated from the fusiform soft tissue swelling of these joints, which is characteristic of rheumatoid arthritis.

Although the degree of inflammatory change (soft tissue swelling and tenderness of the synovium) accompanying osteoarthritis is much less than in rheumatoid arthritis, it is now recognized that some degree of inflammation also accompanies osteoarthritis. Recent identification of immunoglobulins and complement components in osteoarthritic cartilage and adjoining synovium[23-25] has led to the speculation that an autoimmune response to products of cartilage destruction may be at work.

## Diagnosis

Osteoarthritis can be distinguished from other rheumatic diseases by history, physical examination, laboratory findings, and, to a lesser extent, x-ray.

The *history* is very important in making a diagnosis. The specific joints involved provide an initial clue. In the type of osteoarthritis occurring in elderly persons, without known predisposing cause (primary generalized osteoarthritis), the joint involvement, in order of frequency, is as follows: distal interphalangeal joint, carpal metacarpal joint of the thumb, knee, hip, cervical spine, and lumbar spine. Proximal interphalangeal joints and metacarpophalangeal joints, characteristically involved in rheumatoid arthritis, are relatively spared.

Although patients with osteoarthritis may experience stiffness on awakening or rising from a chair after prolonged sitting, the stiffness rarely lasts longer than 10 to 20 minutes.

Patients with osteoarthritis frequently experience moderate pain. This may be of three types: (1) a deep boring pain focused in the involved joint, often occurring at night; (2) a sharp and "jarring" pain, which may occur while walking or placing the joint under stress; (3) pain that may be experienced not in the area of the joint involved but referred elsewhere. Thus, patients with osteoarthritis of the hip may complain of pain in the knee even though this joint may be perfectly normal. Similarly, patients with osteoarthritis of the cervical vertebrae frequently complain of pain in the hands and fingertips.

Patients with osteoarthritis do not experience the fatigue, fever, and other constitutional symptoms that often accompany rheumatoid arthritis and other rheumatic diseases. The erythrocyte sedimentation rate is normal for the given age (unless elevated owing to other causes).

On *physical examination,* the synovium may be noted to be swollen and tender both in patients with rheumatoid arthritis and in those with osteoarthritis. The degree of swelling and tenderness in osteoarthritis is relatively minimal except in the presence of secondary infection or hemarthrosis (the latter condition may occur in people with osteoarthritis secondary to damage to a synovial villus, resulting from being "pinched" by the osteophytic spurs).

*Synovial fluid examination* provides added grounds for differentiation. In patients with osteoarthritis, the fluid is normally viscous and exhibits normal white cell count. In patients with rheumatoid arthritis, the synovial fluid is characteristically thin and watery, and the white cell count is usually elevated (10,000 or more cells per $mm^3$).

*X-rays* have shown that both osteoarthritis and rheumatoid arthritis may be accompanied by generalized osteoporosis, subchondral sclerosis, and narrowing of the joint space. When this occurs in the knee, it can be focused either in the medial or lateral component, resulting in corresponding varus or valgus deformity, respectively. Patients with osteoarthritis exhibit characteristic osteophytes and cystic changes in the bone, beneath the area of denudation. Joints of patients with rheumatoid arthritis may also exhibit osteophytes (since these patients may also have osteoarthritis). In addition, they may exhibit the characteristic erosions and cystic changes especially conspicuous at the point of junction of the synovium and the bone.

The presence of degenerative changes in a joint, even if severe, does not permit one to dismiss the possibility that an additional musculoskeletal disease may be present, either as a preexisting or concomitant disorder. Since the symptoms of osteoarthritis are, as a rule, more resistant to treatment than those of inflammatory joint disease, it is very important to suspect the presence of underlying disease, especially in a large joint such as a hip, before concluding that a patient has idiopathic osteoarthritis.

### Treatment

The treatment of osteoarthritis of any joint, whether it is the hip, knee, or facets of the lumbosacral spine, is guided by several general principles that apply, with some variations, to all areas of involvement (Table 36–3).[26] These will be outlined here. Specific aspects of management of degenerative joint disease of the hips, knees, cervical spine, and lumbosacral spine are referred to in the problem-oriented sections at the end of this chapter. For further details on the important subject of backache, the reader is referred to several excellent reviews on this subject.[27–29]

**Minimization of Predisposing Factors**

The first principle in management is to minimize, insofar as possible, factors that predispose the patient to osteoarthritis. Weight reduction, good posture, avoidance of repetitive trauma, and maintenance of good skeletal strength (through a program of regular exercise) contribute to good health of the joints and to a decrease in the frequency and symptomatology of osteoarthritis and, presumably, its rate of progression. One should be particularly attentive to the possible presence of orthopedic conditions, the correction of which might result in a decrease in overuse of specific joints. For example, in patients with osteoarthritis of the knee one should be certain that the patient has proper shoes so that the leg is not thrown out of position owing to faulty alignment of the foot, arch, or ankle. Stress placed on the joint through poor alignment or hypermobility due to lack of ligamen-

**Table 36–3.** GENERAL PRINCIPLES OF MANAGEMENT OF OSTEOARTHRITIS

1. Minimization of predisposing factors
2. Reduction of pain and muscle spasm
   a. Heat
   b. Rest
   c. Drugs
3. Exercises
4. Orthopedic management
5. Psychologic support

tous or muscular support should be corrected through use of proper braces; surgery, such as tibial osteotomy; and/or exercises.

**Reduction of Pain and Muscle Spasm**

Once the diagnosis of symptomatic osteoarthritis is established, a vigorous program should be instituted to decrease pain and muscle spasm. These two manifestations are closely related, each contributing to the other. Reduction of pain and muscle spasm can be done in three ways: (1) use of heat and other modalities of physical therapy, (2) rest, and (3) use of anti-inflammatory and analgesic drugs.

***Heat.*** Heat can be prescribed in many forms, e.g., deep heat radiation of various types (often expensive) and whirlpool baths. The simplest and least expensive form of heat is as good or nearly as good as the most expensive and elaborate. For hands, a good soak in warm water two to three times daily, preferably accompanied by gentle exercise (as in washing dishes), is helpful. A daily hot bath is comforting and therapeutic for patients with generalized arthritis. For those who experience difficulty in getting into and out of a tub, a hot shower is an adequate substitute. For large joints, such as hip, knee, and shoulder, a Hydrocollator pack is an excellent source of moist heat. It is widely held that moist heat is more beneficial than dry heat in symptomatic treatment of rheumatic diseases. However, this belief has not to our knowledge been proved. Use of cotton nightclothes, with, possibly, cotton sheets as well, contributes substantially to a more relaxed sleep by avoiding the clammy feeling that may accompany the use of pajamas made of synthetic fibers. An electric blanket is also appreciated by many arthritis patients.

***Rest.*** Rest provides an important means of decreasing muscle spasm in an inflamed joint. With arthritis of the spine, large joints, and feet, this is best provided by periods of bed rest, which one should prescribe in detail, just as one does with a pharmacologic agent. The precise program depends on the severity of symptoms and the person's other obligations. It is important to realize that with sufficient rest and use of simple antirheumatic agents, the discomfort of osteoarthritis and, in most cases, rheumatoid arthritis can almost always be alleviated. Failure to respond to these measures should raise the possibility of an alternate diagnosis such as malignancy or sepsis.

With the upper extremities, especially the wrist, application of a light plastic hand splint, for use at intervals during the day and at night, is helpful, permitting localized immobilization.

***Drugs.*** The most important group of drugs for use in patients with osteoarthritis are agents that exert both an anti-inflammatory and an analgesic effect. These are the agents that act by means of prostaglandin inhibition. Aspirin still remains one of the most effective and widely used of these drugs. It may be given in the "plain" form, preferably with meals. Aspirin with an enteric coating may also be used. One should be sure to select a product that has a coating that will be dissolved or removed in the stomach, thus permitting absorption of the salicylate. A preparation such as Enseals (Lilly) is a good example. Alternatively, one may use a form of buffered aspirin. In an elderly person, it is best to limit aspirin dosage to 8 to 10 tablets daily, since elderly people appear to be more sensitive to the central nervous system manifestations of aspirin and may be more sensitive to the gastrointestinal irritation as well. Because of age-related ear problems, elderly people may not exhibit the tinnitus and deafness that are often clues to the presence of salicylate toxicity.

Confirmation that the salicylate is being absorbed but has not reached toxic concentrations can be determined by measuring the serum salicylate level. A range of 12 to 18 mg per dl is a good goal. The use of aspirin and other antirheumatic agents should obviously be prescribed with caution in patients who are receiving warfarin (Coumadin) therapy. In addition, in all elderly patients one must be alert to the possibility that aspirin administration may result in significant bleeding from the gastrointestinal or genitourinary tract.

Although aspirin remains the standard and, in many patients, the best anti-inflammatory and antirheumatic agent, osteoarthritis is a stubborn disease to treat at best, and most physicians will elect a trial of therapy of one of the newer nonsteroidal anti-inflammatory agents.[30-32] No one drug is best for all patients. Therefore, a period of trial, with several agents in series or in combination, is usually indicated. The patient should be alerted before each change that the new program may result in new adverse symptoms and that these should be reported to the physician immediately. Certain of the nonsteroidal anti-inflammatory drugs appear to have a decreased propensity for the induction of gastrointestinal symptoms. However, this is not the case for indomethacin, phenylbutazone, and several other agents in which gastrointestinal toxicity appears to be enhanced.[33]

The overall toxic effect of all these agents has not yet been explored in a sufficiently large number of patients to be certain of the true incidence figures.[33] It is clear, however, that by virtue of their inhibition of prostaglandin synthesis in the kidney, the nonsteroidal agents exert an important effect on renal function.[34,35] The threat of acute or chronic nephropathy due to these agents is a real one.[36] The physician should carefully follow the course of patients receiving these agents, watching for progressive loss of renal function, especially in the presence of volume depletion or congestive heart failure.

Other important side effects of these agents include depression and loss of cognitive function.[37] In view of the high frequency of these central nervous system problems in the elderly, physicians must be alerted to the possibility that changes of this sort in people receiving nonsteroidal anti-inflammatory agents may be due to these agents rather than to simultaneous senile dementia of the Alzheimer type.

Recent studies have shown that these agents may have additional subtle but possibly important effects. These include an influence on cartilage metabolism in patients with osteoarthritis and rheumatoid arthritis.[38,39] Certain of these effects appear to be beneficial, but others are not. These agents have also been shown to suppress immunologic responsiveness.[40] These points are cited here not to discourage use of these agents in patients with disabling symptoms due to osteoarthritis or other rheumatic diseases but to alert the physician that these drugs are not as innocuous as initially hoped and that the possibility of adverse effects must be borne in mind.[41,42]

USE OF A COMBINATION OF ANTIRHEUMATIC AGENTS. Should one utilize a given nonsteroidal agent as the sole mode of anti-inflammatory therapy, or are combinations of agents permissible and, possibly, desirable? The opinion of experts in rheumatology and geriatrics is sharply divided on this issue. Although hazards of polypharmacy and drug interaction are real and must be guarded against, it is our view that a combination of agents may, at least in some cases, produce a better result with less overall toxicity. Thus, we will frequently employ a combination of aspirin, 3.6 or 4.8 gm per day with indomethacin 25 mg or, if necessary, 50 mg daily. Occasionally, a combination of aspirin and ibuprofen may prove effective. We do not combine several of the newer nonsteroidal agents.

In patients with degenerative joint disease, whose pain cannot be relieved by the antirheumatic drugs, analgesic agents may, occasionally, be necessary. In rheumatology, it is a firmly based tradition that one does *not* condone the use of narcotics in a patient with a form of arthritis that is expected to continue over a long term.

Owing to the threat of renal damage, one attempts to avoid the use of phenacetin on a continuing basis. It is not clear whether acetaminophen (Tylenol) carries the same hazard. Nevertheless, all rules may occasionally be broken if one is careful. In patients who are unable to fall asleep as a result of pain, a single tablet of Tylenol with codeine (30 mg) or Empirin compound No. 3 may prove helpful, the benefits outweighing the disadvantages.

**Exercises**

Support to and proper positioning of a joint during normal use depend in part on relatively fixed support structures (such as the ligaments of the knee) but to an even greater extent on support from tendons, the tension of which is controlled by voluntary (and involuntary) muscles. Pain in a given joint and the decrease of normal use of the joint, which almost always accompanies pain, lead immediately to atrophy of these supporting structures. This can usually be identified on physical examination, both by inspection and by feeling the bulk of the muscle when "tensed." When a joint no longer receives support from normal musculature and tendons, it is very susceptible to added injury from very minor trauma, such as stumbling over a stone or curb. This, of course, leads to more pain, more spasm, and more damage to articular surfaces.

The objectives of the exercise program for a patient with osteoarthritis, and also many other forms of arthritis, are listed in Table 36-4. Exercises should be designed with care and prescribed with the same attention to detail that one uses in prescribing a dangerous drug. Overuse can be as bad or worse than no exercise at all. Maintaining a balance between rest and exercise is an essential part of a successful program. It is well for the physician to familiarize himself or herself with simple effective exercises for the back, hip, and knee, as a minimum. Instruction can be obtained from people in a good physical therapy department.

***Types of Exercises.*** In general, exercises can be classified as active exercises, active assistive exercises, resisted exercises, and passive exercises. *Active exercises* are used, primarily, to improve strength and range of motion. They constitute the most important form of exercise for

**Table 36-4.** OBJECTIVES OF THE EXERCISE PROGRAM FOR ARTHRITIC PATIENTS

1. Maintenance or improvement of joint motion
2. Maintenance or improvement of muscle strength
3. Training in the correct or more efficient use of muscles and joints
4. Protection from overuse and misuse
5. Prevention of deformities
6. Attainment of maximal function and independence

most arthritis patients. They are carried out by the patient after he or she has been instructed as to the type and frequency of exercises to be used. They may be in the form of *isometric exercises,* in which a body part remains fixed in one position and the patient contracts a muscle without moving the joint or part, or *isotonic exercises,* in which the patient moves the part and joint through an arc of motion and maintains the tone of the muscles continuously.

In performing both types of exercise the patient should gradually "build up" to a point at which he or she is exercising for periods of 20 to 30 minutes, two or three times daily. Good exercise is often followed by a sense of soreness and fatigue of the muscles. This may last for 5 to 10 minutes. If the exercise is followed by discomfort that lasts for a longer period, it has been too strenuous and should be scaled down to a point that will not yield symptoms of that magnitude. If the patient develops a recurrence of prior symptoms or if new joint complaints develop, he or she should then rest and start again in a day or two but at a more moderate pace. Progress and improvement may take weeks to be apparent.

One set of exercises which, in our view, is seldom given sufficient attention is the quadriceps setting exercises, a form of isometric exercises. Patients with arthritis of the knees and patients who have sustained quadriceps atrophy due to prolonged bed rest should be encouraged to "set" their quadriceps muscles on a regular basis. In our practice, patients usually start with eight to ten "sets" and build up to 40 to 60, three times daily. Ideally speaking, quadriceps setting exercises should be carried out both with the leg flexed and with the leg in a nearly straight position. The reason is that exercising a muscle at a given degree of "stretch" or muscle length will strengthen the muscle at that particular length, but not at other lengths. Thus, quadriceps exercises with the knee at right angle will assist the patient in rising more easily from a chair but will not decrease the likelihood of a fall from the standing position owing to sudden weakening of the quadriceps muscle. To assist in *standing,* the quadriceps exercise should be done in the extended position. This is best accomplished with the patient lying in bed with a coffee can or similar object beneath the knees (Fig. 36–2).

For bedridden patients, isometric exercises, particularly of the quadriceps and gluteal muscles, are often helpful in preserving muscle strength and in preventing rapid muscle atrophy and weakness.

Both isometric and isotonic exercises are also extremely important in many patients who are up and about because normal daily activity does not contribute to muscle strengthening in a fashion comparable with well-designed active exercises focused on specific muscle groups.

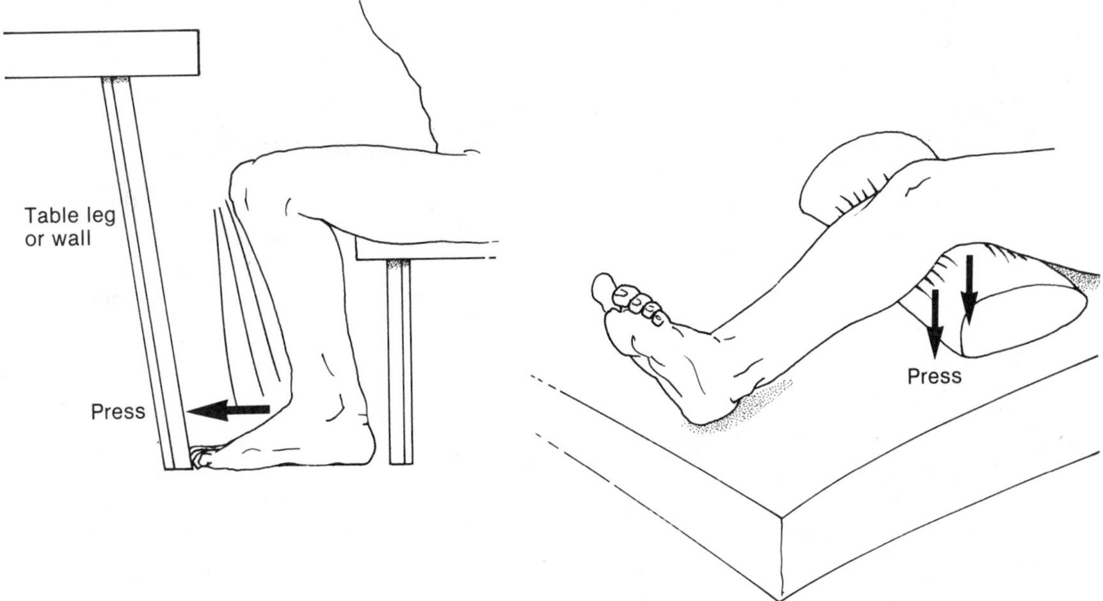


**Figure 36–2.** Quadriceps setting exercises. Quadriceps setting can also be done by raising the leg with weights attached to the shoe. As the patient gets stronger, heavier weights are used. However, the repeated motion of the knee may cause discomfort or pain, and knee motion is not essential for effective exercise to the quadriceps muscle.

*Active assistive exercises* are designed to improve both strength and range of motion but must be used with care in patients with joint inflammation. They are employed when the patient cannot complete the full range of motion of a joint owing to pain or lack of strength. The joint is assisted to move to the point of definite feeling of stretch. The assistance can be given by the patient, a member of the family, or devices, e.g., use of pulley or broomstick for shoulder exercises.

*Resisted exercises* may be needed to maintain or increase muscle strength. The resistance is applied to the part of the body to be moved, and the patient attempts to overcome the resistance. Resisted exercises can be performed manually or by lifting weights, sandbags, and so on. Resisted exercises further increase muscle bulk, strength, and endurance. Muscle bulk is increased by providing maximum resistance, whereas muscle endurance is increased by providing maximum repetitions.

When possible, for fairly active patients, it is helpful to prescribe exercises in a form that is interesting for the patient to do and that involves simultaneous exercise to several joints. Prescribing the use of a "rowing machine" for patients with back pain is an excellent example of this approach. We have found that a number of patients incapacitated by degenerative joint disease of the back can be restored to reasonable function, pain free, through use of a rowing machine and good shoes and avoidance of injurious repetitive trauma.

*Passive exercises* are performed on the patient by someone else, such as a therapist or family member. They consist of passive movements of the joint or part. Such movements help to maintain the available range of motion and to avoid adaptive shortening of muscles and contractures. These exercises do not improve muscle strength, and there is the potential of producing damage by overstretching or tearing. They are infrequently used in patients with inflammatory arthritis and, if used, must be supervised carefully.

Almost all patients benefit from doing their exercises, when appropriate, in a swimming or therapeutic pool. When they are submerged in the pool, the patients can walk and exercise, with the water supporting their body weight. Heat therapy and pain medications should be timed so that the effect of the treatment will occur during exercise.

Both the patient and the family have to be educated about the importance of the program so that they will accept a life-style that moderates stresses and protects the joints from further harm.

**Orthopedic Management**

***Supportive Appliances.*** *Splints* and *braces* are designed to stabilize a joint, relieve pain, and improve function; at times they can be used to prevent or correct deformities of arthritic joints. Long-term use of splints and braces for chronic joint problems usually proves to be impractical, since patient compliance is very low. Lower extremity braces to support an arthritic knee are heavy, cosmetically unappealing, and difficult to put on by the arthritic, elderly person and thus are hardly ever prescribed. On the other hand, elastic knee splints, with or without side hinges, can give symptomatic relief at times. In patients with arthritis of the thumb or wrist, a supportive splint can be beneficial in many instances.

*Canes, crutches,* and *walkers* are practical ambulation assistive devices to support a painful lower extremity and are strongly recommended for patients with arthritis of the hip, knee, or ankle (see Chapter 15). When only one cane or crutch is used, it should be held in the hand opposite to the affected lower extremity in order to achieve the most efficient gait with the least stress on the upper extremity joints. The patient moves the cane at the same time he or she moves the arthritic leg.

***Surgery.*** There are times when disabling pain and functional limitations due to arthritis provide indications for surgery. The decision concerning surgery depends not only on the degree of disability but also on the patient's general outlook on life. Although the risks of surgery are increased by the coexistence of other medical problems in the elderly, orthopedic surgical procedures may be advisable as the only means of maintaining the patient's independence and ability to ambulate. The goals of surgery in these instances are to relieve pain, correct deformity, improve motion, and enhance overall function.

In general, the orthopedic procedures for arthritic joints fall into one of the following four categories:

1. Debridement of a joint involves the removal of inflamed synovium, loose bodies, fragments of cartilage, osteophytes, and so on. In the case of tendon involvement, the tenosynovium is debrided, and tendon sheaths are released, e.g., trigger finger.
2. Osteotomy is used to correct malalignment and eliminate abnormal joint stress, thus slowing the progression of the disease.

3. Arthrodesis, the fusion of a joint, definitely controls pain, but it can interfere with function because of the elimination of motion.

4. Arthroplasty is by far the most effective method of reducing pain and improving function. The clinically applicable methods consist of either resection arthroplasties, in which the damaged joint is removed, or *replacement arthroplasties,* in which artificial materials are used to replace the articular surfaces. Details on the use of arthroplasties are provided later in this chapter.

The preceding types of reconstructive surgery are not equally applicable in the management of arthritis of different joints. In the upper extremity, osteotomy does not have any practical value. Debridement is quite successfully used for the elbow and also the shoulder and hand. Arthroplasty can be used for all joints except the distal interphalangeal (DIP) joint for which arthrodesis is preferred. Arthrodesis of the elbow rarely is practical. In the lower extremity debridement of the knee can be beneficial in relatively early joint involvement. Osteotomies of the hip and knee have proved their value in younger patients, but they are used infrequently in the elderly, who cannot tolerate well the immobilization and rehabilitation required after surgery. Arthrodesis of the ankle and foot can be helpful. Total joint replacement of the hip and total joint replacement of the knee continue to be the most common and successful procedures.

**Psychologic Aspects**

Psychologic stress frequently expresses itself in musculoskeletal symptoms. "He is a pain in the neck!" one might say or "Oh, my aching back!" This association continues to be present and is enhanced in patients who have musculoskeletal disease. In patients with degenerative joint disease, emotional trauma and strain appear to influence the degree of symptoms and, possibly, the course of the disease by exacerbating muscle tension and interfering with free, relaxed joint motion.

In clinical management of patients with osteoarthritis, steps that will give the patient confidence that something *can* be done, that therapeutic possibilities are ahead, and that symptomatic improvement can be achieved, contribute substantially to an improved outlook and morale. The therapeutic program is multifaceted, with each element contributing in a small way to an improved outlook. The physician should capitalize on this broad approach and identify himself or herself with it. A sympathetic ear often contributes as much or more to a patient's mobility and freedom from discomfort as other more expensive and potentially hazardous approaches.

## *Calcium Pyrophosphate Dihydrate (CPPD) Deposition Disease and Pseudogout*

One of the most common of the entities that appear to accentuate the development of degenerative joint disease involves the deposition of calcium pyrophosphate dihydrate (CaPPi) crystals. The gross deposition of these crystals in joint cartilage and periarticular structures,[43] as identified on x-ray or pathologic examination, is designated chondrocalcinosis. This condition may exist in the absence of symptoms of acute inflammation. In approximately 25 per cent of instances, however, it is accompanied by acute inflammatory changes not unlike those seen in gout. This entity is known as pseudogout. The diagnostic criteria for pseudogout, as delineated by McCarty,[44] are shown in Table 36-5.

This condition is more commonly encountered in women than in men. The frequency of CPPD disease increases sharply with advancing age (Fig. 36-3).[45-47] The most frequent site of deposition of CaPPi is in and around the knee

**Table 36-5.** DIAGNOSTIC CRITERIA FOR CALCIUM PYROPHOSPHATE DIHYDRATE DEPOSITION DISEASE (PSEUDOGOUT)*

**Criteria**

I. Demonstration of CaPPi crystals (obtained by biopsy, necropsy, or aspirated synovial fluid) by definitive means (e.g., characteristic "fingerprint" by x-ray diffraction powder pattern)

II. (a) Identification of monoclinic and triclinic crystals showing none or a weakly positive birefringence by compensated polarized light microscopy (see Fig. 36-6)
  (b) Presence of *typical* calcifications in roentgenograms†

III. (a) Acute arthritis, especially of knees or other large joints, with or without concomitant hyperuricemia
  (b) Chronic arthritis, especially of knees and hips and if accompanied by acute exacerbations

**Categories**

A. Definite—Criteria I or II (a) plus (b) must be fulfilled
B. Probable—Criteria II (a) or II (b) must be fulfilled
C. Possible—Criteria III (a) or (b) should alert the clinician to the possibility of the diagnosis

* From McCarty DJ: Pseudogout: Articular chondrocalcinosis calcium phosphate crystal deposition disease. *In* Hollander JL, McCarty DJ (eds.): Arthritis and Allied Conditions, 8th ed. Philadelphia, Lea and Febiger, 1972, p. 1146.

† Occasionally faint and/or atypical calcifications may be the result of $CaHPO_4 \cdot 2H_2O$ deposits or vascular mineralization.

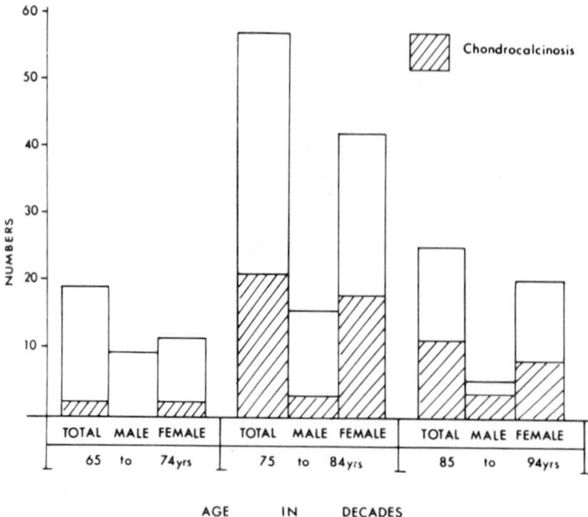


**Figure 36 – 3.** Frequency of evidence of chondrocalcinosis in radiographs of knees, hands, wrists, and pelvis of 100 consecutive admissions to an acute geriatric unit. (Radiographs were taken using special techniques. Positive findings are not always associated with symptoms.) (From Wilkins E, et al: Osteoarthritis and articular chondrocalcinosis in the elderly. Ann Rheum Dis 42:280, 1983. Reproduced with permission.)

(Figs. 36 – 4 and 36 – 5). These deposits are noted in 3 to 5 per cent of persons studied at the time of death.[48] Although this condition occurs predominantly as an isolated entity, numerous familial occurrences have been reported.[49,50] The incidence of CPPD disease appears to be increased in patients with a variety of metabolic diseases, (Table 36 – 6),[51] and the presence of these disorders should be sought in all persons with this condition.

The pathogenesis of CPPD disease is beginning to be understood.[52–54] There is no known reservoir of calcium pyrophosphate in either blood or tissues. Studies of fibroblasts from patients with various forms of sporadic and familial CPPD disease, however, indicate increased intracellular concentrations of pyrophosphate and, in the sporadic group only, of an enzyme ecto-nucleoside triphosphate (NTP) pyrophosphohydrolase.[52,53]

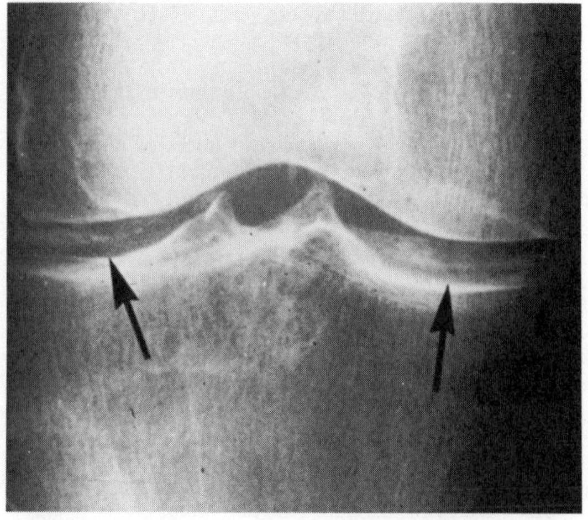

**Figure 36 – 4.** X-ray of knee showing opacification of meniscus due to deposition of calcium pyrophosphate crystals.

The crystals appear to be both formed and deposited in the articular cartilage and are subsequently "shed" into the synovial fluid. Here they are phagocytized by polymorphonuclear leukocytes and synovial cells, resulting in death of the cells and release of lysosomal enzymes in a pattern analogous to that described in gouty arthritis. Acute attacks are accompanied by an increase in synovial fluid leukocytes, and typical calcium pyrophosphate crystals can be identified within the fluid both intracellularly and extracellularly, utilizing the compensated polarized light microscope. The rhomboid-shaped calcium pyrophosphate dihydrate crystals appear blue and weakly positively birefringent (Fig. 36 – 6).[55] They can easily be distinguished from the needle-shaped urate crystals, which, aligned parallel to the compensator, are yellow in color and exhibit strong negative birefringence.

## Pseudogout Versus Gout

The differentiation between attacks of pseudogout and those of gout, on purely clinical grounds, provides an interesting exercise for the clinician. The propensity for involvement of multiple joints is somewhat greater in pseudogout, in which approximately half of the patients exhibit acute inflammatory changes in two or more joints. In contrast to gout, the predominant site of involvement in pseudogout is the knee. Other common areas of involvement in pseudogout, in order of frequency, are the wrists, hips, shoulders, and metacarpophalangeal joints (see Fig. 36 – 5).[56]

Once the attack is underway, the clinical characteristics of the two entities are quite similar and consist of pain, swelling, severe tenderness, warmth, and redness of the involved joints and, often, a joint effusion. These manifestations may be accompanied by fever and constitutional symptoms.[57] The onset of an acute attack in pseudogout often occurs over the course of a day or so, rather than hours as in gout. Although with both gout and, to a lesser extent, pseudogout, an acute attack can be abated by appropriate therapy, acute attacks in both entities are self-limited and will subside in time, even without treatment. Both entities occur in

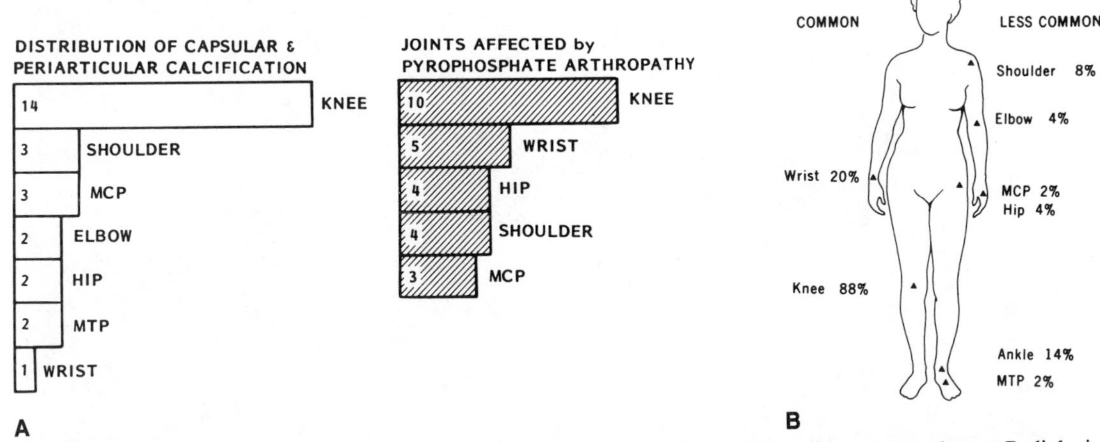


**Figure 36-5.** *A*, Radiologic and *B*, clinical sites of involvement in 50 hospitalized patients with acute pseudogout. Radiologic involvement in this figure refers to involvement of the joint capsule or periarticular structures. Radiologic technique used is not mentioned specifically in report. MCP = metacarpophalangeal; MTP = metatarsophalangeal. (From Fam AG, et al: Clinical and roentgenographic aspects of pseudogout: A study of 50 cases and a review. Can Med Assoc J 124:545, 1981.)

**Table 36-6.** PREDISPOSING FACTORS TO CALCIUM PYROPHOSPHATE DIHYDRATE (CPPD) DISEASE*

| | **Possible Mechanisms Involved** |
|---|---|
| ***Inherited Forms*** | |
| Described from Czechoslovakia, Chile, Netherlands, Sweden, France, USA | Possible abnormality in inorganic pyrophosphate ($PP_1$) metabolism—for example, overproduction of $PP_1$ or decreased degradation of $PP_1$ (possible changes in pyrophosphatases).<br>Reduced inhibitors of crystallization. |
| ***General Associations*** | |
| Aging | Disturbed $PP_1$ metabolism<br>Physical damage to chondrocytes.<br>Release of nucleating agents or decreased inhibitory activity (perhaps via action of released proteases to destroy inhibitors).<br>Increased cartilage permeation by $Ca^{++}$ and $PP_1$. |
| ***Other Joint Disease*** | |
| Osteoarthritis | Epitaxy on apatite crystals; pH may be lowered during inflammation, which promotes crystal transformations to more insoluble forms. |
| Neuropathic joint disease (Charcot joints) | |
| Destructive arthropathy | |
| Ochronosis | |
| Rheumatoid arthritis | |
| Urate gout | Epitaxy on urate crystals |
| ***Metabolic Disorders*** | |
| Hyperparathyroidism | Raised extracellular Ca and/or raised $PP_1$ due to increased adenylate cyclase activity |
| Hypothyroidism | Metabolic changes in cartilage |
| Hypophosphatasia | Raised $PP_1$ due to alkaline phosphatase deficiency |
| Hemochromatosis | Fe as nucleating agent or pyrophosphatase inhibitor |
| Long-term steroid therapy | Secondary hyperparathyroidism |
| ***Possible Associations*** | |
| Hypertension | |
| Renal insufficiency | High $PP_1$ in chronic renal failure: Acidosis promotes crystal transformation to insoluble forms |
| Acromegaly | Metabolic alterations in cartilage |
| Paget's disease | Age related |
| Diabetes mellitus | |
| Wilson's disease | Copper as crystal nucleating agent or pyrophosphatase inhibitor |

*Reproduced by permission from Caswell A, et al: Ann Rheum Dis Suppl 27, 42:27–38, 1983.

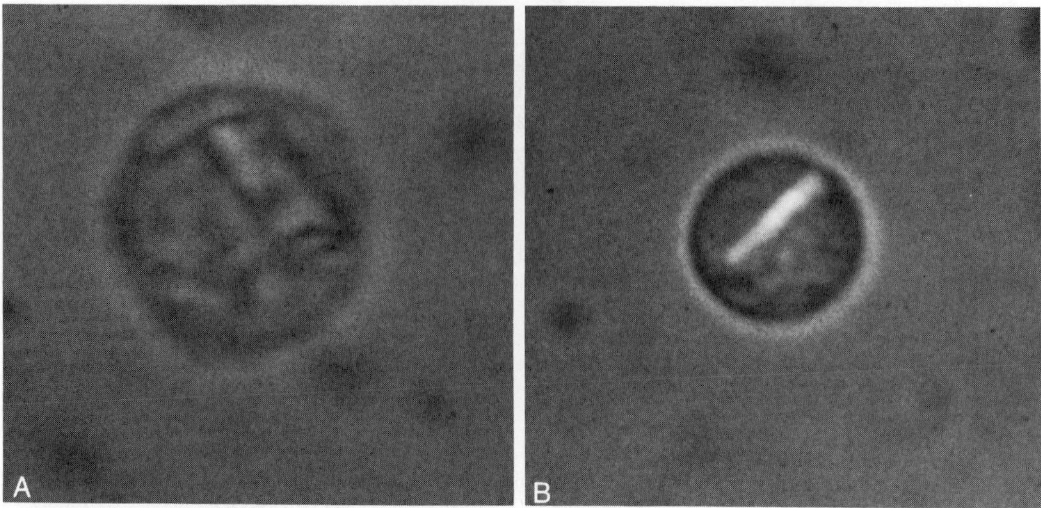


**Figure 36–6.** *A,* Calcium pyrophosphate dihydrate crystal within leukocyte in synovial fluid from a patient with chondrocalcinosis. *B,* Urate crystal within leukocyte in synovial fluid from a patient with gout. (From the Arthritis Foundation. Reproduced with permission.)

increasing frequency in patients with pre-existing joint disease, especially osteoarthritis.

### RELATIONSHIP OF CPPD DISEASE TO OSTEOARTHRITIS

Approximately half the patients with CPPD disease evidence progressive degeneration of multiple joints, whether or not they experience pseudogout. In some instances, the clinical and radiologic manifestations resemble those of generalized "primary" osteoarthritis. In other cases, a particularly destructive form of osteoarthritis may ensue, involving, predominantly, the knees followed by the wrists, hips, shoulder, and metacarpophalangeal joints. In addition to calcification of the meniscus and articular cartilage, x-ray studies reveal severe degenerative changes. This condition has been termed pyrophosphate arthropathy.

In approximately 5 per cent of the patients with CPPD disease the inflammatory changes closely resemble those of rheumatoid arthritis. These patients exhibit morning stiffness and fatigue, mild synovial thickening, and elevation of the erythrocyte sedimentation rate. In some instances this may reflect the simultaneous presence of CPPD disease and rheumatoid arthritis. In others, the presence of normal values for hemolytic complement in the synovial fluid and x-ray changes showing osteophytes and absence of erosions suggest that the entire syndrome is due to CPPD disease itself.

### "MILWAUKEE SHOULDER"

Related to but apparently distinct from CPPD arthritis is a syndrome called Milwaukee shoulder, which has been described in a limited number of elderly women and is characterized by glenohumeral arthritis with calcification and, later, defects of the rotator cuff.[58–61] Involved shoulders may be hypermobile or restricted in motion. X-rays typically show roughening or erosion of the bony cortex of the greater tuberosity of the humerus, cortical cyst formation, and narrowing of the space between the superior aspect of the humeral head and the acromion. The clue to the presence of this disorder is the identification, on x-ray, of a homogeneous "cloud" of very fine crystalline material surrounding the joint. In some cases, calcification of the rotator cuff will be seen (Fig. 36–7). Detailed studies of the synovial fluid obtained from the shoulder joint have shown a crystal population containing partially carbonate-substituted hydroxyapatite, octacalcium pyrophosphate (OCP), and collagen. Approximately half of the patients with Milwaukee shoulder also have knee involvement.[60]

### TREATMENT

The treatment of calcium pyrophosphate deposition disease and related disorders is not as effective as one would like. In those instances in which the disorder is associated with a treatable

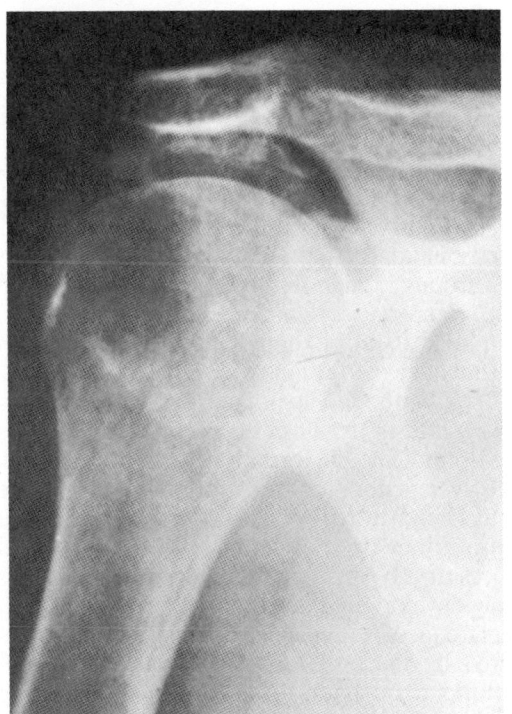

**Figure 36–7.** Calcification of rotator cuff in "Milwaukee shoulder." (From McCarty DJ, et al: Arthritis Rheum 24:464, 1981.)

predisposing condition, such as hypothyroidism or hyperparathyroidism, it is reasonable to treat this condition; however, treatment does not result in resorption of the calcium deposits. In instances of familial or idiopathic disease, there is no known method of halting further deposits.[61]

The treatment of pseudogout is also less effective than one would like. The first step, following confirmation of the diagnosis, is to aspirate the joint, withdrawing as much fluid as possible.[62] Some clinicians favor the injection of corticosteroids (e.g., 5 ml of Depo-Medrol).[62] Physicians should be reminded of recent reports that corticosteroids within a joint may form crystals, which, themselves, contribute to degenerative changes. Joint aspiration may be followed by the oral administration of a nonsteroidal anti-inflammatory agent, such as indomethacin 25 mg three times a day for 2 days, with subsequent stepwise reduction in dosage over the ensuing 3 to 4 days. One must be mindful of the increased toxicity of this and other nonsteroidal anti-inflammatory agents in the elderly, especially in the presence of coincidental disease. Oral colchicine has been reported to be beneficial in the treatment of acute gout in some patients. However, this regimen provides a potentially serious hazard in the elderly patient because of the possible side effects of serious diarrhea and emesis, with attendant dehydration. Faced with this dilemma, at the suggestion of McCarty,[63] it has been our practice, in some elderly individuals, to administer colchicine intravenously in a dose of 1 mg (2 ml) followed by 0.5 ml (0.25 mg) in 12 hours if necessary. This has resulted in a good response in approximately half of the cases. Although one must recognize the potential hazard of hematologic sequelae following administration of colchicine, we have not encountered this to date. In addition to the treatment of pseudogout, careful attention to the management of the degenerative joint disease that frequently accompanies CPPD disease should not be overlooked. Such treatment may decrease significantly the frequency of pseudogout attacks.

Additional readings on crystal deposition diseases are referred to in the bibliography.[64–66]

## *Gout*

The frequency of gouty arthritis increases with advancing age for at least four reasons. First, although the peak age of incidence of primary gout is in the range of 48 to 53 years,[67,68] gout is rarely a lethal condition, and therefore, cases continue to accumulate. Second, because of the increase in serum urate levels in postmenopausal women, women are beginning to constitute a significant segment of gouty patients (15 per cent in one series).[68] Third, a number of drugs commonly used in the elderly, such as thiazide diuretics, are apt to cause or exacerbate already present hyperuricemia. Finally, older persons experience an increased frequency of surgical procedures, which, along with trauma, are among the most common antecedents to attacks of acute gouty arthritis in persons with elevated serum urate levels. Thus, advanced age is accompanied by increased frequency of both primary and secondary hyperuricemia and also acute gouty arthritis. It has been shown, clearly, that hyperuricemia of any cause will predispose to the development of gouty arthritis.[67]

### Diagnosis

The diagnosis of gouty arthritis should never be missed because of the high susceptibility of gout to symptomatic and also preventive therapy. When gouty arthritis manifests itself as classic podagra, the diagnosis can easily be made on clinical grounds. Gout may also be manifested in different ways. One of these is unexplained fever following a surgical procedure. Alternatively, the articular manifestations of gout may involve multiple joints in a fashion somewhat similar to that of rheumatoid arthritis. Therefore, the diagnosis of gout should be considered in any person, especially one in the older age group, who exhibits acute arthritis of one or several joints. In occasional patients, acute gout may be accompanied by the sudden onset of tenosynovitis.[69] When such disorders occur in an individual with elevated serum uric acid concentration, it is best to assume that the inflammatory manifestations are due to gout and initiate treatment accordingly, rather than to conclude that the individual has rheumatoid arthritis or another disorder and incidental hyperuricemia. Occasionally, patients presenting with acute gout will not, at that particular moment, exhibit hyperuricemia. Therefore, it is very important to attempt to obtain synovial fluid in all elderly patients with acute arthritis accompanied by an effusion and to examine the fluid under polarized light for the presence of urate crystals. These can easily be identified by their needlelike shape and strongly negative birefringence. When examined with polarized light microscopy with a first order red plate compensator, urate crystals turn yellow when their long axis is parallel to the direction of slow vibration of light through the compensator and blue when their long axis is lying at right angles to it (see Fig. 36–6).

The patients in whom gout is manifested by tenosynovitis without effusion present a difficult problem in diagnosis.[69] The intermittent nature of the symptoms in the absence of other obvious causes, such as rheumatoid arthritis, provides a clue to this possibility. When gout is suspected, serum urate determinations should be obtained, and if the patient's general condition permits, a therapeutic trial of colchicine should be undertaken.

## TREATMENT

### Drugs

The treatment of hyperuricemia and gout in elderly persons presents special and often perplexing problems. A full course of colchicine (0.6 mg every 2 hours day and night until relief of joint symptoms or diarrhea occurs) is an effective means of therapy, appropriate for use in younger persons, and the development of symptomatic relief provides important confirmation of the diagnosis. However, in an elderly patient one is loath to institute a form of therapy that is apt to produce severe diarrhea and, not infrequently, nausea. Phenylbutazone is another highly effective agent, but the propensity of this drug to cause fluid retention, thus exacerbating congestive failure and hypertension, makes one hesitant to employ it in the elderly. Indomethacin, 150 mg a day, with decreasing doses thereafter, also brings with it the possibility of side effects but appears, in our experience, to be a less hazardous though less effective approach than full courses of colchicine or phenylbutazone. Sulindac (Clinoril) may prove effective in an initial dose of 200 mg twice a day.

In patients who do not respond to the preceding agents, or in whom the use of these agents is contraindicated as a result of their toxic effects, the intravenous administration of colchicine may be indicated. We use this agent in an initial intravenous dose of 1 mg (2 ml), followed, if necessary, by 0.5 mg 12 hours later. Patients may develop mild diarrhea, but it occurs much less frequently than when colchicine is administered by the oral route. We have yet to encounter toxic sequelae following use of this drug in this fashion, although colchicine may induce serious side effects and doses greater than 4 mg intravenously have been fatal.[70]

Once the acute attack has subsided, the patient should be maintained on colchicine in a dose of 0.6 mg orally daily or 0.6 mg alternating with 1.2 mg every other day. Colchicine tablets are available in both a 0.6 mg and 0.5 mg form. The former dose is recommended because it is available as a United States Pharmacopeia preparation, whereas the 0.5 mg tablet is, at present, only available in a proprietary form. Allopurinol or probenecid therapy should also be initiated, in the same way that it is in younger patients, after symptoms of acute gouty arthritis have subsided.

The treatment of *asymptomatic hyperuricemia* has been a subject for debate for some years. In the past, it was deemed important to reduce elevated serum urate levels to normal or near-normal, even in the absence of acute gouty arthritis, in order to prevent the development of urate nephropathy. It is now recognized that renal failure developing in the face of prolonged hyperuricemia is not the result of urate nephropathy but reflects other concomitant conditions[71,72] or the simultaneous presence of lead accumulation (leading to lead nephropathy and "saturnine gout").[73] It is also recognized that the frequency of development of urate stones in persons with hyperuricemia is sufficiently low so that there is no rationale for justifying prophylactic hypouricosuric therapy on this basis.[67] There appear to be three main rheumatologic indications for initiating hypouricosuric therapy. These are tophaceous gout, frequent occurrences of acute gouty arthritis, and radiologic evidence of joint damage due to the preferential accumulation of urate in joint cartilage, despite the absence of tophi.[74] To identify the latter group of patients, persons with hyperuricemia should be followed by having joint x-rays taken at regular intervals.[67] In patients with lymphoproliferative disorders who are receiving cytotoxic therapy, marked hyperuricemia is regarded as an indication for use of allopurinol during periods of therapy.

When one initiates treatment with allopurinol or probenecid in a patient with gout, it is important to stress to the patient that this treatment is not designed to exert an immediate prophylactic effect on the gouty attacks. Indeed, during the first 6 months of therapy with allopurinol, these attacks may be more frequent than before. Unless forewarned, the patient will almost certainly discontinue the allopurinol. In selecting the dose, one should remember that allopurinol itself is excreted by the kidney, and therefore, a somewhat decreased dosage (perhaps 200 mg per day) may yield the desired effect in elderly persons. If probenecid therapy is to be instituted (due perhaps to adverse reaction or failure to respond to allopurinol), it is important to obtain a 24-hour urate determination first, since probenecid therapy in a person who is already excreting large amounts of uric acid (800 mg or more per 24 hours) carries a risk for inducing renal stones. Allopurinol or probenecid therapy should be accompanied by maintenance colchicine during the first 6 months of treatment.

For further details concerning the pathogenesis of the various forms of gout, and their therapy, the reader is referred to references 76 and 77.

**Orthopedic Management**

If treated early and effectively, patients with gout should not develop tophi and the attendant destructive changes to their joints. Older patients, however, may have suffered gout for many years prior to the institution of effective uricosuric therapy, and management must be directed to the destructive changes secondary to gouty arthritis and, in some instances, the continued presence of tophi despite optimal uricosuric treatment. For example, involvement of the metatarsophalangeal area of the big toe will produce local chronic symptoms due to the bunionlike deformity. Wider and deeper shoes with soft (deer skin) uppers and metatarsal bars can be helpful.

When large tophi interfere with function, as in the hand, or when there is danger of ulceration of overlying skin, surgical excision of the tophi may be indicated. If the ulceration is already present then, in addition to the systemic treatment for the gout, local care to avoid infection is of paramount importance. Sometimes, debridement of the deposits and surrounding tissues, usually tendon, is needed to treat infected gouty ulcerations. The effect of hypouricosuric therapy alone should not be discounted.

## *Rheumatoid Arthritis*

### Incidence

Although overshadowed in terms of frequency by osteoarthritis, rheumatoid arthritis is an important disease among the elderly. In part this reflects the survival into old age of patients who developed the disease in youth or young adulthood. Patients with long-standing rheumatoid arthritis who survive until old age tend to have less crippling disease, with fewer constitutional manifestations, than those whose disease was fatal at an earlier age; also, they tend to die of disorders unrelated to the arthritis.[78] These patients constitute one "set" of geriatric patients with rheumatoid arthritis. The clinical and biologic characteristics of this group has been largely ignored in the clinical literature.

Much greater attention has been given to those patients who developed the disease at a relatively advanced age.[79–83] These patients are by no means infrequent. There is a disagreement in the literature concerning the age at which rheumatoid arthritis has its peak incidence and frequency. In a retrospective study of 300 cases from Olmstead County, which surrounds Rochester, Minnesota, Linos and associates,[79] reported that the peak incidence rate in males (99.7 per 100,000) occurred between age 60 and 69; in females (193.5 per 100,000) it occurred in persons age 70 and older. These authors pointed out, however, that the annual incidence varied by a factor of nearly threefold over the course of two decades. Wood and Badley,[5] in a study in Lancashire, England, placed the age of maximal incidence at approximately 50 years. The latter figure is more consistent with the clinical experience of most rheumatologists. The resultant prevalence rates for definite rheumatoid arthritis in the Tecumseh, Michigan, study[4] rose from 0.44 per cent in the fourth decade to 0.79 per cent in the eighth decade for males, and from 1.69 per cent in the fifth decade to 2.47 per cent in the eighth decade for females. In 1966, Adler[80] estimated that 12 to

13 per cent of all cases of rheumatoid arthritis have their onset in people at age 55 and older, and 10 per cent in patients age 60 and above. By 1970, with a larger population of elderly persons, the percentage of patients seen in an arthritis clinic who had their onset at age 60 or over had risen to 15 per cent. Twenty-eight per cent of all rheumatoid patients seen in this clinic were age 60 and older.[81] Race, climate, and geographic location appear to have little effect on the epidemiology of the disease.

## Clinical Aspects

Very few recent objective data are available concerning the clinical and biologic characteristics of rheumatoid arthritis in the elderly. Several publications, written 10 or more years ago, describe two distinct patterns.[82,83] In approximately 75 per cent of the cases, the disease is insidious in onset. It is accompanied by relatively mild constitutional symptoms, with joint involvement, consisting of pain, tenderness, and synovial thickening, focused primarily in the small joints and later spreading to the larger joints. Involvement of the shoulders and cervical spine may be a prominent feature. Synovitis is usually less striking in the elderly than in younger persons. Rheumatoid nodules, extensive joint erosions, and evidences of vasculitis, pulmonary involvement, and neuropathy are also less frequent than in younger persons with this disease. Once established, however, this form of arthritis usually proves to be a continuing problem. Although available data do not permit us to be entirely certain on this point, remissions in this group of patients appear to be much less frequent than in recent-onset rheumatoid arthritis in younger people, two thirds of whom enter a spontaneous remission within 1 year. Therefore, the physician is faced with an elderly person who may have been well all his or her life only to reach retirement age and find himself or herself crippled by a mild but continuously active form of arthritis. Special therapeutic considerations pertaining to this syndrome will be discussed later.

In approximately one quarter of older individuals, the onset of rheumatoid arthritis is precipitous and stormy, occurring over the course of days or even overnight, and accompanied by severe constitutional symptoms. These include malaise, anorexia, weight loss, and, frequently, depression. The patient may be febrile. This is one of the few forms of rheumatoid arthritis that may be accompanied by night sweats. Initially, articular involvement in these patients is usually focused in the shoulders and cervical spine. There is often muscle stiffness, especially in the shoulders and neck, which may last throughout the day. Although these symptoms are alarming to the patient, family, and physician, the patient can receive assurance that in most instances this form of arthritis is self-limited and will enter into a spontaneous remission within a few months.[83]

Findings of rheumatoid factor assay are positive in most elderly patients with rheumatoid arthritis of either type. This fact is of little clinical significance, however, in view of the increasing incidence of positive findings in rheumatoid factor assays among many elderly persons.[7-11] In addition, the presence of rheumatoid factor, even in high titer, in an older person does not appear to convey the same serious prognostic implications that it does in younger individuals. Anti-nuclear antibody and other autoantibodies also occur with increased frequency among the elderly, in comparison with the general population.[7-11]

Assuming that with further clinical study the differentiation of new-onset rheumatoid arthritis in the elderly into two distinct syndromes continues to prove valid, the pathogenetic significance of this differentiation is still obscure. Recent studies concerning the genetics of rheumatoid arthritis, as reflected in the presence of certain histocompatibility antigens,[84] and the presence of immunologic differentiation of a variety of rheumatic diseases[85] represent potentially important breakthroughs in our understanding of the biology of these diseases.

## Treatment

Treatment of rheumatoid arthritis in the elderly presents a therapeutic dilemma. Older persons are, of course, more fragile than younger individuals. There is a marked increase in adverse reaction to drugs due, in part, to age-related changes in pharmacokinetics (see also Chapter 12)[86] and also to multiple drug therapies related to the presence of multiple diseases. Surgical intervention in an elderly person presents a slight but definitely increased risk (see Chapter 47).

Conversely, in an elderly patient, the prevention of joint immobility may represent a major factor in the preservation of independence. As pointed out in Chapters 5, 8, and 14 of this book, preservation of independence in an older person has a major impact on the individual's happiness, longevity, and requirements for care and the happiness of the family. Interestingly, among social factors influencing the likelihood of disability as an outcome of rheumatoid arthritis, age alone has little effect.[87] Nevertheless, because of the importance of mobility in achieving independence and because of the decreased total life expectancy due to age alone, the physician may be justified in undertaking an approach to therapy that may bring inherent long-term hazards in order to achieve the goal of an enhanced ability to enjoy and participate in the activities of life in the more immediate future.

**Rest**

Another way in which the management of an elderly patient with rheumatoid arthritis and many other inflammatory joint diseases differs from that in a younger person is the use of rest. In a younger individual, one may be justified in prescribing periods of several weeks or even months of bed rest, in hopes of increasing the likelihood of remission (although the evidence proving this thesis is not very good). For an older person, this should never be done. Complete bed rest, in the elderly, bringing hazards of osteoporosis, decubitus ulcers, depression, urinary tract difficulties, and permanent loss of mobility, is one long step toward the grave. On the other hand, older persons with rheumatoid arthritis must avoid excessive fatigue and also avoid placing full body weight on inflamed joints. These objectives can be achieved by a carefully worked out daily schedule and by proper use of crutches, walkers, and other supports (see Chapter 15). In addition, a carefully monitored program of exercises is a vital part of treatment of an older person with rheumatoid arthritis.

**Use of Drugs**

A third important principle relates to the use of drugs. The importance of altered pharmacokinetics in elderly persons and of drug interaction has been emphasized in Chapter 12. There are no conditions in which these considerations are more important than rheumatoid arthritis and other musculoskeletal diseases. One reason is that many antirheumatic drugs, notably the nonsteroidal anti-inflammatory agents, act through inhibition of the synthesis of certain prostaglandins involved in the genesis of the inflammatory process. Although inhibition of these prostaglandins exerts a beneficial effect on tissue inflammation, prostaglandins also play an important role in the maintenance of the integrity of the gastric mucosa, in blood pressure regulation, and in sustaining renal function in the face of aging. This explains the high frequency of gastric and renal complications of treatment with this group of antirheumatic agents.

The administration of antirheumatic agents also tends to complicate pharmacologic treatment of concomitant diseases. Many of these drugs, notably phenylbutazone, are cited in the literature as classic examples of agents involved in multiple drug interaction. In addition to these pharmacologic actions, antirheumatic drugs have a tendency to exert important effects on other diseases that the patient may have in addition to the arthritis. Since it is very difficult for a physician to keep in mind all the drug-drug interactions or drug-disease interactions that his or her patient may manifest, it is our practice to start all new drugs in an elderly person in very small doses (approximately one third of the usual daily dose), explaining possible side effects to the patient and family and increasing the dose gradually over the course of approximately 2 weeks to achieve the desired effect. During this time, the possible influence of the antirheumatic drug on other diseases and agents the patient is receiving can be monitored carefully.

Because of the complexity of pharmacotherapy in the elderly, it is all the more important that the physician devote special attention to the *nonpharmacologic* management of the patient through carefully supervised exercises, appropriate use of heat, proper positioning, and psychologic support. None of the preceding has the potential toxic effects of pharmacologic agents.

**Sequential Approach to Management**

With these principles in mind, the treatment of rheumatoid arthritis in the elderly can easily be perceived. The first line of therapy is use of salicylates and/or nonsteroidal anti-inflammatory agents. Detailed suggestions on the use of these agents have been outlined previously (see pages 393–394). If use of these drugs, together with employment of nonpharmacologic management, as outlined previously, proves ineffective after a 2 to 3 months trial, there are several possible routes to follow. One is to institute gold therapy. The principles of gold treatment, including its dosage and effectiveness, in elderly patients are similar to those in younger persons.[88] If a patient has responded to gold salts in the past and has not had this treatment for a number of years a repeat course may prove to be as beneficial as the initial treatment. Indeed, the response of older patients to gold may be even more favorable than that of younger individuals. A major problem with gold therapy in an elderly person, however, is that the treatment involves weekly visits over the course of many months, followed by visits at intervals of 1 month. This follow-up program is essential not only to perform the intramuscular injection of gold but also to obtain a complete blood cell count, urinalysis, and a good history before giving the next dose. The recent introduction of oral gold (auranofin) obviates the need for intramuscular injections. It has proven to be equally effective as intramuscular preparations, but also equally toxic.[89–91] The use of auranofin obviates the need for intramuscular injections, but not the need for careful follow-up and repeated urinalyses and blood cell counts. Since many older persons have difficulty getting to the physician's office frequently enough to ensure safe monitoring of these agents, courses of gold frequently prove impractical. In addition, the continued drawing of blood samples and the atmosphere of concern create an ambiance of invalidism, which is discouraging for the elderly person.

If an elderly patient does not respond favorably to the nonpharmacologic program, plus use of nonsteroidal antirheumatic agents and/or gold, serious consideration should be given to initiating a trial of low-dose corticosteroid therapy (prednisone 7 to 8 mg or, at the most, 10 mg per day).[92,93] Many patients experience considerable symptomatic relief with this dosage and several preliminary controlled trials have indicated that the rate of joint destruction by the rheumatoid process is lessened.[88] The frequency of corticosteroid-induced diabetes mellitus, inadequate wound healing, increased sensitivity to infection, hypertension, and corticoid psychosis does not appear to be greater in elderly persons than it is in the younger individual. These complications are rarely encountered with this dosage schedule.[93] Corticosteroid therapy in the elderly does bring the possibility of an increased likelihood of osteoporosis. For this reason, it is important to be sure that the patient receiving this treatment maintains a systematic program of exercise and has an adequate daily intake of calcium and vitamin D (see Chapter 39).

Penicillamine therapy is an approach that can, at least, be "kept up one's sleeve," but that is where the senior author of this chapter likes to keep it. If used, the drug should be given in a dosage of 125 mg per day for 1 month, followed by 250 mg daily for 3 months, 500 mg daily for 3 to 6 months, and then a maximum dose of 750 mg daily. A complete blood count and urinalysis must be carried out at intervals of 2 to 4 weeks, and the drug should be discontinued if significant changes are noted. Occasional patients will develop a myasthenia gravis–like syndrome, which is reversible if the penicillamine is discontinued. Other toxic effects may include rash, which may be severe, and marked abnormalities in taste. Both these effects are more severe in the elderly than in younger individuals. Because of the toxicity and questionable effectiveness of this agent, we rarely use it in elderly patients, although its use has been advocated by some.[94]

Methotrexate has begun to gain acceptance for use in patients with advanced rheumatoid arthritis resistant to other forms of therapy.[95] The value of this agent as an adjuvant to corticosteroid therapy in polymyositis has been amply demonstrated. Its ease of administration, rapid action, and patient acceptance have led to increased utilization in resistant cases of rheumatoid arthritis, despite the risk of serious toxic sequelae. The drug is particularly hazardous in patients who suffer from obesity, diabetes mellitus, alcohol abuse, and renal disease. It is also said to be hazardous in elderly patients, but this has not been shown clearly. The drug merits more intensive evaluation.

**Orthopedic Management**

Orthopedic management represents an essential part of the treatment of all patients with rheumatoid arthritis. In acute episodes of the disease, temporary splinting of the joints, particularly of the wrist-hand and knee, is helpful in relieving pain and swelling and preventing deformities. Long-term use of splints and braces for chronic joint problems is impractical, and patient compliance is very low. Exception to this is the use of an ankle-foot plastic brace. This brace is comfortable, cosmetically acceptable, and quite effective in reducing ankle pain.

Proper shoes are of paramount importance in relieving foot symptoms. If considerable deformities of the foot and toes have developed, then orthopedic surgical correction and proper supportive shoes give excellent relief for walking. This type of surgery is very reliable and safe, the complication rate being very low; it is the most common type of surgery performed in elderly patients with rheumatoid arthritis. Examples include bunionectomies, hammertoe correction, forefoot plasty, and talonavicular fusion.

Total joint replacements of the hips and knees are very helpful in keeping these patients ambulatory. Please see sections on arthritis of the knee (page 422) and arthritis of the hip (page 423). Arthroplasties of the wrist and fingers improve hand function for activities of daily living. Soft tissue procedures are performed for carpal tunnel syndrome and trigger fingers when nonsurgical methods of treatment fail. In cases of persistent inflammation of the extensor tendons at the wrist, surgery should be seriously considered to prevent tendon rupture because the results from ruptured tendon repair are not very predictable. When both the wrist and fingers are involved, it is generally advisable to operate on the wrist initially and later on the fingers; most of the time a combination of various procedures is needed to improve hand function.

**Psychologic Aspects**

Finally, in caring for patients of any age with rheumatoid arthritis, one must be mindful of the close interaction between emotional factors and the course and manifestations of the disease. The most effective form of treatment lies in careful, thoughtful utilization of all the modalities described previously, coupled with careful explanation to the patient and family of the nature and course of the disease and the goals and expectations from each mode of therapy.

For a more detailed review of recent developments in the pathogenesis and treatment of rheumatoid arthritis, the reader is referred to an excellent review by Decker and associates.[96] Additional information about sources of patient and family education is provided in Chapter 48.

## *Polymyalgia Rheumatica and Giant Cell Arteritis*

Two of the rheumatic diseases that have a unique predeliction for the elderly are polymyalgia rheumatica and giant cell arteritis (also known as temporal arteritis, cranial arteritis, and granulomatous arteritis). The frequent occurrence of both conditions in some individuals had led to the presumption that they constitute different expressions of a single disease.

### POLYMYALGIA RHEUMATICA

Polymyalgia is defined as diffuse muscular stiffness and aching affecting the neck, shoulders, back, and/or pelvic girdle, continuing for 1 month or more, usually accompanied by an elevation of the erythrocyte sedimentation rate, in the absence of other rheumatic disease, such as rheumatoid arthritis, chronic infection, polyarteritis, or malignancy.[97–99] There is as yet no diagnostic test, and the diagnosis is a clinical one; criteria for the diagnosis have recently been proposed,[99a] but are not yet widely accepted.

Rarely encountered in patients under 50 years of age, the disease occurs most frequently in persons 65 years of age and older, twice as often in women than in men. The disease shows a special predeliction for persons of northern European ancestry. Dixon and co-workers[97] have estimated that in patients aged 70 years and older, polymyalgia rheumatica and giant cell arteritis are about half as common as rheumatoid arthritis and that at any age the frequency of these diseases exceeds ankylosing spondylitis and is about equal to that of gout.

**Clinical Manifestations**

Polymyalgia rheumatica is initiated, frequently, by a viral-like illness, consisting of fever and weight loss, usually less than 2 weeks' duration. The patient then experiences, either gradually or acutely, the onset of widespread muscle pain on active motion, involving some or all of the following: neck, shoulders, back and, to a lesser extent, buttocks and thigh. The pain is usually symmetric in distribution but not in extent. It is accompanied by morning stiffness or "jelling," often of several hours' duration. Because of the pain and stiffness, the patient experiences the *sense* of weakness, such as feeling a difficulty in rising from a chair or rolling over in bed.

Constitutional symptoms remain prominent throughout the course of the illness. These include, in addition to the severe morning stiffness, low-grade fever, anorexia, weight loss, depression, and sometimes night sweats.

**Physical Examination**

Examination of the muscles indicates slight tenderness, less than one would expect in patients with a true myositis. There may also be some tenderness over the flexor surfaces of the elbows, wrists, and knees. The consistency of the muscles is normal. Atrophy is minimal or absent, and there is little or no objective evidence of weakness. Examination of the joints shows full range of motion. Synovial thickening or effusion may be present in the knees, shoulders, wrists, and sternoclavicular joints, usually of mild degree. Occasionally, synovial thickening will be evident in the proximal interphalangeal joints and metacarpophalangeal joints, but in these instances the involvement is transient. The joints do not exhibit deformities characteristic of rheumatoid arthritis, and rheumatoid nodules are not present.

**Laboratory Findings**

The erythrocyte sedimentation rate (ESR) is usually, but not always, higher than one would expect from age alone (i.e., in the range of 40 to 110 mm/1 hr Westergren). Total leukocyte and differential counts are normal. There may be moderate hypochromic anemia, with hemoglobin values ranging from 8.5 to 12.5 gm/dl. Assays for rheumatoid factor and antinuclear antibodies yield the same frequency of positive findings as a control elderly population. Serum concentration of creatinine, phosphokinase (CPK), aldolase, and aspartic aminotransferase are normal, as is urinary creatine excretion.

Serum alkaline phosphatase concentration is elevated in 29 per cent of cases, reflecting the presence of concomitant liver involvement. Electromyography of involved muscle is normal.

Radiographs of peripheral joints do not show the periarticular osteopenia nor erosive changes characteristic of rheumatoid arthritis. Technetium pertechnitate joint scan may show increased uptake in the shoulders, elbows, wrists, sternoclavicular joints, sacroiliac joints, and knees. Computed tomography scanning of the sternoclavicular joints and sacroiliac joints frequently shows erosive changes.

Histologic examination of the muscles does not reveal the cellular infiltration or muscle necrosis seen in dermatomyositis, nor the perivascular cellular infiltration often seen in rheumatoid arthritis. Occasionally, mild atrophy of type II muscles will be noted. Histologic examination of clinically involved peripheral joints discloses mild synovial tissue hyperplasia, mild inflammation of periarticular structures, and mixed cellular infiltrate of lymphocytes and plasma cells.

The pathogenesis of the disease is still unknown. The lack of objective evidence of muscle involvement, together with the recent finding of erosive changes in the sternoclavicular and sacroiliac joints, as evidenced by CT scan, has led some investigators to postulate that polymyalgia rheumatica is not primarily a disease of muscle but instead an inflammatory arthropathy of the "central" joints.[100a]

**Differential Diagnosis**

The differentiation between polymyalgia rheumatica and polymyositis is relatively easy. The differentiation between polymyalgia rheumatica and rheumatoid arthritis, however, may be more difficult. Indeed, a number of reports have pointed out that what had been thought to have been long-standing polymyalgia rheumatica ultimately developed or proved to be rheumatoid arthritis in some patients.[102,103]

Although there is no specific diagnostic test for polymyalgia rheumatica, one procedure has been described as being of diagnostic assistance—that is, a dramatic clinical response within a few days following the administration of *prednisone* or its equivalent in a dose of 10 to 30 mg/day, in a single daily dose. Patients with polymyalgia rheumatica will almost always exhibit marked clinical improvement with prednisone therapy in this dosage. Dixon recommends carrying out this procedure as a "single-blind diary monitored trial"—giving the patient, first, aspirin as a placebo, next the corticosteroid, and then returning to aspirin—and asking the patient to record the symptoms throughout.[103a] The symptomatic relief associated with administration of prednisone in this dosage, in patients with polymyalgia rheumatica, is much more dramatic in extent and prompt in its occurrence than is true for patients with rheumatoid arthritis or other rheumatic diseases; the symptoms recur immediately following discontinuation of prednisone therapy.

**Treatment**

Once the diagnosis of polymyalgia rheumatica has been made, therapy should be initiated either with prednisone or with a nonsteroidal inflammatory agent. The excellent response to prednisone, plus the fact that the disease is almost always self-limited, has caused us to favor prednisone therapy. In patients in whom concomitant diagnosis of giant cell arteritis is *not* being entertained (to be discussed), a starting dose of 15 mg daily is sufficient. Assuming that a good clinical response is obtained, the medication should be continued for 2 or 3 months, then tapered very gradually to a dose of 5 to 7.5 mg daily, and maintained at this level for many months. Careful monitoring of clinical manifestations provides the best guide to the rate with which corticosteroid therapy may be "tapered off." Serial determinations of the ESR are less valuable, because in some patients it will remain elevated, even in the presence of significant improvement. The disease is usually self-limited, lasting for approximately 1 to 2 years, and corticosteroid therapy should be continued for this interval.

If a favorable clinical response is not obtained with prednisone 15 mg daily, or if there is a symptomatic relapse, despite continued corticosteroid therapy, one must suspect an alternative diagnosis such as a malignancy or the concomitant presence of giant cell arteritis. A clinical "decision tree," guiding the management of polymyalgia rheumatica, with specific reference to the possibility of concomitant giant cell arteritis, has been proposed by Chang and Fineberg.[103b]

## Giant Cell Arteritis

Giant cell arteritis provides one of the most important mandates for correct diagnosis and treatment of all of the rheumatic diseases. Rarely encountered in whites under age 50 and in blacks at any age, giant cell arteritis exhibits an increasing frequency and prevalence with advancing age.[104-105] The prevalence has been estimated as 0.8 per cent for persons age 80 and older.[106] The disease occurs twice as frequently in females than in males. Increased frequency in certain family clusters has been reported.[107,108]

**Clinical Manifestations**

The onset of the disease, occasionally abrupt, is more frequently insidious, accompanied by fever, malaise, fatigue, anorexia, and weight loss.[99,105,109–114] The fever is usually low grade, but may be more prominent. Headache, characteristically located in the temporal region, is present in approximately 60 per cent of cases. The headache, which may be constant or intermittent, is usually described as "boring" or "shooting" in nature. The patients may complain of some tenderness over the temporal artery itself. This tenderness, and the headache, may be exacerbated by the pressure of a hat or pillow.

Between 25 and 50 per cent of patients experience visual disturbances, often starting in one eye and progressing to the other within a few days or weeks.[115] Initially, these symptoms consist of transient blurring or diplopia. The patient may also experience central scotomas, peripheral field constriction, sector cuts, and blindness, sometimes abrupt in onset. These are a prelude to the total and irreversible blindness that will frequently ensue if the disease is not treated. This is due to ischemia of the optic nerve or, occasionally, occipital infarction. The patient may also evidence ptosis and ophthalmoplegia caused by involvement of the artery supplying the ocular muscles or cranial nerves. Arteritis may also occur in the vertebral, ophthalmic, and posterior ciliary arteries or, occasionally, the carotid, coronary, mesenteric, iliac, femoral and subclavian arteries.[116,117] Ischemia or infarction may ensue in the respective areas of distribution. Aneurysms and/or dissection of the aorta have been recorded.[118] Involvement of intracranial arteries is rare.

Between one half and two thirds of patients with giant cell arteritis experience intermittent claudication of the muscles of mastication. This symptom, caused by involvement of the facial artery, is pathognomonic for this disease. It must be differentiated from the pain of temporomandibular joint disease and from acute dental abscess. Occasionally, the patient may experience claudication of the tongue or swallowing muscles, resulting in dysphagia; claudication of the limbs, abdominal pain, vertigo, and angina pectoris may also occur. The patient may feel depressed, apathetic, and confused. These symptoms are thought to reflect systemic illness rather than intracranial involvement.

**Physical Examination**

Tenderness and swelling of the temporal arteries may or may not be detectable. Rarely the temporal arteries are nodular in character. The presence of diplopia, accompanied by ptosis, is an ominous sign; between 50 and 60 per cent of patients with these manifestations become blind. A careful field examination should be carried out to identify possible scotomas, constriction, or field defects. Funduscopic examination may be normal, however, even during the first 24 to 48 hours after occlusion of the retinal artery. Following this, if retinal artery occlusion has occurred, the retina appears pale and the arteries constricted. The finding of bruits over large peripheral arteries or absence of pulsation in one or several of these arteries provides additional clues to the presence of this disease.

**Laboratory Findings.**

***Pathology.*** By far, the most important laboratory finding is the determination of typical pathologic changes on biopsy. These consist of diffuse mononuclear cell infiltration, throughout the vascular wall, with fragmentation and interruption of the internal elastic lamina. Giant cells are usually found, but their presence is not necessary for diagnosis and is not correlated with the severity or course of the disease. The intima is, characteristically, thickened and frequently thrombosed. These changes are similar to those of Takayasu's arteriopathy ("pulseless disease"), a form of arteritis occurring predominantly in women during the second and third decade, in which the arteritis is confined, primarily, to the arch of the aorta and its branches.[119]

Unfortunately, the clinician who seeks to validate a diagnosis of giant cell arteritis by histologic proof, prior to initiation of therapy, faces several serious problems. One of these is that once the patient begins to exhibit the initial clinical manifestations of this condition, irreversible blindness may ensue at any time and without warning. To delay initiation of therapy while a biopsy is being obtained and interpreted subjects the patient to the hazard of blindness in the meantime, a hazard that would be obviated, almost entirely, by initiation of treatment. The second problem is that the histologic changes may be confined to an isolated segment of an artery.[120] Despite obtaining several biopsies over the course of 4 or 5 cm of artery, there is a considerable likelihood that even in the presence of giant cell arteritis, the biopsy specimens will be negative.

***Other Laboratory Findings.*** These are of interest, in terms of an appreciation of the nature and extent of the disease, but are not of assistance diagnostically, with the possible exception of the ESR. As with patients with polymyalgia rheumatica, an elevated ESR usually accompanies giant cell arteritis. This is not invariably true, however; occasionally patients with biopsy-proven giant cell arteritis have been described in whom the ESR was normal prior to initiation of corticosteroid treatment.

The tests that are of some interest, in terms of pathogenesis, include the presence of immunoglobulin and complement deposits in some involved temporal arteries and identification of increased circulating immune complexes, correlated with disease activity, by means of the Ragji cell immunoassay. It has been suggested that giant cell arteritis develops as the result of cell-mediated granulomatous reaction directed at structures in or near the elastic lamellae in the arterial wall.[121,122]

A particularly disturbing aspect of giant cell arteritis, from the point of view of the clinician, is the important but ill-defined relationship of this entity and polymyalgia rheumatica.[111] A number of investigators have performed routine biopsies of the temporal artery in all members of a series of patients with polymyalgia rheumatica. These studies have shown histologic changes of giant cell arteritis in 20 to 80 per cent of cases of polymyalgia,[111,122] whether or not accompanied by clinical clues suggestive of the presence of arteritis. The true incidence of arteritis in patients with polymyalgia rheumatica must be considerable. This fact provides added urgency, first, to the need to develop improved criteria for the diagnosis of polymyalgia rheumatica and, second, for identification of those patients who also have arteritis.

**Treatment**

Once the presence of giant cell arteritis is suspected, clinically, a regimen should be started, immediately, of prednisone in a dosage of 60 to 100 mg/day. An alternate days-of-dosage schedule is not effective. Biopsy may be carried out after initiation of corticosteroid treatment. The findings will not be altered, substantially, if the biopsy is conducted within a few days. Clinical improvement and a fall in the ESR occur within a few days of initiation of corticosteroid therapy in adequate dosage. The dose should be tapered, gradually, over the ensuing 8 to 12 weeks to a level of approximately 20 mg/day, with further gradual reduction thereafter. Symptoms should be followed closely. If an exacerbation ensues, dosage of corticosteroids should be returned to a level that results in symptomatic relief. Corticosteroid therapy must be continued for at least 2 years.[123]

Additional readings are cited in the bibliography.[124–126]

## *Antinuclear Antibodies*

Tremendous strides have been made in the last few years in the identification of specific patterns of antinuclear antibodies and in the association of these patterns with subsets of the clinically recognized "connective tissue diseases."[85] A list of the nuclear or cytoplasmic antigens to which antibodies have been demonstrated, to date, is cited in Table 36–7. The terms Sm, Ro, La, Ma, Ha, Mi, $Mi_2$, Jo, and Ku refer to the first two initials of the patients in whom these antigens were first identified. SSA and SSB refer to the antigens identified in two subsets of Sjögren's syndrome; PM to an antigen identified in patients with one subset of polymyositis; PM-Scl to patients with a combination of polymyositis and scleroderma; and Scl-O to patients with systemic sclerosis (scleroderma).

From the clinical point of view, application of these immunologic approaches to individual patients has led to significant advances. It is apparent that merely because patients resemble each other clinically does not mean that they are suffering from the same disease. Recognition that a patient may have one or another subset of a given disease state may have major implications as regards course and prognosis. For example, although patients with systemic lupus erythematosis (SLE) may resemble each other clinically, in many respects patients with anti-Ro/SSA have a higher incidence of renal involvement, whereas patients who *also* have

**Table 36–7.** ANTIBODIES TO NUCLEAR OR CYTOPLASMIC ANTIGENS (ANA AND ACA)

| |
|---|
| Anti-DNA-histone |
| Anti-DNA |
| Anti-single-stranded (ss) DNA (denatured) |
| Anti-double-stranded (ds) DNA (native) |
| Anti-histone |
| Anti-nRNP* |
| Anti-Sm* |
| Anti-Ro/SSA* |
| Anti-La/SSB/Ha* |
| Anti-RNA, Poly IC, Poly GC, Poly ADP, Poly A. |
| Anti-Ma |
| Anti-PM-Scl, $PM_1$ |
| Anti-$Mi_1$, $Mi_2$ |
| Anti-Ku |
| Anti-$Jo_1$, $Jo_2$ |
| Anti-$Scl_{70}$ |
| Anti-centromere |
| Anti-nucleosome (cross-reactive with Fc of human IgG) |

*All shown to be RNA-protein conjugates.

*Source:* Reichlin M: Antinuclear antibodies. In Kelley WN, et al (eds.): Textbook of Rheumatology, 2nd ed. Philadelphia, W.B. Saunders Co., 1985, p. 691.

anti-La/SSB rarely develop renal disease. Patients with so-called mixed connective tissue disease who exhibit overlapping clinical features of SLE, scleroderma, and polymyositis all possess antibodies to nuclear ribonucleoprotein (nRNP) in their serum, rarely exhibit renal involvement, and have a relatively benign course. In patients with scleroderma, the presence of the anticentromere antibody has a high specificity for the CREST syndrome, consisting of calcification, Raynaud's phenomenon, esophageal involvement, sclerodactylia, and telangiectasis, and it identifies patients with less severe disease.[127] Almost all patients with polymyositis exhibit some antinuclear antibody, but there is a marked degree of heterogeneity. Several of these antinuclear antibody patterns have been associated with specific histocompatibility loci. The implications of these findings for the elderly have not yet been worked out fully. However, it seems clear that genetic make-up has an important bearing not only on the incidence of these diseases but also on the course of these diseases and, by inference, on the likelihood that patients with these diseases will survive into old age.

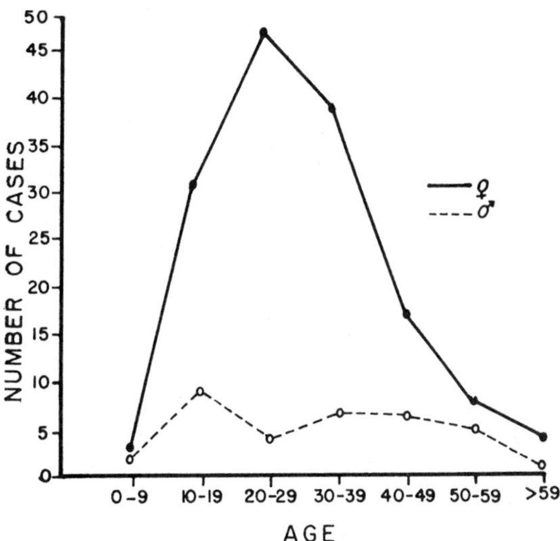


**Figure 36–8.** Age of onset of systemic lupus erythematosus. (From Maddock RK: Incidence of systemic lupus erythematosus by age and sex. JAMA 191:149, 1965. Reproduced with permission.)

## *Disseminated Lupus Erythematosus*

The importance of considering disseminated lupus erythematosus in the geriatric population stems from two facts: First, although the frequency of the disease as an idiopathic or spontaneously occurring entity is much less in the elderly than in the young (Fig. 36–8),[127] it does occur and should be thought of in the differential diagnosis of patients with multisystem involvement and severe constitutional symptoms. Second, with the increasing population of elderly and the numerous drugs many elderly persons are consuming, drug-induced SLE is emerging as an increasingly significant entity and a focus for research, which may have implications for "idiopathic" SLE and for the relationship of genetics to autoimmune disease. (Drug-induced SLE is described in the next subsection.)

The clinical picture of SLE in the elderly has been described in several good clinical studies.[128–134] The number of patients constituting each of these series is quite small, however, ranging from 5 to 31. Not surprisingly, the clinical picture differs in many respects in each of these reports. Only one of these reports[126] addresses the question: Was the onset insidious or acute? In this series, the onset was insidious in all patients. There was general agreement that constitutional manifestations are conspicuous. In one study, the fever and weight loss were frequently of such magnitude as to appear life threatening and suggested the presence of infection or malignancy.[134] Several reports indicate that pleuritis and pericarditis are more conspicuous manifestations of SLE in the elderly than in the young (Table 36–8).[127] In two series[128,134] these changes emerged as the most conspicuous presenting manifestations. Raynaud's phenomenon, lymphadenopathy, and, in most series, arthritis and skin lesions were less frequent in the elderly than in the young. Renal involvement, although less frequent than in younger persons with this disease, is still present in 20 to 50 per cent of elderly patients.[132,134] All authors agree that the prognosis of SLE in the elderly is somewhat more favorable than in the young and that suppression of clinical manifestations can be achieved with a smaller dosage level of anti-inflammatory agents or glucocorticoids than is required for younger patients with this disorder.

## *Drug-Induced Lupus Erythematosus*

Drug-induced SLE has been recognized for the past 30 years. The number of drugs that have been implicated is long.[135] On the other hand, clear-cut association between the drug and the

**Table 36–8.** CLINICAL AND LABORATORY MANIFESTATIONS OF SYSTEMIC LUPUS ERYTHEMATOSUS IN OLDER (AGE 51 AND OLDER) AND YOUNGER (AGE 50 AND UNDER) AGE GROUPS*

| | Younger | Older |
|---|---|---|
| No. of patients | 218 | 16 |
| Mean age (years) | 27 | 60 |
| Average duration of symptoms prior to diagnosis (years) | 1.75 | 1.25 |
| Manifestations (%) | | |
| Malar rash | 61% | 69% |
| Discoid lupus | 21 | 50 |
| Photosensitivity | 13 | 25 |
| Raynaud's phenomena | 44 | 19 |
| Cutaneous vasculitis | 20 | 0 |
| Arthritis or arthralgia | 95 | 94 |
| Pulmonary fibrosis | 5 | 12 |
| Central nervous system involvement | 48 | 19 |
| LE Cells | 61 | 44 |
| Leukopenia | 24 | 13 |
| Thrombocytopenia | 14 | 0 |
| Hemolytic anemia | 17 | 0 |
| Profuse proteinuria (>3.5 gm/24 hr) | 10% | 0% |

* Adapted with permission from Dimant J, et al: Systemic lupus erythematosus in the older age group: Computer analysis. J Am Geriatr Soc 27:58, 1979.

immune disease has been proved for only a small number of agents, notably hydralazine, isoniazid, and procainamide. For the other agents, a question remains: Was the clinical disease truly created by the administration of the drug, or was it an instance of idiopathic SLE that was exacerbated by administration of the drug or by a condition for which the drug was given?[135] As a result, in part, of this uncertainty, little information is available concerning the frequency of drug-induced SLE. For procainamide-induced disease, the mean age is 62 years; for hydralazine, 50.3 years.[136] The preponderance of women is smaller than that for idiopathic SLE.

Clinically, drug-induced SLE resembles idiopathic SLE in the presence of polyarthralgia and arthritis, pleuritis and pericarditis, and positive antinuclear antibody test; there is, however, a notable lack of renal and central nervous system involvement. Antibodies to native DNA are not present. Antibodies to the soluble antigens, nuclear RNP, Sm, Ro and La, typical of idiopathic SLE, are rarely seen. Serum complement values usually are normal.

Antinuclear antibodies develop in 50 to 75 per cent of patients taking procainamide or hydralazine in sufficient doses over 9 to 12 months. Between 20 and 50 per cent of these develop the lupus syndrome.[136] This syndrome may occur as early as 1 month or as late as 5 years following onset of hydralazine therapy. At the time of onset of the lupus syndrome, the hypertension is usually under good control. The lupus syndrome almost always subsides following discontinuation of the drug.

In regard to the pathophysiologic mechanisms, it has recently been shown that the likelihood for the development of the lupus syndrome, following administration of hydralazine, isoniazid, and procainamide depends to a striking extent on whether or not the recipient has the enzymatic mechanism to acetylate these drugs rapidly. The enzyme N acetyl transferase, located in the liver, is genetically controlled. Approximately half of North American and European populations possess the enzyme in sufficient quantity to acetylate, rapidly, drugs that are catabolized in this fashion. The capability of the non-acetylated drug (hydralazine, isoniazid, or procainamide) to stimulate the development of antinuclear antibodies in the recipient is so great that within approximately 6 months all "slow acetylaters" will exhibit circulating antibodies, whereas for the rapid acetylaters 6 years or more of continuous therapy are required. There is also an association between the dose of the lupus-inducing agent and the likelihood that the lupus syndrome will ensue. It has recently been shown that hydralazine-induced lupus patients exhibit an increased frequency of HLA-DR w 4, whereas in idiopathic lupus there is an increased frequency of HLA-DR w 2 and DR w 3. The mechanism by which the non-acetylated drugs hydralazine, isoniazid, and procainamide induce antinuclear antibodies and SLE is not fully understood.

It has recently been shown that many patients with idiopathic SLE also show a defect in the ability to acetylate isoniazid.[137] The ratio of slow acetylaters to rapid in the normal population is 122/105. In a population of patients with idiopathic SLE, the ratio is 150/77. These data have suggested to Reidenberg,[137] who has done much of this work, that some cases of idiopathic lupus may be induced by exposure to chemicals. Hydralazines are present naturally in tobacco smoke and compounds used in agriculture and medicine. The increased incidence of lupus erythematosus in the population of industrialized countries may represent not merely increased recognition but an important environmental problem.[137]

## *Scleroderma*

The term scleroderma is frequently applied to two apparently distinct entities.[138] In one, morphea, the fibrotic changes are confined to the skin, sometimes in localized patches, but in other instances following a more generalized pattern. Since this form of scleroderma does not involve parenchymal organs, the prognosis is good. *Progressive systemic sclerosis* refers to a systemic disease characterized by microvascular abnormalities; collagen deposition in various organs; Raynaud's phenomenon; esophageal dysfunction; sclerotic skin; and, in many instances, pulmonary, cardiac, and renal involvement.[139] Renal involvement is particularly devastating because of the severe hypertension that frequently accompanies it.[140]

In the series of cases studied by Medsger and Masi[141] the age at first diagnosis ranged from between 11 and 83 years, with a median age of 47 years. Females predominated over males in a ratio of approximately 3 to 1. The relationship of scleroderma to the various antinuclear antibody patterns is referred to earlier.[142–144]

The importance of scleroderma in the elderly relates in part to the fact that it *does* occur and, when it does, often results in a serious management problem for physician and patient. In part, it demands attention because the changes of scleroderma resemble, superficially at least, those of aging.[142] Thus, the diagnosis is undoubtedly missed in many elderly patients. Although some authors suggest that scleroderma in the elderly is a more benign condition than in younger persons, others point out that this may reflect the fact that many older persons do not live long enough to experience the full range of manifestations of the disease.[143] There is no clear evidence that scleroderma in the elderly is different from that in younger age groups.

#### Treatment

Management is largely symptomatic. Early use of antibiotics for minor infections of the fingertips may prevent more serious infection. Vasodilator and sympatholytic agents such as guanethidine or reserpine may be helpful symptomatically but must be used with caution in the elderly.[140] The use of angiotensin-converting enzyme blockade (captopril) may be beneficial.[140] Adrenal corticosteroid therapy is not recommended in the belief (not totally proved) that its use will increase the incidence of malignant hypertension. The use of metallic gloves, which are lightweight yet marvelously warming, provides comfort. Penicillamine is sometimes recommended but brings with it the hazard of renal toxicity and its effectiveness is debatable. Hypertension accompanying scleroderma can usually be controlled by the newer antihypertensive agents, such as captopril or nifedipine.

### *Polymyositis and Dermatomyositis*

Polymyositis is an inflammatory myopathy characterized by symmetric weakness, most conspicuous in proximal muscles; tenderness and pain on motion of involved muscle; elevation in serum concentration of sarcoplasmic enzymes; characteristic electromyographic changes; and pathologic findings of lymphocytic inflammation, necrosis of muscle fibers, and regeneration. The condition is known as polymyositis if only skeletal muscles are involved and as dermatomyositis if both muscles and skin are involved.

Although polymyositis may affect persons of any age, the peak incidence is bimodal, with peaks occurring at adolescence and again in later life, in those aged 45 to 54 or 60 to 70, according to different reports.[138,139] In the United States, only 8 per cent of cases occur in persons age 65 and older.[138] Females predominate among patients age 60 or less; above this, the frequency is equal in both sexes. These differences have suggested to some investigators that the polymyositis syndrome may include two separate disease states.

Polymyositis may be accompanied by clinical evidence of other collagen vascular diseases, especially scleroderma, systemic lupus erythematosus, and rheumatoid arthritis. In this case the term overlap syndrome may be applied.[148] In approximately 10 per cent of cases myositis is associated with the development of a visceral malignancy.[149–151] Although either myositis or malignancy may become evident first, both features of the syndrome are usually diagnosed within 1 year of each other.

On physical examination, the condition is characterized by symmetric weakness, primarily of the proximal muscles, accompanied by muscle pain and tenderness. Laboratory workup shows elevation of serum enzymes, especially creatine phosphokinase (CPK) activity. Electromyography shows spontaneous activity and myopathic changes.

Muscle biopsy should be performed to prove the diagnosis. A clamp should be inserted on the muscle in situ, and the muscle should remain within the clamp during surgical removal and subsequent fixation to avoid artifacts. The biopsy will show perivascular and interstitial inflammation; infiltration with lymphocytes; and, occasionally, plasma cells and muscle fiber ne-

**Table 36–9.** CLINICAL AND HISTOLOGIC DIFFERENTIATION OF COMMON MUSCLE DISEASES IN THE ELDERLY

| | Rheumatoid Arthritis | Polymyalgia Rheumatica | Polymyositis | Steroid Myopathy |
|---|---|---|---|---|
| ***Clinical*** | | | | |
| Muscle tenderness | + | – | + to +++ | – |
| Pain on motion | Joints | ++ | 0 to ± | – |
| Generalized weakness | ++ | ++ | ++ to +++ | + |
| Weakness of specific muscle groups | ± to ++ | – | +++ | ++* |
| Muscle enzymes | – | – | +++ | – |
| EMG:† Myositis | – | – | ++ | – |
| Objective evidence of arthritis | + to ++ | ± | ± | – |
| ***Histologic*** | | | | |
| Inflammation | + | ± | ++ | – |
| Muscle necrosis | – | – | ++ | – |
| Atrophy | + | + | – | + |
| Type of fiber involved | II | II | I + II | II |

* Proximal myopathy is classic.
† EMG = electromyogram.

crosis and regeneration. When muscles are characterized histochemically, both type I (oxidative) and type II (glycolytic) are involved.[152,153]

Differential diagnosis includes polymyalgia rheumatica, adult-onset rheumatoid arthritis, and metabolic myopathies (Table 36–9). All three of these syndromes are characterized by symmetric involvement of the shoulders, upper arms, thighs, and hip girdle and by a general sense of weakness. The therapeutic implications of these diagnoses are quite different. If the patient has rheumatoid arthritis, objective evidence of synovial involvement of the shoulder joints and, usually, peripheral joints will begin to appear over the course of several (2 to 6) months. In both rheumatoid arthritis and polymyalgia rheumatica, serum concentration of muscle enzymes will be in a near-normal range and electromyographic studies will show nonspecific findings. Metabolic polymyopathy is most often due either to endogenous or exogenous hypercorticism or to hyperthyroidism. The weakness in this condition is manifested most commonly in the hip girdle. Marked atrophy of the quadriceps is often seen. In thyrotoxic myopathy there is proximal muscle weakness and loss of muscle bulk. The reflexes are brisk. Appropriate laboratory tests will help differentiate these entities.

Cachexia of malignancy, with or without actual myositis, may also simulate polymyositis. Other entities that should be considered in the differential diagnosis include myasthenia gravis; amyotrophic lateral sclerosis; toxic myopathies due to ethanol and certain drugs (penicillamine and clofibrate); proximal neuropathy such as the Guillain-Barré syndrome; and lower limb plexopathies due to diabetes mellitus.

#### Treatment

The treatment of polymyositis in the elderly is similar to that in younger persons. Initial therapy with corticosteroids usually requires a dose of 60 to 80 mg prednisone per day or its equivalent. Clinical response is paralleled by a sharp fall in muscle enzymes, notably CPK. Corticosteroid dosage should be reduced gradually over the course of weeks and months, utilizing serial estimations of CPK as a guide. Therapy is usually continued for at least 2 years.[148] Because of the threat of bleeding or perforation of a duodenal ulcer, which, especially in the elderly, may not be associated with characteristic symptoms, the prednisone should be accompanied by antacid therapy and prophylactic use of cimetidine should be given serious consideration. If prednisone therapy leads to toxic effects or is contraindicated by serious peptic ulcer disease, cytotoxic drugs may be added, thus permitting reduction in the corticosteroid dosage.[154,155]

If the dermatomyositis is accompanied by onset of malignancy, removal or definitive treatment of the malignancy is occasionally followed by improvement in the myositis, but this is not always the case.

## COMMON SYMPTOM COMPLEXES—A PROBLEM-ORIENTED APPROACH

### *Problem 1: Backache*

Pain in the low back is a common and troublesome problem, especially for older people.

Common diagnostic possibilities in elderly persons include the following: osteoarthritis; osteoporosis with compression fractures; herniated intervertebral disc; metastatic malignancy; multiple myeloma; osteomalacia; Paget's disease; "low back strain"; "sacroiliac strain"; and psychosomatic problems, especially depression. In addition, back pain may be referred from an internal organ, such as the kidney, pancreas, and aorta. Carcinoma of the pancreas or dissecting aneurysm of the aorta may yield symptoms suggestive of disease of the spine, even though the spine itself may be uninvolved.

### HISTORY

The history should start with the earliest onset of symptoms. Postural defects that may have congenital origin (such as dysplasia of the hips and scoliosis) will predispose to degenerative changes in later life and increase the likelihood that the back pain is related thereto. Rheumatoid spondylitis developed in a young adult will often result in advanced age in a rigid, deformed spine. The presence of osteoporosis can be suspected in women patients if they are postmenopausal and have not had replacement estrogen therapy, especially if they have not received appropriate calcium intake (see Chapter 39). A history of loss of height, often 2 in. or more, provides added support to the likelihood of severe osteoporosis. Sudden onset of severe low back pain after a sudden but perhaps minor "jolt," such as stepping off a curb, suggests that the patient may have sustained a compression fracture. Symptoms suggestive of malignancy in any organ should be investigated. It should be noted that carcinoma of the prostate is often not accompanied by a history of dysfunction of the urinary tract.

Back pain of any cause is usually intermittent; the precise time sequence may provide clues to diagnosis (Table 36 – 10). The pain accompanying osteoarthritis, compression fracture, or severe osteoporosis (in which the pain usually stems from small fractures) usually becomes more severe late in the day and after standing or sitting in one position for a period of an hour or so. Pain and stiffness on arising in the morning is commonly encountered in osteoarthritis of the spine. It usually subsides or substantially decreases within 5 to 10 minutes. Morning stiffness, extending to mid-day or later, is more characteristic of anklyosing spondylitis or rheumatoid arthritis. Occasionally, persons with osteoarthritis of the spine or functional disorders, such as low back strain, will complain of pain at night, frequently after lying in one position for several hours, especially if the mattress is extremely soft. Very severe "boring" back pain at night is suggestive of malignant disease or Paget's disease but may also be exhibited by patients with incipient dissection of the aorta. Pain on sneezing or straining at stool, a classic symptom of herniated intervertebral disc, may also be exhibited by patients with other conditions, such as epidural tumor or abscess.

The physician in obtaining a history of a patient with back pain should carefully record precisely where the pain focuses and where it radiates. Obviously, pain focused in the region of the sacroiliac joint carries different implications from pain focused in one or more sacral vertebrae.

Finally, the history should include sympathetic inquiry into the patient's life situation and psychologic stresses. These stresses alone constitute the most common mechanism of low back pain; in addition, these factors may play an important role in exacerbating symptoms that also have an organic basis.

### PHYSICAL EXAMINATION

Careful inspection should focus on any asymmetry of alignment or muscular development both in the standing position and as the patient touches fingers to the floor. Inspection from the lateral view should note any abrupt angulation of the spine (suggestive of fracture) and limitation of flexion. Measurement of the degree of "lengthening" of the distance between spinous processes in the dorsal region and lumbosacral region will document limitation in anterior flexion. The "lengthening" in a normal young or middle-aged patient should be at least 2.5 in. in the dorsal region and 2 in. in the lumbosacral area. Loss of flexion may reflect any of the organic processes of the spine cited earlier.

Range of motion of the neck should be assessed carefully. Lesions of the lumbar or dorsal spine, such as fracture, malignancy, or disc disease, do not as a rule lead to limitation of motion of the neck; an exception is rheumatoid spondylitis, in which the neck is characteristically involved. Possible tenderness of each vertebral process should be assessed by firm pressure and/or gentle "pounding" over each process. "Pounding" on the top of the head while the patient is in a sitting position (protecting the skull with one's other hand) may occasionally elicit tenderness in one localized area of the spine, suggestive of an inflammatory or malignant process. A vigorous, sudden squeezing motion of the rib cage may elicit pain in the ribs,

Table 36–10. DIFFERENTIAL DIAGNOSIS OF SOME CAUSES OF BACK PAIN

| | Rheumatoid Arthritis | Osteoporosis (Compression Fracture) | Multiple Myeloma | Osteoarthritis | Paget's Disease | Metastatic Cancer of Prostate |
|---|---|---|---|---|---|---|
| ***Predominant site*** | cervical | D10–L2 | any | any | any* | lumbar |
| ***Time*** | mornings | late day | usually late day | on arising, late day, or night | any | night++ |
| ***Tenderness*** | + | ++ | +++ | ± | + | ± |
| ***Radiating pain*** | ± | no | ± | yes | no | usually no |
| ***X-ray*** | subluxation may be seen | anterior wedging | diffuse or localized osteopenia | spurs | osteoblastic or clastic | some |
| ***CAT scan*** | + | + (if fracture) | no | + (spurs) | +++ | ++ |
| ***Special studies*** | sedimentation rate | NAA*† | serum electrophoresis | | alkaline phosphatase‡ | acid phosphatase |

* Predominant symptomatic sites are long bones, pelvis, and spine.
† NAA = neutron activation analysis.
‡ Also increased urinary hydroxyproline excretion.
*Key:* ± = Equivocally characteristic; + = slightly characteristic; ++ = moderately characteristic; +++ = highly characteristic.

suggestive of the presence of multiple myeloma or metastatic malignancy.

Hips should be examined carefully for rotation, abduction, adduction, and flexion. A deformity or limitation of motion of one or both hips, especially if long-standing, may place an added burden on the spine, leading to back symptoms. This is also true for deformities of the knees or feet. The presence of skeletal deformity in these areas does not, in itself, prove that the back pain is related thereto; a patient may also have, coincidentally, a malignancy or other disease of the spine.

A careful neurologic examination should be performed. The possibility of cord impingement should be borne in mind in all patients with a relatively recent onset of pain in the back. Detection of this condition constitutes a real medical crisis, since failure to correctly identify the problem and institute surgery may result in permanent paraplegia. The search for these important neurologic clues should be conducted even in patients who have other obvious explanations for their back symptoms. Demonstration of absence of "pin prick" sensation or hyperactive deep tendon reflexes provides important clues to the possible presence of serious impingement on the integrity of the spinal column and/or nerve routes. Special attention should be given to eliciting "pin prick" sensation in the perianal region, which may be absent in patients with caudal tumor or other lesions. The abdomen should be percussed to detect the possible presence of a distended bladder; if present, this provides an important additional clue to serious impingement on the cord. The Babinski reaction will not be positive, unless the cord damage is at a high level or there is concomitant disease of the central nervous system.

### Laboratory Examination and Procedures

The first step in dealing with a patient with back pain must be to identify the rare but important instance in which the symptoms reflect potentially serious cord impingement. If this is suspected clinically, immediate performance of appropriate x-rays, followed by a computed axial tomography scan, utilizing the water soluble Amipaque (metrizamide) dye, is indicated. This material is a readily resorbable version of the opaque material (Pantopaque), which used to be employed in myelography. Injection of this material into the intrathecal space, followed by a CT scan, provides, with little morbidity, a finely detailed perspective of the spinal canal, and it has become *the* definitive tool for identifying the presence and extent of the various lesions that cause cord compression.

Unless one's hand is forced by the possibility of an urgent complication of this sort, a more systematic work-up should be undertaken. This should include a complete blood count and determination of erythrocyte sedimentation rate; serum total protein; electrophoretic pattern; and serium calcium, phosphorus, alkaline, and, in men, acid phosphatase levels. Careful anteroposterior, lateral, and, in special situations, spot x-rays of that segment of the spine that appears diseased or injured according to the symptoms should be carried out. There is, however, very little correlation between the extent of degenerative changes, as indicated by osteophytic spurs and erosions, and the extent of symptoms. Many individuals who exhibit x-ray evidence of extensive degeneration of the spine experience, at most, brief, intermittent episodes of backache and are able to continue vigorous active lives, including heavy manual labor, without symptoms. Conversely, other patients with severe back symptoms, which, after considering all other possibilities, appear to be due to degenerative changes in the spine, will exhibit few if any abnormalities by x-ray.

X-ray of the hips, sacroiliac joints, and other bones (so-called bone survey) may be indicated if clinical data point to disease in the hips or pelvis or to more widespread disease such as multiple myeloma, Paget's disease, or metastatic malignancy. Bone scan is helpful in lesions such as Paget's disease, osteoblastic malignancy, or osteomyelitis. By these means, coupled with good clinical work-up, one can almost always differentiate patients with significant organic illness from those with low back strain or with psychosomatic disorders.

### Differential Diagnosis

Differentiation of certain entities, such as degenerative joint disease, metastatic malignancy, and Paget's disease, requires careful integration of all clinical and laboratory data. This is especially true because occasionally a patient will simultaneously have several disorders of the vertebral column, such as senile osteoporosis with perhaps compression fracture, osteoarthritis, plus possible metastatic malignancy, multiple myeloma, and/or Paget's disease. For example, a hypertrophic spur secondary to osteoarthritis may exhibit a positive image on the bone scan, closely resembling metastatic malignancy. It may be necessary to repeat studies and follow the clinical course of a patient for several months before the diagnosis becomes entirely clear. This approach is preferable in most instances to proceeding with more invasive diagnostic procedures, such as bone biopsy, so long as the situation is explained clearly to the patient and family.

### Treatment of Osteoarthritis of the Spine

The most common cause of back pain, other than psychologic stress, is osteoarthritis. Important points to keep in mind in the management of this condition are outlined on pages 392 to 397.

Back exercises are the most important single therapeutic modality (see page 394). The personal physician should assume responsibility either for prescribing these exercises or for monitoring them in a fashion that will indicate to the patient the importance of this form of therapy. A program of back exercises developed by the American Orthopedic Association is available on request (see Chapter 48). Few elderly patients will be able to undertake this full program at the outset. The leg raising and lowering exercise can usually be initiated at the start (two or three times, three sessions each day). Rising to a sitting position may be more attainable at the outset if the patient "starts" from an angle of 40 degrees or so through use of pillows or a slanting board. As the patient gradually builds up strength and confidence, it is helpful to institute a more recreational form of exercise. Use of a rowing machine is ideal. Both the resistance and duration can be increased gradually.

Through psychologic and other mechanisms, exercise permits many patients to maintain comfort with a decreased dosage of antirheumatic agents or none at all.

## *Problem 2: Chronic Neck Pain*

Chronic neck pain, although not as frequent as back pain, is one of the most common and most troublesome concomitants of aging. By far the most frequent cause is cervical spondylosis, i.e., osteoarthritis of the intervertebral joint spaces, with irritation of or compression on the cervical nerve roots. This is frequently exacerbated by emotional factors and trauma. As is the case of osteoarthritis of the lumbodorsal spine, there is no consistent association between the extent of radiographic findings and the severity of clinical symptoms or objective findings. Since this process may involve sympathetic nerves and vertebral arteries and their branches, the clinical manifestations may be widespread, including pain and loss of motion in the neck; numbness, tingling, and weakness in the shoulders and upper extremities; and central nervous system manifestations. In many older persons, the neck becomes thrust forward due, primarily, to kyphosis in the upper dorsal area secondary to osteoporosis. This may or may not be accompanied by limitation of motion of the neck and other symptoms referred to previously.

Other individuals with cervical spondylosis will exhibit limitation in rotation, lateral bending, and, to a lesser extent, anterior flexion. The limitation in motion is due, primarily, to muscle spasm, and spasm of the cervical muscles may be detectable on physical examination. The pain frequently radiates to the posterior occiput and upper extremity, often extending to the fingertips. The pain usually does not follow the distribution of any specific nerve trunk. Painful areas are characteristically tender to palpation. Deep tendon reflexes may be normal, diminished, or absent. There may be striking weakness of shoulder muscles, frequently accompanied by atrophy. Occasionally, glenohumeral motion is limited, owing either to pain or to reflex sympathetic dystrophy. Calcific deposits may be seen in the musculocutaneous cuff (also known as the rotator cuff). Humeral epicondylitis and fibrotic changes in the palmar fascia may develop in association with the reflex dystrophy. Blood pressure readings in the arms may be different. Central nervous system manifestations associated with circulatory changes or reflex dystrophy may include dilation of a pupil, interference with balance, tinnitus, and nausea or vomiting.

### Differential Diagnosis

Symptoms resembling those of cervical spondylosis accompany several other disorders frequently occurring in the elderly. Examples include angina pectoris, shoulder-hand syndrome, polymyalgia rheumatica, and carpal tunnel symdrome.

*Angina pectoris* may be accompanied by numbness and tingling extending down the left arm and occasionally the right. It may occur in patients who also, coincidentally, have limitation in neck motion secondary to cervical spondylosis. Classically, in angina pectoris, the tingling sensation is said to stop at the wrist (unfortunately this is not always true). The history of onset of symptoms at time of stress, relief of symptoms by nitroglycerin, and electrocardiographic changes, if present, will indicate the diagnosis of angina pectoris. This can be confirmed by further cardiac evaluation.

A much more complex differential diagnosis

is provided by the *shoulder-hand syndrome.* This is a reflex dystrophy, resulting from a complex of neurovascular changes, triggered by a variety of conditions, primarily myocardial infarction but also hemiplegia and trauma. Over 90 per cent of patients with this disorder are over 50 years of age. During the first 3 months, the disorder consists of pain, limitation of motion, and diffuse tenderness of the shoulder. X-rays may reveal patchy osteoporosis of the humeral head. This is accompanied by pain in the hand and fingers, dorsal swelling of the hand, diffuse tenderness, and cutaneous hyperesthesia. The skin may be shiny and later exhibit atrophic changes. There may be limitation of flexion of the fingers. During the next 3 to 6 months, there is usually partial or complete resolution of the swelling and vasomotor abnormalities, but trophic changes of the skin and contractures may begin to appear. These may be followed over the course of months to a year by atrophy of the skin of the hand; contractures of the fingers; and "frozen shoulder," accompanied by demineralization of the humerus. The pathogenesis of this disorder is closely related to processes occurring in cervical spondylosis. Occasionally, the latter condition may result in the shoulder-hand syndrome.

*Polymyalgia rheumatica* is not accompanied by numbness or tingling in the hand and forearm. Neck symptoms consist of diffuse muscular stiffness. Limitation of motion of the neck is not seen unless there is coincidental cervical spondylosis. Muscular involvement may extend beyond the cervical area and shoulders, e.g., the pelvic girdle and thighs. The elevated erythrocyte sedimentation rate accompanying polymyalgia may also assist in the diagnosis of this condition.

*Carpal tunnel syndrome* is accompanied by swelling of the wrist and, frequently, a positive Tinel's sign. The numbness and tingling may extend upward to the elbow, but not beyond. Neck symptoms are not present unless the patient has coincidental cervical spondylosis.

### Radiographic Findings

In patients suspected of having cervical spondylosis, x-rays should be studied for the pattern of cervical motion as well as the presence of bony changes. Lateral x-rays, with the neck in flexed, extended, and neutral positions, will show loss of the normal forward curve in the majority of cases and reversal of the curve in 20 per cent of these. The films should be studied for sharp angulation and increased distance between the posterior spinous processes, suggestive of tearing (rupture) of the interspinous ligaments. The lateral films should also be studied for presence or absence of fractures of vertebral bodies, spinous processes, and laminae and for narrowing of the intervertebral disc spaces and hypertrophic spurring. Further definition of the joint spaces and spur formation can be obtained from anteroposterior views, tilted toward the head. Lateral or oblique views may be necessary to obtain a good assessment of the posterior intervertebral joints, interarticular isthmi, and laminae. Myelographic studies should be undertaken if clinical findings suggest a space-occupying lesion or if a conservative therapeutic program fails to give symptomatic relief. The use of the CAT scan and Amipaque dye permits excellent definition without leaving residual.

### Treatment

Treatment of cervical spondylosis involves the use of antirheumatic drugs, hot packs, and gentle exercises. The use of home traction will provide considerable symptomatic relief in approximately two thirds of cases and should be part of the therapeutic armamentarium of every physician providing general care to older patients. A kit can be obtained from most drugstores or medical supply houses. The purpose of neck traction is not to stretch the cervical spine but to carry the weight of the skull for a period of time so that the neck muscles can be relaxed and gentle exercises undertaken. The apparatus should be attached to a doorway (*not* at the top of the cellar stairs) so that the patient can have a pleasant view (Fig. 36–9). The patient should sit in a relaxed position. He or she can regulate the amount of weight by filling the bag to the desired level. A weight of 5 to 7 pounds is sufficient. The procedure should be carried out for 30 minutes three times daily. If relief is not noted within 4 to 6 days, the procedure will probably not prove beneficial. Home neck traction should not be undertaken if the clinical picture suggests the presence of serious disease, such as erosion of the atlanto-occipital joint by rheumatoid granuloma, abscess, or malignancy. If this conservative program does not prove beneficial, referral to a neurologist, orthopedist, or neurosurgeon is indicated.

## Problem 3: Acute Monoarticular Arthritis

Older patients frequently exhibit acute monoarticular arthritis, manifested by pain, swelling, heat, redness, and limitation of motion of joints. This may occur in persons who have no known underlying joint disease or in individ-

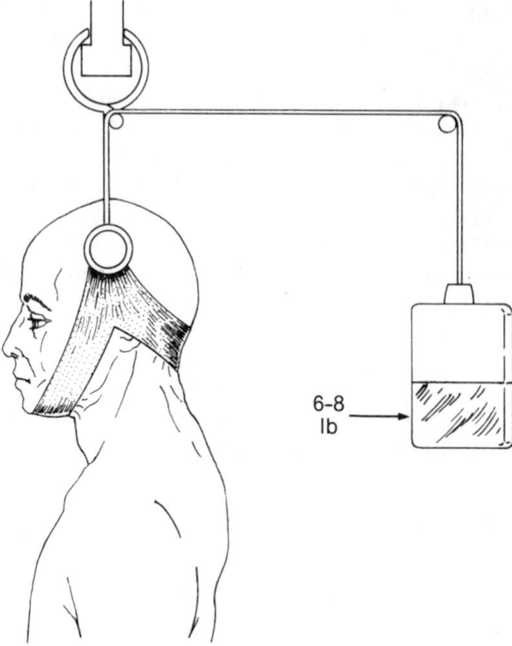


**Figure 36–9.** Neck traction at home.

uals who have one of the many forms of chronic arthritis. Correct and prompt diagnosis will often prevent severe crippling sequelae, which in an older person may make a big difference in the individual's ability to maintain independence.

The major causes of acute monoarticular arthritis in the elderly are sepsis, gout, pseudogout, hemarthrosis, and exacerbation of underlying arthritis. The likelihood that acute arthritis is due to one or another of these conditions varies with individual joints. Gout predominantly involves the first metatarsophalangeal joint. It may, however, involve the knee, ankle, wrist, or other joints. Pseudogout is most apt to involve the knee, a joint that is also a frequent site of hemarthrosis secondary to trauma. Septic arthritis can involve any joint, including any of the larger joints of the extremities, the sternoclavicular joints, and costochondral joints.

When obtaining a careful history, the physician should give special attention to previous episodes of acute arthritis (common in gout and pseudogout) and their course. History of recent dental surgery, previous heart disease, or chills and other constitutional symptoms can be important in the diagnosis of septic arthritis. An acute flare-up of a previously damaged joint is suggestive of septic arthritis or pseudogout. Physical examination should be used to identify the presence of synovial effusion and synovial thickening and to determine whether the point of maximal tenderness is in the synovium, bone, or periarticular tissue. X-rays should always be taken and studied for possible evidence of fracture, previous joint disease, loose bodies, and osteomyelitis. In taking x-rays of one extremity, if there is any question about the diagnosis, one should obtain views of the opposite extremity for comparison, since congenital changes may at times closely mimic fracture or other disease. Other laboratory tests of value include determinations of serum uric acid concentration, white blood cell count and differential, and sedimentation rate. An increased sedimentation rate is indicative of an inflammatory process and provides an index of activity of the disease for future comparison.

By far the most important procedure is joint aspiration. Aspiration of certain joints, such as the knee and wrist, can easily be performed by a general physician. In other instances, it should be entrusted to an orthopedist. Specimens of synovial fluid should always be sent promptly to the bacteriologic laboratory for culture. Since cultures take time, it is of paramount importance to have Gram's stained smears performed immediately. Next in order of priority is examination for the presence of crystals. A drop of fluid should be placed on a slide, with a coverslip, and examined under polarized light for the presence of characteristic crystals of urate or sodium pyrophosphate (see Fig. 36–6). Third in priority is a cell count. For this purpose, fluid should be placed in the same test tube used for blood, when one is obtaining a complete blood count, and counted in a hemocytometer. White cell counts of 20,000 per $mm^2$ or higher are infrequent in patients with rheumatoid arthritis or gout and are suggestive of septic arthritis; cell counts of 100,000 per $mm^2$ are strongly suggestive of infection. The only other examination of clinical importance is the estimation of viscosity. This can be done by drawing a bit of fluid up from a glass slide with a needle and permitting the fluid to drop from the needle. Fluid is normally tenacious and viscous. If it is watery, the physician should suspect the presence of an inflammatory process such as sepsis or rheumatoid arthritis. The presence of grossly bloody fluid may reflect the presence of trauma or spontaneous hemarthrosis in a person with hemorrhagic diathesis or receiving anticoagulant therapy. Alternatively, in persons with osteoarthritis, especially of the knee, one of the osteophytic spurs may "clip off" a synovial villus, leading to hemorrhage.

### Treatment of Septic Arthritis

Treatment includes administration of high doses of parenteral antibiotics, appropriate to the organism, and serial joint aspirations conducted every day until the effusion fails to reaccumulate. The aspirations should be performed using strict sterile technique. Intra-articular administration of antibiotics is not indicated. Immobilization of the joint with a splint or traction (for hip or knee) adds to the comfort of the patient, as does use of moist heat.

Most patients will respond to the preceding treatment in a few days. In a small number of patients, a decision for surgery will have to be made, depending on the progress of the constitutional and local symptoms, the character of the aspirated fluid, the infecting organism, and the joint involved.

## *Problem 4: Arthritis of the Wrist and Hand*

The many joints of the hand may be involved by nearly all forms of arthritis. Several patterns emerge quite clearly.

*Osteoarthritis* involves predominantly the distal interphalangeal joints and, to a lesser extent, the proximal interphalangeal joints. The metacarpophalangeal joints are not involved (except for the first metacarpophalangeal joint of the thumb). In contrast, in *rheumatoid arthritis* the metacarpophalangeal and proximal interphalangeal joints are most frequently involved.

The interphalangeal joints may become disfigured by *Heberden's* and *Bouchard's nodes,* respectively. Joint flexion is frequently limited, and grasping of small objects becomes difficult. Lateral deformities may develop, owing to the stretching of the collateral ligaments. Occasionally mucous cysts develop in association with Heberden's nodes. The overlying skin is very thin and translucent so that the clear mucoid fluid may be seen within the cyst. Aspiration of the cyst, local injection of corticosteroid, and pressure immobilization can prevent rupture of the cyst and secondary joint infection. At times surgical excision of the underlying osteophyte and skin graft are necessary. The majority of the patients with Heberden's and Bouchard's nodes require only symptomatic treatment with antirheumatic medications and gentle exercises.

*Osteoarthritis of the carpometacarpal joint of the thumb* (basal joint of the thumb) is not uncommon in the elderly and produces pain at the base of the thumb with any activity requiring rotation (e.g., sewing, crocheting) or the application of pressure with the thumb (e.g., opening a car door). Gradually the base of the thumb subluxes laterally and the metacarpal becomes adducted; the patient compensates in part by hyperextending the metacarpophalangeal joint of the thumb. It may still be difficult to grasp larger objects (e.g., a water glass). The treatment involves corticosteroid injection (once or twice only) and rest. The latter is facilitated by a splint to maintain the thumb metacarpal in abduction. The preceding measures, if coupled with administration of antirheumatic drugs, usually produce some degree of relief. If this proves only temporary and the patient has increasing difficulties, then surgery in the form of either arthrodesis or arthroplasty (involving either resection or use of Silastic) will produce relief of pain and improve function.

*Wrist pain* is a common complaint in elderly patients. Both rheumatoid arthritis and osteoarthritis can be the cause of pain, accompanied by swelling, tenderness, and limitation of motion of the wrist (radiocarpal) joint. Trauma (e.g., Colles' fracture) can cause similar symptoms and may result in deformity. X-rays can be very helpful. One should initially obtain the standard views and then proceed with a carpal study if needed. Limitation of pronation-supination, with swelling and tenderness over the distal radioulnar joint, is common in rheumatoid arthritis and can also be secondary to an old healed Colles' fracture.

*Swelling of the dorsum of the wrist,* owing to rheumatoid tenosynovitis of the extensor tendons, usually is painless but can result eventually in rupture of some or all of these tendons, with great functional loss. If this occurs, the patient should be referred immediately to an orthopedic surgeon for resuturing of the tendons. Prophylactic management, including use of antirheumatic agents and surgical debridement of the extensor tendons, may delay the development of this complication.

*Stenosing tenosynovitis at the radial styloid,* de Quervain's disease, involves the tendon sheath of the abductor pollicis longus and entensor pollicis brevis muscles and produces pain with any movement of the thumb. If the patient is asked to grasp the thumb firmly in the palm of the hand and then deviate the wrist ulnad, this maneuver will cause severe pain (positive Finkelstein test). This pain may also be produced by arthritis of the basal joint of the thumb, but this can be differentiated by the local tenderness and possible deformity over the basal joint and also by the "grinding test." In this test the thumb metacarpal is pushed proximally against the trapezium and then rotated. The findings are positive if the test causes pain and crepitus at the joint.

If *carpal tunnel syndrome* is suspected, the diagnosis can be confirmed by electromyography and nerve conduction studies. The reduction in nerve conduction velocity is demonstrated by the increase in motor and/or sensory latency. When abnormal, these studies confirm the clinical diagnosis, but a normal study does not necessarily rule out compression.

Because the most common cause of compression of the median nerve at the wrist is flexor tenosynovitis, the usual nonoperative management is (1) splinting, (2) local injection of corticosteroids and (3) administration of nonsteroidal anti-inflammatory medication. A night splint immobilizes the involved wrist in neutral or slight dorsiflexion, thus preventing excessive wrist motion during sleep and attendant pain. Local anesthetic and corticosteroid injection may be given into the tendon sheaths proximal to the transverse carpal ligament. Care must be taken to avoid injecting the medication directly into the median nerve or any of the tendons. This management gives considerable relief to many patients. If the symptoms recur, one additional trial with splint, injection, and anti-inflammatory medication may be recommended. If the patient does not show satisfactory improvement in about 3 months, surgical release is indicated.

*Synovitis of flexor tendons* of the fingers frequently is associated with rheumatoid arthritis but at times is found in patients with osteoarthritis or without any demonstrable disease. The clinical presentation is either swelling or tenderness along the volar aspect of the finger (usually in rheumatoid arthritis) or a painful "locking" and "triggering" of the finger, with a nodular enlargement of the flexor tendon palpable over the metacarpophalangeal joint at the palm. This nodule moves with the flexor tendon when the finger is flexed and extended.

Local corticosteroid injection into the tendon sheath usually relieves the symptoms. In resistant or recurrent cases surgical release using local anesthesia gives predictably good results.

## *Problem 5: Chronic Arthritis of the Knee*

The knee is one of the joints most susceptible to acute and chronic trauma and, often, most difficult to treat. Proper function of the knee joint is essential for normal mobility; conversely; chronic knee dysfunction such as flexion deformity or hypermobility results in serious limitation of a person's ability to walk, arise from a seated position, climb stairs, or even "transfer" from bed to wheelchair. This is accentuated by the fact that a knee that is improperly functioning and exhibits degenerative changes has an increased susceptibility to involvement by pseudogout, gout, and septic arthritis.

Many disabling conditions involving the knee in later life are sequelae of apparently minor congenital deformities or injuries in youth. Proper identification and treatment of conditions such as genu valgum, genu varum, torn menisci, and traumatic injury to the ligaments of the knee early in life are very important in order to minimize painful and serious limitation and mobility at the other end of the age spectrum.

### Diagnosis

When an elderly person enters the physician's office complaining of chronic pain in the knee, the examination should note the presence or absence of synovial thickening and synovial effusion and the degree of atrophy of the quadriceps muscle. Careful palpation, carried out while the knee is put through the full range of motion, should address each individual surface. Palpation of the patella will often reveal fine crepitus, suggestive of chondromalacia of the posterior cartilaginous surface. Palpation of the medial or lateral aspect of the joint space may reveal fine crepitus or the presence of marginal osteophytes and loose bodies moving against one's fingers. The joint should be examined carefully for mediolateral instability, rotational hypermobility, and anteroposterior hypermobility (of the proximal tibia on the femur). The knee joint should be studied while the person is walking to discern the amount of lateral deflection. If the joint exhibits effusion, this should be aspirated and examined (see page 389).

Anteroposterior and lateral x-rays, always taken with the patient in the standing position, should be examined for osteophytic spurs; loss of joint space; subchondral thickening or "sclerosis" of the bone; bony erosions; and, especially, for lack of proper alignment of the joint. The presence of minor degrees of genu varum, for example, may be accompanied by accentuation of degenerative changes of the medial compartment of the joint, as compared with the lateral. In addition, x-rays should be studied for the presence of calcification of the cartilage or periarticular structures, indicative of chondrocalcinosis (see page 397). Arthrography of the knee may be very helpful, particularly in early cases, in which menisceal tear is suspected. Finally, arthroscopy can be used not only to visualize the extent of intra-articular disease but also to debride, partially, the remaining fragments of cartilage, loose bodies, and so on.

### Treatment

Serious damage to the menisci, if present, should be treated surgically. If even minor degrees of genu varum are accompanied by degenerative changes of the medial compartment, consideration should be given to surgical realignment of the tibia (high tibial osteotomy). However, in most cases a conservative approach is appropriate. This includes use of full doses of antirheumatic agents, heat, weight reduction, and exercise. If the joint exhibits any degree of flexion deformity, this must be treated aggressively lest it become worse. In mild cases, graduated leg strengthening exercises may be sufficient. In more advanced cases, serial casting should be considered.

If a joint exhibits severe destructive changes, with pain on walking even for short distances, the options include the use of a sturdy three-point cane, crutches, or walker; use of a walking knee brace with metal supports laterally; or surgical joint replacement. The brace is seldom practical for an older person.

**Arthroplasty.** Total knee arthroplasty has proved effective in relieving pain, providing stability, correcting deformity, and restoring overall function of the knee.[149-156] Elderly patients are considered for this procedure if they have disabling involvement of both compartments of the knee secondary to osteoarthritis, post-traumatic arthritis, rheumatoid arthritis, or certain other arthropathies. It is also used to treat failed knee operations such as arthrodesis, high tibial osteotomy, and synovectomy.

Absolute contraindications for total knee replacement are present or previous joint infection and neurotrophic arthroplasty (Charcot's joint). Relative contraindications, such as osteoporosis, severe instability secondary to the absence of the collateral ligaments, and marked bone loss, depend on the type of implants used.

***Preoperative and Postoperative Care.*** Preoperatively, the patient is evaluated medically, and the nature and extent of postoperative exercises are explained by a therapist. All our patients undergoing total joint replacement receive intraoperative antibiotics (cephalosporin),[155] the use of which continues until the removal of the suction drainage tubes on the second postoperative day.

Although there is a high incidence of thrombophlebitis in total joint surgery,[156,157] it is uncertain whether thrombophlebitis is important enough clinically to justify routine prophylactic use of anticoagulants. Aspirin is routinely used and decreases the incidence of thrombophlebitis, especially in men.

Quadriceps exercises are started during the first postoperative day. The patient is allowed to walk with partial weight using crutches or a walker as soon as muscular control of the leg is achieved. The muscle strength and range of motion usually progress steadily, although manipulation of the knee with the patient under anesthesia to improve flexion is occasionally required. The patient is discharged home during the third postoperative week and continues the exercises and the use of crutches. By the sixth to eighth week the patient usually regains complete extension and a minimum of 90 degrees of flexion, allowing progression to a cane. Further improvement is anticipated for several weeks. Although the final degree of activity depends on the general health of the patient and the involvement of other joints, excellent or good relief of pain and improved function are achieved in up to 90 per cent of cases.

***Complications.*** Poor wound healing can develop after total knee replacement and requires prompt treatment to avoid deep wound infection. Vigorous flexion exercises in the immediate postoperative period can also contribute to poor wound healing.

Deep infection is the most serious local complication. If it cannot be controlled with soft tissue debridement and antibiotics, the treatment is removal of the components and arthrodesis of the knee as a salvage procedure.

Should thrombophlebitis occur, it usually requires that the patient remain on anticoagulant therapy for 9 months or longer. In an older patient, especially one who requires other medications, including nonsteroidal anti-inflammatory agents, close surveillance of prothrombin time and adjustment of dosage of the anticoagulant are required. The possibility of the complications should be explained to the patient and family before surgery.

Mechanical complications with postoperative joint instability; patellar problems (subluxation, dislocation, and pain); and compartment loosening, deformation, and breaking are more common after knee replacement than after hip replacement. Despite these problems, knee replacement may enable an elderly person to maintain or achieve a degree of mobility essential for his or her happiness and/or independence. Therefore, the procedure is an important adjuvant to therapy for chronic arthritis of the knee.

## *Problem 6: Arthritis of the Hip*

Arthritis of the hip is even more disabling than that of the knee, but it is much more susceptible to successful management owing to the effectiveness of surgical replacement.[158–164] Degenerative joint disease of the hip is the sequela to a number of disorders. These include primary osteoarthritis; degenerative changes secondary to congenital lesions; aseptic necrosis secondary to corticosteroid administration or to interference with blood supply due to fracture; rheumatoid arthritis, and ankylosing spondylitis. Severe hip pain, accentuated by walking, loss of motion (especially rotation), and progressive flexion deformity ensue.

#### TREATMENT

Conservative treatment (weight reduction, application of heat, use of anti-rheumatic agents, exercise, and use of a cane or crutches) may alleviate the symptoms for a period of time, but in moderate-to-severe cases, progressive limitation of ambulation ensues and surgery in the form of total hip replacement may be advisable. Diseases that lend themselves to treatment with this procedure include the arthritis conditions mentioned earlier and, occasionally, malignant tumors of the femoral head and neck. In addition, total hip replacement has been used extensively to treat previously unsuccessful hip operations (cup arthroplasty, hemiarthroplasty, femoral osteotomy, fusion, and Girdlestone's procedure) and nonunion of fractures.

Total hip replacement must never be recommended if there is an active infection of the hip. Relative contraindications are neurotrophic arthropathy (Charcot's joint), weak or absent abductor muscles, and inadequate bone stock.

**Preoperative and Postoperative Care.** The principles of preoperative care are similar to those described for surgical replacement of the knee. The advantages and disadvantages of anticoagulant therapy, immediately and postoperatively, are well summarized in a paper by Harris and associates.[164] Our policy in this regard is the same as reported previously for the knee. The operative procedure is followed by a period of intensive rehabilitation, both in-hospital and at home. Activities are increased gradually; the patient is usually able to commence walking with a cane in 6 to 8 weeks.

**Results.** The major advantage of this procedure is the marked decrease or complete elimination of pain. The range of motion, although markedly improved, is still somewhat limited compared with that of a normal hip. Some patients continue to limp after surgery, often because of weak muscles about the hip. These can be strengthened with exercises. Limping can also be caused by inequality in the length of the legs. Usually leg length can be restored during surgery, but if necessary, it can be compensated for by a shoe lift.

**Complications.** *Infection* is the most devastating local complication and often necessitates the removal of the implants because of persistent pain, drainage, or both, leaving the patient with a shortened extremity and an unstable, weak hip. Thereafter, the patient usually must use crutches or a cane, but fortunately, pain is not a prevalent feature.

*Thrombophlebitis* is another complication that, when associated with pulmonary embolism, can be life-threatening. The implications for therapy have been described earlier in the section concerning surgical replacement of the knee.

*Loosening of the components* results in pain on weight bearing and thus necessitates revision and replacement of the implants. The radiographic incidence of loosening of the components, bone resorption, wear of the polyethylene cup, and other signs of potential problems is quite high (25 to 30 per cent) in 4- to 10-year follow-up studies, but these problems appear to have no significant bearing on the quality of the clinical results, as indicated by the reoperation rate of only 5 to 8 per cent.

In addition to the general complications inherent in major surgery in elderly patients, other complications from total hip replacement include dislocation or subluxation, fractures of the upper femur, and nerve and vascular injuries. Despite the possible complications, hip replacement provides the potential for relief of pain and increased mobility to such a degree that it has become an important aspect of therapy in osteoarthritis even in people age 80 and over.

## *Problem 7: Hip Fractures*

Hip fractures occur predominantly in the elderly. It is estimated that more than 20,000 hip fractures occur in the United States each year.[165] One-third are femoral neck fractures and the remaining are intertrochanteric fractures.

Many elderly patients who present with hip fracture also suffer from a multitude of health problems. However, the patient is in his or her best health when the injury occurs; the coincidental problems will most likely become worse with bed confinement. Delay of surgery for more than 3 days after injury results not only in an increased death rate[166] but also in the local complications of fracture healing. Therefore, only life-threatening conditions, such as pulmonary edema, acute myocardial infarction, thyrotoxic crisis, and diabetic coma, should take priority and delay the hip surgery until they are under control.

### Femoral Neck Fractures

The mechanism of injury in femoral neck fractures is external rotation of the femur.[167] These fractures are classified according to the displacement of the femoral neck,[168] the method of treatment and eventual outcome varying with each type.

*Impacted and undisplaced* fractures, if treated nonoperatively, become disimpacted and displaced in 5 to 8 per cent of the cases.[169] Therefore, the preferred treatment is internal fixation in situ with multiple pins or screws. This can be accomplished even using local anesthesia and sedation if need be.

*Displaced* fractures of the femoral neck are always treated surgically. If a good reduction is achieved and the fracture is securely fixed with multiple screws, pins, or sliding compression screws, then most patients will do well. However, about 25 per cent of patients will develop late complications of nonunion and/or avascular necrosis, often necessitating further surgery. If a primary prosthetic replacement is performed, again the majority of the patients will do well. However, if complications develop either early (dislocation, infection) or late (painful migration of the prosthesis, fracture of the femoral shaft), they can be difficult to treat.[170] The present consensus holds that prosthetic replacement is preferable (1) in elderly patients, perhaps over the age of 70 years, with low functional demands; (2) when the fracture is comminuted or reduction is not obtainable or several weeks have elapsed from the time of fracture to the time of examination; and (3) when there are associated conditions such as marked osteoporosis, Paget's disease, or arthritic involvement of the hip joint. Depending on the pathologic condition present in addition to the fractures, various types of prosthetic replacement surgery are performed, e.g., Austin Moore's or Thompson's hemiarthroplasty, biarticular endoprosthesis, and total hip replacement.

### Intertrochanteric Fractures

Intertrochanteric fractures are also predominant in elderly patients, many of whom have other medical problems and limited ability to walk. Therefore, it is of paramount importance to perform early surgical stabilization so that the patients can be mobilized and avoid further deterioration.

The problems encountered in the care of these fractures are (1) appreciable bleeding at the fracture site and (2) instability and deformity, particularly when the fractures are comminuted. Depending on the comminution of the fragments and the concomitant osteoporosis, technique difficulties can be encountered in obtaining reduction and stable fixation. Advances that have contributed to better results are the use of the image intensifier in the operating room (for better control of the reduction of the fracture and insertion of the implant) and improved implants used in internal fixation, such as sliding compression screws or nails and condylocephalic nails (e.g., Enders pins and Harris nail).[171,172] The implants are introduced from the supracondylar area of the femur without opening the fracture site, thus reducing the amount of bleeding and decreasing the incidence of infection.

## References


1. Cobb S: The Frequency of Rheumatic Diseases. Cambridge, Harvard University Press, 1971, pp. 6–16.
2. Barney JL, Neukom JE: Use of arthritis care by the elderly. Gerontologist 19:548, 1979.
3. Hull FM: M.D. Doctoral dissertation. London, University of Cambridge, 1975.
4. Mikkelson WN, et al: Estimates of the prevalence of rheumatic diseases in the population of Tecumseh, Michigan, 1959–60. J Chronic Dis 20:351, 1967.
   *Contains prevalence data for various joint symptoms, positive latex fixation tests, rheumatoid arthritis, ankylosing spondylitis, and osteoarthritis.*
5. Wood PHN, Badley EM: An epidemiological appraisal of bone and joint disease in the elderly. In Wright V (ed.): Bone and Joint Disease in the Elderly. Edinburgh, New York, Churchill Livingstone, 1983.
   *A beautifully written, interesting review by a world recognized authority on rheumatology and epidemiology.*

5a. Hays CS, Stinson IN: Erythrocyte sedimentation rate and age. Arch Ophthalmol 94:939, 1976.

6. Hallgren HM, et al: Lymphocyte phytohemagglutinin responsiveness, immunoglobulins, and autoantibodies in aging humans. J Immunol 111:1101, 1973.
   *One of the better studies delineating increased frequency of rheumatoid and antinuclear factors in apparently normal elderly persons. The population sample, however, was not representative of a normal population.*
7. Whittingham S, et al: Autoantibodies in healthy subjects. Aust Ann Med 18:130, 1969.
8. Pandey J, et al: Autoantibodies in healthy subjects of different age groups. Mech Ageing Dev 10:399, 1979.
9. Gordon J. Rosenthal M: Failure to detect age-related increase of non-pathological autoantibodies. Lancet 1:231, 1984.
   *These recent studies failed to show a relationship be-*

*tween rheumatoid factor and aging in carefully screened cohorts of patients.*

10. Calkins E: Antibodies and aging: A geriatrician looks at the clinical literature. In Milgrom F, Abeyounis CJ, Albini B (eds): Antibodies: Protective, Destructive and Regulatory Role. Basel, Karger, 1985.
*Review and analysis of data relating positive rheumatoid factor tests and antinuclear antibody reactions to aging.*
11. Ryan LM, et al: The radiologic diagnosis of sacroiliitis. A comparison of different views with computed tomograms of the sacroiliac joint. Arthritis Rheum 26:760, 1083.
*Review of published reports of x-ray, computerized tomography, and scintigraphy studies of sacroiliac joints and presentation of original data. Well illustrated.*

## *Osteoarthritis*

12. Kellgren JH, Lawrence JS: Osteo-arthrosis and disc degeneration in an urban population. Ann Rheum Dis 17:388, 1958.
*A classic presentation of epidemiology and antecedents of osteoarthritis and disc degeneration.*
13. Radin EL: The physiology and degeneration of joints. Semin Arthritis Rheum 2:3, 1972–73.
*Although this review is somewhat "dated," it presents an extremely readable review of joint function, with special emphasis on load bearing, the importance of congruity, and the "wear and tear" theory of the pathogenesis of osteoarthritis. Contains 72 references, from 1931 to 1973.*
14. Muir H: Cartilage structure and metabolism and basic changes in degenerative joint disease. Aust NZ J Med 8 (Suppl 1):175, 1978.
*Good, thorough, although somewhat dated, review by a recognized authority. Contains 51 references, from 1958 to 1977.*
15. Peyron JG: Epidemiologic and etiologic approach of osteoarthritis of the knee. Clin Orthop 93:288, 1979.
*A good, complete review presenting the European perspective. There are 224 references, from 1805 to 1978.*
16. Erye DR: Collagen: Molecular diversity in the body's protein scaffold. Science 207:1315, 1980.
*Well-organized, definitive review, in readable English. Contains 113 references, from 1972 to 1980.*
17. Santer V, et al: Proteoglycans from normal and degenerate cartilage of the adult human tibial plateau. Arthritis Rheum 24:691, 1981.
*These investigators fail to identify in cartilage from the human tibial plateau any of the changes associated with glycosaminoglycan synthesis that have been attributed to osteoarthritis, based on studies of the hip. This is an example of the controversy that still exists concerning biochemical changes associated with aging and osteoarthritis. There are 35 references, from 1971 to 1979.*
18. Gardner DL: The nature and causes of osteoarthrosis. Br Med J 286:418, 1983.
*Written in simple, clear terms, this is an excellent review of the anatomic, chemical, and clinical aspects of osteoarthritis.*
19. Hughes GRV: Osteoarthritis. Age Ageing Suppl 1–8, 1979.
20. Bird HA: Osteoarthritis. *In* Wright V (ed.): Bone and Joint Disease in the Elderly. Edinburgh, New York, Churchill Livingstone, 1983.
21. Kellgren JH, et al: Genetic factors in generalized osteo-arthrosis. Ann Rheum Dis 22:237, 1963.
*A careful analysis of genetic factors affecting osteoarthritis, based on a study of joint disease in a random sample of the populations of Leigh and Wensleydale.*
22. Kellgren JH, Moore R: Generalized osteoarthritis and Heberden's nodes. Br Med J 1:181, 1952.
*A classic presentation, well-illustrated.*
23. Cook IDV, et al: The deposition of immunoglobulins and complement components in osteoarthritic cartilage. Int Orthop 4:211, 1980.
24. Solinger AM, Stobo JD: Regulation of immune reactivity to collagen in human beings. Arthritis Rheum 24:1057, 1981.
*Analysis of the genetic and pathogenetic implications of immune reactivity to collagen as related to osteoarthritis, rheumatoid arthritis, and drug-induced lupus erythematosus. Contains 18 references, from 1973 to 1980.*
25. Solinger AM, Hess EV: The role of collagens in rheumatic diseases. Rheumatol 9:491, 1982.
*A review of the immunogenetic role of collagens in pathogenesis of many rheumatic diseases. Contains 17 references from 1975 to 1981.*
26. Moskowitz RW: Management of osteoarthritis. Bull Rheum Dis 31:31, 1981.
*A concise review including references to certain topics (such as the effect of aspirin on cartilage and the effectiveness of acupuncture) are covered in this article.*
27. Resnick D: Diseases of the axial skeleton which are lesser known, poorly recognized, or misunderstood. Bull Rheum Dis 28:932, 1977–78.
*Useful as a guide to the clinical and radiologic literature on osteitis condensans, ochronotic arthropathy, relapsing polychondritis, diffuse idiopathic skeletal hyperostosis (Forestier's disease), and other more common diseases of the spine.*
28. Quinet RJ, Hadler NM: Diagnosis and treatment of backache. Semin Arthritis Rheum 8:261, 1979.
*A highly readable exposition of the pathogenesis, diagnosis, and treatment of regional disease of the low back, with special reference to the intervertebral disc.*
29. Kelsey JL, White AA III: Epidemiology and impact of low-back pain. Spine 5:133, 1980.
*A careful consideration of clinical aspects of prolapsed discs, disc degeneration, osteoarthrosis of the apophyseal joint, fractures and dislocations of the vertebrae, osteoporosis, and spondylolisthesis. Contains 115 references, from 1944 to 1978.*
30. O'Brien WM: Long-term efficacy and safety of tolmetin sodium in treatment of geriatric patients with rheumatoid arthritis and osteoarthritis: A retrospective study. J Clin Pharmacol 23:309, 1983.
31. Barnes CG: A double blind comparison of naproxen with indomethacin in osteoarthritis. J Clin Pharmacol 15:347, 1975.
32. Sack KE: Arthritis: Specifics on long-term management. Geriatrics 35:39, 1980.
33. Clinch D, et al: Nonsteroidal anti-inflammatory drugs and gastrointestinal adverse effects. J R Coll Physicians London 17:228, 1983.
34. Donder ATM, et al: The effect of indomethacin on kidney function and plasma renin activity in man. Nephron 17:288, 1976.
35. Walshe JJ, Venuto RC: Acute organic renal failure induced by indomethacin: Possible mechanism. Ann Intern Med 91:47, 1979.
36. Cove-Smith JR, Knapp MS: Analgesic nephropathy: An important cause of chronic renal failure. Q J. Med 47:46, 1978.

37. Goodwin JS, Regan M: Cognitive dysfunction associated with naproxin and ibuprofen in the elderly. Arthritis Rheum 25:1013, 1982.
38. Herman JH, Hess EV: Nonsteroidal anti-inflammatory drugs and modulation of cartilagenous changes in osteoarthritis and rheumatoid arthritis. Clinical implications. Am J Med Suppl 16, 1984.
*This article is part of an excellent symposium on nonsteroidal anti-inflammatory drugs, published on adjacent pages.*
39. Tornkvist H, et al: Effect of ibuprofen and indomethacin on bone metabolism reflected in bone strength. Clin Orthop 187:255, 1984.
40. Goodwin J, et al: Administration of nonsteroidal anti-inflammatory agents in patients with rheumatoid arthritis. Effects on indexes of cellular immune status and serum rheumatoid levels. JAMA 250:2485, 1983.
41. Brooks PM, et al: Problems of antiarthritis therapy in the elderly. J Am Geriatr Soc 32:229, 1984.
42. Mowat AG: Drug treatment of arthritis in the elderly. Age Ageing. 8:14, 1979.


## *Calcium Phosphate Dihydrate Disease*


43. Resnick D, et al: Rheumatoid arthritis and pseudorheumatoid arthritis in calcium pyrophosphate dihydrate crystal deposition disease. Radiology 140:615, 1980.
*An excellent review of radiologic aspects of calcium phosphate dihydrate disease.*
44. McCarty DJ: Pseudogout: Articular chondrocalcinosis calcium phosphate crystal deposition disease. *In* Hollander JL, McCarty DJ (eds): Arthritis and Allied Conditions. 8th ed. Philadelphia, Lea and Febiger, 1972, p. 1140.
45. Wilkins E, et al: Osteoarthritis and articular chondrocalcinosis in the elderly. Ann Rheum Dis 42:280, 1983.
*One hundred consecutive admissions to an acute geriatric unit were studied radiologically for evidence of chondrocalcinosis. This condition was present in 34 patients. The article delineates demographic and clinical characteristics of this group.*
46. O'Duffy JD: Clinical studies of acute pseudogout attacks. Comments on prevalence, predispositions, and treatment. Arthritis Rheum 19:349, 1976.
*A good brief article from the Mayo Clinic, with helpful information on predisposing factors, symptoms, and response to treatment.*
47. Ellman MH, Levin B: Chondrocalcinosis in elderly persons. Arthritis Rheum 18:43, 1975.
*Brief, informative review of experience with 16 patients with chondrocalcinosis.*
48. McCarty D: Crystals, joints, and consternation. Heberden Oration, 1982. Ann Rheum Dis 43:243, 1983.
*An excellent review of the sequential observations leading to the present state of knowledge concerning CPPD and related disorders. Extensive bibliography.*
49. Bjelle A, Edvinsson U, Hagstam A: Pyrophosphate arthropathy in two Swedish families. Arthritis Rheum 25:66, 1982.
50. Rodriguez-Valverde V, et al: Familial chondrocalcinosis. Prevalence in northern Spain and clinical features in five pedigrees. Arthritis Rheum 23:471, 1980.
51. Caswell A, et al: Pathogenesis of chondrocalcinosis and pseudogout. Metabolism of inorganic pyrophosphate and production of calcium pyrophosphate dihydrate crystals. Ann Rheum Dis 42 (Suppl 1):27, 1983.
*A complete review by British authors, with 105 references.*
52. Ryan LM, et al: Cartilage nucleoside triphosphate (NTP) pyrophosphohydrolase. I. Identification as an ecto-enzyme. Arthritis Rheum 27:404, 1984.
53. Ryan LM, et al: Elevated intracellular pyrophosphate (PPi) and ecto-nucleoside pyrophosphohydrolase activity NTPPPH in fibroblasts of patients with calcium pyrophosphate dihydrate CPPD crystal deposition disease. Clin Res (in press).
*These articles describe important steps toward elucidation of the pathogenesis of this important disorder.*
54. Cheung HS et al: Phagocytosis of hydroxyapatite or calcium pyrophosphate dihydrate crystals by rabbit articular chondrocytes stimulates release of collagenase, neutral protease, and prostaglandins E2 and F2 alpha. Proc Soc Exp Biol Med 173:181, 1983.
55. Rodnan GP (ed.): Primer on the rheumatic diseases. JAMA 224:662, 1973.
56. Fam AG, Topp JR, Stein HB: Clinical and roentgenographic aspects of pseudogout: A study of 50 cases and a review. Can Med Assoc J 124:545, 1981.
*Good clinical study, with excellent "teaching tables" and radiographs.*
57. Bong D, Bennett R: Pseudogout mimicking systemic disease. JAMA 246:1438, 1981.
*Interesting report of five cases in which pseudogout was manifested by conspicuous fever, leading to delay in recognition of the correct diagnosis.*
58. McCarty DJ, et al: "Milwaukee shoulder." Association of microspheroids containing hydroxyapatite crystals, active collagenase, and neutral protease with rotator cuff defects. I. Clinical aspects. Arthritis Rheum 24:464, 1981.
59. Halverson PB, et al: "Milwaukee shoulder." Association of microspheroids containing hydroxyapatite crystals, active collagenase, and neutral protease with rotator cuff defects. II. Synovial fluid studies. Arthritis Rheum 24:474, 1981.
60. Garancis JC, et al: "Milwaukee shoulder." Association of microspheroids containing hydroxyapatite crystals, active collagenase, and neutral protease with rotator cuff defects. III. Morphologic and biochemical studies of an excised synovium showing chondromatosis. Arthritis Rheum 24:484, 1981.
61. Halverson PB, et al: Milwaukee shoulder syndrome. III. Report of 11 additional cases with concomitant involvement of the knee in 7 instances. Semin Arthritis Rheum 14:36, 1984.
*The preceding four articles represent the definitive presentations of this syndrome. Reference includes an excellent summary of clinical aspects, illustrated by instructive, clear radiographs.*
62. O'Duffy JD: Pseudogout syndrome in hospital patients. JAMA 226:42, 1973.
63. McCarty DJ: Pseudogout and pyrophosphate metabolism. Adv Int Med 25:363, 1980.
*An authoritative up-to-date review, with 66 references selected by the expert in this field.*
64. Dieppe PA, et al: Apatite deposition disease. A new arthropathy. Lancet 1:266, 1976.
*Brief description of yet another crystal deposition disease, related to but distinct from chondrocalcinosis.*
65. Martel W, et al: Further observations on the arthropathy of calcium pyrophosphate crystal deposition disease. Radiology 141:1, 1981.
*Outstanding, well-illustrated review of radiologic findings.*

66. Howell DS: Diseases due to the deposition of calcium pyrophosphate and hydroxyapatite. *In* Kelly WN, et al (eds.): Textbook of Rheumatology. Philadelphia, W.B. Saunders Company, 1981, pp. 1438–1454.
*A very good review of the subject by a well-known authority on osteoarthritis, who is a good critic of research on related topics.*

## Gout

67. Hall AP, et al: Epidemiology of gout and hyperuricemia. A long-term population study. Am J Med 43:27, 1967.
*Although old, this classic report based on the Framingham study is definitive.*
68. Currie WJC: The gout patient in general practice. Rheumatol Rehabil 17:205, 1978.
*An excellent British study, carried out by the Wellcome Foundation.*
69. Pasero G: Recurrent gouty phlebitis without articular gout. *In* Muller MM, et al (eds.): Purine Metabolism in Man. New York, Plenum Press, 1977.
*Although the existence of this syndrome is not acknowledged by a number of established rheumatologists, we have seen a number of cases mistakingly diagnosed and inappropriately treated.*
70. Pasero G: Colchicine: Should we still use it? Clin Exp Rheumatol 2:103, 1984.
*I believe this author is mistaken concerning the hazards and value of low-dose maintenance colchicine. In other respects, this is an interesting paper.*
71. Fessel WJ: Renal outcomes of gout and hyperuricemia. Am J Med 67:74, 1979.
72. Yu T, Berger L: Impaired renal function in gout. Its association with hypertensive vascular disease and intrinsic renal disease. Am J Med 72:95, 1982.
73. Batuman V, et al: The role of lead in gout nephropathy. N Engl J Med 304:520, 1981.
74. Nakayama DA, et al: Tophaceous gout: A clinical and radiographic assessment. Brief report. Arthritis Rheum 27:468, 1984.
75. Barthelemy CR, et al: Gouty arthritis: A prospective radiographic evaluation of sixty patients. Skeletal Radiol 11:1, 1984.
*Excellent reproduction of illustrative x-rays.*
76. Boss GR, Seegmiller JE: Hyperuricemia and gout. Classification, complications and management. N Engl J Med 300:1459, 1979.
77. Kelley WN: Gout and related disorders of purine metabolism, *In* Kelley WN, et al (eds.): Textbook of Rheumatology. Philadelphia, W.B. Saunders Company, 1981, pp. 1397–1437.

## Rheumatoid Arthritis

78. Rasker JJ, Cosh JA: Cause and age at death in a prospective study of 100 patients with rheumatoid arthritis. Ann Rheum Dis 40:115, 1981.
79. Linos A, et al: The epidemiology of rheumatoid arthritis in Rochester, Minnesota: A study of incidence, prevalence, and mortality. Am J Epidemiol 111:87, 1980.
80. Adler E: Rheumatoid arthritis in old age. Isr J Med Sci 2:607, 1966.
81. Ehrlich GE, Katz WA, Cohen SH: Rheumatoid arthritis in the aged. Geriatrics 25:103, 1970.
82. Brown, JW, Sones DA: The onset of rheumatoid arthritis in the aged. J Am Geriatr Soc 15:873, 1967.
83. Corrigan AB, Robinson RG, Terenty TR: Benign rheumatoid arthritis of the aged. Br Med J 1:444, 1974.
84. Stastny P: Rheumatoid arthritis. Relationship with HLA-D. Am J Med 75:9, 1983.
*Part of an excellent symposium on oral gold.*
85. Reichlin M: Antinuclear antibodies. *In* Kelley WN, et al (eds.): Textbook of Rheumatology. 2nd ed. Philadelphia, W.B. Saunders Company, 1985.
86. Pickup ME: Drug pharmacokinetics with reference to antirheumatoid drugs. *In* Wright V (ed.): Bone and Joint Disease in the Elderly. Edinburgh, New York, Churchill Livingstone, 1983.
87. Yelin E, et al: Work disability in rheumatoid arthritis: Effects of disease, social, and work factors. Ann Intern Med 93:551, 1980.
88. Kean W, et al: Gold therapy in the elderly rheumatoid arthritis patient. Arthritis Rheum 26:705, 1983.
89. Weisman MH, Hannifin DM: Management of rheumatoid arthritis with oral gold. Arthritis Rheum 22:922, 1979.
90. Blodgett RC Jr: Auranofin: Experience to date. Am J Med 75:86, 1983.
91. Blocka K: Auranofin versus injectable gold. Am J Med 75:114, 1983.
92. Masi AT: Low dose glucocorticoid therapy in rheumatoid arthritis (RA): Transitional or selected add-on therapy. J Rheumatol 10:5, 1983.
93. Lockie LM, et al: Low dose adrenocorticosteroids in the management of elderly patients with rheumatoid arthritis: Selected examples and summary of efficacy in the long term treatment of 97 patients. Semin Arthritis Rheum 8:373, 1983.
94. Kean WF, et al: Efficacy and toxicity of D-penicillamine for rheumatoid disease in the elderly. J Am Geriatr Soc 30:94, 1982.
95. Willkens RF: Methotrexate: A perspective of its use in the treatment of rheumatic diseases. J Lab Clin Med 100:314, 1982.
96. Decker JL, et al: Rheumatoid arthritis: Evolving concepts of pathogenesis and treatment. Ann Intern Med 101:810, 1984.
*An excellent well-illustrated review of recent literature (1973 to 1983).*

## Polymyalgia Rheumatica and Giant Cell Arteritis

97. Dixon AS, et al: Polymyalgia rheumatica and temporal arteritis. Ann Rheum Dis 25:203, 1966.
*One of the earliest and best clinical reports, these authors identified 30 biopsy proven cases among 2222 rheumatologic patients who they had personally studied.*
98. Chuang TY, et al: Polymyalgia rheumatica. A 10-year epidemiologic and clinical study. Ann Intern Med 97:672, 1982.
*An excellent clinical and epidemiologic study, conducted by Mayo Clinic investigators in Olmstead County, Minnesota. A very good analysis of epidemiologic clinical and laboratory data and course of 96 patients.*
99. Hunder GG, Hazlemen BL: Giant cell arteritis and polymyalgia rheumatica. *In* Kelly WN, et al (eds.): Textbook of Rheumatology. Philadelphia, W.B. Saunders Company, 1981, p. 1190.
99a. Bird HA, et al: An evaluation of criteria for polymyalgia rheumatica. Ann Rheum Dis 38:434, 1979.

100. Bruk MI: Articular and vascular manifestations of polymyalgia rheumatica. Ann Rheum Dis 26:103, 1967.
100a. Pierce EW, Wright FW, Hill AGS: Sternoclavicular erosions in polymyalgia rheumatica. Ann Rheum Dis 42:379, 1983.
100b. O'Duffy D, Hunder GG, Wahner HW: A follow-up study of polymyalgia rheumatica: Evidence of chronic axial synovitis. J Rheumatol 7:5, 685, 1980.
101. O'Duffy JD, et al: Joint imaging in polymyalgia rheumatica. Mayo Clin Proc 51:519, 1976.
102. Weinberger K: Rheumatoid arthritis masquerading as polymyalgia rheumatica: Report of two cases. J Am Geriatr Soc 28:523, 1980.
103. Dimant J: Rheumatoid arthritis in the elderly, presenting as polymyalgia rheumatica. J Am Geriatr Soc. 27:183, 1979.
103a. Dixon A St.J: The diagnosis of polymyalgia rheumatica. In Hawkins C, Currey HLF (eds.): Reports on Rheumatic Diseases. Collected Reports 1959–1977. Arth Rheum Council, London, 1978, pp 61–63.
103b. Chang RW, Fineberg H: Risk-benefit considerations in the management of polymyalgia rheumatica. Med Decision Making 3:459, 1983.
104. Bengtsson BA, Malmvall BE: The epidemiology of giant cell arteritis including temporal arteritis and polymyalgia rheumatica. Incidences of different clinical presentations and eye complications. Arthritis Rheum 24:899, 1981.
105. Huston KA, Hunder GG: Giant cell (cranial) arteritis: A clinical review. Am Heart J 100:99, 1980.
106. Hauser WA, et al: Temporal arteritis in Rochester, Minnesota, 1951 to 1967. Mayo Clin Proc 46:596, 1971.
107. Liang GC, et al: Familial aggregation of polymyalgia rheumatica and giant cell arteritis. Arthritis Rheum 17:19, 1974.
108. Granato JE, Abben RP, May WS: Familial association of giant cell arteritis. A case report and brief review. Arch Intern Med 141:115, 1981.
109. Healey LA, Wilske KR: Presentation of occult giant cell arteritis. Arthritis Rheum. 23:641, 1980.
*This excellent clinical study of 74 patients, by one of the two American groups most interested in this topic, emphasizes that 40 per cent of patients will present with few manifestations to suggest the presence of this disease.*
110. Calamia KT, Hunder GG: Giant cell arteritis (temporal arteritis) presenting as fever of undetermined origin. Arthritis Rheum 24:1414, 1981.
*An excellent clinicopathologic review of 100 consecutive biopsy-proven cases collected over a $2\frac{1}{3}$-year period.*
111. Fauchald P, et al: Temporal arteritis and polymyalgia rheumatica. Clinical and biopsy findings. Ann Intern Med 77:845, 1972.
*This clinicopathologic study of 94 patients addresses the question: "How often will temporal artery biopsies be positive in patients with the clinical picture of polymyalgia rheumatica?"*
112. Hunder GG, Allen GL: Giant cell arteritis: A review. Bull Rheum Dis 29:980, 1978–79.
113. Calamia KT, Hunder GG: Clinical manifestations of giant cell (temporal) arteritis. Clin Rheum Dis 6:389, 1980.
114. Goodman BW Jr: Temporal arteritis. Am J Med 67:839, 1979.
*A good literature review from the perspective of a family physician. Contains 165 references on this topic and a "decision chart."*
115. Cohen DN, Damaske MM: Temporal arteritis: A spectrum of ophthalmic complications. Ann Ophthalmol 7:1045, 1975.
116. Klein RG, et al: Large artery involvement in giant cell (temporal) arteritis. Ann Intern Med. 83:806, 1975.
*An excellent clinical and pathologic study of 248 patients with large artery involvement. Contains 46 references.*
117. Wilkinson IMS, Russell RWR: Arteritis of the head and neck in giant cell arteritis. A pathological study to show the pattern of arterial involvement. Arch Neurol 27:378, 1972.
118. McMillan GC: Diffuse granulomatous aortitis with giant cells. Associated with partial rupture and dissection of the aorta. Arch Pathol 49:63, 1973.
119. Vinijchaikul K: Primary arteritis of the aorta and its main branches. (Takayasu's arteriopathy). A clinicopathologic autopsy study of eight cases. Am J Med 43:15, 1967.
120. Klein RG, Campbell RJ, Hunder GG: Skip lesions in temporal arteritis. Mayo Clin Proc 51:504, 1976.
121. Liang GC, Simkin PA, Mannik M: Immunoglobulins in temporal arteritis. An immunofluorescent study. Ann Intern Med 81:19, 1974.
*This excellent group of immunologic investigators studied patients already described by Dr. Healey.*
122. Park JR, Hazleman BL: Immunological and histological study of temporal arteritis. Ann Rheum Dis 37:238, 1978.
123. Jones JG, Hazleman BL: Prognosis and management of polymyalgia rheumatica. Ann Rheum Dis 40:1, 1981.

## *General References*

124. Brooke MH, Kaplan H: Muscle pathology in rheumatoid arthritis, polymyalgia rheumatica, and polymyositis. A histochemical study. Arch Pathol 94:101, 1972.
125. Long R, James O: Polymyalgia rheumatica and liver disease. Lancet 1:77, 1974.
126. Litwack KD, Bohan A, Silverman L: Granulomatous liver disease and giant cell arteritis. Case report and literature review. J Rheumatol 4:307, 1977.

## *Systemic Lupus Erythematosus*

127. Maddock RK: Incidence of systemic lupus erythematosus by age and sex. JAMA 191:149, 1965.
128. Urowitz MB, Stevens MB, Shulman LE: The influence of age on the clinical pattern of systemic lupus erythematosus. Arthritis Rheum 10:319, 1967.
129. Foad BS, Sheon RP, Kirsner AB: Systemic lupus erythematosus in the elderly. Arch Intern Med 130:743, 1972.
130. Dimant J, et al: Systemic lupus erythematosus in the older age group: Computer analysis. J Am Geriatr Soc 27:58, 1971.
131. Baker SB, et al: Late onset systemic lupus erythematosus. Am J Med 66:727, 1979.
132. Ballou SP, Kahn MA, Kushner I: Clinical features of systemic lupus erythematosus. Differences related to race and age of onset. Arthritis Rheum 25:55, 1982.
133. Baer AN, Pincus T: Occult systemic lupus erythematosus in elderly men. JAMA 24:249, 1983.
134. Catoggio LJ, Maddison PJ: Systemic lupus erythematosus in the elderly (abstract). Ann Rheum Dis 41:201, 1982.

135. Harmon CE, Postanova JP: Drug-induced lupus: Clinical and serological studies. Clin Rheum Dis 8:121, 1982.
136. Alarcon-Segovia D: Drug-induced lupus syndromes. Mayo Clin Proc 44:664, 1967.
137. Reidenberg MM: The chemical induction of systemic lupus erythematosus and lupus-like illness. Arthritis Rheum 24:1004, 1981.
*This is part of a symposium on drug-induced lupus, organized by a committee headed by EV Hess. All the publications in this symposium, published in this issue, provide helpful and detailed information on this syndrome.*

## Scleroderma

138. Williams PL, Gumpel JM: Scleroderma in the elderly: Case report. Br Med J 282:948, 198.
*This brief case report and subsequent letter of remonstrance illustrate the extent of disagreement that currently prevails concerning progressive systemic sclerosis in the elderly.*
139. Botstein GR, LeRoy C: Primary heart disease in systemic sclerosis (scleroderma): Advances in clinical and pathologic features, pathogenesis, and new therapeutic approaches. Am Heart J 102:913, 1981.
*This excellent article, with its bibliography of 63 references (1945 to 1979), provides a very good survey of current knowledge in this field, with exception of the more recent immunologic developments.*
140. Traub YM, et al: Hypertension and renal failure (scleroderma renal failure) in progressive systemic sclerosis. Review of a 25 year experience with 68 cases. Medicine 62:335, 1983.
*A clear, detailed review with special emphasis on therapy. Contains 121 references, from 1863 to 1981.*
141. Medsger TA, Masi AT: Epidemiology of systemic sclerosis (scleroderma). Ann Intern Med. 74:714, 1971.
142. Hodkinson HM: Scleroderma in the elderly, with special reference to the CRST syndrome. J Am Geriatr Soc 19:224, 1971.
143. Holti G, Schuster S: Scleroderma in the elderly. Letter to the Editor. Br Med J 282:1400, 1981.
144. Catoggio LJ, et al: Serological markers in progressive systemic sclerosis. Clinical correlations. Ann Rheum Dis. 41:111, 1982.

## Polymyositis

145. Medsger TA Jr, et al: The epidemiology of polymyositis. Am J Med 48:715, 1970.
146. Benbassat J, et al: The epidemiology of polymyositis-dermatomyositis in Israel 1960-76. Isr J Med Sci 16:197, 1980.
147. DeVere R, Bradley WG: Polymyositis: Its presentation, morbidity and mortality. Brain 98:637, 1975.
148. Bohan A, et al: A computer-assisted analysis of 153 patients with polymyositis and dermatomyositis. Medicine 56:255, 1977.
*The preceding two articles, one from Great Britain and the other from Dr. Carl Pearson's unit in the United States, provide thorough reviews of all clinical aspects of polymyositis/dermatomyositis, together with extensive bibliographies.*
149. Barnes BE: Dermatomyositis and malignancy. A review of the literature. Ann Intern Med 84:68, 1976.
150. Vesterager L, et al: Dermatomyositis and malignancy. Clin Exp Dermatol 5:31, 1980.
151. Callen JP, et al: The relationship of dermatomyositis and polymyositis to internal malignancy. Arch Dermatol 116:295, 1980.
152. Möller P, et al: Effect of aging on energy-rich phosphagens in human skeletal muscles. Clin Sci 58:553, 1980.
153. Sirca A, Susec-Michieli M: Selective type II fibre muscular atrophy in patients with osteoarthritis of the hip. J Neurol Sci 44:149, 1980.
154. Metzger AL, et al: Polymyositis and dermatomyositis. Combined methotrexate and corticoid therapy. Ann Intern Med 81:182, 1974.
155. Bunch TW, et al: Azathioprine with prednisone for polymyositis: A controlled clinical trial. Ann Intern Med 92:365, 1980.

## Total Knee Replacement

156. Coventry MB, et al: A new geometric need for total knee arthroplasty. Clin Orthop 83:157, 1972.
157. Gunston FH: Polycentric knee arthroplasty. Prosthetic stimulation of normal knee movement. J Bone Joint Surg 53B:272, 1971.
158. Insall JN, et al: The total condylar knee prosthesis. A report of 220 cases. J Bone Joint Surg 61:173, 1979.
159. Hungersford S, et al: Preliminary experience with a total knee prosthesis with porous coating used without cement. Clin Orthop 176:95, 1983.
160. Insall JN, et al: A comparison of four models of total hip replacement prosthesis. J Bone Joint Surg 55A:754, 1976.
161. Insall JN, et al: The total condylar knee prosthesis and gonarthrosis. A five to nine-year follow-up of the first 100 consecutive replacements. J Bone Joint Surg 65A:619, 1983.
162. Bowers WH: A rational plan for the use of preventive antibiotics in orthopaedic surgery. Instr Course Lect 26:30, 1977.
163. Stulberg BN, et al: Deep vein thrombosis following total knee replacement. J Bone Joint Surg 66A:194, 1984.
164. Evarts CM: Thromboembolic disease. Instr Course Lect 28:67, 1979.
165. Charnley J: Total hip replacement by low-friction arthroplasty. Clin Orthop 72:7, 1970.
166. Charnley J, Cupic Z: The nine and ten year results of the low-friction arthroplasty of the hip. Clin Orthop 95:9, 1973.
167. Muller ME: Total hip prostheses. Clin Orthop 72:46, 1970.
168. Salvati EA, et al: A ten-year follow-up study of our first one hundred consecutive Charnley total hip replacements. J Bone Joint Surg 63A:753, 1981.
169. Stauffer RN: Ten-year follow-up study of total hip replacement. J Bone Joint Surg 64A:983, 1982.
170. Engh CA: Hip arthroplasty with a Moore prosthesis with porous coating—a five-year study. Clin Orthop 176:52, 1983.
171. Harris WH, et al: Comparison of warfarin, low-molecular-weight dextran, aspirin, and subcutaneous heparin in prevention of venous thromboembolism following total hip replacement. J Bone Joint Surg 56A:1552, 1974.

# *Paget's Disease of Bone*

*Stanley Wallach*

## DEMOGRAPHIC CONSIDERATIONS

Paget's disease of bone afflicts approximately 3 per cent of the population over the age of 40 in the United States and is therefore a disease that geriatricians can expect to see frequently. Most often, only one to three bones in nonstrategic areas are involved, with few—or, at most, trivial—symptoms. In approximately 25 per cent of cases, the disease extends over a greater amount of the skeleton, often asymmetrically, with the production of significant symptomatology and disability caused by pain, deformities, and other skeletal disturbances. A variety of manifestations involving the neurologic and cardiovascular systems may also complicate the situation and produce additional disability.

The cause of Paget's disease is unknown, but recent studies suggest a "slow virus" etiology superimposed upon a hereditary disposition. Several different viruses, including the measles virus, respiratory syncytial virus and parainfluenza virus 3, have been suggested, but none has been definitely indicated. Demographic studies suggest a focal incidence, with the highest frequencies in the United Kingdom, New Zealand, Australia, Germany, France, and the United States in that approximate order. A particular area in Lancashire, England, has a frequency of 6 to 8 per cent. Another focus exists in southwest Italy near Naples, where giant cell tumors of bone occur in association. In contrast, the disease is uncommon elsewhere and is especially rare in Scandinavia and the Orient and among the black races. Depending on the series, there is a 15 to 50 per cent incidence of Paget's disease in more than one family member. Both parents and siblings of the patient are ten times likelier to have the condition than are relatives of spouses of the patient. In some families, there is linkage to the human leukocyte antigen (HLA) haplotype.

## PATHOGENESIS

Whatever the etiology, the first pathogenetic event is the stimulation of *osteoclasts,* presumably by an intracellular virus that has lain dormant for a variable period. Such stimulation causes the osteoclasts to increase their size and number, to change their morphology, to acquire an unusually large number of nuclei, and to begin resorbing bone in an accelerated, chaotic fashion. Extremely rapid, disorganized bone resorption ensues, extending radially or linearly from an initial focus. At the same time, *osteoblasts* and their progenitors are signaled to attempt repair by forming new bone. The new bone formation is equally rapid, disorganized, and uncontrolled, and an excessive amount of bone of poor architectural quality is produced. As this process is repeated several times, an enlarged, thickened, structurally inadequate bone is produced; the new bone has low resistance to stress, causes pain, and tends to become deformed and to fracture. Such bone is also highly vascularized and has an extensive low-pressure capillary system.

Rates of bone resorption, formation, and blood flow in afflicted bones may be increased 20-fold over normal, as reflected by increased urinary excretion of hydroxyproline, a marker for bone resorption; an elevated serum alkaline phosphatase, a product of osteoblastic activity; and accelerated turnover of "bone-seeking" elements such as radiotechnetium. Radiotechnetium uptake forms the basis for the use of conventional bone scans to identify pagetic foci in the skeleton, whereas the biochemical abnormalities can be used to quantitate the degree of disturbed skeletal metabolism and the response to treatment.

The explanation for the predilection of Paget's disease for older individuals is unclear, but, again, may be largely a result of the putative slow virus etiology. The condition is unknown to affect individuals in the first decade of life, and patients previously labeled as having "juvenile Paget's disease" actually have been found to have either familial bone dysplasia with hyperphosphatasia or polyostotic fibrous dysplasia. Only rare cases of Paget's disease have been observed in the late second decade. However, many patients presenting with Paget's disease after age 40 can recall significant but disregarded symptomatology extending over a 10- to 20-year period previously; that is, the onset of the condition may require a relatively long "incubation period" followed by an equally long period of mild but progressive symptoms that carries the patient into the second half-century of life before the opportunity for diagnosis arises. Since exposure to the causative agent may presumably occur at any age, a delay in diagnosis of 20 to 40 years would explain the apparent geriatric predisposition. However, it is possible that age-related changes in susceptibility or expression of the causative agent may also be due to an altered immune system.

**Table 36–11.** MUSCULOSKELETAL FEATURES OF PAGET'S DISEASE

| |
|---|
| Pain |
| Skeletal, muscular, osteoarthritic, radicular, headache |
| Deformities |
| Thickening, bowing, enlarged head, kyphosis, acetabular protrusion |
| Fractures |
| Complete fractures, tendon avulsions, fissure fractures, vertebral compression and collapse |
| Neoplasms |
| Osteosarcoma, other sarcomas, giant cell tumors |
| Miscellaneous |
| Osteoporosis circumscripta, osteoarthritis, increased bone vascularity and skin temperature |

## DISEASE COURSE

The natural course of Paget's disease can be summarized as slow but progressive. When the causative agent has invaded relatively few skeletal foci in nonstrategic areas, the condition may remain asymptomatic and trivial throughout life; in such a case, the diagnosis may be made only because of abnormalities accidentally uncovered during multiphasic screening, bone x-ray films, or bone scans taken for unrelated reasons. In other instances, the tempo of the disease may be more rapid and the disease advances measurably from one or more initial foci to involve large portions of bones; in this case, major symptomatology is produced. Nevertheless, the disease course takes decades for full expression, and the overall prognosis for survival is excellent, although moderate to severe disability may be present. Unlike certain other conditions afflicting the older population, Paget's disease usually shows no discernible tendency for the tempo to moderate with advancing age; disabling symptoms, therefore, progress at the same time that degenerative diseases intrude and natural stamina wanes. The incidence of "burned-out" Paget's disease is rarer than portrayed, and it usually occurs in patients with only trivial or moderate involvement.

## CLINICAL FEATURES

The major clinical phenomena seen in Paget's disease are summarized in Tables 36–11 through 36–14.

### *Musculoskeletal Features*

**Pain.** Pain is the most common presenting symptom, but it is variable in both character and cause. Pain may arise from direct neural stimulation in involved bone, muscular injury secondary to improper use of deformed extremities, arthritis secondary to either pagetic changes in subchondral bone or abnormal joint function caused by deformity, or neurologic impingement secondary to involvement of the skull or vertebral column. Headache is particularly common when the skull is affected.

**Deformities and Fractures.** Although deformities and fractures are the most common serious outgrowths of the structural inadequacy of pagetic bones, a variety of other problems can also arise. Deformities of the lower extremities, especially when they cause pain, seriously impair gait and can predispose a person to falls. Spontaneous fractures do not occur in Paget's disease, but fractures with minimal trauma are common. The fractures range from avulsions of tendon insertions, as on the anterior superior iliac spine or tibial tubercle, to complete horizontal or transverse fractures. Small cracks may appear in the cortex of deformed long bones; these fissure fractures may be the site of later complete fractures. Contrary to popular notion, not all pagetic fractures heal uneventfully; moreover, delayed union or non-union can occur in up to 40 per cent of fractures, especially at the upper end of the femora. Paget's disease of the acetabular area or the femoral head is very common and is prone to cause chronic disabling hip joint symptoms simulating osteoarthritis. When acetabular involvement is severe, acetabular protrusion may complicate the picture.

**Neoplasms.** The most dreaded skeletal complication of Paget's disease is malignant conversion to an osteosarcoma or other type of mesenchymal tumor. Sarcoma of the pelvis, humerus, femur, or skull accounts for 80 per cent of the cases. Although malignant degeneration associated with pre-existent Paget's disease accounts for 30 per cent of all bone sarcomas arising after age 40, the complication is actually uncommon, afflicting less than 1 per cent of Paget's disease patients during their lifetimes. The most common event heralding malignant conversion is not a sudden increase in alkaline phosphatase level but worsening pain or a change in previous pain pattern. With rare exceptions, bone malignancies arising in pagetic lesions are rapidly fatal.

## *Neurologic Features*

Neurologic complications of Paget's disease result from a combination of neurologic impingement by a deformed skull or spinal column and the ability of these bones to "steal" blood flow from the neurologic structures they encase. Paget's disease of the skull can affect any cranial nerve, but deficits in visual function, hearing, and balance are particularly disabling to the elderly. In addition to direct optic nerve dysfunction, orbital bone involvement can cause papilledema by obstructing venous return from the retina and may even cause proptosis when extreme. Angioid streaks or mottling of the retina can occur in up to 20 per cent of cases. Visual field defects and loss of visual acuity are sometimes progressive and can lead to blindness.

High-frequency hearing loss is the most common neurologic deficit in Paget's disease and is present in almost all patients with extensive skull involvement. Although of a mixed type, the sensorineural component caused by impingement on, or vascular deprivation of, the cochlea dominates the picture. Unlike the high-frequency hearing loss that is due to presbyacusis, pagetic hearing loss progresses more rapidly, with an average of a 2-decibel loss per year compared with an average 0.5 decibel loss per year in presbyacusis. One recent report suggests that serial audiograms may distinguish the two entities. Annoying tinnitus is much less common than a hearing deficit.

**Table 36–12.** NEUROLOGIC FEATURES OF PAGET'S DISEASE

Cranial nerves
1. Optic atrophy, papilledema, proptosis, angioid streaks, retinal mottling, oculomotor palsies
2. Deafness, tinnitus
3. Facial sensory loss, Bell's palsy, trigeminal neuralgia, hemifacial spasm
4. Dysphagia, dysarthria, pharyngeal, lingual and shoulder muscle weakness

Medulla and cerebellum
Ataxia, cerebellar signs, Valsalva-induced headache, hydrocephalus-dementia syndrome

Spinal cord and nerves
Myelopathy, radiculoneuropathy, corda equina syndrome

Miscellaneous
Pagetic "steal" syndromes, peripheral neuropathy, carpal and tarsal tunnel syndromes

Balance and gait disturbances do not usually arise from vestibular dysfunction, which is rare, but from cerebellar disturbances secondary to posterior skull involvement. Platybasia and basilar impression result from the weakened occiput "sagging" on the cervical spine with consequent lower cranial nerve deficits, ataxia- and Valsalva-induced cranial pain due to partial obstruction of cerebrospinal fluid (CSF) flow in the region of the sylvian aqueduct. A very rare symptom complex known as the *hydrocephalus-dementia syndrome*—consisting of dementia, ataxia, urinary incontinence, and headache—can also result from pagetic skull involvement. The hydrocephalus is either of a high-pressure type caused by obstruction of CSF flow in the region of the basal cisterns or of a low-pressure type of obscure pathogenesis. Defective CSF resorption by the arachnoidal granulations due to Paget's disease of the cranium may contribute.

Neurologic deficits involving the spinal cord, cauda equina, or exiting spinal nerves occur in approximately 3 per cent of Paget's disease patients, although vertebral column involvement occurs five times more frequently. These very disabling deficits may be presaged by a variety of subtle symptoms in the elderly, such as midback pain with or without girdle or sciatic radiation, buttock or hip pain, numbness and weakness of muscle groups in the lower extremities, an ill-defined and inconstant sensory loss that does not follow dermatome distribution, minor sphincter abnormalities, and depressed deep tendon reflexes. Both radiculoneuropathy and myelopathy develop gradually over several months, but the latter sometimes occurs suddenly after sudden collapse of a pagetic vertebra. Radiculopathy is often manifested only by pain of appropriate distribution, but it can also cause muscle weakness, patchy sensory loss, and sphincter abnormalities. Myelopathy is characterized by spastic weakness of the legs, progressing to paraparesis and then paraplegia, a sensory level, and loss of sphincter control. Deep tendon reflexes eventually become hyperactive with a positive Babinski sign.

Two peripheral neurologic problems are also seen in Paget's disease—peripheral neuropathies of various types and carpal and tarsal tunnel syndromes. The pathogenesis of these lesions is not clear, since the lesions usually cannot be ascribed to nerve entrapment by expanding pagetic lesions. A peripheral nerve vascular "steal syndrome" similar to that described for the brain and spinal cord may be responsible, although no clear evidence for this exists.

### *Cardiovascular Features*

Cardiovascular complications derive from a combination of factors, such as (1) increased blood flow through low-pressure capillaries in pagetic bone, (2) calcinosis of major blood vessels and the endocardium, and (3) the severe atherogenesis to which many pagetic patients are prone.

**Increase in Blood Flow.** The increased vascular cross section in pagetic bones can lead to increased blood volume, high cardiac output, cardiomegaly, left ventricular hypertrophy, and depressed myocardial contractibility. Contrary to popular notion, high-output cardiac failure is uncommon, possibly because of the coexistence of vascular calcinosis and coronary atherosclerosis.

**Calcification.** Medial calcinosis of large and medium-sized arteries is common, but it does not seriously impair blood flow. Calcinosis of the aortic valve, the mitral valve annulus, and the perimitral subendocardium occurs in up to 30 per cent of patients, resulting in varying degrees of hemodynamic impairment. The calcinosis may predispose to interventricular conduction defects.

**Atherosclerosis.** Atherosclerotic disease of the coronary and peripheral circulation causes serious problems independently of Paget's disease. Since it reduces total blood flow to the head and spine, it can also intensify deprivation of blood flow to neural structures caused by "steal" to the low-pressure capillary bed of adjacent pagetic bone. These consequences of Paget's disease can be especially serious in the elderly.

**Table 36–13.** CARDIOVASCULAR FEATURES OF PAGET'S DISEASE

| |
|---|
| Increased blood flow in pagetic bone |
| Increased blood volume, high cardiac output, cardiomegaly, left ventricular hypertrophy, depressed myocardial contractility, "steal" syndromes |
| Cardiovascular calcification |
| Arterial medial calcinosis, calcific aortic stenosis, mitral annulus calcification, subendocardial calcification |
| Generalized atherosclerosis |

## LABORATORY AND IMAGING FEATURES

Laboratory and imaging studies in Paget's disease are usually diagnostic. With other than trivial disease, the serum alkaline phosphatase level and urinary hydroxyproline excretion are elevated, sometimes markedly to values greater than 20 times normal. The serum acid phosphatase level may be falsely recorded as slightly elevated when a very high alkaline phosphatase level is present. Urinary hydroxyproline determinations require fastidious attention to detail, and the accuracy of the laboratory must be validated. It is also necessary to have patients restrict their intake of hydroxyproline and gelatin-containing foods such as candy, cakes and pies, jellies, puddings and gelatins, ice cream, marshmallow, fish, gristle and cartilage, sausage, luncheon meats, and creamy salad dressings for 3 days including the day of collection. Because of the difficulties attending accurate hydroxyproline measurements, it is acceptable to use the serum alkaline phosphatase alone as an objective measure of disease activity and response to treatment.

When other multiphasic screening tests are abnormal, they indicate the presence of other diagnoses that either are associated with or are independent of the Paget's disease. Hypercalcemia is rarely seen in Paget's disease, even with extensive immobilization, and usually indicates the presence of associated hyperparathyroidism or an independent hypercalcemic condition. On the other hand, hypercalcuria is common and may predispose to calcium stone formation. Hyperuricemia is also common and indicates either essential hyperuricemia or an associated gouty diathesis, including uric acid stone formation.

Skeletal x-ray films are usually diagnostic, although several different patterns can be seen. In most patients, affected bones are thickened and deformed and show widespread sclerosis of both the cortical and trabecular components. In vertebrae, the sclerosis may ultimately lead to completely opaque vertebrae. At the other end of the

**Table 36–14.** METABOLIC FEATURES OF PAGET'S DISEASE

| |
|---|
| Calcium |
| Hypercalciuria, calcium stones, hyperparathyroidism, hypercalcemia (rare) |
| Uric acid |
| Essential hyperuricemia, gout, uric acid stones |

spectrum, pagetic bones may show almost exclusively resorptive features manifested by a discrete demarcation zone between a resorbing front of pagetic activity and normal bone. This front, usually wedge-shaped in long bones and fan-shaped in the skull, is erroneously named *osteoporosis circumscripta.* In many patients, both sclerotic and resorptive features are present simultaneously with lenticular-shaped areas of resorption interspaced between sclerotic areas. Linear horizontal imperfections called *fissure fractures* are sometimes present along the convex edge of deformed long bones, especially the femora. The combination of Paget's disease and osteoporosis (either spontaneous or due to immobilization from a previous fracture) can be deceptive, since the sclerotic features can then be very subtle.

Bone scans frequently indicate more areas of pagetic activity than do x-ray films, since they depend on increased metabolic turnover, a much earlier event than the final evolution of radiographic abnormalities. In well-established cases, extensive areas of radiotechnetium uptake in a bone distinguish Paget's disease from the more discrete patchy uptake characteristic of metastatic disease. Computed tomography (CT) scanning has recently been applied to pagetic bone lesions and has greatly simplified diagnosis in the occasional difficult case, in malignant degeneration, and in suspected neurologic impingement.

## DIFFERENTIAL DIAGNOSIS

The differential diagnosis of Paget's disease presents little difficulty in the elderly, since pathognomonic sclerotic as well as resorptive features are usually present on x-ray films. The serum alkaline phosphatase level is usually, but not invariably, elevated, depending on the extent and activity of the pagetic lesions. On rare occasions, the diagnosis may be confused with two other entities causing hyperphosphatasia—polyostotic fibrous dysplasia (Albright's disease) and blastic skeletal metastases from nonosseous neoplasms, such as those affecting the prostate, breast, and other organs. Polyostotic fibrous dysplasia almost invariably produces significant skeletal and other symptoms during the first or second decade whereas Paget's disease only rarely begins in the second decade. The x-ray appearance of polyostotic fibrous dysplasia, although having both sclerotic and resorptive features, has a different pattern of involvement, and the two entities are easily distinguished by an experienced radiologist. Skin pigmentation (café au lait spots) and premature menarche are features often present in polyostotic fibrous dysplasia and absent in Paget's disease.

Blastic skeletal metastases may occasionally present a problem in differential diagnosis because the sclerotic bone can resemble that in Paget's disease. In general, blastic metastases are more discrete (although more widespread), do not produce as much sclerosis of cortical bone, and usually do not cause expansion of the cortical envelope of involved bones. However, exceptions to all three characteristics have occurred, resulting in misdiagnosis. The known presence of a neoplasm capable of metastasizing to bone with blastic features should alert the clinician. The only definitive differential test may be a bone marrow or bone biopsy.

In patients with a great deal of distortion of bony architecture, a different type of differential diagnosis may be important, i.e., the determination of whether or not malignant degeneration of a pagetic lesion has occurred. Suspicion of such an event should be based on the x-ray appearance of the lesion and not on clinical, biochemical, or bone scan findings. A large area of resorption in previously sclerotic bone, loss of a reasonably sharp edge to the cortical envelope, and extension of bone fragments beyond the confines of the cortex are all highly suggestive features. Computed tomography has proved very helpful in confirming such suspicions because this modality usually discloses tumor masses not apparent on film. Biopsy is usually required to confirm the diagnosis.

Perhaps the most important differential diagnosis is a determination of whether the pain and disability are due to pagetic activity, to the associated osteoarthritis of joints adjacent to pagetic bones, or to both. It is sometimes impossible to make this distinction, but therapeutic trials with specific drugs for Paget's disease and nonsteroidal anti-inflammatory agents (NSAID) given singly and together may be tried. This problem is common when Paget's disease involves the acetabular region of the pelvis and/or the femoral head. Distortion of the acetabular cup and femoral head and loss of joint space are usually present and do not predict whether or not the patient's symptoms and disability will respond to a specific agent alone, a NSAID alone, or the two in combination or whether it is intractable. The decision to undertake total hip replacement is based on the response to therapy and must be made carefully.

## DIAGNOSIS

The diagnosis of Paget's disease is straightforward and requires a combination of characteristic historical and physical features, typical x-ray changes, and elevated serum alkaline phosphatase and urinary hydroxyproline levels. In many cases, especially in those with minimal or trivial involvement, the clinical and biochemical features may be absent. Even the x-ray evaluation may not reveal abnormalities in very early cases, with only the bone scan positive. However, a positive bone scan alone is not sufficient for diagnosis because any skeletal lesion with increased focal turnover will cause increased radiotechnetium uptake. Also, both benign pagetic lesions and malignant degeneracies will produce the same bone scan pattern so that radiographs must be taken of all parts of the skeleton with positive bone scan uptake to assess structural features. Very rarely, so-called burned-out pagetic lesions will be evident on x-ray examination but have no increased uptake on bone scan because of low residual disease activity. Such lesions, nevertheless, can be symptomatic.

With an adequate workup and knowledge of the variations possible among the diagnostic modalities, the diagnosis of Paget's disease is simple and few errors of commission are likely. However, errors of omission are more common, in that patients may have nonspecific or variant symptoms that suggest an arthritis or functional musculoskeletal disorder and that do not lead to appropriate diagnostic tests. In view of the relatively high frequency of Paget's disease in the geriatric population, a reasonably high index of suspicion should be maintained by physicians who care for older patients with painful syndromes.

**Table 36-15.** INDICATIONS FOR SPECIFIC TREATMENT OF PAGET'S DISEASE

| |
|---|
| Pain — moderate to severe, not relieved by NSAID* |
| Progressive skeletal involvement |
| Fractures, platybasia and basilar invagination, vertebral compression and collapse, moderate to severe acetabular protrusion, progressing deformities |
| Extensive bone resorption |
| Osteoporosis circumscripta, resorptive fronts, lenticular-shaped areas of resorption, fissure fractures |
| Neurologic deficits |
| All types except nonprogressive deafness |
| Progressing visual defects or deafness |
| Preparation for orthopedic surgery |
| Prolonged immobilization |
| Acute fractures, post-surgery, etc. |
| Cardiovascular complications secondary to increased cardiac output |
| Extreme elevations of biochemical parameters |

* NSAID = Nonsteroidal anti-inflammatory drug.

## MANAGEMENT

The management of Paget's disease involves definition of the full extent of the disease, the degree of disability, and the potential for future disability. As indicated earlier, at least 75 per cent of diagnosed cases are of minor consequence and the patient usually needs only reassurance or, at most, the judicious use of safe analgesics or a NSAID. However, in approximately 25 per cent of cases, more intense treatment is needed. The criteria for applying such treatment are given in Table 36-15. Pain is the most common reason for a patient to consult a physician and for treatment to be instituted. A thorough medical history and physical examination, supplemented by skeletal films, a bone scan, and biochemical tests, should enable the physician to determine whether there are features indicating progressive skeletal involvement or predominant bone resorption that can render the patient especially susceptible to fracture. Many authorities believe that fissure fractures predispose to complete fractures, but this point is controversial, since fissure fractures may exist for decades without a complete fracture. Neurologic deficits constitute a most serious complication of Paget's disease and are almost always an indication for treatment. All pagetic patients with skull involvement should have complete ophthalmologic and auditory evaluations. Progressive abnormalities in either the eyes or ears are often pagetic in cause, and treatment may arrest progression. Established hearing loss is seldom if ever improved by treatment, and a stable audiometric deficit is not by itself a reason to treat.

Pagetic bone is highly vascular and may bleed excessively during surgery. Treatment reduces bone blood flow dramatically and lessens the risk of this surgical complication. There is no evidence that healing itself is speeded. However, pagetic bones, when immobilized because of fractures or surgery, manifest a rapid rate of bone loss and severe demineralization, with an added predisposition to further fractures. Treatment started before or at the onset of immobilization may prevent the bone loss because it is due to a further intensification of bone resorption.

The first cardiovascular complication listed in Table 36-14 (increased bone blood flow) can also be ameliorated by treatment. Since the other cardiovascular complications (calcification and atherosclerosis) are not reversible, overall cardiovascular performance will not always improve. Similarly, relief of "steal syndromes" may not improve neurologic phenomena that are due to direct neural impingement or atherosclerotic obstruction to blood flow.

The least clear-cut indication for treatment is the presence of very elevated biochemical parameters (greater than four times the upper limit of normal) in the absence of other indications. There are no data indicating that long-term outcome is improved in such patients by intermittent episodes or prolonged periods of treatment. If clinical features suggest that other indications are imminent, it is best to treat. In completely asymptomatic patients, close observation without treatment is preferred.

Paget's disease that is deemed not to require specific treatment requires much simpler management. Such patients should be seen once or twice a year for an assessment of new skeletal symptoms and physical findings, a neurologic examination if there is cranial or spinal involvement, and a measurement of the serum alkaline phosphatase level. A yearly eye examination, including visual field studies, and yearly audiometry should be done in patients with skull involvement. The bone scan should be repeated approximately every 3 years and radiographs then taken of previously known and newly discovered areas of involvement to ensure that no serious structural defects or x-ray evidence of malignant degeneration has developed in the interim. If only slow progression of the condition is indicated, the patient can be reassured until the next re-evaluation. If there is some pain, a NSAID can be prescribed.

## *Specific Agents*

In patients meeting one or more of the indications in Table 36-15 (excluding item 9), one of the three available specific agents for Paget's disease should be considered. These three agents—calcitonin, disodium etidronate (EHDP), and mithramycin—are described in Table 36-16. These drugs act by inhibition of osteoclastic bone resorption, although their mechanisms differ. As the rapid, chaotic bone resorption characteristic of the disorder is diminished, the vascularity of the involved skeleton decreases and a comparable deceleration in the rate of bone formation occurs with facilitation of normal lamellar bone formation along lines of stress. With continued remodeling, areas of predominant bone resorption disappear

**Table 36-16.** CHARACTERISTICS OF SPECIFIC DRUGS FOR PAGET'S DISEASE

| | Calcitonin | Disodium Etidronate | Mithramycin |
|---|---|---|---|
| Mechanism of action | Hormonal inhibition of bone resorption | Chemisorption to bone surfaces, rendering them inert | Toxic damage to osteoclasts |
| Route of administration | SC, IM | Oral | IV |
| Dose range | 50-100 MRC units daily to tiw | 5-20 mg/kg daily on empty stomach | 25 mcg/kg daily or qod for 9-10 doses |
| Duration of treatment | 6-36 months with subsequent courses as needed | 1-6 month courses with repeat courses 3-6 months afterwards | Repeat courses as needed |
| Side effects | 1. GI (anorexia, nausea, vomiting)<br>2. Dermatologic (nonspecific rash)<br>3. Other: facial flushing | 1. GI (nausea, vomiting, diarrhea)<br>2. Skeletal (increased bone pain) | 1. GI (anorexia, nausea, vomiting)<br>2. Hepatic (abnormal liver function tests)<br>3. Renal (abnormal urinalysis, increased BUN and serum creatinine)<br>4. Hematologic (thrombocytopenia with GI hemorrhage) |
| Potential for resistance | Primary: 15%; secondary: 10-30% | Primary: 15%; secondary: 5-10% | None reported |

Abbreviations: SC = subcutaneous; IM = intramuscular; IV = intravenous; GI = gastrointestinal; MRC = Medical Research Council (U.K.); BUN = blood urea nitrogen; tiw = three times a week; qod = every other day.

or become smaller, the texture of bone improves, and thickened bones may actually become thinner.

There are several forms of calcitonin, but only the synthetic salmon molecule (SCT) is marketed in the United States because of its greater potency. EHDP has an additional skeletal action which is undesirable, the inhibition of bone mineralization with the production of excess unmineralized bone matrix (osteoid). New analogs of EHDP being studied in Europe do not appear to exert this undesirable action at doses that effectively inhibit bone resorption, but these newer analogs are not as yet available for routine use in the United States.

In most patients with Paget's disease that is severe enough to treat, the sclerotic features of the disease predominate over the resorptive ones and there are no unusual conditions, such as a recent fracture or a requirement for orthopedic surgery. In such patients, each of the drugs just mentioned will produce approximately the same beneficial effects on relief of symptoms, neurologic status, and serum alkaline phosphatase and urinary hydroxyproline levels. Mithramycin and EHDP may produce a greater decrease in biochemical parameters than SCT, which will last longer after the course of treatment is completed, but symptomatic improvement is the same and the data demonstrating improved neurologic status are strongest for SCT.

In general, the choice of an agent will be between SCT and EHDP, both of which can be given on an outpatient basis; mithramycin will be held in reserve for resistant cases because it is the most toxic of the treatments and generally requires hospitalization. Some experience with outpatient intravenous mithramycin has been reported. EHDP is more convenient than SCT since it can be given orally. However, it must be given as a single daily dose on an empty stomach. Recent experimentation with SCT nasal spray suggests it may be effective, obviating the need for parenteral administration.

Side effects of SCT treatment occur in approximately 30 per cent of patients, are usually mild, and regress as treatment continues (Table 36–16). Gastrointestinal side effects with EHDP are rare, but increased bone pain resulting from the production of excess osteoid occurs in approximately 20 per cent of patients given 5 mg/kg and in a higher fraction of patients given higher doses for more than a month. Increased rates of fracture and worsening resorptive features have been reported at doses above 5 mg/kg, but it is unclear whether the 5 mg/kg dose has ever caused such serious side effects.

Both SCT and EHDP fail to affect either symptoms or biochemical parameters in approximately 15 per cent of cases. Fortunately, most patients with primary resistance to one agent will respond to the other. Secondary resistance can occur with both agents, but is more common with SCT. Antibodies to the salmon molecule will develop in 30 to 60 per cent of patients, but they are generally of low titer and do not block the therapeutic effect. In 5 to 10 per cent of patients, high titers of anti-salmon calcitonin antibody appear with a return of symptoms and biochemical parameters to pretreatment levels. In such patients, human calcitonin, still a research drug in the United States, can be used to reinduce a therapeutic effect. However, in a larger number of resistant patients, antibody titers remain low and an unexplained escape from the therapeutic effect occurs. A similar "escape phenomenon" occurs with human calcitonin in a comparable number of patients. A common conceptual error in the course of calcitonin treatment, regardless of the type used, is to regard as resistance the usual plateau achieved by the biochemical parameters at some level above the normal range but significantly below pretreatment levels. Even a small rebound in these levels during the latter part of a treatment course is satisfactory as long as the clinical features continue to improve or maintain previously attained improvement.

There are no satisfactory long-term comparative studies with any of the calcitonins to indicate the desired duration of courses of treatment. Some therapists treat for as long as 36 months without respite even though maximal clinical and biochemical improvement is usually achieved in the first 12 months. Others treat for 6 months at a time or until maximal clinical and biochemical improvement occurs. The major problem is that the longer the course of treatment or the more intermittent the treatment, the more likely resistance to calcitonin is to appear. Therapeutic periods of approximately 18 months' duration may minimize resistance, but this is by no means certain.

Generally, EHDP is given in 6-month courses at a dose of 5 mg/kg daily. Higher doses are rarely justified. Such courses can be repeated relatively early, after 3 to 6 month rest periods, should there be an early return of symptoms. Recently, 1-month courses of 20 mg/kg daily have been employed, but it is unclear whether the overall results are superior. Intravenous EHDP and newer analogues are being researched in Europe and appear to offer a more rapid induction of the therapeutic effect.

After a course of SCT is completed, it is expected that the biochemical parameters will return to pretreatment levels by 6 to 12 months, whereas EHDP may have a prolonged inhibitory effect. In most patients, however, clinical improvement will last considerably longer, and it is loss of clinical effect rather than biochemical regression that should indicate a repeat course of treatment. With EHDP, the reverse has also been observed, i.e., clinical regression with continued inhibition of biochemical parameters. In such patients the results of retreatment are more difficult to assess because of the loss of objective parameters of response. As patient experience mounts and patients receive a large number of retreatment courses, doubly resistant patients who will respond only to mithramycin are beginning to appear in increasing numbers. It is nevertheless advisable not to withhold treatment with SCT or EHDP when a clear indication exists, since mithramycin is an option when needed and newer, more effective agents will undoubtedly appear during the next few years.

As noted earlier, osteoarthritis is almost always present in moderate to severe Paget's disease. In many instances, it is impossible to distinguish osteoarthritic from pagetic pain. Since NSAID are not innocuous in the elderly and may contribute to renal failure from other insults such as radiographic dyes, nephrotoxic drugs, and hypovolemia, it is generally best to treat Paget's disease first and if there is residual pain despite a good biochemical response, add a NSAID. On occasion, this maneuver has been necessary to achieve a good clinical response and avert therapeutic defeat.

## *Operative Treatment*

The availability of specific medical therapy for Paget's disease has greatly lessened the indications for orthopedic or neurosurgical operations and also has helped clarify their proper place in present-day therapy. In general, such surgery should be avoided if at all possible. Contrary to common belief, pagetic bone does not necessarily heal well after fractures and surgical procedures, and the frequency of non-union, infection, periarticular calcification and ossification are similar to those to be expected in elderly patients in general. More importantly, the consequent immobilization of the patient causes marked loss of bone and may result in greater disability than the original problem. Finally, the surgical complications unique to pagetic bone—excessive bleeding, sufficient sclerosis to interfere with the procedure itself, and later loosening of prosthetic materials—must be considered.

Nevertheless, operative procedures should not be delayed when they are clearly indicated. The most common need is total hip replacement in patients with severe acetabular and/or femoral head involvement who have failed to respond to both SCT and EHDP with a NSAID added. Operative repair of fractures is also a clear indication. Rapidly advancing neurologic deficits constitute a third indication, since there may not be sufficient time to assess the effects of medical therapy. Whenever possible, osteotomies to correct deformities should be avoided and other means should be undertaken to help the patient, such as shoe lifts. Braces also cause immobilization and should not be used except as a last resort. Post-operative casts should be removed as early as possible, and active rehabilitative programs should be started as soon after surgery as possible.

Except in emergencies, SCT in usual therapeutic doses should be given preoperatively to reduce bone vascularity and lessen the rate of skeletal turnover. A recent study indicates that as little as 1 week of SCT therapy can decrease blood flow; however, a 3- to 6-month course of treatment is preferable. In some cases, SCT treatment may initiate a clinical response that will obviate the need for surgery. This is particularly true with Paget's disease of the hip and neurologic deficits involving the lower cranial nerves and the spinal cord and nerves. These neurologic deficits generally progress slowly enough to permit a trial of medical therapy before determining the need for neurosurgical intervention. The rare hydrocephalus-dementia syndrome will always require ventricular shunting in addition to drug therapy. Although EHDP will also reduce bone vascularity and improve structure, it should not be used preoperatively when the patient is responsive to SCT because the additional inhibitory effect on bone mineralization could impede healing. In fact, it is better to keep the patient off EHDP for 6 months before elective but necessary orthopedic surgery.

## *Family Considerations*

With an illness as chronic and disabling as Paget's disease, the family most often plays a critical role in patient support (Table 36–17). Family members must be aware of the clinical features of the disease and their impact on the patient. Fortunately, pagetic patients usually manifest no loss of mental ability as a result of

**Table 36–17.** IMPACT OF PAGET'S DISEASE ON THE PATIENT AND FAMILY

| |
|---|
| Creation of hazard-free home environment |
| Reduction of stairs and number of living levels |
| Surveillance of analgesic use |
| Adjustment of slowed locomotion |
| Adjustment to visual and auditory impairment |
| Acceptance of physical deformity |

their disease (except in hydrocephalus-dementia syndrome) and manage to control the outward manifestations of their symptoms sufficiently to retain status within the family. To ensure an adequate adjustment to a chronic disabling condition, the family should design their living space to spare the patient undue trauma, which can cause fractures, and to allow the patient a normal range of daily activities. A home or apartment on one floor with easy access to the street level is preferred. Nevertheless, the patient's locomotion will usually show some impairment and adequate allowance should be made for this. When specific therapy plus a NSAID is unavailing, the judicious use of analgesics will lessen pain and disability. Visual impairment is seldom a serious problem, but loss of hearing can be severe. Family members must learn to cope with an intelligent and loved relative who cannot hear. Finally, should Paget's disease be very severe, significant deformities such as a huge head, kyphosis, and bowlegs may develop, diminishing the patient's self-image. The family should provide emotional support and reassurance that the individual is loved.

Satisfactory adaptations by the family are the rule rather than the exception, and the majority of pagetic patients appear to enjoy a normal family life that is hampered only by the purely somatic aspects of their disease. However, patients who have a solitary life or are estranged from their family may receive little outside support to bolster their waning vitality and mobility or to compensate for their pain, hearing loss, and deformities. It is this latter group that deserves attention and support above and beyond pure therapeutics from the health care team.

## References


1. Arnalich F, Plaza I, Sobrino JA, et al: Cardiac size and function in Paget's disease of bone. Int J Cardiol 5:491, 1984.
   *The full range of cardiovascular complications of Paget's disease is discussed.*
2. Baraka ME: Rate of progression of hearing loss in Paget's disease. J Laryngol Otol 98:573, 1984.
   *This article demonstrates that progressive hearing loss in Paget's disease can be distinguished from presbyacusis by serial audiography and may thereby justify treatment.*
3. Boudreau RJ, Lisbona R, Hadjipavlou A: Observations on serial radionuclide blood-flow studies in Paget's disease: Concise communication. J Nucl Med 24:880, 1983.
   *This article documents increased bone blood flow in Paget's disease and the rapid response to treatment.*
4. Cawley MI: Complications of Paget's disease of bone. Gerontology 29:276, 1983.
   *A geriatrician reviews the complications of Paget's disease.*
5. Dohrmann PJ, Elrick WL: Dementia and hydrocephalus in Paget's disease: A case report. J Neurol Neurosurg Psychiatry 45:835, 1982.
   *This article illustrates the hydrocephalus-dementia syndrome in Paget's disease and the dramatic response to ventricular shunting.*
6. Douglas DL, Duckworth T, Kanis JA, et al: Spinal cord dysfunction in Paget's disease of bone. J Bone Joint Surg 63B:495, 1981.
   *The range of spinal cord dysfunction seen in Paget's disease and the response to nonoperative treatment are reviewed.*
7. Eretto P, Krohel GB, Shihab ZM, et al: Optic neuropathy in Paget's disease. Am J Ophthalmol 97:505, 1984.
   *This study shows that visual complications of Paget's disease are relatively common but progressive changes leading to blindness are less common. The data support the need for serial ophthalmologic examinations in patients with skull involvement.*
8. Flores EG, Joo KG, Baeumler GR: Radionuclide cerebral angiographic findings in Paget's disease of the skull. Clin Nucl Med 7:77, 1982.
   *Vascular "steal" from the internal to external carotid system is demonstrated.*
9. Merkow RL, Lane JM: Current concepts of Paget's disease of bone. Orthop Clin North Am 15:747, 1984.
   *Written from the viewpoint of the orthopedist, this article updates some of the material in reference 13.*
10. Merkow RL, Pellicci PM, Hely DP, Salvati EA: Total hip replacement for Paget's disease of the hip. J Bone Joint Surg 66A:752, 1984.
    *This excellent article details the indications, results, and complications of total hip replacement for Paget's disease of the acetabular region and/or femoral head.*
11. Mills BG, Singer FR, Weiner LP: Evidence for both respiratory syncytial virus and measles virus antigens in the osteoclasts of patients with Paget's disease of bone. Clin Orthop 183:303, 1984.
    *This article cites ultrastructural and immunohistochemical evidence for a "slow virus" etiology of Paget's disease.*
12. Smith J, Botet JF, Yeh SD: Bone sarcomas in Paget disease: A study of 85 patients. Radiology 152:583, 1984.
    *A review of 85 cases of sarcomatous degeneration in Paget's disease seen at Memorial Sloan-Kettering Cancer Center over a 55-year period. The discussion also reviews other data on this subject.*
13. Wallach S: Treatment of Paget's disease. Adv Intern Med 27:1, 1982.
    *Written from the viewpoint of the endocrinologist, this article presents a comprehensive review of Paget's disease and its treatment.*
14. Wootton R, Tellez M, Green JR, Reeve J: Skeletal blood flow in Paget's disease of bone. Metab Bone Dis Relat Res 3:263, 1981.
    *This article documents increased bone blood flow in Paget's disease and the rapid response to treatment.*

Chapter 37

# Common Foot Problems in the Elderly

Charles J. Gudas

It has been estimated that, at one time or another, approximately 50 per cent of the general population will be affected by a foot problem. The incidence and severity usually increase with age until, after the age of 65 years, three of every four individuals complain of foot pain. Among individuals over 55 years old, 88 per cent of women and 83 per cent of men show radiographic evidence of arthritis involving the foot. Of these individuals, 25 per cent have symptomatic foot problems, including heel spur deformities, hammertoes, bunions (hallux valgus), generalized foot weakness, and misalignment.[1] Two per cent of all visits to physicians each year are for foot problems, and foot problems are the primary reason for 500,000 hospital admissions per year.[2]

The foot is a complex organ which can mirror a variety of systemic diseases in the body, including diabetes, gout, rheumatoid arthritis, ankylosing spondylitis, Paget's disease, and osteoporosis. Diabetic foot complications are most common after the age of 50 years. Levin[3] estimates that 20 per cent of all diabetics who enter the hospital are admitted for complications secondary to a foot disorder. An increased incidence of neurocirculatory problems is encountered in diabetics with foot disorders. According to Warren[4] to about 70 per cent of all foot amputations in the United States are performed on diabetic patients.

Musculoskeletal foot problems also increase with advancing age. Hallux valgus formation, whether the cause is hereditary or functional, becomes particularly prevalent after the age of 55 years. Hammertoes, mallet toes, callus formation, heel spur formation, and various bony exostoses commonly become symptomatic with increasing age and increasing changes in foot shape. The foot begins to change shape in females after childbirth and in males during their early forties. The altered shape, combined with a gradual loss of fat padding, subjects the foot to greater stress and increases the potential for age-related musculoskeletal disorders.

Dermatologic foot problems, such as formation of corns, calluses, and various other hyperkeratoses also become more prevalent with age. Nail atrophy, hypertrophy, and incurvation are common. Each of these may cause ulceration or infection, which can become disastrous in patients with vascular insufficiency.

Fungus (tinea pedis) infections account for a fairly large percentage of dermatologic disorders. With increasing age, a greater number of individuals become afflicted with tinea pedis, so that approximately 70 per cent of the general shoe-wearing population past the age of 60 years has chronic fungal infections of the feet. Viral infections with herpes simplex and herpes zoster are two of the many forms of blistering that can lead to foot problems in the elderly patient.[5]

There is a large group of erythematosquamous disorders that may affect the foot, such as psoriasis and pityriasis rubra pilaris. This group of skin diseases can lead to fissures, breakdown, and infection of the soles of the feet, thus causing potentially dangerous complications in the elderly patient.

Some neoplastic diseases have a predilection for the foot in elderly individuals. These include Kaposi's sarcoma, squamous cell carcinoma, and malignant melanoma.

Neurologic deficits that affect the motor and sensory nerves in the elderly may produce a wide variety of disorders that can have serious consequences for the patient. Motor nerve derangements may be secondary to trauma or to metabolic or ischemic mechanisms. Peroneal nerve injury may cause partial or complete loss of the extensor and pronator apparatus of the foot, creating a progressive cavus foot deformity. The polyneuropathy that occurs secondary to diabetes mellitus or alcoholism may cause a combined motor and sensory loss leading to either hyperesthesia or hypoesthesia of the foot. This may hasten ulceration of a portion of the foot and result in infection, osteomyelitis, gangrene, and the need for amputation (Fig. 37–1). Ischemic neuropathy also may cause hyperesthesia or hypoesthesia of the foot, with burning night pain or decreased sensation in the feet of elderly patients.

Arteriosclerosis obliterans causing chronic occlusive arterial disease becomes prevalent between the ages of 50 and 70 years. In diabetics, however, the disease usually begins about 10 years earlier. Segmental occlusion affecting the foot can occur at any level of the vascular system including the common femoral bifurcation and the common iliac bifurcation.[6] In diabetics, degeneration of the tibial artery, along with segmental degeneration of small vessels and microangiopathy, occurs with much greater frequency than is observed in the general population. Age-related disturbance in the blood supply must be considered and investigated before any invasive procedure on the foot is attempted. Seemingly minor foot procedures can lead to disaster in the elderly patient if the local and general conditions of the arteries are not analyzed accurately.

Infections of the foot can be greatly exacerbated in older patients because of coexisting metabolic, neurologic, and musculoskeletal problems. Musculoskeletal abnormalities such as hammertoes, bunions, and calluses can become irritated and subsequently infected much more rapidly in elderly patients than in younger individuals. Puncture wounds, chronic fissures, fungal infections, or ingrown toenails can be the inciting factor for a variety of infections caused by many different agents. Metabolic diseases resulting in neuropathic and hemodynamic abnormalities may transform a minor irritation into a major infection. Treatment of local foot infections requires skill, patience, and a thorough understanding of the complicating factors that may affect the older patient.

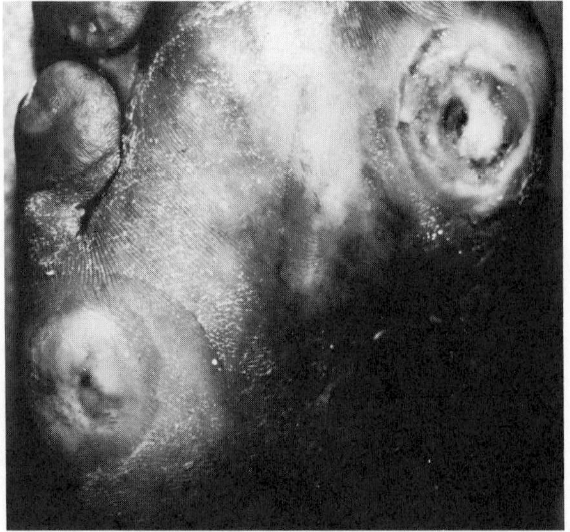

Figure 37–1. Diabetic polyneuropathy with associated superficial ulcerations.

The diagnosis and treatment of gerontologic foot problems are thus interesting, but complex subjects. This chapter is intended to serve as a reference point for further study of geriatric foot disorders.

## METHODS OF ASSESSMENT OF FOOT DISORDERS

### *Vascular Analysis of Pedal Blood Flow*

Pedal blood flow should be analyzed in the following sequence: noninvasive physical assessment, noninvasive laboratory procedures, and finally invasive arteriographic procedures. In some instances, it may only be necessary to do a physical evaluation. Noninvasive physical assessment of the elderly patient's pedal flow should include palpation of the dorsalis pedis, posterior tibial, popliteal, and femoral pulses. The blanch test, consisting of digital compression of the tip of the toe, is easily performed. In a healthy individual the skin should return to its normal color in 3 to 4 seconds. When blood flow is decreased, the skin will not return to its normal color within 6 seconds. Absence of hair growth on the dorsum of the toes, in combination with absent or weak pulses, may indicate decreased blood flow. Thickened hypertrophic, mycotic nails may also indicate a decrease in circulation. Skin pallor, if present, and skin temperature should be noted. Trophic changes in the skin and lack of skin turgor are additional means by which distal pedial blood flow is analyzed. It is also helpful to question the patient about claudication and night cramps. It may be necessary to have the patient walk vigorously before the examination in order to determine more accurately whether there are impediments to segmental arterial blood flow. The presence of burning night pain may also indicate a neurocirculatory disturbance.

Noninvasive laboratory analysis should be undertaken in (1) patients with open lesions, (2) those in whom physical examination indicates decreased blood flow, (3) those with metabolic disease (diabetes) in combination with open ulcerations or infections, and (4) patients who have patchy or digital gangrene. This analysis usually includes (1) segmental pressure analysis, (2) pulse wave analysis, and (3) blood flow studies (Fig. 37-2). Segmental pressure analysis is performed with the use of a Doppler ultrasound device and various-sized blood pressure cuffs. Segmental pressure ratios are determined by comparing the pressures above the ankle, at the midfoot, and at the hallux, with the brachial blood pressure reading taken as a baseline. The ratio of the distal pressure divided by the brachial pressure has been termed the ischemic index by Wagner and associates.[7] Wagner states that 93 per cent of patients with indices above 0.45 and with pulsatile flow will heal. Indices below 0.45 may necessitate vascular reconstruction or amputation. Patients experiencing intermittent claudication usually have ratios of 0.5 to 0.6. Elderly patients with impending gangrene or with rest pain often have an ankle brachial ratio below 0.5.[8] Pulse wave analysis is a routine test performed in vascular laboratories with the use of a pulse volume recorder. With this device, the pulse wave can be analyzed serially in regard to its contour and amplitude. Blood flow is analyzed with a Doppler ultrasound instrument, using transcutaneous, wide-angle, and miniature probe devices. Other devices currently under investigation are the photplethysmograph and thermocouples for skin and core temperature analysis. Noninvasive testing is important for the determination of segmental blockages as well as healing levels in debilitated elderly patients when complications arise from a foot problem.

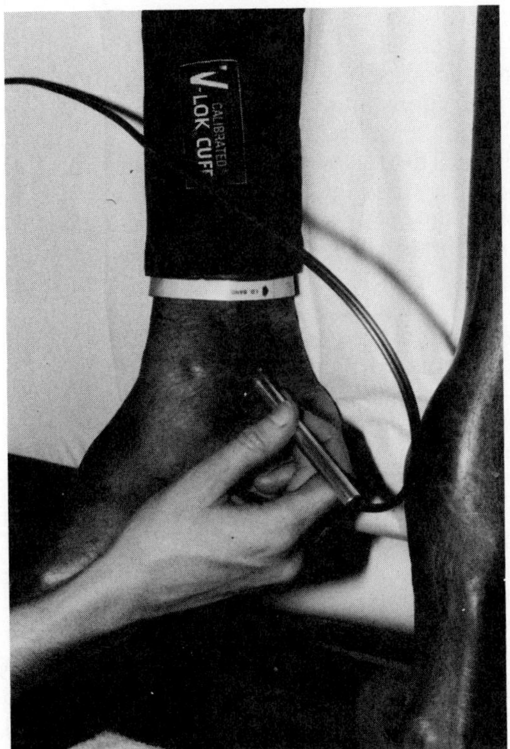


**Figure 37-2.** Doppler determination of the brachial pedal segmental ratio.

Invasive (arteriographic) procedures should be performed if the noninvasive tests indicate the presence of occlusion of major arteries and if endartectomy is contemplated.

## *Neurologic Examination*

Evaluation of the peripheral neurologic status of the elderly patient is important for the determination of the effects of sensory and motor degeneration on the formation and progression of foot disorders. Local evaluation of the sensory nerves includes the use of a tuning fork at 128 vibrations per second; two-point discrimination; and pinch, prick, pain, and temperature assessments. Motor function can be tested easily by the presence or absence of patellar and Achilles reflexes in comparison with the reflexes of the upper extremity. Determination of proprioception, muscle strength, and gait analysis provides important additional information. A painful hip or knee may contribute to the foot deformity. Atrophy or wasting of any muscle or muscle groups in the lower extremity should be noted. Electrodiagnostic tests of sensory and motor nerve conduction and electromyographic analysis[9,10] may be helpful in pinpointing the nature of the pathologic process.

## *Radiographic Examination*

Radiographic evaluation of the foot in the elderly patient should include baseline anteroposterior and lateral weight-bearing views. These should be taken while the patient is standing. Non-weight-bearing radiographs often yield little or no quantitative information. Misalignment of joints, erosions, bone loss, and soft-tissue problems are often overlooked. Further studies may include special views such as axial sesamoid, axial calcaneal, Harris and Beath, lateral oblique, and stress views. In addition, soft tissue radiography, tomography, magnification views, and computed tomography scans may be indicated.

### *Dermatologic Examination*

Dermatologic evaluation of the older patient includes recognition and treatment of skin atrophy; ulcerations; sinus tracts; fissures; hyperkeratic lesions overlying bony prominences, such as soft and hard corns/calluses; and primary skin lesions including hemorrhagic lesions. Systemic diseases that may have dermatologic manifestations in the foot include discoid lupus erythematosus, erythema multiforme, psoriasis, Kaposi's sarcoma, scleroderma, and sarcoidosis. Fungal infections of both the skin and nails are the rule rather than the exception in the elderly. Minor nail or skin problems often become severe in the older patient; therefore, careful assessment and treatment are necessary.

## DISORDERS OF THE FOOT

### *Musculoskeletal Disorders*

Musculoskeletal foot disorders in elderly patients are usually a result of aging-associated degeneration of muscles, tendons, ligaments, and joints.

### *Corns (Clavi)*

Corns occur in more than 50 per cent of the geriatric population and can develop on or between the toes. Corns may be secondary to hallux valgus formation, which pushes the lesser toes upward, resulting in a flexor extensor imbalance (Fig. 37–3). Corns are due to the formation of hyperkeratotic tissue over underlying bony prominences, upon which pressure is exerted by an ill-fitting or loose shoe. There are two main types of corns. The first occur on a hammertoe over the proximal interphalangeal joint; the second type occurs over a mallet toe, which is a plantar deviation of the distal phalanx that results in formation of hyperkeratotic tissue on the distal tips of the toes. In the elderly patient, these lesions often become infected, with sinus tract formation extending down to the bone. A soft corn is a bony prominence between two toes that produces keratotic tissue that is macerated and moist.

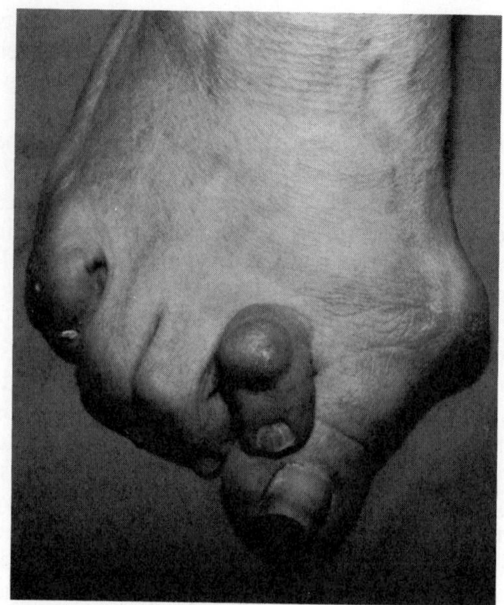

**Figure 37–3.** Hallux valgus with severe hammertoe formation.

Treatment includes careful debridement and padding. Incision and drainage of the sinus tract are often necessary, with padding and gentle lukewarm Domeboro soaks. Padding is best achieved by careful application of soft sponge pads held in place by tape or self-adhering gauze. Care must be taken not to decrease the digital circulation with the tape or gauze. If the infection is severe, antibiotic coverage and hospitalization may be indicated. The patient should be advised to wear wider and softer shoes. If distal clavi are present, a soft insole (Dr. Scholl's air pillow or sports cushion) may be utilized. If simple treatment does not effect relief, surgical intervention may be indicated. This is possible only if the patient's circulatory status is adequate. The procedure consists of resection of the proximal or distal interphalangeal joints, with or without pin fixation.

### *Neuroma*

Neuroma affects between 8 and 10 per cent of the over-65 population and is often seen in combination with a chronic interdigital bursitis or inflammation. Neuroma usually occurs between the third and fourth toes but can occur between the second and third toes as well. Pain may set in at any time but usually becomes worse when shoes are worn. The painful area can be palpated between the metatarsal heads. Nonoperative treatment includes injections of local anesthetic between the metatarsal heads. The patient is advised to wear wide, open-toed shoes, if possible. Arch supports with a metatarsal rise are often helpful. Temporary padding is achieved with a $\frac{1}{8}$-in. moleskin or $\frac{1}{4}$-in. felt Mayo pad placed slightly posterior to the metatarsal heads. In rare instances, when surgical removal is indicated, the neuroma is removed through a dorsal incision.

## *Calluses*

Callosities (plantar keratoses) in the elderly patient often present a severe problem because of the fat pad atrophy associated with aging (Fig. 37–4). Calluses may be found under any of the metatarsal heads; however, the most common site is beneath the second and third metatarsal heads in conjunction with metatarsal-phalangeal dorsal dislocation secondary to hallux valgus. Plantar calluses affect about 50 per cent of the geriatric population to some extent. Progressive loss of toe function probably contributes to callus formation. The treatment of plantar keratoses ranges from use of a wide variety of over-the-counter medications to physician-prescribed measures. Over-the-counter devices include metatarsal-head pads with or without salicylic acid. Salicylic-acid pads and plasters *should be avoided* in the elderly patient. Soft-soled shoes with the insertion of soft $\frac{1}{8}$-in. insoles are very helpful. Soft insoles such as Dr. Scholl's System III may also be of benefit. If these measures are not effective, the patient should be referred to a podiatrist for gentle debridement and padding around the affected metatarsal head. In some cases, an orthotic (arch support) with a metatarsal rise may be indicated. Surgical intervention for metatarsal-head lesions is rarely advisable because of an extremely high incidence (40 per cent) of transfer lesions (recurrent calluses) to an adjacent metatarsal. Currently, investigations are being undertaken to determine whether an injectable colloid substance is of use in the reconstruction of atrophied fat pads.

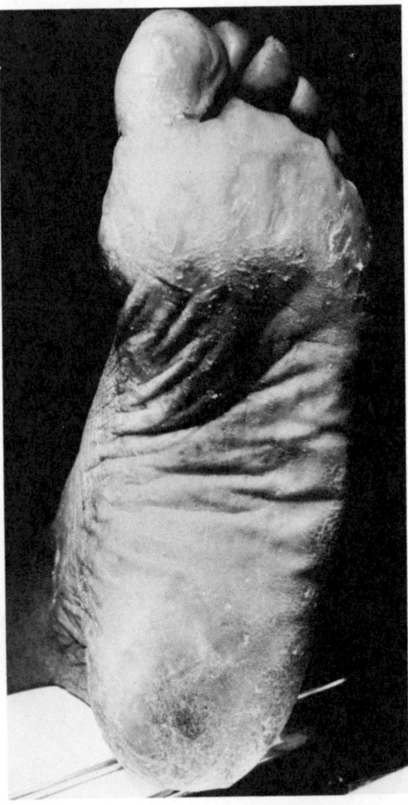

**Figure 37–4.** Calluses associated with fat pad atrophy.

## *Hallux Valgus (Bunions)*

Hallux valgus is one of the most common afflictions of the human foot. The deformity may appear at any age, but becomes more prevalent after the age of 50 years. A recent analysis of more than 200 patients indicated that 25 per cent of all patients seen for hallux valgus were more than 65 years old. Bunions are more prevalent in women than in men, in a ratio of 4 to 1. In the elderly patient, atrophy of muscles, ligaments, and tendons often complicates the problem. Progressive hallux valgus often leads to subluxation or dislocation of the second metatarsophalangeal joint, leading to severe hammertoe and callus formation. These deformities are often severe; however, the severity of the deviation is not a realistic indicator of pain. Often, shoe fitting will be a greater problem than pain (Fig. 37–5).

Nonsurgical treatment is aimed at giving the forefoot enough space both laterally and dorsally. This can be achieved simply by the use of a running shoe with a wide toe box. Depth inlay shoes manufactured by the Alden Shoe Company may give significant relief. The Miller Shoe Company offers an extra-depth shoe for women. Custom-made shoes can be obtained at great expense to the patient. Simpler and less expensive shoe therapy involves the use of a running shoe or an ultralight walking shoe.

Surgical treatment of hallux valgus in the older patient is indicated if pain and shoe-fitting difficulties persist after nonoperative treatment. Procedures should be kept as simple as possible and should be designed to allow ambulation as quickly as possible. It is rarely necessary nowadays to keep a patient nonambulatory for more than 24 hours after hallux valgus surgery. Large resections of the first metatarsal head should be avoided because of the high probability of transfer lesions to the lesser metatarsals.

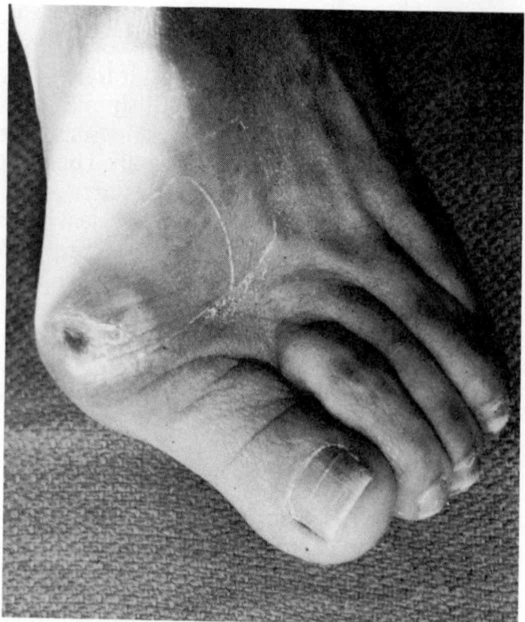

**Figure 37–5.** Hallux valgus with associated shoe irritation.

## *Heel Spurs*

Heel spurs are usually localized around the inferior and posterior aspects of the heel. This problem can be a source of great pain in the elderly patient (Fig. 37–6). In some instances, heel pain is associated with systemic diseases such as rheumatoid arthritis. In some instances, inferior heel pain is the major complaint in this disease. In older patients, the cause may be heel pad atrophy, inferior spur formation, or plantar fasciitis. The pain usually occurs early in the morning when the patient arises, or after the patient has been sitting for a long period, but gradually disappears after 15 or 20 minutes of walking. Posterior heel pain is usually associated with calcification of the insertion of the Achilles tendon.

Treatment of inferior heel pain consists of corticosteroid and local anesthetic injections, slightly inferior to the heel spur, directly into the most painful area. Three injections over a 3-month period are the maximum that should be given in 1 year; injections repeated more frequently may cause increased atrophy of the heel pad. After the injection, the plantar fascia should be supported with a Mayo pad and tape or with a specially molded arch support device. The heel should be padded. Cutting an accommodation in the sponge or felt should be avoided, as this may concentrate the stress and increase the pain. One can achieve relief of inferior heel pain in 85 per cent of the cases by using injections and arch support devices. Posterior heel pain is usually treated with oral anti-inflammatory agents and heel elevation with a pad or arch support. Corticosteroid injections should be avoided in the posterior heel because of the risk of rupture of the Achilles complex.

## *Arthritic Disorders*

### OSTEOARTHRITIS

Osteoarthritis in the foot is usually localized to the first metatarsophalangeal joint, where bony hypertrophy occurs (Fig. 37–7). The condition may also be termed hallux limitus or rigidus, and it may be accompanied by hallux valgus formation.

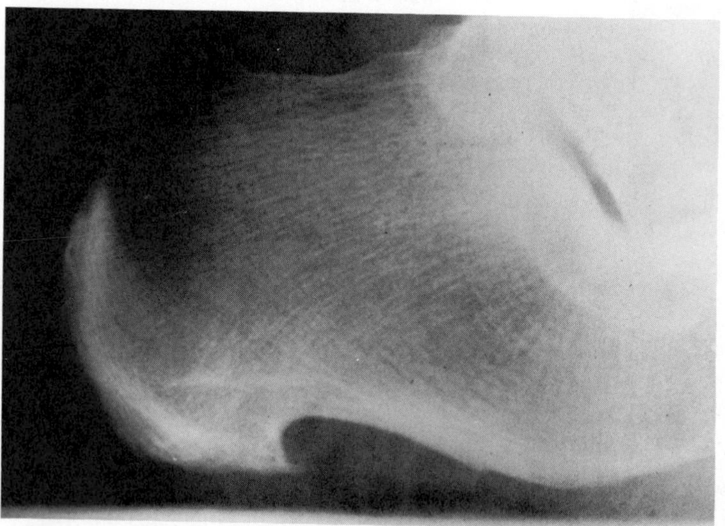

**Figure 37–6.** Inferior heel spur formation.

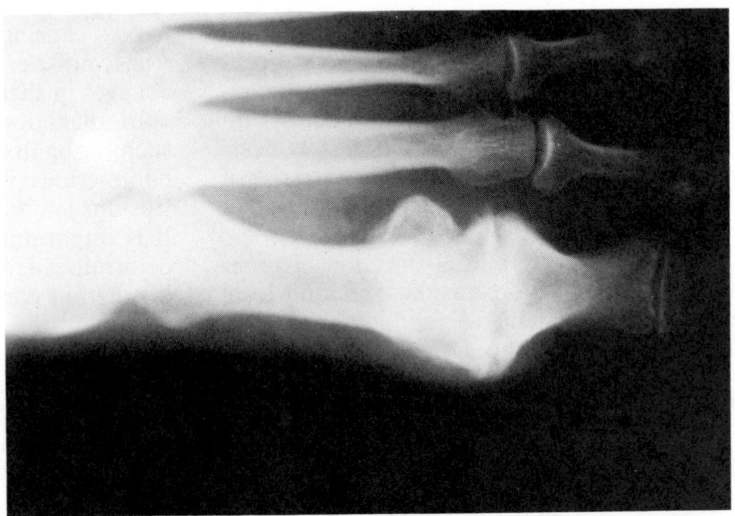

**Figure 37–7.** Hypertrophic osteoarthritis of the first metatarsophalangeal joint.

Treatment involves measures to limit motion of the joint or surgical excision of the hypertrophic bone. Nonoperative treatment includes wearing of a stiff, solid shoe or extended arch support device, which limits motion of the first metatarsophalangeal joint. If the circulation is adequate and nonoperative treatment has failed, the surgical procedures of choice are a Keller bunionectomy with a Silastic prosthesis, Keller bunionectomy without a Silastic prosthesis, and a combination cheilectomy exostectomy for removal of the hypertrophic bone.

## Gout

Up to 80 per cent of all patients with gout will, at one time or another, have an inflamed first metatarsophalangeal joint.[11] Treatment includes systemic management with anti-inflammatory drugs, uricosuric agents, or xanthine oxidase inhibitors (see Chapter 36). Because trauma can be an initiating factor, nonoperative therapy should be directed at controlling excess motion around the joint with the use of arch supports or stiff-soled shoes. Surgical treatment may be contemplated if the patient has (1) a painful and deformed joint; (2) an open sinus tract to the joint; (3) multiple tophaceous deposits and severe joint deformity, which make shoe-wearing impossible; and (4) breakdown of the skin over the joint. The procedures of choice are the Mayo and Keller bunionectomies with or without a Silastic prosthesis.[12] Care must be taken not to cause an acute attack of gout by surgical intervention. The patient should be placed on cholchicine 0.6 mg per day to help avert an acute attack of gout in the postoperative period.

## Rheumatoid Arthritis

Rheumatoid arthritis frequently involves the forefoot, yielding a symmetric, bilateral polyarthritis (Fig. 37–8). The major structures in-

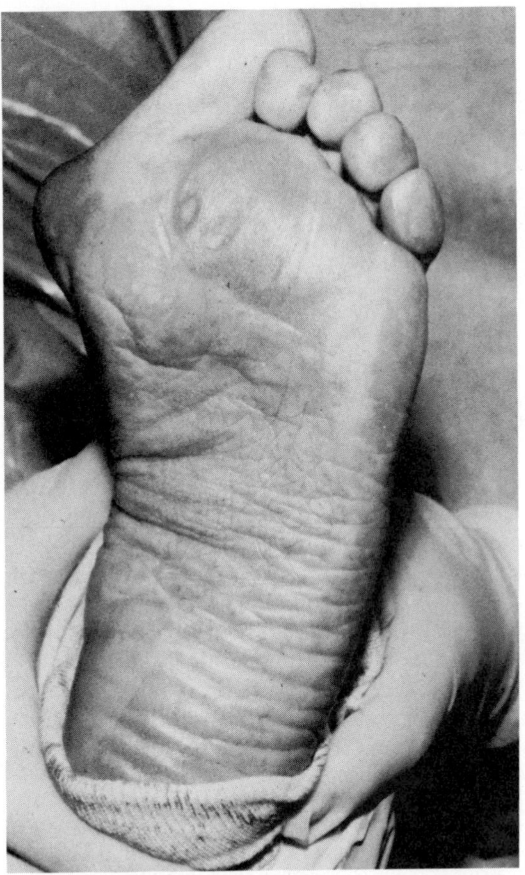

**Figure 37–8.** Rheumatoid foot with severe forefoot deformities.

volved are the metatarsophalangeal joints of the forefoot. It has been estimated that 85 per cent of all patients with rheumatoid arthritis manifest some form of foot disease.[13] Patients with rheumatoid vasculitis may manifest skin ulceration and digital ischemia with increased risk of infection, especially those receiving long-term corticosteroid therapy.

Treatment includes local injection of water soluble cortisone* (dexamethasone) and local anesthetic into inflamed areas and use of depth inlay shoes, molded shoes, plastizote shoes, arch supports, and decompression padding. The most common surgical procedure is complete removal of the metatarsal heads. Approximately 70 per cent of these patients can subsequently wear a fairly regular shoe with minimal pain. However, 25 per cent of the patients require additional surgery at a later date. Surgery should only be undertaken in an elderly patient with rheumatoid arthritis after a careful assessment of the degree of vascular insufficiency, since the presence of severe vasculitis will predispose to postoperative complications.

## *Metabolic (Diabetic) Disorders*

In a 1960 study, 29 per cent of diabetic patients were found to have gangrene in the lower extremities.[4] According to a National Institutes of Health study,[14] diabetes mellitus is the most common disease resulting in foot disorders. Arterial disease and neuropathy are common parts of the disease and are major causes of diabetic foot complications.

Diabetic polyneuropathy usually results in hypoesthesia. This process takes from 2 to 7 years to develop fully, depending upon the sensitivity of the test used. Clinical evidence of a decreased sensorium develops over 15 years. Repetitive stress on the insensate foot causes inflammation, which, if prolonged, leads to necrosis and ulceration. Brand[15] has shown that intermittent low to moderate stress of 1 to 5 lb per in.$^2$ for 5 to 10 hours can cause breakdown of the skin in the neuropathic foot. This can result in infection, which may be accompanied by a two- to fivefold increase in local blood flow.[16] Unfortunately, the diabetic may not be able to adapt to increased blood flow requirements because of tissue-level end-stage occlusion of small vessels. Neuropathy may also affect the motor nerves, causing weakness and wasting of the intrinsic muscles and thus predisposing the foot to changes in shape upon increased pressure.

In diabetics, pre-existing foot deformities such as hallux valgus, depressed metatarsals, hammertoes, ingrown toenails, and bony protrusions are prone to breakdown and infection. It is important to categorize pre-existing foot deformities accurately in order to pinpoint areas of potential complication. It is also important to document the neurovascular status of the diabetic foot by a combination of clinical and laboratory studies for diagnosis and treatment of the complications of neurovascular dysfunction. Studies have shown that routine podiatric care in compliant elderly diabetic patients can significantly decrease the morbidity caused by foot problems.

Prophylaxis and patient education are essential if complications of foot problems are to be prevented in the elderly diabetic patient. The following simple procedures should be followed:

1. Have someone with *good eyesight* check the feet daily for blisters, inflammation, and ulcerations.
2. Use good hygiene of the feet and toes—wash feet daily in lukewarm water.
3. Avoid heating pads or hot-water bottles.
4. Avoid extreme cold.
5. Avoid wet shoes and socks if possible.
6. Wear properly fitted stockings without seams.
7. Wear soft leather shoes with wide toes, snug heels, and soft soles.
8. Do not use salicylic acid or caustic agents on any portion of the foot.
9. Never walk barefoot.
10. Check insides of shoes for foreign objects or protruding nails.
11. Cut nails straight across—*never* cut into the corner of a nail.
12. Make periodic visits to the podiatrist for routine foot care—*never* cut corns or calluses.
13. Change shoes daily.
14. Walk slowly.
15. Do not smoke.
16. Keep the diabetes under control with regular checkups by the physician.

Once a breakdown occurs over an existing foot deformity, it is graded according to severity. Meggitt[17] devised a simple grading system for diabetic ulcers. The ulcers are graded from 0 (no open lesions—healed ulcer) to V (total-foot gangrene). Treatment regimens can be tailored to the degree of disruption of the skin, soft tissue, and bone.

* Repeated corticosteroid injections into joints carry increased risk of infection and, in all probability, increase the likelihood of the development of subsequent degenerative changes.

Treatment of Grade 0 ulcers includes periodic debridement; use of padding, decompressive insoles, and space shoes; and prophylactic reduction of the deformity. Before prophylactic surgery can be performed, the surgeon must carefully analyze the patient's vascular status to ascertain whether the surgical site will heal. Simple toenail, digital, and forefoot procedures can be performed that reduce the localized stress caused by pre-existing musculoskeletal deformities. These procedures include simple bunionectomies, metatarsal osteotomies about the metatarsal heads, arthroplastic resections of the digital joints, and removal of ingrown toenails. Improper surgery may lead to destruction of fragile arterioles, with development of gangrene.

Grade I ulcers (superficial) may require extensive treatment, including debridement, incision and drainage, antibiotic therapy, physical therapy, depressurization by casting or use of plastizote shoes, and surgical intervention, if necessary, with bony debridement and skin grafting.

Grade II ulcers are deeper and may penetrate through soft tissue to bone. These lesions require aggressive treatment, including incision and drainage, bed rest, physical therapy, debridement, antibiotic therapy, toe amputations, ray resections, secondary wound closure, skin grafting, and use of walking pressure-reduction casts and healing shoes. Localized pressure reduction around ulcerated areas enhances healing and reduces tissue-level anoxia.

Grade III lesions are complicated by the presence of osteomyelitis, one of the most serious problems of foot care in elderly diabetic patients. These lesions are infected by a variety of aerobic and anaerobic bacteria, including staphylococci, streptococci, and enterobacteria. Multiple superficial and deep cultures as well as aggressive incision and drainage techniques are necessary. Repeated debridement of infected bone and soft tissue is often required; debridement should be combined with whirlpool therapy. Quantitative wound cultures should be performed before closure or skin grafting is attempted. Digital amputations and ray resections are often indicated. Pressure reduction casts and healing shoes help to reduce the lesions to Grade 0. Antibiotics include intravenous mixtures of aminoglycosides and semisynthetic penicillin. Appropriate renal and auditory function studies are mandatory during aminoglycoside therapy. The drugs of choice in bacteroides or anaerobic streptococcal infections are clindamycin or metronidazole penicillin G.

Patients with Grade IV lesions have digital or forefoot gangrene. Careful vascular analysis is mandatory for determination of amputation levels. For patients with these lesions, an attempt is made to keep the amputation as far distal as possible. Amputations used include digital resections; medial, lateral, or central ray resections; transmetatarsal resections; and the two-stage Syme procedure. Wounds are often left open until quantitative wound culture methods show that the bacterial count is less than $10_5$. Delayed primary closure or skin grafting is then permissible. Meticulous cast and shoe fitting is necessary after forefoot amputations. After Syme's amputation, a special prosthesis should be fitted that helps maximize patient comfort.

Grade V lesions consist of total-foot gangrene. Accurate calculation of the extent of ischemia is important for precise determination of the level of the below-the-knee amputation. The patient should receive a well-fitted below-the-knee prosthesis, which will help maintain independent ambulation.

Treatment of diabetic foot complications in elderly patients is a complex and frustrating art. New methods of analysis, combined with more aggressive and definitive treatment regimens than were available previously, are radically changing the outlook for these patients. Continued efforts in the future may bring even more success in the diagnosis and treatment of this difficult problem.

## *Skin and Nail Disorders*

### SKIN

Most individuals experience a gradual drying and thinning of the skin with advancing age. This can lead to cracking, fissures, inflammation, and infection. Cancers of the skin also show an increased incidence with age. Skin atrophy and diffuse keratosis are the rule in the older patient. Ichthyosis becomes more pronounced. Stasis dermatitis related to venous insufficiency often affects the lower extremities of the elderly. Localized neurodermatitis may manifest itself on the dorsum of the foot. Exfoliative dermatitis on the dorsum of the foot and distal portion of the leg may predate mycosis fungoides.

Treatment of dry skin and fissures centers on hydration of the skin. Good emollient skin lotions or petrolatum jelly may be beneficial. Occlusion with petrolatum jelly for one or two nights is an excellent treatment for fissured heels. Local corticosteroid preparations are indicated for neurodermatitis and exfoliative dermatitis. If exfoliative dermatitis is severe, various forms of lymphomas must be ruled out. Keratosis formation can be treated by gentle debridement; application of emollient creams; and use of pressure-reducing insoles made of poron, plastizote, or latex. A depth inlay shoe may be helpful.

### Nails

According to Evanski,[18] approximately one third of all geriatric patients complain of toenail problems. The most common geriatric nail disorders are incurvated nail borders, onychauxis (hypertrophy) (Fig. 37–9), onychogryphosis (ram's horn) and onychomycosis. Severely hypertrophic nails can cause nail bed ulcerations in the elderly. Incurvated nail borders can lead to irritation, inflammation, and infection and result in pain. Treatment of nail disorders in the elderly should be kept as simple as possible. Inappropriate procedures on a dysvascular digit may be dangerous because of the risk of gangrene and amputation. Incurvated nails should be debrided gently with or without the use of local anesthesia. Surgical treatment is rarely indicated. Debridement of hypertrophic and mycotic nails should be performed by a podiatrist or orthopedist with the proper instruments for nail cutting and grinding. Debridement with sharp scissors may cause a puncture wound with accompanying bacterial infiltration. When subungual infections persist, the nail plate should be avulsed gently with the patient under local anesthesia if his or her circulatory status permits it. Gentle lukewarm Domeboro or Betadine soaks are indicated. One must be careful not to overtreat nail problems because new problems may arise.

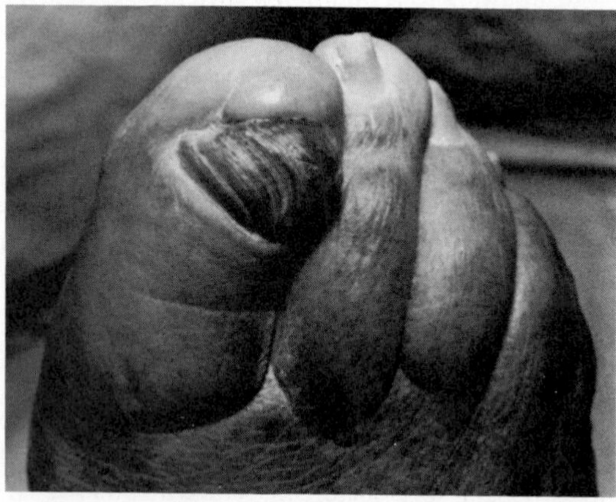

**Figure 37–9.** Hypertrophied hallux nail.

## CONCLUSION

The diagnosis and treatment of geriatric foot problems present an interesting challenge. Complex diagnostic procedures are often necessary prior to adequate treatment of a routine geriatric foot problem that is easily cured in a younger patient. Often, simple treatment may bring lasting relief. Care must be taken not to overtreat geriatric foot disorders and thus incur iatrogenic complications.

### References


1. Helfand AE: At the foot of South Mountain: A five-year longitudinal study of foot problems and screening in an elderly population. J Am Podiatry Assoc 63:512, 1973.
2. U.S. Department of Health, Education and Welfare, Public Health Service: Diabetes Data—Compiled 1977. Washington, DC, National Center for Health Studies Publication #79-1468, Reprinted August 1979.
3. Levin ME, O'Neal LW: The Diabetic Foot. St. Louis, C.V. Mosby Company, 1983, pp. ix–xiii.
   *An excellent reference on the diabetic foot.*
4. Warren R, Kihn RB: A survey of lower extremity amputation for ischemia. Surgery 63:107, 1968.
5. Laros GS: Chicago, Workshop on Advancement of Foot Care. October 23, 24, 25, 1981, pp. 2–95.
6. Warren S, LeCompte PM, and Legg MA: The Pathology of Diabetic Mellitus. Philadelphia, Lea and Febiger, 1966.
7. Wagner FW: The dysvascular foot: A system for diagnosis and treatment. Foot Ankle 2:64, 1981.
8. Yao JST: New techniques in objective arterial evaluation. Arch Surg 106:600, 1973.
9. Dorfman LJ, Cummins KL: Nerve fiber conduction velocity distributions in normal and diabetic human nerves. Neurology 30:126, 1980.
10. Jahss MH: Disorders of the Foot. Philadelphia, W.B. Saunders Company, 1982, pp. 68–80.
11. Yu TF, Katz WA: Gout and pseudogout. *In* Katz WA (ed.): Rheumatic Diseases: Diagnosis and Management. Philadelphia, J.B. Lippincott Company, 1977, pp. 697–730.
12. Kurtz JF: Surgery of tophaceous gout in the lower extremity. Surg Clin North Am 45:217, 1965.
13. Vainio K: The rheumatoid foot. A clinical study with pathological and roentgenological comments. Ann Chir Gynaecol 45(Suppl 1):1, 1956.
14. Crofford OB: Report of the National Commission on Diabetes to the Congress of the United States. U.S. Department of Health and Education Publication No. (NIH) 67-1018, Washington, DC, Government Printing Office, 1975.
15. Brand PW: Pathomechanics of pressure ulceration. *In* Fredericks S, Brody OS (eds.): Symposium on the Neurologic Aspects of Plastic Surgery. Vol. 17. St. Louis, C.V. Mosby Company, 1978, pp. 185–189.
16. Lippman HI, Farrar R: Prevention of amputation in diabetes. Angiology 30:649, 1979.
17. Meggitt BF: Orthopedic Management of Foot Breakdown Problems in the Diabetic Patient. Orthopedic resident proceedings, UCLA, May 1972.
18. Evanski PM: The geriatric foot. *In* Jahss MH (ed.): Disorders of the Foot. Philadelphia, W.B. Saunders Company, 1982, pp. 964–978.

Chapter 38

# Endocrine Diseases

Paul J. Davis
Faith B. Davis

The practice of endocrinology applied to the elderly patient population requires that we distinguish among three states: (1) endocrine function that is altered relative to young subjects but is an expected consequence of normal aging, (2) altered endocrine function that is secondary to the presence of nonendocrine disease and is of no pathologic consequence, and (3) endocrinopathy. The patterns of change in endocrine function in the course of normal aging are several and are summarized in Table 38–1. Certain of these changes materially affect diagnostic evaluations, e.g., the relative nonresponsiveness of the renin-aldosterone axis in normal elderly subjects, the failure of a subpopulation of normal elderly men to respond to the administration of thyrotropin-releasing hormone (TRH), and the alteration in carbohydrate tolerance. In the course of normal aging such changes can create the impression of the presence of endocrine disease. These changes are discussed in more detail in subsequent sections. There is no unifying pathophysiologic mechanism to explain these alterations in endocrine function in the course of normal aging. Rather, these changes appear to have different and specific mechanisms within each hormonal axis.

The impact of nonendocrine disease states on endocrine physiology in subjects of all ages can also lead to the misimpression of endocrinopathy. Interesting examples of such changes are the reduction in serum triiodothyronine ($T_3$) and thyroxine ($T_4$) levels in patients with nonthyroidal illness and the fall in serum testosterone concentration that occurs in men in the course of serious systemic (nonendocrine) diseases, such as cancer and heart disease. Endocrine evaluation carried out on multisystemically ill elderly is an exercise in cautious interpretation of laboratory test results.

Finally, bona fide endocrinopathies in the elderly need not present in conventional patterns observed in younger patients. For example, the presentations of hyperthyroidism or hyperparathyroidism in older patients may be muted or monosystemic or obscured by the coincidence of unrelated heart, lung, or nervous system diseases that have life-threatening implications. The epidemiology of the various endocrinopathies is also different in the elderly (Fig. 38–1). For example, in older patients, diabetes mellitus is of the Type II variety, and adrenocortical disease is very rare. The aggressiveness of endocrine tumors, notably thyroid cancer, is different in the elderly compared with the younger population, despite histologically identical lesions. The treatment of endocrinopathies may also require modification in older patients.

## PITUITARY-THYROID FUNCTION

### Physiology

The concentration in serum of the metabolically important forms of thyroid hormone, thyroxine ($T_4$) and triiodothyronine ($T_3$) does not significantly change over the life span.[1,2] Although several reports suggest that serum $T_3$ levels fall progressively with age, the changes are trivial, or the study populations upon which these conclusions were based included subjects with nonthyroidal illness. Systemic (nonthyroidal) illness is usually associated with impaired extrathyroidal conversion of $T_4$ to $T_3$ and depressed serum concentrations of $T_3$. The specific serum thyroid hormone–binding proteins, i.e., thyroxine-binding globulin (TBG) and thyroxine-binding prealbumin (TBPA), are not

**Table 38-1.** PATTERNS OF CHANGE IN ENDOCRINE FUNCTION WITH NORMAL AGING*

| Change | Example |
|---|---|
| Endocrine gland failure | Ovary |
| Reduction in target organ sensitivity | Peripheral tissue response to insulin |
| | Renal collecting tubule response to AVP† |
| Failure of adaptive response | Renin-aldosterone response to change in posture |
| | AVP response to change in posture |
| Heightened sensitivity within endocrine axis | AVP response to increase in plasma osmolality |

* Examples of endocrine axes in which no physiologically substantive change in function occurs with aging are the pituitary-thyroid system and the pituitary-cortisol axis.

† AVP = arginine vasopressin (antidiuretic hormone).

importantly affected by age.[2,3] The concentration of free $T_4$ in serum is also unaffected by normal aging.[1] Basal levels of thyrotropin, or thyroid-stimulating hormone (TSH) also appear to be unchanged by aging,[1,4] and the responsiveness of the thyroid gland to exogenous TSH stimulation remains intact over the life span.

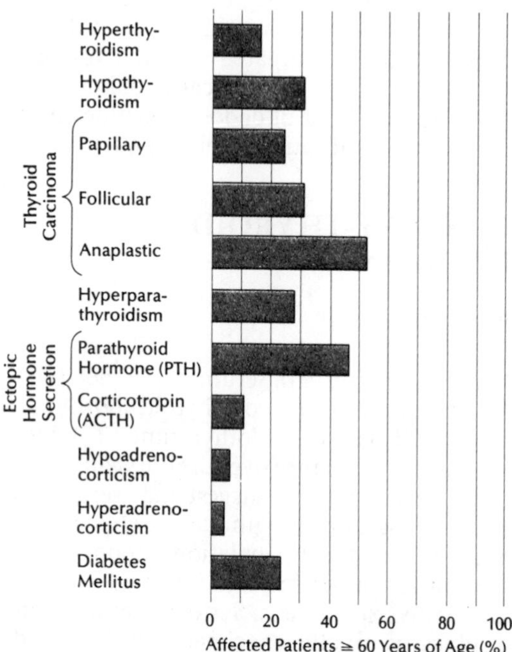


**Figure 38-1.** Percentage of patients with a variety of endocrinopathies who are aged 60 years or more. For example, 45 per cent of patients with ectopic parathyroid hormone secretion are 60 years of age or older. (From Davis PJ: Endocrines and aging. Hosp Pract 12:113, 1977. Rendered by Albert Miller. Reproduced with permission.)

On the other hand, age-dependent alteration in pituitary response to the administration of thyrotropin-releasing hormone (TRH) has been reported.[4,5] TRH is a hypothalamic principle, the administration of which stimulates the secretion of both TSH and prolactin.[6] In some normal elderly men, the ability of the pituitary gland to secrete TSH in response to TRH is significantly damped. The frequency of this finding is not clear.[2] In contrast, TRH responsiveness in women is reported to be unchanged over the life span.[7] No physiologic consequences appear to result from the sex-dependent difference, but the observation is clinically relevant because TRH administration is a frequently used assessment of pituitary-thyroid function. An absent or decreased response of TSH release to TRH administration is consistent in younger patients, regardless of sex, with several endocrinopathies: (1) hypopituitarism, (2) hyperthyroidism, and (3) excessive thyroid hormone therapy in patients with goiter or thyroidal hypothyroidism. In patients with untreated thyroidal, or primary, hypothyroidism, exaggerated TSH secretion occurs in response to TRH administration. Decreased or absent TRH responsiveness in men over 60 years of age is diagnostically ambiguous because it may reflect nothing more than normal aging. Nonetheless, we are assured that the pituitary-thyroid gland axis is intact when an elderly man demonstrates normal TRH response.

Despite the fact that serum levels of $T_4$ and $T_3$ are stable over the life span, changes in hormone half-lives do occur as a function of aging, as noted in Table 38-1. The prolonged metabolic half-life ($T\frac{1}{2}$) of $T_4$ in elderly subjects is a nonendocrine function; that is, it is due to the altered disposal rate of thyroid hormone in nonendocrine tissues. Given that $T_4$ levels are constant with age while the $T\frac{1}{2}$ is increased, it follows that the thyroidal secretion of $T_4$ must be decreased. The decrease is presumed to occur through a small downward adjustment in basal TSH levels, a change that is imperceptible using conventional radioimmunoassays for TSH.

The putative interrelationships of thyroid hormone and catecholamines have been studied extensively. Many clinical manifestations of hyperthyroidism appear to represent a hyperadrenergic state, and many of the clinical manifestations of thyrotoxicosis may be suppressed with administration of drugs that produce blockade of tissue beta-adrenergic binding sites.

Studies in animal models suggest that thyroid hormone may affect adrenergic receptor sites and thus could modulate sympathetic activity in the face of constant circulating levels of catecholamines.

## *Clinical*

### HYPERTHYROIDISM

The clinical symptoms and signs encountered in a large group of hyperthyroid patients are summarized in Table 38-2. Most aged hyperthyroid patients demonstrate classical findings of thyrotoxicosis.[8] When findings of thyrotoxicosis are mild and occur in the setting of high-morbidity syndromes such as heart failure, systemic infection, and cerebrovascular disease, they may be overlooked ("masked" hyperthyroidism).

Occasionally, primary involvement of a single organ, such as the heart, is encountered in thyrotoxicosis. Patients may present with a phlegmatic or apathetic mien. Masked monosystemic or apathetic syndromes account for 25 per cent of the presentations in elderly thyrotoxic subjects. Crescendo angina pectoris may herald the appearance of thyroid hyperfunction, but paradoxically, myocardial infarction has occurred infrequently in the setting of hyperthyroidism and coronary artery disease. The constellation of weight loss, anorexia, and constipation occurs in as many as 15 per cent of elderly hyperthyroid patients, and anorexia, alone, is present in one quarter of the older thyrotoxic population. New hypertension or accentuation of pre-existent systolic hypertension may occur without a decrease in diastolic pressure in older patients with hyperthyroidism. Atrial fibrillation is eight times more frequent in elderly hyperthyroid individuals than in younger patients. Atrial fibrillation in young thyrotoxic patients usually reverts to a normal sinus mechanism spontaneously in the course of primary treatment of thyrotoxicosis. In contrast, in only 50 per cent of elderly thyrotoxic patients with atrial fibrillation does the arrhythmia spontaneously revert to sinus mechanism in the course of antithyroid therapy. It is also important to recognize that atrial fibrillation in the older thyrotoxic patient may be associated with a slow ventricular response (ventricular rate, 50 to 60 beats per minute). This atrioventricular conduction block relates to the concomitant presence of arteriosclerotic disease in the conducting system or the use of digitalis or both.

Goiter is absent in as many as 40 per cent of older patients with thyrotoxicosis.[8] Insistence by the physician upon the presence of goiter before obtaining tests of thyroid function will therefore lead to underdiagnosis of hyperthyroidism in the elderly. Although toxic multinodular goiter and hyperthyroidism associated with an autonomous thyroid nodule are more common in older hyperthyroid patients than in younger subjects, one third or more of older patients with thyroid hyperfunction present with a thyroid gland in which no thyroid nodularity can be discerned.

Serious ophthalmopathy is infrequent in the elderly. On the other hand, stare and lid lag are not uncommon. These findings, however, are nonspecific, since they are encountered in the settings of nonendocrine diseases such as chronic congestive heart failure, renal failure, liver decompensation, and chronic obstructive pulmonary disease.

Diffuse lymphadenopathy is virtually never encountered in elderly thyrotoxic patients, although it may be seen in younger patients with

**Table 38-2.** CLINICAL FEATURES OF HYPERTHYROIDISM IN THE ELDERLY*

| Symptom | Frequency (%) |
|---|---|
| Hyperhidrosis | 38 |
| Heat intolerance | 63 |
| Weight loss | 69 |
| Palpitation | 63 |
| Angina pectoris | 20 |
| Respiratory symptoms consistent with congestive heart failure | 66 |
| Polyphagia | 11 |
| Anorexia | 36 |
| Increased stool frequency | 12 |
| Constipation | 26 |
| Tremor/nervousness | 55 |
| **Sign** | |
| Hyperkinesis | 25 |
| Apathy | 16 |
| Cachexia/chronically ill appearance | 39 |
| Classical skin changes (warm, fine, moist) | 81 |
| Proptosis | 8 |
| Lid lag | 35 |
| Extraocular muscle palsy | 22 |
| Impalpable or normal-sized thyroid gland | 37 |
| Multinodular thyroid gland | 20 |
| Solitary thyroid nodule | 21 |
| Diffuse thyroid enlargement | 22 |
| Atrial fibrillation (AF) | 39 |
| Supraventricular tachycardia (rate > 120 beats/minute) | 11 |
| Brisk deep tendon reflexes, shortened relaxation phase | 26 |

*Adapted from Davis PJ, Davis FB: Hyperthyroidism in patients over the age of 60. Medicine 53:161, 1974.

diffuse toxic goiter (Graves' disease). Although splenomegaly may occur in as many as 10 per cent of younger patients with hyperthyroidism, splenic enlargement in the older patient with thyroid hyperfunction is usually accounted for by the concomitant presence of a nonendocrine disease, for example, cirrhosis. Although hepatomegaly may be an isolated finding attributed to thyrotoxicosis in the elderly patient, concomitant nonendocrine disease (cirrhosis, cor pulmonale) usually explains liver enlargement.

In the vast majority of elderly hyperthyroid patients, the laboratory profile includes elevations of the conventional parameters of thyroid function. These include serum $T_4$ concentration, resin $T_3$ uptake, serum free $T_4$, and the thyroidal radioactive iodide uptake. The screening of elderly patients for the presence of hyperthyroidism, as in younger patients, involves measurement of serum $T_4$ level and resin $T_3$ uptake. The latter test allows us to detect abnormalities of serum TBG concentration. When a high serum $T_4$ level is due to the presence of elevated serum TBG concentration and not to thyroid disease, the resin $T_3$ uptake is low. A variety of combinations of serum $T_4$ and estimations of serum TBG content are available ("free thyroxine index," "$T_7$"). These combinations correct for the contribution of abnormalities in serum TBG to serum $T_4$ measurements. As many as 20 per cent of elderly thyrotoxic individuals may have normal or only slightly elevated serum $T_4$ levels and $T_3$ resin uptake. In most of these patients the clinical findings of hypermetabolism relate to the presence of $T_3$-toxicosis,[9] a hyperthyroid state in which serum $T_3$ levels are elevated, but serum $T_4$, free $T_4$, and resin $T_3$ uptake are normal.

Occasionally, in patients with minimal elevations of serum $T_4$ and $T_3$ values, it is useful to resort to a TRH stimulation test to confirm the diagnosis of hyperthyroidism. As pointed out earlier, the test is valid in women throughout their lives. The test may not be useful in elderly men if there is little or no TSH response to TRH. However, a normal TRH test in elderly males is helpful in ruling out the presence of thyrotoxicosis. Except as part of a TRH stimulation test, serum TSH measurements by conventional radioimmunoassay are *not* indicated in cases of thyrotoxicosis. There are two clinical settings in which serum TSH should be obtained in the presence of hyperthyroxinemia: (1) excessive TSH secretion by a pituitary tumor and (2) peripheral resistance to thyroid hormone action.[10] In the near future, highly sensitive radioimmunoassays for TSH will become commercially available and will enable the physician to distinguish between normal levels of TSH in euthyroidism and suppressed levels of this pituitary hormone in the setting of hyperthyroidism due to autonomy of the thyroid gland.

There are no accurate, cost-effective tests of the effects of thyroid hormone on peripheral target tissues, such as the heart and nervous system. Estimations of pulse wave arrival time or Q-$K_d$ interval have not been widely applied to the problem of diagnosis of hyperthyroidism in older subjects. Laboratory measurements such as serum cholesterol concentration, serum alkaline phosphatase activity, and serum calcium level may be abnormal in patients with thyrotoxicosis, but none of these parameters is helpful in establishing the diagnosis of thyrotoxicosis.

Therapeutic alternatives in the acute therapy of hyperthyroidism in the elderly are summarized in Table 38–3. Acute management requires control of the symptoms of thyroid dysfunction, anticipation of life-threatening complications of thyrotoxicosis, and preparation of the patient for definitive therapy, usually radioactive iodide ablation of the thyroid gland. Age-specific guidelines for adjusting the dose of thioamide therapy—propyl thiouracil (PTU) or methimazole—in elderly thyrotoxics are not available. It appears that thioamide suppression of granulocyte production is more likely to develop in patients over age 40 years than in younger subjects when conventional doses of methimazole (30 mg per day) are exceeded.[11] Many of the manifestations of hyperthyroidism in the elderly can be controlled with the cautious administration of propranolol. As little as 40 mg of propranolol daily in four divided doses of 10 mg may be effective in controlling tachycardia in elderly hyperthyroid subjects, although total daily doses of 80 to 120 mg are usually required. It is important to recognize that as the patient is rendered euthyroid by the use of radioactive iodide or thioamide drugs, the dose of propranolol that initially was therapeutic may in fact become toxic. Impressive sinus bradycardia may sometimes emerge as thyrotoxicosis remits and relatively high doses of propranolol are continued.

It is widely acknowledged that propranolol may exacerbate congestive heart failure in patients with thyrotoxicosis; however, cautious slowing of heart rate with small doses of propranolol may improve patients with heart failure. We recommend a careful trial of propranolol in patients with thyrotoxicosis and ventricular rates of greater than 140 beats per minute. Titration is carried out to a heart rate of 100 to 110 beats per minute. In patients with

**Table 38-3.** ACUTE THERAPY OF HYPERTHYROIDISM

| Modality | Dosage | Therapeutic Goal | Onset of Clinical Effect |
|---|---|---|---|
| Propylthiouracil* | 300–450 mg orally daily | Inhibition of thyroid hormonogenesis† | 2–8 weeks |
| Iodide | 1–3 drops SSKI‡ orally 1–3 times daily§ | Inhibition of thyroid hormone release<br>Inhibition of thyroid hormonogenesis | Hours |
| Propranolol‖ | 10–40 mg orally** 4 times a day | Damping of peripheral manifestations of hyperthyroidism | Hours to days, depending upon dose |

* Methimazole may be substituted (30 to 45 mg orally daily). Either thioamide drug may be administered as a single daily dose or in divided dosage.

† Propylthiouracil also acts to inhibit conversion in extrathyroidal tissues of thyroxine ($T_4$) to triiodothyronine ($T_3$); whether this is a clinically significant action is unclear. Methimazole does not affect conversion of $T_4$ to $T_3$.

‡ SSKI = supersaturated solution of potassium iodide.

§ In situations in which oral administration is impractical, iodide may be administered intravenously as sodium iodide, 250 to 500 mg bolus daily.

‖ Caution is advised in treating thyrotoxicosis in the setting of heart failure with beta-blocking agents (see text). Experience with other beta-blockers in managing hyperthyroidism is limited. Dosage is titrated against heart rate.

** In situations in which oral administration is impractical, propranolol may be administered intravenously, 0.5 to 1.0 mg bolus, titrating against heart rate (e.g., maintenance of rate at 120 per minute or less).

thyrotoxicosis and heart failure who present with heart rates under 140 beats per minute, we withhold beta-blockade. In the inpatient setting, reserpine may be employed as an emergent agent for control of peripheral signs of hyperthyroidism and tachycardia. The depressant actions of reserpine on the central nervous system can be carefully monitored in inpatients. Reserpine will not worsen congestive heart failure.

The life-threatening phase of hyperthyroidism is termed "thyroid storm." This state is ambiguously defined as fever, tachycardia, and "exaggerated symptoms of hyperthyroidism." Sometimes "apathetic thyroid storm" may occur; this may result in coma and death with very few signs of thyrotoxicosis—except for fever or tachycardia—having been manifest. We look upon elderly thyrotoxic patients with heart rates of 120 beats per minute or greater, those with a previous history of congestive heart failure unrelated to thyroid disease, and those with significant fever (greater than 100.6° F rectally) as "prestorm" patients who should be aggressively treated with beta-blockade (or reserpine, if heart failure is a major consideration), iodide administration, and a thioamide drug, as would be the case in younger patients.

## HYPOTHYROIDISM

Because younger patients do not tolerate the major symptom complex of hypothyroidism—lassitude, constipation, ambient cold intolerance, and dry skin—moderately advanced and severe hypothyroidism are disease states found almost exclusively in the elderly. Thus, myxedema stupor and coma are rare in patients under the age of 50 years. The subtlety of early hypothyroidism in elderly subjects is easily confused with the progression of "normal aging," and a low diagnostic threshold for the possibility of hypothyroidism should be maintained by the physician in dealing with this age group. The incidence of subclinical or incipient hypothyroidism in the elderly is appreciable.[12]

The classical clinical features of hypothyroidism are well known. Several features of thyroid hypofunction may be emphasized, however, as they herald findings of hypothyroidism. As many as one third of the hypothyroid population are hypertensive, and one third of these patients will normalize their blood pressure with thyroid hormone replacement therapy alone.[13]

Gait disorders, apparently due to cerebellar dysfunction, occur in hypothyroidism; voluntary muscle myopathy, usually in a proximal muscle distribution, can also be prominent. Asymmetric septal hypertrophy of the myocardium is also an occasional feature of hypothyroidism. Although pericardial effusion is recognized to be common in this disease state, pleural effusion and ascites are sometimes observed in the absence of prominent pericardial fluid accumulation. Such patients appear to have the nephrotic syndrome. Carbon dioxide retention occurs in hypothyroid patients who may have little or no intrinsic pulmonary disease. Difficulties experienced by the physician in weaning elderly patients from mechanical ventilatory support should raise the possibility of hypothyroid myopathy and/or medullary insensitivity to hypercarbia.

Thyroid gland failure, spontaneous or iatrogenic, explains 95 per cent of the hypothyroidism encountered. The residual minority reflects pituitary or hypothalamic-pituitary disease. Distinguishing between primary thyroid gland failure and secondary or hypothalamic-pituitary origin hypothyroidism is important therapeutically, as will be discussed later. Patients with marginal thyroid function and minimal symptoms of hypothyroidism may become more severely hypothyroid in an accelerated manner when serious systemic, nonthyroidal illness supervenes. Unexplained medical deterioration of patients with serious but appropriately treated nonthyroidal illness should cause the physician to consider the possibility that previously unappreciated thyroid hypofunction may have preceded the onset of the systemic disease.

A diagnosis of thyroidal or primary hypothyroidism is secured by the finding of an elevated serum TSH level and a low serum thyroid hormone ($T_4$) concentration. Measurement of serum resin $T_3$ uptake or one of the several "thyroxine indexes" permits correction for the contribution of low serum TBG levels to the serum $T_4$. In contrast, the patient with low serum $T_4$ and low TSH levels has either hypopituitary hypothyroidism or the "euthyroid sick" syndrome. The latter is a state that accompanies serious systemic nonthyroidal illness of diverse etiologies. Serum TSH results are variable in this syndrome. The resin $T_3$ uptake is normal or borderline elevated in such patients. There is no indication for measurement of antithyroid antibody titers in elderly patients with spontaneous hypothyroidism; although thyroid gland failure is presumed to be autoimmune in such patients, antibody levels are rarely elevated. The possibility of hypopituitarism can be evaluated further with TRH testing of the pituitary-thyroid axis and measurement of serum cortisol levels. Roentgenographic evaluation of the sella turcica to assess the possibility of pituitary tumor (computer-assisted sellar tomography) is also indicated.

A number of other laboratory test abnormalities can accompany hypothyroidism. These include macrocytic anemia (due either to concomitant pernicious anemia or to erythroid maturation arrest of unknown etiology), elevated serum creatine phosphokinase (CPK) activity, hyponatremia, and hyperuricemia. When present, CPK elevations are usually of skeletal muscle origin (MM isoenzyme) and are stable from day to day until thyroid hormone replacement therapy is instituted.[14] Hyponatremia in the hypothyroid population represents a decrease in free water clearance resulting from excessive antidiuretic hormone (ADH, arginine vasopressin [AVP]) secretion of central origin[15] or from intrarenal abnormalities. Institution of effective thyroid hormone replacement normalizes the serum sodium concentration. In patients with rheumatic complaints of myxedematous origin, the finding of hyperuricemia suggests the presence of gout, but hypothyroidism alone can account for both elevated serum uric acid and musculoskeletal symptoms.

Treatment of thyroidal hypothyroidism in older patients involves oral thyroid hormone replacement ($T_4$) in graded dosage. In many elderly subjects, the concomitant presence of heart disease (usually arteriosclerotic, but occasionally cardiomyopathic on a hypothyroid basis) mandates meticulous attention to the rate of incremental increase in hormone dosage. Operationally, the presence of clinically significant heart disease in the setting of hypothyroidism is defined as any one or more of the following: cardiomegaly, evidence of heart failure, prior history of myocardial infarction, angina pectoris, or cardiac arrhythmia. Initial hormone replacement therapy in such patients consists of 0.025 mg L-thyroxine daily. After 2 to 4 weeks the dose is raised to 0.050 mg per day and then the daily dose is increased by 0.025 mg at 2 to 6 week intervals to 0.125 to 0.150 mg per day. It should be emphasized that total daily replacement dosage in elderly patients may amount to no more than 0.075 to 0.125 mg,[16] and the definition of full replacement therapy in hypothyroid older subjects is occasionally rather difficult. However, the lowering of previously elevated serum levels of TSH into the normal range is one widely accepted criterion. The issue becomes whether the TSH concentration is, in fact, normal or suppressed by excessive amounts of replacement hormone. Most TSH radioimmunoassays currently do not adequately distinguish between normal and suppressed serum TSH levels. TRH testing, particularly in elderly women, will reliably indicate whether the dose of thyroid hormone used is excessive.

An alternative test of sufficiency of hormone replacement is measurement of serum TSH by a recently described, highly sensitive method that is able to distinguish between normal and suppressed levels of this trophic hormone.[17] Metabolic equilibration at a given dose of thyroid hormone is sometimes incomplete for months.

Thus, in treating the elderly patient, adjustments in thyroid hormone replacement dosage should be considered if symptoms suggestive of the thyrotoxic state develop months after a "stable" replacement dose of thyroxine has been achieved. There is no role for the use of triiodothyronine ($T_3$) in the management of hypothyroidism in elderly patients. Replacement preparations that contain mixtures of $T_4$ and $T_3$ also offer no advantages over the use of $T_4$ alone. Nonthyroidal illness that may accompany hypothyroidism obviously requires specific and effective treatment at the same time that hypothyroidism is managed.

Severe hypothyroidism (myxedema stupor or coma) is a medical emergency and requires treatment with parenteral $T_4$.[18] The diagnosis is entertained when profound alteration of sensorium is complicated by hypothermia (body core temperature less than 95° F) and/or hypotension in a patient with already established or presumptively diagnosed hypothyroidism. Management should be carried out in an intensive care unit setting. L-thyroxine, 0.250 to 0.400 mg (250 to 400 mcg), is administered over 1 minute as a bolus intravenously. The dose is repeated in 12 hours if no change in sensorium, blood pressure, or body temperature ensues. If improvement in any of these features results after one or two doses of thyroid hormone, low-dose maintenance therapy is then instituted (0.0125 to 0.025 mg [12.5 to 25 mcg] intravenously, daily). High-dose thyroid hormone replacement therapy is indicated in the setting of myxedema stupor or coma even when evidence exists for the presence of concomitant heart disease.

When hypotension or hyponatremia is present in the patient with myxedema stupor or coma, stress level corticosteroid replacement therapy should also be instituted because of the possibility of relative adrenocortical insufficiency in the early phase of thyroid hormone replacement. Stress level steroid replacement consists of 150 mg of hydrocortisone or its equivalent daily, administered in divided intravenous bolus doses or as an infusion. Parameters that are useful to monitor during the early phase of management of myxedema coma include pulmonary capillary wedge pressure and cardiac output (both via a Swan-Ganz catheter) and the myocardial (MB) fraction of serum CPK activity, in addition to arterial blood pH, $PCO_2$ and $PO_2$. These measurements are used to anticipate the possible development of congestive heart failure, myocardial dysfunction, and decreased peripheral tissue oxygen delivery with development of lactic acidosis.

# PITUITARY-ADRENAL FUNCTION

## *Physiology*

Basal levels of serum cortisol and the response of cortisol secretion by the adrenal cortex to exogenous adrenocorticotropic hormone (ACTH) are unaffected by normal aging in humans.[19] The provocative stimulus of insulin-induced hypoglycemia (and attendant release of endogenous ACTH) is not diminished in effectiveness over the life span.[20] On the other hand, sensitivity of aldosterone secretion to the conventional stimuli of sodium restriction and prolonged assumption of the upright posture is diminished in normal elderly subjects.[21] Response of plasma renin to the same stimuli is also decreased in older subjects. The physiologic significance, if any, of these changes in control of aldosterone secretion in the course of normal aging is unknown. Whether the stimulation by hyperkalemia of aldosterone release is also diminished in older individuals is not known. The diagnosis of hyporeninemic hypoaldosteronism as a cause of hyperkalemia should be applied cautiously to elderly subjects because of the diminished sensitivity of the renin-aldosterone axis to provocative testing in these patients.

## *Clinical*

### HYPOADRENOCORTICISM

The clinical syndrome of adrenocortical hypofunction is unaltered by aging. Because weakness and easy fatigability may be associated with the stereotype of "normal aging," these symptoms as heralds of hypoadrenocorticism may attract insufficient medical attention in the elderly. Hyponatremic and hyperkalemic syndromes of various etiologies are relatively common in the elderly patient. In the majority of elderly patients with hyponatremia, however, euvolemia is present and the hyponatremia relates to "decreased free water clearance." "Free water" represents water excretion beyond that obligated by solute excretion by the kidney. The settings in which this abnormality is seen include tumoral secretion of antidiuretic hormone (ADH, AVP, vasopressin) and the administration of various drugs, including diuretics, oral sulfonylureas, carbamazepine, and large doses of cyclophosphamide. Although adrenocortical insufficiency may also be associated with decreased free water clearance, the major explanation for hyponatremia is the inability to retain sodium due to loss of mineralocorticoid secretion.

In addition to hypoadrenocorticism, hyperkalemic syndromes in older patients may relate to decreased renal function, the excessive use of potassium-sparing diuretics (particularly when oral potassium intake is high), and hypoaldosteronism. The last-named condition may reflect an isolated biochemical abnormality in the adrenal cortex or may be due to inadequate production of renin by the kidney (hyporeninemic hypoaldosteronism). The frequency of hyporeninemic hypoaldosteronism is increased in patients with maturity-onset diabetes (Type II), with minimal decreases in glomerular filtration rate. The diagnosis is difficult to establish in elderly subjects, however, because of the changes in renin and aldosterone secretion expected in the course of normal aging (see Physiology, above).

The treatment of adrenocortical hypofunction in the elderly is identical to that in younger patients. The prescription of mineralocorticoid replacement (in addition to glucocorticoid) in older subjects should not be routine but individualized, since this therapy occasionally promotes hypertension and edema formation.

#### Hyperadrenocorticism

Except when caused by ectopic ACTH secretion, hyperadrenocorticism is very uncommon in the elderly. The finding of severe hypokalemia (serum potassium concentration less than 3.0 mEq per L) usually relates to diuretic administration or gastrointestinal potassium loss, as seen with laxative abuse. The decreased incidence in the elderly of nonendocrine syndromes requiring high-dose anti-inflammatory corticosteroid use results in a relatively small number of elderly patients who are iatrogenically cushingoid. Expected age-related decreases in bone mineral content and in cell-mediated immunity increase the risk of long-term glucocorticoid therapy in this population.

## CATECHOLAMINES

### *Physiology*

The ability of the adrenal medulla to release catecholamines remains intact over the life span. There is a heightened capacity of nerve terminals to release norepinephrine (NE) in aged subjects in response to mental stress.[22] Whether target tissue responses to epinephrine (adrenal medullary origin) and NE change with age is not clear.

### *Clinical*

The incidence of pheochromocytoma does not decline with age. More than 40 per cent of autopsy-proved pheochromocytomas occurred in patients over age 60 years in one series.[23] The symptom complex of pheochromocytoma does not change over the life span, and diagnostic evaluation is similar in young and old subjects.

## PARATHYROID GLAND AND VITAMIN D

### *Physiology*

In the course of normal aging, circulating levels of immunoreactive parathyroid hormone (PTH) increase.[24,25] The changes are small and appear to be due to the progressive decrease in glomerular filtration rate that accompanies aging.[26] That is, a decline in glomerular filtration rate results in a decrease in phosphate excretion, an increase in serum phosphate concentration, and a nonsteady-state fall in blood calcium, provoking increased PTH secretion. The phosphaturic action of increased levels of the hormone normalizes serum phosphate, and the stimulus of hypocalcemia remits. A new steady-state is achieved, however, in which the price paid for normocalcemia is a small increase in circulating levels of PTH. It can be assumed that a series of subtle upward adjustments in serum PTH levels contributes to bone demineralization over the life span. Despite the modest increases in circulating PTH with age, the PTH-responsive activation of vitamin D, that is, conversion of liver source 25-OH-vitamin $D_3$ by the kidney to 1,25-$(OH)_2$-$D_3$, is not increased with aging. Although studies of vitamin D metabolism in the elderly are flawed by inclusion of sick or institutionalized patients exposed infrequently to sunlight, the conclusion of most studies is that levels of vitamin D (including 1,25-$(OH)_2$-$D_3$) do, in fact, fall with age.[25,27] Vitamin D levels vary seasonally, and isolated determinations should be interpreted cautiously. Inexorable declines in serum vitamin D contribute to the decrease in gastrointestinal tract absorption of calcium over the life span.[25] Decreased absorption of calcium may also contribute to the rise of PTH with advancing age, mentioned earlier.

### *Clinical*

Loss of the capacity of the parafollicular cells of the thyroid gland to secrete calcitonin in response to hypercalcemic stress has been observed in the elderly.[28] It is doubtful that decreased responsiveness of calcitonin secretion contributes to bone demineralization. Calcitonin does oppose PTH action on bone.

### Hyperparathyroidism and Hypercalcemia

The extensive and traditional differential diagnosis of hypercalcemia is, in practical terms, composed of a small group of disease entities in the elderly. These diseases include primary hyperparathyroidism, cancer-related hypercalcemia, and drug-induced hypercalcemias. Conditions such as sarcoidosis and hypercalcemia due to thyrotoxicosis, Addison's disease, and the diuretic phase of post-rhabdomyolytic renal failure are uncommon in older patients. Occasionally encountered are hypercalcemic states consequent to immobilization of patients with widespread Paget's disease of bone or to the initiation of estrogen therapy in women with breast carcinoma widely metastatic to bone. Self-administration of large doses of vitamin A, as well as vitamin D, may cause significant hypercalcemia.

Primary hyperparathyroidism has been recognized with increased frequency in elderly patients, and as much as 20 per cent of the hyperparathyroid patient population is over the age of 60 years. The prevalence of hyperparathyroidism in geriatric hospitals is high.[29] The increased frequency with which primary hyperparathyroidism is recognized in the geriatric population is a reflection of the now routine measurement (sequential multiple analysis [SMA]-12, or equivalent survey) of serum calcium concentration in inpatients and outpatients who have no symptoms attributable to parathyroid disease. Thiazide diuretic administration promotes hypercalcemia in a small minority of patients; in our view, hypercalcemia that develops during thiazide use reflects previously latent primary hyperparathyroidism.[30] In contrast to thiazides, loop diuretics (furosemide, ethacrynic acid, bumetanide) are calciuretic agents and do not provoke hypercalcemia.

When symptomatic, primary hyperparathyroidism in the elderly is not different from that in younger patients. That is, constipation, increased urinary frequency, urinary tract stone formation, and symptomatic myopathy or arthralgias may occur. In asymptomatic patients, mild hyperparathyroidism is regarded as a factor promoting demineralizing bone disease in old and young patients alike.

The diagnosis of primary hyperparathyroidism is based on the finding of elevated serum immunoreactive PTH levels. If hypercalcemia has developed on a basis other than primary hyperparathyroidism, PTH levels should be suppressed. A group of patients with hypercalcemia due to production of a hypercalcemic principle by nonparathyroid tumors has been shown to have serum PTH concentrations in the normal range, rather than suppressed. Presumably this finding represents the release by nonparathyroid tumor tissue of a biologically active polypeptide hormone that partially cross-reacts with the antibody used in conventional PTH radioimmunoassays. Beyond the scope of this discussion are experimental methods currently in use for distinguishing between authentic PTH and non-PTH hypercalcemic peptides of cancer origin.

Aside from primary hyperparathyroidism, the major differential diagnostic considerations as causes of hypercalcemia in the elderly patient population are squamous cell carcinomas, which elaborate hypercalcemic hormones; multiple myeloma; and use of certain drugs. In addition to thiazide diuretics, several other agents in use in the elderly patient population promote hypercalcemia. These include estrogens in breast carcinoma patients (mentioned earlier) and vitamin D, an agent that may find favor as an adjunctive approach to osteoporosis in postmenopausal women.

Therapeutic approaches to the management of hypercalcemia in the elderly are, of course, etiology specific. The issue frequently encountered in elderly patients with asymptomatic primary hyperparathyroidism is when, if ever, to endorse surgical exploration of the neck to remove a parathyroid adenoma or hyperplastic parathyroid glands. The tendency for hyperparathyroidism in this age group to be indolent and the presence of concomitant nonendocrine illnesses that heighten the risk of anesthesia in surgery (e.g., chronic obstructive lung disease and arteriosclerotic heart disease) cause us to be conservative with many patients and not recommend surgery if the serum calcium is minimally elevated. Twenty per cent or more of these patients will require parathyroidectomy in 5 to 10 years, usually for relief of hypercalcemia.[31] We follow such asymptomatic patients with annual measurements of bone mineral content by photon absorptiometry in a search for accelerated loss of bone mass. Serum calcium levels greater than 11.5 mg per dl, accelerated bone demineralization, and increased rate of decline in glomerular filtration rate are factors that cause us to recommend parathyroid surgery in patients in whom the diagnosis of primary hyperparathyroidism has been confirmed by serum PTH assay. Length of hospitalization after neck exploration and permanent complication rates (hypocalcemia, vocal cord paralysis) are identical in young patients with hyperparathyroidism and elderly patients who have no systemic illnesses other than parathyroid hyperfunction.

The hazards of conventional medical management of hypercalcemia are increased in older patients. Expansion of intravascular volume by saline diuresis in patients with impaired left ventricular function may worsen heart failure, and the concomitant intravenous administration of large doses of furosemide may lead to hypokalemia and its attendant risks. When treatment of hypercalcemia in an elderly patient with heart disease involves saline administration and loop diuretic use, the insertion of a Swan-Ganz catheter to monitor pulmonary capillary wedge pressure is judicious. Alternative strategies to induction of a saline diuresis include calcitonin administration (e.g., 2 to 8 Medical Research Council [MRC] units per kg body weight subcutaneously daily in divided doses) or mithramycin (25 mcg per kg body weight intravenously). Either of these approaches requires 12 to 24 hours to reduce serum calcium significantly. Calcitonin is a particularly attractive agent for use in the elderly patient population because of its low toxicity and lack of dependence upon the kidney for its effect. The administration of corticosteroids is useful in the management of patients with tumoral hypercalcemia due to multiple myeloma or breast carcinoma, but several days are required before the calcium-lowering effect of steroids will be seen.

Chronic management of the patient with hypercalcemia may involve the use of a loop diuretic (for its calciuretic effect), with frequent monitoring of serum potassium levels, or agents such as calcitonin or oral phosphate administration. Calcitonin may be self-administered subcutaneously by patients daily or at less frequent intervals. Oral phosphate use, e.g., Neutra Phos, is of low risk in patients with adequate renal function. Diarrhea is a limiting factor with larger doses of phosphate.

## ANTIDIURETIC HORMONE

### *Physiology*

Normal aging is characterized by progressive resistance of the renal collecting tubules to the action of antidiuretic hormone (ADH, AVP). As a result, basal levels of AVP increase slightly over the life span. Central osmoreceptor sensitivity, that is, the amount of AVP secreted for a given increase in plasma osmolality, is increased in older subjects compared with young individuals.[32]

### *Clinical*

Primary disorders of AVP secretion are uncommon in the older patient population. Management of diabetes insipidus in older subjects is made more difficult by the presence of concomitant nonendocrine diseases (notably, heart disease) in which intravascular volume expansion and contraction are both of particular risk. Both states can be experienced by patients who incorrectly dose themselves with antidiuretic hormone replacement. The administration of 1-desamino-8-D-arginine vasopressin (dDAVP)[33] in older subjects with diabetes insipidus is attractive because of its short biologic half-life and intranasal route of administration. Thus, the possibility of prolonged antidiuresis sometimes seen with subcutaneous administration of vasopressin tannate in peanut oil is minimized. On the other hand, dDAVP must be administered several times daily, and noncompliance is unavoidable in patients with memory loss.

Water intoxication syndromes in older subjects result from the inappropriate secretion of AVP by nonendocrine tumors or from the administration of a variety of drugs. Most common among the latter are diuretics (which promote saluresis, but, paradoxically, water antidiuresis), chlorpropamide, and carbamazepine. Although a large number of other pharmacologic agents are cited in reviews of water intoxication as factors leading to hyponatremia, only the three preceding agents are of well-documented clinical significance. In the elderly population we most commonly encounter hyponatremia in the euvolemic or hypervolemic patient whose serum sodium concentration has fallen with the introduction of diuretic therapy. Drug-related urinary sodium loss contributes minimally to the hyponatremia observed in this situation, i.e., the decrease in free water clearance is more important than the saluresis. Except for chlorpropamide, oral sulfonylureas used in the management of Type II diabetes mellitus have either an insignificant antidiuretic effect (tolbutamide) or are, in fact, promoters of free water clearance (water diuresis) (tolazamide, glyburide).[34] Additional discussion of water and sodium excretion is found in Chapter 31.

## GROWTH HORMONE

### Physiology

The response of pituitary secretion of growth hormone (GH) to provocative stimulation declines over the life span.[20] Provocative stimuli under controlled diagnostic circumstances are insulin-induced hypoglycemia and intravenous arginine administration. The functional role of GH in the adult population is unclear, except for its participation in the counter-regulatory response to spontaneous or drug-induced hypoglycemic states.

### Clinical

Disorders of GH secretion are uncommon in the geriatric population. Acromegaly that occurs in the older subject has no features that distinguish the syndrome from that in younger individuals. Pituitary deficiency of GH release in the mature adult is not clinically apparent and is recognized only by laboratory testing.

## PROLACTIN

### Physiology

The control of prolactin (PRL) release is unaltered with aging.[35] PRL secretion is provoked under diagnostic conditions by the administration intravenously of thyrotropin-releasing hormone (TRH). The biologic role of PRL in men and in women beyond reproductive age is unclear.

### Clinical

Abnormalities of PRL in older subjects are uncommon. Hyperprolactinemia may provoke galactorrhea in women of virtually any age. The common presentation of hyperprolactinemia in premenopausal women is amenorrhea and infertility, a syndrome obviously not expressed beyond the reproductive age. A small minority of breast cancers in women appear to be prolactin-dependent, but it is not known whether longstanding hyperprolactinemia in any age group is a risk factor for breast carcinoma.

## GONADAL FUNCTION

### Physiology

The inevitable loss of ovarian function in women is of unknown mechanism. Progressive loss of ovarian estrogen secretory capacity is accompanied by increases in circulating levels and urinary secretion of gonadotropins (follicle-stimulating hormone [FSH], luteinizing hormone [LH]), loss of pulsatile release of gonadotropins by the pituitary, and preservation of adrenocortical secretion of androgens. The functional ovary is, during active reproductive life, a second source of androgens. Ovarian secretion of androgens persists into the menopause as estrogen secretory capacity is lost. Thus the ratio of circulating estrogens to androgens in menopausal women declines not only as a result of decreased estrogen release but also as a result of relative preservation of androgen secretion. Administration of exogenous gonadotropins to menopausal women reveals little or no end organ response in terms of estrogen release. Intravenous administration of luteinizing hormone–releasing hormone (LHRH) to menopausal women results in an exaggerated LH response superimposed on elevated basal levels of LH and FSH.

Controversy surrounds the concept of a clinically significant and inevitable decline in testosterone secretion in men over the life span. Studies that have contended that androgen secretion in men declines with age have usually included institutionalized or chronically ill males. Studies in which there has been scrupulous exclusion of sick subjects suggest that there is little substantive change in testosterone secretory capacity over the life span in men.[36,37] The circadian rhythm of serum testosterone levels is lost in elderly men. On the other hand, serum gonadotropin levels in aging males are increased even in those studies in which serum testosterone levels have been stable into the eighth decade of life.[36] These observations indicate that the testis in older men is less responsive to pituitary gonadotropin than is that of younger men. In those reports in which circulating levels of androgens are decreased in aged men, the range of levels is great. Thus, no studies mandate routine administration of testosterone to elderly men.

### Clinical

#### Menopause

The indications for hormonal replacement therapy in menopausal women are discussed in

Chapters 35 and 39.[38] From the point of view of the endocrinologist, indications for estrogen replacement are several. These include (1) vasomotor symptoms, the severity of which interferes with activities of daily living; (2) surgical menopause before the age of 30 years; and (3) genetic states of hypoestrogenism (e.g., Turner's syndrome). Accelerated loss of bone mass in appendicular or axial skeleton—documented either by long bone or vertebral fracture or by serial photon absorptiometry—is also a criterion for estrogen replacement therapy in the postmenopausal woman. The management of metabolic bone disease in the elderly is discussed in Chapter 39.

## CARBOHYDRATE METABOLISM AND DIABETES MELLITUS

### Physiology

Fasting serum or plasma glucose concentration does not change over the life span. Regardless of age, the patient who has a fasting serum or plasma glucose level greater than 140 mg per dl is classified as diabetic, according to the criteria established by the National Diabetes Data Group.[39] An extensive literature has documented a decrease in carbohydrate tolerance in the course of normal aging, defined in terms of serial blood sugar levels obtained during a 2-hour period following oral glucose ingestion.[40] The clinical significance of this change in carbohydrate tolerance is unknown, and the National Diabetes Data Group ignored age-specific changes in performance in classifying results of oral glucose tolerance testing: that is, changes in carbohydrate tolerance resulting in blood sugar values between 140 and 200 mg per dl 2 hours after a standard oral glucose load are classified as "impaired glucose tolerance."[39] This performance range encompasses the changes in glucose tolerance that have been reported previously as characteristic of normal aging. Recent evidence suggests that changes in glucose tolerance with age reflect decreased peripheral tissue sensitivity to insulin.[41] That is, insulin-responsive tissues such as fat cells and muscle take up less glucose in response to a given amount of insulin in the course of aging. Interestingly, this alteration in target organ sensitivity to insulin appears to be expressed by middle age[41] and occurs at a cellular level beyond the insulin receptor.[42]

Hypoglycemia provokes release of counter-regulatory hormones—epinephrine, glucagon, growth hormone, and cortisol. The course of normal aging appears to have little effect on the response of cortisol levels to hypoglycemia; in contrast, GH release in response to hypoglycemia is significantly reduced in elderly subjects,[20] as pointed out earlier. Because GH is an adjunctive contributor to the counter-regulatory response, it is unlikely that this age-dependent change in GH release is clinically significant. Fasting levels of immunoreactive glucagon have been shown to rise within the third and fourth decades but do not rise further thereafter.[43]

### Clinical

Diabetes mellitus with onset in middle-aged or elderly subjects has a clinical pattern of hyperglycemia uncomplicated by significant ketosis or acidosis (Type II diabetes mellitus).[39] Type II diabetics are usually overweight, and more than 20 per cent have a family history that is positive for maturity-onset diabetes mellitus. Although such patients have frequently been described as "non–insulin-dependent" because of failure to exhibit ketosis in the absence of exogenous insulin therapy, they may in fact require exogenous insulin therapy to control hyperglycemia. Type I diabetes mellitus is that which is prone to result in ketoacidosis when exogenous insulin therapy is omitted. Occasionally, Type I diabetes occurs in elderly patients, and in these patients, episodes of diabetic ketoacidosis are observed that are indistinguishable from those occurring in patients with so-called juvenile-onset diabetes mellitus.

In the past decade a number of studies have supported the concept that maintenance of normoglycemia in the diabetic patient population prevents or postpones complications of this disease.[44,45] Longitudinal studies have not been carried out in elderly diabetics to prove this point, but it is clear that Type II diabetics are subject to the same complications that are acknowledged to occur in young diabetics. The alternative strategies that the physician may consider in managing the elderly diabetic include (1) "tight" control, based on repeated injections postprandially of regular insulin or use of the insulin pump; (2) avoidance of substantive hyperglycemia (blood sugar concentrations at any time of day greater than 250 mg per dl), and maintenance of fasting blood sugar levels below 160 mg per dl with one or two doses daily of intermediate-acting insulin; (3) oral sulfonylurea management with variable degrees of control of blood sugar; (4) dietary strictures designed to provoke weight loss and attendant improvement in peripheral tissue sensitivity to insulin; and (5) a permissive approach—applied to asymptomatic hyperglycemic patients—in which control of blood sugar is not attempted. Combinations of these strategies are obviously possible. We do not believe a permissive approach can be justified in any cohort of diabetic patients. Weight loss is a desirable goal in all overweight diabetic patients; it may result in a lowering of blood sugar by improving insulin responsiveness of peripheral tissues and also may improve control of blood pressure in those individuals with concomitant hypertension.[46] Weight loss also treats the increased mortality rate associated with obesity, at least in those subjects who are 30 per cent or more above ideal body weight.[47] The safety of "semistarvation" regimens (300 kcal daily) has not been established in Type II diabetics over the age of 60 years. Modest weight loss may be achieved with limitation of total daily caloric intake to 800 to 1000 kcal.

The wisdom of restricting carbohydrate calories in any diabetic population is subject to question. High carbohydrate intake (up to 70 per cent carbohydrate) may actually improve carbohydrate tolerance in subjects with mild Type II diabetes; whether dietary carbohydrate composition is complex or simple also appears to be irrelevant in terms of impact on blood sugar levels.[48] Thus, we endorse in the elderly diabetic patient a conventional diet (50 per cent or more carbohydrate in composition), which in overweight subjects is restricted in terms of total caloric content.

The desirability of oral sulfonylurea therapy for Type II diabetics has been tempered by the apparent risks of this approach. Hepatotoxicity may be seen in a small minority of patients in the course of treatment with any of the sulfonylureas. Hypoglycemia is an uncommon side effect unless alcoholic beverage abuse occurs concomitant with sulfonylurea administration. Because alcohol inhibits hepatic gluconeogenesis, patients who are alcohol-dependent may be unable to restore euglycemia after sulfonylurea-induced hypoglycemia. The desirable potency of chlorpropamide as a blood sugar–lowering agent is accompanied by the risk of hyponatremia,[34] mentioned earlier. Other sulfonylureas have either trivial antidiuretic effects or are, in fact, capable of inducing water diuresis (tolazamide, glyburide).

An issue of greater importance than these side effects of oral sulfonylureas is the possibility of increased cardiovascular mortality associated with administration of these agents. The controversy springs from a longitudinal study of sulfonylurea use,[49] the design of which was subsequently subjected to repeated criticism and defense. Additional studies of long-term sulfonylurea use have been published that found no increase in risk of sudden death.[50] In addition, it is now appreciated that sulfonylurea therapy is effective primarily because of insulin-potentiating effects on peripheral tissue, rather than on islet cell release of endogenous insulin.[51] In Type II diabetic patients who are not candidates for insulin therapy because of advanced age or unwillingness to self-administer insulin, oral sulfonylurea therapy must be regarded as a reasonable alternative. The selection of a specific sulfonylurea should be based upon potency of the agent and relative freedom from side effects. In our view, the most potent available oral hypoglycemic agent is chlorpropamide; we have pointed out, however, that the risk of hyponatremia with this drug is substantial, particularly when patients are receiving diuretic therapy for management of hypertension or congestive heart failure.[52] Tolazamide appears to be a less potent hypoglycemic agent than chlorpropamide but does not promote hyponatremia. Glyburide and glipizide are agents that have recently been approved for use in the United States and offer the advantages of potency and a positive, rather than negative, effect on free water clearance.

The diabetic patient between the ages of 60 and 70 years faces the prospect of 10 to 20 years survival. Patients in this age group should be seriously considered for insulin therapy if they are compliant and functional. Our experience with Type II diabetics indicates that 25 per cent of these patients maintain normal fasting blood sugar and glycosylated hemoglobin levels on one or two injections of intermediate-acting and regular insulin daily. Glycosylated hemoglobin is a summational record of glycemia.[53] Reasonable therapeutic goals are (1) freedom from symptoms, that is, absence of polyuria, polydipsia, and weight loss attributable to poor diabetic control; (2) fasting blood sugar concentrations below 140 mg per dl; and (3) glycosylated hemoglobin levels close to or below the upper limit of the normal range.

As in younger diabetics, the management of older subjects with this disease is based on systematic surveillance and anticipation of complications of the illness. Surveillance is designed to detect large blood vessel disease, nephropathy, and neuropathy. Peripheral neuropathy (polyneuropathy) and peripheral vascular disease are particularly devastating in elderly patients when these complications lead to limb loss; rehabilitation of the elderly subject who has undergone lower extremity amputation is frequently unsuccessful because of coincident syndromes, such as angina pectoris and dizziness, which forestall gait re-education.

Extreme loss of control of hyperglycemia in the elderly patient results in the syndrome of hyperglycemic nonketotic stupor or coma. The absence of ketosis in Type II diabetics, regardless of the severity of hyperglycemia, is believed to be due to the residual capacity of pancreatic islet cells to secrete enough insulin to suppress lipolysis (and the free fatty acid liberation that ultimately leads to hepatic ketone production), but inadequate amounts of insulin to control the level of blood sugar. The acute management of this syndrome is discussed in detail in standard textbooks of endocrinology and involves re-expansion of intravascular volume, intravenous low-dose insulin administration (regular insulin, 5 to 10 units per hour), and potassium administration. Potassium replacement is indicated as blood sugar levels begin to fall and serum creatinine levels, which are almost invariably elevated in this syndrome, also decline, indicating improvement in glomerular filtration rate.

The devastating complications of management of hyperglycemic nonketotic coma include (1) over-replacement of intravascular volume with resultant pulmonary edema; (2) precipitous decline in serum potassium concentration, particularly in the already digitalized patient, resulting in refractory cardiac tachyarrhythmias; (3) failure to identify a treatable precipitating cause for the syndrome, particularly infections of the lower respiratory tract, biliary tree, and urinary tract; and (4) failure to acknowledge the presence of unrelated metabolic acidosis. Arterial pH in the patient with hyperglycemic nonketotic stupor should be 7.35 or higher and venous bicarbonate levels 18 or more mEq per L. When significant metabolic acidosis is seen in the setting of nonketotic stupor or coma, sources of lactic acid production should be sought, such as infection or tissue ischemia, both of which are amenable to specific therapy. As stated earlier, hyperglycemic nonketotic stupor or coma is a syndrome in which administration of 5 to 10 units of regular insulin intravenously per hour is usually adequate; doses up to 20 to 30 units per hour may occasionally be required in patients whose hyperosmolar syndrome is complicated by lactic acidosis. The mortality rates in this syndrome remain high in many centers, with deaths 3 to 5 days after admission attributable to inadequately treated infections, myocardial infarction, or a stroke that occurred during the episode of uncontrolled diabetes mellitus with volume depletion and hypotension.

## References


1. Olsen TP, et al: Low serum triiodothyronine and high serum reverse triiodothyronine in old age: An effect of disease not age. J Clin Endocrinol Metab 47:1111, 1978.
2. Harman SM, et al: Pituitary-thyroid hormone economy in healthy aging men: Basal indices of thyroid function and thyrotropin responses to constant infusions of thyrotropin releasing hormone. J Clin Endocrinol Metab 58:320, 1984.
3. Braverman LE, et al: Observations concerning the binding of thyroid hormones in sera of normal subjects of varying ages. J Clin Invest 45:1273, 1966.
4. Snyder PJ, Utiger RD: Response to thyrotropin releasing hormone (TRH) in normal man. J Clin Endocrinol Metab 34:380, 1972.
5. Ordene KW, et al: Variable thyrotropin response to thyrotropin-releasing hormone after small decreases in plasma thyroid hormone concentration in patients of advanced age. Metabolism 32:881, 1983.
6. Hershman JM: Clinical application of thyrotropin-releasing hormone. New Engl J Med 290:886, 1974.
7. Snyder PJ, Utiger RD: Thyrotropin response to thyrotropin releasing hormone in normal females over forty. J Clin Endocrinol Metab 34:1096, 1972.
8. Davis PJ, Davis FB: Hyperthyroidism in patients over the age of 60. Medicine 53:161, 1974.
9. Sterling K, et al: $T_3$-thyrotoxicosis. Thyrotoxicosis due to elevated serum triiodothyronine levels. JAMA 213:571, 1970.
10. Gershengorn MC: Inappropriate thyroid-stimulating hormone secretion: Description and classification. *In* Weintraub BD (moderator): Inappropriate secretion of thyroid-stimulating hormone. Ann Intern Med 95:339, 1981.
11. Cooper DS, et al: Agranulocytosis associated with antithyroid drugs. Effects of patient age and drug dose. Ann Intern Med 98:26, 1983.
12. Bagchi N, et al: Thyroid function in older persons. Ann Intern Med 101:718, 1984.
13. Attarian E: Myxedema and hypertension. NY State J Med 63:2801, 1963.
14. Ladenson PW, et al: Early peripheral responses to intravenous L-thyroxine in primary hypothyroidism. Am J Med 73:467, 1982.
15. Skowsky WR, Kikuchi TA: The role of vasopressin in the impaired water excretion of myxedema. Am J Med 64:613, 1978.
16. Davis FB, et al: Estimation of a physiologic thyroxine replacement dose in elderly hypothyroid patients. Arch Intern Med 144:1752, 1984.
17. Wehmann RE, et al: Extended clinical utility of a sensitive and reliable radioimmunoassay of thyroid-stimulating hormone. South Med J 76:969, 1983.
18. Holvey DN, et al: Treatment of myxedema coma with intravenous thyroxine. Arch Intern Med 113:89, 1964.
19. Gherondache CN, et al: Steroid hormones in aging men. *In* Gitman L (ed.): Endocrines and Aging. Springfield, Ill., Charles C Thomas, 1967.
20. Muggeo M, et al: Human growth hormone and cortisol response to insulin stimulation in aging. J Gerontol 30:546, 1975.
21. Weidman P, et al: Effect of aging on plasma renin and aldosterone in normal man. Kidney Int 8:325, 1975.

22. Barnes RF, et al: The effects of age on the plasma catecholamine response to mental stress in man. J Clin Endocrinol Metab 54:64, 1982.
23. St. John Sutton MG, et al: Prevalence of clinically unsuspected pheochromocytoma. Review of a 50-year autopsy series. Mayo Clin Proc 56:354, 1981.
24. Insogna KL, et al: Effect of age on serum immunoreactive parathyroid hormone and its biological effect. J Clin Endocrinol Metab 53:1072, 1981.
25. Chapuy M-C, et al: Age-related changes in parathyroid hormone and 25 hydroxycholecalciferol levels. J Gerontol 38:19, 1983.
26. Marcus R, et al: Age-related changes in parathyroid hormone and parathyroid hormone action in normal humans. J Clin Endocrinol Metab 58:223, 1984.
27. Corless D, et al: Vitamin-D status in long-stay geriatric patients. Lancet 1:1404, 1975.
28. Deftos LJ, et al: Influence of age and sex on plasma calcitonin in human beings. New Engl J Med 302: 1351, 1980.
29. Tibblin S, et al: Hyperparathyroidism in the elderly. Ann Surg 197:135, 1983.
30. Christensson T, et al: Hypercalcemia and primary hyperparathyroidism. Prevalence in patients receiving thiazides as detected in a health screen. Arch Intern Med 137:1138, 1977.
31. Scholz DA, Purnell DC: Asymptomatic primary hyperparathyroidism. 10-year prospective study. Mayo Clin Proc 56:473, 1981.
32. Helderman JH, et al: The response of arginine vasopressin to intravenous alcohol and hypertonic saline in man: The impact of aging. J Gerontol 33:39, 1978.
33. Robinson AG: DDAVP in the treatment of central diabetes insipidus. New Engl J Med 294:507, 1976.
34. Moses AM, et al: Diuretic action of three sulfonylurea drugs. Ann Intern Med 78:541, 1973.
35. Jacobs LS, et al: Prolactin response to thyrotropin-releasing hormone in normal subjects. J Clin Endocrinol Metab 36:1069, 1973.
36. Harman SM, Tsitouras PD: Reproductive hormones in aging men. I. Measurement of sex steroids, basal luteinizing hormone, and Leydig cell response to human chorionic gonadotropin. J Clin Endocrinol Metab 51:35, 1980.
37. Zumoff B, et al: Age variation of the 24-hour mean plasma concentrations of androgens, estrogens, and gonadotropins in normal adult men. J Clin Endocrinol Metab 54:534, 1982.
38. Council on Scientific Affairs: Estrogen replacement in the menopause. JAMA 249:359, 1983.
39. National Diabetes Data Group: Classification and diagnosis of diabetes mellitus and other categories of glucose intolerance. Diabetes 28:1039, 1979.
40. Andres R: Aging and diabetes. Med Clin N Am 55:835, 1971.
41. DeFronzo RA: Glucose intolerance and aging. Evidence for tissue insensitivity to insulin. Diabetes 28:1095, 1979.
42. Fink RI, et al: Mechanisms of insulin resistance in aging. J Clin Invest 71:1523, 1983.
43. Berger D, et al: Effect of age on fasting plasma levels of pancreatic hormones in man. J Clin Endocrinol Metab 47:1183, 1978.
44. Pirart J: Diabetes mellitus and its degenerative complications: A prospective study of 4,400 patients observed between 1947 and 1973. Diabetes Care 1:168, 1978.
45. Raskin P, et al: The effect of diabetic control on the width of skeletal-muscle capillary basement membrane in patients with Type I diabetes mellitus. New Engl J Med 309:1546, 1983.
46. Reisin E, et al: Cardiovascular changes after weight reduction in obesity hypertension. Ann Intern Med 98:315, 1983.
47. Bierman EL, Hirsch J: Obesity. *In* Williams RH (ed.): Textbook of Endocrinology. Philadelphia, W.B. Saunders Company, 1981.
48. Bantle JP, et al: Postprandial glucose and insulin responses to meals containing different carbohydrates in normal and diabetic subjects. New Engl J Med 309:7, 1983.
49. The University Group Diabetes Program: A study of the effects of hypoglycemic agents on vascular complications in patients with adult-onset diabetes. II. Mortality results. Diabetes 19 (Suppl. 2):789, 1970.
50. Paasikivi J: Long-term tolbutamide treatment after myocardial infarction. Acta Med Scand 507 (Suppl.): 1, 1970.
51. Olefsky JM, Reaven GM: Effects of sulfonylurea therapy on insulin binding to mononuclear leukocytes of diabetic patients. Am J Med 60:89, 1976.
52. Davis FB, et al: Factors moderating the effect of oral sulfonylureas on free water clearance. J Clin Pharmacol 22:652, 1982.
53. Bunn HF: Evaluation of glycosylated hemoglobin in diabetic patients. Diabetes 30:613, 1981.

Chapter 39

# Osteoporosis

*John Jennings*
*David Baylink*

Osteoporosis is a generalized reduction of bone mass. It is a group of disorders with heterogeneous etiologies, which can be divided into two major forms, primary and secondary. In primary osteoporosis there is a reduction of histologically normal bone, whereas in secondary osteoporosis, the bone may or may not be morphologically normal. The cause of the loss of bone in primary osteoporosis is not readily identifiable. Cases of primary osteoporosis can be classified on the basis of age and sex (Table 39–1). We have not included genetic forms of osteoporosis in this classification because the initial diagnosis of these genetic diseases is usually made prior to middle age. Loss of bone appears to be a consequence of aging and may begin as early as the third decade.[6] The loss involves cortical and trabecular bone, with subsequent hip and vertebral fractures occurring after age 70. This condition is called "senile" osteoporosis.[24] Premature trabecular bone loss in adults, leading primarily to vertebral compression fractures, is called (1) idiopathic osteoporosis in females under 50 years and in males under 70 years or (2) postmenopausal osteoporosis in females over 50 years. More than 85 per cent of patients with primary osteoporosis are in the postmenopausal and senile groups. Secondary osteoporosis occurs in association with well-defined inherited or acquired disorders or with the administration of certain drugs, and it accounts for approximately 10 to 15 per cent of cases of osteoporosis (Table 39–2).

The clinical complications of osteoporosis are a major source of disability in the elderly. Twenty-five per cent of females over the age of 65 have back pain, deformity, or loss of height due to vertebral compression fractures.[18] Although these fractures are seldom catastrophic, the continued pain may significantly alter lifestyle. Hip fractures, which occur with a cumulative incidence of 30 per cent in white females by age 90,[18] not only cause pain and disability but also may cause death within 6 months of the acute fracture in as many as 15 per cent of patients. To further illustrate the extent of this problem, 5.3 per cent of hospitalized patients over 65 and 10.2 per cent of hospitalized patients over 85 have the diagnosis of fracture.[31] In the United States, the cost of acute health care for hip fractures alone is estimated to exceed 1 billion dollars annually.[18]

Several factors have contributed to the limited clinical initiative of physicians in dealing with these disorders despite their major health impact: (1) The pathophysiology is not clearly understood. (2) Guidelines and techniques for diagnosis are not widely available. (3) There is no simple and rapidly effective therapy. In this chapter we will summarize the techniques for diagnosis and outline current modes of therapy. Our comments will focus on primary osteoporosis, but the different causes of secondary osteoporosis will be presented, since one must exclude secondary osteoporosis to make the diagnosis of primary osteoporosis.

## PATHOPHYSIOLOGY OF PRIMARY OSTEOPOROSIS

Bone volume is determined by the rates of bone formation and bone resorption. The loss of skeletal mass in osteoporosis implies that resorption exceeds formation. According to studies using current techniques of measurement, the rates of formation and resorption are normal in almost 90 per cent of patients with primary osteoporosis.[9] The available evidence supports the concept that the pathogenesis of

**Table 39-1.** CLASSIFICATION OF PRIMARY OSTEOPOROSIS

| Subgroups of Osteoporosis | Sex | Age |
|---|---|---|
| Juvenile | Both | Puberty |
| Idiopathic | Female | Puberty to 50 years |
| | Male | Puberty to 70 years |
| Postmenopausal | Female | 50-70 years |
| Senile | Female | >70 years |
| | Male | |

primary osteoporosis is not homogeneous and that subgroups exist with normal, increased, or decreased bone turnover.[30]

Extensive studies have attempted to determine the mechanisms by which bone is lost with aging and in osteoporosis. Calcium absorption and the serum concentrations of calcitonin and 1,25-$(OH)_2D$ (basal or after provocative stimuli) decrease with aging.[4,5] These age-related changes are exaggerated in postmenopausal osteoporosis.[4,19,28,29] Parathyroid hormone (PTH) concentration increases with aging,[13] but the increase is less in subjects with osteoporosis and vertebral fracture.[22a] The increase in PTH with aging is probably due to changes in renal function,[16] whereas the relative decrease in PTH in osteoporosis may be due to accelerated bone loss.[22a] In individual patients, PTH concentrations are usually within the normal range. The changes in these calcium-regulating hormone concentrations or reserves are small and may not fully account for the development of osteoporosis.

**Table 39-2.** COMMON CAUSES OF SECONDARY OSTEOPOROSIS IN GERIATRIC SUBJECTS

1. Excess glucocorticoids—endogenous or exogenous source
2. Hypogonadism—male and female; acquired, iatrogenic, inherited
3. Immobilization
4. Hyperthyroidism
5. Vitamin D deficiency states*
   a. Decreased vitamin D intake
   b. Decreased vitamin D absorption
   c. Increased 25-OHD degradation
6. Idiopathic hypercalciuria†
7. Multiple myeloma
8. Primary hyperparathyroidism

* In these disorders, mild reductions in vitamin D intake lead to secondary osteoporosis, whereas more severe decreases lead to osteomalacia (see text).

† This disease may be associated with hypophosphatemia, and chronic hypophosphatemia of any cause, as with vitamin D deficiency, will produce osteoporosis when mild and osteomalacia when severe.

The majority of patients with primary osteoporosis are postmenopausal women. The effects of estrogen deficiency upon bone are very similar to the changes seen with aging; calcium absorption and calcitonin reserve are reduced.[4,10] The mechanism by which estrogen acts upon bone is unknown and may be indirect, since bone cells do not appear to possess estrogen receptors.[21] Two lines of evidence suggest that the increase in bone resorption seen with estrogen deficiency[9] is not solely responsible for the development of osteoporosis: (1) The onset of bone loss in females precedes the onset of menopause by a number of years. (2) Like estrogen deficiency, thyrotoxicosis and mild hyperparathyroidism are associated with an increase in bone resorption. Although estrogen deficiency is associated with bone loss, the resorption in these two disorders is often accompanied by a proportionate increase in bone formation, which preserves skeletal mass. Evidence has been presented that this coupling of bone resorption to bone formation is defective in osteoporosis, but the importance of this abnormality to bone loss is unknown.[2,14]

Estrogen deficiency is associated with increased (i.e., above basal) bone resorption;[9] other evidence suggests that some patients, women aged 50 to 83 years, with primary osteoporosis have decreased bone formation.[30] *In vitro* studies of bone metabolism suggest that growth hormone and the growth hormone-dependent peptides, somatomedins (insulin-like growth factors), may play a role in bone formation.[22] Both growth hormone and somatomedins are reduced with aging.[25] It has been suggested that these might be involved in the pathogenesis of osteoporosis, but there is currently no direct evidence to support this hypothesis.

Genetic, nutritional, and local factors within bone may also be involved in the pathogenesis.[22] Blacks have a greater bone mass and a lower incidence of osteoporosis than age-matched Whites. There is a high concordance of bone mass in identical twins. Thus, bone mass may be, in part, genetically determined. Obese females are less likely to develop osteoporosis than matched thin controls. This may be mediated by increased estrogen produced by conversion of androgens in adipose tissue and increased load-bearing in the obese subjects. Immobilization and exercise have substantial and opposite effects upon bone volume. Such effects could be mediated through stress-induced changes in local piezoelectric currents reported to be present in bone.

It appears likely that the loss of bone with age

and the additional loss seen in primary osteoporosis are multifactoral and that the combination of hormonal, genetic, nutritional, and local factors will be different in individual patients.

## CLINICAL FEATURES

Patients with primary osteoporosis generally present with acute or chronic back pain or deformity. The pain of new vertebral compression fractures is acute in onset and may occur with or without significant trauma or stress. The pain is sharp and centered over the vertebra, which may be tender to palpation. Pain may be accompanied by substantial muscle spasm. The pain is generally relieved with rest and disappears spontaneously within 4 to 12 weeks. Causes other than primary osteoporosis (e.g., metastatic disease, degenerative joint disease) should be investigated if the pain is not relieved by rest or if it is prolonged. The second type of pain is chronic, paraspinal in location, not associated with spinal tenderness, and relieved partially with rest. The pathogenesis of this pain is not clear, but it may result from mechanical abnormalities induced by the fracture or from bone deformation without an identifiable fracture.

Pain in a radicular pattern or signs of spinal cord compression are very rarely caused by simple compression fractures due to primary osteoporosis.

Patients may present with chronic pain without an identifiable acute episode. Other individuals may have radiologic evidence of compression fractures but no symptoms. Thus, lack of pain does not preclude the presence of significant osteoporosis. Back pain in elderly individuals has many etiologies and could result from any one or a combination of disorders. For example, a patient may have compression fractures and degenerative joint disease and pain owing to only one or to both.

The most common physical signs of primary osteoporosis are a loss of height and kyphosis of the dorsal spine (dowager's hump). Other signs may include a deformed wrist, an abnormal gait due to previous hip fracture, or pain on breathing with a rib fracture. The physical examination is also useful in identifying secondary causes for osteoporosis (Table 39–2).

New compression fractures may occur at a highly variable rate within an individual patient. For example, a patient may have two fractures per month for 2 months and then have no fractures for another year or longer. The onset and duration of and disability from back pain are also variable and do not always correlate well with the number of compression fractures.

Although vertebral compression fractures may first occur in the early postmenopausal period, hip fractures are usually seen at a later age (over 70 years).[18] Unlike in vertebral fractures, a fall frequently accompanies a hip fracture either as a cause or as a consequence.

## DIAGNOSIS

The two major goals of diagnostic procedures are (1) to establish the presence and severity of reduced skeletal mass and (2) to distinguish between primary and secondary etiologies, that is, differential diagnosis.[8]

### *Determination of the Presence and Severity of Osteoporosis*

#### Radiographs

Despite their limitations, plain spinal radiographs are the principal diagnostic tool for the evaluation of osteoporosis. They are most useful for determining the presence and distribution of compression fractures and the presence of other bone or joint lesions, such as metastases or degenerative arthritis, which may cause back pain.

Loss of the horizontal trabeculae, thinning of the cortex, collapse or wedging of the anterior portion of the vertebra, and biconcavity (codfishing) of the lumbar vertebrae are characteristic of osteoporosis. Radiologic features that are *not* characteristic of primary osteoporosis include posterior wedging or total collapse (particularly if no other vertebrae are involved) of a vertebra; isolated compression fractures of cervical or upper thoracic spine, even if only anterior collapse is present; erosion of the vertebra, particularly of the pedicles; expansion of the periosteum; and atraumatic fractures of the long bones, except in the hip and Colles' fracture of the wrist. In the geriatric population, these changes are most likely to be due to causes other than primary osteoporosis, such as trauma, metastases, or Paget's disease of bone. It must be remembered that other bone disorders may coexist with typical osteoporosis.

The sensitivity for radiologic density of the plain x-ray is low; 20 to 25 per cent of bone mineral must be lost before unequivocal changes are seen on back films. Thus, "normal" density does not preclude the presence of significant loss of bone mass. Owing to the low sensitivity as well as to differences in density due only to changes in technique, the x-ray cannot be used to quantify bone mineral content.

To avoid the technical problems, but to still

use the widely available plain radiograph, a number of investigators have measured cortical bone thickness, particularly of the metacarpals.[12] As with some other techniques (see later), this has one significant drawback. Although primary osteoporosis is defined as a generalized loss of bone mass, in the postmenopausal form the loss occurs mostly in the axial skeleton and involves mostly trabecular bone. Cortical bone in the appendicular skeleton is involved to a lesser degree.[24] The mechanism for this partially selective bone loss is not known.[27] As a general guideline, loss of cortical bone (a decrease in cortical width) is almost always accompanied by similar or more severe osteoporosis in the axial skeleton. In contrast, significant axial osteoporosis may occur in the presence of normal cortical width.

#### Bone Scan

After a few days, new compression fractures will appear as areas of increased isotope uptake on a bone scan. The scan cannot differentiate new compression fractures from other lesions (e.g., metastases, osteomyelitis) associated with increased uptake. We do not routinely do bone scans in patients with typical compression fractures. If spinal lesions are atypical, such as an isolated compression fracture in the upper thoracic spine, a bone scan may be helpful, since the presence of a "hot" area in the skull or long bones would suggest metastases or Paget's disease.

#### Osteodensitometry

Bone mineral content (BMC) measured by photon absorptiometry of the distal radius and ulna correlates well with measurements of total body calcium,[3] an index of total bone mass. These sites contain approximately 80 per cent cortical bone and 20 per cent trabecular bone. Thus, this technique has the same problem as the measure of cortical width described previously: Reduced BMC at these sites is almost always associated with lower BMC of the axial skeleton, whereas normal BMC of the radius may still be associated with spinal osteoporosis.

#### Dual Photon Absorptiometry/ Quantitative Computerized Axial Tomography

Two new techniques to measure BMC, one a modification of the absorptiometry, described previously,[17] and the other an extension of computerized axial tomography (CAT) scanning[7] have recently been described. Both are sensitive and provide reproducible results, and more importantly, both can quantify BMC in the vertebrae. The dual photon method can also measure BMC of the hip. Neither method is widely available at this time. Nonetheless, noninvasive and quantitative methods for measuring changes in the axial skeleton, the site of most bone loss in postmenopausal/idiopathic osteoporosis, should improve our ability to diagnose and evaluate the treatment of these disorders. The ability to determine bone density of the femoral neck and intertrochanteric region of the femur may improve the ability to predict which individuals are at greatest risk for hip fractures.

#### Bone Biopsy

Bone biopsies with quantitative histomorphometry yield important data concerning the pathogenesis of primary osteoporosis.[30] However, a bone biopsy is seldom necessary for the clinical diagnosis of osteoporosis. A biopsy should be considered when there are radiographically atypical lesions and less invasive techniques do not yield a definitive diagnosis. A biopsy may also be used to rule out osteomalacia.

#### Laboratory Studies

Serum and urine chemistries are generally normal in primary osteoporosis. Although the mean levels of calcitonin and 1,25-$(OH)_2D_3$ are reduced in groups of patients with postmenopausal osteoporosis, measurement of these regulatory hormones in individual patients is seldom useful. They may be used to differentiate primary from secondary etiologies and will be discussed in the following section.

### *Differential Diagnosis: Secondary Osteoporosis*

No radiologic pattern or laboratory test result is sufficiently characteristic of primary osteoporosis to make a definitive diagnosis. Thus, the diagnosis is one of exclusion of secondary etiologies of spontaneous fractures. Osteoporosis may occur in association with a wide variety of acquired or inherited disorders. Although secondary causes account for only a small percentage of cases, their recognition is important for several reasons. In most types of secondary osteoporosis, specific therapy for the underlying disorder will lead to improvement of the osteoporosis. In addition, if it is incorrectly assumed that the patient has primary osteoporosis, the proper therapy of the secondary disorder may be delayed. In this section, we will discuss the diagnostic features and also the management of the major secondary causes of spontaneous fractures. The most common secondary causes of osteoporosis likely to be encountered in the geriatric patient are listed in Table 39–2 and are presented individually below.

### Glucocorticoid Excess

Administration of pharmacologic doses of glucocorticoids is the most common cause of secondary osteoporosis. Vertebral compression fractures and hip fractures may be the most significant late consequence of their use. Glucocorticoids reduce calcium absorption by acting directly upon the intestine, increase PTH, reduce calcitonin, inhibit collagen synthesis, and reduce proliferation of osteoblast precursors. Any or all of these changes may contribute to the development of osteoporosis. Preliminary observations suggest that the combination of calcium, vitamin D, and sodium fluoride may increase bone mass and decrease bone pain in some, although perhaps not all of these patients.[1,23] Whether this therapy will prevent glucocorticoid osteoporosis is not yet known. The incidence and severity of steroid-induced osteoporosis should be reduced by use of glucocorticoids only when clear benefit can be demonstrated. They should be used (1) in the lowest possible dose, (2) every other day when this will control the underlying disorder, and (3) for the shortest possible duration. As in all forms of osteoporosis, we recommend that immobilization be avoided and physical activity be encouraged.

### Hypogonadism

Osteoporosis may occur in acquired or hereditary hypogonadism in either sex. All geriatric females are physiologically estrogen deficient, and the relationship of estrogens to bone loss is considered with primary osteoporosis elsewhere in this chapter. The fact that androgen deficiency causes osteoporosis is less well appreciated. Nevertheless, testosterone deficiency is clearly associated with premature and/or increased severity of bone loss. Elderly males with reduced testosterone may have no symptoms or signs of this deficiency. Thus, we measure plasma testosterone of all males with compression fractures. If testosterone is low and gonadotropins are also reduced or not appropriately elevated, the patient should be evaluated for hypothalamic/pituitary disorders. The diagnosis of hypogonadism in elderly males may be difficult. This problem is discussed in Chapter 38.

Parenteral testosterone ethanate (200 to 300 mg intramuscularly every 2 to 3 weeks) should be used as replacement therapy. Oral methyltestosterone (25 to 50 mg every day, buccal) may be substituted but is not preferred, since it may cause hepatic dysfunction.

### Immobilization

Immobilization may decrease bone formation and increase bone resorption, with a substantial and often rapid loss of bone mineral. This is accompanied by increased urine calcium and occasionally by hypercalcemia. Elevated serum calcium is most likely to occur when bone turnover is elevated, such as in Paget's disease. Thus, urine and serum calcium should be monitored in patients at complete bed rest for more than a few days. When the patient is obligatorily immobilized, an attempt should be made to simulate load-bearing as soon as possible in a physical therapy program. Use of hydrochlorothiazide will reduce urine calcium and use of diphosphonates will lower the elevated bone resorption.

### Hyperthyroidism

Thyroid hormone excess appears to increase bone resorption directly, independent of other calcium regulatory hormones. Clinical osteoporosis is not seen in hyperthyroid patients unless the disease has been chronic. Measurement of serum $T_4$ and $T_3$ resin uptake (the product of which is the free thyroxine index) will establish the diagnosis in the majority of cases. In the geriatric population the clinical presentation and laboratory evaluation of hyperthryroidism may be different from those in younger patients. These problems are discussed in Chapter 38.

### Vitamin D–Related Disorders: Osteoporosis/Osteomalacia

In mild vitamin D deficiency there is a reduction in histologically normal bone; i.e., secondary osteoporosis. In more severe cases there is an increase in unmineralized matrix and an increase in the mineralization lag time, i.e., osteomalacia.[20] Although osteomalacia occurs in only a small portion (less than 5 per cent) of patients with spontaneous fractures, it is important to recognize, since the condition is readily treated.

Vitamin D deficiency is most likely to occur in geriatric patients with poor nutrition and little exposure to sunlight and in institutionalized patients taking more than one anticonvulsant. In severe deficiency states serum alkaline phosphatase is increased and serum $PO_4$ and serum calcium are reduced as is the urine calcium (less than 50 mg per day). In mild vitamin D deficiency there may be none of these changes. In both mild and severe deficiency, serum levels of 25-OHD are decreased. The treatment of these disorders involves the administration of vitamin $D_2$ 5000 units per day for 1 to 2 months. In nutritional vitamin D deficiency, therapy should be discontinued when urine calcium exceeds 200 mg per day. Vitamin D may need to be given continuously in patients with malabsorption, but the dose must be individualized. Patients should receive chronic vitamin D supplements (5000 units every day) while continuing anticonvulsant therapy.

#### Idiopathic Hypercalciuria

At least 5 per cent of males or females presenting with vertebral compression fractures exhibit hypercalciuria (i.e., a 24-hour urine calcium of 300 mg or more in males and 250 mg or more in females). These patients usually do not exhibit features of secondary causes of hypercalciuria (e.g., sarcoidosis, immobilization, or hypercalciuria secondary to increased bone resorption) and thus are considered to have idiopathic hypercalciuria. We cannot further classify their condition into the calcium leak versus the phosphate leak type of idiopathic hypercalciuria because current methods fail to consistently accomplish this separation. Some patients with idiopathic hypercalciuria have obvious hypophosphatemia, and chronic hypophosphatemia associated with this disease or any other disease is associated with metabolic alterations in bone. Accordingly, patients with mild hypophosphatemia develop osteoporosis, whereas those with severe hypophosphatemia develop osteomalacia. All patients with idiopathic hypercalciuria and osteoporosis are treated with a thiazide to correct the high urine calcium, and then they are treated with the same approach outlined below for patients with primary osteoporosis.

#### Multiple Myeloma

Myeloma generally presents with discrete lytic lesions on bone x-rays. However, a diffuse decrease in bone density without focal lesions may occur, and in such patients, the clinical presentation may be indistinguishable from that of osteoporosis. The pattern of diffuse bone loss is frequently, but not invariably, associated with elevated serum calcium. The probability of a diagnosis of myeloma is increased in the presence of an abnormal hemogram (decreased red blood cells, white blood cells, and/or platelets) and confirmed by quantitatively or qualitatively abnormal globulins in the serum or urine and abnormal plasma cells in the marrow.

#### Primary Hyperparathyroidism

The radiographic findings of osteitis fibrosa cystica and subperiosteal bone resorption are features of chronic severe primary hyperparathyroidism, which was seen a decade ago but seldom now because of current capabilities in early detection and treatment of this disease. Currently, primary hyperparathyroidism usually presents with no abnormalities or a diffuse loss of bone density with no focal abnormalities on plain radiographs. In the latter situation, serum calcium will always be elevated, and in many patients, it will be accompanied by an increased alkaline phosphatase and reduced serum phosphate.

Although many of the preceding diagnoses can be made on the basis of a thorough history and physical examination; laboratory studies are an important part of the osteoporosis workup. Screening laboratory tests in patients with osteoporosis should include a complete blood count; assays of serum calcium, phosphate, and alkaline phosphatase; and a 24-hour urinary excretion of calcium. Plasma testosterone is obtained in all males. Measurement of PTH, adrenal steroids, vitamin D metabolites, and thyroid hormones should be reserved for cases in which the history and physical examination or the screening tests give clues to the potential diagnosis. It should be emphasized that all these parameters used to evaluate for secondary osteoporosis are within the normal range in primary osteoporosis.

If specific treatment for secondary osteoporosis is not effective in restoring the depleted skeleton, patients with this condition are then treated with the same approach outlined below for patients with primary osteoporosis.

## THERAPY OF PRIMARY OSTEOPOROSIS

### *General Measures*

For patients with acute compression fractures, bed rest for short periods is the most effective therapy for pain relief. Common minor analgesics, aspirin or acetaminophen, and muscle relaxants (including heat) are added when rest is not effective, or for periods of mobilization. Nonsteroidal analgesics such as ibuprofen and piroxicam may be tried when aspirin is not effective, but they are not as a general rule superior to aspirin. Drugs inhibiting prostaglandin synthesis do not appear to be superior to those that do not have this action. If the preceding measures are not effective, codeine alone or in combination with one of the drugs mentioned above may be used for short periods (4 to 6 weeks). If codeine does not relieve the pain or is needed for more than 6 weeks, we re-evaluate the patient for pathologic fractures, particularly as a result of metastatic disease. If no other causes are found we refer patients to a pain clinic for evaluation of the use of newer techniques such as transcutaneous electrical nerve stimulation. Measures similar to those described previously are also used for chronic pain. We do not recommend long periods of immobilization, since this may aggravate the underlying bone loss and increase the risk of new fractures.

## *Exercise*

Little emphasis has been placed on the role of weight bearing and mechanical stress in osteoporosis.[15] Immobilization and weightlessness result in bone loss. Conversely, moderate exercise can reduce bone loss. Whenever possible, immobilization should be avoided. Exercise or a physical therapy program with an emphasis on impact loading (e.g., walking rather than swimming or passive movement) should be encouraged.

## *Pharmacologic Measures*

Effective therapy for primary osteoporosis should increase bone mass and reduce fracture frequency. The results from clinical trials for agents in which these criteria were examined are given in Table 39–3 and a general outline of therapy is provided in Table 39–4.

**Table 39–3.** TREATMENT OF PRIMARY OSTEOPOROSIS*

| | Osteodensitometry | | Fracture Frequency |
|---|---|---|---|
| | *Appendicular* | *Axial* | |
| Calcium supplements | ↑ | ↑ | ↓ |
| Estrogen | ↑ | ↑ | ↓ |
| Sodium fluoride | →/sl ↑ | ↑ | ↓ ↓ |

* This analysis does not include other agents, not because the above three are the only agents considered to be effective in osteoporosis but because this type of information is not available for other agents.

↑ = increased; ↓ = decreased; → = no change.

### Calcium

In postmenopausal osteoporosis, increasing calcium intake to 1200 to 1500 mg per day corrects the negative calcium balance and reduces bone loss. More importantly, several investigators have reported that calcium supplementation alone decreases fractures.[23] We recommend that all patients with osteoporosis increase their total elemental calcium intake to 1500 mg per day. This can be done by drinking an 8-oz glass of milk (290 mg of elemental calcium) two times daily and taking 800 mg of calcium via calcium supplement. A normal daily diet excluding milk contains from 100 to 200 mg of calcium. All forms of oral calcium should be equally effective, but it should be remembered that the quantity of elemental calcium in the supplements differs for each preparation (Table 39–5). This level of calcium intake will not produce hypercalcemia but may aggravate pre-existing hypercalciuria. Therefore, urine calcium should be measured prior to and during therapy to detect individuals with hypercalciuria. In patients with a history of recurrent nephrolithiasis and pre-existing hypercalciuria, we correct the hypercalciuria, usually with thiazide diuretics, prior to starting calcium supplements.

### Vitamin D

Vitamin D metabolites will correct the negative calcium balance by increasing calcium absorption but do not appear to independently increase bone volume or decrease the fracture rate.[23] Vitamin D supplements in large doses can produce hypercalciuria and hypercalcemia. Thus, we only use vitamin D in large doses for secondary osteoporosis due to deficiency states documented by a reduced serum 25-OHD.

### Estrogen

Estrogen replacement improves results of indirect and direct measures of bone volume. Conjugated estrogens and ethinyl estradiol are equally effective. Doses of conjugated estrogens lower than 0.625 mg per day or of ethinyl estradiol less than 0.05 μg per day are less effective.[7,11] Continued administration of estrogens appears to afford persistent benefit. Bone loss accelerates when estrogen is discontinued. Estrogens are less effective in preventing bone loss when they are started more than 5 years after

**Table 39-4.** GENERAL GUIDELINES FOR TREATMENT AND PREVENTION OF OSTEOPOROSIS*

| | Normal BMC | | | |
|---|---|---|---|---|
| **Agent/Patient Group** | ***Low Risk*** | ***High Risk*** | **Reduced BMC** | **Compression Fractures** |
| Exercise | + | + | + | + |
| Calcium | + | + | + | + |
| Estrogen/testosterone† | +/− | + | + | + |
| Anabolic steroids | − | − | + | + |
| Sodium fluoride | − | − | +/− | + |
| Vitamin D‡ | ~ | ~ | ~ | ~ |

* Patients may be classified into three groups: those with compression fractures, those with reduced bone mineral content (BMC) without fractures, and those with normal (within two standard deviations of the age adjusted mean) BMC. Subjects with normal BMC are further divided into high- and low-risk groups. Higher risk may be estimated from the actual BMC and from the factors listed in Table 39-6. The agents and modalities used for prevention and treatment of primary osteoporosis are listed in approximate order of potential toxicity. As a general principle of prevention and treatment, the lower risk or the less severe the bone disease, the less justifiable the employment of agents with serious side effects. Thus, exercise and calcium supplements, which present minimal side effects, may be used in all groups. Sodium fluoride (NaF), which has significant adverse effects, is routinely used only in patients with compression fractures. In subjects with reduced BMC (greater than 2 standard deviations below mean) and no fractures, NaF is used if (1) other risk factors are present and/or (2) agents ranked before NaF in the table do not stabilize or increase BMC.

† Estrogens and anabolic steroids are used only in females, whereas testosterone is used exclusively in males.

‡ Vitamin D is included in the table, since it has been frequently used in combination with other agents. We prescribe vitamin D only for patients with documented vitamin D deficiency or with proven osteomalacia.

menopause compared with when they are started at menopause.

Use of estrogens increases the risk of developing endometrial carcinoma, benign breast lesions, and gallbladder disease and may aggravate hyperlipidemia. It is not clear whether postmenopausal estrogen administration increases the risk of thromboembolic phenomena or atherosclerotic vascular disease. The effect upon endometrial proliferation is reduced by giving estrogens cyclically and adding a progestogen during the last 10 to 14 days of the cycle. At higher doses of estrogen (i.e., greater than 0.625 mg per day of conjugated estrogens) cyclic therapy may induce menses. Cyclic therapy is effective, and there is some evidence that progestogens may have a positive independent effect on bone volume.

We recommend that all women with compression fractures who do not have a specific contraindication (see below) to estrogens be treated with conjugated estrogen (0.625 to 1.25 mg per day) or ethinyl estradiol (0.05 mg per day) in a cyclic fashion as described previously. Estrogens should not be given to females with a history of endometrial carcinoma or hyperplasia or breast carcinoma and should be avoided if possible in patients with cholelithiasis or severe atherosclerotic vascular disease. Patients on estrogens should undergo regular breast and gynecologic examinations. However, since gynecologic examinations and PAP smears are not adequate for the diagnosis of endometrial carcinoma, abnormal uterine bleeding must be investigated with endometrial biopsy.

**Table 39-5.** CALCIUM PREPARATIONS

| | mg Ca/gm of Compound | |
|---|---|---|
| Calcium gluconate | 100 | |
| Calcium lactate | 130 | |
| Calcium carbonate | 400 | |
| | **mg Compound** | **mg Elemental Ca** |
| OsCal* | 625 | 250 |
| OsCal 500 | 1250 | 500 |
| Tums | tablet | 200 |
| Titralac | tablet 420 mg | 168 |
| | liquid 5 ml | 400 |

* Contains 125 units of Vitamin $D_2$.

### FLUORIDE

In postmenopausal osteoporosis, large doses of fluoride increase new bone formation and decrease fracture frequency. In combination with calcium and estrogen, fluoride significantly decreases the rate of vertebral compression fractures to a greater degree than calcium or calcium plus estrogen.[23,26] Forty to 90 mg per day have been used in most studies, but the minimally effective and optimally effective doses have not been established.

The use of fluoride has several important drawbacks: (1) Side effects, including gastrointestinal complications (nausea, vomiting, epigastric pain, and peptic ulceration with or without blood loss), periostitis, and osteomalacia, require discontinuation or a reduction in the dose in a substantial percentage of patients. Gastrointestinal distress is reduced by giving fluoride after meals. A history of recent peptic ulceration is a relative contraindication to its use. (2) A substantial number of patients do not respond, or respond only after a delay of 2 to 5 years. The mechanism for the lack of or delay in response is unknown, and consequently, it is not possible to predict which patients will have an early response. (3) Sodium fluoride has not been approved by the Food and Drug Administration (FDA) for general use in the treatment of primary osteoporosis. At this time, patients with osteoporosis who do not respond adequately to calcium and estrogen should be referred to specialized centers conducting clinical trials with fluoride.

### Anabolic Steroids

Stanozolol is an anabolic steroid with weak virilizing properties. In patients with postmenopausal osteoporosis, 6 mg per day for 3 of 4 weeks increases total body calcium and may increase bone formation. The effect on total body calcium is sustained during 2 years of administration. There is insufficient information to know whether stanozolol is as effective as calcium, estrogen, or fluoride in the treatment of postmenopausal osteoporosis. Carcinoma of the breast is a contraindication to the use of stanozolol. This compound may cause mild virilization and liver function abnormalities. Although cyclic therapy reduces liver abnormalities, liver enzymes should be monitored during therapy and the drug discontinued if these rise significantly.

### Calcitonin

Synthetic salmon calcitonin has been approved by the FDA as an adjunctive treatment for osteoporosis. Since the major action of calcitonin is to reduce bone resorption, it should be most useful in states in which bone resorption is elevated. The subgroup of primary osteoporosis with high bone turnover rates (with increased urinary calcium and hydroxyproline) would be expected to show a positive response to this agent, but this has not been adequately documented. In general, however, calcitonin does not appear to be as effective as calcium, estrogen, or fluoride in the treatment of postmenopausal osteoporosis.[26] Systemic allergy and idiopathic hypercalciuria with nephrolithiasis (calcitonin decreases calcium reabsorption in the kidney) are contraindications to the use of calcitonin.

### Other Agents

Progestogens (alone), PTH, and several diphosphonates have been used for short-term studies and assessed for possible effectiveness in the treatment of osteoporosis. Thus far, insufficient information has accumulated to conclude whether these agents will be effective in increasing bone mass and decreasing fracture rate.[26] None of these agents are currently approved by the FDA for the treatment of primary or secondary osteoporosis.

Continued patient acceptance of any drug regimen depends, in part, upon the perceived long-term benefit and the rapidity of relief of symptoms. This is a particular problem in primary osteoporosis in which pre-existing structural damage is not usually corrected. Patients should be advised that the response to the medication may be delayed and that new fractures early in the course of therapy do not mean that the drugs are ineffective. Individuals with chronic back pain should be advised that even if new fractures do not occur, back pain may not be totally eradicated in spite of successful therapy to increase bone volume.

## PREVENTION

The ultimate goal in the management of osteoporosis is prevention. The risk for the development of bone loss, osteoporosis, and fractures can be estimated on the basis of pre-existing factors (Table 39–6) and upon bone density of the axial and appendicular skeleton. BMC of the radius, measurement of cortical thickness, or an estimate of bone density from plain radiographs

**Table 39–6.** RISK FACTORS OF OSTEOPOROSIS

| Parameter | High-Risk Group |
|---|---|
| Sex | Female |
| | Male or female with hypogonadism |
| Race | White |
| Body weight | Thin |
| Nutrition | Reduced calcium intake |
| | Malabsorption |
| | Diabetes mellitus |
| | Chronic alcoholism |
| Physical activity | Immobilization, inactive |
| Tobacco | Smoker |
| Drug therapy | Glucocorticoids |
| | Anticonvulsants |
| | Chronic heparin therapy |
| Other diseases | Chronic obstructive pulmonary disease |
| | Cirrhosis |

should be substituted when axial measurements and densitometry of the hip are not available.

Scientifically based recommendations for the prevention of fractures are not available, since there are no prospective, randomized, longitudinal studies testing agents alone or in combination in people with normal axial bone mineral content. A rational program would include the same modalities described previously for the treatment of patients with compression fractures (see Table 39–4).

Avoidance of immobilization and an active physical therapy or exercise program should be used in all groups unless there are specific contraindications. Calcium supplementation in the geriatric population in which there is reduced calcium absorption is reasonable and safe as long as urine calcium is monitored during therapy.

The use of estrogen in the postmenopausal patient will undoubtedly reduce bone loss. It is equally clear that the use of estrogens involves known and also poorly defined risks (see earlier). The risk of endometrial proliferation is reduced by cycling the estrogen, and we recommend that estrogen be given in this manner. The greater the risk of fractures, that is, the lower the BMC and the more risk factors present (see Table 39–6), the more likely we are to prescribe estrogen. One way to determine if patients in the moderate- to high-risk groups should receive estrogens is to repeat BMC measurements at 6 to 12 month intervals, and if BMC falls, estrogen may be added to the prevention program.

In males, the effect of aging on the pituitary-gonadal axis is controversial. Thus, it may be difficult to distinguish changes of normal aging from gonadal failure. In males with borderline plasma testosterone, our policy is to treat the high-risk group with testosterone and follow the others with serial BMC determinations, as described in the previous paragraph.

Elderly patients may have subclinical vitamin D deficiency, with normal serum calcium, phosphate, and alkaline phosphatase. Serum 25-OHD concentrations should be determined in patients with poor milk intake and/or little exposure to sunlight. One thousand units of vitamin D per day should prevent vitamin D deficiency, but larger doses (5000 units for several weeks) may be required at the beginning of therapy in order to replete body stores. When larger doses are used, serum and urine calcium should be determined to avoid overtreatment.

Recent data suggest that determination of BMC of the hip will prove helpful in determining patients at high risk for developing hip fractures. There is only limited data on the efficacy of the previously described measures and agents in preventing hip fractures. Because it appears to preferentially act upon trabecular bone, primarily in the axial skeleton, fluoride may be less effective in preventing hip than in preventing spine fractures. Estrogen may be particularly effective, since it acts upon both trabecular and cortical bone. Hip fractures are almost always associated with falls. Environmental precautions should be taken, such as installment of rails to prevent falls.

## References


1. Baylink DJ, Duane PB, Farley SM, Farley JR: Monofluorophosphate physiology: The effects of fluoride on bone. Caries Res 17(Suppl 1):56, 1983.
2. Baylink DJ, Ivey JL: Sodium fluoride for osteoporosis—some unanswered questions. JAMA 243:463, 1980.
3. Cameron JR, Mazess RB, Sorenson JA: Precision and accuracy of bone mineral determination by direct photon absorptiometry. Invest Radiol 3:11, 1968.
4. Deftos LJ, Weisman MH, Williams GW, et al: Influence of age and sex on plasma calcitonin in human beings. N Engl J Med 302:1351, 1981.
5. Gallagher JC, Riggs BL, Eisman J, et al: Intestinal calcium absorption and serum vitamin D metabolites in normal subjects and osteoporotic patients: Effect of age and dietary calcium. J Clin Invest 64:729, 1979.
6. Garn SM: The earlier gain and the latter loss of cortical bone. Springfield, IL, Charles C Thomas, 1970.
7. Genant KH, Cann CE, Ettinger B, Gordan GS: Quantitative computed tomography of vertebral spongiosa: A sensitive method for detecting early bone loss after oophorectomy. Ann Intern Med 97:699, 1982.
   *Briefly describes the technique for measurement of bone density using computed tomography.*
8. Gruber HE, Baylink DJ: The diagnosis of osteoporosis. J Am Geriatr Soc 29:490, 1981.
   *Review of clinical and laboratory diagnoses of primary and secondary osteoporosis.*
9. Heaney RP, Recker RR, Saville PD: Menopausal changes in bone remodelling. J Lab Clin Med 92:964, 1978.
10. Heath H III, Sizemore GW: Plasma calcitonin in normal man: Differences between men and women. J Clin Invest 60:1135, 1977.
11. Horsman A, Jones M, Francis R, Nordin C: The effect of estrogen dose on postmenopausal bone loss. N Engl J Med 309:1405, 1983.
12. Horsman A, Simpson M: The measurement of sequential changes in cortical bone geometry. Br J Radiol 48:470, 1975.
13. Insogna KL, Lewis AM, Lipinski BA, et al: Effect of age on serum immunoreactive parathyroid hormone and its biological effects. J Clin Endocrinol Metab 53:1072, 1981.
14. Ivey JL, Baylink DJ: Postmenopausal osteoporosis: Proposed roles of defective coupling and estrogen deficiency. Metab Bone Dis Rel Res 3:3, 1981.
15. Leader: An overview of osteoporosis. Lancet 2:423, 1982.
16. Marcus R, Madvig P, and Young G: Age-related changes in parathyroid hormone and parathyroid hormone action in normal humans. J Clin Endocrinol Metab 58:223, 1984.

17. Mazess RB: Noninvasive methods for quantitating trabecular bone. *In* Avioli, LV (ed): The Osteoporotic Syndrome. New York, Grune & Stratton, 1983, pp 85–114.
18. Melton LJ, and Rigs BL: Epidemiology of age-related fractures. *In* Avioli, LV (ed): The Osteoporotic Syndrome. New York, Grune & Stratton, 1983, pp 45–72.
19. Morimoto S, Tsuji M, Okada Y, et al: The effect of oestrogens on human calcitonin secretion after calcium infusion in elderly female subjects. Clin Endocrinol 13:135, 1980.
20. Nordin BEC, Heyburn PJ, Peacock M, et al: Osteoporosis and osteomalacia. Clin Endocrinol Metab 9:177, 1980.
*General review of osteoporosis and osteomalacia including some aspects of treatment of osteomalacia.*
21. Nutik G, and Cruess RL: Estrogen receptors in bone. An evaluation of the uptake of estrogen into bone cells. Proc Soc Exp Biol Med 146:265, 1974.
22. Raisz LG: Osteoporosis. J Am Geriatrics Soc 30:127, 1982.
*General review of bone metabolism as well as osteoporosis.*
22a. Riggs BL and Melton LJ: Evidence for two distinct syndromes of involutional osteoporosis. Amer J Med 75:899, 1983.
23. Riggs BL, Seeman E, Hodgson SF, et al: Effect of the fluoride/calcium regimen on vertebral fracture occurrence in postmenopausal osteoporosis. N Engl J Med 306:446, 1982.
24. Riggs BL, Wahner HW, Seeman E, et al: Changes in bone mineral density of the proximal femur and spine with aging. Differences between postmenopausal and senile osteoporosis syndromes. J Clin Invest 70:716, 1982.
*Description of the technique of dual photon absorptiometry for bone density of vertebral and proximal femur. Data presented here suggest that postmenopausal and senile osteoporosis are separate entities.*
25. Rudman D, Kutner MH, Rogers CM, et al: Impaired growth hormone secretion in the adult population: Relation to age and adiposity. J Clin Invest 67:1361, 1981.
26. Seeman E, Riggs BL: The treatment of postmenopausal and senile osteoporosis. *In* Heath DA, and Marx SJ (eds): Clinical Endocrinology 2: Calcium Disorders. London, Butterworth Scientific, 1982, p 69.
*Comprehensive review of the treatment of osteoporosis including more recent experimental drugs.*
27. Seeman E, Wahner HW, Offord KP, et al: Differential effects of endocrine dysfunction on the axial and the appendicular skeleton. J Clin Invest 69:1302, 1982.
28. Slovik DM, Adams JS, Neer RM, et al: Deficient production of 1,25-dihydroxyvitamin D in elderly osteoporotic patients. N Engl J Med 305:372, 1981.
29. Taggart HM, Chesnut CH III, Ivey JL, et al: Deficient calcitonin response to calcium stimulation in postmenopausal osteoporosis? Lancet 1:475, 1982.
30. Whyte MP, Bergfeld MA, Murphy WA, et al: Postmenopausal osteoporosis: A heterogeneous disorder as assessed by histomorphometric analysis of iliac crest bone from untreated patients. Am J Med 72:193, 1982.
31. Wylie CM: Hospitalization for fractures and bone loss in adults. Public Health Rep 92:33, 1977.

## Chapter 40

# Oral Aspects of Aging

*Sheldon Winkler*
*Maury Massler*

It is unfortunate that the geriatric patient needs essential and complex dental services at an age when he or she is least able to tolerate and, possibly, afford these services. Degenerative, physiologic, and biologic changes (and associated chronic diseases and disorders, directly or indirectly resulting from this deterioration) make the elderly patient a greater endodontic risk and a poor candidate for oral rehabilitation. Although fluoridation and other preventive measures will undoubtedly have an effect on lowering the incidence of dental caries and the resultant tooth loss in the young, their benefits are negligible for geriatric patients. The amount of tooth loss due to periodontal disease and the prosthetic needs of the geriatric population are monumental.

On the positive side, recent years have witnessed a shift in emphasis from a restorative orientation to a preventive approach. Contrary to the belief of many patients and, unfortunately, some health professionals, the loss of teeth is not an inevitable consequence of growing old. People can and should keep their teeth all their lives. However, there is more to prevention than the control of dental plaque. Prevention includes *all* procedures for preventing oral disease. It starts with the child and continues throughout the life of the individual.

Dental care includes not only regular professional care, but also daily oral hygiene procedures. Poor oral health can contribute to systemic disease, malnutrition, speech defects, and facial deformity. Unfortunately, a great many elderly patients have had no dental care for a number of years and have had little or no instruction in the importance of and procedures for caring for their teeth or prostheses.

Lack of motivation, forgetfulness, and physical disabilities such as arthritis can contribute to the neglect of daily oral hygiene. This neglect can result in serious oral disorders, which could compound the oral health problems that accompany aging.

If an elderly patient is unable to care for his mouth or is afraid to try to care for his dentures because of the fear of dropping and breaking them, oral hygiene will be entirely dependent upon another person. The responsible person, usually a close relative or friend or a nursing staff member if the patient is in a home or institution, must receive the proper cleansing instructions. If oral hygiene procedures cannot be demonstrated personally by the dentist, it is imperative that the responsible person receive specific, detailed written instructions.

To a great number of elderly patients, aesthetics is paramount. Fortunately, today it is possible for the dental profession to fabricate virtually undetectable complete dentures for the edentulous that simulate the harmonious positions and relationships of the lost natural teeth during speech, mastication, and rest. The emotional and psychologic effects of improved appearance can create a new outlook on life for many patients.

## ORAL MANIFESTATIONS OF AGING

The oral tissues, like the tissues in other parts of the body, change markedly as a person grows older (Table 40–1). The teeth wear down (Fig. 40–1), the rate depending on the occlusion, the muscular pattern and muscular strength, and, above all, the abrasiveness of the diet (although the latter is generally low in the elderly).

**Table 40–1.** ORAL MANIFESTATIONS OF AGING*

| | |
|---|---|
| Loss of teeth | Due primarily to degeneration of periodontal structures. |
| Attrition | Rate is influenced by diet and masticatory habits (bruxism). |
| Oral mucosa | Loss of elasticity with dryness and atrophy. Tendency to hyperkeratosis. |
| Gingivae | Loss of stippling. Edematous appearance. Keratinized layer thin or absent. Tissue friable and easily injured. |
| Saliva | Diminished function of salivary glands with relative or absolute xerostomia due to atrophy of cells lining the intermediate ducts. Xerostomia also results in abnormal taste sensations and stomatodynia. |
| Tongue | Atrophic glossitis, probably due to concurrent vitamin B complex deficiency. |
| Lips | Angular cheilosis is very common and probably is related to concurrent vitamin B deficiency and close bite. Cheilitis and "purse-string" mouth due to dehydration. |

* From Massler M: Oral aspects of aging. Postgrad Med 49:179, 1971. Reproduced with permission.

## *Periodontal Disease and Tooth Loss*

Loss of teeth, usually through periodontal disease, leads to dietary restrictions, with increased ingestion of soft, nondetergent foods (usually carbohydrates) and resultant poor nutrition. As a result, aging of tissue is accelerated. Loss of skin tone, depleted subcutaneous reserves, and further periodontal breakdown are evidence of tissue aging.

The periodontal structures (the gingivae, the alveolar bone, the periodontal membrane, and probably also the cementum) become ischemic and undergo typical fibrotic changes. Various cells become less active. Because the osteoblasts and fibroblasts are able to repair the wear and tear of daily function less rapidly and less completely as age advances, the periodontium becomes atrophic and breaks down more easily than in the young. In addition, since the periodontal tissues are subject to more trauma and stresses than other tissues of the body, including the joints, atrophy is seen earliest in these tissues.

Most loss of teeth occurring during middle and later age is the result of degenerative changes in the periodontium. It is not uncommon for a person to become edentulous before the age of 50 years because of progressive atrophy of the periodontal tissues, usually associated with secondary infection.

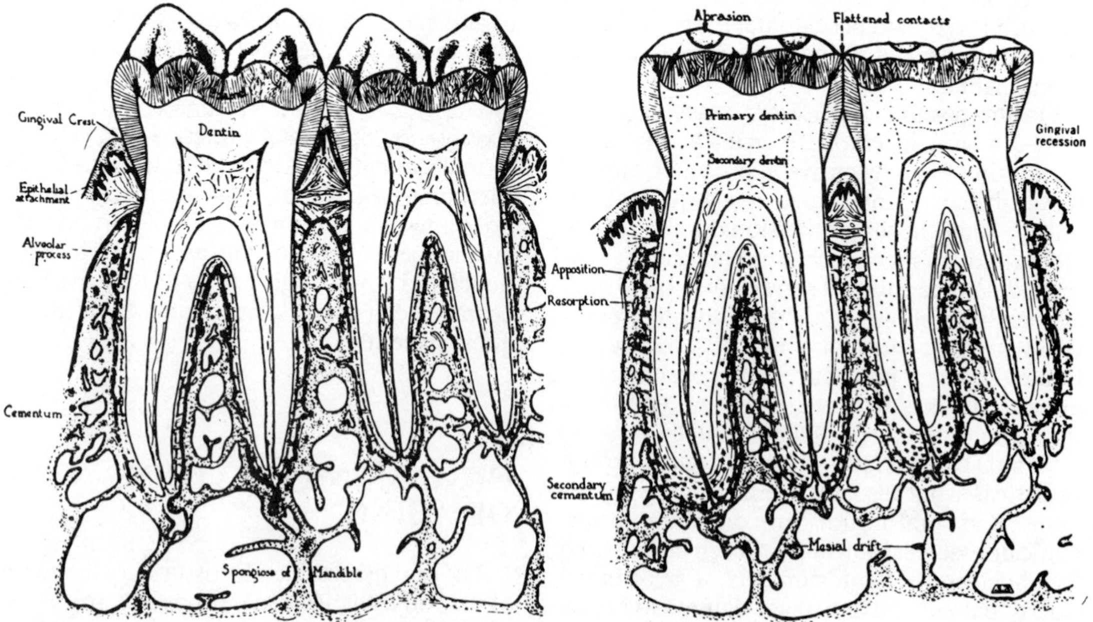


**Figure 40–1.** Diagram of the effects of attrition and mesial drift on the dental tissues. Note changes in cusp height and angulation, increase in contact areas, formation of secondary dentin, decrease in pulp size, apposition of cementum, and alterations in bone. (From Schour I: Noyes' Oral Histology and Embryology. 8th ed. Philadelphia, Lea & Febiger, 1960. Reproduced with permission.)

## *Changes in the Oral Mucosa*

The most common complaints by the elderly stem from the friability of the oral mucosa. Traumatic ulcers developing under new or even old dentures are probably the most frequent direct cause of inability to tolerate the prosthesis. Tissue friability arises from three distinct sources: (1) It arises from progressive dehydration of the oral mucosa, which results from diminished kidney function and the shift in water balance from the intracellular to the extracellular compartment. This is aggravated by (2) a progressive thinning of the epithelial layer as age advances. This thinning is associated with a reduction in the number of component cells, with a resultant decrease in thickness of both the mucosa and submucosa.[1] Since the mucosa, particularly at the transitional borders, is not covered with a layer of keratinized cells, the thinning of the epithelium leaves the unprotected tissue vulnerable even to mild stresses. (3) Finally, the cells are usually nutritionally deficient.[3] Even under the best circumstances, with age, these cells lose the optimal nourishment and vitality of youthful cells. Therefore, although denture adaptation may be good, tissue resistance is reduced, so that inflammation and even ulceration are common results.

Deficiencies in the nutrition of cells are the rule rather than the exception in the elderly. Vitamin B deficiency reduces the metabolism of these cells. Vitamin A deficiency reduces cohesiveness and integrity of the epithelial layer. Vitamin C deficiency results in poorly differentiated connective tissue cells and fibers. Clinically, nutritional deficiencies are reflected in easily torn epithelium and slow-to-heal connective tissue. Canker sores, traumatic ulcers, and angular cheilosis commonly occur with mild emotional stress or even when stress is not clinically apparent.

Other frequent complaints are abnormal taste and burning sensations in the mouth. Eighty per cent of postmenopausal women complain of these symptoms during the period of "hot flashes."[2] The symptoms are caused by the low estrogenic levels and possibly also by vitamin B complex deficiencies.

## *Bone Resorption*

Bone is the storehouse of calcium. When the intake of calcium is deficient, as it frequently is in the elderly, and the ability to digest raw milk is markedly reduced due to lactase enzyme deficiency (almost universal in the elderly),[3] the calcium must be withdrawn from the bones to keep the blood level at 10 mg per cent. Osteoporosis is also aggravated by decreased use and, in women, by the postmenopausal state. It is seen early in the weight-bearing bony structures, such as the vertebral column and the alveolar bone (see Chapter 39).[4-6] As the supporting bony tissues undergo resorption, the crest of the residual alveolar ridge is usually found to be flat or even concave and can terminate in a "knife edge." In some geriatric patients, extensive resorption of the mandibular alveolar ridge may expose the mental foramen at or near the crest, with consequent pain when the denture presses on the exposed nerve. In extreme cases, the layer of bone overlying the mandibular canal may have resorbed completely, leaving a thin layer of oral epithelium as the only protection for the contents of the exposed nerve canal (Fig. 40-2).

As a result of senile atrophy, the geriatric mandible decreases in circumference, with a corresponding reduction of denture-bearing area. The attachments of the mentalis and buccinator muscles appear to migrate toward the receding crest of the ridge. The attachments of the mylohyoid and buccinator muscles can sometimes be found at the crest of the ridge when extreme atrophy has occurred (Fig. 40-3).

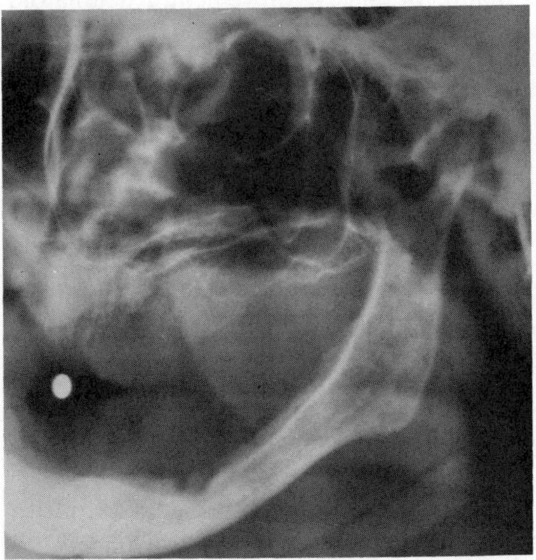

**Figure 40-2.** Radiograph of a resorbed mandible. Resorption of the alveolar bone has caused the mental foramen to be at the crest of the ridge instead of at the lateral border of the mandible.

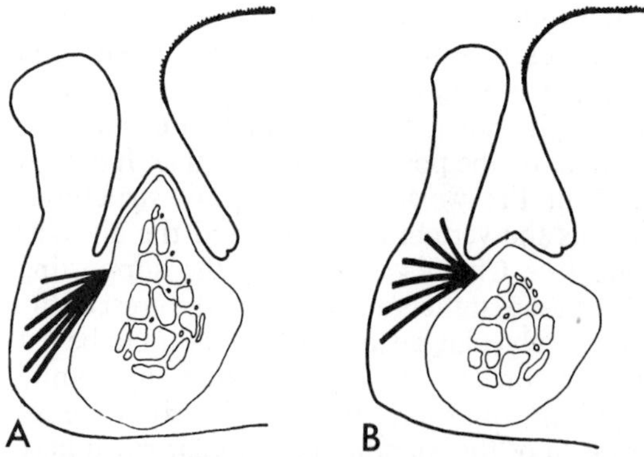


Figure 40-3. A diagrammatic representation of the effect of changes due to age in the lower anterior region of the mandible. *A,* The ridge is well formed, the lip is supported, and the origin of the mentalis muscle is low. *B,* The ridge has suffered severe resorption, the lip inclines inward, and the origin of the mentalis muscle is near the crest of the ridge. (From Anderson JN, Storer R: Immediate and Replacement Dentures. 3rd ed. Oxford, Blackwell Scientific Publications, 1981. Reproduced with permission.)

## *Temporomandibular Joint*

The temporomandibular joint of the elderly patient exhibits many changes of a degenerative nature. Many of these changes are associated with degenerative changes in other joints of the body. Osteoarthritis or degenerative joint disease is the most common form of inflammatory process affecting the temporomandibular joint. It causes splitting of the articular surfaces and even perforation of the articular disc and, therefore, manifests itself clinically with pain and limitation of range of movement. Rheumatoid arthritis, prevalent among the older members of our population, may also erode bone and cartilage and cause serious malfunction and malocclusion.

It has been difficult to single out those changes in the temporomandibular joint that are age related. Studies have shown that the condyles and fossae of older people tend to remodel to conform closely to each other. The fossae also appear to become shallower with age, and there are decreases in the inclinations of the anterior fossa wall and condyle.

## *Changes in the Tongue*

The tongue seems to increase in size in the edentulous mouth. Therefore, the elderly show this hypertrophy with greater frequency. This may possibly be a result of transference of some masticatory and phonetic functions to the tongue. This enlargement has a negative effect on denture retention.

Probably the most common manifestation of aging of the tongue is depapillation (loss of papillae), which usually begins at the apex and lateral borders. Fissuring is also common (Fig. 40-4). Both of these characteristics are also associated with various diseases (e.g., anemia, chronic fevers) and deficiency states (e.g., vitamin B deficiencies) (Fig. 40-5).

With age, the undersurface of the tongue shows an increasing number of "caviar" lesions. These are small, roughly spherical or dome-shaped varicose enlargements of the poorly supported veins in the collecting system (Fig. 40-6). The smaller ones develop as outpouchings of a communicating vein near the ranine veins. Pressure with a glass slide causes them to empty. Knots and clusters of such vessels are dark blue or black, resembling caviar or buckshot. The lesions are venous dilations, with thick walls, and hypoplastic endothelium, but with no inflammatory changes.

## *Xerostomia*

As a result of regressive changes in the salivary glands, particularly atrophy of the cells lining the intermediate ducts, there is a decrease in salivary flow in the aged.[7] The diminished function of the glands also results in a change in the quality of the saliva. Saliva shows a decrease in ptyalin content and increase in mucin content and becomes more viscous and ropy. This change in the character of saliva contributes to plaque formation and creates a favorable environment for the growth of cariogenic bacteria.

A decrease in salivary flow can also be the result of illness (e.g., diabetes mellitus and insipidus, nephritis, pernicious anemia), administration of certain medications (phenothiazine, chlorpromazine, belladonna, atropine, ephedrine, scopolamine, rauwolfia derivatives), and

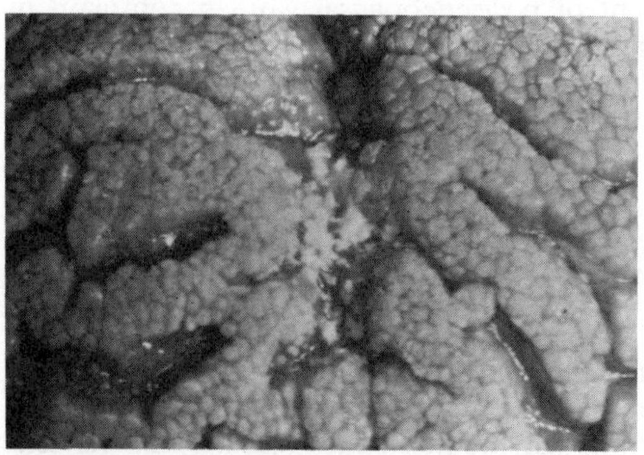

Figure 40-4. Section of a fissured tongue.

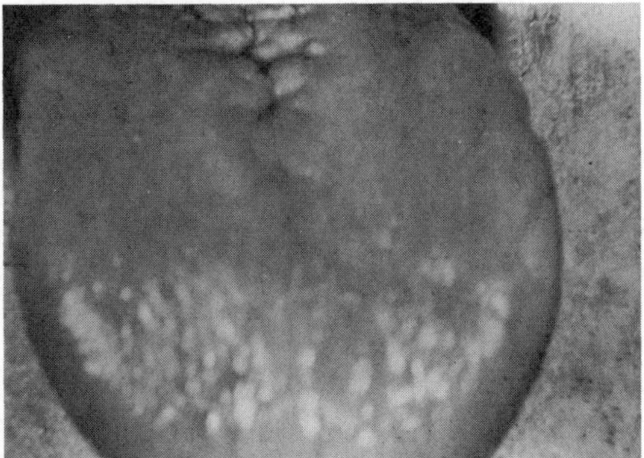

**Figure 40–5.** Tongue of a patient with vitamin B deficiency.

conditions such as menopause, x-ray irradiation, and vitamin deficiencies. A temporary decrease in salivation can be caused by a severe emotional reaction or blockage of a salivary duct by calculus (sialolithiasis).

The resulting dryness of the oral cavity (xerostomia) can lead to other symptoms.[7] Among them are abnormal taste sensations, "burning" of the oral tissues and tongue, cracking of the lips, and fissuring of the tongue. The oral mucosa becomes dry, smooth, and translucent, and the tongue can acquire a thick, white, foul-smelling coating (Fig. 40–7).

The adhesive action of a thin film of saliva between the denture base and the underlying soft tissues is considered to be one of the principal factors in denture retention. The thin film of saliva also acts as a lubricant and cushion between the denture base and the tissues and tends to eliminate irritating friction. A decrease in salivary flow interferes with denture retention as well as makes mastication and deglutition difficult. (A moist bolus of food is essential to swallowing.) The mechanical protection of the denture-supporting tissues by the saliva film is lost in patients with xerostomia, leading to irritation of the tissues. The antibacterial action of the saliva is reduced proportionally to the decrease in salivary flow.

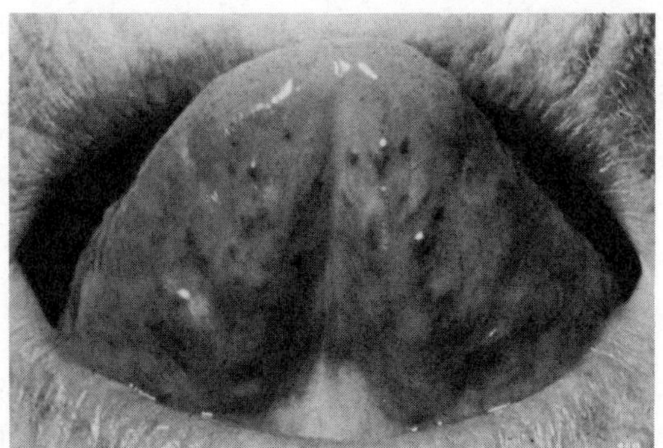

**Figure 40–6.** "Caviar" lesions on the undersurface of the tongue. (Courtesy of Dr. Samuel Driezen.)

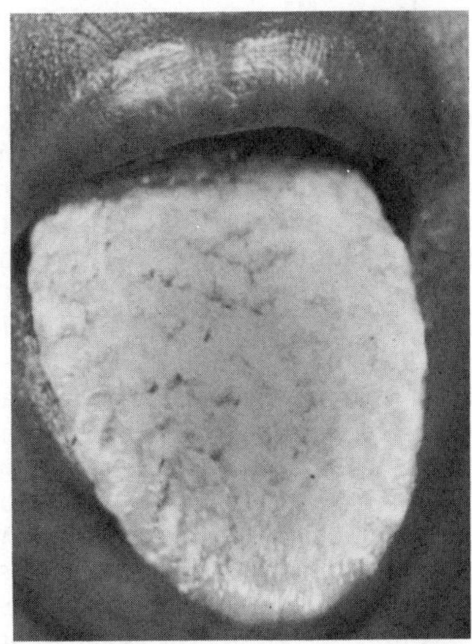

**Figure 40–7.** Coated fissured tongue.

## *Muscle Weakness*

The diminished vigor seen in many muscles of the body in elderly individuals is also evident in the masticatory and facial muscles. The facial muscles sag and become imbalanced. Learning how to manipulate these flaccid muscles is difficult for the elderly, especially when a new, and therefore foreign, denture is inserted into the oral cavity. As a result, new dentures are often rejected by the elderly, who claim they are uncomfortable and "don't fit."

## *Pain*

A potential source of discomfort after severe atrophy of the mandibular ridge is the compression of nerve endings between sharp vertical bony projections and the thin mucosal covering by the hard artificial denture base. This is particularly likely to occur in the anterior mandibular region. The soft tissues are unable to absorb or evenly distribute forces applied during mastication. This pressure on the pain receptors in the mucosa can cause severe discomfort. The pressure of a denture on an exposed mental nerve emerging from the mental foramen can cause extreme pain and even paresthesia of the lower lip and chin.

Obviously, the best treatment is relief of the

overlying denture. However, in the case of advanced bony atrophy, the amount of necessary relief in many cases would mutilate the patient's prosthesis and make it impossible to function. A more logical approach would be to try to replace the lost resilient mucosal tissue covering the residual ridge with a layer of soft resin on the tissue surface of the denture. Besides absorbing a part of the masticatory load, it could distribute the force throughout the resorbed ridge to minimize the pressure at any one particular spot.[8]

Causalgia arising in an area where a painful tooth was extracted some years previously is not uncommon in the aged.[9–11] Many flap operations and bone scrapings have been done to alleviate these characteristic pains, especially when they interfere with the wearing of dentures, but these procedures have not been successful. Causalgias may be referred to facial areas and diagnosed as atypical facial neuralgias. Causalgias are often related to emotional disturbances. Thus, treatment is often difficult.

## *Depressed Taste and Smell*

A major reason for denture failure in the elderly is deficient tissue tolerance resulting from inadequate nutrition. This stems, in part, from poor appetite, attributable in part to a depressed sense of smell and taste common in the elderly.[12] The dimming of taste results from degeneration of taste buds and reduction in their total number. Taste buds in youth are renewed approximately every 10 days. Renewal is slow in the elderly, especially in postmenopausal women suffering from estrogen deficiency. Shortages of protein and zinc also retard taste bud renewal.[13] In addition, the gustatory and olfactory nuclei in the brain decline, and the olfactory receptors in the roof of the nasal cavity regress. Elderly patients may not be aware of these changes until their attention is drawn to the mouth during the fabrication of new dentures. When they realize foods do not taste as they used to, they may blame it on the dentures and complain to the dentist.

## *Calcium Deficiency*

Calcium deficiencies and even negative calcium balance are common in elderly people (see Chapter 39). Maintenance of normal bone metabolism and structure cannot be expected in these circumstances. Osteoporosis occurs earlier and more predominently in stress-bearing areas, such as the vertebrae, and in the mandible and maxilla. Further study is necessary to determine whether the changes in the jaw bones are related to negative calcium balance or to a lack of function, or both. Pocket formation as a result of alveolar crest resorption can hasten tooth loss in partially edentulous patients. The rapid ridge resorption sometimes seen under what appears to be an excellent prosthesis (and often occurring without a prosthesis) also suggests the presence of a systemic factor, such as negative calcium balance. The relationship between excessive alveolar bone and ridge resorption and negative calcium balance merits further research.

## *Prosthetic Failures in Postmenopausal Women*

Most of the gerodontic problems already mentioned, including prosthetic failures, are more frequent and more severe in postmenopausal women. Menopause results in a number of endocrine changes, metabolic disturbances, and emotional upsets. The frequent prosthetic failures occurring in this period of life must be assessed carefully. In many instances, gross tissue deficiencies are present. These can be partially corrected by judicious dietary adjustments and vitamin supplements (especially B complex). Referral to a competent gynecologist for hormone therapy in severe cases is advised. (see Chapter 39). In other cases, tissue deficiencies may be relatively mild and unimportant but be greatly exaggerated in emotionally disturbed patients.

It is not a simple matter, therefore, to single out the basic cause of inability to wear dentures. A complete examination of (1) the prosthesis, (2) the integrity of oral tissues, and (3) the physical and emotional status of the patient *must* be undertaken. Prosthetic failure may be due to inadequacies in the denture, tissue deficiencies,[14] emotional disturbances, or, usually, a combination of these factors. In view of recent improvements in materials and techniques, it would seem that one should look more carefully for tissue deficiencies and emotional upsets than for technical defects when prosthetic failures do occur in this age group.

## *Oral Neoplasms*

The physician performing a routine physical examination is in a unique position to detect oral cancer at an early and curable stage. The mouth may be the site of development of a wide variety of neoplastic growths. As a general rule, the older the patient, the more likely that the neoplasm is malignant.

The examiner should use a good source of light, ask the patient to first remove any removable prostheses, and thoroughly explore both the oral and pharyngeal cavities. A dental or laryngeal mirror can be used to advantage to see otherwise inaccessible areas. The base of the tongue and the nasopharynx must not be overlooked. Every physician should be familiar with a method of examining the oral cavity and with the appearance of benign and malignant tumors. Biopsy of any suspicious lesion is generally a simple procedure.

### *Emotional Problems*

Finally, the vague fears and pains characteristic of insecure people of any age are exaggerated in the elderly. These call for patience, understanding, and empathy on the part of the dentist. The aged can be helped considerably by those who understand the problems of the aging person and are willing to grapple with them.[15,16]

## THE MANAGEMENT OF DENTAL PROBLEMS

### *Dental Caries and Preventive Procedures*

Dental caries is an infection that attacks the hard tissues of the teeth.[17] Caries cannot be produced in germ-free animals. A carious lesion can only occur when a mass of cariogenic microorganisms colonize on the tooth surface (bacterial plaque). These bacteria then produce acids to demineralize the underlying mineralized tooth tissues (enamel, dentin, or cementum), after which the organic matrix is digested and cavitation results.

The oral flora, like the pharyngeal, gastrointestinal, and skin floras, changes with every decade of life. The reasons are not clear, but the indigenous bacterial flora in the mouth does change in the elderly. There are three classes of carious lesions, produced by three different classes of cariogenic microorganisms, in three different age periods (Fig. 40–8).

1. Pit and fissure caries occurs primarily in newly erupted teeth and are usually produced in

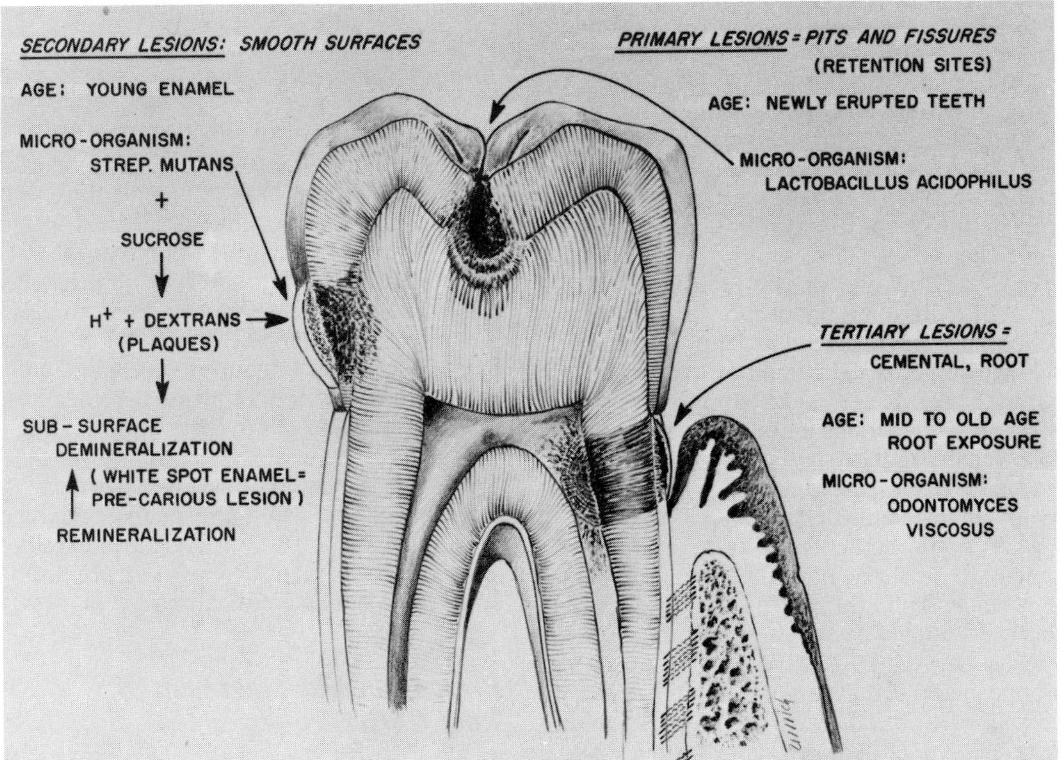


**Figure 40–8.** Diagram showing the types of carious lesions, their incidence by age, and the microorganisms responsible for these lesions.

young children by cariogenic *Lactobacillus acidophilus* organisms. Lactobacilli cannot produce extracellular dextrans (bacterial glue) from sucrose, as do the streptococci, and therefore do not form "plaques" on smooth surfaces. Instead, they invade and colonize retention sites such as pits and fissures and the leaky margins of restorations. Pits and fissures in newly erupted teeth contain *biodegradable* glycoproteins upon which these organisms can grow and produce acids.

2. Smooth-surface (enamel) caries occurs primarily in young adults while the enamel and dentin are still permeable and immature. The organism responsible for most if not all carious lesions in adults is *Streptococcus mutans.* This organism can appear in the oral environment at any time from infancy to old age. It is a destructive organism and deeply invasive in the young. It acts more slowly and intermittently in older age groups, probably because enamel and dentin become more resistant with age. Enamel caries are much less frequent after age 35 because the enamel becomes much more dense and acquires a much higher surface fluoride content.

3. Cemental caries in the patient past age 50 is probably produced primarily by the *Odontomyces viscosus.* The normal habitat of the *O. viscosus* is among the filiform papillae of the tongue, where they grow, coating the dorsum of the tongue with a viscous, white nonadherent material. The organisms then spread to the exposed cementum and are particularly prone to invade and grow within gingival pockets, where they can form a bacterial plaque. Under this plaque, a carious lesion is produced, extending through the porous cementum and into the dentin (Fig. 40–9). The lesion, when exposed to view, is shallow and deeply pigmented (dark brown). Cavitation is not deep as under a streptococcal plaque. Instead, the dentin is softened and discolored. A radiograph will show the lesion in the dentin as a vague radiolucent streak. Progress of the carious lesion is generally slow. However, in irradiated patients with xerostomia and friable tissues, the cemental lesion develops rapidly and is highly destructive.

With age, the contents of pits and fissures become hard, leathery, dark brown, and *nonbiodegradable.* Thus the pits and fissures in the elderly eventually become resistant to caries.

In people past 70 years, *O. viscosus* tend to disappear, and *Candida albicans* begin to infest the oral cavity. *Candida* grow in moist, stagnant areas, e.g., under dentures. They form a white, cheesy colony under which the mucosal tissue becomes raw, red, and painful.

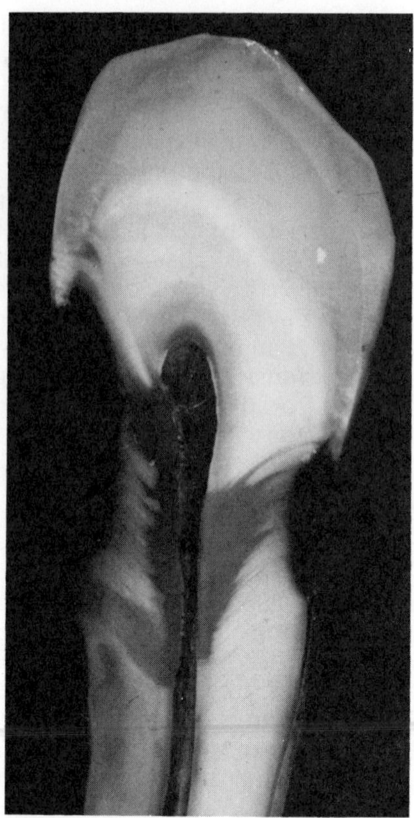

**Figure 40–9.** Cemental lesions. Typical shallow lesion on the right; older lesion on the left.

## *Tongue Cleaning*

The practice of regular tongue brushing should be initiated in the elderly as soon as the tongue shows signs of developing a thick white mucoid coat, evident upon arising and persisting after breakfast. This coating can be easily removed using a soft toothbrush (or a dry gauze pad in the bedridden). The coating can also be removed by "detergent" foods such as hard bread, dry cereal, uncooked vegetables, and fibrous meats. In some countries, the elderly use a tongue scraper to remove the thick coating on the tongue.

The tongue should be cleansed twice daily, in the morning on rising and in the evening on retiring (Fig. 40–10). Oral hygiene in the elderly is essential to prevent *O. viscosus* from proliferating and forming a critical mass.

## *Prevention and Treatment of Root Caries*

Topical applications of stannous fluoride solutions to the demineralized cementum and

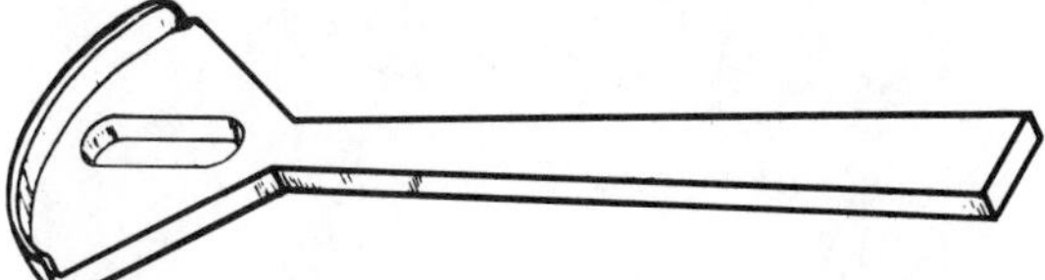

**Figure 40–10.** Diagram of a commercially available tongue cleaner.

dentin remineralizes these tissues and increases their resistance to further demineralization after the surface bacterial plaque is removed. Cementum absorbs the fluoride much more rapidly and in much higher concentration than enamel and dentin do. Stannous fluoride 4 per cent is generally preferred, although no scientific evidence is yet available to compare its effectiveness with that of sodium fluoride or the acidulated fluorophosphate.

## *Elimination of Gingival Pockets*

Gingival pockets are the sites of predilection for cemental caries caused by *O. viscosus.* These organisms are strict anaerobes and prefer deep pockets for their growth. Exposure of the cementum to the washing action of the saliva and the cleansing action of detergent foods will cause even active cemental lesions to become arrested. The tissue will become partially remineralized, hard and leathery, and deeply pigmented. These arrested lesions can remain in status quo for many years, without restorations, if the area is smoothed and kept free of bacterial plaque by brushing. If the cavitation is deep, restoration of tooth contour to protect the gingivae is indicated after application of a stannous fluoride solution.

## *Nutrition*

Nutrition is one of the factors under human control that can influence the health of the aging. A good general diet is essential to the supporting tissues of the teeth and to the health of the elderly. A lack of essential nutrients can cause tissue friability and depress the potential for repair. The diets of elderly individuals are often nutritionally inadequate (see Chapter 13). It is essential for the geriatric patient to retain an interest in food. He or she must be prevented, because of dental difficulties, from gradually changing his or her diet to softer foods that require little or no chewing and are easy to swallow. A great many elderly people exist on inadequate diets, not realizing or caring about the effects on their overall health. Although the aged require fewer calories than do the young, the diet must include the proper amounts of protein, fats, carbohydrates, vitamins and minerals, and even more important—water. Unhealthy (nutritionally deficient) oral tissues will not provide a satisfactory foundation for successful denture service, no matter how carefully the procedure is executed.

Delayed healing of extraction wounds, with excessive and painful postoperative swelling, may be related to relative or absolute vitamin C deficiency found so often in aged people. A number of reports indicate that ascorbic acid in high dosages (500 to 1000 mg per day) given before and after surgical procedures promotes healing and seems to reduce the postoperative morbidity.[18]

"Denture sore mouth" (pain and burning of the denture-supporting tissues, with the resultant inability to wear dentures) has been treated successfully by Payne and others by flooding the body and, therefore, the mouth with vitamin C (ascorbic acid). Payne recommends 1500 mg per day, two tablets of 250 mg taken with each meal, for a 4-week period. He then reduces the dosage to 750 mg per day, one tablet of 250 mg with each meal, which is continued indefinitely.[19] However, it should be stressed that vitamin therapy by itself is not a substitute for a well-balanced diet.

The elderly should be encouraged to add flavoring agents and condiments to their food, rather than relying on excessive salt and sugar to maintain taste. Seasoning must be added to foods to preserve the stimuli that taste and smell add to the enjoyment of food.

## *Treatment of Xerostomia*

The treatment of xerostomia has been generally unsatisfactory. If the dry mouth is a result of the diminution of salivary gland secretion, the use of artificial saliva and frequent mouth rinses, particularly during meals, may be helpful.[20] Coating the tissue surface of the denture with petrolatum or lubricating jelly, silicone fluid, or one of the commercial semisolid denture adhesive preparations can *temporarily* increase denture retention and decrease irritation of the underlying soft tissues.

Sialogogues, drugs that stimulate the flow of

saliva without affecting the ptyalin content, can be tried if some glandular function is still present. Pilocarpine hydrochloride in 5-mg doses (10 drops of a 10 per cent solution) before meals will cause a pronounced flow for 2 to 5 hours. Because it also causes excessive sweating and discomfort, pilocarpine is seldom prescribed or used. Sucking on a sour hard candy is often just as effective as the administration of sialogogues. If the decrease in salivary flow is due to nutritional deficiencies, a therapeutic dose of nicotinamide (250 to 400 mg three times daily) for a period of up to 2 weeks can be used.

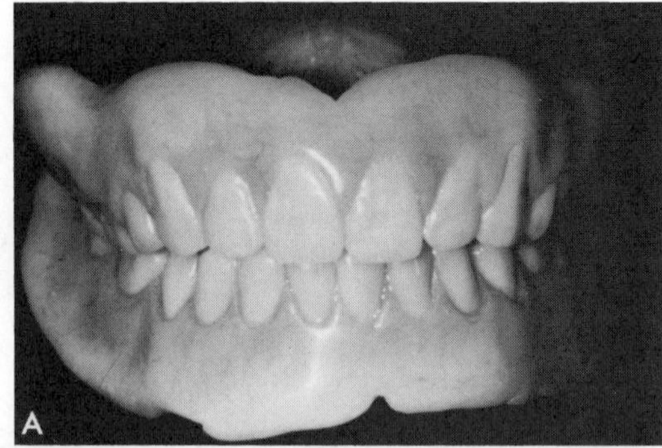


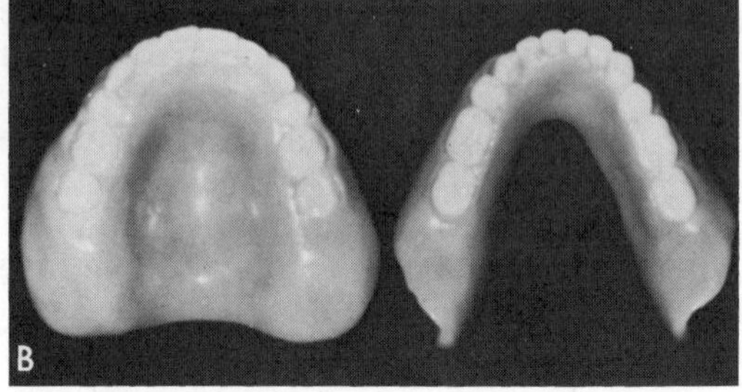


**Figure 40–11.** Upper and lower complete dentures. *A*, Front (labial or facial) view. *B*, Top (occlusal) view.

## *Complete Denture Prosthodontics*

Complete denture prosthodontics involves the replacement of the lost natural teeth and associated structures of the maxilla and mandible in patients who have lost all their remaining natural teeth or are soon to lose them. As complete dentures are the last consideration for the patient, arrived at only when all other avenues have been closed, they must be designed and constructed with an emphasis on the preservation of the remaining oral structures.

In 1971, an estimated 22.6 million Americans were edentulous. About half of these people were over 65 years of age. Approximately 1.8 million had either an incomplete set of dentures (upper or lower only) or no dentures at all.[8] The Bureau of Economic Research and Statistics of the American Dental Association reported that, in 1975 in the United States, of a total civilian population of 211,445,000, 23,500,000 people were edentulous. Although no later figures are available at the time of writing, it is safe to say that the number is slowly increasing.

The basic objectives of complete dentures (Fig. 40–11) are the restoration of function and facial appearance and the maintenance of the patient's health. The person wearing complete dentures should be able to speak distinctly and experience oral comfort. The patient should also be educated in the importance of periodic examination and subsequent treatment when necessitated by changes in the supporting tissues.

The mastication of food with complete dentures assists the edentulous patient in obtaining adequate nutrition. However, complete dentures constructed even under the most ideal conditions will have a chewing efficiency of only a fraction of that of the natural dentition. The elderly patient must understand and accept the reduced efficiency of the artificial dentition.

Elderly people who have been without teeth for many years and have no desire for complete dentures are best left alone. If facial appearance is unimportant to these patients and being without teeth does not alter their personalities, it is an error to try to convince them to have complete dentures constructed. Some of these patients get along very well nutritionally without teeth—in fact, much better than some people with inadequate dentures.

## *Soft Denture Liners*

The indications for soft denture liners were discussed previously. Soft denture liners would be more widely used if better products were available. Unfortunately, the dental profession has witnessed the introduction and subsequent withdrawal from the market of numerous unsatisfactory soft lining materials. In spite of their shortcomings, some of them do give a degree of comfort to geriatric patients for a short time.

The gradual hardening of soft denture liners over a moderate period of time occurs at a slow rate and is barely perceptible to some geriatric patients. By the time the soft liner has completely lost its resiliency, the patient may become used to the masticatory forces transmitted by a hard denture base. The oral mucosa and underlying bone may have become more resistant to occlusal stress. Dentures with a soft liner can be replaced at this time with a new denture, or the liner can be removed and the prosthesis relined or rebased. At best, soft denture liners should be considered temporary and should be re-examined at regular intervals.

# CONCLUSION

Dental care of the aging patient (gerodontics) presents a number of problems not encountered in younger patients. Most of these problems result from tissue changes that occur during aging. The dentist, especially the prosthodontist, is in a strategic position to evaluate and correct many of the dietary and nutritional deficiencies that promote premature aging of tissues. In particular, the prosthodontist is in a position to reduce the number of prosthetic failures through application of knowledge of the physical, metabolic, and endocrine changes associated with aging, as well as the nutritional deficiencies and emotional disturbances common among the aged. Geriatric patients can be helped toward optimal health and happiness by those who are willing to study their problems.

## References

1. Shklar G: Oral pathology in the aging individual. *In* Toga CJ, Nandy K, Chauncey HH (eds.): Geriatric Dentistry. Lexington, Massachusetts, D. C. Heath & Co., 1979, pp. 127-145.
2. Albright F, Smith PH, Richardson AM: Postmenopausal osteoporosis. JAMA 171:1637, 1941.
3. Birge SJ Jr, Keutmann HT, Cuatrecasas P, Whedon GD: Osteoporosis, intestinal lactase deficiency and low dietary calcium intake. N Engl J Med 276:445, 1967.
4. Albanese AA, Edelson AH, Lorenze EJ, Wein EH: Quantitative radiographic survey technique for detection of bone loss. J Am Geriatr Soc 17:142, 1969.
5. Jowsey J: Why is mineral nutrition important in osteoporosis? Geriatrics 33:39, 1978.
6. Massler M: Geriatric nutrition. I. Osteoporosis. J Prosthet Dent 42:252, 1979.
7. Massler M: Geriatric nutrition. II. Dehydration in the elderly. J Prosthet Dent 42:489, 1979.
8. Winkler S: The geriatric complete denture patient. Dent Clin North Am 21:403, 1977.
9. Marbach JJ, Hulbrock J, Holm C, Segal AG: Incidence of phantom tooth pain: An atypical facial neuralgia. Oral Surg Oral Med Oral Path 53:190, 1982.
10. Massler M: Dental causalgia. Quintessence Int 12:341, 1981.
11. Melzack R: The Puzzle of Pain: Revolution in Theory and Treatment. New York, Basic Books, 1973.
12. Hyde RJ, Feller RP, Sharon IM: Tongue brushing, dentifrice, and age effects on taste and smell. J Dent Res 60:1730, 1981.
13. Massler M: Geriatric nutrition. III. The role of taste and smell in appetite. J Prosthet Dent 43:247, 1980.
14. Langer A: Oral signs of aging and their clinical significance. Geriatrics 31:63, 1976.
15. Pfeiffer E: Handling the distressed older patient. Geriatrics 34:24, 1979.
16. Pitt BM: Psychogeriatrics: An Introduction to the Psychiatry of Old Age. London, Churchill Livingstone, 1974.
17. Massler M: Geriatric dentistry: Root caries in the elderly. J Prosthet Dent 44:147, 1980.
18. Miller JM, Stare FJ: Nutritional problems and dietary requirements. *In* Powers JH (ed.): Surgery of the Aged and Debilitated Patient. Philadelphia, W. B. Saunders Co., 1968, p. 132.
19. Payne SH: Personal communication, 1972.
20. Shannon IL: A saliva substitute for dry mouth relief. *In* Toga CJ, Nandy K, Chauncey HH (eds.): Geriatric Dentistry. Lexington, Massachusetts, D. C. Heath & Co., 1979, pp. 161-173.

### *Additional Reading*

1. Davidoff A, Winkler S, Lee MHM: Dentistry for the Special Patient: The Aged, Chronically Ill and Handicapped. Philadelphia, W. B. Saunders Co., 1972.
*This book, the first United States textbook on geriatric dentistry, presented the combined efforts of many individuals representing disciplines dedicated to serving the dental and medical needs of the aged, chronically ill, and handicapped. The introduction is by Howard A. Rusk, M. D. This is the standard reference on geriatric dentistry.*
2. Fishman N, Bikofsky CG (eds.): Proceedings of the Conference on Dentistry and the Geriatric Patient. Boston, Harvard School of Dental Medicine, April 10-12, 1972.
*Proceedings of a conference dedicated to providing the general dentist with proper medical, nutritional, psychologic, and social background to be better able to approach the delivery of dental care to the aged. The many areas of availability and accessibility of comprehensive dental care to the elderly in varying environments are explored.*
3. Kutscher AH, Goldberg IK (eds.): Oral Care of the Aging and Dying Patient. Springfield, Illinois, Charles C Thomas, 1973.
*An overview of the oral problems inherent in the treatment of geriatric and terminally ill patients. Various modalities of therapy are examined not only in general terms but also in relation to specific oral conditions and disease entities specific to these patients.*

## Chapter 41

# Skin Diseases in the Elderly

*Barbara A. Gilchrest*

Skin is the interface between people and their environment that protects the other organs of the body from excessive temperature changes, mechanical injury, ultraviolet irradiation, toxic chemicals, and microbial pathogens. It is also a tactile organ through which individuals receive pleasurable stimuli and assess their physical surroundings. With age, the skin performs each of these vital functions less well. Skin is also readily visible and hence of great psychologic and social, as well as physiologic, importance. For this reason the morphologic changes that accompany aging in the skin often affect an individual as greatly as do the functional changes.

Dermatologic problems are exceedingly common, especially among old people, and are frequently among the chief complaints that bring geriatric patients to the physician. It has been estimated that at least 7 per cent of all physician visits are prompted exclusively by disorders of the skin.[1] Moreover, examination of more than 20,000 noninstitutionalized Americans revealed that 40 per cent of those beyond age 65 suffered from a dermatologic disease sufficiently severe in the opinion of the consultant dermatologist to justify at least one physician visit and that the average affected individual had 1.5 such disorders.[2] These figures do not include the nearly universal "cosmetic" changes in aging skin, which may lower self-esteem and which may have a measurable negative impact on society's perception of the elderly.[3]

Morphologic and probably even physiologic age-associated cutaneous changes are most pronounced in fair-skinned individuals in whom sun damage is superimposed on intrinsic aging. The major stigmata of aging in the skin—wrinkling, "dryness" (roughness), uneven pigmentation, and cancer—are indeed virtually restricted to habitually sun-exposed areas. However, these sun-induced changes, which have dominated the public and even medical perception of cutaneous aging, are only one aspect of a subtle but undoubtedly biologically significant process that gradually alters the function of normal skin and its response to a large number of disease states. The following sections review the age-associated changes now recognized in normal skin and discuss selected disorders of the skin with special relevance to the elderly.

## AGE-ASSOCIATED CHANGES IN NORMAL SKIN

A detailed well-referenced discussion of the age-associated changes in normal skin is beyond the scope of this chapter, but is available in other recent reviews (see reference 4 and Additional Reading, page 498).

Histologic features associated with aging in human skin are shown schematically in Figure 41–1. The most striking and consistent change is flattening of the dermoepidermal junction, with effacement of both the dermal papillae and the epidermal rete pegs. This results in a considerably smaller contiguous surface between the two compartments, presumably less "communication" and nutrient transfer, and less resistance to shearing forces.

Loss of dermal thickness approaches 20 per cent in elderly individuals and may account for the paper-thin, sometimes nearly transparent quality of their skin. The remaining dermis is relatively acellular and avascular. Precise histologic concomitants of wrinkling, if any, are unknown, although age-related loss of normal elastin fibers may be contributory.

Table 41–1 lists the major functions of the skin that decline with age. Many of the entities are necessarily interrelated or overlapping.

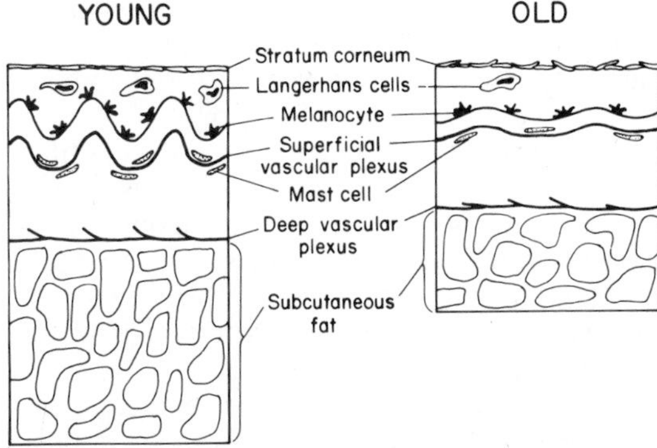


**Figure 41-1.** Histologic changes in aging normal skin. Schematic drawings emphasize the age-associated flattening of the dermoepidermal junction (basement membrane zone [BMZ]); loss of dermal and subcutaneous mass; shortened capillary loops; and reduced numbers of melanocytes, Langerhans cells, and mast cells. Note that average thickness of the stratum corneum (barrier layer) and viable epidermis (area above the BMZ) does not vary with age. In most body areas, epidermal thickness is approximately 0.1 mm; dermal thicknesses range from 0.1 to 4.0 mm, depending on body site. Melanocyte densities range from 1000/mm$^2$ to 2000/mm$^2$ surface area in most body areas; Langerhans cell density is approximately 500/mm$^2$. (From Gilchrest BA: Age-associated changes in the skin. J Am Geriatr Soc 30:139, 1982.)

An age-associated decrease in epidermal turnover rate of approximately 30 to 50 per cent between the third and eighth decades has been determined by a study of desquamation rates for corneocytes (cells of the stratum corneum) at selected body sites; other investigators have reported a corresponding 100 per cent prolongation in stratum corneum replacement rate in old versus young men. Linear growth rates for hair and nails also decrease by approximately 30 to 50 per cent between early and late adulthood. Repair rate in the skin likewise declines with age, whether measured as development of wound tensile strength, collagen deposition, regeneration of excised blister roofs, or excision of thymine dimers in ultraviolet-irradiated DNA of cultured dermal fibroblasts.

Neoplasia is associated with aging in virtually all organ systems but is especially characteristic of skin. One or more benign proliferative growths (Table 41-2) are present in nearly every adult beyond age 65 years, and most individuals have dozens of lesions. In the United States, basal cell carcinoma and squamous cell carcinoma outnumber all other human malignancies combined. These benign and malignant neoplasms almost certainly reflect in part the loss of proliferative homeostasis with age and perhaps an over-responsiveness to appropriate growth stimuli. Other factors may include the decrease in enzymatically active melanocytes per unit surface area of the skin (approximately 10 to 20 per cent of the remaining cell population each decade), since these cells constitute the body's major defense against ultraviolet radiation, to which more than 90 per cent of cutaneous malignancies can be attributed.

Although stratum corneum thickness and degree of compaction remain constant, an age-related decrease in surface barrier function as measured by percutaneous absorption of at least some substances has been reported. This increased absorption is accompanied by a decreased dermal clearance rate for the materials, possibly increasing the risk of an irritant or allergic contact dermatitis.

Decreased sensory perception was documented in old skin more than three decades ago, using several techniques: optimal stimulus in grams for light touch, vibratory sensation, and corneal sensation. Pacinian and Meissner's corpuscles, the cutaneous end organs responsible for pressure perception and light touch, progressively decrease to approximately one third their initial average density between the second and ninth decades of life.

Early studies demonstrated that eccrine sweating is markedly impaired with age. Spontaneous sweating in response to dry heat, measured on digital pads, was reduced more than 70 per cent in healthy old subjects as compared with young control subjects. This response is

**Table 41-1.** PHYSIOLOGIC PARAMETERS IN HUMAN SKIN THAT DECLINE WITH AGE*

| | |
|---|---|
| Growth rate | Immunosurveillance |
| Injury response | Vascular responsiveness |
| Barrier function | Thermoregulation |
| Chemical clearance rates | Sweat production |
| Sensory perception | Sebum production |

* Adapted from Gilchrest BA: Age-associated changes in the skin. J Am Geriatr Soc 30:139, 1982.

**Table 41-2.** PROLIFERATIVE GROWTHS ASSOCIATED WITH AGING IN HUMAN SKIN*

| Lesion | Participating cells or tissue |
|---|---|
| Acrochordon (skin tag) | Dermis, keratinocytes, melanocytes |
| Cherry angioma | Capillaries |
| Seborrheic keratosis | Dermis, keratinocytes, melanocytes |
| Lentigo | Melanocytes |
| Sebaceous hyperplasia | Sebaceous glands |

* From Gilchrest BA: Age-associated changes in the skin. J Am Geriatr Soc 30:139, 1982. Reproduced with permission.

attributable primarily to a decreased output per gland, although the number of eccrine glands also decreases approximately 15 per cent during adulthood in most body sites.

Decreased vascular responsiveness in the normal skin of old versus young individuals has been documented by measuring vasodilation and transudation after application of standardized chemical irritants and exposure to a standardized ultraviolet dose. The decreased erythematous response is probably attributable in part to the striking age-associated loss of dermal venules, although decreased responsiveness of individual vessels may also be responsible. Compromised thermoregulation, which predisposes the elderly to hypothermia and possibly heat stroke, may be due in part to reduced vasodilation or vasoconstriction of dermal arterioles, in part to decreased eccrine sweat production, and in part to loss of subcutaneous fat, all of which occur with advancing age.

Dermoepidermal separation has been reported to occur more readily in the elderly under experimental conditions, as might be anticipated from the histologic finding of reduced interdigitation between the dermis and epidermis. The poor adhesion between these two cutaneous compartments in the elderly undoubtedly explains the propensity of elderly people to "torn" skin and superficial abrasions following minor trauma, such as bandage removal, and to bulla formation in edematous sites. It may also contribute to the increased prevalence of certain bullous dermatoses in the elderly.

An age-associated decrease in delayed hypersensitivity reactions in human skin is manifested by a relative inability of healthy older subjects to develop sensitivity to dinitrochlorobenzene (DNCB) and by their lower rate of positivity for standard test antigens compared with young adult controls. In one study comparing two groups of 45 healthy volunteers, 70 per cent of those younger than 80 years reacted to at least one of five standard recall antigens, whereas only 24 per cent of the octogenarians did. The positivity rates for candidin and trichophytin decreased by 67 per cent and 85 per cent, respectively. In another group of 116 healthy subjects, 94 per cent of those below age 70 years could be sensitized to DNCB, versus 69 per cent of those older than 70 years. This decrease undoubtedly reflects in part the well-documented reduction in total number of circulating thymus-derived lymphocytes and their decreased responsiveness to standard mitogens. The nearly 50 per cent reduction in morphologically identifiable epidermal Langerhans' cells, the cell population believed to be responsible for recognition of foreign antigens in the skin, that occurs between early and late adulthood may also contribute to this decrease in immune function.

The decrease with age in cutaneous manifestations of immediate hypersensitivity is equally pronounced. In one well-controlled epidermiologic study of over 3000 subjects, the percentage of people with at least one positive wheal-and-flare reaction to a standard battery of potential allergens fell from 52 per cent at age 20 years to 16 per cent at age 75 years. The smaller groups of subjects with at least three, seven, or 11 positive test results showed parallel reductions with advancing adult age. The investigators were unable to determine the relative contributions of systemic versus local cutaneous changes in this decline. However, in one study, there was approximately a 50 per cent reduction in mast cells, the source of histamine in the skin, in the papillary dermis of buttock skin in old compared with young adults. This reduction is associated with a corresponding reduction in stimulated histamine release.

A decrease in sebum production of approximately 60 per cent accompanies advancing age in both men and women and has been attributed to the concomitant decrease in production of gonadal or adrenal androgen to which sebaceous glands are exquisitely sensitive. The clinical effects of decreased sebum production, if any, are unknown. There is no direct relationship to xerosis or seborrheic dermatitis.

## *Herpes Zoster*

Herpes zoster or "shingles" is a familiar vesicular dermatomal eruption due to reactivation of latent varicella virus in the dorsal sensory ganglia of a partially immune host. More than two thirds of cases occur in patients older than 50 years, with age-adjusted annual incidence rates per 1000 population less than 1 at age 0 to 10 years, approximately 2.5 at age 20 to 50 years, and more than 10 at age 80 years.[5] It has been estimated that by age 85 an individual has a 50 per cent risk of having had at least one attack of herpes zoster and a 10 per cent risk of having had two attacks. Immunosuppressed patients have an annual incidence of herpes zoster 20 to 100 times that of the general population and often have much more severe disease.

Herpes zoster usually begins with dysesthesia or paresthesia of the involved dermatome. These symptoms persist for days, but rarely longer than a week, before the appearance of vesicles and may mimic angina, spinal cord compression, renal or biliary colic, muscle sprains, or many other disorders. Constitutional symptoms are rare.

The rash of herpes zoster is virtually pathognomic (Fig. 41–2). Clusters of vesicles, sometimes superimposed on an erythematous plaque, erupt in a dermatomal distribution. Lesions do not cross the midline, and the eruption is unilateral in at least 98 per cent of patients, although occasional individual "disseminated" vesicles occur frequently. The diagnosis of herpes virus infection may be confirmed by a Tzanck test of material scraped from the base of an intact vesicle. The initially clear vesicles may become pustular or, especially in the elderly, hemorrhagic within a few days. New lesions continue to appear for several days, often progressing distally along the dermatome. Widespread dissemination, if it is to occur, usually does so during this period. Pain and hyperesthesia are frequently prominent during the first days of the eruption, although their severity is unrelated to either the risk or the severity of post-herpetic neuralgia in individual patients. Vesicles usually begin to crust in the second week and resolve within 4 weeks in most patients; the eruption tends to persist longer and to be more severe in the elderly. Vesicle fluid is contagious, but the attack rate (cases of varicella) in susceptible household contacts is much less than for chicken pox (primary varicella infection).

The course of herpes zoster infection in young and old adults differs primarily in the incidence and severity of post-herpetic neuralgia. This problem occurs in approximately 10 per cent of cases overall but is uncommon in patients less than 40 years old. In one survey of 916 patients, more than half of those above 60 years old experienced pain lasting at least 1 year.[6] The increase in severity and duration of post-herpetic neuralgia with age is even more marked than the increase in incidence. Persistent pain is especially common in those patients with trigeminal involvement (10 to 15 per cent of reported cases) or immunosuppression.

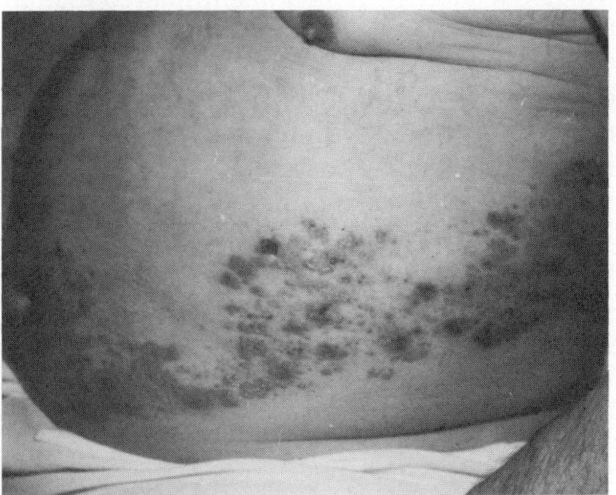

**Figure 41–2.** Herpes zoster involving the left T10 dermatome. Eruption consists of clear grouped vesicles and hemorrhagic crusts superimposed on erythematous plaques. Note sharp cutoff at the umbilicus.

Persistent hyperpigmentation or true scarring of involved skin is a less important complication of herpes zoster that is also more common in the elderly. Fortunately, patients with herpes zoster appear not to be at increased risk for the subsequent development of malignancy.[7]

During the acute phase of the infection, some patients require narcotic analgesics for adequate relief of pain. These agents should be prescribed cautiously in the elderly to avoid overmedication and adverse systemic effects.

Early skin lesions are best treated with local compresses of Burow's solution (1:20 in cool water) or other hypertonic soaks for 10 minutes 3 to 4 times daily, followed by gentle washing with Hibiclens or other antibacterial soap to hasten drying and prevent bacterial superinfection. Topical antibiotic ointment may be applied twice daily to already crusted lesions. Systemically administered corticosteroids may dramatically reduce the pain and inflammation associated with acute herpes zoster, especially herpes zoster ophthalmicus, apparently without adverse effects on healing. Relative contraindications to the use of steroids, such as diabetes, hypertension, and certain psychiatric disorders, must be weighed for each patient.

Several forms of treatment have been proposed for the devastating problem of post-herpetic neuralgia. The best established and most readily available therapy is systemically administered corticosteroids.[8–10] In a recent study,[10] 40 otherwise healthy patients at least 50 years old with early severe herpes zoster were randomly allocated to two groups of similar composition and average age (66.4 years and 68.5 years) for treatment with either prednisolone or carbamazepine (as a placebo). The eruption had been present an average of approximately 5 days in both groups before therapy began. Skin lesions healed significantly faster in the prednisolone group (3.65 versus 5.25 weeks), and the incidence of post-herpetic neuralgia was 15 per cent (3 of 20), versus 65 per cent (13 of 20) in the control group. Pain in the three prednisolone-treated patients lasted 4 to 6 months, whereas in 4 of the 13 control patients, pain persisted for at least 1 year. No patient in either group had viral dissemination or other major complications of therapy. The prednisolone was administered orally, 40 mg per day (equivalent to prednisone 40 mg per day) for 10 days; the dosage was then tapered over 3 weeks. Other dosage schedules were not investigated.

In Europe, pain associated with herpes zoster has been successfully treated with L-dopa, an anti-parkinsonian agent previously demonstrated effective in relieving the pain associated with bony metastases. In a double-blind study,[11] 47 outpatients were randomly assigned to treatment with L-dopa (100 mg) and benserazide (25 mg), a peripheral decarboxylase inhibitor, or a lactose placebo in capsular form, administered orally 3 times daily for 10 days. The two groups were quite comparable in all regards, including average age, duration of lesions before treatment, and number of "high-risk" patients, either older than 65 years or afflicted with herpes zoster ophthalmicus. Healing time for the cutaneous eruption averaged slightly greater than 2 weeks in both groups overall, but among high-risk patients (including the elderly), average healing time was significantly reduced in the L-dopa group (14 versus 22 days). After 2 days, average pain intensity was significantly less in the high-risk L-dopa-treated patients than in controls; after 3 days it was significantly less in the entire group compared with controls. Overall, post-herpetic neuralgia was present after 60 days in 5 of 15 patients in the placebo group and in only 1 of 16 patients in the levodopa group for whom complete data were available: in the high risk groups, these ratios were 4 of 7 patients and 1 of 8 patients, respectively. Although not statistically significant, these differences suggest that L-dopa may reduce the incidence and/or duration of post-herpetic neuralgia. Scarring of the skin was statistically less frequent among the high-risk L-dopa-treated patients. The only adverse effect of therapy was vomiting, which occurred in 4 patients with a mean age of 81 years (as well as in 2 young placebo-treated patients). The authors postulated that this side effect could be avoided by initiating L-dopa therapy at lower dosage.

More rapid healing and decreased pain during herpes zoster infection have also been reported for non-immunosuppressed patients treated with the guanine derivative acyclovir.[12] Consecutive patients hospitalized for herpes zoster were treated either with acyclovir 5 mg per kg or mannitol 100 mg (placebo) as an intravenous bolus every 8 hours for 5 days in a randomized double-blind trial. Using a somewhat complicated weighted clinical and photographic assessment, the investigators determined that the 20 acyclovir-treated patients had statistically more rapid improvement than did the 22 controls. During the second week of the eruption, the proportion of patients in the acyclovir group reporting pain was statistically reduced by approximately half compared with the proportion of patients in the control group reporting pain; this beneficial effect was more prominent for patients older than 67 years (approximately 10 per cent in the acyclovir group versus 65 per cent in the control group) and for those beginning therapy within 3 days of the onset of symptoms. The authors do not state the overlap between these groups (the elderly and those seeking hospitalization within 3 days). However, despite the initial differences, at 1 and 3 months after discharge, there was no effect of treatment on the persistence of pain. No patient had adverse effects attributable to acyclovir. Improvements seen during the acute phase of the infection were attributed to the known antiviral effect of acyclovir.

Successful treatment of already established post-herpetic neuralgia has been reported for both chlorprothixene[13] and a combination of psychotropic drugs,[14] although the anecdoctal, unreported experience with these drugs has been disappointing. Patients with severe, long-standing neuralgia not responsive to the preceding measures should consider less "conventional" approaches, such as transcutaneous electrical stimulation.

## *Pruritus*

Elderly people often experience localized or generalized pruritus. For some, it is a minor annoyance; for others the pruritus leads to extensive slow-healing excoriations or loss of sleep with associated irritability and impaired mental function.

Many patients presenting to the physician because of pruritus in fact have an eruption that is responsible for the symptom, although its other manifestations may be so subtle that the patient or even the physician does not notice the rash. Because cutaneous inflammatory responses may be muted in the elderly, a careful history and physical examination are necessary before excluding primary disorders of the skin such as eczema, early bullous pemphigoid, urticaria, scabies, or pediculosis. Proper identification of a causative dermatosis leads to effective treatment in most patients and enables the patient to avoid the hematologic, radiographic, and other laboratory procedures that constitute the work-up for unexplained generalized pruritus.

Table 41 – 3 lists the systemic disorders asso-

**Table 41-3.** SYSTEMIC DISORDERS SOMETIMES ASSOCIATED WITH PRURITUS IN THE ELDERLY*

| | |
|---|---|
| Renal | Chronic renal failure |
| Hepatic | Extrahepatic biliary obstruction<br>Hepatitis<br>Drug ingestion |
| Hematopoietic | Polycythemia vera<br>Hodgkin's disease<br>Other lymphomas and leukemias<br>Multiple myeloma<br>Iron deficiency anemia |
| Endocrine | Hyperthyroidism<br>Diabetes mellitus |
| Miscellaneous | Visceral malignancies<br>Opiate ingestion<br>Drug ingestion<br>Psychosis |

* Adapted from Gilchrest BA: Pruritus: Pathogenesis, therapy and significance in systemic disease states. Arch Intern Med 142:101, 1982.

ciated with generalized pruritus. Among all patients seeking medical attention for pruritus, the prevalence of underlying systemic disease has been reported as 10 per cent to 50 per cent,[16,17] the percentage depending on patient selection, diagnostic evaluation, and period of follow-up.

Numerically, perhaps the most important known cause of persistent generalized pruritus is chronic renal failure. However, the degree of renal failure necessary to cause pruritus is unknown, complicating interpretation of this symptom in the elderly patient with mild to moderate renal insufficiency. From a practical viewpoint, it is probably unwise to attribute pruritus to otherwise asymptomatic renal failure, or equivalently, to renal insufficiency not requiring specific therapy for any metabolic imbalance.

Pruritus is probably the most distressing and consistent symptom of chronic cholestasis, which underlies all the hepatic disorders listed in Table 41-3. Overall, pruritus occurs in approximately 20 to 25 per cent of jaundiced patients, but it is rare in those lacking cholestasis. Drugs that can cause pruritus by inducing cholestasis include phenothiazines, tolbutamide, erythromycin estolate, anabolic hormones, estrogens, and progestins.[18]

Approximately 30 to 50 per cent of patients with polycythemia vera[19,20] and up to 20 per cent of patients with Hodgkin's disease[21,22] experience pruritus. The incidence and significance of pruritus in other lymphomas and leukemias are unknown, but the occasional association cannot be disputed.[21] Generalized pruritus has been reported as an initial symptom in patients with multiple myeloma, Waldenström's macroglobulinemia, and benign gammopathies.[23,24] Iron deficiency anemia has been reported as the cause of generalized pruritus in more than 50 patients,[25,26] including six with polycythemia,[27] although this phenomenon is apparently rare.

Pruritus attributable to endocrine or specific "miscellaneous" causes is rare,[15] and many elderly people experience generalized pruritus for which there is no apparent explanation. Hence, one must either accept a higher incidence of idiopathic pruritus with advancing age or infer the existence of "senile pruritus," the result perhaps of age-associated degenerative changes in peripheral nerve endings.

The appropriate laboratory evaluation for the patient with unexplained generalized pruritus remains a matter of opinion because cost/benefit ratios for individual procedures have not been determined. Measurement of serum creatinine, blood urea nitrogen, bilirubin, and hepatic enzymes and a complete blood count seem to constitute a reasonable survey; a chest x-ray may also be justified as a screening for malignancy.

The pathophysiology of pruritus associated with these systemic diseases is incompletely understood, and the optimal therapy is that for the underlying disease, whenever possible. Specific approaches to the treatment of the pruritus itself are available in a few instances,[15] but for most patients, nonspecific therapies must be employed.

Often it is worthwhile to prescribe an emollient even in the absence of clinical xerosis because minimal or intermittent "dryness," present in virtually all elderly individuals, may notably exacerbate pruritus of another cause. Patients should specifically be cautioned against topical application of alcohol or hot water (both of which may temporarily relieve but ultimately exacerbate pruritus) or excessive washing, especially with soap. Topical application of menthol, 0.25 to 0.5 per cent, or the anesthetic phenol, 0.5 to 1.0 per cent, in an appropriate vehicle may provide considerable temporary relief; other topical anesthetics can be used only at the risk of allergic sensitization.[28] Oral antihistamines are widely prescribed for pruritus of all causes, although their efficacy is slight in most instances,[28] even when combinations of $H_1$ and $H_2$ blockers are used. Use of antihistamines by the elderly may result in the additional problems of paradoxical restlessness or significantly impaired psychomotor function.[29]

## *Xerosis*

Xerosis is the term used to describe the "dry" or rough quality of skin that is almost universal among the elderly. The condition may be generalized but is especially prominent on the lower legs and is exacerbated by low humidity environments classically found in overheated rooms during cold weather. "Xerosis" is a misnomer; the initial assumption that the disorder resulted from a lack of water in the skin has been disproved.[30] The occasional classification of xerosis as a disorder of sebaceous (oil) glands is similarly without experimental basis.[2] Xerosis probably reflects minor abnormalities in the epidermal maturation process that in turn result in an irregular surface for the stratum corneum (SC); to date it has not been investigated experimentally.

Whatever its cause, xerotic skin in the elderly is often pruritic and may show evidence of inflammation, probably due to defects in the SC, with secondary entry of irritating substances into the dermis. The resulting condition, called erythema craquélé or winter eczema, responds promptly to topical corticosteroid ointment and/or emollients, although these preparations do not correct the xerosis itself.

"Dry skin" is best treated prophylactically by avoidance of sun exposure and other cumulative injuries ultimately reflected in abnormal epidermal maturation. Once xerosis is present, frequent regular use of a topical emollient makes the skin more attractive and more comfortable and prevents the complications discussed previously.

The mechanism of action of emollients is so poorly understood by most physicians and virtually all patients and so misrepresented by current advertisements that some discussion is warranted. Figure 41–3 schematically represents normal, "dry," and treated "dry" skin. In normal skin, there is an orderly progression of keratinocytes from the viable epidermis to the overlying SC. The morphologic transition occurs abruptly, although the process of terminal differentiation is gradual. The keratinocytes or corneocytes in the SC are flattened discs composed of keratin proteins, enclosed by permeable cross-linked protein envelopes. The water content is quite low, dropping abruptly from approximately 70 per cent in the viable epidermis, in equilibrium with the rest of the internal milieu, to near zero at the skin surface. The number of cell layers in the SC is similar to that in the epidermis, approximately 7 to 10 in most sites under normal conditions, and the corneocytes are arranged in an orderly fashion parallel to the skin surface. The result is skin that looks and feels smooth. In "dry skin" the situation differs in that the corneocyte arrangement is less orderly, with many cells disposed at an angle to the surface; the water content of the viable epidermis and the water gradient within the SC are normal. The rather rigid disc-like corneocytes projecting from the skin surface refract incident light unevenly, causing a scaly or dull appearance and feel rough to touch. Immersing the skin in water rapidly hydrates the SC and causes individual corneocytes to swell. Corneocyte edges are thus rounded, and the skin surface is smoother. However, in a low humidity environment, the SC quickly loses this water by evaporation, restoring the original morphology. Repeated cycles of hydration and dehydration further disrupt the cutaneous barrier and induce "chapping." Water loss from the SC can be slowed markedly by application of a greasy (hydrophobic) substance to the surface. This is the function of an emollient. From the preceding considerations, it is clear that emollients are most effective when applied to already moistened skin, e.g., immediately after the bath or shower. Emollients applied to nonhydrated skin act by trapping within the SC the water constantly entering it from below. However, transepidermal water loss is a slow process, and emollients have frequently worn off the skin surface before hydration is complete. "Heavy," frankly greasy emollients have the additional property of perceptibly coating the skin, producing a smooth surface film, and are usually better barriers against evaporation than are more cosmetically elegant preparations.

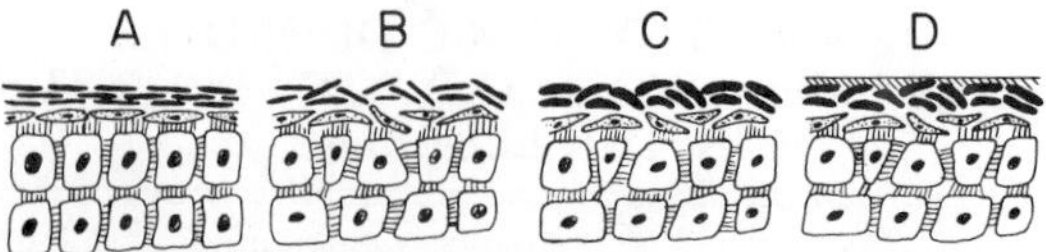


**Figure 41–3.** Schematic representation of normal, "dry," and treated "dry" skin. *A*, Normal skin. Note disc-like corneocytes in parallel array at the skin surface above the granular and malpighian layers. *B*, "Dry" skin. Corneocytes are irregularly aligned, with many cells projecting above the skin surface. *C*, "Dry" skin after immersion in water. Corneocytes are swollen, lacking sharp projections. There is virtually no change in the viable epidermis. *D*, "Dry" skin after immersion in water and topical application of an emollient. A hydrophobic film overlies the swollen corneocytes, slowing water loss and further smoothing the surface.

Finally, it should be noted that emollients applied to the skin immediately after bathing retain water more effectively than gels or oils added to the bath water and that such additives may coat the bathtub as well as the skin, producing a dangerously slippery and difficult-to-clean surface.

## *Malignancy*

Malignant neoplasms are strongly age-associated in most organ systems, as discussed in Chapter 42. This section briefly reviews the clinical features of the most common cutaneous malignancies: basal cell carcinoma, squamous cell carcinoma, and malignant melanoma. The *annual* incidence of these potentially life-threatening cutaneous disorders increases from 3.2 per 100,000 population at age 35 to 40 years to 36.4 per 100,000 population at age 65 to 74 years,[2] with a much higher regional incidence in the South and Southwest.

Skin cancer is common, and unlike most malignancies, virtually all lesions can be recognized early in their course, at a time when cure is easily and reliably effected.[31] The great majority of skin cancers are basal cell epitheliomas. Early lesions are asymptomatic, firm, opalescent or "pearly" papules with fine telangiectases on the surface (Fig. 41-4). More than 90 per cent occur on the habitually sun-exposed areas of the face and neck, usually in fair-skinned individuals with extensive sun damage.[32] Basal cell epitheliomas enlarge very slowly, and patients frequently insist that 4-mm lesions have been present for years. The classic neglected "rodent ulcer" is much less common today but can still be identified by its firm, opalescent telangiectatic rolled border. Differential diagnosis of basal cell epithelioma includes dermal nevi, which are flesh-colored but not as firm, and sebaceous hyperplasia, which is also less firm and is characterized by a slightly yellow color and a central punctum, the sebaceous orifice.

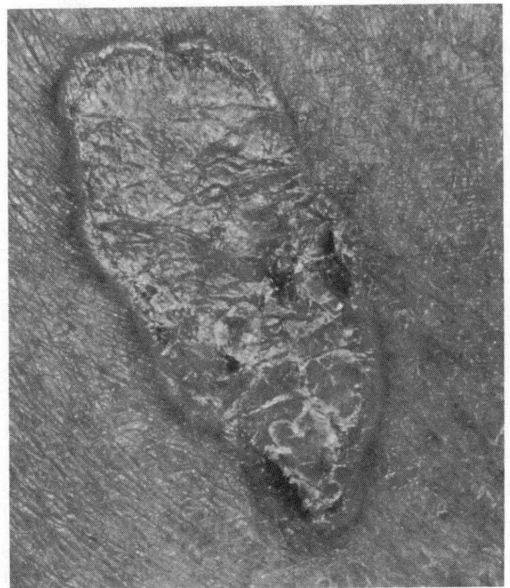

**Figure 41-4.** Basal cell carcinoma (epithelioma) on the midback of an elderly woman. The center is flat and scaly, but the firm, rolled telangiectatic border is diagnostic.

Squamous cell carcinomas occur in the same fair-skinned patient population as basal cell epitheliomas, primarily in habitually sun-exposed areas, but occasionally in sites of chronic ulceration or other skin damage. Early lesions are asymptomatic firm red papules or plaques, usually with scale; more advanced lesions are often ulcerated (Fig. 41-5). Differential diagnosis usually involves various premalignancies, which require similar treatment in any case; verrucous lesions occasionally resemble viral warts, rare among older adults. Biopsy of suspect lesions is always warranted.

Malignant melanoma is rare in comparison with nonmelanoma skin cancer but is now more common than Hodgkin's disease or thyroid carcinoma[33] and is increasing in incidence at an alarming 6 per cent annually, approximately sixfold over the past four decades.[34] Depending on the subtype, peak incidences occur in the fifth to eighth decade of life.[35] Unlike the situation with other cutaneous malignancies, successful treatment depends on early recognition. Clinical criteria for the diagnosis of melanoma have been extensively reviewed[35,37] and include diameter greater than 7 mm, variation in color (red, white, and blue areas within a brown-black lesion), irregular border, and irregular surface topography. The extremely common seborrheic or senile keratoses can usually be easily differentiated by their "stuck on" quality, even brown pigmentation, and "regularly irregular" surface.

Treatment of any cancer must be directed primarily at *cure*. However, because recurrence rates even for neglected nonmelanoma skin cancers rarely exceed 5 per cent in large patient series regardless of therapeutic approach,[31] the physician can consider other factors such as cosmetic result, cost, and patient comfort and convenience. Excision, liquid nitrogen cryotherapy, electrodessication and curettage, Mohs' chemosurgery, and x-irradiation provide a wide range of effective therapies to consider for individual patients with basal cell or squamous cell carcinoma.[31] Prompt surgical excision remains the only acceptable therapy for malignant melanoma, although controversy persists concerning

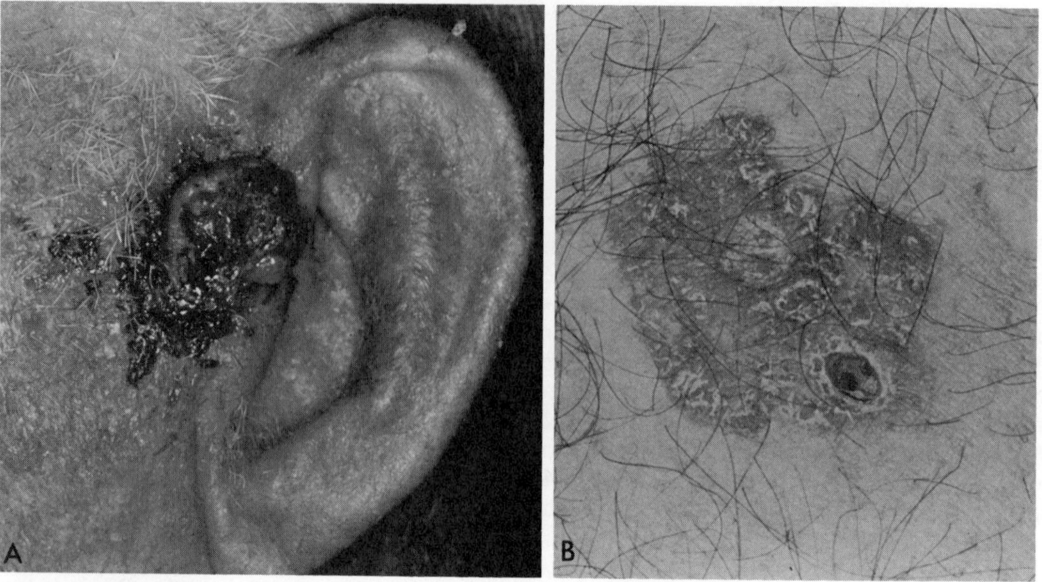


**Figure 41–5.** *A*, Squamous cell carcinoma of the preauricular area. There is central ulceration and hemorrhage. *B*, Squamous cell carcinoma in situ (Bowen's disease). The lesion is a sharply demarcated scaly plaque; circular crusted area at the lower pole is a biopsy site. (Courtesy of M. Pugliese, M.D.)

the exact procedure.[36] All skin cancer patients require frequent follow-up examinations to permit early detection of subsequent or recurrent lesions.

## *Bullous Pemphigoid*

For nondermatologists, blistering disorders of the skin frequently evoke confused and confusing differential diagnoses of entities that they have rarely seen and possibly never managed. However, of these disorders, only bullous pemphigoid (BP) is strikingly more common in the elderly than in middle-aged adults. This seems at first anomalous, since, like young children, the elderly appear to have a lower threshold for experimental blister formation than young and middle-aged adults in response to standardized stimuli,[38] and young children frequently develop blisters in the course of certain infections and inflammatory disorders of the skin that do not cause blisters in adults. Perhaps the increased propensity for dermal-epidermal separation in the elderly is counterbalanced by reduction of the cutaneous inflammatory response or by failure of those patients at high risk for blister formation due to underlying systemic disease to survive into old age.

Bullous pemphigoid is an idiopathic, immunoglobulin-mediated disease, first differentiated clinically and histologically from the much less common pemphigus vulgaris approximately 20 years ago. Although its pathogenesis has since been extensively studied,[40] many questions remain. The elderly are affected most commonly,[41] and conversely, BP is almost certainly the most common blistering disease affecting older patients. Untreated, this disease varies in severity from mild to disabling, and the prolonged loss of an effective cutaneous barrier may be fatal. The disease is self-limited, lasting months to years,[42] with recurrences following disease-free periods in a substantial minority of patients.[43]

Bullous pemphigoid is characterized clinically by large, tense bullae arising on either erythematous or normal-appearing skin (Fig. 41–6); preceding or accompanying pruritus is common and may be intense. Crusted erosions and urticarial wheals may coexist with intact bullae; hemorrhagic bullae are not unusual. Lesions occur most often on the trunk and proximal extremities; approximately one third of patients have oral blisters,[39,42] although unlike pemphigus vulgaris, the mouth is rarely the initial site of involvement. In some patients, bullae remain localized to one area for several months, and in a few, the lesions never become widespread.

The diagnosis is confirmed by skin biopsy of an early lesion.[41] In most cases, routine sections stained with hematoxylin and eosin allow definitive diagnosis. Immunofluorescent staining of perilesional skin is virtually pathognomic, showing linear deposition along the basement

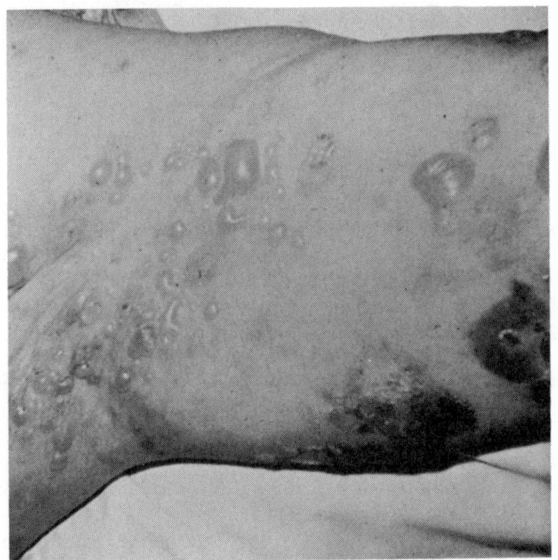

**Figure 41-6.** Bullous pemphigoid involving the axilla and medial arm. Note numerous tense bullae and scattered hemorrhagic erosions. (Courtesy of K. Arndt, M.D.)

membrane zone (BMZ) of $C_3$ (third component of complement) in all patients and of IgG in most.[44] Linear deposition of IgA or IgM in addition to $C_3$ and IgG is present in approximately 25 per cent of patients with this disorder. Indirect immunofluorescent studies utilizing patient serum and monkey esophagus or other cutaneous preparation demonstrate anti-BMZ antibodies of the IgG class in approximately two thirds of patients, and probably more often if the disease is widespread.[44] Referral to a dermatologist for the biopsy procedure is advisable because special handling of the tissue is required.

Corticosteroids are the mainstay of therapy.[41,44] In mild or localized cases, topical application of a potent steroid cream once or twice daily may control the lesions, but almost all patients require prednisone or its equivalent. Dosage and schedule of administration are determined by the extent, severity, and rate of progression of the disease as well as by patient age and the presence or absence of contraindications, such as hypertension, diabetes, and osteoporosis.

Patients with extensive or rapidly progressive, disabling BP should begin therapy with prednisone, 60 to 100 mg daily (some authors recommend 2 to 3 times this dose). They should be re-evaluated at weekly intervals, and the prednisone reduced rapidly (e.g., 10 to 20 mg per week) as new blisters cease forming and clinical remission is achieved. An immunosuppressant such as azothioprine (150 mg daily)[45] or cyclophosphamide (100 mg)[46] may be added to the regimen initially or at the time of remission in order to reduce the eventual maintenance level of prednisone; 6 to 8 weeks are required for full expression of the steroid-sparing effect. Patients with less severe BP may initiate therapy with 40 to 60 mg of prednisone on alternate days and/or daily use of an immunosuppressant. Drug dosages are decreased gradually to zero over many months, provided the disease remains in remission. Sulfapyridine or sulfones may be valuable alternative therapies for patients with major contraindications to systemic steroids.[39,47]

Most patients achieve prolonged remissions, and at least half can ultimately discontinue treatment without recurrence of lesions.[41] However, frequent exacerbation of the BP and potential complications of therapy require close monitoring of all patients throughout the course of their disease. Early reports of an association between BP and internal malignancy (beyond that expected on statistical grounds in an elderly population) have not been confirmed.[48]

## References


1. Stern RS, Johnson ML, DeLozier J: Ultilization of physician services for dermatologic complaints. Arch Dermatol 113:1062, 1977.
2. Johnson MLT, Roberts J: Prevalence of dermatological disease among persons 1-74 years of age: United States. Advance Data No. 4. USDHEW, 1977.
3. Lutsky NS: Attitudes toward old age and elderly persons. *In* Eisdorfer C (ed.): Annual Review of Gerontology and Geriatrics. New York, Springer Publishing Co, 1980.
4. Gilchrest BA: Age-associated changes in the skin. J Am Geriatr Soc 30:139, 1982.
   *Brief, referenced discussion on age-associated changes in skin, with emphasis on the clinical relevance to geriatric medicine.*
5. Oxman MN: Varicella and herpes zoster. *In* Fitzpatrick TB, Eisen AZ, Wolff K, et al (eds.): Dermatology in General Medicine, New York, McGraw-Hill, 1979, p. 1600.
   *Excellent general discussion of herpes zoster infections.*
6. de Moragas JM, Kierland RR: The outcome of patients with herpes zoster. Arch Dermatol 75:193, 1957.
7. Ragozzino MW, Melton LJ, Kurland LT, et al: Risk of cancer after herpes zoster: A population-based study. N Engl J Med 307:393, 1982.
8. Sultzberger MB, Sauter GC, Herrmann F, et al: Effects of ACTH and cortisone on certain diseases and physiological functions of the skin. I. Effects of ACTH. J Invest Dermatol 16:323, 1951.
9. Eaglstein WH, Katz R, Brown JA: The effects of corticosteroid therapy on the skin eruption and pain of herpes zoster. JAMA 211:1681, 1970.
10. Keczkes K, Basheer AM: Do corticosteroids prevent post-herpetic neuralgia? Br J Dermatol 102:551, 1980.
11. Kernbaum S, Hauchecorne J: Administration of levodopa for relief of herpes zoster pain. JAMA 246:132, 1981.
12. Peterslund NA, Ipsen J, Schonheyder H, et al: Acyclovir in herpes zoster. Lancet 2:827, 1981.

13. Farber GA, Burks JW: Chlorprothixene therapy for herpes zoster neuralgia. South Med J 67:808, 1974.
14. Taub A: Relief of postherpetic neuralgia with psychotropic drugs. J Neurosurg 39:235, 1973.
15. Gilchrest BA: Pruritus: Pathogenesis, therapy and significance in systemic disease states. Arch Intern Med 142:101, 1982.
16. Rajka G: Investigation of patients suffering from generalized pruritus with special reference to systemic disease. Acta Derm Venereol 49:190, 1966.
17. Lyell A: The itching patient: A review of the causes of pruritus. Scott Med J 17:324, 1972.
18. Thorne EG: Coping with pruritus: A common geriatric complaint. Geriatrics 33:47, 1978.
19. Easton P, Gailbraith PR: Cimetidine treatment of pruritus in polycythemia vera. N Engl J Med 229:1134, 1978.
20. Klein H: Polycythemia: Theory and Management. Springfield IL, Charles C. Thomas Publishers, 1973, p. 96.
21. Winkelmann RK: Dermatologic clinics. I. Comments on pruritus related to systemic disease. Proc Staff Meetings Mayo Clin 36:187, 1961.
22. Bluefarb SM: Cutaneous Manifestations of Malignant Lymphomas. Springfield IL, Charles C. Thomas Publishers, 1959, p. 534.
23. Erskine JG, Rowna RM, Alexander JO, et al: Pruritus as a presentation of myelomatosis. Br J Med 1:687, 1977.
24. Zelicovici A: Pruritus as a possible early sign of paraproteinemia. Isr J Med Sci 5:1079, 1969.
25. Lewiecki EM, Rahman F: Pruritus: A manifestation of iron deficiency. JAMA 236:2319, 1976.
26. Vickers CF: Iron-deficiency pruritus. JAMA 238:129, 1977.
27. Salem AH, van der Weyden MB, Young IF, Wiley JS: Pruritus and severe iron deficiency in polycythaemia vera. Br Med J 285:91, 1982.
28. Arndt KA: Manual of Dermatologic Therapeutics. 2nd ed. Boston, Little, Brown & Co., 1978, p. 263.
29. Vestal RE: Drug use in the elderly: A review of problems and special considerations. Drugs 16:358, 1978.
30. Kligman AM: Perspectives and problems in cutaneous gerontology. J Invest Dermatol 73:39, 1979.
31. Albright SD III: Treatment of skin cancer using multiple modalities. J Am Acad Dermatol 7:143, 1982.
32. Emmett EA: Ultraviolet radiation as a cause of skin tumors. CRC Crit Rev Toxicol 2:211, 1973.
33. Silverberg E: Cancer statistics 1979. Cancer 29:6, 1979.
34. Elwood JM, Lee JAH: Recent data on epidemiology of malignant melanoma. Semin Oncol 2:149, 1975.
35. Sober AJ, Mihm MC Jr, Fitzpatrick TB, et al: Malignant melanoma of the skin, and benign neoplasms and hyperplasias of melanocytes in the skin. *In* Fitzpatrick TB, Eisen AZ, Wolff Y, et al (eds.): Dermatology in General Medicine. New York, McGraw-Hill, 1979, p. 630.
36. Sober AJ, Fitzpatrick TB, Mihm MC Jr: Primary melanoma of the skin: Recognition and management. J Am Acad Dermatol 2:179, 1980.
37. Mihm MC Jr, Fitzpatrick TB, Lane-Brown MM: Early detection of primary cutaneous malignant melanoma: A color atlas. N Engl J Med 289:989, 1973.
38. Kiistala U: Dermal-epidermal separation. I. The influence of age, sex, and body region on suction blister formation in human skin. Ann Clin Res 4:10, 1972.
39. Lever WF: Pemphigus and Bullous Pemphigoid. Springfield IL, Charles C. Thomas Publishers, 1965.
40. Sams WM, Gammon WR: Mechanism of lesion production in pemphigus and pemphigoid. J Am Acad Dermatol 6:431, 1982.
41. Jordon RE: Pemphigus. *In* Fitzpatrick TB, Eisen AZ, Wolff Y, et al: (eds.): Dermatology in General Medicine. New York, McGraw-Hill, 1979.
42. Person JR, Rogers RS III: Bullous and cicatricial pemphigoid. Clinical, histopathologic, and immunopathologic correlations. Mayo Clin Proc 52:54, 1977.
43. Ahmed AR, Maize JC, Provost TT: Bullous pemphigoid. Clinical and immunologic follow-up after successful therapy. Arch Dermatol 113:1043, 1977.
44. Lever WF: Pemphigus and pemphigoid: A review of the advances made since 1964. J Am Acad Dermatol 1:2, 1979.
45. Burton JL, Greaves MW: Azathioprine for pemphigus and pemphigoid: A four-year study follow-up. Br J Dermatol 91:103, 1974.
46. Krain LS, et al: Cyclophosphamide in the treatment of pemphigus vulgaris and bullous pemphigoid. Arch Dermatol 106:657, 1972.
47. Person JR, Rogers RS III: Bullous pemphigoid responding to sulfapyridine and the sulfones. Arch Dermatol 113:610, 1977.
48. Stone SP, Schroeter AL: Bullous pemphigoid and associated malignant neoplasm. Arch Dermatol 111:991, 1975.

## *Additional Reading*

1. Gilchrest BA: Aging of the skin. *In* Baden HP, Soter NA (eds.): Pathophysiology of the Skin. New York, McGraw-Hill, 1983, p. 44.
*Completely referenced, detailed discussion of the known morphologic, physiologic, and biochemical changes associated with aging in human skin.*
2. Gilchrest BA: Skin and Aging Processes, Boca Raton, Florida, CRC Press, 1984.
*Detailed, exhaustively referenced discussion of age-associated changes in normal and diseased skin.*
3. Montagna W: Advances in the Biology of Skin. Vol. 6. Aging. Oxford Pergamon Press, 1965.
*This is a compilation of the proceedings of the 1962 Annual Symposium on the Biology of the Skin. It is an excellent survey of work in the field through the early 1960s. Primarily of historical interest, but some of the papers remain "state of the art."*
4. Montagna W, Kligman AM, Wuepper KD, Bentley JP: Special issue of aging. Proceedings of the 28th Symposium on the Biology of the Skin. J Invest Dermatol 73:1, 1979.
*The Proceedings of the 1978 Annual Symposium on the Biology of Skin were again devoted to aging after a 16-year hiatus. A broad cross-section of introductory papers by gerontologists and more focused papers of varying quality and relevance by dermatologists and others interested in cutaneous aging.*
5. Selmanowitz VJ, Rizer RL, Orentreich N: Aging of the skin and its appendages. *In* Finch CE, Hayflick L (eds.): Handbook of the Biology of Aging. New York, Van Nostrand Reinhold Co., 1977.
*First "modern" attempt to review the field, with emphasis on morphologic changes.*

Chapter 42

# Malignant Diseases

*W. Bradford Patterson*
*Rosemary Yancik*
*Paul Carbone*

Cancer is a group of diseases that attacks all organs of the body and strikes at any age. But because the risk of developing cancer increases as individuals advance in age, it is among the most serious of the chronic diseases affecting older people. As data from the Surveillance, Epidemiology, and End Results (SEER) program of the National Cancer Institute show, more than 50 per cent of all cancers are diagnosed in people 65 years and older. The SEER data set, which consists of 10 selected population-based cancer reporting areas, represents 10 per cent of our nation's population. It is interesting to note that cancer incidence is significantly greater among elderly men than among elderly women. Figure 42–1 shows the differences according to age and sex. The incidence of malignant neoplasms is slightly higher for females than males between the ages of 20 and 60 years. A change then occurs with male incidence rates accelerating more rapidly than female, culminating in a rate that is almost twice as high for males than for females in the last years of life, i.e., 3381 per 100,000 males at age 85 compared with 1795 per 100,000 females.

Mortality data from the SEER program areas disclose that 58 per cent of people dying of cancer were 65 years or older. The median age for all deaths for both sexes was 67.9. Figure 42–2 presents leading causes of cancer deaths by sex for people 65 years and older. For women, breast, colorectal, and pancreas cancer death rates are observed to increase continuously as age increases. Similarly, a ladderlike progressive pattern is observed for colorectal, prostate, pancreas, and stomach cancer death rates for males. However, cancer of the lung and bronchus is the leading cause of cancer deaths for most age groups of males, except prostate cancer in people 85 years or older.

These observations, when coupled with the demographic changes that have been discussed in earlier chapters, create some sense of the increasing medical and social impact of cancer in the elderly. What do these data mean for the primary care physician? In this chapter, an attempt is made to cover a variety of concerns that occur when problems of aging are associated with the problems of cancer.

The age of the patient does not affect the behavior of the cancer. Although data on this point are still being gathered, present information suggests that cancers in elderly patients grow at about the same rate, metastasize to similar organs, and yield to treatment in about the same ratio as cancers in adults of younger age. Yet treatment objectives for elderly patients may vary, partly in relation to the fact that the elderly may have a large burden of associated nonmalignant diseases, which hamper their defenses, as well as a limited reserve capacity of bodily function.

At the outset, it may be wise to point out that there exist some prevailing, but unproven, assertions about cancer in the elderly. For example, a belief that patients with cancer can be "too old to treat" is unsubstantiated. Also, the contention that cancers in the elderly host are slow to grow and invade is not supported by data. Moreover, so little is known about the interface between the fields of cancer and aging that both the National Cancer Institute and the National Institute on Aging of the National Institutes of Health are encouraging research initiatives in these areas.

Physicians in primary care have a key role to play in the prevention, detection, and treatment of cancer in the elderly. Through their knowledge of cancer etiology, they can steer patients and their families away from avoidable causes of cancer; by being aware of risk factors, they can detect cancer earlier through appropriate exam-

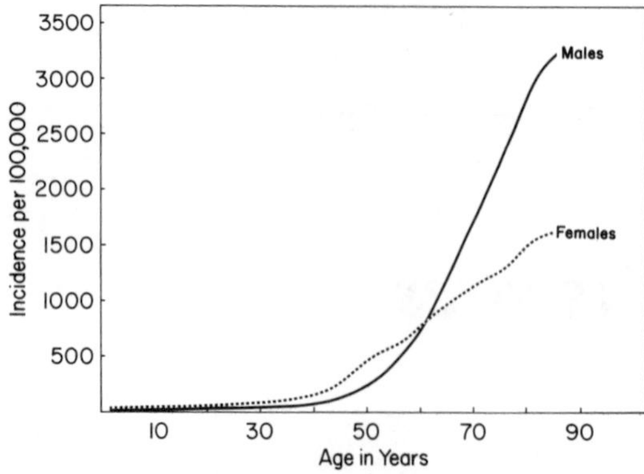


**Figure 42–1.** Cancer incidence rates per 100,000 population, by age and sex. (From SEER Incidence and Mortality Data, 1973–77. National Cancer Institute Monograph 57, NIH Publication No. 81-2330, 1981.)

inations; they can guide patients to the most appropriate oncologic specialist for treatment and can greatly assist patients in completing therapy successfully. Finally, they can carry out long-term follow-up and when prognosis is poor, they can prescribe drugs for the relief of pain and distress (in elderly patients, this can be the most significant challenge). These interventions are described in greater detail in later portions of this chapter.

When cancer is suspected, the required approach to the aged patient is usually straightforward: A good history and a directed physical examination are the tools with the greatest payoff and far outweigh complex "tests" in their diagnostic importance at the outset. It is important to identify some possible distinctions between the age groups that affect cancer management; these distinctions have been discussed and should be considered by the family physician.

## DISTINGUISHING CHARACTERISTICS OF ELDERLY CANCER PATIENTS

### *Presentation*

There is some speculation that older people may have atypical presentations of certain kinds of cancer. It has also been suggested that older people more often come to medical attention when the cancer is advanced. These assertions are still being tested, and the information that we have is conflicting. Prognosis and treatment requirements for breast cancer in younger and older women, for example, are receiving much attention. Some of the issues being studied are

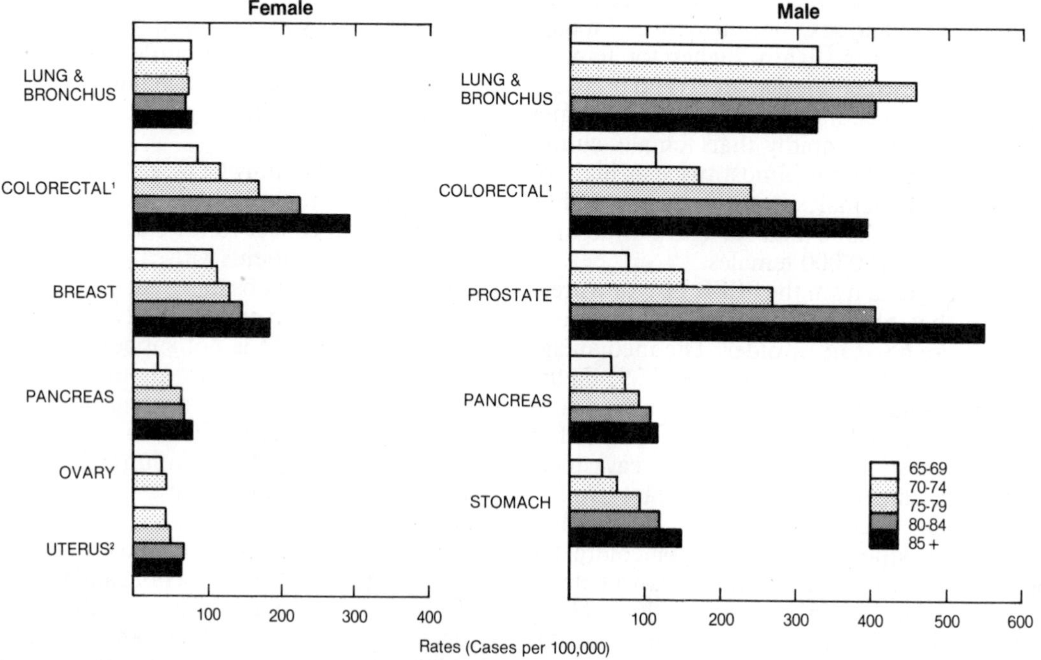


[1] Categories of Colon, Rectum, and Rectosigmoid cancers collapsed for this display.
[2] Categories of Cervis Uteri, Corpus Uteri, and Uterus (NOS) cancers collapsed for this display.

**Figure 42–2.** Leading cancer death rates by age and sex for people over 65 years of age. (From SEER Incidence and Mortality Data, 1973–77. National Cancer Institute. Monograph 57, NIH Publication No. 81-2330, 1981.)

age-related influences on treatment and stage of disease at the time of presentation,[1,2,3] whether premenopausal and postmenopausal breast cancers are the same disease,[4] and aggressiveness and indolence of cancer in younger and older patients.[5,6]

Since older people are at greater risk for developing cancer, the age/stage relationship is an important factor to consider. There are some indications that older people have more advanced local disease, higher incidences of metastatic disease at presentation, and lower survival rates.[7] These findings may reflect delayed detection of cancer in the elderly rather than biologic differences. Serpick[8] suggests that older people may not be able to "verbalize their complaints" and may accept certain symptoms as normal concomitants of old age. Thus, primary care physicians must actively seek information to find and treat cancer in the elderly. Physicians should also be conscious of the possibility that atypical presentations of cancer may arise in older people whose other handicaps such as failing vision or stiff joints prevent them from seeing or feeling a lesion.

### *Coexisting Diseases*

Geriatric patients have a higher incidence of chronic conditions such as cardiovascular disease, diabetes, and chronic obstructive pulmonary disease. This fact has major implications in cancer management, since these other diseases may confuse diagnostic studies and cause major problems during therapy.

### *Tolerance to Therapy*

Because there is a steady decline in the capacity of organ systems during aging, older patients are less able to withstand the stresses that treatment may inflict on their heart, lungs, kidneys, liver, and bone marrow. The problem of compromising therapy in order not to cause irreparable damage to normal organs is a real one.

### *Treatment Goals*

In young patients, the major goal of cancer therapy is to extend useful life by eradicating cancer or causing a remission. As patients age, the importance of extending life gradually diminishes while the importance of relieving symptoms and preserving function gradually increases. Consider the following case report:

**Case Study.** K.C., an 82-year-old woman, was found to have cancer of the rectum. Her son and daughter-in-law reported that the patient had a long history of depression, with repeated hospitalizations and electroconvulsive therapy. They doubted her ability to tolerate colostomy and supported her refusal to accept an abdominoperineal resection. Consultation at a cancer center led to development of a treatment plan using local electrocoagulation plus external beam radiotherapy. Family and physicians agreed that control of bleeding and diarrhea was more important than choosing a treatment that might offer greater prolongation of life. Two years later, the patient is fully functional, free of symptoms, and, thus far, grateful for the decision.

## GENERAL MANAGEMENT CONSIDERATIONS

Of the many critical decisions made by primary physicians for elderly cancer patients, none is more important than determining the need for haste or the wisdom of delay. Guidelines shown in Figure 42–3 for common oncologic situations may be useful.

Once there is a strong suspicion of cancer, the primary physician should make a conscientious effort to establish a tissue diagnosis. He or she can then decide whether an early referral to a specialist in oncology is indicated or whether further diagnostic tests should be done. This decision, which will be discussed in greater detail later in the chapter, depends on multiple factors, such as the size and location of the cancer, state of health of the patient, and special skills of the primary physician. In general, the rationale for referring a patient should be unaffected by the patient's age.

Decisions about referral are critical. For example, by choice of a surgeon, the primary physician may determine whether an aged patient with rectal cancer is spared a permanent colostomy. Some surgeons believe that an abdominoperineal resection should be used for all rectal cancers, whereas others use sphincter-saving procedures extensively (see later). Whether to refer the patient to a hospital within the community or to a cancer center outside the community is another decision often made by the primary physician that may be of great importance to the health or comfort of the aged patient. Some patients are better managed close to home, whereas others may profit psychologically and physically from the expertise available at a cancer center.

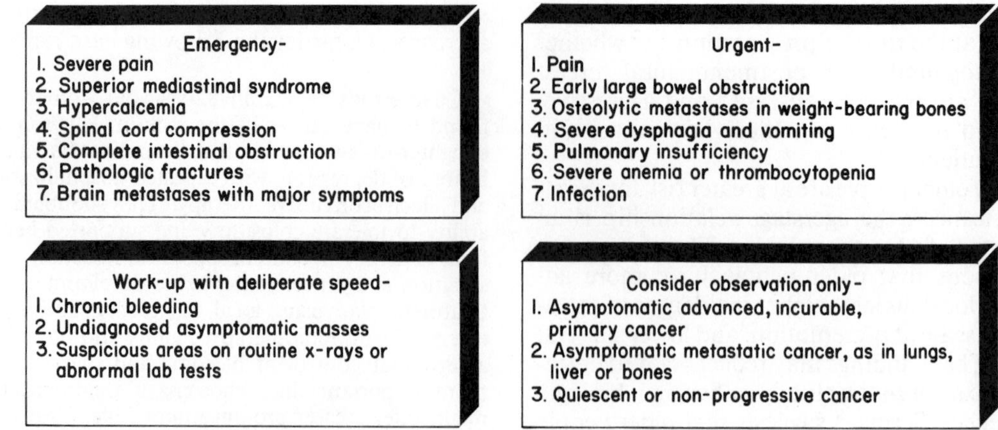

Emergency-
I. Severe pain
2. Superior mediastinal syndrome
3. Hypercalcemia
4. Spinal cord compression
5. Complete intestinal obstruction
6. Pathologic fractures
7. Brain metastases with major symptoms
Urgent-
I. Pain
2. Early large bowel obstruction
3. Osteolytic metastases in weight-bearing bones
4. Severe dysphagia and vomiting
5. Pulmonary insufficiency
6. Severe anemia or thrombocytopenia
7. Infection
Work-up with deliberate speed-
I. Chronic bleeding
2. Undiagnosed asymptomatic masses
3. Suspicious areas on routine x-rays or abnormal lab tests
Consider observation only-
I. Asymptomatic advanced, incurable, primary cancer
2. Asymptomatic metastatic cancer, as in lungs, liver or bones
3. Quiescent or non-progressive cancer


**Figure 42–3.** Examples of clinical situations requiring different response times.

We propose that referral to a cancer center should be strongly considered when

1. there is a competitive edge at the cancer center as a result of rarity of the cancer, or there is a need for particularly skilled management in a fragile patient.
2. there are special diagnostic or therapeutic resources not available at the community hospital.
3. the possibility exists for substantial benefit by aggressive treatment, whether in symptom relief or useful prolongation of life.
4. the patient and family have considered the pros and cons and desire to have a cancer center referral.

Because primary physicians have such a critical role in detecting cancer, making referrals, and initiating a treatment plan, they should also be aware of certain pitfalls. These include the following:

1. Precipitous decisions. Except in the few emergencies, examples of which are given above, thoughtful deliberation and involvement of family as well as professional consultation are greatly preferred over an immediate decision that a cancer diagnosis needs standard, urgent treatment.
2. Unreviewed pathology reports. Unless the clinician sits down and examines the slide with a pathologist, the distinction between a truly life-threatening cancer and a barely-invasive equivocal lesion may be missed, leading to more or less treatment than is appropriate, particularly in a geriatric patient.
3. Options for management not being considered. In developing the best cancer management plan, the physician considers a number of options, some aggressive, others perhaps safer, before selecting one that best balances the risks and benefits for an individual patient.
4. Excessive diagnostic staging work-up. If the patient is to be referred for treatment, most of the expensive staging procedures, such as scans, may be better left for the consultant to obtain, rather than risk that they will have to be done twice.

# THE ETIOLOGY OF CANCER

## *Relation of Cancer to Age*

Is cancer a disease of aging or a disease that is common in the aged? In a textbook written by James Ewing in 1940, an answer to this question appears that is as good today as it was then: "The most important element determining the high incidence of cancer in old age is the lapse of time. The disease must always be regarded as pathological and not as a natural termination of the life history of tissues."[9] The relationship between cancer and age has been explained by several interrelated hypotheses:

1. Cancers arise from a series of chance mutations. Most mutations are not viable. As people age, the rather rare chance that the necessary number of viable mutations will develop into a clinical cancer gradually increases.[10]
2. Environmental causes. Since most cancers are due to environmental causes (diet, cigarettes, external carcinogens), the chance of developing cancer increases steadily with years of exposure.
3. Immune surveillance. Burnet[11] has advanced the hypothesis that natural immunity to cancer wears out and the ability to fight off cancer diminishes with age. Data indicate that

immune competence decreases with age, but whether this relates to the frequency of cancer incidence in the aged is not known.

There are no satisfactory explanations for the cancers that do not show an increased incidence with aging. Those cancers common to children are the best known examples, and most of these, such as Wilms' tumor and neuroblastoma, are rarely seen in adults. Another group of cancers, including those of the testes and Hodgkin's disease, has a peak incidence in the third and fourth decades of life. Finally, the incidence of some cancers, such as soft tissue sarcoma, does not appear to vary with age.

### *Causes of Cancer*

"Life-style" encompasses habits, tastes, and activities. We will describe the separate components of life-style that are considered to be cancer-related.

#### Tobacco

Tobacco use is the most common cause of cancer in the elderly. There is strong epidemiologic evidence that cancer of the oral cavity, larynx, lung, esophagus, pancreas, kidney, and bladder is increased in cigarette smokers.[12] All these cancers are age-related. When smokers of any age stop smoking, their risk of cancer falls, and although it may never be as low as that of a nonsmoker, it becomes appreciably lower than in continuing smokers.[13] Smoking is also a factor in the carcinogenic effect of asbestos. Workers exposed to asbestos are at increased risk of lung cancer and mesothelioma, even if they are nonsmokers, but the risk escalates dramatically with increased use of tobacco.[14]

#### Alcohol

Although it is difficult to separate the effects of tobacco from those of alcohol, since excessive drinkers are so often smokers, many epidemiologic studies implicate alcohol as a causative agent in cancer of the oral cavity, esophagus,[15] and liver.[16]

#### Obesity or High-Fat Diets

It has been known for many years that overweight rats are prone to cancer, but only recently has it become evident that a diet high in saturated fat, usually linked to overweight, is associated with a higher incidence of certain human cancers. These include cancer of the breast,[17,18] endometrium,[19] and colorectum.[20]

#### External Environment

Sunlight or actinic exposure is the primary risk factor for the common skin cancers, i.e., basal cell carcinoma and squamous carcinoma. Whether it is also a factor in melanoma is disputed. People who have worked outdoors, such as farmers and fishermen, show an increased incidence of basal cell carcinoma and squamous carcinoma. These cancers appear on parts of the body most directly exposed to the sun, such as the forehead, nose, and dorsum of the hands. Fortunately, such cancers are highly curable with conventional techniques.

Although industrial wastes, toxic fumes, and other forms of pollution contain carcinogens, studies indicate that they contribute less to the cancer risk than popular belief suggests. Most of the excess cancer reported from highly industrialized areas can be attributed to an older-than-average population with high smoking rates.

#### Occupation

On the other hand, occupation may lead to significant cancer risk due to specific exposures. Well-established relationships between cancers and specific agents or industrial processes are described in Table 42–1.

#### Family History

This item is intentionally placed last on the list because we are discussing cancer in geriatric patients. Those cancers that are hereditary characteristically occur at earlier ages, with a median age as young as 45 years, and are thus not important causes of cancer in the aged patient.

## PREVENTION OF CANCER

Cancers are generally slow to develop, whatever the cause. Latent periods for carcinogenesis have a median of about 20 years. Although a 65-year-old patient is reaching the age when cancers due to chronic exposures may appear, he or she has an opportunity to prevent later cancers by voluntary changes in life-style. Table 42–2 lists important cancers for which there is some evidence that voluntary preventive measures may be useful. Although some of the evidence is still controversial, we believe that scientific fact will eventually support the prudent course that is also dictated by common sense.

**Table 42–1.** CANCER SITES FOR WHICH RELATIONSHIPS WITH OCCUPATIONAL EXPOSURES ARE WELL-ESTABLISHED IN HUMAN STUDIES*

| Site | Agent or Industrial Process |
|---|---|
| Bladder | Benzidine, β-naphthylamine, 4-Aminobiphenyl (xenylamine) |
| | Manufacture of certain dyes (e.g., auramine and magenta) |
| Blood (leukemia) | Gas retorts |
| | Rubber and cable making industries |
| | Benzene |
| | X-radiation |
| Bone | Radium, Mesothorium |
| Larynx | Ethanol (ethyl alcohol) manufactured by strong acid process (diethyl sulfate?) |
| | Isopropyl alcohol manufacture by strong acid process (diisopropyl sulfate?) |
| | Mustard gas |
| Liver (angiosarcoma) | Arsenic (inorganic compounds) |
| | Vinyl chloride |
| Lung, Bronchus | Arsenic (inorganic compounds) |
| | Asbestos |
| | Bis(chloromethyl) ether |
| | Chromium compounds |
| | Coal carbonization processes (coke ovens, gas retorts, producer gas manufacture) |
| | Coal tar pitch volatiles (roofing materials, aluminum reduction plants) |
| | Iron ore (hematite) mining |
| | Mustard gas |
| | Nickel refining |
| | Radiation (radioactive ores) |
| Nasal Cavity, Sinuses | Isopropanol (isopropyl alcohol) manufacture by strong acid process (diisopropyl sulfate?) |
| | Mustard gas |
| | Nickel refining |
| | Radium, Mesothorium |
| | Shoe manufacturing (leather dust?) |
| | Woodworking (wood dust?) |
| Peritoneum (mesothelioma) | Asbestos |
| Pharnyx | Mustard gas |
| Pleura (mesothelioma) | Asbestos |
| Skin (including scrotum) (Epitheliomas) | Arsenic (inorganic compounds) |
| | Coal tar products (mainly coal tar, creosote, pitch, soot) |
| | Coal hydrogenation |
| | Mineral oils (from coal, petroleum, shale) |
| | X-radiation |

* Adapted from Decouflé P: Occupation. *In* Schottenfeld D, Fraumeni J (eds.): Cancer Epidemiology and Prevention. Philadelphia, W.B. Saunders Co., 1982, pp. 321–322.

**Table 42–2.** PREVENTABLE CANCERS

| Causative Factor | Cancer Site | Preventive Measures |
|---|---|---|
| Cigarette Smoking | Lung, oral cavity, larynx, esophagus, pancreas, kidney and bladder | Stop smoking; cancer risk diminishes |
| Alcohol | Oral cavity, esophagus, liver | Cancer danger is from excessive use, not moderate drinking |
| Diet | Colon and rectum, breast, endometrium | Reduce saturated fats (i.e., lower meat consumption); increase intake of grains and vegetables for more roughage and for vitamins A and C |
| Sunlight | Skin | Use sunscreen lotions and avoid midday exposure |

## SCREENING

The concept of screening for cancer has been attractive; theoretically, one could periodically examine and test the well population and find malignant disease before it was symptomatic, before it metastasized, and while it was curable. Sadly enough, serious obstacles have appeared in the way of each step described above, and screening is now considered to have proven efficacy only for cancers of the breast and the cervix.[21,22]

Screening a high-risk population such as the elderly will, in fact, bring to light occult cancers, and these will be found somewhat earlier than if they are left to become symptomatic. But differences in survival rate between screened and unscreened groups are small, since even early cancers will occasionally have metastasized and death will then occur on schedule. For such patients, early detection may only mean a longer period of living without a breast or with a colostomy and not more years of life. This and other negative results from screening have recently been elaborated by more careful biostatistical analysis.[23]

To be effective, a screening test should have high sensitivity and specificity, be relatively cheap and noninvasive, and find cancers for which treatment is highly effective. (Cancers of the lung and pancreas are examples of cancers that fail to meet these criteria.) For the primary physician, no screening test for cancer in the elderly patient should replace the targeted physical examination, which can be done quickly and effectively as part of the regular routine. This examination is summarized in Table 42–3. One is cautioned to maintain a high index of suspicion, remembering that with geriatric patients, the skin lesion, anemia, or weakness can be due to an occult malignancy.

A good cancer detection examination can be carried out in 15 to 20 minutes by an experienced physician. Nevertheless, it is not a routine with many primary care physicians because positive findings are uncommon and studies have discredited the cost-effectiveness of most routine examinations. With geriatric patients the payoff is higher, and regular examinations can be strongly recommended. Examples of elderly patients in whom a cancer detection examination is particularly indicated include (1) new pa-

**Table 42–3.** PHYSICAL EXAMINATION FOR CANCER DETECTION

| Site | Usual Type of Cancer Found | How to Examine |
|---|---|---|
| Skin | Basal cell, squamous, melanoma | Observe and palpate entire skin surface, including palms, soles and interdigital areas |
| Oral cavity | Squamous | Seek ulceration or mass<br>Use throat stick, light, and finger cot; remove dentures; observe and palpate |
| Thyroid | Papillary, follicular, anaplastic | Observe while patient is swallowing and palpate |
| Salivary glands (parotid and submaxillary) | Mixed tumors | Firm or hard nodules in substance of gland |
| Lymph nodes (cervical, axillary, and inguinal) | | Palpate for nodes over 1 cm in size, particularly watching for roundness, firmness, and fixation |
| Breasts (female *and* male) | Invasive intraductal carcinoma | Observation with arms up and at sides; look for dimpling or distortion; palpate for hard masses of any size |
| Muscle masses in extremities | Soft tissue sarcomas | Any mass deeper than subcutaneous tissue is suspicious |
| Liver | Metastatic carcinoma<br>Hepatoma | Look for enlargement plus hardness and irregular edge |
| Spleen | Lymphoma<br>Chronic leukemia | Bimanual exam in left upper quadrant on inspiration |
| External genitalia | Squamous (vulva, penis)<br>Germ cell tumors (testis) | Inspection and palpation |
| Internal genitalia (pelvic exam) | Squamous (vagina and cervix)<br>Adenocarcinoma (fundus of uterus)<br>Germ cell (ovary) | Bimanual pelvic exam with speculum, light (and Pap, if indicated) |
| Rectum | Squamous (anus)<br>Adenocarcinoma (rectum and prostate) | Inspection of anal area<br>Digital exam is possible to 8–10 cm; feel size and shape of prostate and surface of rectal wall. |

tients, (2) patients requesting a cancer checkup, (3) patients at high risk because of previous cancer, family history, or other factors.

Are there other tests that conscientious physicians should use in order to find cancers early in geriatric patients? Many are proposed, but very few have been demonstrated to influence patient survival in well-designed trials. The following are examples of these cancer tests:

**Chest X-Rays.** Recent trials in screening for lung cancer have shown marginal or no benefit even in patients at high risk. In several clinical trials, frequent chest x-rays, with or without sputum cytology, have not improved survival as compared with ordinary follow-up procedures.[24]

**Mammograms.** One important randomized trial has shown a clear survival benefit for asymptomatic women over age 50 who have annual mammograms, compared with those followed only by physical examination.[25] Mammograms, or xerograms, are therefore recommended at regular intervals of 1 to 3 years in women over 65, so long as the radiographic equipment used is of high quality. Physicians and patients should ask questions of the radiologist about the equipment. It is no longer necessary to expose the breast to more than 1 rad per examination, and the newest equipment requires only a 0.1 to 0.5 rad exposure. Also, the breast should be compressed during the procedure to increase clarity. It is less important whether a film mammogram or a xerogram is used.

**Pap Smears (Cervical Cytology).** This examination is of minor importance as a screening test in women over 65, except for those who have never had a Pap test or who have demonstrated dysplasia (benign but premalignant). Older women who have had normal Pap smears over the years have a very low risk of cervix cancer. Many older women have already had a total hysterectomy and have no cervix. Although endometrial cancer is more common in the older population, the Pap test cannot be recommended as a screening test for this cancer, since it is quite insensitive, i.e., there is a high percentage of false-negatives for endometrial cancer.*

**Hemoccult.** This patented test for occult blood in the stool has most of the characteristics one would want in a good cancer screening test. It is cheap, noninvasive, and possesses reasonable sensitivity and specificity. On these grounds, its use as a screening test for early colorectal cancer is very attractive. Unfortunately, no clinical trials have been completed that prove that patients who have regular Hemoccult testing have an increased chance of living longer. Nevertheless, primary physicians can hardly go wrong in using Hemoccult testing liberally in their geriatric patients who are at high risk of colorectal cancer simply because of their age. In a project designed to check the ability of older people to test their own stool for blood, we offered Hemoccult kits to 237 members of senior citizen groups, along with instructions. These were accepted by 136, and 86 of these submitted at least one correctly tested set of Hemoccult slides over the following 6 months.[26] For the early detection of colorectal cancer in geriatric patients, we agree with Winawer[27] in recommending annual testing with Hemoccult slides.

**Sigmoidoscopy.** One study, often quoted, describes a group of patients who had annual sigmoidoscopy with removal of any polyps encountered. Over many years of follow-up, this group showed a very low incidence of rectal cancer compared with the expected incidence.[28] This study seems to justify routine use of sigmoidoscopy for screening. Unfortunately, the need for highly skilled technique, expense, and poor patient acceptance weigh heavily against its widespread use as a screening test in well patients.

**Prostatic Acid Phosphatase (the "Male Pap").** Promoted commercially as useful in screening for prostate cancer in older men, this test fails because of its low sensitivity for early prostate cancer.[29]

## DIAGNOSIS AND STAGING

In a patient with signs or symptoms of cancer, the primary physician should stop and consider the following before embarking on tests or consultation.

1. Is there good palliative or curative treatment for the suspected condition? For example, an elderly patient with a history of colon cancer who develops asymptomatic jaundice and is found to have a huge hard liver is certainly in-

* Readers will note differences in these recommendations compared with those in Chapter 35 on geriatric gynecology. In their chapter, Dr. Schinfeld and Dr. Ryan recommend that physicians find cancer before symptoms bring patients in and suggest that an annual Pap smear is "mandatory." Our more conservative recommendations reflect statements found at the beginning of this section on cancer screening. A policy on screening of asymptomatic people to find early cancer must rely on hard data proving that such screening saves lives and is reasonably cost-effective.

curable and does not require palliative intervention if there are no symptoms.

2. Will the patient and family be interested in diagnosis and treatment?

3. Where will treatment be best carried out: at home, in the community, or at a regional cancer center?

The choice of consultants should then be considered. For example, a correct diagnosis of a colorectal or breast biopsy is rarely a challenge for the community hospital pathologist, but in cases of lymphoproliferative diseases, such as non-Hodgkin's lymphoma, review by experts in the field is a necessity. Even the national cooperative groups that conduct large clinical trials require a "pathologists' panel" to review these histologies. When rare malignant diseases are involved and when optimal treatment can make a difference in outcome, it is often preferable to refer the patient to a cancer center. Examples of these are cancer of the anus and a lung cancer with Pancoast's syndrome. Finally, decisions about referral may be influenced because one knows that a local medical oncologist tends to be very conservative or very aggressive, and a particular patient may be inappropriate for one philosophy or the other.

Staging a cancer has become one of the hallmarks of modern cancer management. Staging means a determination of the extent of spread. Staging may involve clinical findings (palpating enlarged nodes), laboratory tests (an elevated carcinoembryonic antigen [CEA]), surgical findings (liver metastases), or pathologic findings (lymph nodes that are microscopically positive although they were not initially thought suspicious). With careful staging, a much more accurate prognosis is possible, which may be of enormous help to the patient and family. Staging also helps to direct therapy. For example, a bone scan in an elderly woman with an operable breast cancer might reveal diffuse skeletal metastases, which might change the plan of treatment from mastectomy to biopsy plus treatment with tamoxifen.

It is becoming as important today to avoid unnecessary staging because of attendant costs, discomfort, and wasted resources as to do adequate staging. Recent studies have called attention to excessive staging procedures done in cases with an unknown primary cancer,[30] even when possible therapeutic interventions are lacking. Therefore, it is usually preferable that staging procedures be deferred until expert advice is available and until decisions are reached about what will be done and where, in the event that staging contributes new information.

## TREATMENT OF CANCER

### *General*

Although the primary physician usually does not carry out cancer therapy, he or she retains responsibility for deciding on referrals, advising on acceptance or rejection of a specialist's recommendations, supporting patient and family during therapy and convalescence, relieving symptoms, and conducting follow-up. It is now rarely indicated for the primary physician to give low-dose "safe" outpatient chemotherapy, since the evidence is convincing that full doses, with attendant risks of leukopenia and other side-effects, are necessary in chemotherapy if anything more than a placebo effect is wanted. Hormonal treatment in breast or prostatic cancer may, on the other hand, be safely carried out by primary physicians.

With many geriatric cancer patients, the objective of treatment is palliation of symptoms rather than cure, and the skills of primary care may in this instance be equal to or exceed those of the oncology specialist. Since cancer is a chronic disease, skilled palliation is often required repeatedly during the years of an elderly patient's battle with cancer.

### *Surgery*

Surgery is still the technique most frequently used to treat cancer (1) because cancer more often occurs as a solid tumor than as a systemic disease like leukemia and (2) because surgical procedures are still needed to palliate obstruction, remove bulky disease, or relieve pain. Elderly patients tolerate cancer operations well if lungs, kidneys, and blood vessels have sufficient reserves. For example, in a recent study of 142 mastectomies for breast cancer in patients over 75, no operative deaths were reported.[31] However, older patients may not easily adapt to severe functional limitations that follow operations such as amputations or total gastrectomy.

### *Radiation Therapy*

Radiation therapy, like surgery, can be used in older patients; there will be a tolerable level of complications if nutrition can be maintained and careful attention to skin dose and other factors is given.[32] The megavoltage units used in most radiotherapy units today expend their greatest energy several centimeters below the skin and thus do not produce the skin damage and radiation ulcers that used to be seen with conventional voltage. There are two general dose ranges used by radiotherapists. For curative intent, use of 5000 to 6000 rads over 5 to 6 weeks is a general standard. For relief of pain or obstruction of a hollow viscus when symptomatic relief is the goal and the outcome beyond 6 to 12 months cannot be predicted; use of 3000 to 3600 rads given in approximately 3 weeks is equally standard.

## *Chemotherapy and Hormone Therapy*

The management of systemic cancer metastases is the major obstacle to the control of cancer in most patients. Most common lethal cancers present with or develop metastatic disease during their clinical course. Over the past 3 decades, 80 different drugs have become available for the treatment of cancer. The enumeration of the exact dosages and schedules of the use of each drug in specific cancers is beyond the scope of this chapter. However, certain principles relating to the treatment of cancer in the elderly with drugs can be proposed.

The expected impact of drugs in the treatment of specific cancers is shown in Table 42–4. In general, the response to treatment in older patients is the same as in younger individuals. In patients with breast and prostate cancers, a major element of therapy involves the use of sex hormones. Elderly patients with breast cancer are more likely to be estrogen receptor (ER) and/or progesterone receptor (PR) positive and thus more likely to respond to hormonal manipulations. Patients with prostate cancer respond frequently to endocrine treatments, such as estrogens or orchiectomy.

The use of adjuvant chemotherapy or hormone therapy, i.e., combining drugs with surgical and/or radiation treatment in an attempt to destroy occult micrometastases, is still experimental in the treatment of most cancers. In breast cancer patients, the results appear encouraging with the use of tamoxifen alone or in combination with chemotherapy and can be recommended in patients who are at high risk of recurrence. In other common solid tumors the routine use of adjuvant therapy is not warranted.

The anticipated toxicity of chemotherapeutic drugs in the elderly patient occurs in the bone marrow, gastrointestinal tract, central nervous system, and lung. These side-effects have deterred the use of drugs or have caused arbitrary dosage reductions because of age. In the state of Wisconsin, where cancer is a reportable disease, patients over 70 years old with cancer are less likely to receive chemotherapy when compared to younger patients with the same disease.[33] It has also been found that older patients are less likely to be referred to oncology centers.[34] The reasons for denying therapy or access to therapy are obviously complex, but one of the major concerns of patients and physicians relates to the anticipated enhanced toxicity of drugs in the elderly patient.

**Table 42–4.** DRUG EFFECTIVENESS IN CANCER

| Degree of Effectiveness | Type of Cancer |
|---|---|
| Cure | Hodgkin's disease<br>Histiocytic lymphoma<br>Seminoma<br>Breast (?) |
| Significant palliation with drugs | Breast<br>Prostate<br>Ovary<br>Head and neck<br>Small cell carcinoma of the lung<br>Lymphocytic lymphoma |
| Some effect | Colon and rectum<br>Soft tissue sarcoma<br>Cervix<br>Thyroid<br>Stomach<br>Non-small cell carcinoma of the lung<br>Glioma |
| Little or no effect | Pancreas<br>Hepatoma<br>Gallbladder and bile ducts<br>Kidney<br>Adrenal |

In a study by Begg and Carbone[35] patients on cooperative group trials were analyzed for a variety of response, toxicity, and clinical parameters relating to age. Major toxicity did not occur more often in the patient over 70 and there was no evidence that response or survival rates were adversely affected by age. Regarding the impact of specific drugs, methotrexate and methyl CCNU were the only drugs for which reported toxicities were different in the two age-group populations. This was entirely due to more hematologic toxicity for both drugs. One might expect that methotrexate would be more toxic to the elderly kidney if adjustments for renal function were not made. Serum measurements of blood urea nitrogen (BUN) and creatinine do not predict for renal function. There is no explanation for the enhanced bone marrow toxicity of methyl CCNU.

In the elderly cancer patient other significant medical problems are more likely to be present. The Begg study did not suggest that all elderly patients should receive chemotherapy irrespective of these associated problems, but rather that excessive toxicity could be avoided by selecting patients with good performance status and physiologic function. Therefore, elderly patients should not arbitrarily be excluded from chemotherapy trials on the basis of chronologic age, but rather physiologic parameters should determine protocol treatment assignments.

## THERAPY OF SPECIFIC TUMORS*

### *Breast Cancer*

Breast cancer incidence increases with age. More than half the women affected with this disease are over age 55. The principles of management are the same in the elderly as they are in younger patients. Surgery is the primary mode of therapy in most patients; its extent does not influence patient survival. Even limited surgery, with or without postoperative radiotherapy, can sometimes be curative. Thus, most patients with localized breast cancer should be offered curative therapy, even though they may have other medical problems. Modified radical mastectomy is now the operation used in most women. This operation is more conservatively done today, and skin grafts are rarely needed. Axillary nodes now are removed primarily for staging information, rather than with the conviction that they must all be removed to increase survival. As a result, arm swelling is less frequently seen. Postoperative radiotherapy is now used infrequently, since studies have shown that it does not increase survival. At the time of primary surgical treatment, samples of tissue should be taken for ER analysis. A recent case history in which mastectomy was used in a fragile older patient may be illustrative.

**Case Study.** M.M. is a single, 68-year-old woman who lives with her two unmarried sisters. When a breast cancer was discovered by the physician who treats her long-standing asthma, she was sent to the regional cancer center to see if a conservative, nonsurgical treatment could be recommended, since her pulmonary reserve was so limited. She was seen in a breast evaluation clinic by a surgeon, a radiotherapist, and a medical oncologist. There was no clinical or radiologic evidence that the cancer had spread beyond the breast. It was concluded that a modified radical mastectomy under general anesthesia with good control of airway and ventilation would be better tolerated by M.M. than 6 weeks of x-ray therapy with the attendant necessary travel and stress. She did not object to losing her breast. There was no justification for treatment with hormones or chemotherapy. Therefore, she received 5 days of preoperative therapy with bronchodilators, positive pressure ventilation, and antibiotics. The operation, lasting 2 hours, was well tolerated, and her convalescence was uneventful. She is now feeling as well as she did prior to the surgery and continues under regular follow-up.

A recent trend is to offer breast-sparing treatment for primary breast cancer to older as well as to younger women. Since many women over 65 care greatly about losing a breast, this therapeutic option is appropriate if certain conditions are met:

1. The cancer is small in relation to the size of the breast, so that a satisfactory cosmetic result is possible.
2. The kind of special expertise in radiation therapy necessary for satisfactory treatment is available.
3. Full explanation is given to the patient of the pros and cons of this treatment compared with conventional, radical mastectomy.

In this technique, a segmental excision of the breast cancer, or lumpectomy, replaces the mastectomy. An axillary staging dissection is done, if patient and physician have agreed that adjuvant chemotherapy is appropriate in the event that lymph nodes are positive. Later, external beam radiotherapy to a total dose of approximately 5000 rads is given to the breast and the regional lymph nodes. Finally, the site of the cancer receives a boost of about 2000 rads by means of an electron beam or iridium implant.[36]

In the elderly postmastectomy patient in whom the lymph nodes are not involved, the ER is positive, and the primary lesion is small (<3.0 cm), no additional therapy is recommended. If the tumor is larger (>3.0 cm) or the estrogen receptor test is negative, then the probability of systemic relapse is approximately 25 to 40 per cent in 10 years. These patients may be candidates for adjuvant treatment with tamoxifen alone or in association with chemotherapy.

For the elderly patient with one or more lymph nodes involved by cancer, the use of adjuvant therapy may be warranted. The best

* For cancer sites not covered here, readers are referred to Chapter 35 (gynecologic), Chapter 34 (prostate), Chapter 43 (hematologic), Chapter 41 (skin).

combination or duration of therapy is not precisely known but would potentially include tamoxifen alone or in combination with cyclophosphamide, methotrexate, 5-fluorouracil, and prednisone, depending on ER status and the number of nodes involved.

Locally advanced breast cancer (primary and/or lymph nodes large and fixed) often is not treated by mastectomy first; only enough tissue is removed surgically to make a diagnosis and obtain a sample for ER determination. Attempts to remove extensive or fixed cancers of the breast have been known to be misguided since Haagensen[37] first elaborated criteria of inoperability in the 1940s. Whether to use radiotherapy, chemotherapy, mastectomy or all three in these patients is a matter for careful individualization. Radiotherapy can successfully control local ulceration and growth in a high percentage of patients, although the 5-year survival of this group is less than 50 per cent.

## *Colon and Rectum*

Large bowel cancer is a major problem in the elderly. The symptoms may masquerade as weakness, fatigue, weight loss, or change in bowel habits. Presenting symptoms and signs in geriatric patients are more likely to be acute than in younger patients. Vowles[38] reports that in patients over 65, two thirds with cancer of the right colon and over half with cancer of the left colon first presented as emergencies, usually with bleeding or obstruction. Irrespective of age, anemia may be the first presenting symptom of right colon cancer, whereas in the distal colon, passage of blood per rectum or change in bowel habits is more common. Bleeding and tenesmus are the most common complaints for cancer of the rectum.

Patients who are at particularly high risk for colorectal cancer include those with a history of a rectal or a colonic polyp. A few of these patients will belong to cancer-prone families. In cancer-prone families there is a true genetic susceptibility to colorectal, endometrial, and other cancers.[39]

The syndromes of familial polyposis will not be discussed here because the transition from polyps to cancer or total colectomy will essentially have already occurred before patients who express the genetic trait for polyposis reach 65 years of age. Ulcerative colitis, chronic and long continued, also places patients at high risk for colorectal cancer, but this sequence also usually runs its course before old age.

With few exceptions, colorectal cancers both in young and old are adenocarcinomas arising from colonic mucosa. Other histologic types are most often metastatic and cause symptoms because of bleeding or obstruction.

Work-up of the geriatric patient suspected of having colorectal cancer should always start with rectal examination. Sigmoidoscopy and then barium enema should follow. If this sequence is reversed, the barium mixture used during radiologic examination may unwisely be allowed to flow past a nearly obstructing rectal lesion, creating possible danger and certain delay while it is removed. Even though a mass or other signs point to a more proximal cancer, the frequency of multiple lesions in the colorectum is sufficient to mandate checking the rectum first.

Surgical treatment of colon cancer has not changed significantly in the past several decades, except in technical details such as bowel preparation and the use of mechanical staplers. Right and left colectomy and sigmoid resections, with or without temporary colostomy, are regularly done in patients over age 65 with acceptable low mortality. With cancers of the rectum that are too low to permit a surgical anastomosis, the operative risks of surgical treatment in all patients, and particularly the elderly, are higher. Morbidity from abdominoperineal resection is substantially greater than from other colonic resections, probably because of factors such as longer operating time, interference with urinary function, and tendency to thrombosis of pelvic veins and development of pulmonary emboli. Fortunately, resection and anastomosis are now possible for about two thirds of rectal cancers. This includes cancers in the upper rectum and as low as 5 to 7 cm from the anus,[40] which can be treated using a variety of surgical techniques to do a safe low anastomosis. Small rectal cancers, even those that are very close to the anus, can sometimes be managed by conservative procedures including electrocoagulation[41] or endocavitary irradiation,[42] which have very little morbidity and mortality yet can achieve a respectable rate of local disease control. Efforts should be made to avoid colostomy in aged patients, but if a colostomy is necessary, the availability of improved stoma appliances and of enterostomal therapists adds greatly to quality of life.[43]

Radiation therapy has become a valuable adjunct in the management of rectal cancer. Used preoperatively and postoperatively, external irradiation has been shown to reduce the incidence of perineal recurrence, one of the more painful and disabling forms of recurrent rectal cancer. However, several large trials have failed to prove that radiation prolongs survival. For inoperable rectal cancer, radiotherapy often provides useful palliation, and the new technique of intraoperative radiotherapy may be used in the future in conjunction with resection to reduce local recurrence rates even further.[44] These techniques are equally appropriate for young and old patients.

Adjuvant chemotherapy of colorectal cancer has not been shown to be effective. In disseminated colorectal cancer, 5-fluorouracil has long been used, either by intravenous injection or via intra-arterial catheter for hepatic infusion, but its use is really confined to providing occasional symptomatic relief.

Recurrent, advanced cancer of the colon and rectum in geriatric patients occurs in at least three common patterns, each requiring different palliative strategies:

1. Hepatic metastases are common. Resection of solitary metastases in good risk patients is occasionally justifiable. Intra-arterial chemotherapy by infusion, either using a peripheral artery or the new implantable infusion pump, is an option regarded by some specialists as valuable and by others as an experimental technique of dubious benefit. There are wide differences of opinion regarding the cost-effectiveness of such complex and experimental treatment when the gain in useful life is seldom more than 6 months.

2. Intraperitoneal recurrence with intestinal obstruction occasionally responds to aggressive chemotherapy or to a single operative procedure, but more often only temporary relief is obtained. Eventually, persistent obstruction may require nasogastric suction for relief and leave no other alternative than providing high enough levels of narcotics to permit pain relief during the final days or weeks of life.

The primary physician can sometimes manage incomplete large bowel obstruction conservatively. The best regimen here requires a very low residue diet coupled with a laxative such as magnesium citrate, which assures a semiliquid stool, and a nonabsorbable sulfa drug to eliminate that part of the bulky residue in the stool that is made of bacteria. With this regimen, a nearly obstructed patient may have only an occasional small stool and be nursed along through a terminal period without needing a colostomy.

3. Perineal metastasis refers to recurrent rectal cancer in the presacral and perineal area. This syndrome is well known to oncologists because of the frequency with which it produces severe pain and discomfort. Occasionally surgical resection of large, slowly growing, and symptomatic lesions in this area is justifiable, sometimes including the lower half of the sacrum.[45] More often, resection is not possible and radiotherapy becomes the treatment of choice.

Follow-up for colorectal cancer patients requires not only abdominal and rectal examinations but also a routine of Hemoccult testing and interval sigmoidoscopy for the remainder of the patient's life. These patients are at increased risk for both cancer recurrence at suture lines and elsewhere and for additional cancers in other parts of the large bowel. Many reports of three or more cancers spread over a long follow-up period can be found in the literature. The use of periodic CEA determinations in follow-up is more controversial. If the CEA is normal after a colorectal cancer is first resected and rises to abnormal levels during the next year or so, recurrent cancer is a strong possibility. Twenty per cent of patients with this finding who have no metastases found outside the abdomen will potentially be helped by a second look procedure.[46] Most of those who undergo re-exploration will not have resectable cancer and, in the absence of other curative treatment, cannot be said to have profited from this operation.

## *Lung Cancer*

It is ironic that the cancer that is increasing most rapidly in frequency and that is almost solely responsible for the public concern about an epidemic of cancer is one of the few for which the cause is largely known and avoidable. The increase of cigarette smoking in men after World War I and in women after World War II has been linked not only to heart disease but also to cancers of the lung and other tissues, as described earlier. Both the total number of lung cancers seen and the incidence rate will inevitably continue to increase for the next few years, although there is some reason to hope that a peak in incidence rates may be near.[47] Whether low-tar cigarettes and filters will lessen the carcinogenic effects so that the rate will fall is uncertain. Cancer of the lung is important in the geriatric patient because it is strongly age-related, with a peak incidence past 80 years. Although previously uncommon in women, it is now increasing so rapidly that it is expected to pass breast cancer as the most common lethal cancer in women during this decade. Both squamous carcinomas and adenocarcinomas are common histologic types, whereas small cell lung cancer (previously called oat cell), once relatively rare, now makes up 20 per cent or more of the total.

Older people may neglect to seek medical help for early symptoms of lung cancer. A cigarette cough is often part of their everyday experience. Hemoptysis, shortness of breath, and chest pain can also be brushed off as inconsequential. In many instances, only the signs of advanced disease, such as hoarseness due to recurrent nerve paralysis or pneumonia following obstruction of a major bronchus, force these patients to seek help. Paraneoplastic syndromes such as clubbing of the fingers or Cushing's syndrome may occur. A most tragic first sign of advanced lung cancer is the abrupt onset of headache, convulsions, or coma, which signals a cerebral metastasis from an unsuspected bronchogenic primary tumor.

The diagnosis of cancer of the lung is often almost pathognomonic on a chest x-ray. A mass, either in the peripheral or central area, in an otherwise normal patient who gives a 20+ pack per year history of cigarette smoking is lung cancer until proved otherwise. Tissue diagnosis is needed early on. For central lesions, bronchoscopy, which can be done safely in most geriatric patients under local or light general anesthesia, provides tissue for the pathologist and permits the assessment of surgical resectability. Shadows in the more peripheral lung field used to require exploratory thoracotomy to establish the diagnosis, but with the advent of new techniques, including bronchial brushing* and transthoracic needle aspiration under fluoroscopic control, this is rarely necessary.

Although the overall survival statistics for cancer of the lung at any age are dismal, the physician in primary care need not adopt a nihilistic attitude toward all older patients with this disease. Rather, there should be a careful exercise of judgment to find those patients who have a chance for cure or disease remission. Examples include the following:

1. Adenocarcinoma primary in the periphery of the lung, with the mediastinum normal by x-ray and CT scan. Pulmonary function and not age is the determinant that will dictate whether lobectomy is possible. In Stage I lung cancer (limited to small cancers with or without hilar node involvement), 40 to 50 per cent of patients may survive for 5 years.[48]

2. Small cell lung cancer response rates to chemotherapy are now regularly seen in the 60 to 80 per cent range. Radiotherapy to the brain, to prevent metastases, is usually given also. For patients with symptomatic disease, this may result in significant relief of symptoms and knowledge that some regression has occurred. Remissions lasting from 3 months to 2 years are possible. Although the median duration of remission is not over 12 months,[49] even this length of improvement will be chosen by many patients.

3. Palliation of the pain and other symptoms that occur with lung cancer is a challenge both for the primary physician and oncologic specialist. Invasion of the mediastinal structures, chest wall, and spine are often best treated by radiotherapy. Thoracic surgeons have long argued that if resection of a primary cancer can be done, better palliation results even though survival may not be improved. Patients with disseminated lung cancer have a high probability of adrenal metastases with overt or subtle symptoms of hypoadrenalism. Treatment of this complication is relatively simple and may lead to great symptomatic improvement.

## CONTROL OF PAIN

Of all the unwanted symptoms that occur in cancer patients, pain is the most common and troublesome. Some pain occurs in about 50 per cent of cancer patients, but there is no systematic data that quantifies the frequency or severity of pain in geriatric patients who are under the care of their primary physicians. Even in patients at a cancer center, not more than 10 per cent have severe pain requiring a specific pain consultation.[50] There is also no evidence that cancer pain is age-related. However, chronic pain of cancer is a different problem from acute pain. As pointed out by Beecher[51] years ago, the ominous meaning of pain from a disease such as cancer adds greatly to its symptomatology, and he emphasizes that psychic suffering must be regarded as an important pain component.

The cause of pain in a cancer patient may be either benign or malignant and may result either from growing cancer or from cancer treatment. Foley found that in 397 cancer patients, 79 per cent had pain "caused by tumor invasion or compression of pain-sensitive structures (bone, nerve, and hollow viscus), 19 per cent had pain caused by or associated with cancer therapy."[50] Practitioners should first seek simple, treatable reasons for pain. An example might be the elderly patient already on codeine therapy who begins to complain of a dull, diffuse abdominal discomfort. This is often due to severe constipation and will respond much better to disimpac-

* Bronchoscopes are now flexible, and tissue samples sufficient for histologic diagnosis can often be obtained even from the small segmental bronchi by the use of a fine brush inserted through the scope.

tion, laxatives, and enemas than to a stronger narcotic. Another benign cause can be arthritis, which is made worse by inactivity and loss of muscle tone in depleted cancer patients. Common causes of treatment pain include post-thoracotomy syndromes, peripheral neuropathy related to vincristine and other drugs, and radiation fibrosis in the brachial or lumbar plexus.[52]

In making a differential diagnosis of cancer pain, nothing can be substituted for a careful history and physical examination. For example, sensing the importance of anxiety in a particular patient may lead to a supportive discussion instead of medication. On the other hand, cancer regrowth may be diagnosed by repeated palpation in an axilla where postradiation fibrosis would otherwise be blamed for the pain. Subsequently, careful x-rays of bones, computerized tomography (CT scans), and myelograms may all be needed to document whether pain is or is not due to an occult focus of cancer. If pain is diagnosed as due to local invasion or obstruction by cancer, the most effective relief will be achieved when cancer-directed therapy is available and appropriate, as described earlier in this chapter.

Medical treatment for cancer pain in the elderly, as in younger patients, begins with mild analgesics. As pain becomes more severe, the narcotics including codeine and related compounds are first used (in combination with aspirin or its substitutes), followed by morphine and methadone. Of greatest importance in management is knowledge of the comparable analgesic potency of various narcotics and the recognition that many can be equally well given by mouth if dose is appropriately increased. Oral morphine at 20 mg is approximately equal to 10 mg intramuscularly. Houde[53] has tested and described these equianalgesic doses in great detail. The use of oral morphine administered "by the clock" to treat severe pain in patients with advanced cancer has been a major contribution of the hospice movement and needs wider adoption both in hospitals and home care situations. The principles are as follows:

1. Regular doses of narcotics given every 4 hours, as opposed to "prn" orders, help patients to achieve a pain-free state (i.e., patients no longer have to try to endure pain as long as possible).

2. Oral, self-administered medication is less costly, reduces nursing time, and is safe. Hospice experience has shown that medication abuse does not occur and that side-effects such as excessive drowsiness can be easily controlled by careful monitoring.[54]

3. Dose should be escalated if needed to relieve pain. Although a few patients will require large amounts of narcotic, most will not, and there is no evidence that addiction or mental deterioration results when the drug is given in this way for cancer pain.[55]

Some additive benefit may be achieved by the use of phenothiazines and the tricyclic antidepressants, although controlled studies have not been carried out. Chlorpromazine in doses of 100 to 500 mg per day for cancer patients with chronic pain has been recommended to avoid the necessity of increasing narcotic doses, for example. When depression and anxiety accompany cancer pain, as is often the case, drugs such as amitriptyline may be useful.

Until very recently, pain that could not be controlled with narcotics was usually considered a neurosurgical problem. Temporary nerve blocks were sometimes used for testing, but anterior rhizotomy or spinothalamic tractotomy (cordotomy) were commonly used for treatment. These procedures are less common now, as specific therapy has become more effective and as alternatives have been developed. These alternatives include transcutaneous nerve stimulation, hypnosis, biofeedback, and acupuncture. All these techniques have their proponents and are clearly useful for some patients.[56] Finally, a major advance in the neurosurgical approach to pain has been the use of percutaneous localization of appropriate nerve targets under x-ray control, which may permit nerve blocks and thermocoagulation of nerve fibers to be done without the risk of general anesthesia and long postoperative recovery periods.

## CONTINUING CARE FOR THE CANCER PATIENT

A perception that cancer is an overwhelming rapidly fatal illness affecting healthy adults is misleading. For the majority of patients, cancer is a chronic disease with an average range of survival not very different from that seen with congestive heart failure or alcoholic cirrhosis. After a hospital admission, when the diagnosis of cancer is established and primary treatment is carried out, patients require advice and instruction about their future care. Discharge planning is therefore an important part of modern cancer management. In Table 42–5, referral groups are listed. These have been drawn together by the Office of Cancer Communication of the National Cancer Institute.

Primary care physicians often need to be involved in the big decisions that have to be made

**Table 42–5.** ORGANIZATIONS AND PROGRAMS OFFERING SERVICES TO THE CANCER PATIENT AND THE FAMILY

| | General Description | Psychological and Emotional Support; Education | Medical, Physical, Logistical Support | Financial and Employment Assistance |
|---|---|---|---|---|
| National organizations and affiliates | | | | |
| American Cancer Society* 777 Third Ave New York, NY 10017 | Voluntary organization offering programs of cancer research, education, and patient service and rehabilitation | Programs to support psychological and physical rehabilitation of patients<br>Patient education and information | Equipment loans for care of homebound, blood programs, surgical dressings, medication<br>Transportation to and from treatment. e.g., volunteer drivers or taxi fare reimbursement | Financial counseling<br>Assistance with employment problems |
| CanSurmount | Composed of patient, family member, trained volunteer (also a cancer patient), health professional<br>Volunteers visit hospitals and homes | Patient and family education and information | | |
| I Can Cope | Addresses the educational and psychological needs of people with cancer | Educational program to provide information and psychological support | | |
| International Association of Laryngectomees | Voluntary umbrella organization of 225 local clubs (varying names) that promote and support total rehabilitation program<br>Volunteers visit hospitals | Support and education programs for persons who have had laryngectomees | | Program to inform employees about reemployability of laryngectomees |
| Reach to Recover (Breast cancer) | Provides rehabilitation support for women who have had mastectomies<br>Volunteers visit hospitals | Information on rehabilitative exercises<br>Psychological support | Demonstrates rehabilitative exercises<br>Provides temporary prosthesis | |
| Cancer Information Service† | Telephone information and referral service, supplemented by printed materials | Information on local and regional resources and programs | Information on local and regional resources and programs | Information on local and regional resources and programs |
| The Concern for Dying 250 W 57th St New York, NY 10019 | Nonprofit educational organization distributes the living will, a document that records patient wishes concerning treatment | Provides copies of living will and referral to local sources of same | | |

| | | | | |
|---|---|---|---|---|
| Leukemia Society of America<br>211 E 43rd St<br>New York, NY 10017 | Offers financial assistance and consultation services for referrals to other means of local support to cancer patients with leukemia and allied disorders | | | Financial assistance to outpatients for drugs, laboratory costs associated with blood transfusions, transportation, and radiation therapy |
| Make Today Count<br>PO Box 303<br>Burlington, IA 52601 | More than 200 chapters made up of patients and family members, with the general goal of living each day as fully and completely as possible | Peer emotional support | | |
| The National Hospice Organization<br>1311A Dolly Madison Blvd.<br>McLean, VA 22101 | Membership organization consisting of groups providing or preparing to provide hospice care; institutions concerned with care of the terminally ill and their families | Literature, information, and referral to local and regional resources | Literature, information, and referral to local and regional resources | |
| United Cancer Council, Inc<br>1803 N Meridian St<br>Indianapolis, IN 46202 | Federation of voluntary cancer agencies that seek the control of cancer through a three-point program of service, education, and research<br>Agencies are funded by the United Way | Health promotion and education programs and therapy groups | Screening, nursing, homemaking, medication, prostheses | |
| United Ostomy Association<br>1111 Wilshire Blvd<br>Los Angeles, CA 90017 | Nonprofit organization with more than 500 chapters in United States and Canada. General goal is to provide ostomy patients with mutual aid, moral support, and education.<br>Members visit hospitals | Publish ostomy information<br>Peer support | Encourage development of better equipment and supplies<br>Promote better management techniques | Insurance programs for members include hospital income plan and major medical plan |
| Regional organization and programs | | | | |
| Cancer Call PAC (People Against Cancer)<br>American Cancer Society<br>37 S Wabash Ave<br>Chicago, IL 60603 | Emotional support via telephone service; volunteers are recovered cancer patients and family members | Trained volunteers provide emotional support, information, and appropriate referrals | | |

*Table continued on following page*

**Table 42–5.** Continued

| | General Description | Psychological and Emotional Support; Education | Medical, Physical, Logistical Support | Financial and Employment Assistance |
|---|---|---|---|---|
| Cancer Care, Inc. of the National Cancer Foundation‡<br>One Part Ave<br>New York, NY 10016 | Voluntary social service agency providing professional counseling and planning to patients with advanced cancer and their families | Programs of professional consultation and education<br>Public education | Nursing care, homemaker, home health aids, housekeepers | Financial assistance offered |
| TOUCH, Coordinator, Cancer Control Program<br>University of Alabama in Birmingham<br>104 Old Hillman Bldg<br>Birmingham, AL 35294 | General goal is to provide assistance to cancer patients and their families in forming realistic, positive attitudes toward cancer and its treatment | Peer emotional support<br>Continuing education on treatment methods | | |
| Psychosocial Counseling Service<br>UCLA-Jonsson Comprehensive Cancer Center<br>1100 Glenson Ave<br>Suite 844<br>Los Angeles, CA 90024 | Telephone counseling service directed to psychosocial needs of patients and care givers | Trained mental health professionals directly counsel cancer patients, family members, and friends<br>Provide referrals to other sources of assistance | | |

* For information on the following programs, contact the American Cancer Society.

† See list of telephone numbers and areas served.

‡ Direct services in tristate metropolitan areas of New York, New Jersey, and Connecticut.

when cancer treatment is failing and death appears to be an assured outcome. Should aggressive treatment against the cancer be stopped and when? Who should make the decision? Where should the patient be cared for? What symptoms will occur and how can they be relieved?

One should not "stop treating" a cancer patient, but one may redirect the objectives of treatment. Early on, when the objectives are to achieve a remission or cure, patients put up with painful drug injections, uncomfortable diagnostic studies, and being awakened every 4 hours at night so that vital signs may be kept. But, if an agreement has been reached among the patient, family, and physician that cure or remission is not the objective, treatment can focus on relieving symptoms, and many of the actions that caused discomfort and pain can be omitted. The art of providing care under these circumstances has become known as hospice, which should be understood as a concept rather than a place. The concept recognizes that many patients pass through a phase when medical efforts to fight the disease are less important than efforts to keep patients comfortable, to reduce emotional strain, and to help the patient live his or her last days of life at home, if appropriate and desired. A decision to redirect patient care and to omit aggressive cancer therapy is often made by permitting the patient and family gradually to accept the inevitable. At this point, the chief players in this drama (patient, physician, family member, or other significant person) should have an open discussion during which the physician can describe what can be done to relieve symptoms, what is apt to happen, and the options for placement. It should also be explained that any decisions made at this time are not irrevocable but can be changed if the patient's condition warrants or if new therapy becomes available.

Our clinical observations suggest that elderly patients dying of cancer are generally less worried that their life is going to end than about the process of dying. They worry that they will strangle, that pain will become unbearable, and that the process is horrible. If reassured that nature usually makes dying relatively easy and that the physicians and nurses will stand by so that none of these symptoms occur, many patients are greatly relieved. Families also worry unnecessarily that a cancer patient who dies at home will present some awful responsibility for action at the last moment. They need reassurance that the time of death is usually very quiet and that when it occurs there is no need for hurried action.

## CONCLUSION

The primary care physician should not be daunted by a diagnosis of cancer in an elderly patient. Cancer is simply another chronic disease, and it is often possible with judicious treatment for the cancer patient to continue life with function unimpaired for as long as other chronic illnesses permit.

### References

1. Albert S, Belle S, Swanson GM: Recent trends in the treatment of primary breast cancer. Cancer 41:2399, 1978.
2. Donegan WL: Treatment of breast cancer in the elderly. *In* Yancik R et al (eds.): Perspective on Prevention and Treatment of Cancer in the Elderly. New York, Raven Press, 1983, p. 83.
3. Noyes RD et al: Breast cancer in women aged 30 and under. Cancer 49:1302, 1982.
4. de Waard F: Premenopausal and postmenopausal breast cancer: One disease or two? JNCI 63:549, 1979.
5. Devitt JE: The influence of age on the behavior of carcinoma of the breast. Can Med Assoc J 103:923, 1970.
6. Lubin JH et al: Risk factors for breast cancer in women in Northern Alberta, Canada, as related to age at diagnosis. JNCI 68:211, 1982.
7. Redding WH et al: Age and prognosis in breast cancer. Br Med J 1:1465, 1979.
8. Serpick AA: Cancer in the elderly. Hosp Pract 13:101, 1978.
9. Ewing J: Neoplastic Diseases. Philadelphia, W.B. Saunders Co., 1940.
10. Cairns J: Cancer: Science and Society. San Francisco, W.H. Freeman and Company, 1978.
11. Burnet FM: Immunologic Surveillance. Oxford, Pergamon Press, 1970.
12. U. S. Department of Health and Human Services: The Health Consequences of Smoking: A Report of the Surgeon General. Washington DC, US Government Printing Office, 1982.
13. Doll R, Peto R: Mortality in relation to smoking: 20 years' observations on male British doctors. Br Med J 2:1525, 1976.
14. Hammond EC et al: Asbestos exposure, cigarette smoking and death rates. Ann NY Acad Sci 330:473, 1979.
15. Wynder EL et al: A study of the etiologic factors in cancer of the mouth. Cancer 10:1300, 1957.
16. Purtilo DB, Gottlieb LS: Cirrhosis and hepatoma occurring at Boston City Hospital (1917–1968). Cancer 32:458, 1973.
17. de Waard F, Baanders-Van Halewijn EA: A prospective study in general practice of breast cancer risk in postmenopausal women. Int J Cancer 14:153, 1974.
18. Staszewski J: Breast cancer and body build. Prev Med 6:410, 1977.
19. Armstrong BK: The role of diet in human carcinogenesis with special reference to endometrial cancer. *In* Hiatt HH, Watson JD, Winsten JA (eds.): Origins of Human Cancer. New York, Cold Spring Harbor Laboratory, 1977, p. 557.
20. Wynder EL, Reddy BS: Colon cancer prevention:

Today's challenge to biomedical scientists and clinical investigators. Cancer 40:2565, 1977.
21. Love RR, Camilli AE: The value of screening. Cancer 48:489, 1981.
22. Eddy DM: Screening for Cancer. Englewood Cliffs, New Jersey, Prentice-Hall, 1980.
23. Cole P, Morrison AS: Basic issues in cancer screening. *In* Miller EB (ed.): Screening in Cancer. Geneva, International Union Against Cancer, 1978.
24. American Cancer Society: Guidelines for the cancer-related checkup: recommendations and rationale. Cancer of the lung. CA 30:199, 1980.
25. Shapiro S et al: Changes in 5-year breast cancer mortality in a breast cancer screening program. *In* Seventh National Cancer Conference Proceedings. Philadelphia, J.B. Lippincott Co., 1973, p. 63.
26. Patterson WB, Pardo JR: Self-testing for colon cancer among senior citizens using the Hemoccult slide. 1978 (unpublished).
27. Winawer SJ: Screening for colorectal cancer: An overview. Cancer 45:1093, 1980.
28. Gilbertsen VA: Proctosigmoidoscopy and polypectomy in reducing the incidence of rectal cancer. Cancer 34:936, 1974.
29. Goldenberg SL et al: A critical evaluation of a specific radioimmunoassay for prostatic acid phosphatase. Cancer 50:1847, 1982.
30. Stewart JF et al: Unknown primary adenocarcinoma: Incidence of overinvestigation and natural history. Br Med J 1:1530, 1979.
31. Cortese AF, Cornell GN: Radical mastectomy in the aged female. J Am Geriatr Soc 23:337, 1975.
32. Gunn WG: Radiation therapy for the aging patient. CA 30:337, 1980.
33. Carbone PP et al: Oncology perspective on breast cancer in the elderly. *In* Yancik R et al (eds.): Perspective on Prevention and Treatment of Cancer in the Elderly. New York, Raven Press, 1983, p. 63.
34. Begg CB et al: Cooperative groups and community hospitals: Measurement of impact in the community hospitals. Cancer 52:1760, 1983.
35. Begg CB, Carbone PP: Clinical trials and drug toxicity in the elderly: The experience of the Eastern Cooperative Oncology Group. Cancer 52:1986, 1983.
36. Harris JR et al: Primary radiation therapy without mastectomy for early carcinoma of the breast. *In* Kreger WP (ed.): Annual Review of Medicine. California, Annual Review, 1981, p. 387.
37. Haagensen CD: Diseases of the Breast. 2nd ed. Philadelphia, W.B. Saunders Co., 1971.
38. Vowles KDJ: Surgical Problems in the Aged. Bristol, John Wright and Sons, 1979.
39. Anderson DE: Familial cancer and cancer families. Semin Oncol 5:11, 1978.
40. Goligher JC: Current trends in the use of sphincter-saving excision in the treatment of carcinoma of the rectum. Cancer 50:2627, 1982.
41. Madden JL, Kandalaft S: Electrocoagulation and the treatment of cancer of the rectum: A continuing study. Ann Surg 174:530, 1971.
42. Sischy B, Remmington JH, Sobel SH: Treatment of rectum carcinomas by means of endocavitary irradiation: A progress report. Cancer 46:1957, 1980.
43. Rowbotham JL: Managing colostomies. CA 30:336, 1981.
44. Gunderson LL et al: Intraoperative irradiation: A pilot study combining external beam photons with "boost" dose intraoperative electrons. Cancer 49:2259, 1982.
45. Wanebo HJ, Marcove RC: Abdominal sacral resection of locally recurrent rectal cancer. Ann Surg 194:471, 1981.
46. Steele G Jr et al: Results of CEA-initiated second-look surgery for recurrent colorectal cancer. Am J Surg 139:544, 1980.
47. Fraumeni JF Jr, Blot WJ: Lung and pleura. *In* Schottenfeld D, Fraumeni JF (eds.): Cancer Epidemiology and Prevention. Philadelphia, W.B. Saunders Co., 1982, p. 564.
48. Beahrs OH, Myers MH (eds.): American Joint Committee on Cancer, Manual for Staging of Cancer, 2nd Edition. Philadelphia, JB Lippincott Co, 1983.
49. Bunn PA Jr, Cohen MH, Ihde CD, et al: Advances in small cell bronchogenic carcinoma. Cancer Treat Rep 61:333, 1977.
50. Foley KM: Pain syndromes in patients with cancer. *In* Bonica JJ, Ventafridda V (eds.): Advances in Pain Research and Therapy. Vol. 2. New York, Raven Press, 1979, p. 59.
51. Beecher HK: Relationship of significance of wound to pain experience. JAMA 161:1609, 1956.
52. Black P: Management of cancer pain: An overview. Neurosurgery 5:507, 1979.
53. Houde RW: Medical treatment of oncological pain. *In* Bonica JJ et al (eds.): Recent Advances on Pain: Pathology and Clinical Aspects. Springfield, Illinois, C.C. Thomas, 1974, p. 168.
54. Saunders C: Principles of symptom control in terminal care. Med Clin North Am 66:1169, 1982.
55. Walsh TD, Saunders CM: Oral morphine for relief of chronic pain from cancer (Letter to the Editor). N Engl J Med 305:1417, 1981.
56. Bonica JJ, Ventrafridda V (eds.): Advances in Pain Research and Therapy. Vol. 2. New York, Raven Press, 1979.

*Chapter 43*

# Hematologic Problems

*Harvey Jay Cohen*
*Jeffrey Crawford*

Hematologic disorders in the elderly individual often present difficult diagnostic and therapeutic dilemmas to the practitioner. One is frequently faced with laboratory abnormalities generated from screening studies or during the evaluation of other problems. The practitioner must decide whether these results represent a true disease state and how aggressively such findings should be pursued. Alternatively, many symptoms of hematologic disorders are relatively nonspecific and may be quite vague. Thus, the potential of ascribing such changes to "getting older" must be avoided lest correctable disease states be missed.

Diagnostic vigor in the elderly patient must be tempered by the functional status of the patient, the benefit/risk ratio of the diagnostic intervention, and the potential for the outcome to influence management of the patient in a meaningful way. Coexistent diseases, but not age alone, may limit the value of an aggressive diagnostic work-up. Evaluation for reversible causes of anemia may be warranted in almost all elderly patients to try to prevent the consequences of falls, confusion, or ischemic events. However, an exhaustive search for occult gastrointestinal bleeding in the bedridden, severely demented patient may be inhumane.

## CHANGES IN NORMAL HEMATOPOIESIS WITH AGE

Red blood cells, granulocytes, monocytes, platelets, lymphocytes, and plasma cells are produced in the bone marrow from a common stem cell. Estimations of the normal senescence of the bone marrow are complicated by its diversity and are at this point quite imperfect. Although bone marrow activity shows a great deal of individual variation, anatomic studies of the bone marrow suggest that overall, bone marrow cellularity decreases by approximately one-third during adult life, and bone marrow scans utilizing iron labeling of erythroid elements also indicate decline in marrow activity with advancing age.[1]

Renewal of peripheral blood cells remains normal with advancing age, except in circumstances of excess stress. In mice, there is a reduction in bone marrow stem cell reserve and proliferative capacity with age;[2] this limited murine bone marrow reserve with age may have a clinical corollary in the observation that elderly patients may not respond to infection with the same degree of leukocytosis or to bleeding with the same degree of reticulocytosis as younger patients. Whether these blunted responses in man are secondary to aging alone or to coexistent diseases has not been rigorously studied.

A number of studies have suggested that the mean hemoglobin level is 1gm/dl lower in elderly females compared with younger females and 2gm/dl lower in elderly males (with a much wider standard deviation) compared with younger males.[3–6] However, most of these studies are flawed by not clearly distinguishing healthy from unhealthy individuals. Most are cross-sectional, and longitudinal data have not been available. A number of subclinical alterations have been noted in the aged including slight increases in red cell size and membrane viscosity and a somewhat shortened red blood cell life span.[5,7] In addition, there are slight decrements in enzyme content and metabolic activity.[5,8] From a clinical standpoint, whether or not slight defects in production or destruction rates exist, if there is a significant decline in hemoglobin below the normal adult range in an elderly individual, one must assume a pathologic process is present until proven otherwise.

Decreased leukocyte counts in the peripheral blood of elderly patients have been reported in cross-sectional studies.[9] However, recent longitudinal study data suggest that no such alteration in leukocyte numbers occurs.[10,11] The leukocytes present in elderly individuals may, however, be less readily mobilized by a stressful challenge, such as bacterial pyrogen and corticosteroids.[6] This is of considerable clinical relevance, since infection in some older people may not be recognized if the physician relies on the white blood cell count. Studies of granulocyte function with age have produced somewhat conflicting results. In general, polymorphonuclear leukocytes and monocytes from elderly individuals maintain their ability to phagocytose and kill bacteria. However, certain responses of neutrophils, such as production of superoxide, may be deficient.[10] Peripheral blood lymphocyte numbers appear to be maintained throughout life, although cross-sectional studies have suggested that T cell numbers may decrease, with an increase in the ratio of helper to suppresser cells.[11,12] Platelet counts appear to be maintained in a normal range throughout the age span.

Another area of confusion has been the erythrocyte sedimentation rate (ESR) in the aged. Although multiple studies show an increase in the ESR above the normal range in 20 to 40 per cent of the elderly, the etiology is not clear.[13–15] In many instances, this elevation may be due to associated chronic disease and/or subclinical alterations in plasma proteins. Since the majority of the elderly maintain a normal sedimentation rate, it is hard to ascribe an elevated ESR to normal aging. However, because of the prevalence of an elevated sedimentation rate in the elderly, its utility as a screening test is limited, although the ESR may be useful in following disease activity in selected patients.

## CLINICAL PROBLEMS OF THE HEMATOPOIETIC SYSTEM

### *Anemia*

Anemia is the most frequently encountered hematologic problem in the elderly. It must be remembered that this is not a disease, but simply a sign of an underlying problem of either a primary or a secondary nature. The definition of the "limits of normal" for the elderly population with respect to hemoglobin and hematocrit values has been controversial. The "normal" adult values used routinely in hematology cite a mean hemoglobin level of 15.5 gm/per dl (13.3 to 17.7 gm per dl) for men and 13.6 gm per dl (11.7 to 15.7 gm per dl) for women. The World Health Organization (WHO) established the criteria for anemia as a hemoglobin level of less than 13 gm per dl in men and 12 gm per dl in women.[5] A number of surveys have attempted to determine whether these limits are applicable to the elderly population as well, with varying results. One study of active, presumably healthy, individuals over the age of 65 demonstrated only a minor fall in mean hemoglobin level from the values previously cited.[16] However, in other surveys of presumably well ambulatory patients, 12 to 20 per cent of the population had hemoglobin levels below the usual limits. Such values are even more common in surveys of nursing home populations and of people over age 75. This may be at least partially explained by the increased prevalence of chronic diseases in these groups.[5] In Lipschitz's study of 222 presumably healthy individuals over the age of 65, over 25 per cent of the group fell into the anemic range. Very few could be demonstrated to have specific causes for their anemia, even following a therapeutic trial of iron, prompting the term "anemia of senescence."[17] The low socioeconomic status and unknown nutritional status of these patients raise other possibilities, however. Another study of 292 elderly ambulatory patients also found 25 per cent with a hemoglobin in the anemic range.[18,19] However, in the subgroup evaluated for anemia, an etiology was determined in the majority of cases. In summary, the majority of healthy elderly maintain a hemoglobin in the normal adult range. Those who do not should undergo evaluation for possible reversible causes of anemia.

The classic signs and symptoms of pallor, weakness, and fatigue may be present in the anemic elderly patient. However, unlike younger patients, the initial manifestations may be those of specific end-organ dysfunction. Thus, behavioral changes and confusional states, ischemic chest pain, congestive heart failure, pulmonary decompensation, syncope, and falls may all be initial presenting complaints of the older patient with anemia. A relatively small improvement in hemoglobin level may produce dramatic symptomatic improvement in the elderly individual. This is additional impetus toward appropriate evaluation of anemia in the elderly.

When anemia is diagnosed, initial information should be obtained, including hemoglobin and hematocrit values, red cell indices, white blood cell and platelet counts, peripheral blood film, and reticulocyte count. Multiple etiologies for anemia may exist in the same individual, so careful description and analysis of the anemia are important. An elevated reticulocyte count represents an appropriate response to anemia by the bone marrow and should suggest a hemolytic process, blood loss, or recent recovery from a toxin or nutritional deficiency. However, failure to mount an appropriate reticulocyte response may be due to complicating diseases and does not exclude the preceding possibilities. By definition, a hypoproliferative anemia is accompanied by a low reticulocyte count. The anemia can be further categorized morphologically as microcytic, normocytic, or macrocytic.

### Microcytic Anemia

Iron deficiency anemia and the anemia of chronic disease are commonly microcytic but may be normocytic in earlier phases. Serum iron and total iron binding capacity are not reliable indices of iron deficiency in the elderly, owing to their wide fluctuations in disease states and a tendency for serum iron to decrease with age in the absence of true iron deficiency.[20] On the other hand, a low serum ferritin is diagnostic of iron deficiency. It may be falsely raised into the normal range by liver disease or inflammatory disorders.[21] If the serum ferritin is nondiagnostic, iron stores can be directly assessed by bone marrow aspiration.

A diagnosis of iron deficiency requires the identification of a cause for this deficiency. Absorption of iron decreases in the elderly, and is perhaps associated with the age-related increase in gastric achlorhydria. However, dietary iron deficiency is rare except in strict vegetarians. Overwhelmingly, iron deficiency in the elderly is a result of blood loss, most often from the gastrointestinal tract. Multiple drugs, such as aspirin and other nonsteroidal anti-inflammatory agents, may frequently produce low-grade gastrointestinal blood loss. Peptic ulcer disease, colon carcinoma, diverticulitis, and vascular abnormalities must be considered. Past history should be assessed, since many patients may have had prior partial gastrectomies resulting in abnormal iron absorption secondary to achlorhydria.

Treatment of the iron deficiency per se can generally be accomplished with ferrous sulfate, 300 mg three times a day for 6 months. However, increased gastric sensitivity in elderly individuals may produce many complaints and failures in compliance. One 300-mg tablet per day, if compulsively taken, can result in adequate correction of anemia.[22] This may require a longer period of therapy in order to replete iron stores. Use of pediatric liquid suspension of ferrous sulfate is an alternative approach. Because of the prevalence of achlorhydria in the aged, some physicians have advocated use of supplemental ascorbic acid to enhance iron absorption. In rare instances, oral supplementation is not adequate to keep up with iron loss (e.g., chronic gastrointestinal bleeding), and intramuscular or intravenous iron dextran is necessary. In the elderly individual with decreased muscle mass, intravenous administration may be preferable.[23] Anaphylaxis is an uncommon reaction, but when it occurs in the elderly, it is often fatal. More commonly arthralgia, myalgia, pyrexia, malaise, nausea, and vomiting have been noted during large infusions. Current recommendations are to limit single doses to 2 ml (100 mg); these may be repeated daily or weekly until iron stores are repleted.[24]

Some symptoms of iron deficiency, such as fatigue, may result from iron depletion at the tissue level in addition to changes brought about by anemia per se. One may see a symptomatic improvement before the hemoglobin rises 10 days to 2 weeks following initiation on therapy. Reticulocyte response and/or hemoglobin level can be followed to ensure adequacy of response. If a complete response is not obtained, compliance should be evaluated and other causes for anemia reconsidered.

The anemia of chronic disease, also known as simple chronic anemia or secondary anemia, can be difficult to distinguish from the anemia of iron deficiency. When mild, it may be normocytic, but often it is microcytic and somewhat hypochromic. This anemia is due in part to a block in release of iron from the reticuloendothelial system, which creates an abnormality in iron utilization, simulating an iron deficient state in the developing red blood cell precursors.[19] This is complicated by a shortened red cell life span in the face of a decreased marrow response to stress. This type of anemia is quite common in the elderly, owing to the high incidence of chronic inflammatory diseases in this age group. Measurement of serum iron and total iron capacity does not distinguish reliably the anemia of chronic disease from that of iron deficiency. A normal level of serum ferritin would make the possibility of iron deficiency less likely. However, an unequivocal diagnosis can only be established by bone marrow examination to document iron stores and to exclude other causes of hypoproliferative anemia. This anemia may be responsible for some of the diagnoses of "anemia of senescence" in elderly individuals. Once the diagnosis is made, correction of underlying problems, such as chronic inflammatory states, infections, neoplastic disorders, and soon, can result in improvement of the anemia. When the anemia is mild, it is generally well tolerated and requires no specific therapy.

Another microcytic anemia that may present initially in older age is thalassemia minor, a group of disorders characterized by genetically determined imbalanced globin chain synthesis, resulting in decreased hemoglobin production. This condition is compatible with long life, and symptoms are very mild in the heterozygous state.[25] Such patients may escape detection until they develop another illness or disease in later life that leads to exacerbation of their anemia or to screening blood studies. The blood film differs from iron deficiency, with a more uniform population of cells, often with basophilic stippling and more prominent target cells. Unlike iron deficiency, hemoglobinopathies may show severe microcytosis when the anemia is mild and will often be accompanied by reticulocytosis. The diagnosis can be confirmed by studies of family members. Distinguishing this from iron deficiency is of some importance, since iron overload can result from inappropriate iron treatment and is to be avoided.

The fourth anemia that may be microcytic is sideroblastic anemia. These anemias are seen with increasing frequency in elderly individuals and are uncommon in younger individuals.[25] They are characterized by the presence of increased serum iron and increased saturation of iron binding capacity, or an elevated serum ferritin. Bone marrow aspiration and examination are necessary for diagnosis, since the characteristic finding is that of iron-laden mitochondria in the red cell precursors, or ringed sideroblasts. Sideroblastic anemia may be secondary to use of drugs, alcohol, or pyridoxine deficiency, but more frequently, in the elderly it occurs as an acquired idiopathic form. It may be accompanied by thrombocytopenia and leukopenia. Sideroblastic anemia is often considered a preleukemic syndrome, which may develop into a form of acute granulocytic or myelomonocytic leukemia in 10 per cent of patients. In some instances it will evolve into multiple myeloma. Once the diagnosis is made, treatment is symptomatic. Transfusion therapy is often required. Accurate diagnosis will allow the avoidance of iron therapy, which could cause further damage to such patients.

### Macrocytic Anemia

In the elderly, macrocytic anemias resulting from megaloblastic erythropoiesis are most frequently produced by a deficiency of folic acid or vitamin $B_{12}$. Although such anemias constitute a small percentage of the total in the elderly population, they are of considerable importance because of their correctability.

Nutritional folic acid deficiency is probably found more often than vitamin $B_{12}$ deficiency in elderly individuals.[21] The main dietary sources of folic acid are green vegetables and fresh fruit. Elderly people often fail to meet the daily requirement of 50 mg of folic acid because they decrease markedly their intake of such foodstuffs. Body stores of folate are limited and may be exhausted within weeks to months by a deficient diet. Moreover, folate metabolism may be affected adversely by alcohol ingestion. The continuing and often unsuspected problem of alcoholism in the elderly is being recognized more frequently as a contributor to such a problem.[26] In addition to macrocytic anemia, thrombocytopenia and leukopenia may be seen. Clinical symptoms are nonspecific, although they may include glossitis. Serum folate levels are not helpful, since as many as ten per cent of presumably healthy aged individuals have been found to have levels below the normal limit.[5] Red cell folate levels are a more reliable indicator of tissue folate deficiency, but assays to provide this information are not widely available. Deficiency of vitamin C in elderly undernourished patients may complicate the situation further, since vitamin C is necessary for the reduction of folic acid to its metabolically active form. Folic acid deficiency is corrected readily by the administration of 1 mg of folic acid per day orally, unless a malabsorptive process is present.

Vitamin $B_{12}$ deficiency in the elderly is most commonly caused by pernicious anemia, a failure of absorption of vitamin $B_{12}$ due to a lack of intrinsic factor normally produced by the gastric parietal cells. This lack of intrinsic factor is secondary to chronic atrophic gastritis, an idiopathic disease that increases in frequency with age.[27] In the absence of this type of malabsorptive defect or other defects to be described later, the very large body stores of vitamin $B_{12}$ (predominantly in the liver) and the high content of vitamin $B_{12}$ in much of the American diet make it unlikely for this deficiency to be produced by lack of dietary intake. However, in the elderly, other forms of malabsorption, including previous total gastrectomy or disease of the terminal ileum (final site of absorption of vitamin $B_{12}$), can also produce vitamin $B_{12}$ deficiency. The initial approach to diagnosis involves serum $B_{12}$ measurement (normal range is 200 to 900/ng per ml). The lower limit of normal in the elderly is uncertain because of the progressive fall in serum $B_{12}$ levels with advancing age.[28] It is not clear that those low serum levels reflect depleted tissue stores of $B_{12}$ in all cases. If in doubt, a Schilling test can be performed. The patient is given radioactive $B_{12}$, and the 24-hour urinary excretion of this compound is determined. Normal individuals excrete at least 8 per cent of the administered dose, whereas patients with pernicious anemia excrete less than 2 to 3 per cent in the absence of intrinsic factor and normal amounts when intrinsic factor is supplied. Failure of $B_{12}$ absorption at the ileal site can also be determined by this mechanism.

The role of folic acid in the production of neurologic symptoms in the elderly individual has long been debated. Although some neurologic signs have been described in folic acid deficiency, a direct relationship has not been clearly established. On the other hand, vitamin $B_{12}$ deficiency can produce a variety of neurologic changes, including paresthesias, dysesthesias, difficulty in proprioception, and personality changes. Although it has been claimed that subnormal vitamin $B_{12}$ levels may be related to dementia in elderly patients, attempts at screening large numbers of patients in psychiatric institutions for previously undiagnosed vitamin $B_{12}$ deficiency have been generally unproductive.[29] Descriptions of dementia and other mental symptoms in association with vitamin $B_{12}$ deficiency, in the absence of hematologic manifestations, are unusual.[30] In the patient with neuropathy due to $B_{12}$ deficiency, the hematologic manifestations may be mild (e.g., macrocytosis without anemia) or vice versa.

The treatment of vitamin $B_{12}$ deficiency can generally be accomplished with use of intramuscular injections of vitamin $B_{12}$. Initially, weekly doses of from 100 to 1000 $\mu$gm are given. For maintenance, a dosage of 100 $\mu$gm per month is quite adequate. A brisk reticulocyte response can generally be seen within 5 to 7 days following initial therapy. The same time of response is generally seen in treatment of folic acid deficiency with oral folic acid as well.

One note of caution concerning nutritional deficiency is especially pertinent in the elderly individual. It is not uncommon to see combined nutritional deficiencies involving both vitamin $B_{12}$ and folic acid or a megaloblastic process complicated by iron deficiency. Thus, a patient with documented $B_{12}$ deficiency may appear to respond initially to therapy, but fail to correct. In some instances, there may have been limited iron present in the bone marrow prior to therapy. The initial burst of red cell production may have exhausted these stores, resulting in a subsequent state of iron deficiency. Such patients will require iron replacement in order to complete the hematologic response. In addition, once this phenomenon is revealed, the previously described approach to determining the cause of the iron deficiency should be followed.

## Normochromic or Normocytic Anemia

Blood loss must always be suspected first in patients in this category. Do not depend upon the elderly patient to report melena. There is no substitute for several negative tests for occult blood in the stool. Beyond this, the blood film and reticulocyte count are essential in subclassification of these anemias, because most anemias may present with normal indices. Early iron deficiency anemia or anemia of chronic disease may be normocytic. $B_{12}$ and folate deficiency may not be associated with macrocytosis if iron deficiency coexists. A dimorphic population of cells is helpful in diagnosing this combined deficiency as well as sideroblastic anemia.

A blood film with microspherocytes should suggest autoimmune hemolytic anemia. Warm antibody autoimmune hemolytic anemia, especially the drug-induced type, is more common in elderly individuals, presumably because of the increased incidence of drug utilization in this age group.[31] Moreover, the occurrence of autoimmune hemolytic anemia in patients with chronic lymphocytic leukemia (to be described later) contributes to the incidence of this disorder in the elderly population. In elderly patients with other chronic illnesses, the absence of a marked reticulocytosis should not blunt further inquiry when hemolysis is suspected, and a Coombs test should be obtained. The test should be done for both IgG and C3 on the surface, since in some instances of cold agglutinin hemolysis, the only remaining evidence of hemolysis is the presence of C3 on the red blood cells. Chronic cold agglutinin disease, characterized by both agglutination and hemolysis due to cold-reacting IgM antibodies, is predominantly a disease of the elderly. Since red cell destruction is often complete in cold agglutinin hemolysis, the blood film may be normal. However, signs of hemolysis often exist, including increased reticulocyte count, bilirubin, and urinary hemoglobin/hemosiderin level.[25]

The possibility of a mild hereditary anemia that has escaped attention until old age must always be considered. Hereditary spherocytosis may mimic autoimmune hemolytic anemia on blood film but can be differentiated by a negative Coombs test, a positive family history, and the presence of splenomegaly. G6PD deficiency is generally associated with acute self-limited hemolysis in the setting of an oxidant stress, generally drug-related. The blood film may be normal, but the signs of intravasular hemolysis noted previously for cold agglutinin disease are generally present.

A normocytic hypoproliferative anemia with a normal blood film may be the initial clue to coexistent renal or endocrine disease. Renal insufficiency is common in the elderly and may be associated with decreased erythropoietin. Endocrine disease, particularly hyper- and hypothyroidism and other endocrine insufficiency states, is commonly associated with anemia.[25]

### Pancytopenia

When anemia is accompanied by leukopenia and thrombocytopenia, other diagnostic possibilities should be considered. An elevated reticulocyte count in this setting suggests peripheral destruction of cells, as might occur with splenomegaly of any etiology. Less commonly, immune pancytopenia may occur. More often the reticulocyte count is low, and the pancytopenia is secondary to a lack of production. Although this may be due to a nutritional deficiency of vitamin $B_{12}$, folate, or even iron, intrinsic bone marrow failure must be considered. Aplastic anemia is uncommon but increases in frequency with age.[32] The presence of immature red cell or white cell precursors on blood film should suggest the possibility of a myeloproliferative or myelodysplastic process or cancer or other infiltrative disease. Bone marrow aspirate and biopsy are essential in this setting. The myeloproliferative and myelodysplastic syndromes will be discussed in a subsequent section.

### Concluding Remarks

In summary, anemia is common in the elderly, and the number of possible diagnoses are large. By use of basic laboratory data, history, and examination, work-up can be directed simply, inexpensively, and generally noninvasively. Evaluation is often rewarded by finding a reversible etiology. In other settings, transfusions may be necessary on an acute or chronic basis. In the elderly patient with symptomatic anemia, appropriate studies should be obtained and transfusion initiated to avoid a major ischemic event or fall. Each unit of packed red cells should be transfused over 3 to 4 hours to avoid precipitation of angina or congestive heart failure. If these conditions already exist, careful transfusion should reverse them.

## *Myeloproliferative Disorders*

### Polycythemia

The elderly patient with primary and secondary polycythemia generally presents vague symptoms such as dizziness, headaches, or thrombocclusive events. An elevated hemoglobin and hematocrit level are noted. Absolute erythrocytosis may be confirmed by measurement of the red cell mass and plasma volume by radioisotopic techniques, but these formal studies are not generally necessary. A medical history should be taken to identify "spurious" polycythemia by finding such causes of a decreased plasma volume as hypertension, diuretics, and cigarette smoking. *Secondary polycythemia* is most frequently associated with cigarette smoking, an elevated carbon monoxide level, and/or chronic pulmonary disease, with decreased arterial oxygen saturation. Less commonly, secondary polycythemia may be associated with renal tumors, cysts, or hydronephrosis, hepatomas, ovarian, or cerebellar tumors.

Primary polycythemia, or polycythemia vera, is a proliferative disorder involving red cells, granulocytes, and platelets. In primary polycythemia, splenomegaly, leukocytosis, and thrombocytosis are frequently present. Symptoms may include those created by the elevated blood viscosity, as well as the paradoxical association of thromboembolic and bleeding events produced by the increased number of platelets that are functionally defective.[25,27]

Treatment of secondary polycythemia depends on accurate diagnosis and treatment of the primary illness. When the primary problem is not correctable, such as chronic pulmonary disease, consideration should be given to lowering the hematocrit level, since hematocrit levels above 60 per cent are associated with reduced cerebral blood flow, to which the elderly patient may be most susceptible. Thus, cautious, staged phlebotomy, with the goal of maintaining the hematocrit level below 50 per cent, is indicated.[33]

The treatment of polycythemia vera has undergone shifts in emphasis over the past few years. A recent cooperative study group studied the side effects of radiophosphorus ($^{32}$P) versus chlorambucil versus phlebotomy alone.[34] In this study, the overall survival rate was similar for all three treatment modalities, but the incidence of acute leukemia as a complication of treatment was considerably higher in the chlorambucil group than in the other groups. On the other hand, patients receiving phlebotomy alone were susceptible to increased number and severity of thromboembolic and bleeding events. Thus, at this time, use of $^{32}$P may be the treatment of choice if given by an experienced hematologist. Ultimately, many patients with polycythemia vera will exhibit a "burned out" or "spent" phase in which myelofibrosis supervenes and hepatosplenomegaly and marked cytopenias become the major problems. It is ironic that such patients who earlier required phlebotomy may now require transfusion therapy. At this stage of the disease, cytotoxic therapy does not appear to be very useful.

### Agnogenic Myeloid Metaplasia with Myelofibrosis

Patients with myeloid metaplasia with myelofibrosis will frequently present with symptoms of anemia, hepatosplenomegaly, and lymph node enlargement. There is frequently leukocytosis, with variable platelet counts. The peripheral blood film characteristically shows teardrop erythrocytes and immature granulocyte precursors, although these are fewer than in acute leukemia. The bone marrow may be variably cellular, with variable degrees of fibrosis. This disorder may overlap with the rest of the spectrum of the myeloproliferative disorders, including polycythemia vera, essential thrombocytosis, chronic granulocytic leukemia, and acute myelogenous leukemia. In general, this disorder is treated symptomatically, with attention to specific cytopenias. Thus, folic acid deficiency or iron deficiency, when they exist, may be corrected and blood transfusions utilized when anemia is predominant. Chemotherapy should be used judiciously, since the hematologic balance of patients with this condition is often precarious and therapy can potentially do more harm than good. Splenectomy may be useful when the spleen is the source of major complications, such as splenic infarction, portal hypertension, or severe cytopenia. Since this disease may be indolent for long periods of time, a cautious approach is generally warranted.[27]

### Chronic Granulocytic Leukemia (CGL)

Although often considered a disease of middle age, CGL, like all leukemias, continues to increase in incidence with advancing age (Fig. 43–1).[35,36] In early stages, patients have minimal symptoms, including fatigue, and occasionally, symptoms related to splenomegaly. The blood film characteristically shows a leukocytosis with an increase in granulocytes and myelocytes, but generally without blasts. As a rule the bone marrow cannot be distinguished from a benign increase in myeloid activity, except by chromosomal studies, which reveal the presence of a Philadelphia chromosome in 95 per cent of cases. Occasionally, thrombocytosis can be prominent, causing confusion with essential thrombocytosis. The stable phase of CGL is best treated with intermittent alkylating agents, such as melphalan, to control spleen size, white blood count, and systemic systems. The terminal phase of CGL, or blast crisis, is heralded by a fall in peripheral counts, rapid splenic growth, fever, marked systemic symptoms, and a conversion of the bone marrow to acute leukemia. This is often accompanied by further chromosomal abnormalities. The median time from CGL to blast crisis is 3 years, with a mean survival of 2 months after blast crisis. Approximately 20 per cent of patients with CGL in blast crisis will respond to treatment for acute lymphoblastic leukemia with vincristine and prednisone. High-dose cytosine arabinoside,[37] bone marrow transplantation, and other experimental protocols are being evaluated for patients with acute myeloblastic leukemia arising from CGL.

### Acute Myeloblastic Leukemia (AML)

AML poses one of the most difficult problems in clinical decision making in relation to elderly patients.[38] Although AML constitutes only a small proportion of neoplasia in the elderly, it is often one of the more dramatic events, with a rapid clinical course and short survival when untreated. Over one half of all patients with AML are over the age of 60 years. Acute leukemia in the elderly may present with large numbers of circulating myeloblasts. However, more commonly, elderly patients will present with nonspecific symptoms, including fatigue, ano-

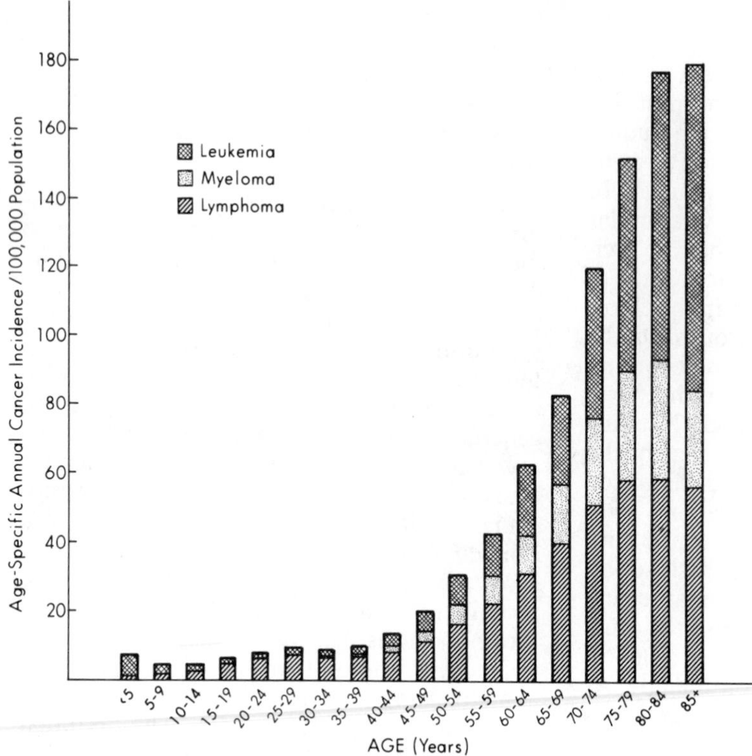


**Figure 43–1.** Age-specific incidence of hematologic malignancies.

rexia, weakness, loss of weight, and so forth. On examination of the peripheral blood, cytopenia may be noted, with few or no characteristic myeloblasts present. In such a situation, the index of suspicion must be high, since the only way to establish the diagnosis is through bone marrow aspiration and/or biopsy. In this circumstance, the marrow will generally be hypercellular, with extensive replacement by immature myeloid cells, especially myeloblasts. Such patients will often have a characteristically rapid, severe course of acute leukemia. Another presentation may be similar to that described previously, but with a bone marrow containing a lower percentage of blast cells and less severe cytopenias. Such patients may have indolent or smoldering leukemia. Finally, there is a group of elderly patients with AML, perhaps as high as one third, who will have had a preleukemic phase.[38] Such patients may have a previous history of cytopenias, refractory anemia, sideroblastic anemia, or other so-called myelodysplastic syndromes that although sometimes characterized by slightly increased numbers of myeloblasts or other immature myeloid cells, are not fully consistent with the diagnosis of acute leukemia. Such patients may have chromosomal abnormalities, as well as other qualitative abnormalities of their myeloid cells, but may continue in a fairly stable situation for a period of years before developing a more characteristic picture of acute leukemia. Once again, only careful clinical follow-up can be used as the guideline for appropriate treatment for such patients.

Given these variabilities in presentation, treatment decisions are difficult. In general, it is suggested that most patients with indolent or smoldering leukemia or the "preleukemic" myelodysplastic syndrome who do not have life-threatening complications be followed carefully with symptomatic treatment, including blood transfusions. In such situations, attempts to treat with cytotoxic chemotherapy in the face of decreased total marrow reserve may be fraught with considerable difficulty. On the other hand, when the patient clearly develops overt acute leukemia or the clinical situation suggests that a prolonged or indolent course is not likely, a decision to treat with chemotherapy must be faced. The usual approach to chemotherapy of acute leukemia in younger individuals utilizes a combination of agents, generally including cytosine arabinoside and an anthracycline (either doxorubicin hydrochloride [Adriamycin] or daunomycin). The goal is to achieve complete bone marrow aplasia and then allow cellular regrowth, with the hope that normal myeloid elements will repopulate the marrow to the exclusion of the previous leukemic cells. In using this approach and the supportive and ancillary therapy currently available, approximately 50 to 70 percent of patients can achieve a complete remission, with an increase in overall survival for such patients.[38]

Earlier clinical series suggested that older patients (older than 50 years) with acute leukemia responded to this form of therapy with remission rates ranging from 20 to 40 per cent.[39–41] However, many older patients were unable to tolerate prolonged bone marrow aplasia and succumbed to infection and other complications during the initial phases of treatment. Even in such clinical series, however, some elderly patients who were able to achieve remission had prolonged survival. In more recent clinical series, elderly patients whose acute leukemia evolved from a preleukemic syndrome appeared to have a particularly poor response rate and shorter survival. On the other hand, elderly patients without a prior preleukemic syndrome had response and survival rates comparable to those of younger patients.[42] Furthermore, other recent studies, using quite aggressive induction chemotherapy, have now reported response rates for individuals over 50 years of age comparable to those in younger patients.[43–45] Thus, it appears that despite the tendency toward decreased marrow reserve and the more precarious homeostatic balance of elderly patients, intense chemotherapeutic regimens can be successful in appropriately selected individuals. Physiologic status, rather than chronologic age, should be considered carefully in this situation , and other organ systems, such as cardiovascular and pulmonary, should be assessed before final decisions are made.

This is an area in which a specialist and a physician experienced in dealing with geriatric patients can have a fruitful collaboration. For example, awareness of potential alterations in renal function that can affect chemotherapeutic drug excretion in this age group will have a major impact upon design of appropriate therapy for such patients. In situations in which the patient has major physiologic deficits that would seriously compromise the ability to respond to and/or recover from therapy, alternative approaches involving less intense therapy may be needed. Such decisions should involve discussions with the patient and family. Optimal care is best provided by a team of health professionals who can work to maintain the functional level of the elderly patient during treatment.

## *Lymphoproliferative Disorders*

### Acute Lymphoblastic Leukemia (ALL)

ALL is a disorder with two peaks of incidence at the extremes of age (Fig. 43–1). These may or may not represent two different disorders. Both are characterized by proliferation of blastic cells of similar morphology, which are generally null cell, but occasionally have B, T, or pre-B cell phenotypes. The clinical presentation of ALL in the elderly is similar to that described for AML, and although this disorder is less responsive than ALL of childhood, it appears to be more responsive than AML in the adult.[46] This disorder can be treated with a combination of vincristine and prednisone without necessarily producing complete bone marrow aplasia. It is thus important to establish whether acute leukemia in an elderly patient is lymphoblastic or myeloblastic, utilizing currently available enzymatic, histochemical, morphologic, and immunologic techniques.

### Chronic Lymphocytic Leukemia (CLL)

The most prevalent lymphoid neoplasias in the elderly are those of B cell origin. Most characteristic among these is CLL, occurring generally in patients over the age of 60.[47] CLL is characterized by the accumulation of large numbers of mature-appearing small B cells in the bone marrow, peripheral blood, and other lymphoid organs. These are both qualitatively and quantitatively abnormal cells, and there is resultant hypogammaglobulinemia, cytopenias, and frequent association with Coombs' positive hemolytic anemia. Patients with Stage I and II disease, predominantly involving cellular accumulation in peripheral blood, lymph nodes, and bone marrow without cytopenias, have a good prognosis. There is the expectation of many years of good quality survival often without specific therapy. On the other hand, patients with advanced disease, generally with bone marrow involvement sufficient to produce cytopenias, have a median survival of less than 2 years and need treatment.[47] This generally involves use of an alkylating agent such as chlorambucil, frequently given in combination with prednisone. This approach has been well tolerated, and complete responses or partial control of disease can usually be obtained. In some instances, radiation therapy, splenectomy, and leukopheresis can be helpful adjuncts for specific symptomatic problems.

Other variants of CLL, including prolymphocytic leukemia, hairy cell leukemia, and lymphosarcoma cell leukemia, are less common but also occur predominantly in the elderly population. These disorders are characterized by proliferations of lymphoid cells presumed to be of different B cell subtypes or differentiation stages. Cells have characteristic morphologic and surface immunoglobulin fluorescence characteristics, which can aid in diagnosis. Lymphosarcoma cell leukemia most often is derived from a previously existing tissue phase lymphoma, whereas hairy cell leukemia is often dominated by marked splenomegaly and peripheral cytopenia. Alkylating agent therapy has been successful in these situations, but in hairy cell leukemia, splenectomy may be the preferred first treatment.

## Lymphoma

The non-Hodgkin's lymphomas are predominantly B cell tumors in the elderly. Nodular, poorly differentiated lymphoma is frequently seen and may follow a relatively indolent course. In many elderly patients with such a disorder, initial therapy can be withheld until the pace of the disease is determined. Diffuse, poorly differentiated lymphocytic and histiocytic lymphomas, on the other hand, are more aggressive and require immediate therapy. Occasionally, histiocytic lymphoma may present in the elderly individual as a more localized disease, involving only one lymph node or organ site. In such cases, local therapy with surgery or radiation may suffice. For the more indolent lymphomas, even when widely disseminated, initial treatment with a single alkylating agent is suggested. More aggressive forms of combination chemotherapy should be reserved for nonlocalized diffuse lymphomas, after careful consideration of the physiologic status of the individual patient. Hodgkin's disease, which is usually considered a disease of the young population, has a bimodal incidence, with a second peak occurring in the elderly population. In general, the response and survival rates of patients in the older group with Hodgkin's disease are worse than those in the younger population.[48,49] This may be explained by differences in stage and histology of Hodgkin's disease in the elderly. In addition, full-dose radiotherapy and chemotherapy have been poorly tolerated in such elderly individuals, and careful attention to treatment design must again be given.[49]

## Monoclonal Gammopathies

These disorders also show a striking age incidence relationship (Fig. 43–1). They range from benign to malignant clonal proliferations of plasma cells, producing protein of a single immunoglobulin class, as detected by serum and/or urine protein electrophoresis and immunoelectrophoresis. Idiopathic monoclonal gammopathy is the most common of these disorders, with a prevalence of 1 per cent in people over the age of 50 and 5 per cent in people over the age of 80. In most cases, this is not truly a disease state. However, with long term followup, one third of these individuals may progress to multiple myeloma or another related disease. Unfortunately, no reliable criteria exist to determine, prospectively, which patients will progress and which will remain asymptomatic for prolonged periods of time.[50]

Multiple myeloma is characterized by marked proliferation of plasma cells within the bone marrow and, occasionally, in extramedullary organs, with resultant bone destruction and bone pain, anemia and other cytopenias, hypercalcemia, renal failure, and increased tendency toward infection.[51] In such patients, one must be careful not to dismiss the weakness and aches and pains as simply symptoms of "old age." Serum and urine protein electrophoresis will demonstrate the monoclonal protein abnormality in approximately 99 per cent of such patients. Bone marrow aspiration and demonstration of plasma cell proliferation will then be confirmatory. The abnormal protein is most frequently IgG or IgA. Approximately 20 per cent of myeloma patients produce only free light chains (Bence-Jones proteins). Thus, even in the absence of an obvious serum protein abnormality, urine light chains should be sought first by a sulfosalicylic acid precipitation test of the urine (light chain immunoglobulins are not detected on dipstick) and then by urine protein electrophoresis. Although most of the symptoms of this disease are produced by malignant plasma cell proliferation, the serum proteins themselves may produce abnormalities in the form of the hyperviscosity syndrome.[52] This syndrome may be treated symptomatically by plasmapheresis, but ultimately, control of the cellular proliferation must be achieved with specific chemotherapy. Recent studies have indicated that elderly patients with myeloma can be treated with combination chemotherapy, with resultant response and survival rates equivalent to those of younger patients and with little increase in toxicity.[51]

Waldenstrom's macroglobulinemia presents a clinical syndrome more related to the lymphomas, with organomegaly and lymphoid enlargement, accompanied by a monoclonal IgM serum protein abnormality. Because of the higher intrinsic viscosity of IgM, hyperviscosity may be problematic, especially in the elderly patient with a tenuously balanced microcirculatory system.[52] Since plasma volume expansion occurs in this situation, the elderly patient with reduced cardiovascular reserve may be more prone to congestive heart failure and require earlier symptomatic therapy. For ultimate control of the proliferative process, alkylating agent therapy has been most frequently utilized and appears well tolerated in the elderly patient.

## Disorders of Hemostasis

### Purpura

The most frequent clinical disorder of hemostasis in the elderly is senile purpura, occurring in 10 to 20 per cent of geriatric patients.[53] The purpura occurs as purple-red lesions generally on the extensor surfaces of the forearms and hands. The etiology is presumably related to age-related loss of subcutaneous fat and weakening of supporting structures of small blood vessels, often with no history of trauma. Qualitative platelet dysfunction may coexist in the elderly patient with senile purpura.[53]

Steroid purpura can have the same appearance as senile purpura. Thus the clinician must always be aware of the other manifestations of Cushing's syndrome. Purpura secondary to thrombocytopenia or vasculitis should be considered with the coexistence of petechiae, or dotlike hemorrhages. The purpura of vasculitis is often palpable and accompanied by other clinical or labortory features.

### Thrombocytopenia

Thrombocytopenia may be one of the presenting signs of a myeloproliferative, myelodysplastic, or lymphoproliferative disorder but may also exist independently. Immune thrombocytopenia occurs in the elderly but is not seen as an acute event as frequently as in the younger age group.[25] Its onset appears to be somewhat more insidious and its course more chronic when it does occur. Depending upon the patient's physiologic status, however, the approach is similar to that in the younger individual, with consideration of splenectomy, steroid treatment, and/or cytotoxic therapy. Because of the hazard of prolonged steroid therapy in the elderly, splenectomy should be done promptly in patients who do not achieve a complete response within a few weeks of prednisone therapy.[25]

Drug-induced thrombocytopenia is of special concern in the elderly patient and should always be considered, since many of the drugs known to cause thrombocytopenia are in common use in the elderly population. Drugs such as barbiturates, quinidine, diuretics, and digoxin are frequently being taken by elderly patients presenting with thrombocytopenia. Moreover, several of these are often used simultaneously, thus presenting especially difficult diagnostic situations. Whenever possible, use of such drugs should be discontinued in order to determine whether they played a role in the disease process, and restarted only if specifically required and/or if alternative drugs are not available. Discontinuation of the use of these drugs is the only practical way to establish the diagnosis, since assays for drug-related antiplatelet antibodies are not yet widely available.

### Thrombocytosis

Thrombocytosis is most often secondary to iron deficiency, chronic inflammatory and infectious disorders, and malignancies, all of which are frequent in the elderly population. The level to which the platelet count rises may be indistinguishable from that level found in patients with essential thrombocytosis or other myeloproliferative disorders. The latter patients may have thrombotic or bleeding complications, but those with secondary thrombocytosis will have normal platelet function. The possibility of iron deficiency should be considered, since treatment of this disorder can readily reverse the associated thrombocytosis.

## Coagulation Disorders

Clotting factors, like other elements of the hematopoietic system, do not vary to a major degree with age in the absence of associated disease states.[54] Congenital factor deficiencies are generally detected at an early age, with the possible exceptions of a mild Factor XI deficiency and von Willebrand's disease. The latter condition, associated with a decreased factor VIII level and/or abnormal platelet function, is manifested by a prolonged bleeding time or impaired platelet aggregation with ristocetin in vitro. In addition to the usual spectrum of acquired clotting factor deficiencies, Factor V or VIII deficiency can occur secondary to the presence of spontaneous antibody-like inhibitors, especially in the aged and in postpartum women. Nonspecific inhibitors, such as the lupus anticoagulant, also occur more frequently in the elderly. The presence of an inhibitor may be suggested by a prolonged partial thromboplastin time that does not correct after mixture with normal plasma.

Thrombosis is common in the geriatric population because of the high prevalence of venous stasis and insufficiency as well as limited mobility. Whether fibrinolytic activity is altered in the elderly is often debated. Anticoagulation therapy, although necessary for deep venous thrombosis above the calf and/or pulmonary embolism, is associated with increased bleeding complications in the elderly, due to altered vascular integrity and complicating drug regimens, which may make therapeutic control difficult. The list of drug interactions is extensive, but nonsteroidal anti-inflammatory agents, antibiotics, and barbiturates are major offenders. In addition, the problem of falls in the elderly, as well as cerebrovascular accidents, leads to the potential for life-threatening central nervous system bleeding. However, in the elderly patient with a well-documented thrombotic event, age should not be a barrier to use of anticoagulation agents as long as it is accompanied by careful clinical and laboratory monitoring.

## CONCLUSION

The diagnosis and treatment of hematologic disorders in the elderly present major challenges to the practitioner. Utilizing currently available clinical and laboratory tools, most of the diagnostic challenges can be met without undue risk or expense to the patient. Furthermore, by working together with the patient and family, the physician may resolve therapeutic dilemmas by individualizing the approach to the elderly patient.

### References


1. Hartsock RJ, Smith EB, Petty CS: Normal variation with aging of the amount of hematopoietic tissue in the bone marrow from the anterior iliac crest. Am J Clin Pathol 43:326, 1965.
2. Mauch P, Botnik LE, Hannon EC, et al: Decline in bone marrow proliferative capacity as a function of age. Blood 60:245, 1982.
3. MacLennan WJ, Andrews GR, MacLeod C, Caird FI: Anemia in the elderly. Q J Med 42:1, 1973.
4. Myers AM, Saunders CR, Chalmers DG: The haemoglobin level of fit elderly people. Lancet 2:261, 1968.
5. Vogel JM: Hematologic problems of the aged. Mt. Sinai J Med 47:150, 1980.
*Excellent review, with emphasis on red blood cell and coagulation problems.*
6. Seligman PA: Hematologic and oncologic problems in the elderly. *In* Schrier RW (ed.): Clinical Internal Medicine in the Elderly. Philadelphia, W.B. Saunders Co., 1982, p. 280.
*Fine overall review, including attention to neoplastic problems.*
7. Butterfield DA, Ordaz FE, Markesbery WR: Spin label studies of human erythrocyte membranes in aging. J Gerontol 37:535, 1982.
8. Okabe, R, Ishizawa S, Ishii T, et al: Erythrocyte aging changes evaluated by the deoxyuridine suppression test. J Am Geriatr Soc 30:626, 1982.
9. Caird FI, Andrews GR, Gallie TB: The leukocyte count in old age. Age Aging 1:239, 1972.
10. Nagel JE, Pyle RS, Chrest FJ, Adler WH: Oxidative metabolism and bactericidal capacity of polymorphonuclear leukocytes from normal young and aged adults. J Gerontol 37:529, 1982.
11. Sparrow D, Silbert JE, Rowe JW: The influence of age on peripheral lymphocyte count in men: A cross-sectional and longitudinal study. J Gerontol 35:163, 1980.
12. Van de Griend RJ, Carreno M, Van Door E, et al: Changes in human T lymphocytes after thymectomy and during senescence. J Clin Immunol 2:289, 1982.
13. Bottiger LE, Svendberg CA: Normal erythrocyte sedimentation rate and age. Br Med J 2:85, 1967.
14. Sharland DE: Erythrocyte sedimentation rate: The normal range in the elderly. J Am Geriatr Soc 28:346, 1980.
15. Sparrow D, Rowe JW, Silbert JE: Cross-sectional and longitudinal changes in the erythrocyte sedimentation rate in men. J Gerontol 36:180, 1981.
16. Pincherle G, Shanks S: Hemoglobin values in business executives. Br J Prev Soc Med 21:40, 1967.
17. Lipschitz DA, Mitchell CO, Thompson C: The anemia of senescence. Am J Hematol 11:47, 1981.
18. Freedman ML, Marcus DI: Anemia and the elderly: Is it physiology or pathology? Am J Med Sci 280:81, 1980.
*Addresses in depth the issue of whether or not there is "normal anemia" in the elderly.*
19. Freedman ML: Anemias in the elderly: Physiologic or pathologic? Hosp Pract 17:121, 1982.
20. Caird FI: Problems of interpretation of laboratory findings in the old. Br Med J 4:348, 1973.
21. Walsh JR: Hematologic disorders in the elderly. West J Med 135:446, 1981.
*Excellent overall review, including attention to neoplastic as well as other disorders.*
22. Fulcher RA, Hyland CM: Effectiveness of once daily oral iron in the elderly. Age Ageing 10:44, 1981.
23. Wright WB: Iron deficiency anemia of the elderly treated by total dose infusion. Gerontol Clin 9:107, 1967.
24. Merrell Dow Inc: Iron Dextran Information (od). 1982.
25. Williams, W, Beuther E, Erslev A, Rundles RW: Hematology. New York, McGraw Hill, 1983.
*Excellent resource for general hematologic information.*
26. Hartford JT, Samorajski T: Alcoholism in the geriatric population. J Am Geriatr Soc 30:18, 1982.
27. Wintrobe W: Clinical Hematology. Philadelphia, Lea and Febiger, 1981.
*Excellent resource for general hematologic information.*
28. Fairbanks VF, Elveback LR: Tests for pernicious ane-

mia: Serum vitamin $B_{12}$ assay. Mayo Clin Proc 58:135, 1983.
29. Murphy F, Srivastava PC, Voradi S, Eluis A: Screening of psychiatric patients for hypovitaminosis $B_{12}$. Br Med J 3:559, 1969.
30. Strachan RW, Henderson JG: Psychiatric syndromes due to avitaminosis $B_{12}$ with normal blood and marrow. Q J Med 34:303, 1965.
31. Sokol RJ, Hewitt S, Stamps BK: Autoimmune haemolysis: An 18-year study of 865 cases referred to a regional transfusion centre. Br Med J 282:2023, 1981.
32. Bottiger LE, Bottiger B: Incidence and cause of aplastic anemia, hemolytic anemia, agranulocytosis and thrombocytopenia. Acta Med Scand 210:475, 1981.
33. York EL, Jones RL, Menon D, et al: Effects of secondary polycythemia on cerebral blood flow in chronic obstructive pulmonary disease. Am Rev Resp Dis 121:813, 1980.
34. Beck PD, Goldberg JD, Silverstein MN, et al: Increased incidence of acute leukemia in polycythemia vera associated with chlorambucil therapy. N Eng J Med 304:441, 1981.
35. Crawford J, Cohen HJ: Aging and neoplasia. Annu Rev Gerontol Geriatr *4*:3, 1984.
*General review stressing epidemiology, etiology, and approaches to treatment.*
36. Crawford J, Cohen HJ: Cancer in the aged: Myths and realities. Gerontologist 22:197, 1982.
37. Priesler HO, Early AP, Raza A, et al: Therapy of secondary acute nonlymphocytic leukemia with cytarabine. N Engl J Med 305:21, 1983.
38. Peterson BA: Acute nonlymphocytic leukemia in the elderly: Biology and treatment. *In* Bloomfield CP (ed.): Adult Leukemias I. The Hague, Martinus Nijhoff Publishers, 1982.
*Excellent recent review of entire subject of acute leukemia in the elderly.*
39. Grann V, Erichson R, Flannery J, et al: The therapy of acute granulocytic leukemia in patients more than 50 years old. Ann Intern Med 80:15, 1974.
40. Cosby WH: Acute granulocytic leukemia (AGL) in the elderly. Arch Intern 136:493, 1976.
41. Barbui T, Bassan R, Chisesi T, et al: Retrospective analysis of treatment of acute myeloblastic leukemia in patients more than 55 years old. Acta Haematol 67:170, 1982.
42. Keating MJ. McCredie, RB, Benjamin RS, et al: Treatment of patients over 50 years of age with acute myelogenous leukemia with a combination of rubidazone and cytosine arabinoside, vincristine, and prednisone (ROAP). Blood 58:584, 1981.
43. Foon KA, Zighelboim J, Yale C, Gale RP: Intensive chemotherapy is the treatment of choice for elderly patients with acute myelogenous leukemia. Blood 58:467, 1981.
44. Peterson BA, Bloomfield CD: Treatment of acute non-lymphocytic leukemia in elderly patients. Cancer 40:647, 1977.
45. Reiffers J, Raynal F, Broustet A: Acute myeloblastic leukemia in elderly patients—treatment and prognostic factors. Cancer 45:2816, 1980.
46. Woodruff R: The management of adult acute lymphoblastic leukemia. Cancer Treat Rev 5:95, 1978.
47. Silber R: Chronic lymphocytic leukemia in the elderly. Hosp Pract 17:131, 1982.
*Fine review of overall approach to a disorder frequently seen in elderly people.*
48. Lokich JJ, Pinkus GS, Moloney WC: Hodgkin's disease in the elderly. Oncology 29:484, 1974.
49. Peterson BA, Pajak TF, Cooper MR, et al: Effect of age on therapeutic response and survival in advanced Hodgkin's Disease. Cancer Treat Rep 66:889, 1982.
50. Kyle R: Monoclonal gammopathy of unknown significance. Am J Med 64:814, 1978.
51. Crawford J, Cohen HJ: An approach to monoclonal gammopathies in the elderly. Geriatrics 37:97, 1982.
*General review of background and approach to treatment.*
52. Crawford J, Cohen HJ: Hyperviscosity syndromes. *In* Ritzman SE (ed.): Protein Abnormalities. Vol. 2. Pathology of Immunoglobulins: Diagnostic and Clinical Aspects. New York, Alan Liss, 1982.
53. Hyams DE: The blood. *In* Brocklehurst JC (ed.): Textbook of Geriatric Medicine and Gerontology. London, Churchill Livingstone, 1978.
54. Ratnoff OD: The diagnosis of hemostatic defects in older individuals. *In* Smith I (ed.): Medical Care for the Elderly. New York, Spectrum Publications, 1982.

## Chapter 44

# Host Resistance Impairment and Protection Against Infection

*Ian M. Smith*

## NATURAL BARRIERS TO INFECTION

The body is protected against infection by circulating antibodies, which in combination with antigens encourage the elimination or destruction of infecting organisms by a variety of mechanisms. Examples include activation of the complement system, thereby recruiting inflammatory cells and encouraging phagocytosis. In addition, each system of the body, in health, has efficient mechanical and chemical protective mechanisms, many of which are rendered less effective by the process of aging.

The respiratory tract is an important example. Incoming air is filtered through the nasal vibrissae, and much of the incoming debris impinges on the fluids of the mouth and pharynx. These fluids are enriched with *Streptococcus viridans* and other normal flora, which are ready to compete with incoming pathogenic bacteria. In healthy elderly people, a system of continuously beating cilia moves a blanket of mucus upwards from the lower respiratory tract, thereby preventing the lodgment of foreign bacteria and viruses. Breathing is normally interrupted by deep sighing once or twice every 15 minutes. This helps to keep the alveoli open. Coughing is also a defense against incoming irritants. In normal aged people, the esophagus is closed off by peristalsis or by the lower esophageal sphincter, or both, thereby preventing aspiration of chemicals and bacteria from the gastrointestinal tract. Should invading microbes pass these barriers, there are alveolar macrophages and polymorphonuclear leukocytes to phagocytose and kill bacteria and viruses. There are probably other chemicals as yet unidentified, such as surfactant, that will also kill invading microbes.

Other systems of the body have specific natural barriers to infection. For example, in the skin there is an acid mantle with a pH of 5 to 6. The secretions contain lysozyme, immunoglobulin (Ig), and secretory IgA, which are antibacterial in nature. In the intestinal tract, the pH of the stomach is protective, but acid secretion declines with age. Similarly, pancreatic enzymes are protective; however, the number of these enzymes also declines with age. Perhaps the most specific protection against pathogens in the gastrointestinal tract is provided by the $10^{10}$ organisms per gram of feces, which constitute the normal flora. Inappropriate use of antibiotics can destroy this protection and even lead to diarrhea. In the urinary tract, the acidity of the urine and the rapidity of the urine flow are protective. In the male, the long urethra protects against bacterial invasion. Vaginal and prostatic fluids are antibacterial. Systemically, the immunologic properties of the blood are protective; these too have been shown to change with age. In the elderly, a healthy nutritional state contributes in an important way to an individual's defense against infection. This can be assessed roughly by determining the serum albumin concentration or the urinary creatinine/height ratio. Aging is accompanied by changes in the nature of the T-cell population, with the result that in some elderly patients, diagnostic skin tests are no longer effective and the surveillance activity by T-cells against infection and cancer is compromised (Table 44–1).

**Table 44-1.** SKIN REACTION TO FIVE COMMON SKIN TESTS AND SUBSEQUENT DEATH IN THE "HEALTHY" ELDERLY AGE 80 AND OVER*

| No. of Positive Reactors | No. of Subjects | Per Cent Dead After 2 Years |
|---|---|---|
| 0–1 | 35 | 80 |
| 2–5 | 17 | 35 |

* Data from Roberts-Thomson IC, Whittineham S, Youngchaiyud U, Mackay IR: Ageing, immune response and mortality. Lancet 2:368, 1974.

Thus each system has a complex and efficient method of avoiding invasion by pathogenic microbes. All these protective mechanisms are susceptible to decline with aging, but are even more susceptible to disruption by the physician.[1-3]

# VACCINATION[4]

Because of failing host defenses, any artificial means of increasing protection is very useful in the survival of the elderly population. Certain vaccines are available that can favorably affect the individual's anti-infection armamentarium.

## *Influenza Vaccine*

The use of influenza vaccine is very important in the elderly and is the only means of preventing influenza recommended without reservation by the Canadian Task Force studying periodic health examinations. This vaccine is effective in 80 to 85 per cent of those inoculated, provided that the influenza virus currently circulating was correctly predicted when making the vaccine. It is a trivalent vaccine containing two A viruses (H1N1 and H3N2) and one B virus. The virus is grown in chick embryos and then is concentrated, purified, and (in a significant proportion) split into smaller subvirus units (split-virus). The nonvirus preparative chemicals are for the most part removed.

This virus vaccine is recommended for older people, particularly those over 65. It is also recommended for people of all ages with heart disease, chronic lung disease, chronic renal disease, chronic severe anemia such as sickle cell disease, and a compromised immune system caused by, for example, malignancies or immunosuppressive therapy. Contraindications are allergy to chicken egg (indicated by signs of anaphylaxis such as swelling of the lips and larynx or dyspnea on eating eggs) or a past history of Guillain-Barré syndrome. Epinephrine 1/1000 must be immediately available in a loaded syringe during inoculation sessions. The intramuscular route is preferred over the subcutaneous route for the vaccine. The vaccine should *not* be given intravenously. A moderate number of people experience slight to moderate tenderness or redness, occurring 6 to 8 hours after injection and lasting for one to 2 days. Use of influenza vaccine will decrease hospitalization for influenza by 72 per cent and mortality by 80 per cent in the elderly.[5]

### Pneumococcal Vaccine

Pneumococcal vaccine consists of a mixture of purified capsular polysaccharides from the 23 most prevalent serotypes that cause pneumonia and septicemia in the community. Use of this vaccine will produce resistance to the vaccine types of pneumococcal pneumonia for life. In at least 90 per cent of adults, the vaccine will produce a fourfold or greater increase in the antibody titer. In adults over 65, the overall antibody titer following vaccination is on the average lower than in younger people but is none the less satisfactory against the strains in the vaccine.

About 1 to 2 per cent of the recipients develop a fever of over 100° F and 6 to 10 per cent develop local reactions. In people over 65 the pneumococcal pneumonia rate was reduced by at least 35 per cent (compared with a reduction of 80 per cent in younger adults)[6] by the 14 antigen-vaccine (in use until 1983). The protective effect of the new 23-antigen vaccine is expected to be greater. Studies of long-term care have noted an institutionally acquired pneumococcal pneumonia rate of 13 to 23 per thousand patient years. This rate is much higher than the 2 to 5 cases per thousand patient years for community-acquired pneumococcal pneumonia in adults. The vaccine is recommended for people with functional (sickle cell disease) or anatomic asplenia and for those with congenital or acquired immunodeficiency. Patients with hematologic disorders such as multiple myeloma, lymphatic leukemia, and Hodgkin's disease and patients treated with intensive radiotherapy or chemotherapy are at increased risk of developing or succumbing to pneumococcal infection. They may not respond to the vaccine, but it may be offered to them with appropriate explanation.[7] Administration before the outset of intensive treatment is recommended.

Use of the vaccine is recommended in people with other chronic illnesses (e.g., diabetes mellitus and functional impairment of the heart, liver, or kidney) in whom there is an increased risk of pneumococcal infection. I use it in all patients age 65 and over. The vaccines do not have to be prepared every year because, to date, no obvious shifts in the distribution of pneumococcal serotypes have occurred from one year to the next.[8] This vaccine is given only once in the patient's lifetime.

### *Tetanus Immunization*

Tetanus organisms are omnipresent in nature, and man is the most susceptible of all species to the potent neurotoxin produced by *Clostridium tetani.* No one is born with natural immunity against tetanus nor can it be acquired except by immunization. Tetanus must be considered as a possibility with any wound. Tetanus toxoid administered at the right time prevents tetanus. Even with modern treatment, tetanus is at least 25 per cent fatal, so vaccination is very worthwhile. The incidence and mortality increase approximately eight- to tenfold between the ages of 20 and 70. It is, therefore, advisable that all elderly, particularly rural elderly, be immunized against tetanus. A dose of 0.5 ml is given intramuscularly twice 4 to 6 weeks apart. A third dose of 0.5 ml given approximately 1 year after the second injection is required for permanent immunization.[4] Following vaccination, the patient may develop local redness, tenderness, edema, and transient fever. Persistent nodules have been described, and in rare cases, a neuropathy may ensue. Immunization lasts for approximately 10 years. However, if a tetanus-prone wound occurs 5 or more years after primary vaccination, a booster dose of 0.5 ml should be given. Patients with special susceptibility, such as those who garden as a hobby and use manure to fertilize their gardens, should receive a booster immunization if within 5 years of the primary vaccination.

### *Hepatitis B Vaccine*

The lifetime risk of developing hepatitis B in the United States is 5 per cent,[10] but certain populations have an increased risk. Approximately 5000 people die directly from hepatitis B or from its complications yearly. People at increased risk include those traveling to the Near and Far East; immigrants from Southeast Asia and Africa, south of the Sahara Desert; clients in institutions for the mentally retarded, homosexually active males, and patients, especially the elderly, in hemodialysis units. Medical technologists and other people exposed to human blood are particularly at risk, as are dental professionals, blood bank technicians, morticians, and other professionals exposed to human blood. Prisoners also require protection. Long-term care personnel probably would benefit from hepatitis B vaccination.[10] Hepatitis B virus vaccine is the suspension of inactivated surface antigen particles that have been purified from human plasma. A series of three intramuscular doses of hepatitis B vaccine produces protective antibody in an average of over 90 per cent of healthy adults. Special trials in the elderly have not yet been made. Primary adult dosage consists of three intramuscular doses of 1 ml of vaccine. The second and third doses should be given 1 and 6 months later. The duration of protection is not yet known, but it is at least 3 years. This vaccine is expensive.

## OTHER TYPES OF PROTECTION

### *Amantadine*

Immunocompromised people may not respond adequately to influenza vaccine. Included in this group are patients with the following conditions: abnormalities in the white cell host defense system, such as neutropenia; complement system diseases (inherited or acquired); structural and functional abnormalities of the immunoglobulins; congenital and acquired disorders of B- and T-lymphocyte function; drug induced B- and T-lymphocyte malfunctions, such as those due to corticosteroids and cytotoxic agents; severe malnutrition; and certain diseases, such as uremia, cardiopulmonary disease, and cancer. Many elderly people are in this group.

When the antibody status of a patient is uncertain, amantadine prophylaxis may be indicated. The rate of efficacy of amantadine as a chemoprophylactic drug against influenza A is approximately 70 per cent and is comparable to that reported for inactivated influenza virus vaccine. This form of prophylaxis is also useful for long-term care personnel and is essential for public servants such as policemen, firemen, and hospital personnel who have been exposed to influenza under epidemic conditions and have not been immunized. Amantadine does not suppress the antibody formation from an influenza vaccine and can be given at the same time as the vaccine and can be discontinued after 10 days when active immunity takes over. The adult dose is 200 mg given as 100 mg capsules twice a day, as one teaspoon-full of syrup four times a day, or as a single dose daily. Lightheadedness, nervousness, difficulty in concentration, or drowsiness has been observed in 7 per cent of people taking amantadine. These side effects tend to occur within the first several hours of treatment. If they do not develop within 48 hours, they are not likely to occur.

To be effective as a *treatment* of infuenza A, amantadine hydrochloride must be administered as soon as possible and not later than 48 hours after the onset of symptoms. This form of therapy is particularly useful in patients with life-threatening primary influenza pneumonia. It should be pointed out that influenza is a mild disease in almost all otherwise healthy patients. However, many elderly patients have cardiopulmonary disease, which is adversely affected by influenza. Preliminary evidence indicates that the abnormalities in pulmonary function caused by influenza return to normal more rapidly in amantadine-treated patients than in untreated patients.

## *Travel and the Elderly*

Many elderly people travel extensively and need protection against malaria, hepatitis, and diarrhea (Table 44–2).

Gammaglobulin for the *prevention of hepatitis A* is recommended for all travelers planning to stay 3 or more months in tropical areas or in developing countries where hepatitis A is common and where they may be exposed to infected people and contaminated food and water.[9] It should be given close to the time of departure in a dose of 2 ml intramuscularly for a visit of less than 3 months and 5 ml intramuscularly for a longer stay. If possible, immunoglobulin should not be administered for 3 months before or at least 2 weeks after live viral vaccine is given.

Most commonly, *traveler's diarrhea* is caused by enterotoxigenic *Escherichia coli*. Shigellae or salmonellae sometimes cause this syndrome. The traveler should drink only bottled or carbonated water and avoid ice, salads, and unpeeled fruit. A single dose of 200 mg of doxycycline followed by a 100-mg capsule daily for several days after the onset of a single diarrheal stool will usually take care of the problem. The generic drug tetracycline is cheaper, approximately one tenth the price of the proprietary drug. One tablet daily of double strength trimethoprim sulfamethoxazole can also prevent or treat traveler's diarrhea.[11] Pepto-Bismol liquid has some antidiarrheal effects, but the dose needed is quite high.

## *Antibiotic Prophylaxis in Surgical Patients*

The elderly are being admitted to acute-care hospitals in increasing numbers (see below). The prevention of wound infections is very important.[12] Each postoperative wound infection adds about 1 week to the patient's hospitalization and over $1000 to the bill. From the time of incision until 5 to 6 hours later the patient is most susceptible to wound infection. In clean surgery, in which there is no entry into the respiratory, genital, urinary, or alimentary tract, the expected rate of postoperative infection is only 2 to 5 per cent. This rate can not be improved by antibiotic prophylaxis. "Clean" surgery makes up about 75 per cent of all surgery. Surgical procedures involving insertion of prosthetic heart valves, artificial joints, and vascular grafts, even though "clean" should be accompanied by antibiotic prophylaxis. "Clean-contaminated" procedures are, broadly speaking, those involving entrance into the respiratory, genital, urinary, or gastrointestinal tract. Representing about 15 per cent of surgical procedures, they account for 10 per cent of postoperative infection. "Contaminated and dirty" procedures are those in which there is an abnormal source of severe contamination. Although these procedures make up 5 per cent of operations, they account for 20 to 40 per cent of postoperative infection.

The use of antibiotic therapy or prophylaxis before and during surgery will be effective if the following three rules are strictly adhered to:

1. Antibiotic therapy is used only for clean-contaminated or contaminated and dirty operations.
2. The antibiotic level is reached before the skin is incised.
3. The antibiotics are used for less than 24 to 48 hours; preferably only in a single dose, provided that the operation does not last longer than 4 hours.

The details of indications and regimens for antimicrobial prophylaxis in surgery are contained in Table 44–2.[13,14]

### Prophylaxis Against Infective Endocarditis in Patients with Valvular Disease

The need for prophylaxis at surgery in patients with valve disease is suggested by the fact that patients with undetectable serum levels of cephalosporins at the end of surgery had an infection rate of 27 per cent, whereas those with measurable levels had a rate of postoperative

**Table 44-2.** CHEMOPROPHYLAXIS IN THE ELDERLY*

| | Indications | Antibacterial Regimen |
|---|---|---|
| ***Almost Always Beneficial*** | | |
| Single organism—short-term treatment | Meningococcal exposure<br>Same house or room | Rifampin 600 mg bid† for 2 days<br>Minocycline 50 mgm qid** 4 days |
| | Implant surgery<br>Prosthetic valve surgery, etc. | Cefazolin |
| | Positive urine culture at time of urologic operation for specific pathogen | Laboratory-directed antibiotics |
| Single organism—long-term treatment | Tuberculosis contacts<br>Over 35 *only* in damaged host | INH‡ 300 mg daily for 1 year§ |
| | Influenza A<br>Unvaccinated population | Amantadine 200 mg daily for 9 days (give vaccine on day 1) |
| | Malaria chloroquine sensitive<br>For travelers | Chloroquine 500 mg weekly from 2 weeks before until 7 weeks after |
| | Malaria chloroquine resistant<br>For travelers to certain areas‖ | 25 mg pyrimethamine + 500 mg sulfadoxine (Fansidar), 500 mg chloroquine 2 weeks before until 7 weeks after |
| | Traveler's diarrhea<br>Foreign travel | Tetracycline 250 mg qid** for 4 days at onset of first diarrheal stool |
| Multiple organisms—similar antibiotic susceptibility, short-term treatment | Bacterial endocarditis<br>High-risk patients with prosthetic heart valves | 1.2 million units aqueous penicillin IM†† + 1 gm streptomycin IM |
| | Patients allergic to penicillin | Vancomycin 1 gm IV twice on day of operation |
| | Other endocarditis patients | Penicillin V 2 gm orally 60 minutes before operation, then 3 doses 0.5 gm penicillin V po‡‡ every 6 hours |
| | Same endocarditis patients, but allergic to penicillin | Erythromycin 1 gm po 60 minutes preoperation then 3 doses 500 mg po every 6 hours |
| Multiple organisms—variable antibiotic sensitivity, short-term treatment | High-risk prosthetic valve patients | 1.2 million units aqueous procaine penicillin IM + 1.0 gm streptomycin IM |
| | Genitourinary and gastrointestinal instrumental invasion | Same |
| | Peritoneal cavity contamination<br>Trauma or spillage of intestinal contents at operation | Cephalosporin + clindamycin single or three doses |
| | Colorectal operations | Oral metronidazole single or three doses |
| ***Usually Beneficial*** | | |
| Few organisms—short-term treatment | Biliary surgery<br>Especially for patients age 70 and over | Cephalosporin |
| | Traumatic contaminated wounds | Cephalosporin |
| | Extremity amputation | Cephalosporin; possibly add clindamycin |
| ***Uncertain Benefit*** | | |
| Few organisms—long-term treatment | Leukopenic patients<br>PMN§§ count of 1000 or less | One-half tablet trimsulfa (40 mg trimethoprim and 200 mg sulfamethoxazole) |
| | Recurrent urinary tract infections | Once weekly at bedtime for 6 months |
| | Recurrent pulmonary infections<br>Emphysema or chronic bronchitis | Ampicillin, tetracycline or trimsulfa when sputum is purulent |
| ***Useless or Harmful*** | | |
| Use local prophylaxis only | Indwelling cathethers<br>Hospital-acquired pneumonia<br>Burns | |

* Adapted from inactivated hepatitis B virus vaccine. MMWR 31:317, 1982 and from Anonymous: Immunization and chemoprophylaxis for travellers. Med Lett 25:37, 1983 and Quintiliani R: Modern approaches to antibiotic chemoprophylaxis. Infect Dis Pract 3:1, 1979.
† bid = twice daily.
‡ INH = isonizad.
§ Not truly prophylaxis. This is suppressive treatment.
‖ South America, Southeast Asia, Western Pacific, East Africa.
** qid = four times a day.
†† IM = intramuscularly.
‡‡ po = orally.
§§ PMN = polymorphonuclear neutrophil leukocytes.

infection of only 1 per cent. Nonetheless, the efficacy of prophylaxis in this type of surgery is unproved. At this time, prophylaxis is used for patients with most congenital heart disease, acquired valvular disease, idiopathic hypertrophic subaortic stenosis, or mitral valve prolapse with mitral insufficiency or with prosthetic heart valves. Different regimens are indicated according to whether a dental, an upper respiratory tract, a genitourinary, or a gastrointestinal procedure is being undertaken. These are summarized in Table 44–2.[14,15]

### *Medical Antibiotic Prophylaxis*[12–14]

In contrast to surgical prophylaxis, medical prophylaxis usually involves repeated or relatively extended exposure to antibiotics, so that the prophylaxis has to be maintained for days or weeks. Effective prophylaxis is required for patients with traveler's diarrhea, influenza (i.e., amantadine), and recurrent urinary infection as well as for treatment of household contacts of patients with meningococcal meningitis, and patients undergoing therapy for cancer and other diseases who have developed severe neutropenia.

Hirschmann[13] said, "Some physicians tend to be guided by the maxim it can't do any harm and it may do good. Of course antibiotics can do harm, both directly through side effects or by opening the way to superinfection with resistant organisms. They can also cause problems indirectly by encouraging the development of drug resistant pathogens that can complicate the treatment of future patients." This is particularly true in nursing homes where prophylactic antibiotics have been used in patients with indwelling bladder catheters. This has resulted in the spread throughout the institution of antibiotic resistant infections, which in some patients lead to septicemia.

## EPIDEMIOLOGY OF INFECTIONS IN THE ELDERLY

Elderly people who live alone but are independent in an apartment or house or live with family or friends have the same probability of developing infections as the general population, with the possible exception of an increase in respiratory infection due to subclinical or clinical chronic respiratory and chronic cardiac diseases. Patients at high risk either at home or in an institution are those age 70 and over who are confined and living alone; the recently bereaved; people with an ill spouse; mentally retarded or mentally diseased elderly; the immobilized; the loners; and people recently discharged from acute care hospitals. Failure to provide an adequate program of home care for ill elderly confined to their homes contributes to increased immobility, lack of bladder and bowel control, and inability to care for personal needs, all of which increase the likelihood of infection. In the mobile elderly living at home, great benefits can be gained by patient education in regard to behavior modification. This applies particularly to exercise, alcohol, and smoking.

There are about 1.5 million elderly in acute-care hospital beds at any one time. There are more elderly in acute-care beds than there are in long-term care beds. Whereas the admission rate of all age groups to acute-care hospitals has risen approximately 5 to 7 per cent in 10 years, admission of the elderly has increased by 35 to 40 per cent. The median nosocomial infection rate is 341 per 10,000 patients discharged. This rate has declined from 358 to 329 with the employment of hospital epidemiologists. This has been particularly true on surgical services. Patients with infections stay in hospitals an average of 13 to 35 days longer than matched controls, and the outcome is worse in these nosocomially infected patients. Nosocomial infections occur in the urinary tract in 40 per cent of patients, surgical wounds in 25 per cent, the respiratory tract in 16 per cent, the skin in 5 per cent, and the blood stream in 3 per cent. About 1 per cent of urinary tract and surgical wound infections and about 2 per cent of respiratory tract and skin infections become septicemic. One of the most striking predisposing factors in nosocomial infections is the increase in elderly patients in hospitals. From 30 to 70 per cent of hospital-acquired infections in the respiratory tract are fatal; 50 to 80 per cent of those in the blood stream are fatal.[16]

The 1.3 million beds in 18,300 extended-care facilities are used annually by over 2 million patients in the United States. Five per cent of the elderly reside in extended-care facilities, and about 25 per cent of elderly individuals spend at least 3 weeks in an extended-care facility at some time after the age of 65. On the average, these residents have between two and three chronic clinical conditions. Approximately one third are identified as having chronic urinary tract infection. One third of admissions to all extended-care facilities come from acute-care hospitals; in skilled nursing facilities, two thirds of the patients are admitted through transfer from the acute-care hospital. Among those admitted from a hospital, whose stay there exceeded 30 days, 75 per cent developed a nosocomial infection. Nearly one half of those admitted from the hospital or from home have an active infection at the time of admission. At any given time between 5 and 20 per cent of residents of extended-care facilities have a current infection.

Urinary tract infections are the most common infections in the elderly in extended-care facilities. One third of these infections are present at admission; 50 per cent are related to catheter use. Indwelling catheters are more dangerous than suprapubic catheters; the latter are more dangerous than condom catheters, and these, in turn, cause more trouble than no catheter at all. *Proteus* is a frequent isolate but so is *E. coli.* The rate of urinary tract infection increases with the dependency status of the patient.[17]

Approximately 10 per cent of infections in long-term care patients involve skin and soft tissue. Up to 30 per cent of immobilized bed patients have skin or soft tissue infection. *Staphlyococcus aureus* is the most common etiologic agent, but gram-negative rods and anaerobic agents are also common in infections of anatomic areas below the waist.

Respiratory illness is a less common cause of endemic infection in extended-care facilities, but it is a common cause of epidemic illness. Over one half of febrile patients in long-term care centers have a respiratory cause of their fever. Gram-negative rod organisms are frequent causative agents in these patients. Gram-negative bacilli are usually carried in the throat of these patients before active pneumonia. Less than 10 per cent of independent apartment-dwelling elderly or young people have gram-negative rods colonizing their respiratory tracts, whereas approximately 25 per cent of nursing home residents, over one third of patients in skilled nursing facilities, and 60 per cent of elderly patients in acute-care hospitals have gram-negative bacilli colonizing their respiratory tracts. This colonization is associated with a sevenfold increase in gram-negative pneumonias when these patients are hospitalized. Mortality in this group of pneumonia patients exceeds 40 per cent and often reaches 70 per cent.

Certain important recommendations for control of infections in extended-care facility patients include the following[18]:

1. Surveillance for infection on admission.
   A. Determine temperatures and respiratory rates for at least 48 hours.
   B. Perform culture of any infected site, including any skin lesions; urine culture in persons with indwelling catheters, together with culture of exudate around catheter, if present.
   C. Institute bed or room segregation or both of new admissions during the surveillance period.
2. Segregation of identified infected people to single rooms with sinks.
3. Documentation in writing of what good skin care, catheter care, and handwashing programs are recommended.
4. Discontinuation of all bladder irrigation unless specific medical need is redocumented by the physician.
5. Performance of cultures before therapy.
6. Routine involvement of physicians in supervision of the program.
7. Routine reporting of all infection data to attending physicians.
8. Provision of routine orientation and in-service education on nosocomial infection to all extended-care personnel.
9. Arrangement of appropriate immunization for all patients and staff, including influenza vaccination and pneumococcal vaccination.[15,16]

## References


1. Mandell GL, Douglas RG Jr, Bennett JE: Principles and Practice of Infectious Diseases. 2nd ed. New York, John Wiley and Sons, 1984.
2. Phair J, Kauffman CA, Bjornson A, et al: Host defenses in the aged. Evaluation of the components of the inflammatory and immune responses. J Infect Dis 138:67, 1978.
3. Roberts-Thomson IC, Whittineham S, Youngchaiyud U, Mackay IR: Ageing, immune response and mortality. Lancet 2:368, 1974.
4. Goodman RA, Orenstein WA, Hinman AR: Vaccination and disease prevention for adults. JAMA 248:1607, 1982.
5. Ruben FL: Prevention of influenza in the elderly. J Am Geriatr Soc 30:577, 1982.
6. Bentley DW, Ha K, Mamot K, et al: Pneumococcal vaccine in the institutionalized elderly. Rev Infect Dis 3:S71, 1981.
7. American College of Physicians: Pneumococcal vaccine recommendation. Ann Intern Med 96:206, 1982.
8. Broome CV, Facklam RR, Allen JR, et al: Epidemiology of pneumococcal serotypes in the United States, 1978–79. J Infect Dis 141:119, 1980.
9. Health Information for International Travel. 1981 MMWR HHS Publication No. 81-8280 CDC (HEW Publication), Atlanta, GA.

10. Anonymous: Inactivated hepatitis B virus vaccine. MMWR 31:317, 1982 CDC (HEW Publication), Atlanta, GA.
11. Anonymous: Immunization and chemoprophylaxis for travellers. Med Lett 23:105, 1981.
12. Anonymous: Antimicrobial prophylaxis for surgery. Med Lett 23:77, 1981.
13. Hirschmann JV: Rational antibiotic prophylaxis. Hosp Pract, 105:123, 1981.
14. Quintiliani R: Modern approaches to antibiotic chemoprophylaxis. Infect Dis Pract 3:1, 1979.
15. Petersdorf RG: Antimicrobial prophylaxis of bacterial endocarditis. Am J Med 65:220, 1978.
16. Garibaldi RA, Brodine S, Matsomiya S: Infections among patients in nursing homes. Policies, prevalence and problems. N Engl J Med 305:731, 1981.
17. Kaye D: Urinary tract infections in the elderly. Bull NY Acad Med 50:209, 1980.
18. Cohen ED, Hierholzer WJ Jr, Schilling CR, Snydman DR: Nosocomial infections in skilled nursing facilities. A preliminary survey. Public Health Rep 94:162, 1979.

*Chapter 45*

# Prevalence, Diagnosis, and Treatment of Infectious Diseases

*Ian M. Smith*

Fever is an exaggeration of the normal diurnal swing of temperature in normal, healthy elderly individuals. Normal temperature is highest at 6 to 8 PM in the evening and lowest at 2 to 3 AM in the morning. There is a 1° C (2° F) difference between these two temperatures. When the temperature is abnormally elevated ("fever"), this swing is exaggerated, so initially there is a spiking fever, which rises in the evening. When it becomes more marked, the fever becomes plateau in type. Apart from this, there are no other characteristic fever charts except for the obvious malaria charts. Fever is caused by a proteinaceous material called endogenous pyrogen, which is secreted by polymorphonuclear leukocytes and macrophages that have engulfed foreign material. Although this foreign material is most frequently derived from bacteria and next most often from viruses, antigen antibody complexes or dead tissue may play this role. Shaking chills or rigors, headache, anorexia, and weight loss may be associated with fever. Rigors usually indicate septicemia, and blood cultures should be performed. Danger signals are the development of septic shock, with reduced renal and cerebral flow causing oliguria, confusion, disseminated petechiae, or all of these phenomena.

In the elderly patient with fever, one must answer the following four questions;

1. Is an infection present?
2. What is the site of the primary infection (for example, in the lung or in the blood stream)?
3. What is the pathogen? With practice at performing adequate cultures, one learns to recognize that certain organisms are located in certain anatomic areas, as shown in Table 45–1.
4. How much underlying disease is present?

This last question is very important because infection is the immediate cause of death in only about half of the elderly. The others die as a result of an exacerbation of the underlying disease.

When patients have a temperature of 102° F or higher for 2 weeks or longer and have undergone a careful work-up for a week without a cause of the fever being found, the fever will be attributable to cancer in 20 per cent of the cases.[1] Therefore, very careful investigation of the causes of fever is important in the elderly. Connective tissue diseases can also cause fever.[2]

Fever may be missed in the elderly for a variety of reasons. The temperature may be taken in the morning only and a significant evening fever missed. Some elderly people have a low basal temperature, and there is some evidence that patients with orthostatic hypotension (and probably disease of the autonomic nervous system) are more likely to have this type of low basal temperature than other healthy elderly people. Steroid therapy can eliminate any fever; therefore, any patient on steroid therapy with an unexplained tachycardia must be investigated carefully to rule out infection. It is possible but not certain that continuous therapy using aspirin or other nonsteroidal anti-inflammatory agents may do the same. Patients of any age with renal failure respond to febrile illness with a rise in temperature that is approximately 50 per cent less than that of patients without renal failure.

**Table 45–1.** PROBABILITIES OF BACTERIAL INVOLVEMENTS IN INFECTIONS

| Infectious Disease | Organism | Age 70 Years and Over (%) | Age 30 to 49 Years (%) |
|---|---|---|---|
| Septicemia | *Staphylococcus aureus* | 24 | 13 |
| | Polymicrobes | 21 | 10 |
| | *Streptococcus pneumoniae* | 15 | 7 |
| | *Escherichia coli* | 10 | 15 |
| | *Klebsiella-Enterobacter* | 8 | 18 |
| | Bacteroides | 6 | 8 |
| Endocarditis | *Streptococcus viridans* | 32 | 33 |
| | *Staphylococcus aureus* | 24 | 15 |
| | *Staphylococcus epidermidis* | 10 | 5 |
| | Other streptococci | 20 | 11 |
| Urinary tract infections | *Escherichia coli* | 62 | 62 |
| | *Proteus* | 31 | 31 |
| | *Pseudomonas* | 4 | 4 |
| Pneumonia | *Streptococcus pneumoniae* | 70 | 83 |
| | Gram-negative rods | 21 | 8 |
| | *Legionella pneumophila* | 8 | 2 |
| | *Staphylococcus aureus* | 1 | 2 |
| Meningitis | *Streptococcus pneumoniae* | 46 | 20 |
| | *Listeria* | 21 | 2 |
| | Gram-negative rods | 14 | 4 |
| | *Neisseria meningitidis* | 10 | 32 |

Many elderly patients exhibit decline in renal function. There are probably other unknown factors that prevent the infected elderly from being febrile that are as yet unidentified.

## INFLUENZA[3]

*Influenza* usually has an abrupt onset after an incubation period of 1 to 2 days. The patient complains of feverishness, chilliness, or a frank shaking chill. There are headaches, myalgias, and low back pain. The patient has a dry cough with deep substernal pain but no actual pleurisy. There may be abundant nasal discharge but very little or no sputum. The patient has a temperature of 100 to 104° F, lasting about 3 days. The diagnosis should be made easily once the influenza virus has been isolated in a single patient in the community. The virus is isolated from throat specimens obtained through garglings which are inoculated into monkey or canine kidney cell cultures. Some laboratories isolate the virus by inoculation of embryonated hens' eggs. About two thirds of the positive cultures can be detected within 3 days of inoculation and the remainder by 5 to 7 days. Acute- and convalescent-care serum specimens can be used to make the diagosis on the basis of complement-fixating antibodies, or hemagglutinating antibodies, but these are less useful in day-to-day practice. After the first case is diagnosed, further laboratory diagnostic tests are unnecessary, and diagnosis can be made on a clinical basis with 85 per cent certainty.

In addition to its role in prophylaxis (see page 534), amantadine may be useful in the treatment of influenza A, particularly in elderly people who have a severe influenza-like illness, with temperatures over 100° F. A dose of 200 mg initially and 100 mg twice a day for 3 to 5 days thereafter is recommended.

Influenza will strip off the ciliated surface epithelium of the bronchi and allow bacteria to invade. The affected patients are most often elderly individuals who have chronic pulmonary, cardiac, metabolic, or other diseases. After the first few days of fever, there may be an exacerbation of fever, with signs and symptoms of bacterial pneumonia such as cough, rapid respiratory rate, sputum production, and an area of consolidation on physical examination and x-ray. Gram stain should be performed to rule out rapidly progressive staphylococcal pneumonia. Other patients are infected with pneumococci or *Hemophilus influenzae.* Here one sees patchy, widely scattered infiltrates with pleural reaction and sometimes pleural fluid formation. About 25 per cent of these patients develop lung abscess and 10 per cent have empyema. Therefore, in elderly patients with influenza and pneumonia, it is important to perform one or, better, two blood cultures, which, when positive, will identify the presence of bacterial infection. Treatment should be with penicillin G, ampicillin, or nafcillin, depending on the pathogen.

It is important to remember that respiratory syncytial virus infection occurs in the elderly and can mimic influenza. In both diseases patients have cough, sore throat, occasional pneumonia, fever, malaise, myalgia, anorexia, headache, and chills. The only significant clinical difference is the greater occurrence of rhinorrhea in respiratory syncytial virus disease compared with influenza. Influenza can occur as an epidemic in 20 per cent of all the patients in a family practice and in 30 per cent of all the residents of a nursing home.[4]

## PNEUMONIA

### *Incidence*

The incidence of pneumonia has not been adequately determined but death rates are well categorized. In 1900, approximately 1500 people per 100,000 aged 70 and over died of pneumonia. This rate fell to 700 in 1940 and to 439 in 1965. Since that time the rate has fallen very little, staying around 400 people per 100,000 in 1980, with slightly more cases in males than in females.

### *Pathophysiology*

Most pneumonias, if not all, are preceded by an asymptomatic state, during which the carrier harbors the organisms in the nasal pharynx. This has been well studied with pneumococci and *H. influenzae.* Only recently has this phase been examined in regard to gram-negative rods. Nine per cent of elderly individuals living independently (e.g., in apartments) are carriers of gram-negative rods, compared with 8 per cent of young controls. Gram-negative organisms are carried in the throats of 12 per cent of the elderly in nursing homes, 30 per cent in skilled nursing facilities, and 60 per cent in acute-care hospitals.[5] This asymptomatic state can be transformed into active infection of the lung (pneumonia) by the introduction of nasal tubing for oxygen delivery, nasal-tracheal suction, and so forth, or by aspiration following induction of anesthesia or as a result of oversedation. Both in long-term care units and in hospitals, those who most commonly are carriers of gram-negative rods are patients with respiratory disease and patients who are bedridden or chair-fast. The brain-damaged elderly are more apt to be carriers and to develop pneumonia. The mechanism for this is not clear. In the throat *Streptococcus viridans* is a potential inhibitor of the growth of gram-negative bacilli, but careless use of antibiotic chemotherapy can interfere with this dynamic ecosystem. Additionally, the nasal vibrissae, the sinuses, and the mucociliary blanket protect the lung. The mucociliary blanket is most commonly destroyed by influenza. Forced vital capacity of an adequate degree and an efficient cough are protective, as is closure of the esophagus from the lung by peristalsis or by the lower esophageal sphincter. The majority of the pathogens of the lung are acquired by person-to-person transmission. The exception to this is *Legionella pneumophila,* which is acquired from the environment, such as from soil or water.

### *Clinical Findings*[6]

Typically, pneumonia in the elderly person develops suddenly, and sputum production is associated with pleurisy, shaking chills, and fever. The sputum may be purulent, bloody, or rusty. Although the onset of pneumonia is usually abrupt, approximately 25 per cent of patients have a preceding viral illness. Unfortunately many elderly people have pre-existing cough and are somewhat less sensitive to the pain of pleurisy. They may also be afebrile. In fact, in certain elderly people, the pneumonia can be totally asymptomatic, and patients who appear well one day can die within 2 to 3 days of a fulminating pneumonia. Perhaps the most reliable indicator of pneumonia is the respiratory rate; however, this is too frequently ignored. Infection may divert energy, or oxygen, or both, from essential organs in elderly patients with pneumonia. This may well result in a confused state. Patients with Legionnaires' pneumonia are especially apt to exhibit confusion. It is present on admission to the hospital in 30 per cent of patients with this disorder and develops at some time during the course of the illness in half of the patients. Thus the prevalence of confusion in this disorder is greater than in pneumococcal pneumonia.[7]

### *Diagnosis*

Having established that an infection is present and having localized it to the lung, it is important to make some decisions about the likely etiology. In Iowa, in patients aged 40 to 59 years, 9 per cent of community-acquired pneumonia is due to legionellae, 7 per cent due to mycoplasmas, and the rest probably due to pneumococci. In people age 60 years and over, these figures are 4.4 per cent due to legionellae and 5.3 per cent due to mycoplasmas.[8]

Pneumonia acquired in a long-term care hospital is likely to be due to a gram-negative rod or staphylocci. Pneumonia occurring after a well-defined attack of influenza is likely to be caused by pneumococci, staphylococci, or *H. influenzae,* with pneumococcal pneumonia being more frequent, but with staphylococcal pneumonia more apt to be fatal. The Gram stain is useful primarily in ruling out gram-negative rod pneumonia. If gram-negative rod pneumonia can be ruled out, the use of erythromycin is justified because it is effective against both pneumococci and legionella organisms.

The next clinical assessment to make is how extensive the pneumonia is. One-lobe pneumonias are much less lethal than pneumonias involving two or more lobes. One should also look for a pleural effusion, occurring in about 25 per cent of patients with pneumonia. This can be used to obtain an uncontaminated culture. A positive blood culture indicates extensive disease.

Aspiration pneumonia must be ruled out. It differs from spontaneous bacterial pneumonia in that it occurs in patients who have reduced levels of consciousness, absent gag and cough reflexes, esophageal disorders, intratracheal intubation, or nasogastric intubation. The organisms aspirated are the normal, predominantly anaerobic flora of the mouth. This, together with the chemical destruction of tissue caused by gastric acid, leads to a particularly rapidly advancing form of pneumonia associated with a decreased aterial $Po_2$.

The next diagnostic assessment relates to underlying disease, which is present in 50 to 80 per cent of elderly patients with pneumonia. Predisposing diseases are primarily emphysema, congestive cardiac failure, diabetes mellitus, and chronic renal disease. For example, one third of elderly people who develop pneumococcal pneumonias have congestive cardiac failure.[5]

If a condition is clinically suspicious, particularly when the patient has a respiratory rate of over 24 breaths per minute, a chest x-ray should be taken. It is important to take a lateral as well as a posteroanterior view because 20 per cent of the lung hides behind the heart. A sputum Gram stain will help to rule out gram-negative rod pneumonia, and if pus cells are present without organisms, the diagnosis of Legionnaires' disease should be considered. Sputum specimens, to be suitable for culture, should contain 25 or more white blood cells per high power field and 10 or less epithelial cells. Blood culture is positive in 15 to 30 per cent of cases of pneumonia and is helpful in determining treatment. Pleural fluid, found in 25 per cent of cases of pneumonia, provides an uncontaminated source of the causative organism. The white cell count in pneumonia is elevated in only 60 per cent of elderly people, but the differential white cell count shows a shift to the left in 95 per cent. The differential count should always be obtained. In elderly patients, particularly in males, infiltrate seen on chest x-ray may be scanty, because of the frequent presence of underlying emphysema, it may be hard to recognize as a single-lobe infiltrate. Empyema is a complication of 32 per cent of gram-negative rod pneumonias, and lung abscess occurs in 11 per cent. If empyema is suspected on x-ray, it should be confirmed by aspiration. In patients doing poorly, a bronchoscopic culture and biopsy, transtracheal aspiration, or direct-needle aspiration of the lung should be considered. Each of these procedures has a complication rate, but the consequences of not performing them are vastly more serious. Serologic tests for Legionnaires' disease and for mycoplasmal pneumonia should also be carried out. A fourfold rise in titer, or a titer of greater than 1 to 128, is diagnostic.

**Differential Diagnosis.** The main differential diagnoses are pulmonary embolus and cancer. The former can be ruled out by history, clinical presentation, and a negative ventilation/perfusion scan. If the ventilation/perfusion scan is positive, it can be followed by an angiogram to make an accurate diagnosis. Three negative sputum cytologies indicate that cancer is not present.

## *Treatment*

Treatment of pneumonia is directed at finding the proper antibiotic for the etiologic agent, drainage of abscess or empyema, maintenance of oxygenation, and support of other systems of the body. In treatment of pneumococcal pneumonia, penicillin G is the antibiotic of choice. In our experience, aqueous penicillin is more effective than procaine penicillin or benzathine penicillin G (Bicillin). Intramuscular penicillin is better than oral penicillin, but only initially. After the first intramuscular dose to provide the early high blood concentration necessary for proper treatment, a switch can be made to oral penicillin. Erythromycin is the treatment of choice for pneumonia caused by legionellae. Aspiration or anaerobic infection is treated with clindamycin. In pneumococcal pneumonia, treatment should be continued for 72 hours after the last evidence of infection, whether it is abnormal temperature, white cell count, or clinical signs and symptoms. X-ray changes, which will still be present in 25 per cent of patients 1 month following treatment, do not indicate a need for further treatment. In 25 per cent of patients with underlying emphysema, the pneumonia will still be unresolved, according to x-ray, 3 months after treatment. Follow-up x-rays are useful in the deteriorating patient but are not helpful in the patient who is doing well.

Pneumonia due to infection with gram-negative rods is treated with aminoglycosides; if due to pseudomonas organisms, carbenicillin should be added. Trimethoprim sulfamethoxazole is also useful against some gram-negative rods[10]. In all patients undergoing antibiotic treatment, a rough calculation should be made of the creatinine clearance using the following formula:

$$\frac{140 - \text{age of patient}}{\text{serum creatinine level}}$$

The dosage of antibiotics that are eliminated predominantly through renal excretion should be reduced accordingly.

Any very large pulmonary abscesses will need draining, but the smaller ones will respond to antibiotic treatment. Empyema is a kind of abscess and should be drained. Empyemas can contain 500 to 1000 ml of fluid, usually with $10^5$ or more bacteria per milliliter. This constitutes a population of $10^8$ organisms that can be removed mechanically. This takes the patient away from the point of death, which usually occurs after the accumulation of $10^{13}$ organisms (this figure is extrapolated from data from experimental studies using animals).[9] If two or more lobes are involved, the patient should have blood gases analyzed, and the $Po_2$ should be increased to 60 torr by whatever means necessary. The concentration of oxygen delivered by nasal prongs should be 15 to 20 per cent at most; delivered intratracheally, the concentration should be up to 60 to 100 per cent. One hundred per cent oxygen should rarely be used for more than 1 day. Patients who accumulate carbon dioxide should be placed on the respirator if their $PCO_2$ rises acutely to more than 55 mm.

Because infection interferes with the production of energy and diverts it for the production of new proteins and white cells, the cardiovascular, renal, or pulmonary system may fail. A great deal of attention should be paid to analyzing how much underlying disease is present and in supporting those systems that are failing.

In the patient who is seriously ill with pneumonia, for whom no bacterial diagnosis can be made or approximated, the following approach is suggested: If the overall risk is judged to be relatively low, use of cephalosporin together with an aminoglycoside is recommended. If *Pseudomonas* is judged to be a likely etiologic agent (i.e., in the presence of assisted respiration or, possibly, contaminated intravenous lines), carbenicillin should be added. Carbenicillin contains 5 mEq of sodium per gram, and the amount given daily contains an amount of sodium equivalent to that found in 1 L of normal saline. Ticarcillin and piperacillin contain half the amount of sodium, and their use is preferable in patients requiring sodium restriction. If aspiration pneumonia is suspected, clindamycin should be used along with the cephalosporin and aminoglycoside.[10]

### *Prognosis*

In elderly patients in hospitals, pneumonia is the primary cause of death in 8 per cent and a contributory cause in 20 per cent. In the nursing home it is the primary cause of death in 15 per cent; the degree to which it contributes to death is unknown but may well be 30 per cent or higher. Pneumococcal pneumonia has a 20 per cent fatality rate in the elderly, and Legionnaires' disease a 30 per cent case fatality rate.[11] Case fatality rates in gram-negative rod pneumonia are higher, but precise data are not available. It should always be remembered that half the deaths in the elderly are due to failure of other organ systems with underlying disease rather than due to overwhelming pneumonia.

## TUBERCULOSIS

### *Incidence*

In the United States, tuberculosis occurs in patients under 25 years at a rate of 18 per 100,000 population; at ages 25 to 64, 52 per 100,000; and over age 65, 75 per 100,000. Tuberculosis occurs particularly in the elderly male and is frequently a reactivation of previous subclinical infection.

### *Pathophysiology*

Initial infection can occur anywhere in the lung and sensitizes the patient to subsequent reinfection. This initial infection changes the tuberculin skin test from negative to positive. At a later time, the initial "healed" lesion, which nonetheless has live tubercle bacilli in it, may break down and cause dissemination. Less commonly, reinfection from outside can occur and cause typical granulomatous-type inflammation. Tubercle bacilli need a high $Po_2$ of approximately 140 mm Hg (torr). Therefore the bacilli localize in areas where the $Po_2$ is in the range of 120 to 130 mm Hg (torr), such as the apices of lungs, the kidney, or the growing end of long bones. The usual infecting organism is *Mycobacterium tuberculosis.* Two closely related organisms, *M. avium-intracellulare* and *M. kansasii,* can cause very similar diseases. It is not certain where these rare types of mycobacteria come from, but *M. tuberculosis* is a human-to-human transmitted infection. Bovine tuberculosis probably does not account for more than 10 per cent of the cases. If tuberculous infection goes untreated, necrosis of tissues with cavitation occurs, most commonly in the lungs, but occasionally in the kidneys, bones, lymph nodes, or meninges.

## *Clinical Findings*[12]

Tuberculosis in the elderly may be misleadingly benign or may be almost entirely asymptomatic. Screening of all admissions to long-term care facilities is strongly recommended.[12] Intermediate tuberculin should be used and injected intradermally. A positive reaction is indicated by *induration* of 10 mm or more. Patients with negative reactions should be retested within 1 week with the same test material.[13] All individuals who have positive reactions should be x-rayed and re-x-rayed at yearly intervals.[14]

Approximately 4 per cent of all tuberculin-positive patients will break down with active tuberculosis during their lifetime.[13] The characteristic manifestations of the active disease are fever, weight loss, cough, and debility. Sputum is purulent and frequently contains blood. Sixty to 90 per cent of cases of tuberculosis in the elderly result from a recrudescence of tuberculosis acquired at an earlier age. It is characterized by absence of recent exposure to tuberculosis, a tendency to chronicity and cavitation, and production of scar tissue during repair. Tubercle bacilli are found in solid caseous material, in liquid caseous material within tuberculous cavities, and also in white cells. The numerous bacilli in the liquid caseous material can lead to drug resistance, but the other tubercle bacilli are harder to kill and are responsible for relapse after treatment.

Although post-tussive rales may be present on inspiration, early tuberculosis is usually undetectable by physical examination. It is usually obvious on x-ray. If the chest x-ray is difficult to interpret, it can be very helpful to compare it with x-rays taken at an earlier date. In evaluating a patient with possible tuberculosis, it is very important to obtain a history of any illness resembling tuberculosis that the patient had at ages 15 to 30 years, for example, a pleural effusion.

## *Diagnosis*

Diagnosis depends on the tuberculin skin test, chest x-ray, and bacteriologic diagnosis. The tuberculin skin test, as noted previously, indicates the presence of tuberculous infection but does not distinguish between clinical and dormant infections. The chest x-ray indicating infiltration of the subclavicular region of the lung, particularly in the posterior aspect, is highly suggestive of tuberculosis. In the elderly and, frequently, in diabetics, lesions can be limited to the lower lobes. Pleural effusions as the initial pulmonary involvement of tuberculosis are being seen with increasing frequency in the elderly. Cavities should be looked for in the routine films and also on tomograms.

Tuberculosis can only be diagnosed definitively on the basis of isolation of *M. tuberculosis* from the sputum. The more tubercle bacilli there are in the sputum, the more likely that a direct smear of the sputum, stained with Ziehl-Neelsen or equivalent stain, will be positive. Three specimens of morning sputum should be sent for culture. Sputum should not be collected over a period of time, as this increases the yield of nonrelevant atypical mycobacteria. With fewer organisms in the sputum, the culture will be positive, but the direct smear will be negative.

Cultures, unfortunately, take about 4 to 6 weeks to become positive. The patient should be treated in the meantime. All cultures must be tested for drug sensitivity because approximately 5 to 10 per cent of cultures of specimens from patients from the United States are antibiotic resistant. This is true for between 25 to 55 per cent of cultures of specimens from patients from Asia or Mexico. In patients who have had previous treatment, the resistance rate to standard drugs is approximately three times that of people with no previous treatment.

Patients with positive direct smear require

isolation. With modern treatment the direct smears become negative in approximately 2 weeks, and the patient can then be removed from isolation.

**Differential Diagnosis.** Differential diagnosis has to be made from carcinoma of the lung. The best differentiation is made on three fresh sputum specimens studied for cytology and compared with three sputum specimens studied for tubercle bacilli. The two diseases can coexist. Bronchial brushing bronchoscopy and even thoracotomy may be necessary. Tuberculosis has to be differentiated from mycotic infections, particularly histoplasmosis and blastomycosis. Also, it must be distinguished from actinomycosis and nocardiosis. These diagnoses are based on the appropriate cultures. Aspiration pneumonia with or without lung abscess may also sometimes be confused with tuberculosis. The occurrence of tuberculosis is ten times greater in patients with chronic renal failure, many of whom are elderly, compared with age-matched controls. The involvement in these cases is predominantly extrapulmonary. These patients may be tuberculin negative, and biopsy diagnosis may be necessary.[5]

## *Treatment*

Tuberculosis is eminently treatable. It is also preventable. Isoniazid (INH) prophylaxis (300 mg in a single dose daily for 12 months) should be used in patients over age 35 who are tuberculin positive when they develop a new reaction and have additional risk factors, such as immunosuppression or a large, positive skin test and an abnormal chest x-ray, which although not diagnostic of tuberculosis, is highly suggestive. Daily users of alcohol should not receive this prophylaxis nor should patients with current chronic or subacute liver disease because it could predispose to hepatic toxicity. The drug should be dispensed at monthly intervals to monitor toxicity.

The drugs primarily used in the treatment of tuberculosis are isoniazid and rifampin; other drugs that may be used are listed in Table 45–2. The standard short-course chemotherapy is isoniazid (300 mg) and rifampin (600 mg) once daily for 9 months for adults.[16] This regimen is appropriate only in cases in which there is no drug resistance on culture and the disease is not extrapulmonary. Ethambutol is added if the patient is from an area with high drug resistance, primarily Asia, or has had previous treatment for tuberculosis. In patients who are poor compliers, such as alcoholics, one can change to supervised twice-weekly treatment at month two or month three through month nine. All patients are treated for 6 months after the last negative sputum *culture;* this usually involves a total course of 9 months. Patients should be followed for 12 months after the course of treatment. In patients undergoing supervised treatment twice weekly or three times weekly because of poor compliance, the doses used after 2 months of daily treatment should be as follows: isoniazid, 5 mg per kilogram orally; rifapin, 600 mg orally; and ethambutol, 15 mg per kilogram orally or streptomycin, 1 gm intramuscularly. Pyridoxine (Vitamin $B_6$), 50 mg daily, can be used for malnourished, very old, alcoholic, uremic, and diabetic patients and for patients with chronic neurologic disease, except epilepsy.

The most common mistake made in treating tuberculosis is to use INH and one other antituberculosis drug for Asian patients.[17] The next most common error is to use a single drug in patients from whom tubercle bacilli have been isolated. It is also an error to add a single drug to a failing regimen. At least two drugs must be added when results are unfavorable.

**Table 45–2.** PRIMARY AND SECONDARY ANTITUBERCULOSIS DRUGS—DAILY DOSES FOR ADULTS

| Primary Drugs | | Secondary Drugs* | |
|---|---|---|---|
| Isoniazid | 300 mg p.o.† | Kanamycin | 15 mg/kg IM‡§ |
| Ethambutol | 15 mg/kg p.o. | Ethionamide | 750 mg p.o. |
| Rifampin | 600 mg p.o. | Cycloserine | 500 mg p.o. |
| Streptomycin | 1 gm IM§‖ | Capreomycin | 1 gm IM daily for 120 days then 1 gm twice weekly§ |

Adapted from Kasik JE, Schuldt S: Why tuberculosis is still a health problem in the aged. Geriatrics 32:63, 1977; Centers for Disease Control: Guidelines for short-course tuberculosis chemotherapy. MMWR 29:97–105, 1980.

* These drugs are used for resistant or treatment failure patients.

† p.o. = by mouth.

‡ IM = intramuscularly.

§ Always check renal function before use and at intervals during treatment.

‖ Up to 8 weeks of therapy.

In *genitourinary tuberculosis* the best results are obtained with isoniazid, ethambutol, and streptomycin for 12 months. The results from using rifampin as one of the drugs are not yet available. Two drugs for 18 months have been used for *tuberculosis of the spine;* the results for three drugs are not yet available. Bed rest, mechanical restraint, or surgical debridement are of no benefit. Three-drug treatment is recommended for *tuberculous meningitis.*

### *Prognosis*

Before the availability of chemotherapy, approximately 30 per cent of tuberculosis patients were cured; another 30 per cent continued with positive sputum for 2 or more years; and about 40 per cent died of the disease. With modern treatment, 92 to 98 per cent of patients are cured. Death from tuberculosis is extremely rare.

## DIARRHEA

### *Incidence*

Diarrhea can be mild but is often severe in the elderly. Severe diarrhea can threaten life. The incidence of diarrhea in the elderly is greater than in young adults, but exact rates are not available. On a 1-day survey of a nursing home, one will find that a total of 16 per cent of patients will have infections and 1.5 per cent will have diarrhea. Outbreaks occurring in the closed population of a long-term care unit can be devastating.

### *Pathophysiology*

The elderly are particularly susceptible because of decreased gastric hydrochloric acid, decreased intestinal motility, and decreased mucosal immunity. The fecal flora in old people is very susceptible to change by antibiotics and to the overgrowth of toxin-producing organisms normally suppressed by the *Escherichia coli* and *Bacteroides* species of the gut. Certain diarrheas, such as those due to salmonellae, shigellae, and *Campylobacter* organisms, produce an outpouring of polymorphonuclear leukocytes that can be recognized on a Gram stain of the stool; others such as those due to viruses, do not.

### *Clinical Findings*

The clinical findings[18] in the elderly are similar in many respects to those encountered in younger adults but differ according to whether the cause of the diarrhea is a virus, a bacterium, or a toxin. Thirty-four per cent of diarrheas in the elderly are caused by viruses and 14 per cent by bacteria. A rare cause of diarrhea occurring in institutions is amebiasis.[19]

The viral diarrheas, caused by rotaviruses or parvoviruses, tend to have an abrupt onset and to be short-lived (1 to 5 days). The patient usually experiences malaise, anorexia, abdominal cramps, and voluminous watery stools without blood or mucus. Dehydration can be severe.

Thirty per cent of patients with bacterial diarrheas, as typified by shigellosis, have bloody stools; others have occult blood in the stool. The temperature usually rises sharply and there is tenesmus. Diarrheas caused by salmonellae usually follow a similar pattern. Enteritis due to *Campylobacter* organisms, in addition, causes severe abdominal pain. In these three diseases, the peripheral white cell count may or may not be raised. White blood cells are observed in the stool in 66 per cent of cases.

Patients with diarrhea associated with bacterial toxins are usually afebrile. Most typical of this type of diarrhea is traveler's diarrhea. It is usually caused by the toxins of enteropathogenic *E. coli* and occurs about 5 to 15 days after arrival in a foreign country. This disorder affects between 7 and 50 per cent of travelers, depending on the country visited. The lower figures relate to the northern, colder climates, and the higher figures to the more tropical climates. There is evidence that traveler's diarrhea can be reduced by prophylactic use of tetracycline or trimethoprim sulfamethoxazole, but many physicians prefer to wait to give the medication promptly on the occurrence of the first diarrheal stool. A similar type of diarrhea can occur after the use of antibiotics, especially clindamycin, tetracycline, or erythromycin but also, less frequently, ampicillin or penicillin. The normal flora are reduced, and there is an overgrowth of *Clostridium difficile,* which produces a toxin that induces diarrhea. A more severe toxic type of diarrhea occurs when food is contaminated with *Staphylococcus aureus,* which produces an enterotoxin. This is characterized by the very sudden onset of nausea and vomiting and, very shortly thereafter, a profuse watery diarrhea. So much fluid can be lost that the patient may faint or collapse. Toxin-associated diarrheas are not characteristically associated with peripheral leukocytosis, and leukocytes are not found in the Gram stain of the stool.

### *Diagnosis*

The diagnosis is made on the basis of the nature of the stool and Gram stain and stool culture for viruses and bacteria. When a large and spreading outbreak of diarrhea occurs in a nursing home, stool specimens should be sent quickly for culture to the state's public health laboratory. Some of these laboratories, but not all, are able to isolate viruses. All of them should be able to characterize salmonellae, shigellae, and *Campylobacter* organisms.

**Differential Diagnosis.** The differential diagnosis also involves ruling out fecal impaction (occurring in 16 per cent of diarrheas), laxative abuse (in 6 per cent), antibiotic use (in 11 per cent), and inflammatory bowel disease (in 4 per cent).

### *Treatment*

Treatment involves nonspecific therapy and the use of the appropriate antibiotic. It is therefore important to perform stool culture and sensitivity tests, and if faced with an outbreak of diarrhea in an institutional setting, to diagnose at least one patient carefully, using appropriate laboratory procedures.

Diarrhea caused by *Campylobacter* organisms will respond to erythromycin or tetracycline. Diarrhea caused by salmonellae and shigellae will respond to treatment with trimethobrim sulfamethoxazole, ampicillin, tetracycline, or chloramphenicol, according to the sensitivities of the local organisms. Patients should be monitored very carefully for fluid intake and output and for fever. An ideal mixture for oral replacement of fluids is 3.5 gm of sodium chloride (1 teaspoonful), 2.5 gm of sodium bicarbonate (1 heaping teaspoonful baking soda), 2.5 gm potassium chloride (1 teaspoon) and 20 gm glucose (4 heaping teaspoonfuls). A pharmacist can make up this mixture in a foil packet. The contents are added to a liter or a quart of water when needed. When elderly people travel, they can take packets of this salt mixture with them. If five to ten stools occur per day, at least 1 L of this fluid should be taken daily. If ten or more stools occur per day, 2 L should be given daily. Opiates and diphenoxylate (Lomotil) should be avoided because they prevent the excretion of toxins and bacteria.

### *Prognosis*

The prognosis of diarrhea in the elderly is variable. It is known that the mortality of elderly people with enteritis resulting from rotaviruses is 2 per cent. Fatality rates from shigellosis or salmonellosis average 2 to 5 per cent in the population as a whole but are probably higher in the elderly (approximately 10 per cent). Two thirds of all diarrheas subside within 7 days, and three quarters within 14 days. About 5 per cent of elderly diarrhea patients will develop cardiovascular or respiratory complications. An outbreak of diarrhea in a long-term care unit usually lasts for from 4 to 6 weeks. General hygienic and isolation procedures are indicated. Sanitary disposal of human feces and the maintenance of clean bathrooms are essential. Provision should be made for suitable handwashing facilities. Scrupulous cleanliness in the preparation and handling of all foods is necessary. Infected patients should be isolated until a diagnosis is made. Patients with diarrhea in a nursing home should be kept in one area of the home. Attendants with diarrhea should be given sick leave.

## APPENDICITIS

Because appendicitis is considered to be a disease of children, it is frequently missed in the elderly, in whom it evolves more rapidly. Appropriate surgical care is urgently needed to treat this condition.

### *Incidence*

The incidence in children is 140 per 100,000, and in patients over 65 it is approximately 20 per 100,000. Therefore, appendicitis accounts for about 1.64 per 1000 hospital admissions of elderly patients. The pathophysiology of the disease in the elderly does not differ from that in children except for the more rapid course.

### *Clinical Findings*

Although 75 per cent of elderly patients with appendicitis present with typical clinical findings, the 25 per cent with unusual clinical pictures are difficult to diagnose.[20] Vomiting occurs in 33 per cent (compared with 72 per cent in children). Shaking chills occur in 21 per cent (compared with 8 per cent in children). Nausea and vomiting may be absent. Only about 70 per cent of elderly patients are tender over McBurney's point. Still fewer exhibit tenderness on rectal examination. About 40 per cent have rebound tenderness only. Guarding is present in 71 per cent (compared with 77 per cent in children). Thirteen per cent of elderly patients with appendicitis fail to develop peripheral leukocytosis. Because of these problems, there is a lapse of 72 hours in making the diagnosis in 18 per cent of the elderly compared with 6 per cent of children. Related to this, perforation occurs in 46 per cent of elderly patients with appendicitis (compared with 18 per cent of children) and abscess in 30 per cent (compared with 10 per cent in children). Drains are needed in 37 per cent of elderly patients (compared with 14 per cent of children).

Although the clinical manifestations of appendicitis are attenuated in a number of elderly people, as noted previously, others will exhibit more classic manifestations. The differential diagnosis includes renal disease, diverticulitis, and obstruction associated with neoplasm. Twenty-six per cent of appendicitis cases are misdiagnosed in the elderly compared with 6 per cent of cases in the young.

### *Treatment*

The treatment is primarily surgical. Because of the frequency of perforation in the elderly, surgery should be combined with an antibiotic regimen likely to cover the bowel flora, such as a cephalosporin with clindamycin.[21] The earlier the operation is performed, the better the prognosis. Peritoneal lavage is required in 30 per cent of the elderly compared with 14 per cent of children. It is very important to identify underlying disease, such as unrecognized congestive cardiac failure or pulmonary embolus. The overall fatality rate in the elderly is 5 to 10 per cent compared with 0.1 to 0.3 per cent in children.

## DIVERTICULITIS[22]

Please see Chapter 46, page 566, for information on diverticulitis.

## HEPATITIS[23]

Although 60 to 85 per cent of the elderly have antibodies to hepatitis A and 32 per cent to hepatitis B,[24,25] hepatitis can occur in the elderly. About half the cases are caused by the B virus; about one third by the A virus; and about one fifth by the non-A, non-B virus. The presentation of hepatitis in the elderly is very similar to that in young people, but other diseases are usually suspected rather than hepatitis. Women particularly may have a severe form of hepatitis. Up to 40 per cent of cases in women are of the severe form, and 15 per cent of these severe cases die. Weight loss and jaundice may lead one to think of cancer, but an exploratory laparotomy in hepatitis is extremely dangerous, having a 66 per cent fatality rate. Hepatitis antigen and antibodies should be looked for in the serum. The aims of treatment are adequate nutrition, relief of symptoms, and avoidance of further liver injury by inappropriate drugs. In a nursing home outbreak of hepatitis B it must be remembered that discharges from decubitis ulcers and materials contaminated with blood are infectious. (Nail brushes, for example, can spread the disease.)

## SEPTICEMIA AND BACTERIAL ENDOCARDITIS IN THE ELDERLY

### *Incidence*

The annual admission rate in an acute-care hospital for septicemia is 35 or less per 1000 for patients age 50 and younger, 40 per 1000 for patients age 50 to 59, 48 per 1000 for persons 60 to 69 years, and 50 per 1000 for individuals age 70 and over. Patients aged 65 and over make up approximately 50 per cent of all people with septicemia. Septicemia occurs in twice as many men as women. Endocarditis in the elderly makes up approximately 25 per cent of all endocarditis cases. It occurs in four times as many men as women.

### *Pathophysiology*

About 50 per cent of patients with septicemia have a severe underlying disease. This may be cancer or neutropenia, or both. It can also be rheumatoid arthritis, an infected urinary tract, pneumonia, or biliary tract disease. Patients who are particularly susceptible are those whose white cell count has fallen below 500 polymorphonuclear leukocytes per cubic millimeter. In younger patients, the majority of those who develop endocarditis have underlying heart disease, but in the elderly this disease occurs on apparently normal heart valves in 30 per cent. In the elderly, calcified valves are found in 30 per cent, rheumatic valves in 35 per cent, and a floppy mitral valve in 5 per cent. About one third of cases involve the aortic valve, one third the mitral valve, and one third both.

## *Clinical Findings*

In 70 to 85 per cent of elderly patients, the onset of these diseases is typical. That is, the patient frequently complains of a shaking chill and fever, and leukocytosis is found. There may be a history of a preceding illness such as pneumonia or urinary tract infection. Endocarditis presents with the same symptom complex as septicemia, with the added finding of embolization, often manifested by petechiae in the conjuctivae or subcutaneous hemorrhages in the hands and feet. The classic finding of Osler's nodes or Janeway lesions is rare. About half the patients with endocarditis develop congestive heart failure. Patients may suddenly develop uremia, caused by embolization of the kidney and indicated by red blood cells in the urine.[26-33]

In both endocarditis and septicemia, perhaps 20 to 30 per cent of elderly patients present atypically. In both diseases, confusion is common in elderly patients. Fever is absent in 12 per cent of the elderly, compared with 4 per cent of younger patients. Fifteen to thirty per cent of older patients with endocarditis do not have a heart murmur. Therefore, any patient who is confused or febrile, or both, for longer than a week should have blood cultures performed. The blood culture bottle is a useful piece of apparatus to carry in one's professional bag. One should suspect endocarditis particularly in elderly patients who do poorly after surgical operations, especially when they are febrile or confused. In any patient with a bed sore who develops shaking chills, blood cultures should be performed. The same is true in diabetics with ulcers or gangrene and shaking chills. Endocarditis is suspected clinically in only 30 per cent of elderly patients in whom the diagnosis is eventually made, compared with 90 per cent accuracy of suspicion in younger patients.

The examination of a patient suspected of having endocarditis includes a careful search for septic foci in the skin or elsewhere. In addition, one should look carefully for rashes, large lymph nodes, petechiae (particularly in the conjuctivae), and red blood cells in the urine. The patient should be monitored carefully in regard to mental clarity, blood pressure, and urinary output. The survival of the patient depends on careful and accurate diagnosis and treatment with the correct antibiotics for an adequate time. If adequate investigation cannot be done, for example in the long-term care unit, the patient should be transferred promptly to an acute-care hospital.

## *Diagnosis*

Patients who have a temperature of 101° F or higher for 7 days or longer should have blood drawn for culture.[32] If there is no evidence of endocarditis, three blood cultures taken 2 hours apart are adequate. If a heart murmur is heard or embolization is suspected, then five should be taken at 2-hour intervals. There is no benefit to be derived from drawing blood for culture at times of rising or falling temperature. The number of bacteria in the blood stream are always adequate for growth, although the total numbers may vary. Any patient who has two or more lobes involved with pneumonia should have a blood culture performed, as does any patient with meningitis or peritonitis. A single blood culture is accurate in 80 per cent of patients not on antibiotics, three blood cultures will accurately diagnose 96 per cent of all cases of septicemia and five blood cultures will accurately diagnose 96 per cent of all endocarditis cases. The cultures usually become positive within 3 days. However, with modern radioactive blood culture techniques, a diagnosis can be made in 12 to 24 hours.

Misdiagnoses occur in approximately one third of patients with endocarditis or septicemia, and late diagnoses are made in about one fifth. In 10 to 25 per cent of patients, no source of origin for the septicemia will be found. It is important to differentiate between septicemia and endocarditis because the organisms that cause each disease are different from one another and the length of treatment is different.[31,32]

**Differential Diagnosis.** Life-threatening septicemia or endocarditis has to be recognized among patients with fever from various causes. For example, the prognosis of the patient with pneumococcal pneumonia *with* septicemia is significantly worse than that of a similar patient with pneumonia *without* septicemia. Patients with endocarditis may be treated mistakenly for congestive cardiac failure of undetermined type. In endocarditis, hematuria may make the physician think that the patient has renal disease. With renal failure (which is common in the elderly and particularly common in those with endocarditis), fever may be lessened. Weight loss can occur over a period of weeks and may confuse the physician, who may diagnose cancer of undetermined origin.

## *Treatment*

It is important to treat the patient on the basis of reasonable clinical suspicion after adequate cultures have been taken as detailed earlier. If a serious illness like endocarditis or septicemia occurs in a nursing home, there are certain ways to avoid delay in treatment. Cultures can be performed and the patient started on treatment while both the culture bottle and the patient are sent to the acute-care hospital. If the patient has septicemia, the most common organisms causing this condition are *E. coli, S. aureus, Klebsiella* species, and *Bacteroides* species. The first three would be covered by nafcillin and gentamicin, and the last would require the addition of clindamycin. In contrast, the common organisms causing endocarditis are *S. viridans, S. aureus,* and *S. epidermidis* (Table 45–1). If the disease is due to *S. viridans,* there is usually a minor degree of anemia, with hemoglobin around 12 to 13 gm, and a white blood cell count usually under 14,000. In contrast to this, the patient with staphylococcal endocarditis usually has a hemoglobin of 10 gm or less and a white cell count of 15,000 or higher.[33] In patients suspected of having endocarditis due to *S. viridans,* penicillin G (20 million units intravenous daily) is indicated. If the endocarditis is due to a staphylococcus, methicillin or nafcillin (12 gm daily intravenously) is used, with or without gentamicin for the first week of treatment.[34,35] If the patient is allergic to penicillin, there are two courses that can be followed: a cephalosporin can be substituted (if the adverse reaction is other than an anaphylactic type of response); alternatively, the patient can undergo a skin test for sensitivity to the penicillins using penicilloic acid and aged penicillin (penicillin stored in the refrigerator for 3 months or longer). If the skin test is positive and yet penicillin still appears to be the drug of choice, the patient may be treated with the administration at half-hour intervals of 1 unit of penicillin G intradermally, 10 units intradermally, 10 intramuscularly, and then 100 or 1000 units intramuscularly, while monitoring the systolic blood pressure. Any fall of systolic pressure greater than 20 mm indicates the need for treatment with 0.3 ml epinephrine subcutaneously for anaphylaxis.[10] The antibiotic sensitivities of commonly occurring organisms are shown in Table 45–3.

Abscesses should be incised and drained because death from overwhelming infection occurs when the total number of organisms approximates $10^{13}$ per a 70 kg patient. About $10^{8}$ organisms can be removed by incising and draining a large abscess. Any underlying disease must also be treated, as the diversion of energy by a serious infection can cause organ systems with borderline function to fail (i.e., heart, respiratory, or renal failure). The temperature should be followed, particularly in the evening. If the patient is receiving appropriate treatment, there should be no rise of temperature after 24 to 48 hours, and preferably a fall. Serum bactericidal levels must be determined; that is, the patient's own organisms from the blood culture bottle should be titrated against the patient's own antibiotic-containing serum.

## *Prognosis*

The main complications that worsen the prognosis of patients with endocarditis or septicemia are the development of septic shock, as demonstrated by a fall in blood pressure; reduction in urinary output; and the development of confusion and drowsiness. Congestive cardiac failure or an arrhythmia may also develop. Embolization can also occur in endocarditis, but it is usually not as severe as the preceding complications. Untreated septicemia is 90 to 95 per cent fatal in all age groups and probably 100 per cent fatal in elderly patients. If untreated, endocarditis is probably 100 per cent fatal in all age groups. With appropriate treatment for the appropriate length of time, patients over 65 years of age with endocarditis, without underlying complicating disease, still have a 20 to 30 per cent fatality rate. If underlying disease is present and is likely to cause death within a year, the fatality rate is likely to be 80 per cent; if death is likely to occur from underlying disease within 5 years, the fatality rate is approximately 40 per cent. If the physician has inadequate experience in treating these diseases, the patient should be transferred rapidly to someone who does have this experience.

## *Prevention*

Prompt treatment of any septic condition in the skin or urinary tract is a prophylactic measure against the development of complicating septicemia. Because endocarditis is so difficult to diagnose and cure, prophylaxis is particularly important.

The duration of treatment for uncomplicated septicemia with highly sensitive organisms such as pneumococcus is 2 weeks. If staphylococcal infection follows infection caused by an indwelling catheter, which can be removed easily,

**Table 45–3.** ANTIBIOTIC SENSITIVITIES OF COMMONLY OCCURRING ORGANISMS*

| | Ampicillin | Cephalothin | Gentamicin/ Tobramycin | Tetracycline | Carbeni-cillin | Chloram-phenicol | Amikacin | Trimetho-prim-Sulfa-methox-azole | Clindamycin | Erythro-mycin | Methicillin | Penicillin G | Vancomycin |
|---|---|---|---|---|---|---|---|---|---|---|---|---|---|
| *Escherichia coli* | I[†] | I | S[‡] | I | I | S | S | S | | | | | |
| *Pseudomonas aeruginosa* | R[§] | R | S | R | S | R | S | R | | | | | |
| *Klebsiella pneumoniae* | R | I | S | I | R | S | S | S | | | | | |
| *Enterobacter* | R | R | S | I | I | S | S | S | | | | | |
| *Proteus mirabilis* | S | S | S | I | S | S | S | S | | | | | |
| Other *Proteus* species | R | R | S | R | I | I | S | S | | | | | |
| *Hemophilus influenzae* | I | I | S | S | S | S | S | S | | | | | |
| *Serratia* | R | R | S | R | I | R | S | I | | | | | |
| *Salmonella* | I | I | I | I | | S | S | I | | | | | |
| *Shigella* | I | I | S | | | I | | S | | | | | |
| *Staphylococcus aureus* | R | S | S | I | R | I | | | S | S | S | R | S |
| *Staphylococcus epidermidis* | R | S | I | R | R | S | I | S | R | R | R | R | S |
| *Enterococcus*[‖] | S | R | R | R | S | S | R | | R | R | R | I | S |
| *Streptococcus pyogenes* | S | S | R | R | S | S | R | | S | S | S | S | S |
| *Streptococcus pneumoniae* | S | S | R | R | S | S | R | | S | I | R | S | S |
| *Bacteroides fragilis* | R | R | R | I | I | S | R | | S | I | R | R | |

* This table is constructed from a combination of my personal experience and a survey of the literature. It is very important for physicians to correct the table to conform to their own experience and laboratory results.
[†] I = intermediate (75–90 per cent of strains susceptible).
[‡] S = sensitive (90 per cent of strains susceptible).
[§] R = resistant (less than 75 per cent of strains susceptible).
[‖] Usually responds to a penicillin aminoglycoside combination.

a 2-week course is also adequate; most other septicemias require 4 weeks of treatment.[36–38] In contrast to this, endocarditis on a natural valve requires 6 weeks for treatment and endocarditis on a prosthetic valve requires at least 6 to 12 weeks of treatment.[39–42]

## SKIN INFECTIONS

The incidence of wound infections increases with age. Rates of 10 per cent have been described after colon resection and 15 per cent after hysterectomy.[32]

Elderly dependent patients are predisposed to burns, and 25 per cent of all deaths from burns are due to infection. Applications of 0.5 per cent silver nitrate or mafenide (Sulfamylon) or silver sulfadizine cream are applied locally. Systemic antibiotics should be used primarily to combat infections indicated by positive cultures from the blood or other sources.

Skin infections in diabetics are frequent and can be serious.[43] Pulses in the legs are often absent and the skin may be anesthetic. Injuries or nail cuttings can become infected easily and are usually infected by stool on the patient's hands after defecating. This results in a polymicrobial infection with two or three aerobes, such as *E. coli* and *S. aureus,* and two or three anaerobes such as bacteroides, anaerobic streptococci, or anaerobic staphylococci. About half these diabetics are on insulin, and increased insulin requirements will develop with the infection. Most of these patients have had diabetes for 13 or more years, and therefore, renal function should be monitored when administering antibiotics. A suitable antibiotic combination to treat them with would be gentamicin and clindamycin.

Decubitus ulcers or pressure sores occur frequently in the frail elderly, 70 per cent of them being found in people over age 70.[44–48] Again, the infection is usually polymicrobial and of fecal derivation. Septicemia often develops, and when it does, the fatality rate is about 50 per cent. All patients with decubitus ulcers and shaking chills should have a blood culture performed. Local treatment is important, as well as systemic therapy with antianaerobic antibiotics such as clindamycin. Enzymatic methods of debridement can be useful. Antipressure padding and water mattresses are also helpful.

Herpes zoster occurs primarily in the elderly, particularly in patients over 80 years. A unilateral, painful vesicular eruption develops in one or two dermatomes. Scraping of the base and staining will show multinuclear giant cells. A bandlike pattern of grouped papules is topped by clear vesicles within 12 to 24 hours. These progress to pustules in 72 hours. In 7 to 8 days the pustules begin to crust and dry up; they fall off in 2 to 3 weeks. The dermatomes involved are in a thoracic area in half the patients, the neck area in 15 per cent, the lumbar area in 10 per cent, and the sacral area in 5 per cent. The incidence of postherpetic neuralgia increases with age, occurring in about 75 per cent of untreated elderly patients, but in only 30 per cent of those treated with steroids, such as prednisone 60 mg per day for the first week, 30 mg per day for the second week, and 20 mg per day for the third week.[48–50] Herpes zoster in the trigeminal area represents a hazard to the eye. Patients with vesicles on the tip of their nose should be examined carefully for corneal damage and referred to an ophthalmologist.

## USE OF ANTIBIOTICS

When confronted with an infection, the physician should ask himself or herself whether the infectious agent will respond to penicillin G (pneumococci, streptococci, gonococci, meningococci or gram-positive rods, and spirochetes). Is it a staphylococcal infection, such as boils or wound infections, and will it respond to the semisynthetic penicillins? Is it a mild gram-negative rod infection, such as urinary tract infection or wound infection, and therefore, will it respond to ampicillin, the cephalosporins, or trimethoprim sulfamethoxazole? Is it a severe life-threatening gram-negative rod infection of the blood stream or lung, requiring more toxic medications such as gentamicin, trimethoprim sulfamethoxazole, or carbenicillin? And finally, does the patient have an anaerobic infection, such as abscesses of the brain, lung, abdomen, or female genital tract; decubitus ulcers; or diabetic ulcers, requiring clindamycin, chloramphenicol, or carbenicillin?[10,30]

### References


1. Esposito AL, Gleckman RA: Fever of unknown origin in the elderly. J Am Geriatr Soc 26:498, 1978.
2. Smith IM: Infections in the elderly. *In* Steinberg FU (ed.): Care of the Geriatric Patient in the Tradition of E.V. Cowdry. St. Louis, C.V. Mosby Co, 1983.
3. Gowda HT: Influenza in a geriatric unit. Postgrad Med J 55:188, 1979.
4. Mathur U, Bentley DW, Hall CV: Concurrent respiratory syncytial virus in influenza A infections in the institutionalized elderly and clinically ill. Ann Intern Med 93:49, 1980.
5. Valenti WM, Trudell RG, Bentley DW: Factors predisposing to oropharyngeal colonization with gram-

negative bacilli in the aged. New Engl J Med 298:1108, 1978.

6. Ebright JR, Rytel MW. Bacterial pneumonia in the elderly. J Am Geriatr Soc 28:220, 1980.
7. Helms M, Vines JP, Sturm RH, et al: Comparative features of pneumococcal, mycoplasmal, and Legionnaires' disease pneumonias. Ann Intern Med 90:543, 1979.
8. Helms CM, Renner ED, Viner JP, et al: Legionnaires' disease among pneumonias in Iowa (FY 1972–1978). J Iowa Med Soc 71:335, 1981.
9. Smith IM, Wilson AP, Hazard EC, et al: Death from staphylococci in mice. J Infect Dis 107:369, 1960.
10. Smith IM, Habte-Gabr E: Life-threatening infections: How to choose the right antibiotics. Geriatrics 32:83, 1977.
11. Frazier DW: Tsai TR, Orenstein W, et al: Legionnaires' disease: description of an epidemic of pneumonia. N Engl J Med 297:1189, 1977.
12. Stead WW: Tuberculosis among elderly persons: An outbreak in a nursing home. Ann Intern Med 94:606, 1981.
13. Kasik JE, Schuldt S: Why tuberculosis is still a health problem in the aged. Geriatrics 32:63, 1977.
14. Thompson NL: The booster phenomenon in serial tuberculin testing. Am Rev Resp Dis 119:587, 1979.
15. Anonymous: Tuberculosis in chronic renal failure. Lancet 1:909, 1980.
16. Centers for Disease Control: Guidelines for short-course tuberculosis chemotherapy. MMWR 29:97–105, 1980.
17. Byrd RB, Horn BR, Solomon DA, Griggs GA, Wilder NJ: Treatment of tuberculosis by nonpulmonary physician. Ann Intern Med 86:799, 1977.
18. Dusdieker NS: Diarrhea in the elderly. *In* Smith IM (ed.): Medical Care for the Elderly. New York, Spectrum Publishers, 1982.
19. Pentlund B, Penington CR: Acute diarrhea in the elderly. Age Ageing 9:90, 1980.
20. Yusuf MF, Dunn E: Appendicitis in the elderly: Learn to discern the untypical picture. Geriatrics 34:73, 1979.
21. Berne TV, Yellin AW, Eppleman MD, Haseltine PNR: Antibiotic management of surgically treated gangrenous or perforated appendicitis. Am J Surg 144:8, 1982.
22. Burakoff R: An up-dated look at diverticular disease. Geriatrics 36:83, 1981.
23. Soltis RD: New concepts in viral hepatitis. Geriatrics 36:62, 1981.
24. Weiland O, Berg JV, Böttinger M, et al: Prevalence of antibody against hepatitis A in Sweden in relation to age and type of community. Scand J Infect Dis 12:171, 1980.
25. Finkelstein MS, Freedman ML, Shenckman L, Krugman S: Evidence of prior hepatitis B and hepatitis A virus infections in an ambulatory geriatric population. J Gerontol 35:302, 1981.
26. Esposito AL, Gleckman RA, Cram S, et al: Community-acquired bacteremia in the elderly: Analysis of 100 consecutive episodes. J Am Geriatr Soc 28:315, 1980.
27. Robbins N, Demaria A, Miller MH: Infective endocarditis in the elderly. South Med J 73:1335, 1980.
28. Habte-Gabr E, January LE, Smith IM: Bacterial endocarditis: The need for early diagnosis. Geriatrics 28:164, 1973.
29. Madden JW, Croker JR, Beynon GPJ: Septicemia in the elderly. Postgrad Med J 57:502, 1981.
30. Gleckman R, Hibert D: Afebrile bacteremia: A phenomenon in geriatric patients. JAMA 248:1478, 1982.
31. Denham MJ, Goodwin GS: The value of blood cultures in geriatric practice. Age Ageing 6:85, 1977.
32. Smith IM: Infections in the elderly. Hosp Pract 17:69, 1982.
33. Smith IM, Vickers AB: Natural history of 338 treated and untreated patients with staphylococcal septicaemia (1936–1955). Lancet 1:1318, 1960.
34. Sande MA: Experimental endocarditis. *In* Kaye D (ed.): Infective Endocarditis. Baltimore, University Park Press, 1976.
35. Wright AJN, Wilson WR: Experimental animal endocarditis. Mayo Clin Proc 57:10, 1982.
36. Deralgie H, Garrod JP: Secondary septicemia from intravenous cannulae. Br Med J 2:481, 1969.
37. Bentley DW, Leher MH: Septicemia therapy of staphylococcus aureus. Bacteremias associated with removable focus of infection. Ann Intern Med 84:558, 1976.
38. Watanakunakorn C, Baird IM: Staphylococcus aureus bacteremia and endocarditis associated with a removable infected intravenous device. Am J Med 63:253, 1977.
39. Slaughter L, Morris JE, Star A: Prosthetic valve endocarditis. A twelve-year review. Circulation 47:1319, 1973.
40. Wilson WR, Danielson GK, Giuliani ER, et al: Prosthetic valve endocarditis. Mayo Clin Proc 57:155, 1982.
41. McCabe WR: Gram-negative bacteremia. Medical Microbiology and Infectious Diseases. Philadelphia, W.B. Saunders Co., 1981.
42. Perry M, Neu HC: A comparative study of ticarcillin plus tobramycin or carbenicillin plus gentamycin for the treatment of serious infections due to gram-negative bacilli. Am J Med 64:961, 1978.
43. Bessman AN, Wagner W: Nonclostridial gas gangrene: Report 48 cases and a review of the literature. JAMA 233:958, 1975.
44. Lowe TJ, Bartlett JG, Talley FP, Gorbach SL: Aerobic and anaerobic bacteria in diabetic foot ulcers. Ann Intern Med 85:461, 1976.
45. Peromet M, Labbe M, Yourarsowski E, Schoutens E: Anaerobic Bacteria Isolated from Decubitus Ulcers. Infection I. 205, 1973.
46. Galpin JE, Chou AW, Bayer AS, Guze LB: Sepsis associated with decubitus ulcers. Am J Med 61:346, 1976.
47. Russing JP, Crowder JG, Dunfee T, White A: Bacteroides bacteremia from decubitus ulcers. South Med J 67:1179, 1974.
48. Eaglestein WH, Katz R, Brown JA: The effects of early corticosteroid therapy on the skin eruption and pain of herpes zoster. JAMA 211:1681, 1970.
49. Gafland ML: Treatment of herpes zoster with cortisone. JAMA 154:911, 1954.
50. Elliott FA: Treatment of herpes zoster with high doses of prednisone. Lancet 2:610, 1954.

## Chapter 46

# Gastrointestinal Diseases

*Manuel Sklar*

Aging is associated with many morphologic and physiologic changes in the gastrointestinal (GI) tract. These lead to increased vulnerability to cancer of the GI tract, diverticular disease of the colon, and mesenteric vascular insufficiency with persistent liability to hiatal hernia disease, peptic ulcer, and functional bowel distress. Each of these conditions is influenced in its course, presentation, and management by nutritional, psychologic, social, and economic factors, many of which are age related. These factors are often found in the context of other diseases, conditions involving other body systems. Symptoms may be atypical or blunted. Treatment may be complicated by unpredictable sensitivity to drugs or other drug reactions as well as by lack of patient compliance. Thus, the aged patient with gastrointestinal disease offers a great challenge to the physician.

The true prevalence of GI disorders in the geriatric age group can only be estimated. In Table 46-1 the eight most frequent diagnoses established in a group of 900 patients over the age of 65 are listed.[1] These patients constitute three separate population groups of 300 each, personally managed in a private office, university outpatient clinic, and community hospital, respectively. The most frequent diagnosis established after a thorough investigation and follow-up of a year or more was functional bowel distress. The most common indication for admission to the hospital was upper GI hemorrhage; cancer of the gastrointestinal tract was the most common gastrointestinal diagnosis at the time of discharge from the hospital.

## CHANGES ASSOCIATED WITH NORMAL AGING

Physiologic and morphologic changes associated with aging have been reported for many years, but in general, the information is sketchy, and there has been a paucity of good studies in recent years. In addition, it has been difficult to differentiate whether the changes observed were due to aging per se or to coincidental disease.

Gradual deterioration in the morphology and physiology of many oral structures is characteristic of the aging process (see Chapter 40).[2] These changes may lead to nutritional and digestive difficulties. Changes in esophageal function include a decreased peristaltic response and often increased nonperistaltic response as well. Transit time is delayed, and the lower esophageal sphincter often becomes incompetent,[3] resulting in reflux esophagitis. The so-called corkscrew esophagus, or presbyesophagus, results from a prolonged spastic contraction of ringlike segments of the distal two thirds of the esophagus. There is increased frequency of hiatal hernia in the elderly, but most individuals are asymptomatic. Gastric motility is impaired and gastric secretion usually associated with atrophic mucosa is reduced, with decrease in acid and pepsin concentration. The low acid environment may impair absorption of iron and vitamin $B_{12}$. The small intestine may also atrophy, fibrous tissue replacing parenchyma and villi becoming broader and shorter, contributing to subclinical degrees of malabsorption. It has been suggested that selective defects in amino acid absorption occurs, and there is evidence of impaired carbohydrate absorption as measured by the D-xylose study. Absorption of fat may be impaired, and in some instances this abnormality can be modified by adding lipase to the diet, suggesting a decrease in pancreatic function.

Fecal incontinence may become a problem. Manometric studies of the reflex responses of the internal and external sphincters have demonstrated that aged incontinent patients have a normal internal sphincter reflex but lack exter-

**Table 46-1.** MOST COMMON DIAGNOSES IN 900 PATIENTS OVER 65

| | |
|---|---|
| Functional bowel distress | 31% |
| Peptic ulcer disease | 16% |
| Neoplasm | 15% |
| Diverticular disease | 7% |
| Inflammatory bowel disease | 7% |
| Hiatal hernia | 6% |
| Cholelithiasis | 5% |
| Liver disease | 4% |
| Miscellaneous (achalasia, anorectal disease, pancreatitis, intestinal obstruction, post-gastrectomy syndrome, ischemic bowel disease, etc.) | 9% |

nal sphincter response. Normally, these two sphincters function in a coordinated fashion, controlling the passage of gas without loss of stool. The failure of this competency may lead to fecal incontinence.[4]

Aging is associated with a decrease in the weight and size of the liver. There is a decrease in the number of hepatic cells and their mitochondria, but it has been established that there is also a compensatory increase in the volume of both. As their mitochondria age, cells seem to function more actively but have a more limited reserve power, becoming more readily exhausted. These changes are due to reduced ability of regeneration, modified by environmental and possibly nutritional conditions. Decreasing functional capacity of the liver is demonstrated by impairment in uptake of Bromsulphalein (BSP) dye in part related to a decrease in hepatic blood flow, capacity to metabolize various drugs, and ability to synthesize free cholesterol.[5]

## FUNCTIONAL DISORDERS OF THE GASTROINTESTINAL TRACT

### *Functional Bowel Syndrome*

Diseases of the GI tract manifest themselves in many ways. Insidious anorexia and weight loss may result from a malignancy of the stomach or pancreas but also may be a manifestation of depression. Conversely, an acute onset of depression may be associated with the development of an occult malignancy. Difficulty in swallowing must always be considered a signal of organic disease, but it may also result from neurologic or functional causes. Although upper abdominal discomfort, heartburn, nausea and vomiting, lower abdominal distress, bloating, distention, flatulence and bowel irregularity, constipation, or diarrhea may herald a serious GI disorder, in many instances, no organic cause can be established. These patients must be diagnosed as having a functional bowel disorder. This is the most common gastrointestinal illness found in all patients, including those in the geriatric age group.

A functional bowel disorder is a syndrome characterized by symptoms of apparent gastrointestinal origin, occurring in the absence of demonstrable organic disease. Functional bowel distress, psychophysiologic gastrointestinal disturbance, spastic colon, mucous colitis, and irritable bowel syndrome are commonly employed synonyms. The irritable bowel syndrome is associated with an increase in sigmoid colonic pressures, which correlate with abdominal pain and constipation, and an increase in manometric response to cholinergic agents, cholecystokinin, and feeding. Patients with irritable bowel syndrome have also been shown to have abnormal basal electrical activity compared with controls. Furthermore, it has been demonstrated that the infusion of gas into the rectum of patients with irritable bowel syndrome produces pain with lesser pressure than in control patients.[6]

The diagnosis of functional bowel syndrome is often suspected by history. Symptoms may be continuous and long-standing, or recurrent over years. The abdominal discomfort is often diffuse and vague and often related to dietary indiscretion or stress. Recent onset of symptoms is often correlated with an illness or death of a friend or family member. Poverty, estrangement from children, moving from an old home, and recognition of mortality are factors that frequently precipitate symptoms. Often, somatic feelings that were never before a concern assume life-threatening proportions in the mind of the patient. Organic brain syndromes related to cerebrovascular diseases or senile dementia of the Alzheimer type may also be associated with functional GI symptoms.

The physician may make a provisional diagnosis of this condition after taking a careful history; performing a thorough physical examination, including sigmoidoscopy; and performing laboratory studies, including a complete blood count, sequential multichannel autoanalyzer (SMA) 12, sedimentation rate, and at least three stool tests for occult blood. At this point, the physician may be faced with a dilemma. Should he or she subject this elderly patient to a complete GI investigation (an abdominal ultrasound and upper GI and lower GI series) or should he or she undertake a therapeutic trial? Clinical wisdom suggests that the more conservative approach is usually correct. If, after several weeks, satisfactory improvement does not occur, a thorough investigation is mandatory, and in the old and infirm, hospitalization may be justified in many instances. At this time, endoscopic examination of the upper gastrointestinal tract and colon must be included if radiologic findings are negative and the significant symptoms such as upper abdominal pain or diarrhea persist. Computerized tomography of the abdomen may also be helpful.

Management of the functional bowel syndrome includes reassurance, supportive psychotherapy, dietary regulation, and judicious administration of medication such as antacids, anti-spasmodics, bulk agents such as Metamucil, and, if required, psychoactive agents. Reassurance as to the innocent nature of the illness is the best type of psychotherapy. This includes a careful explanation of the nature of the disorder and physiologic mechanisms involved and the relationship of the symptoms to dietary and emotional factors. It must be emphasized that the symptoms experienced are real and not imaginary. Never is the patient to be told "it's all in your head." Air swallowing can explain belching, acid reflux is an easily understood cause of heartburn, increase in sigmoid pressures can explain the lower abdominal pain and constipation. Patients appreciate and usually accept thoughtful and rational explanations expressed in a confident manner.

Dietary manipulation should include the prescription of a nutritious and tasteful diet high in fiber and low in roughage (Table 46–2). The concept of a bland diet is to be avoided. The diet should be nutritious and tasteful. It is reasonable to eliminate any foods that the patient recognizes as causing symptoms. The theory that a high fiber diet is beneficial has been widely endorsed since the classic work of Painter and Burkitt.[7] The physiologic function of fiber includes increasing fecal bulk, shortening transit time, and altering bile metabolism.[8] Clinical experience, however, indicates that not all forms of fiber are well tolerated in the patient with irritable bowel syndrome. Raw fruits and raw vegetables may produce discomfort in such patients and should be restricted. These foods consist largely of cellulose, a linear polysaccharide, as opposed to bran and cereal products, which are composed largely of hemicellulose, whose structure is that of a complex branched carbohydrate polymer. Bran has been shown to increase the bulk and wet content of the stool significantly, compared with fruits and vegetables. Bran and the cereal grains are well tolerated in patients with irritable bowel syndrome and assist in normalizing bowel function. Cooking raw fruit or vegetables does change their physical and chemical structure, so that they may be included in the diet. Thus the concept has evolved of a high fiber, low roughage diet. As the patient's condition improves, the diet should be liberalized with the gradual addition of other foods. Basically, patients must learn for themselves what foods they can best tolerate.

**Table 46–2.** THERAPEUTIC GASTROINTESTINAL DIET*

**Cereals**
All cooked and cold cereals except sugar-coated; bran cereals especially recommended for constipation (miller's bran, obtainable in health food stores may be an excellent supplement); pasta (no tomato-based sauce); rice

**Breads**
White, whole-wheat, or rye without seeds; crackers without seeds; bagels; plain rolls

**Eggs**
All forms except fried

**Dairy Products†**
Cheeses: cream, cottage, Swiss, American, and nonaged soft cheeses; yoghurt; milk; cream; ice cream

**Fats**
Butter, margarine, vegetable† oils, mayonnaise†

**Soups**
All soups except bean and cabbage; chili

**Fish**
Poached, broiled, or baked; all except shellfish

**Meats**
Roast, broiled, or boiled beef; veal; lamb; chicken; turkey; liver; crisp bacon

**Potatoes**
All except fried

**Beverages**
Decaffeinated coffee,† cocoa,† tea,† citrus juices, prune juice, ginger ale,† 7-Up,† club soda†

**Vegetables**
***Cooked or Canned Only***
Asparagus, string beans, carrots, spinach, sweet potatoes, peas, tomatoes, beets

**Fruits**
***Cooked or Canned Only***
Prunes, peaches, applesauce, apricots, pears, grapes, raisins, baked apples

**Condiments†**
Pepper, salt, spices, ketchup, mustard

**General Exclusions**
Raw fruits and raw vegetables. Fried, highly spiced, highly seasoned, or "fast" foods
Alcoholic, carbonated cola, or fruit-based beverages
Potato chips, corn chips, popcorn

* This is a general description of foods that may be included in your diet. Some of these foods may be troublesome based on your experience or the physician's practice. These are to be avoided. Many foods not mentioned here may be well-tolerated. As you improve, the diet may be expanded, as advised by your physician.

† Use with caution; poorly tolerated by some patients.

Medications may be useful. Antacids are usually effective in relieving heartburn or postcibal epigastric discomfort. The commonly available aluminum-magnesium mixtures taken in the dose recommended by the manufacturer is usually adequate. The particular combination selected, however, should depend upon cost; taste; side effects, such as diarrhea or constipation; and sodium content. The antacid mixtures containing simethicone, especially recommended for gas or belching, do little more than the less expensive, simpler, conventional mixtures. Antispasmodics are useful adjuncts in the control of bloating, cramping, lower abdominal discomfort, and bowel irregularity. Simple phenobarbital-belladonna mixtures such as Donnatal offer an excellent starting point for therapy. Alternatively, one may use tincture of belladonna in doses of 5 to 10 drops three times a day or dicyclomine 10 to 20 mg before meals and at night. Side effects similar to those caused by atropine may occur and under these circumstances medication should be decreased or withdrawn. More potent anticholinergic agents should not be employed in the aged patient, since their side effects (dryness of the mouth, constipation, urinary retention, and glaucoma) may be more severe than in the younger patient. Psychoactive drugs, such as the benzodiazepines or haloperidol, in small doses may be helpful in the agitated patient. Antidepressant medication may be tried where indicated, but the anticholinergic side effects often limit their usefulness. In general, the patient with a functional bowel disorder responds to the physician who is patient, attentive, and alert and who insists upon an intensive investigation to search for a serious occult disease in those patients who do not respond satisfactorily to the preceding program.[9]

## *Constipation*

Constipation is a common symptom in the elderly patient and presents a most difficult and often frustrating management problem. Constipation in most patients is a chronic symptom. When it is of recent onset, an organic cause such as carcinoma of the colon must be excluded by radiologic and endoscopic examination. The patient usually complains that his bowels move with difficulty and less frequently or are harder than desirable. Constipation is not a disease but a symptom of significance only if viewed as such by the patient. The patient with constipation may also complain of headache, foul breath, furred tongue, fatigability, irritability, and insomnia. He or she may have a vague sense of uneasiness and ill health, relieved by defecation. Symptoms are believed to be caused by distention and mechanical irritation of the colon.

Constipation may be classified into two classic types: spastic and atonic. The spastic type is characterized by small hard stools and lower abdominal discomfort, and upon digital examination of the rectum, the ampulla is empty. Intermittent episodes of diarrhea are common. This results from excessive segmental contraction of the lower colon as well as increase in sigmoid tone. The atonic form of constipation appears to be more frequent in the elderly and is associated with a hypotonic colon. It is thought that repeatedly ignoring the urge to defecate causes the rectum to accommodate, and there is loss of the awareness of a full rectum. Examination of the rectum reveals considerable stool, sometimes puttylike, and a dilated colon often filled with feces is observed on plain films of the abdomen. Laxative abuse, commonly associated with all forms of constipation, is particularly frequent in patients with this condition.

Many factors contribute to constipation in the aged. These include decreased physical activity, inadequate intake of fluid, faulty eating habits (especially inadequate intake of fiber), and use of constipating drugs such as codeine, opiates, aluminum-containing antacids, anticholinergics, antidepressants, and antiparkinsonian drugs. Psychologic factors may also contribute to symptoms, especially anxiety and depression. Many elderly center their lives on the need for a daily bowel movement, with great concern and anxiety arising when this bowel movement does not occur.

The proper management of constipation involves a comprehensive, coordinated approach designed to remedy the contributing factors. The program should include a careful explanation of normal bowel function, instruction to avoid laxatives, and a plea for patience. Restoration of normal bowel function takes much time and initially may be discouraging. The patient must be encouraged at all times. He must be convinced that normal bowel function may vary from three bowel movements a week to three bowel movements a day.

The diet should include a generous intake of cooked fruits and vegetables and whole grain breads and cereals, supplemented by unprocessed miller's bran. Although 2 to 4 tablespoonfuls (10 to 20 gm) a day of coarse bran may suffice, as much as 8 to 12 may be necessary in some circumstances.[17] Bran, which looks and tastes like sawdust, can be made more palatable by sprinkling it in cereals, mixing it with juice, or incorporating it into many foods. The patient must be cautioned that bran may produce bloating, gas, and cramps; these symptoms usually subside within a matter of a few weeks. Abundant intake of liquids is necessary, with a minimum of 2 L of fluid a day. In those patients who cannot tolerate the bran program, hydrophilic mucilloids, such as Metamucil, 1 or 2 tablespoonfuls a day, may be used. Irritant laxatives are to be avoided. The patient should regularly attempt a bowel movement shortly after breakfast and supper, sitting on the toilet for at least 10 minutes. If, after 2 days, a bowel movement is not forthcoming, stimulation from below is advised, using either glycerin suppositories or enemas, which may be either of the hypertonic phosphate type or plain tap water. In truly resistant cases, it may be useful to give a 2-oz oil retention enema at night, followed by a saline or tap water enema in the morning. Regular exercise is beneficial and is to be encouraged in the constipated patient.

A particular problem related to severe constipation is fecal impaction. This condition may produce a paradoxical effect of overflow diarrhea, and fecal incontinence may occur. A common error in the nursing home and hospitalized patient is to treat diarrhea without a rectal examination, administering antidiarrheal drugs when a digital examination of the rectum will provide the proper diagnosis. Manual disimpaction, followed by the enema regimen outlined in the previous paragraph, can often control the problem.

## *Diarrhea*

Diarrhea, defined as increased frequency or increased water content in the stool, occurs far less frequently than constipation in the elderly patient and is usually easier to manage. The common causes of acute diarrhea include infections related to the ingestion of contaminated food by staphylococcal toxins, *Salmonella* organisms, and, especially significant in these days of travel, strains of *Escherichia coli.* Management in the elderly person is not significantly different from treatment of younger individuals. Most patients with typical infectious diarrhea related to food ingestion require only supportive therapy to prevent dehydration and antidiarrheal drugs for comfort and relief of symptoms.

Traveler's diarrhea, usually due to toxogenic strains of *E. coli,* is usually a self-limited disease and may be best managed by large doses of bismuth subsalicylate (Pepto-Bismol) given in doses of 30 to 60 ml every four hours. Individuals may take doxycycline or trimethoprim-sulfamethoxazole to prevent diarrhea when traveling to endemic areas.

Antibiotic-associated diarrhea is commonly encountered in the aged person. The milder case is usually associated with normal sigmoidoscopic findings and is usually terminated upon withdrawal of the antibiotic. The more severe cases, usually with rectal mucosal changes or pseudomembranes, require therapy against the usual causative bacteria, *Clostridium difficile.*[10] The most extensively studied drug used in the treatment of this condition is vancomyin, which is almost universally effective.[11] It has, however, some disadvantages. These include expense (a course of treatment usually costs between $200 and $350) and a 20 per cent relapse rate. More recent reports indicate that metronidazole may also be effective. This drug is less expensive and is universally available. The usual dose is 250 mg three to four times a day over a 7- to 10-day period. An alternate to antibiotic therapy is the use of cholestyramine, an anion-exchanging resin that binds the *C. difficile* toxins until their normal flow in the gut regenerate. Because of the availability, cost, and ease of administration, cholestyramine and metronidiazole should be the drugs of first choice in the nonhospitalized patient, whereas vancomycin is indicated in the seriously ill hospitalized patient or the patient who fails to respond to the less expensive drugs.

Chronic diarrhea may be of functional or organic origin. The functional type is characterized by a lack of nocturnal movements, small stool volume, and absence of blood, pus, or mucus in the stool. After a careful history and physical, the next diagnostic measure should be an unprepared sigmoidoscopic examination, allowing for easy collection of fresh fecal material for bacteriologic study, mucosal smear for methylene blue stain for leukocytes, and direct examination of the mucosa with biopsy, if indicated.[12] Barium studies should not be done prior to the sigmoidoscopic examination and, when done, should include a barium enema, upper GI, and small bowel series. In patients with very high volume diarrhea, a determination of stool pH may differentiate diarrhea as a consequence of carbohydrate malabsorption from secretory diarrhea. In the former situation, the pH is acidic whereas in the latter it is alkaline.

High volume diarrheas, those characterized by copious liquid bowel movements, may further be subdivided into those caused by increased osmotic forces acting within the lumen of the bowel and those caused by increased secretion of electrolytes and water. These conditions can be differentiated by stopping feeding for 24 hours. Osmotic diarrhea will stop when the patient fasts in contrast with secretory diarrhea, which persists in spite of fasting. The best example of an osmotic diarrhea is that caused by lactose intolerance. This condition is not uncommon in middle-age and older people. It tends to occur in individuals with no prior history of diarrhea. Careful history reveals that the diarrhea tends to occur promptly after ingestion of foods that are high in lactose content and subsides completely during fasting. Treatment consists of partial or complete removal of lactose from the diet. Chronic secretory diarrheas are rare, but it should be stressed that the chronic abuse of certain laxatives can result in this type of problem. These patients are particularly troublesome because some will deny the use of laxatives and may require hospitalization and many tests before the diagnosis can be established. Small volume diarrheas associated with organic causes, characterized by fecal leukocytes and blood and pus in the stool are due to inflammatory or ischemic disease of the colon, diverticulitis, or cancer (see subsequent discussion).

Malabsorption syndromes are not common in the elderly but, if present, may lead to severe nutritional problems. Their hallmark is the presence of steatorrhea, due to failure to digest or absorb dietary fat. The causes of steatorrhea are multiple. In patients suspected of the malabsorption syndrome, serum carotene levels, prothrombin time, blood calcium studies and stool examinations for quantitative and qualitative fat are useful in the verification of malabsorption. Once preliminary evidence of malabsorption has been obtained, the next step is to distinguish maldigestion from true malabsorption. The most commonly used method is the D-xylose test. When the patient is given a 25-gram load of D-xylose, the normal 5-hour urinary secretion is greater than 4.5 gm. In the elderly patient, however, it is probably prudent to correlate urinary with blood D-xylose levels in order to eliminate renal factors and delayed gastric emptying. In almost all patients with malabsorption caused by diffuse mucosal disease of the proximal small bowel, the test is clearly abnormal. In patients with normal D-xylose secretion and steatorrhea, the diagnosis of pancreatic exocrine insufficiency is most likely, and pancreatic extract may be given a therapeutic trial. Other studies to evaluate pancreatic function include the secretin test, abdominal sonography, computerized tomography, and endoscopic retrograde pancreatography, all of which may be helpful in resolving a diagnostic dilemma. If pancreatic function is found to be normal in the patient with steatorrhea, the next diagnostic test should be the bile salt breath test. This measures the radionuclide $^{14}CO_2$ in expired air after oral administration of $^{14}C$-labeled glycocholate. If the diagnosis is still uncertain, small bowel biopsy is indicated. Giardiasis may be detected in the biliary drainage.

Once a specific diagnosis has been made, management is usually effective. Maldigestion caused by pancreatic insufficiency responds to pancreatic supplements. Broad spectrum antibiotics, most often tetracycline, may control upper small bowel bacterial overgrowth. Of the specific mucosal causes of malabsorption, theoretically the easiest to treat should be celiac disease, which, in the younger person, responds dramatically to a gluten-free diet. However, the response in elderly patients with celiac disease may be slow and not infrequently incomplete. Some patients may benefit from prednisone therapy as well as tetracycline. If such a patient fails to respond to these measures, one must consider the presence of a small bowel lymphoma.

Diarrhea associated with fecal incontinence is a major problem in the care of the geriatric patient, especially the patient with senile dementia.[13] It is an unpleasant problem for both patient and nursing staff and the most difficult problem in management. Most common causes of fecal incontinence include fecal impaction, as previously described; underlying disease of the colon, rectum, or anal sphincter as a consequence of cancer of the bowel; diverticular disease; diabetic neuropathy; destruction of the anal sphincter as a result of hemorrhoidal surgery; prolapsed rectum; ingestion of drugs such as iron- and magnesium-containing antacids and laxatives, and many neurogenic disorders. The physiologic disturbance in many of these conditions is that the distention of the rectum resulting from mass movement of feces is followed by an intrusive rectal contraction and by inhibition of contraction of the anal sphincter so that the bolus of the stool is passed spontaneously. A treatment of planned bowel evacuation utilizing bisacodyl (Dulcolax) suppositories or enemas is often useful in controlling this most distressing problem.

## *Esophageal Disease*

Dysphagia, frequently encountered in elderly patients, is a serious manifestation not only because of the diseases that underlie it but also because of its implications as regards nutrition and aspiration. The causes of dysphagia may be divided into two broad groups: (1) motor abnormalities and (2) mechanical obstruction. These groups can, as a rule, be differentiated by a careful history. When a difficulty in swallowing "progresses" from solids to liquids, the problem is invariably mechanical or organic; if the onset involves difficulty with liquids and solids simultaneously, motor abnormalities are more likely the cause.

### Motor Abnormalities

One of the more frequent motor abnormalities is pseudobulbar palsy due to cerebrovascular accident. This may result in oropharyngeal paralysis, with misdirection of food, particularly liquids, into the nose and respiratory passages. A careful barium swallow is essential for proper diagnosis. Unfortunately, there is no satisfactory treatment for pseudobulbar palsy secondary to cerebrovascular disease. In some patients, however, this condition is due to myasthenia gravis or polymyositis. In these instances, the dysphagia may respond to appropriate medical therapy.

Occasionally, a lateral x-ray, taken during swallowing, will reveal a prominent cricopharyngeal muscle on the posterior esophageal wall. The demonstration of this finding in a patient with dysphagia leads to the diagnosis of cricopharyngeal achalasia. This problem may represent paradoxical contracture or lack of relaxation of the cricopharyngeal muscle during the pharyngeal phase of swallowing. This condition may be associated with Zenker's diverticulum. Cricopharyngeal achalasia may be treated by cricopharyngeal myotomy and Zenker's diverticulum may also benefit from surgical extirpation.

Occasionally patients with scleroderma or, in some instances, disseminated lupus erythematosus will exhibit a form of swallowing difficulty that is posture related. This can be demonstrated by having the patient swallow liquids in the recumbent position. Patients with scleroderma may also exhibit reflux and peptic esophagitis, secondary to intermittent lower esophageal sphincter incompetence. Occasionally this results in stricture.

Intermittent dysphagia for both solids and liquids, often accompanied by chest pain, is a characteristic manifestation of diffuse esophageal spasm. The chest pain may mimic angina pectoris. Its cause is highly variable. It is often precipitated by certain foods or hot and cold beverages. Sometimes it occurs spontaneously, with no relation to any bodily activities or functions. Further confusion with angina may exist because the pain of esophageal spasm may be relieved by nitroglycerin. Radiographic characteristics of this condition include spontaneous nonpropulsive contractions of the esophagus, producing the picture of a corkscrew esophagus. It should be emphasized, however, that because the symptoms are intermittent, a routinely performed barium swallow may not reveal the abnormality. The cine-esophagram is a better means of evaluating esophageal motility. The most sensitive test available is esophageal manometry.

Treatment of diffuse esophageal spasm includes use of anticholinergics and long-acting nitroglycerin and avoidance of exogenous precipitating factors such as cold, liquids, or emotional distress; reassurance is also important in treatment. Nifedipine and hydralazine have recently been reported to have been useful in the management of this condition. In intractable cases, bouginage, pneumatic dilatation, and surgical treatment may be considered. Achalasia is a severe disorder of esophageal motility, characterized by aperistalsis, elevated lower esophageal sphincter pressure, and impaired lower esophageal sphincter relaxation. Patients experience progressive dysphagia for solids and liquids, with frequent regurgitation of undigested material. Pulmonary aspiration is not uncommon. Although achalasia is usually painless, in some patients this disorder may resemble diffuse esophageal spasm with substernal pain associated with hypermotility of the esophagus. The diagnosis of achalasia is confirmed by barium swallow, which reveals a smooth, tapered narrowing at the distal end of the esophagus, and/or by manometry. The esophagus usually is dilated and demonstrates no peristalsis. Endoscopy should always be performed on patients with suspected achalasia to rule out a carcinoma involving the esophagogastric junction, which may produce similar manometric and radiographic findings. Failure to pass the endoscope through the esophagogastric junction indicates an organic obstruction, either a tumor or stricture, and is not a feature of achalasia. Furthermore, since esophageal carcinoma is a well-documented complication of achalasia, the endoscopic examination is helpful in ruling out this disease. The treatment for achalasia is aimed at reducing the pressure gradient between the esophagus and stomach. Pneumatic dilatation or surgery offers the patient the best opportunity for relief.[14]

### Mechanical Causes of Dysphagia

Of the mechanical causes of dysphagia, the two most common are benign strictures secondary to reflux and carcinoma of the esophagus. Benign stricture is usually the result of longstanding reflux esophagitis as a consequence of gastroesophageal incompetence. Although bouginage is helpful, control of reflux is paramount in patients with reflux esophagitis. Gastroesophageal reflux is a well-recognized clinical disorder characterized by the familiar symptoms of heartburn and regurgitation. These symptoms may reflect hiatal hernia or incompetency of the lower esophageal sphincter. Reflux esophagitis is strongly suspected on the basis of a history of classic heartburn and regurgitation. When these symptoms are associated with radiologic evidence of hiatal hernia, the clinician may embark on a therapeutic program without the use of the more complex tests of reflux that are sometimes required to confirm this diagnosis (upper GI endoscopy, esophageal intubation for demonstration of acid reflux or acid sensitivity, the so-called Bernstein test, and esophageal manometry).[15] Sliding-type hiatal hernia can be demonstrated in many patients over 65 years. In most instances, other than producing mild heartburn after dietary indiscretion, this condition is not clinically significant. The paraesophageal or rolling form of hiatal hernia is very uncommon, particularly in the younger patient. Although causing upper abdominal and chest pain, it usually does not produce reflux.

The aim of therapy in the management of hiatal hernia is to reduce the frequency and volume of acid reflux. The mainstay of therapy is control of gastric acidity. This control may be achieved by the regular use of an antacid, 15 to 30 ml 1 hour after each meal and at night. Cimetidine or ranitidine may be helpful in the very symptomatic patient. Diet similar to that indicated in Table 46–2, modified by specific advice to avoid juices, chocolate, peppermint, fat, and alcohol, is prescribed. The patient is further advised not to overdistend the stomach by eating excessively or by drinking large quantities of fluid with meals. The diet should be relatively dry. Smoking must be discontinued. Elevation of the head of the bed 4 to 8 in. is advised, and if this is not possible, the patient should sleep with a support or pillow placed so that the shoulders are elevated at least 30 degrees. Tight garments should be avoided and weight loss, when indicated, is mandatory. Agents to increase lower esophageal sphincter pressure, such as bethanechol chloride (Urecholine) and metoclopramide, may be employed in resistant cases. The dose of Urecholine is 25 mg three times a day, before meals and at night, and metoclopramide is prescribed 10 mg three times daily before meals. Urecholine is usually well tolerated in this dose with few side effects, whereas metoclopramide may be associated with restlessness, anxiety, insomnia, and acute extrapyramidal reactions, which necessitate its discontinuation in a small number of patients. Anticholinergic drugs are to be avoided as they decrease lower esophageal sphincter pressure and inhibit gastric emptying. Antireflux surgery may be an effective means for treating complicated intractable gastroesophageal reflux, but it should be a last resort in the elderly patient. Indications for surgical intervention include hemorrhage secondary to erosive esophagitis, peptic stricture, peptic ulcer of the esophagus, recurrent aspiration pneumonia, and intractability of symptoms.[16]

Squamous cell carcinoma of the esophagus is the fifth most common cancer in adult males, occurring twice as often in men as in women. Although squamous cell carcinoma may involve any part of the esophagus, its most common location is just proximal to the esophagogastric junction. Adenocarcinoma of the stomach may involve the distal esophagus and may be confused with a primary carcinoma of the esophagus, but squamous cell carcinoma does not involve the stomach. The classical presentation of this cancer is progressive dysphagia associated with weight loss. Dysphagia implies that the esophageal lumen has already lost at least 50 per cent of its normal diameter, and thus, the tumor is usually far advanced by the time that it has produced symptoms. The prognosis in esophageal cancer, regardless of the mode of therapy, is extremely poor, with survival beyond 5 years reported to be less than 3 per cent. Radiation and chemotherapy are the preferred treatments for squamous cell carcinoma involving the upper thoracic and cervical esophagus. Use of radiation with or without surgical resection is the usual therapy for squamous cell carcinoma of the lower esophagus. In adenocarcinoma, when it arises from the stomach, a brief course of preoperative irradiation therapy has been reported to improve the prognosis. Adenocarcinoma, whether it arises from the stomach or Barrett's epithelium within the esophagus, is best treated surgically when feasible. The role of chemotherapeutic agents in treatment of all forms of esophageal cancer has not been established. Esophageal bouginage and esophageal prosthesis (Celestin's tube) may be helpful as palliative measures in maintaining swallow function in selective cases.[17]

## *Diseases of the Stomach and Esophagus*

Just as in younger patients, the incidence of peptic ulcer disease in the elderly is about 10 per cent.[18] Gastric and duodenal ulcer diseases, however, occur with about equal frequency in the elderly. Interestingly, there is a higher incidence of both gastric and duodenal ulcer diseases in elderly women than in younger ones. The symptoms of both duodenal ulcer and gastric ulcer diseases may be characteristic, including gnawing or burning epigastric or left upper quadrant pain, which occurs 1 to 4 hours after eating and is relieved by antacids or food. Symptoms, however, are frequently atypical and nonspecific, and the first manifestation may be an upper gastrointestinal hemorrhage or an acute perforation. In patients with a long history of peptic ulcer disease, nocturnal pain may occur, usually signifying intramural penetration of the ulcer or low-grade gastric retention. Symptoms of pain, and especially bleeding, often occur in relation to ingestion of medication such as aspirin or nonsteroidal anti-inflammatory drugs. Alcohol may also be a precipitating factor. Giant duodenal and benign gastric ulcers are not uncommon in the elderly. Radiographic examination of the upper gastrointestinal tract may miss as many as a quarter of peptic ulcers. Therefore, when a patient has chronic ulcer disease with duodenal bulb deformity, the presence of an active ulcer can only be established by direct visualization by means of fiberoptic endoscopy. This is a useful and safe technique in the elderly. In the presence of upper GI bleeding, it probably should be the first procedure attempted.

The management of peptic ulcer disease is based primarily on the control or neutralization of the secretion of acid.[19–21] This goal can be achieved adequately and most appropriately so in the elderly by a good antacid regimen.[19] The usual dose of antacid, as recommended by the manufacturer (see Table 46–3), taken seven times a day, will usually relieve symptoms and allow proper healing of the ulcer. The choice of a particular antacid should be based on potency, cost, taste, ease of administration, effect on bowel function, and sodium content. Compliance with the ideal antacid program is often not achieved but most ulcers tend to heal with lesser adherence to therapeutic recommendations.[21] With the advent of cimetidine, there has been a shift in the routine management of ulcer disease to the employment of this drug 300 mg four times a day.[22] Because in elderly patients cimetidine may lead to adverse reactions such as confusional states,[23] it should be given with caution and its adverse effects specifically described to patients and their families.

A new histamine $H_2$ receptor antagonist, ranitidine hydrochloride (Zantac), is now available. This drug has increased potency and longer duration of action (twice-a-day dosage) and has been associated with fewer side effects and drug interactions than cimetidine. Another drug that has been shown to be of value is sucralfate. This drug, which is not absorbed, has been demonstrated to coat and protect the ulcer crater by binding to necrotic ulcer tissue. The agent is believed to have protective and antipeptic activity. Its primary side effect is constipation.

Restrictive ulcer diets are no longer in vogue in the management of ulcer disease. The patient should be encouraged to eat regular meals and not go for long periods without eating. The patient should avoid foods that have produced gastrointestinal symptoms in the past. It must be stressed that many patients with peptic ulcer disease often suffer from an irritable bowel and may benefit from the high fiber, low roughage diet described previously. Smoking should be prohibited. The management of gastric ulcer disease, although similar to that of duodenal ulcer disease as far as diet and antacid therapy are concerned, does differ in that follow-up to complete healing of the ulcer is essential because of a significant incidence of malignancy. Upper GI endoscopy with biopsy of the gastric ulcer and gastric brushing should be an essential procedure in the diagnostic evaluation of any gastric ulcer to avoid this error. However, the most important criteria is complete healing of the gastric ulcer. If this fails to occur within a given period of 6 to 12 weeks, then gastric resection must be considered.

Upper gastrointestinal hemorrhage is a major problem in the elderly, associated with a high mortality, ranging from 10 to 25 per cent.[24] Azotemia, peripheral vascular failure, and dehydration appear quickly and are often difficult to reverse. Upper GI fiberoptic endoscopy has revolutionalized diagnosis of upper gastrointestinal hemorrhage, and emergency endoscopy performed by a skilled endoscopist usually will delineate the bleeding site in about 90 per cent of patients with active hemorrhage. For the optimal management of any patient with upper GI

**Table 46-3.** SOME LIQUID ANTACIDS

| | Ingredients/5 ml | Usual Dose* | Acid-Neutralizing Capacity | High-Dosage Regimen | Sodium (mg/5 ml) | Cost of High-Dosage Regimen |
|---|---|---|---|---|---|---|
| ALternaGEL—*Stuart* | 600 mg aluminum hydroxide | 5–10 ml | 12 mEq | 60 ml | 2 | $ 89.44 |
| Aludrox—*Wyeth* | 307 mg aluminum hydroxide<br>103 mg magnesium hydroxide | 10 ml | 28 mEq | 50 ml | 1 | 76.61 |
| Amphojel—*Wyeth* | 320 mg aluminum hydroxide | 10 ml | 13 mEq | 110 ml | 7 | 168.53 |
| Basaljel—*Wyeth* | 400 mg aluminum hydroxide | 10 ml | 28 mEq | 50 ml | 2 | 76.61 |
| (Extra Strength) | 1000 mg aluminum hydroxide | 5 ml | 22 mEq | 30 ml | 23 | 84.30 |
| Bisodol—*Whitehall* | 644 mg sodium bicarbonate<br>475 mg magnesium carbonate | 5 ml | 15 mEq | 45 ml | 196 | 170.43 |
| Camalox—*Rorer* | 200 mg magnesium hydroxide<br>225 mg aluminum hydroxide<br>250 mg calcium carbonate | 10–20 ml | 36 mEq | 40 ml | 3 | 78.40 |
| Delcid—*Merrell Dow* | 600 mg aluminum hydroxide<br>665 mg magnesium hydroxide | 5 ml | 42 mEq | 15 ml | 15 | 45.72 |
| Di-Gel—*Plough* | 282 mg aluminum hydroxide<br>87 mg magnesium hydroxide<br>20 mg simethicone | 10 ml | 18 mEq | 80 ml | 9 | 99.06 |
| Gelusil—*Parke-Davis* | 200 mg aluminum hydroxide<br>200 mg magnesium hydroxide<br>25 mg simethicone | 10 ml | 24 mEq | 60 ml | <1 | 78.79 |
| Gelusil-II—*Parke-Davis* | 400 mg aluminum hydroxide<br>400 mg magnesium hydroxide<br>30 mg simethicone | 10 ml | 48 mEq | 30 ml | 1 | 60.52 |
| Kolantyl—*Merrell Dow* | 150 mg aluminum hydroxide<br>150 mg magnesium hydroxide | 5–20 ml | 10.5 mEq | 65 ml | <5 | 98.43 |
| Maalox—*Rorer* | 225 mg aluminum hydroxide<br>200 mg magnesium hydroxide | 10–20 ml | 27 mEq | 50 ml | 1 | 66.25 |
| Maalox Plus—*Rorer* | 200 mg magnesium hydroxide<br>225 mg aluminum hydroxide<br>25 mg simethicone | 10–20 ml | 27 mEq | 50 ml | 1 | 71.28 |
| Maalox T.C.—*Rorer* | 300 mg magnesium hydroxide<br>600 mg aluminum hydroxide | 5–10 ml | 28.3 mEq | 25 ml | <1 | 46.58 |
| Mylanta—*Stuart* | 200 mg aluminum hydroxide<br>200 mg magnesium hydroxide<br>20 mg simethicone | 5–10 ml | 12.7 mEq | 55 ml | <1 | 73.53 |
| Mylanta-II—*Stuart* | 400 mg aluminum hydroxide<br>400 mg magnesium hydroxide<br>30 mg simethicone | 5–10 ml | 25.4 mEq | 30 ml | 1 | 58.39 |
| Riopan—*Ayerst* | 480 mg magaldrate | 5–10 ml | 13.5 mEq | 50 ml | <1 | 60.93 |
| Simeco—*Wyeth* | 365 mg aluminum hydroxide<br>300 mg magnesium hydroxide<br>30 mg simethicone | 5–10 ml | 22 mEq | 30 ml | 7–14 | 47.92 |
| Tritralac—*Riker* | 1000 mg calcium carbonate | 5 ml | 20 mEq | 35 ml | 11 | 40.99 |

* Recommended by the manufacturer.

bleeding, it is advised that this procedure be performed within the first 24 hours of the patient's admission to the hospital. Endoscopic hemostatic techniques, including electrocautery and laser therapy, may be of value in some cases. Therapy for major upper gastrointestinal hemorrhage in the elderly is similar to that in younger persons and involves nasogastric suction; careful monitoring of intravascular volume with central venous pressure or Swan-Ganz lines in place; and the judicious use of crystalloid solutions, albumin, and blood. Surgical intervention must be considered if bleeding is prolonged or massive (i.e., when the patient requires transfusions of more than 1500 ml of blood within the first 12 to 24 hours or requires transfusions beyond 48 hours because of the continuing hemorrhage). Although antrectomy with vagotomy is probably the most commonly applied surgical procedure for the management of duodenal ulcer disease, and gastrectomy with or without vagotomy for gastric hemorrhage, less invasive procedures such as vagotomy combined with pyloroplasty with oversewing of the ulcer may be adequate in the poor-risk patient.

In patients with nonhealing gastric ulcer disease, gastric resection with or without vagotomy is the operation of choice. In the patient with duodenal ulcer disease complicated by unresponsiveness to treatment, frequent occurrences, and repeated hemorrhages, vagotomy with antrectomy is usually recommended. The most important innovation in the elective surgical management of duodenal ulcer disease has been use of proximal gastric vagotomy. This operation may be performed without a drainage procedure, such as pyloroplasty or gastroenterostomy, and is associated with a low risk and reduced incidence of side effects. Zollinger-Ellison syndrome,[25] although extremely rare, should be considered when peptic ulcer disease is associated with diarrhea; when there is a family or personal history of endocrine adenomatosis; and when there are atypical ulcer features such as unusual location, multiple or large ulcers, intractability to management, early complications, or recurrence postoperatively. If fasting serum gastrin level is elevated, then a gastric analysis should be performed to determine whether or not there is hyperchlorhydria. Hypergastrinemia occurs in patients with atrophic gastritis, especially in patients with pernicious anemia; thus, it is not an unusual finding in the elderly. These conditions are characterized by achlorhydria. The diagnosis of Zollinger-Ellison syndrome is virtually assured when hyperchlorhydria and serum gastrin levels exceeding 1000 pg per milliliter are encountered in the patient with peptic ulcer disease. The therapeutic approach to the management of the Zollinger-Ellison syndrome is usually medical, consisting of use of $H_2$ receptor blocking agents, but in intractable cases, surgical therapy may be necessary.

Chronic gastric atrophy is a feature of old age and is readily identifiable histologically and endoscopically; it has little or no clinical significance until pernicious anemia or cancer develops. Strickland and McKay[25a] have classified chronic atrophic gastritis into types A and B. Type A is characterized by the presence of antibodies against parietal cells and is associated with pernicious anemia and other autoimmune phenomena such as thyroiditis. Type B is not associated with pernicious anemia but is associated with a higher incidence of vague digestive tract symptoms, gastric ulcer, and hemorrhage. Both types may predispose the patient to cancer. Currently, there is no treatment for these conditions, and their presence may have implications for nutrition and drug absorption.

Gastric cancer, although it has declined in overall incidence during the past decade, is still a serious problem among the elderly. The death rate from cancer of the stomach in 1930 was 38 per 100,000 male population. In 1978 the overall incidence had fallen to below 10 per 100,000. The high incidence of this disease occurs after the sixth decade; among males it is the fifth leading cause of cancer deaths after the age of 55. It occurs twice as commonly in men as women. The cause of the decline in the overall incidence of this disease in the United States and Western Europe is unknown. The symptoms commonly associated with gastric carcinoma include anorexia, weight loss, early satiety, distaste for meat, and vague upper abdominal discomfort occurring immediately after meals and unrelieved by antacids. Blood loss anemia is commonly present at the time of diagnosis. Physical examination is rarely of value early in the course of this cancer. The diagnosis is usually based upon the x-ray demonstration of a fungating mass, with ulceration and infiltration of the gastric wall. Upper GI endoscopy is usually employed to confirm the diagnosis, both visually and by biopsy and brush cytologic studies. Gastric resection is the only therapeutic modality of any value. The overall 5-year survival rate is about 12 per cent. The value of radiation and chemotherapy in gastric cancer is uncertain; at best these modalities are of palliative value. The risks, side effects, and cost of these modalities must be weighed against the limited benefits expected.

# COLONIC DISEASES

## Diverticulosis

Diverticulosis is a disease of advancing age, occurring in about 40 per cent of all individuals over 70 years.[26] The most common location is in the sigmoid colon, but diverticula may be found throughout the colon.

The classic work of Painter and Burkitt[7] has suggested that this disease is related to the changing character of the Western diet, characterized by decreasing amounts of fiber consumed. The fiber deficiency results in an altered motility state in the colon, characterized by high resting intraluminal pressures and increased pressure responses to meals, especially in the sigmoid colon. Clinically, diverticulosis can be classified as (1) asymptomatic diverticulosis, the most prevalent form; (2) diverticular disease characterized by a complex of lower abdominal pain and bowel disturbance (constipation more commonly than diarrhea) without evidence of inflammation; (3) acute diverticulitis and its complications of abscess formation, fistulization, perforation, and obstruction; and (4) bleeding diverticulosis.[27]

The concept of painful diverticular disease without inflammation (see earlier) is controversial, and indeed, the clinical picture of this condition cannot be separated from that of the irritable bowel syndrome. Management includes a high-fiber, low-roughage diet and mild antispasmodic therapy. Bulk-producing laxatives may be useful in selected cases.

The incidence of diverticulitis is difficult to assess but is said to occur in anywhere from 10 to 25 per cent of all patients with diverticulosis coli. Lower abdominal pain, often with obstructive features, marked left lower quadrant tenderness; fever; and leukocytosis characterize this complication. Abscess formation, fistulization, perforation, and obstruction may ensue. Treatment of serious diverticular disease includes use of intravenous fluids (or, sometimes, a clear liquid diet) and parenteral antibiotics, such as amino glycosides, ampicillin, cephalosporins, and clindamycin. Milder forms of diverticulitis can be treated with a high-fiber diet, antispasmodics, and oral antibiotics such as tetracycline or ampicillin. Long-term antibiotic therapy, or serial courses of antibiotics, may be helpful in patients with a tendency to frequent recurrences. Surgery should be reserved for those with severe complications.[28] Fistulization or perforation usually requires a multiple-stage procedure, consisting of initial diversion and colostomy formation, with subsequent resection and closure of the colostomy. Bowel resection may be necessary as a primary procedure for intractable or recurrent disease. A bout of diverticulitis responding to medical management is not an indication for elective surgery.[29] Lower gastrointestinal hemorrhage may occur in as few as 5 per cent or as many as 20 per cent of patients. This complication is thought to be related to the juxta-arteriolar course of the diverticula. Bleeding usually appears to be brisk and profuse, but characteristically, the blood count does not seem to fall in proportion to the apparent magnitude of the hemorrhage. In most instances, bleeding terminates spontaneously. Surgery may be necessary in a small percentage of cases but should be preceded by angiography or colonoscopy for precise location of the site of blood loss because the bleeding may arise from anywhere within the colon and from sources other than diverticula.

## Angiodysplasia

With the advent of these newer diagnostic techniques, lower gastrointestinal hemorrhages, which in years past were largely attributed to diverticulosis, are often found to be due to angiodysplasia, a relatively new term referring to a type of arteriovenous malformation in the GI tract.[30] This abnormality can only be demonstrated angiographically or endoscopically. It has been found that angiodysplasia causes lower GI bleeding in the elderly as frequently as does diverticulosis. Together, both conditions account for 75 per cent of all lower GI hemorrhages in older people.

In angiodysplasia, bleeding is venous and tends to be recurrent, in contrast to the brisk arterial hemorrhage of diverticular disease, which is usually not recurrent. Aortic stenosis may be present in the patient with angiodysplasia. During the acute phase of bleeding, the diagnosis can be made by angiography, and surgical resection must be undertaken if bleeding does not cease. In most instances, however, the bleeding will spontaneously stop; colonoscopy should be performed to localize the lesions and, possibly, to cauterize them. There is no effective medical management of this condition. Iron therapy may be necessary to maintain the blood count in patients who have recurrent minor episodes of bleeding.[30]

### Other Causes of Rectal Bleeding

Although diverticulosis coli and angiodysplasia produce the most dramatic type of rectal bleeding, other lesions such as polyps, carcinomas, and, especially, anorectal diseases are common causes of rectal bleeding. If the patient presents with stools streaked with blood or reports blood on the toilet paper or in the toilet bowl alone and demonstrates obvious hemorrhoids with fissures upon sigmoidoscopic examination, a 2-week trial of local therapy should be prescribed. This consists of sitz baths and rectal suppositories twice a day. If bleeding ceases after such a regimen and does not recur, further diagnostic tests are unnecessary. If, however, bleeding continues, colonoscopy should be performed. Barium enema studies are of less value.

## *Intestinal Ischemia*

Ischemic bowel disease is characteristically a disorder of the elderly. Diagnosis is difficult and seldom made, however, and the treatment of this condition is unsatisfactory. Intestinal ischemia may be either acute or chronic, occlusive or nonocclusive. Occlusive intestinal ischemia, which produces the acute syndrome, is caused by a complete or very high-grade obstruction of the major mesenteric artery or one or more of its principle segmental branches, usually by a thrombus or an embolus. Nonocclusive ischemia, which may be either chronic or acute, is associated with low flow states, mesenteric vasoconstriction, and mucosal hypoperfusion without actual mechanical obstruction to arterial flow. It frequently coexists with congestive heart failure and generalized arteriosclerotic vascular disease. Intestinal ischemia may involve either the small intestine or colon. Acute ischemia of the small intestine is associated with a poor prognosis leading in some cases to fatal circulatory shock. The clinical picture is characterized by sudden onset of severe abdominal pain with the signs of an acute abdomen. Rectal bleeding may occur. Initially the abdomen may be soft, with hyperactive bowel sounds, but subsequently the picture is one of typical acute peritonitis. Immediate surgical exploration with appropriate bowel resection is mandatory, although the outcome is usually poor.

In contrast, ischemia of the colon, when it occurs without concomitant small intestinal ischemia, is rarely of a catastrophic nature. Abdominal pain and rectal bleeding may occur. This condition is frequently reversible, rarely requires surgical resection, and is rarely the principle cause of a patient's death.

*Chronic intestinal ischemia* produces the syndrome of intestinal angina. The symptoms include diffuse abdominal pain, weight loss, and either constipation or diarrhea. Patients develop an aversion to eating because of the pain and also may show evidence of malabsorption. Although it has been said that chronic intestinal ischemia is associated invariably with involvement of more than one vessel, a recent study of 203 unselected autopsy specimens disclosed that there was no relationship between the degree of stenosis and the presence of previous gastrointestinal symptoms.[31] Medical management includes small feedings and discontinuation of digitalis preparations, which have been demonstrated to decrease mesenteric blood flow. The extent of the disease may be confirmed by angiography. Recent reports indicate satisfactory results may be obtained in some cases by restoration of normal flow, either by endarterectomy or bypass graft. The long-term efficacy of these procedures has not been determined, however, and progress in this area has yet to be convincingly established.[32]

## *Colitis*

Inflammatory bowel disease, usually identified as ulcerative or granulomatous colitis, exhibits a bimodal age distribution, with the peak incidence in the third and fourth decades and a small subsequent peak in the sixth and seventh decades. The explanation is that there appear to be two different disease processes at work. Kirsner and co-workers,[33] and others, suggest that ischemia may account for the secondary rise, whereas Burch and associates[33a] postulate immunologic factors.

In a recent review of 81 patients with colitis, over age 65, half of whom had been classified as having either ulcerative or granulomatous colitis, the conclusion was reached that 75 per cent were suffering from ischemic colitis, 14 per cent from ulcerative colitis, and 5 per cent from Crohn's disease.[34] In this series, patients with ischemic colitis were more likely to have abdominal pain, distention, and constipation than persons with ulcerative colitis or Crohn's disease. Although bloody diarrhea was common in all patients, sparing of the rectum and sigmoid is more common in the ischemic group. X-ray changes are characteristically segmental in distribution, often associated with thumb-printing or stricture. At times, complete resolution may be seen. Patients with ulcerative colitis and intermittent exacerbations usually respond to sulfasalazine or steroid therapy. Surgery, however, is required in all patients with Crohn's disease and more than half of those with ischemic colitis. Thus, the differentiation of the form of colitis in these elderly patients presenting with abdominal pain and/or bloody diarrhea now appears possible and is important diagnostically from a therapeutic and prognostic viewpoint. Colitis, whether it is ischemic or inflammatory, appears to be a more serious disease in the elderly, responding less well to medical therapy and often requiring surgery, especially in the granulomatous form. Ischemic colitis and inflammatory colitis are associated with a significant mortality, which may be related to other coincidental diseases of aging rather than to the colitis per se.

A unique problem in older patients is that of granulomatous colitis masquerading as diverticulosis coli. The clinical picture is characterized by abdominal pain and diarrhea, with radiologic evidence of diverticulosis or diverticulitis. These patients fail to respond to antibiotic therapy and, following sigmoid resection for what appears to be intractable diverticulitis coli, frequently develop fistulas and abscesses. The disease may then extend to involve the more proximal and distal colon. The diagnosis is established by discovering granuloma in the surgical specimen or occasionally on rectal biopsy. Prednisone therapy may be helpful in these patients, but the course is usually unsatisfactory and a colostomy or ileostomy usually becomes necessary.

## Colorectal Cancer and Polyps

Colorectal cancer is the most common malignancy of the gastrointestinal tract, reaching its highest incidence after the age of 70.[35] Most colorectal cancers occur in the distal colon, although there is an increasing distribution of these tumors in the right colon. Tumors of the left colon manifest themselves with rectal bleeding, constipation, and abdominal pain, whereas those in the right colon are secretive, with patients usually presenting with anemia. The diagnosis is usually made by barium enema study. Colonoscopy is helpful in confirming the diagnosis and is often of value in primarily diagnosing the condition in patients with occult blood loss and normal x-rays. Early diagnosis is essential because the 5-year survival rate depends upon finding the tumor before it spreads beyond the muscularis mucosa. Routine stool examination for occult blood is a useful screening method for the early detection of this cancer. When patients evidence change of bowel habits, lower abdominal distress, and occult or gross blood in the stool, sigmoidoscopic examination and barium enema study should be performed. When these are undertaken, approximately 10 per cent of patients will be found to have polyps of the rectum or proximal colon. The presence of a polyp places a patient at risk for colorectal cancer and is an indication for colonoscopy and polypectomy, utilizing electrocautery snare or hot biopsy forceps. It is widely recognized that adenomatous polyps are premalignant lesions, often multiple, and, when larger than 2 cm, have a high probability of malignancy.

Aggressive management of these lesions is well tolerated in the older patient. The treatment of colon and rectal cancer is surgical removal of the lesions, even if the procedure is only palliative. In patients with nonresectable lesions, a diverting colostomy must be done. Chemotherapy for colorectal cancer has, as yet, not proved to be effective, and radiation therapy is of questionable value. The place of adjuvant chemotherapy in patients who have had a curative resection has not been established and it is probably not applicable in the elderly patient. The 5-year survival rate of patients with colorectal cancer is approximately 50 per cent, and thus, early diagnosis and early surgical treatment should be encouraged regardless of the patient's age.

## Gallbladder Disease

The incidence of cholelithiasis increases with advancing age, and this condition has been reported to be present in as many as 50 per cent of autopsied patients over the age of 70. The vast majority of stones found in the elderly are composed of cholesterol and result from formation of bile that is supersaturated with cholesterol. This high incidence is thought to be related to alterations in gallbladder emptying and mucous production and an increase in the secretion of cholesterol into the bile by the liver. In many instances, the condition is asymptomatic. Indigestion, belching, and flatulence are common complaints in the elderly and are not necessarily related to gallbladder diseases. Cholelithiasis may result in acute cholecystitis, in which the cystic duct is almost always obstructed. Biliary colic and jaundice occur if the stone migrates through the common bile duct. Acute pancreatitis may also be a complication. Cholecystectomy is the operation of choice. In the very debilitated, a cholecystostomy may be necessary, with the patient under local anesthesia. Stones in the common ducts, in the absence of cholecystitis, may now be managed by endoscopic papillotomy.

The management of silent stones remains controversial, but there is evidence that the majority of these gallstones remain silent.[36] Thus, in the nondiabetic elderly the consensus would favor expectant rather than surgical therapy. The use of gallstone-dissolving drugs chenodeoxycholic acid and ursodeoxycholic acid would seem ideal for this type of patient, but experience with these drugs is still very limited and the stones do recur when use of the drugs is stopped.[37,38]

Although classically the diagnosis of gallbladder disease has rested upon oral cholecystographic demonstration of a stone or stones or nonvisualization of the gallbladder, abdominal ultrasonography has assumed a role equal to if not greater than oral cholecystography in the diagnosis of cholelithiasis. This technique has permitted visualization of stones in the presence of jaundice or a nonfunctioning gallbladder, as well as occasionally demonstrating stone or gravel in the so-called "normal gallbladder." Ultrasonography can also be used reliably in the patient who is acutely ill. Further diagnostic studies that may be of value include the intravenous cholangiogram and scintigraphy utilizing technetium-labeled HIDA or PIPIDA. Intravenous cholangiography is rarely indicated in the patient with an intact gallbladder and should be reserved for the cholecystectomized patient with recurrent symptoms. The intraoperative cholangiogram is a far more accurate and reliable study. Cholescintigraphy, performed utilizing isotope-labeled aminodiacetic acid, may be helpful in the establishment of the diagnosis of acute cholecystitis, demonstrating cystic duct obstruction in the acutely ill, slightly icteric patient whose serum bilirubin is below 8 dl. When all these studies are normal in the patient with suggestive or equivocal symptoms, biliary drainage for cholesterol crystals and endoscopic retrograde cholangiopancreatography may be helpful in establishing the presence of cholelithiasis. Liver function tests, including measurement of serum bilirubin, serum alkaline phosphatase, serum aspartate immunotransferase, and glutamic transferase levels, may provide the objective evidence of disease in the acutely symptomatic patient whose test results might otherwise be negative.

## *Choledocholithiasis*

The incidence of common bile duct stones at cholecystectomy is about 10 per cent, with an increasing likelihood of the complication occurring in the aged as a result of a greater chance of stone migration. The rate of recurrence of stones following cholecystectomy has been reported to vary from 0.8 to 4 per cent, depending upon the skill of the surgeon and whether common duct exploration was performed at the time of cholecystectomy. Classically, the patient with a stone impacted in the common bile duct presents with severe mid-epigastric and right upper quadrant pain, often radiating through to the back, accompanied by chills, fever, and jaundice, the so-called Charcot's triad. A more insidious presentation may occur, with vague or minimal discomfort and persistent obstructive jaundice, and cannot be differentiated clinically from the other causes of extrahepatic biliary tract obstruction such as carcinoma of the pancreas. Ultrasonography may demonstrate stones in the acute case and dilatation of the intrahepatic ducts in the more chronic situation. Intravenous antibiotic therapy is indicated in the case of ascending cholangitis, and emergency surgery is necessary if the clinical picture fails to improve within a relatively short time.

In cases of obstructive jaundice with dilated ducts, a percutaneous transhepatic cholangiogram should be performed to define the nature and location of the obstructive process. Should there be no evidence of a stone or dilated intrahepatic duct, then endoscopic retrograde cholangiopancreatography should be performed. When the diagnosis of choledocholithiasis is established, removal of the calculi becomes mandatory. Such removal may be accomplished by a common duct exploration, choledochostomy, and surgical sphincteroplasty procedures or by a relatively new procedure using endoscopic techniques. These techniques consist of cannulation of the ampulla of Vater with a fiberoptic duodenoscope and performance of a papillotomy using electric current. First reported in Germany and Japan in 1974, this procedure is now being performed at many medical centers throughout the United States.[39] The procedure is basically a diathermy sphincterotomy, thus resulting in a larger orifice at the ampulla, allowing many stones to pass spontaneously. Stones may also be extracted utilizing balloon catheters or baskets. This transendoscopic procedure is particularly suited for patients who are frail owing to age or intercurrent disease. The application of endoscopic sphincterotomy in patients with an intact gallbladder with a common duct obstruction has not been established clearly. Another problem occurring in about 5 per cent of patients undergoing cholecystectomy and choledochotomy is that of retained stones in the bile duct, demonstrated by T-tube cholangiography. Until recently, re-exploration was required to remove such retained duct stones. This procedure can now be avoided by utilizing steerable bile duct catheters through the T-tube, extracting the retained stone or stones with minimal risk.

## *Pancreatic Cancer*

Carcinoma of the pancreas is the second most common gastrointestinal malignancy, with its highest incidence in the ninth decade of life. Once diagnosed, the median survival of patients with this disease is 4.5 months, and the 5-year survival rate is less than 1 per cent. The clinical picture is one of insidious onset of vague discomfort and loss of appetite. Anxiety and depression are common early in its course. Patients with lesions located in the head of the pancreas commonly present with obstructive jaundice; the lesions are sometimes painless, but often they are associated with upper abdominal or back pain occurring shortly after the patient has eaten or been awakened during the night. There is often a history of relief from aspirin. Tumors of the tail and body of the pancreas may also produce this type of pain. Not uncommonly, carcinoma of the pancreas presents as a migratory thrombophlebitis or with metastasis in the liver or elsewhere.

The diagnosis of carcinoma of the pancreas has become simpler and more accurate in recent years, although the outcome of this disease has not improved. With the advent of ultrasonography and computerized tomography, the demonstration of dilated intrahepatic bile ducts or a mass in the pancreas, or both, can be accomplished in virtually every symptomatic case.[40] If a mass is demonstrated within the pancreas, a percutaneous fine needle pancreatic biopsy under imaging control may yield the correct diagnosis in many cases.[41] Furthermore, in the very elderly or markedly debilitated patient with deep jaundice, decompression of the liver may be accomplished by the insertion of an endoprosthesis into the liver for decompression purposes, thus avoiding surgery.[42]

The usual treatment for pancreatic cancer is surgical; the most common operation is of a palliative nature to bypass the obstructed common duct; a cholecystojejunostomy is performed, and to prevent gastric outlet obstruction a gastrojejunostomy is carried out. Radical pancreatectomy, such as a Whipple procedure, is rarely indicated in the elderly patient. Radiation and chemotherapy have yet to be established as useful. The relief of pain, however, can sometimes be accomplished by celiac or splanchnic block.

## *Pancreatitis*

When acute pancreatitis occurs in the elderly, it is most likely to be related to gallstones rather than to alcoholism. The disease is more likely to be associated with amylase levels greater than 1000 units, and to have a greater mortality in the elderly compared with younger people. It tends not to recur when the biliary tract disease is corrected. Although the clinical presentation in the elderly may be identical to the classic presentation seen in young adults, it is occasionally atypical. The pain may be more prominent in the lower abdomen than in the epigastrium, and loss of consciousness is not uncommon. Of great interest is the frequency of unrecognized or painless episodes of pancreatitis. These attacks may be fatal and are diagnosed only at autopsy. Hypotension, shock, hypoxia, and respiratory failure, which are frequent complications of acute pancreatitis, are poorly tolerated by the elderly patient. Pre-existent cardiac, pulmonary, or renal diseases are responsible for the relative high mortality. Other causes of pancreatitis include postoperative pancreatitis and drug-induced pancreatitis, such as that associated with use of thiazides, sulfonamides, azathioprine, furosemides, and other drugs.[43]

Although elevations in serum amylase, lipase, or urine amylase levels are usually present, acute severe pancreatitis may occur without increase of serum amylase, and conversely, striking elevations of serum amylase may occur without pancreatitis. The latter may be due to renal failure, peritonitis, macroamylasemia, intestinal obstruction, infarction or perforation, diabetic ketoacidosis, drugs, or acute alcoholic intoxication. The amylase-creatinine ratio is now recognized as being of questionable significance. Classical radiologic changes are those of a sentinel loop found on the plain film of the abdomen, with gaseous distention of various portions of the ascending and transverse colon, with no gas evident beyond the splenic flexure or the so-called colon cutoff sign. Abdominal ultrasonography may reveal an enlarged pancreas or cholelithiasis. Management includes the relief of pain, primarily utilizing meperidine, and, at times, epidural block. Measures to arrest shock are of utmost importance. The necessity for nasogastric suction, long an integral part of the medical treatment for acute pancreatitis, has been questioned and, in the absence of severe nausea and vomiting, may not be necessary. Although antacid therapy has been advocated to decrease pancreatic secretion, the use of intravenous cimetidine has not been shown to be helpful. Anticholinergic drugs should be avoided because they affect the serial assessment of vital signs and may cause urinary retention. Surgical intervention has been advocated in the desperately ill patient with acute pancreatitis who does not respond to the conservative approach. Certainly, in the presence of known gallstones, such intervention would appear indicated.

### Chronic Pancreatitis

The prevalence of chronic pancreatitis in the elderly is unknown. Alcohol-induced pancreatitis is the dominant form of this disease. Classically, patients present with recurrent attacks of pain, but in some patients, the clinical picture may be dominated by pancreatic insufficiency. Secondary diabetes is almost invariably present.The radiologic hallmark of this disease is calcification of the pancreas.

The major problem clinically is to differentiate chronic pancreatitis from carcinoma of the pancreas. Ultrasonography and computerized tomography may not discriminate these entities. Endoscopic retrograde cholangiopancreatography may prove helpful. Duodenal drainage studies requiring intubation of the small bowel and injection of secretin to measure pancreatic function have been shown to be of limited value.[44]

## *Liver Disease*

Jaundice in the aged is due to obstructive disease in the majority of cases, but intrinsic liver disease is not rare. The common causes of intrinsic liver disease include drug-induced disease, post-transfusional hepatitis, and various forms of cirrhosis. Drug-induced liver disease may be due to direct and predictable toxicity-causing necrosis or fatty changes within the liver. Examples of drugs that may have these effects include halogenated hydrocarbons, heavy metals, cytotoxic drugs, acetaminophen, intravenous tetracycline, and alcohol. Hepatocellular-type reactions due to hypersensitivity are also common and are caused by such drugs as monoamine oxidase inhibitors, antidepressants, anticonvulsants, isoniazid, halothane, and methyldopa. In these instances, the clinical picture may include either insidious or acute onset of jaundice and liver function studies are characterized primarily by elevation of the serum aminotransferase level.[45] The clinical picture of this form of hepatitis cannot be differentiated from that of post-transfusional hepatitis other than by history. Type A hepatitis is rare in the elderly. Serum hepatitis, which is more commonly of the non-A, non-B type rather than B type, is a frequent illness in the aged patient who is subject to multiple surgical procedures.[46] This disease is characterized by a long incubation period, usually 6 weeks or more. Chronic persistent or active hepatitis is a not an infrequent sequel to serum hepatitis, occurring more commonly after the non-A, non-B type. The prognosis of all forms of hepatitis is more serious in the elderly patient because of debility and concomitant diseases.

Intrahepatic cholestasis is another form of drug-related liver disease. This condition may be due to hypersensitivity to various drugs, the classical ones being of the phenothiazine group, antidepressants, oral hypoglycemics, and thiazides. Nonhypersensitive cholestasis (that is, cholestasis related to dose and duration of drug use) is caused by methyltestosterones and similar compounds. The clinical picture of intrahepatic cholestasis is characterized by insidious painless jaundice, pruritus, and acholic stools. The alkaline phosphatase level is usually markedly elevated, with a lesser rise in amino transferase level. Although this form of cholestasis usually resolves upon the withdrawal of the offending drug, rarely chronic biliary cirrhosis can result. Although steroid therapy can result in a decrease of the serum bilirubin level, it is not likely that these drugs alter the course of the disease.

Cirrhosis, the end stage of chronic hepatitis, has been reported to be an increasing problem in the elderly patient. Alcohol is a common cause of cirrhosis, but many cases have no known cause and are classified as cryptogenic cirrhosis. The clinical features and management of this entity are the same as in younger patients and will not be considered further here. Although there is no effective treatment for cirrhosis per se, its complications do require skilled management. Upper GI hemorrhage requires emergency endoscopy to ascertain the cause of blood loss. In cirrhotic patients, peptic ulcer disease and ulcerative gastritis are more common causes of hemorrhage than are esophageal varices, and they respond to nasogastric suction and antacid therapy. Bleeding esophageal varices are sometimes controlled by intravenous vasopressin; if this fails, sclerotherapy should be employed. Surgical decompression of the portal system may be undertaken electively, but is associated with a high mortality in the elderly and an even higher incidence of encephalopathy following the procedure. Portal encephalopathy requires protein restriction and lactulose therapy. Neomycin may also be helpful. The management of ascites includes sodium restriction and, at times, fluid restriction with judicious use of diuretics, initiating such therapy with spironolactone followed by more potent diuretics in resistant cases. Renal failure, the so-called hepatorenal syndrome, may be a complication of this type of therapy. Paracentesis is to be decried except in cases of uncertain diagnosis or severe respiratory distress. The insertion of a peritoneovenous shunt may be of value in refractory cases (the so-called LeVeen shunt).

Primary biliary cirrhosis, classically a disease of middle-aged females, is rarely found in patients older than 70 years. It is a chronic, nonsuppurative, destructive cholangitis, which early in its course is silent and often discovered following a routine blood chemistry profile that demonstrates an elevated alkaline phosphatase. Pruritus may be present initially, with or without jaundice. Immunologic disturbances are characteristic, and these include an elevated serum antimitochondrial antibody titer and elevated IgM levels. Hypercholesterolemia is common. The serum amino transferase levels are minimally elevated. Hepatosplenomegaly, skin pigmentation, xanthelasma, and xanthoma are found on physical examination. Skeletal thinning and pathologic fractures are common. The disease usually runs a long, although inexorable course, leading to death either as a result of hepatic failure or GI hemorrhage secondary to portal hypertension. Because patients with primary biliary cirrhosis have elevated hepatic and serum copper levels, D-penicillamine, a copper-binding agent, has been used to treat this disease, but its value has not been established.[47]

The most common malignancy to involve the liver is metastatic carcinoma. Classically, the liver is enlarged and irregular. Sometimes the primary tumor is not apparent. Laboratory studies usually reveal significant elevations of aminotransferase and alkaline phosphatase levels. If these values are normal, the likelihood of metastatic cancer in the liver is small. Hepatic imaging techniques, including hepatic scintigraphy, ultrasonography, and CT scanning, reveal the character of the abnormal liver. Liver biopsy confirms the diagnosis.

## CONCLUSION

The human digestive tract ages well. Digestion rarely fails; absorption usually diminishes insignificantly, although excretion does often become a major problem. In most cases, carefully listening to the patient's history will provide enough clues for the correct working diagnosis, and reassurance, proper dietary instruction, and judicious administration of medication will provide adequate treatment. Catering to the emotional needs of patients and tending to their physical ills in a diligent but human fashion should be the basic approach of the physician. In patients in whom organic disease is probable, use of noninvasive studies should be the initial step in diagnosis. The elderly are to be treated gingerly although not neglected. Organic disease, when found, is often treatable. As a result of treatment, many patients will be provided with many happy and healthy additional years. When a poor outcome is a foregone conclusion, heroic measures that offer only small hope of cure should be avoided. The physician must always weigh the risks of diagnostic and therapeutic measures not necessarily against the longevity of life but, rather, against the quality of life that is likely to follow.

"It is as much the business of the physician to alleviate pain and to smooth the avenues of death when unavoidable as to cure disease" (John Gregory [1725–1773], Lectures on the Duties and Qualifications of the Physician).[48]

## References

1. Sklar M: Gastrointestinal diseases in the aged. *In* Reichel W (ed.): Clinical Aspects of Aging. 2nd ed. Baltimore, Williams and Wilkins, 1983.
*A review of a large number of elderly patients, emphasizing the clinical features of gastrointestinal disease in those over the age 65.*
2. Zack L: The oral cavity. *In* Rossman I (ed.): Clinical Geriatrics. 2nd ed. Philadelphia, J.B. Lippincott Company, 1979, pp. 618–627.
*An excellent review of the changes that occur in the oral cavity during the aging process.*
3. Soergel KH, Zboralske FF, Amberg JR: Esophageal motility in nonagenarians. J Clin Invest 43:1472, 1964.
*A classic article discussing the functional esophageal abnormalities occurring in the aged.*
4. Keighley MRB: Anal function and fecal incontinence. *In* Jewell DP, Amanoell P (eds.): Topics in Gastroenterology. Vol. 9. Oxford, Blackwell Scientific Publications, 1982, pp. 305–322.
*A well-written current review of anal function and fecal incontinence, dealing with the physiology, pathology, and management of this most perplexing problem.*
5. Tauchi H, Sato T: Hepatic cells of the aged. *In* Kitane K (ed.): Liver in Aging. Amsterdam, Elsevier-North Holland Cryomedical Press, 1978, pp. 3–20.
*This article, and the many other articles in this excellent monograph, provides the most recent authoritative information related to the morphologic, pathologic,*

*and physiologic changes that occur in the aging liver. The material is discussed in a highly technical fashion.*

6. Snape WJ Jr, Carlson GM, Matarazzo SA, Cohen S: Evidence that abnormal myoelectrical activity produces colonic motor dysfunction in the irritable bowel syndrome. Gastroenterology 72:383, 1977.
*This study of 20 patients with irritable bowel syndrome suggests that increased colonic 3 cycle per minute slow wave activity may be the basic abnormality that leads to colonic motor dysfunction.*
7. Painter NS, Burkitt DP: Diverticular disease of the colon: A deficiency disease of Western civilization. Br Med J 22:450, 1971.
*A hypothesis is presented of the cause of diverticulosis coli that is consistent with its geographical distribution, its recent emergence as a medical problem, and its changing incidence. Classic work suggesting the importance of fiber in the diet.*
8. Floch MH: Nutrition and Diet Therapy in Gastrointestinal Diseases. Medical Book Company, 1981.
*An excellent review of the physiologic and chemical characteristics of fiber. The best textbook on diet therapy in gastrointestinal disease. In an extremely readable and authoritative manner, the author has covered most types of diet as they affect the gastrointestinal tract.*
9. Thompson WG: The Irritable Gut. Baltimore, University Park Press, 1979.
*This text is the best available source for information regarding this syndrome. The student as well as the experienced gastroenterologist will find this book interesting and informative.*
10. Bartlett JG, Chang T, Gurwith M, et al: Antibiotic associated pseudomembranous colitis due to toxin-producing clostridia. N Engl J Med 298:531, 1978.
*The observations in this study lead to the incrimination of toxogenic clostridia as the cause of pseudomembranous colitis.*
11. Chang T: Antimicrobial-associated diarrhea and enterocolitis. Drug Therapy, September 1981, pp. 117–124.
*An excellent presentation of the etiology, clinical features, and treatment of this relatively common illness. The value of vancomycin and cholestyramine is emphasized.*
12. Harris JC, Dupont HL, Hornig RB: Fecal leukocytes in diarrheal disease. Ann Intern Med 76:697, 1972.
*A very simple test utilizing a rectal smear, which is then stained for fecal leukocytes; this test is of great value in differentiating infectious and inflammatory-induced diarrhea from functional illness.*
13. Brockelhurst JC: Textbook of Geriatric Medicine and Gerontology. 2nd ed. Edinburgh, Churchill and Livingstone, 1978, pp. 377–380.
*Pragmatic and comprehensive review of fecal incontinence written by a physician with wide experience with the problem. The entire chapter on the gastrointestinal system is to be commended in this textbook of geriatric medicine.*
14. Tucker H, Cohn S: Management of esophageal disorders. Drug Therapy, January 1979.
*A pragmatic discussion of esophageal disorders designed for the primary physician, with concise description of the most common disorders and their management.*
15. Rixter JE, Castell DO: Gastroesophageal reflux; pathogenesis, diagnosis, and therapy. Ann Intern Med 97:93, 1982.
*This article presents an overview of the current therapy of reflux disease and summarizes the controlled studies in the medical literature.*
16. Ellis FH: Controversies regarding the management of hiatus hernia. Am J Surg 139:782, 1980.
*Differences of opinion regarding the nature of hiatus hernias and their management are discussed, and the author presents the advantages of various fundal plication procedures.*
17. Ellis FH Jr, Lane FW Jr, Boyce HW Jr: Management of esophageal cancer: Three viewpoints. Hosp Pract 11:63, 1982.
*The cases for surgery, irradiation, and palliation are presented for the management of this disease, the prognosis of which, regardless of treatment, is very poor.*
18. Grossman MI, Kurata JH, Rotter JI, et al: Peptic ulcer: new therapies, new diseases. Ann Intern Med 95:609, 1981.
*This article presents a sampling of the present state of knowledge about ulcer disease. Sections dealing with gastric motility, cytoprotection, and endoscopic treatment of GI bleeding are of special interest.*
19. Hollander D, Harlan J: Antacids versus placebos in peptic ulcer therapy. JAMA 226:1181, 1973.
*Ability of an antacid preparation to relieve discomfort and to promote healing of peptic ulcer was compared with that of a placebo in a controlled double-blind outpatient study. Antacids were demonstrated to be more effective than placebos in the promotion of healing and relief of discomfort.*
20. Ippoliti AF, Sturdevant RAL, Isenberg JI, et al: Cimetidine versus intensive antacid therapy for duodenal ulcer. Gastroenterology 74:383, 1978.
*In a randomized double-blind multicenter trial, patients treated with cimetidine and those treated with an intensive regimen of antacids had similar rates of duodenal ulcer healing and pain relief. Both methods of therapy are superior to placebo.*
21. Drake D, Hollander D: Neutralizing capacity and cost effectiveness of antacids. Ann Intern Med 94:215, 1981.
*Commonly available antacids were tested for their acid neutralizing capacity. Excellent advice is offered the prescribing physician who is faced with this wide choice of antacid preparations.*
22. Freston JW: Cimetidine: Its development, pharmacology and efficacy. Ann Intern Med 97:573, 1982.
23. Freston JW: Cimetidine: Adverse reactions and patterns of use. Ann Intern Med 97:728–734.
*Both articles provide excellent reviews of the current state of cimetidine therapy. The indications for the use of this drug are clearly indicated as well as unapproved conditions for which it is being used. The numerous adverse reactions are also clearly described and their low frequency emphasized.*
24. Chang FC, Drake JE, Farha GJ: Massive upper gastrointestinal hemorrhage in the elderly. Am J Surg 134:721, 1977.
*This study evaluates the effectiveness of early and aggressive diagnosis and therapy in elderly patients with massive upper gastrointestinal bleeding. The study supports a concept of early diagnosis with fiberoptic endoscopy and prompt surgical intervention in patients with continued bleeding.*
25. Jansen RT, Gardner JD, Raufman JP, et al: Zollinger-Ellison syndrome, current concepts in management. Ann Intern Med 98:59, 1983.
*A review of advances in the diagnosis and treatment of the Zollinger-Ellison syndrome, as well as progress in the understanding of its natural history, is presented. The results of a recent 7-year-experience with 42 patients and the experience of others are reported.*

25a. Strickland RG, Mackay IR: A Reappraisal of the Nature and Significance of Chronic Atrophic Gastritis. Dig Dis 18:426, 1973.

26. Almay TP, Howell DA: Diverticular disease of the colon. N Engl J Med 302:324, 1980.
*Epidemiologic, clinical, pathologic, radiologic, and physiologic data regarding diverticular disease of the colon are discussed and correlated. The rationale for currently accepted medical management and for hypotheses regarding the prevention of this condition is presented.*

27. Berardi RS: Diverticular disorders of the colon, a need for standard clinical classification. American Journal of Proctology, Gastroenterology and Colon and Rectal Surgery, May–June 1978, pp. 11–16.
*A study of patients with diverticular disorders of the colon was analyzed from the point of view of clinical manifestations. An excellent clinical classification is presented, which allows for a better understanding of the disease process as well as provides information of therapeutic usefulness.*

28. Larson DM, Masters FS, Spiro HM: Medical and surgical therapy of diverticular disease. Gastroenterology 71:734, 1976.
*A large group of patients with documented acute diverticulitis was treated medically and a smaller group was treated surgically, with a long follow-up. The rationale for the medical treatment of an episode of diverticulitis is presented.*

29. Ulin AW, Pearce AF, Weinstein SM: Diverticular disease of the colon: Surgical perspectives in the past decade. American Society of Colon and Rectal Surgeons, May–June 1981, pp. 276–281.
*This article provides a rational, coherent clinical view of some of the medical and surgical problems associated with diverticular disease and focuses on the determination of the various therapeutic groups (e.g., medical, surgery advisable, and surgery inevitable).*

30. Marks FW Jr, Gray RK, Duncan AM, Bakhtia RL: Angiodysplasia as a source of intestinal bleeding. Am J Surg 134:125, 1977.
*Cases of angiodysplasia identified angiographically are reported, and it is suggested that this abnormality may not be as rare as commonly assumed because it may escape detection even angiographically, at least initially. The character and clinical behavior of these lesions are well described.*

31. Croft RJ, Mennen GP, Marston A: Does "intestinal angina" exist? A critical study of obstructed visural arteries. Br J Surg 68:316, 1981.
*The study calls into question the clinical significance of radiologic demonstration of stenosed or blocked visceral arteries and discusses the lack of any method that predicts which patients with abdominal pain and visceral arterial disease are at risk of developing intestinal infarction.*

32. Lottinger LW: Mesenteric ischemia. N Engl J Med 307:335, 1982.
*The complexity of the various presentations, multiple causes, and high mortality rate of acute mesenteric ischemia is presented. The short-term results of surgery in the management of chronic intestinal ischemia, as well as the potential of transluminal angioplasty, are discussed.*

33. Kirsner JB, Schroeder RG: Inflammatory Bowel Disease. Philadelphia, Lea and Feiberger, 1980, pp. 13–15.
*This is the authoritative text on the subject of inflammatory bowel disease. All aspects of this difficult clinical problem are covered with clarity and accuracy.*

33a. Burch PEJ, DeDombal FT, Watkinson C: Etiology of ulcerative colitis. II, A new hypothesis. Gut 10:277, 1969.

34. Brandt LJ, Boley SJ, Migsudo S: Clinical characteristics and natural history of colitis in the elderly. Am J Gastroenterol 77:382, 1982.
*The clinical behavior and course of ischemic, ulcerative, and Crohn's colitis in the elderly are analyzed. The various clinical features differentiating these forms of colitis are presented.*

35. Winowar SJ: Colorectal cancer. Clinical Roundtables. Vols. 1 and 2, June 1982.
*The discussions contained in these roundtables by authorities in the field of colorectal cancer provide the most up-to-date information regarding the prevention and management of this common gastrointestinal cancer.*

36. Gracy WA, Ranslhoff DF: The natural history of silent gallstones. N Engl J Med 307:798, 1982.
*In a series of patients with silent stones, a benign course is reported.*

37. Isselbacher KJ: Chenodiol for gallstones: Dissolution or disillusion. Ann Intern Med 95:377, 1981.

38. McSherry CK: The national cooperative gallstone study report: A surgeon's perspective. Ann Intern Med 95:379, 1981.
*The present status of chenodiol therapy from the medical and surgical points of view is discussed with the conclusion that cholecystectomy continues to be the treatment of choice for a great majority of patients with cholelithiasis. The role of chenodiol is very limited.*

39. Cotton TB: In Burke JE (ed.): Developments in Digestive Diseases. Vol. 2. Philadelphia, Lea and Feibeger, 1979, pp. 127–139.
*Excellent results of endoscopic sphincterotomy in removing calculi from the common bile duct are presented. Complication rate and mortality appear to be extremely low, and this technique would be applicable in the high-risk elderly patient.*

40. Cello JP: Diagnostic approaches to jaundice. Hosp Pract 17:49, 1982.
*A rational diagnostic approach is presented that differentiates intrahepatic from extrahepatic cholestasis by defining the nature and site of the pathologic process without use of surgery.*

41. Mueller PR, van Sonnenberg E, Cemone JF: Fine needle transhepatic cholangiography: Indications and usefulness. Ann Intern Med 97:567, 1982.
*Fine needle transhepatic cholangiography is reported as a diagnostic tool valuable for evaluating the biliary tree because of its wide availability and relatively low complication rate. The central role that fine needle cholangiography plays in the finding of the site and cause of biliary obstruction is emphasized.*

42. MacCarty RL: Non-surgical management of obstructive jaundice in the patient with advanced cancer. JAMA 244:1976, 1980.
*Most patients with malignant biliary obstruction have incurable disease. A method is described in which adequate drainage of the obstructed biliary system is carried out without major surgery.*

43. Berk JE: Acute pancreatitis: clinical features, diagnosis and management. Curr Concepts Gastroenterol 2:14, 1977.
*Acute pancreatitis is a challenging disease that commands respect. A summary of the important developments in the diagnosis and treatment of this disorder is presented.*

44. Marks IN, Bank S: Chronic pancreatitis; classification, clinical aspects, diagnosis and management. Curr Concepts Gastroenterol 2:21, 1977.

*Major advances in the diagnosis and classification of chronic pancreatitis and in the understanding of the pathogenesis, endocrine aspects, clinical features, and natural history of the disease are discussed.*

45. Klatskin G: Toxic and drug induced hepatitis. *In* Shiff Leon (ed.): Diseases of the Liver. 4th ed. Philadelphia, J.B. Lippincott Company, 1975, pp. 605–681.
*An excellent review dealing with drug metabolism and drug-induced liver disease in an authoritative textbook that covers the entire field of hepatology.*

46. Rakela J, Redeker AG: Chronic liver disease after acute non-A, non-B viral hepatitis. Gastroenterology 77:1200, 1979.
*It appears that chronic hepatitis is more commonly a complication of non-A, non-B viral hepatitis than of B hepatitis, contrary to what was thought in the past. The problem is emphasized in this article.*

47. Christiansen E, Crowe J, Boniach D: Clinical patterns in the course of disease in primary biliary cirrhosis, based on analysis of 236 patients. Gastroenterology 78:236, 1978.
*An excellent review of primary biliary cirrhosis, stressing the indolent although inexorable course of this condition, for which treatment is still experimental and of inconclusive value.*

48. Hollander W Jr, Williams TF: Dr. Strauss' last teaching session. Arch Intern Med 135:1391, 1975.
*A touching article describing the humane, dignified management of a distinguished physician dying of esophageal carcinoma.*

# Chapter 47

# Anesthesiology

*Jonathan M. Stein*
*John Hedley-Whyte*

During the nearly 140 years since the first successful demonstration of general anesthesia, the scope of anesthesiology has grown far beyond the mere provision of unconsciousness during surgery to encompass the diagnosis, minimization, and treatment of major organ impairment during the perioperative period. This trend has had the most impact on the elderly, who are more prone than the young to failure of every major organ. The development of potent anesthetics with minimal cardiac depressant effects, the elaboration of the causes of perioperative respiratory and circulatory failure and the means of treating them for prolonged periods, and the development of sophisticated cardiopulmonary monitoring techniques for routine use have revolutionized geriatric anesthetic practice. Virtually any elderly patient can now be anesthetized for any operation with relative safety if proper technology and personnel are at hand. Extension of the means of vital organ monitoring and support from the intraoperative to the postoperative periods has spawned modern intensive care, which is increasingly utilized by the elderly at ever-increasing cost. Indeed, our technical ability to ensure indefinite vegetative survival in critically ill aged patients may be outpacing our ability to pay for it.

At the same time, analysis of demographic trends has led to the conclusion that a limit to the natural life span at about 85 years will be realized sometime early in the next century, barring any unforeseen breakthrough in the fundamental biology of aging itself.[1] In a time of increasing realization of the finite nature of our medical resources, we are thus led to a paradox that is already familiar to those working in intensive care units. Indiscriminate application of the full armamentarium of anesthetic and intensive care support systems to all elderly patients who satisfy physiologic criteria for their application inevitably leads to few years of useful patient life span gained at prohibitive cost. Furthermore, the physician must take account of the possibility of suffering induced by technologically advanced care, often with questionable benefit. Both from humanitarian and economic points of view, it is imperative, therefore, that those caring for the elderly during and after operation concentrate on the preoperative *prophylaxis* of organ failure and on the recognition of the potential for *reversibility* of organ failure if it does occur. This chapter will focus on those aspects of predictable perioperative morbidity, which, on the basis of geriatric physiology, can most effectively be avoided or reversed by the primary physician, anesthesiologist, and surgeon.

## TRENDS IN GERIATRIC POSTOPERATIVE MORTALITY

Examination of results of geriatric surgery over the last three decades reveals that the incidence as well as the leading causes of postoperative mortality have changed markedly. Overall surgical death rates have generally declined (Table 47–1).[2–6] In 1961, Wilder and Fishbein[3] at the Baltimore City Hospital reported a 33 per cent 30-day postoperative mortality after all surgical procedures in 207 patients over age 80. Marshall and Fahey,[4] in 1964 at the University of Louisville, achieved a 22 per cent postoperative mortality after 500 operations on 443 octogenarians. By 1979, we were able to report a 6 per cent postoperative mortality in 500 consecutively operated patients over the age of 80.[6]

**Table 47–1.** MORTALITY BY OPERATION AND SERIES

| | Series | | | | | | | | | | | |
|---|---|---|---|---|---|---|---|---|---|---|---|---|
| | *Anglem (1953)*[2] | | *Wilder (1961)*[3] | | *Marshall (1964)*[4] | | *Palmberg (1979)*[5] | | | | *Djokovic (1979)*[6] | |
| Number of Patients | 500 | | 207 | | 443 | | 289 | | 77 | | 500 | |
| Age of patients | >70 | | >80 | | >80 | | >70 | | >80 | | >80 | |
| Number of procedures | 621 | | 284 | | 500 | | 289 | | 77 | | 644 | |
| *Procedure* | | | | | | | | | | | | |
| Peripheral vascular | — | | (2/3) | 67% | (4/8) | 50% | — | | — | | (0/20) | 0% |
| Laparotomy, colostomy, lysis of adhesion, small bowel resection | (5/35) | 14% | (6/19) | 32% | (20/57) | 35% | (7/39) | 17% | (3/8) | 37% | (7/37) | 19% |
| Gastric | (7/53) | 13% | (4/8) | 50% | (7/18) | 39% | — | | — | | (1/9) | 11% |
| Amputation | (6/25) | 24% | (7/16) | 44% | (12/60) | 20% | (6/48) | 12% | (3/16) | 19% | (4/53) | 7% |
| Colectomy | (29/206) | 14% | (2/4) | 50% | (5/24) | 21% | (2/16) | 12% | (1/2) | 50% | (4/53) | 7% |
| Thoracotomy | — | | (1/1) | 100% | — | | — | | — | | (1/5) | 20% |
| Cholecystectomy with or without duct exploration | (7/81) | 8% | (1/2) | 50% | (1/14) | 7% | (1/44) | 2% | (0/6) | 0% | (0/47) | 0% |
| Hip procedures | | | (26/78) | 33% | (30/148) | 20% | (9/66) | 13% | (5/24) | 21% | (6/115) | 5% |
| Open prostatectomy | | | (4/20) | 20% | (6/40) | 15% | — | | — | | (0/17) | 0% |
| Herniorrhaphy | (3/36) | 8% | (1/24) | 4% | (2/46) | 4% | (0/10) | 0% | (0/6) | 0% | (1/27) | 4% |
| Gynecologic | (0/35) | 0% | — | | (0/4) | 0% | — | | — | | (0/18) | 0% |
| Breast procedures | (0/31) | 0% | (0/3) | 0% | (0/4) | 0% | (1/12) | 8% | (0/4) | 0% | (0/18) | 0% |
| Transurethral prostatectomy | — | | (8/31) | 26% | (6/56) | 11% | (0/7) | 0% | (0/1) | 0% | — | |
| Head and neck | (4/54) | 7% | — | | (1/5) | 20% | — | | — | | (0/22) | 0% |
| All other | (1/65) | 2% | (7/75) | 9% | (3/16) | 9% | (2/47) | 4% | (0/12) | 0% | (7/203) | 3% |
| *Total Patient Mortality* | (62/500) | 12% | (69/207) | 33% | (97/443) | 22% | (28/289) | 10% | (12/77) | 16% | (31/500) | 6% |

The decline in fatal complications has been uneven (Table 47–2). Pneumonia, which caused 26 per cent of fatalities in Palmberg's series and 29 per cent of fatalities in Wilder's series, had declined to a 7 per cent proportion of fatal events in Djokovic's series. We believe that the decrease in the lethality of pneumonia resulted from earlier postoperative mobilization, vigorous application of postoperative chest physiotherapy, greater anesthetic attention to the problem of pulmonary aspiration, better surveillance of the bacterial flora of the upper and lower airway, the development of new potent antibiotics, and, finally, the vastly increased ability to safely maintain mechanical ventilation for prolonged periods in patients with pneumonia and respiratory failure. With assiduous application of these developments and practices in the elderly, pneumonia should rarely cause a postoperative fatality.

Postoperative pulmonary embolus is largely a geriatric disease. The tendency of elderly individuals toward lower extremity venous incompetence, their decreased ability to ambulate rapidly after major surgery, and the increased incidence of associated conditions, such as malignancy, render the elderly especially vulnerable to this complication. Nevertheless, in the geriatric postoperative population, the absolute incidence of, as well as the proportion of fatalities from, postoperative pulmonary embolism has sharply declined. This is probably due to widespread use of heparin prophylaxis. In our institution, all surgical patients except those having neurosurgical procedures receive 5000 units of heparin subcutaneously 1 to 2 hours prior to surgery, repeated every 12 hours after surgery until ambulation is achieved. This regimen has been shown by Kakkar and associates to reduce dramatically the incidence of fatal postoperative pulmonary embolism.[7] A slight increase in the incidence of wound hematoma is the only significantly increased complication. Of the 18 patients in Kakkar's series who developed fatal embolism, the mean age was 70 years, whereas the mean age of all the 4021 patients was significantly less, thus demonstrating the geriatric predilection for this catastrophe.

In contrast to the marked decline in the rates of fatal postoperative pneumonias and pulmonary emboli, the raw fatility rates of myocardial events and strokes have not dramatically changed in 30 years. Myocardial and mesenteric infarction have emerged as the major causes of postoperative death in the elderly, together accounting for over 50 per cent of the mortality in the Beth Israel series.[6] Although it is likely that the increasing presentation for surgery of patients with more advanced vascular disease has concealed statistically those improvements in management that have occurred, it is clear that prevention of heart and bowel infarction must become a major priority.

Certain operations have been fairly safe to perform on the elderly for decades. These include herniorrhaphy, gynecologic procedures, and breast surgery. Modern care has not significantly improved mortality for these procedures, which rarely cause cardiopulmonary compromise, prolonged immobilization, or septic complications. Conversely, exploratory laparotomy and colectomy, especially when performed on an emergency basis, have remained high-risk undertakings (Table 47–3).[8] Death rates for

**Table 47–2.** CAUSES OF GERIATRIC POSTOPERATIVE DEATHS

| | Series | | | | | |
|---|---|---|---|---|---|---|
| | *Anglem (1953)*[2] | *Wilder (1961)*[3] | *Marshall (1964)*[4] | *Palmberg (1979)*[5] | *Djokovic (1979)*[6] | *Blake (1976)*[8†] |
| Age | >70 | >80 | >80 | >70 | >80 | >75 |
| *Cause of Death* | | | | | | |
| Pneumonia | 13% | 29% | 38% | 26% | 7% | 17% |
| Pulmonary embolus | 11% | 6% | 14% | 33%* | 3% | 7% |
| Myocardial infarction and heart failure | 29% | 12% | 17% | 13% | 32% | 19% |
| Sepsis and primary surgical disease | 16% | 14% | 13% | 9% | 19% | 43% |
| Stroke | 2% | 9% | 2% | 6% | 7% | 2% |
| Mesenteric infarction | — | — | — | — | 23% | — |
| Renal failure | — | 4% | 8% | — | 3% | — |
| Other (suicide, trauma, "shock," unexplained) | 29% | 26% | 8% | 13% | 6% | 12% |
| *Total Number of Patients* | 500 | 207 | 443 | 289 | 500 | 375 |
| *Total Patient Mortality* | 12% | 33% | 22% | 10% | 6% | 32% |

* Heparin prophylaxis not used.
† Emergencies only.

**Table 47-3.** EMERGENCY SURGICAL MORTALITY IN 375 PATIENTS OLDER THAN 75 YEARS*

| Diagnosis | Mortality | Rate |
|---|---|---|
| Ruptured abdominal aortic aneurysm | 7/9 | 78% |
| Small bowel ischemia | 6/9 | 67% |
| Colonic perforation | 14/22 | 64% |
| Gastrointestinal hemorrhage | 12/27 | 44% |
| Colonic obstruction | 24/60 | 40% |
| Miscellaneous | 5/13 | 38% |
| Small bowel obstruction | 15/43 | 35% |
| Biliary disease | 4/21 | 19% |
| Strangulated hernia | 19/115 | 16% |
| Appendicitis | 4/34 | 12% |
| All diagnoses | 119/375 | 32% |
| **Causes of death** | | |
| Peritonitis and septicemia | 25/119 | 21% |
| Pneumonia or other thoracic infection | 20/119 | 17% |
| Hemorrhage and shock | 14/119 | 12% |
| Heart failure | 13/119 | 11% |
| Undefined | 12/119 | 10% |
| Myocardial infarction | 10/119 | 8% |
| Pulmonary embolus | 8/119 | 7% |
| Carcinomatosis | 8/119 | 7% |
| Other (related to surgical disease) | 4/119 | 3% |
| Other (unrelated to surgical disease) | 3/119 | 2% |
| Stroke | 2/119 | 2% |

* Data from Blake R, Lynn J: Emergency abdominal surgery in the aged. Br J Surg 63:956, 1976.

elective gastric, biliary, hip, vascular, and urologic procedures have improved most, as a result of improvements in care over the last 30 years.

## GERIATRIC PHYSIOLOGY AND ANESTHESIA

### *Respiratory Morbidity*

Major functional and structural alterations of the upper airway and lungs occur in the fit elderly, which render them at increased risk of developing perioperative respiratory complications. There is a progressive and dramatic loss of protective laryngeal reflexes in healthy old people, even in the absence of nervous system disease.[9] Thus, they have a predisposition to pulmonary aspiration, which is aggravated by use of central nervous system depressants preoperatively and residual anesthetic after surgery. Elderly patients frequently have full stomachs, thus providing a reservoir of acidic material for potential aspiration. The mean half time of gastric emptying increases from 50 to 123 minutes from the third to eighth decade in healthy volunteers. Moreover, there is tremendous variation in gastric emptying times, some being much longer than the stated mean.[10] It is therefore imperative to avoid sedative premedication in all but the hardiest and most anxious elderly patients and to delay emergency surgery as long as is feasible after the last ingestion of food or drink. If the surgical situation precludes reasonable delay, consideration should be given to partial emptying of the stomach via a nasogastric tube prior to induction of anesthesia. In such cases, the anesthesiologist may wish to perform endotracheal intubation while the patient is awake. This procedure is usually well tolerated if skillful performance is preceded by careful explanation to the patient and family.

Neutralization of the stomach contents will decrease the severity of pulmonary damage if aspiration does occur. Both antacid and single-dose parenteral or oral cimetidine effectively and rapidly reduce gastric acidity in preoperative patients.[11] All elderly patients undergoing emergency surgery should receive one or the other therapy. If symptoms of gastroesophageal sphincter incompetence or hiatal hernia are present, gastric buffering should be ordered prior to elective surgery as well. However, the use of antacids and cimetidine on a chronic basis is not without disadvantage, as the bacterial count of the stomach is positively correlated with pH. Airway colonization and pneumonia may result from microaspiration of these organisms.[12]

Normal changes in the properties of the pulmonary parenchyma and chest wall render the elderly at increased risk of postoperative respiratory failure. With aging, there is an increase in the ratio of elastin to collagen in lung tissue, increasing lung compliance and decreasing elastic recoil.[13] Thoracic compliance decreases with age, as the chest wall becomes more rigid and increases its resting anteroposterior diameter. As a result, the equilibrium between the chest wall and lung shifts, with residual volume increasing markedly while total lung capacity remains roughly constant.[14] Thus, vital capacity is limited by the enhanced residual volume, and maximal breathing capacity falls. Airway resistance increases with aging even in the absence of pulmonary disease, thereby increasing the metabolic cost of breathing.[15]

Arterial $Pa_{O_2}$ falls with normal aging. This is due to impaired efficiency of the matching of ventilation and perfusion and to an increase in lung closing volume. The closing volume is defined as that lung volume at which small airway closure and shunting begin to occur. It is increased when the patient is supine, which is the most common position postoperatively. Hypoxemia from ventilation-perfusion mismatch and closure of small airways can be corrected through administration of oxygen via mask or, if severe, via positive pressure mechanical ventilation. Positive end-expiratory pressure (PEEP) may play a role in maintaining patency of compromised small airways if hypoxemia is severe.[16]

Upper abdominal and thoracic incisions reduce the vital capacity and functional residual capacity drastically, owing to reflex muscular splinting secondary to pain. This causes the postoperative patient to breathe at low lung volumes, increasing the tendency toward airway closure, atelectasis, and hypoxemia. This tendency toward postoperative hypoxemia is exaggerated in old patients.[17] Furthermore, residual anesthetic and narcotic drugs, whose elimination is delayed in the elderly, depress the ventilatory responses to hypercapnia and hypoxia to a greater degree in older than in younger patients. Excretion of muscle relaxants via the liver and kidney is also delayed in the elderly, and hence, respiratory neuromuscular function may be grossly impaired in the first postoperative hours. Hypovolemia impairs pulmonary function by causing a diminution of blood flow to superior portions of the pulmonary vascular bed, thus increasing pulmonary dead space and the cost of breathing.

Overall, both the gas exchange efficiency and the maximal oxygen uptake capacity are reduced in normal aging. Therefore, the respiratory stresses of anesthesia and operation are especially liable to produce respiratory failure in the geriatric age group. In order to minimize pulmonary perioperative morbidity and mortality, we advocate the following in patients aged 70 or above:

1. Performance of preoperative pulmonary function testing before all thoracic or abdominal procedures. Vital capacity less than 1.5 L or an $FEV_1$ of less than 1 L is associated with postoperative respiratory failure, especially if thoracic or abdominal surgery is to be performed.
2. Instruction of patients as to the potential need for postoperative intubation and ventilation, with consequent temporary loss of voice during intubation. Patients should be assured that nurses will anticipate their needs without vocal cues.
3. Familiarization of high-risk patients with the chest physical therapist and his or her treatments before operation.
4. Optimization of preoperative pulmonary function by treatment of bronchospasm, congestive heart failure, and hypovolemia before operation.
5. Maintenance of postoperative intubation and mechanically assisted ventilation until an inspiratory force of −25 cm of water and a vital capacity of 15 ml per kg are demonstrated. If advanced obstructive airways disease is present, the criteria for extubation should be more rigorous, as the associated increased airway resistance may produce exhaustion and eventual respiratory failure if function is borderline.
6. Consideration of perioperative placement of an indwelling radial artery catheter to facilitate blood gas sampling.
7. Maintenance of continuous surveillance cultures of airway bacteria and a vigilant search for evidence of pneumonia, such as fever, pulmonary infiltrates, or leukocytosis in high-risk elderly postoperative patients.
8. Placement of spontaneously breathing postoperative patients with borderline respiratory function in a semi- or fully sitting position, if possible.
9. Provision of adequate pain relief after surgery to reduce splinting of ventilatory muscles, either with small intravenous (IV) doses of narcotic that are "titrated" to the patient's needs, or with regional analgesic techniques.
10. Encouragement of early ambulation, deep breathing, and coughing after surgery as part of a "stir-up" regimen.
11. Provision of supplemental oxygen via face mask for at least 72 hours after major procedures and for at least 12 to 24 hours after any general anesthetic.

## *Cardiac Morbidity*

Postoperative myocardial infarction is a highly lethal event and is more likely to occur in those over the age of 70. In recent series, mortality from postoperative myocardial infarction ranged from 44 to 62 per cent, roughly twice that of infarctions occurring outside the surgical setting.[18,19] The problem is compounded by the fact that the presentation of postoperative infarctions may be subtle, with only half of them causing pain. Often, these events are heralded by T-wave changes in the electrocardiogram; congestive heart failure; hypotension; or arrhythmias, such as supraventricular tachycardia, nodal rhythm, and ventricular ectopy.[18] Only a minority of postoperative infarctions occur in the recovery room, probably because of low myocardial oxygen demand during the immediate postoperative period, intensive monitoring, and immediate availability of IV drugs such as nitroglycerin and propranolol. Rather, the period of maximal infarction risk occurs during the third through the fifth postoperative days. During this time, ambulation, wound healing, fluid mobilization, and postoperative pain impose significant demands upon the myocardium, while, for the reasons stated previously, pulmonary efficiency is still grossly impaired. Thus, myocardial oxygenation is jeopardized, as demand may exceed supply. Because of the highly lethal nature of the postoperative infarction and the limited efficacy of postinfarction interventions in reducing mortality, it behooves the clinician to maintain vigilance for the development of untoward cardiac events for a prolonged period after surgery and to correct them quickly if they occur. The maintenance of maximal oxygen supply and minimal demand of the elderly heart is the paramount consideration.

Several predictable myocardial changes that occur in many aged patients directly increase the risk of infarction. Not surprisingly, the increased incidence of ischemic coronary disease in the elderly renders age itself a major risk factor. In addition, aging produces a linear increase in left ventricular wall thickness and thus ventricular mass. Between the ages of 30 and 80 years, left ventricular thickness increases by approximately 8 mm. The stimulus for this hypertrophy is believed to be the elevated peripheral vascular impedance characteristic of aging.[20] Since neovascularization of the myocardium probably does not keep pace with the growth of the myocardium, the hypertrophied muscle is at increased risk for ischemia during stress. Decreased myocardial compliance and impaired ability of elderly cardiac muscle to relax during diastole increase the average diastolic wall tension. Since coronary flow occurs chiefly during diastole, increases in wall tension inhibit intramyocardial flow, thus favoring the development of ischemia, especially in subendocardial regions.

The occurrence of frequent premature atrial and ventricular contractions and of atrial fibrillation is more common in the elderly than in the young and is correlated with postoperative cardiac death.[18] In a study of ambulatory electrocardiography in the elderly, Camm and associates[21] found an extraordinarily high incidence of asymptomatic arrhythmias. Supraventricular ectopic rhythms and atrial fibrillation occurred in 27 per cent and 10 per cent of the subjects, respectively. Serious ventricular arrhythmias, including frequent ventricular ectopic beats, couplets, bigeminy, and even ventricular tachycardia occurred in 13 per cent of those studied. These arrhythmias are probably significant as markers of serious coronary disease and degeneration of the cardiac conduction system, and their presence should alert the physician accordingly.

The presence of severe heart failure preoperatively greatly increases the risk of postoperative death.[17] Heart failure is a frequent occurrence in the elderly immediately after termination of use of an anesthetic. Although it is especially likely to occur in patients who have manifested a prior history of failure, it may emerge in those who have had no symptoms. Not infrequently, heart failure may progress to full-blown pulmonary edema in the recovery room, requiring vigorous resuscitative maneuvers if respiratory arrest is to be avoided.

There are several reasons why congestive failure occurs during emergence from anesthesia. First, cessation of positive pressure ventilation at extubation causes an abrupt reduction of mean intrathoracic pressure, which suddenly increases venous return to the heart. Under stress, hearts of elderly people tend to perform less well than those of young people and may thus fail.[22] Second, upon extubation, the patient must assume the metabolic work of breathing, which places an added strain on the circulation. Third, residual anesthetic drugs, particularly inhalational agents, depress myocardial contractility. Fourth, if pain is severe upon resumption of consciousness, sympathetic tone and norepinephrine levels rise quickly and increase peripheral resistance and cardiac inotropy, and thus the workload of the heart. Fifth, if the patient has become hypothermic during surgery, he or she may shiver upon emergence, further increasing circulatory demand. Sixth, if there has been fluid overload during surgery, preload will be increased accordingly and congestive failure may be precipitated.

Aside from interfering with pulmonary function, congestive heart failure also tends to favor the development of myocardial ischemia and thus increase the risk of infarction. This is a consequence of Laplace's law, which states that the tension in the wall of a vessel is proportional to the pressure of the contained fluid times the radius of the vessel. Since congestive failure elevates both ventricular diastolic pressure and size, it greatly elevates ventricular wall tension, thus impairing perfusion. At the same time, pulmonary congestion may produce a decline in arterial oxygen saturation, further threatening myocardial oxygen delivery. Therefore, if postoperative heart failure occurs, it must be quickly corrected. Intubation and controlled ventilation should be utilized in severe cases.

Other important risk factors for postoperative infarction and cardiac death include emergency operation, abdominal or thoracic operation, recent (within 6 months) myocardial infarction, significant aortic stenosis, and serious intraoperative hypotension. Interestingly, preoperative controlled hypertension, duration of use of anesthetic during surgery, presence of stable angina, and history of previous coronary artery bypass grafting are *not* risk factors for postoperative cardiac death.[18] Performance of successful coronary artery bypass grafting in patients with severe angina, left main coronary artery disease, ventricular aneurysm, and impaired left ventricular function prior to major surgery decreases the risk of postoperative myocardial infarction and should be considered for high-risk elderly patients prior to major elective surgery.[23]

Clearly, benefit can be obtained in the preoperative identification of those elderly at high risk for infarction and in taking measures aimed at prevention. If signs or symptoms of infarction occur, accurate diagnosis and rapid, vigorous monitoring and treatment of complications must be instituted. The following may be useful in the minimization of cardiac mortality in the elderly:

1. Insertion of preoperative monitoring catheters, such as central venous pressure catheters, pulmonary artery catheters, and radial artery lines, to facilitate real-time hemodynamic monitoring, accurate fluid management, and continuous blood gas sampling.
2. Thorough treatment of congestive heart failure preoperatively, including the maintenance of digoxin and oxygen therapy, and achievement of a well-tolerated fluid volume status. Excessive plasma volume contraction resulting from preoperative diuretic therapy is to be avoided, however, since significant intraoperative fluid demands are likely to produce hypovolemia.
3. Treatment of preoperative arrhythmias with therapeutic levels of antiarrhythmic agents, including digoxin, up to the time of anesthetic induction.
4. Consideration of cardiac catheterization and coronary artery bypass grafting in patients with unstable or high-grade angina who require abdominal or thoracic surgery.
5. Maintenance of therapy with beta-blocking agents through the day of surgery.
6. Intensive monitoring of high-risk elderly patients for the development of arrhythmias, heart failure, T-wave changes, and hypotension while in the recovery room and afterward. Extremely high-risk patients should undergo pulmonary and radial artery catheterization for monitoring for several days postoperatively in an intensive care unit.
7. Vigorous management of congestive heart failure in the recovery room. This includes possible continuation of positive pressure ventilation after emergence if cardiac performance is marginal, administration of inotropic agents such as digoxin or dopamine, provision of adequate analgesia with narcotic or regional techniques, and cautious use of diuretic agents in the event of severe fluid overload. If intra-arterial blood pressure monitoring is being performed, IV nitroglycerin and nitroprusside are excellent agents for reducing both preload and afterload.

## *Cerebrovascular Morbidity*

The perioperative period is a time of high risk for the development of stroke, which causes between 2 and 9 per cent of postoperative deaths among the elderly. As in myocardial infarction, both physiologic and pathologic changes with age contribute to the problem. Since post-stroke interventions are of extremely limited efficacy, emphasis has been on prevention by way of long-term modification of risk factors, particularly hypertension. Treatment of risk factors over a prolonged period is associated with decreased risk of stroke; however, short-term therapy prior to surgery does not affect the risk of perioperative stroke.[24] Therefore, when surgery is urgent, we do not insist on normal levels of blood pressure in elderly hypertensives because therapy to obtain these levels entails the risk of inducing hypoperfusion.

In the general population, atherothrombotic and embolic strokes each cause about a third of cerebrovascular accidents, with the rest attributable to hypertensive hemorrhage, lacunar infarction, and rupture of intracranial aneurysms. In the elderly population, a greater proportion of strokes are atherosclerotic in origin. Thus, maintenance of sufficient flow of fully oxygenated blood through narrowed vessels is a prime physiologic consideration in elderly surgical patients, particularly those with identifiable stroke risk factors.

Cerebral blood flow is remarkably well regulated in health, such that if mean arterial pressure is between 60 and 170 mm Hg cerebral blood flow is constant at 55 ml per minute per 100 gm of brain tissue, as seen in Fig. 47–1.[25] Since neurons do not begin to die until flow falls below 10 ml per minute per 100 gm of brain tissue, a considerable margin of safety exists, even if mean blood pressure should fall below the critical level of 60 mm Hg, the level at which resistance is minimized. With aging, vascular changes occur that decrease this margin of safety. Cerebral blood flow diminishes linearly

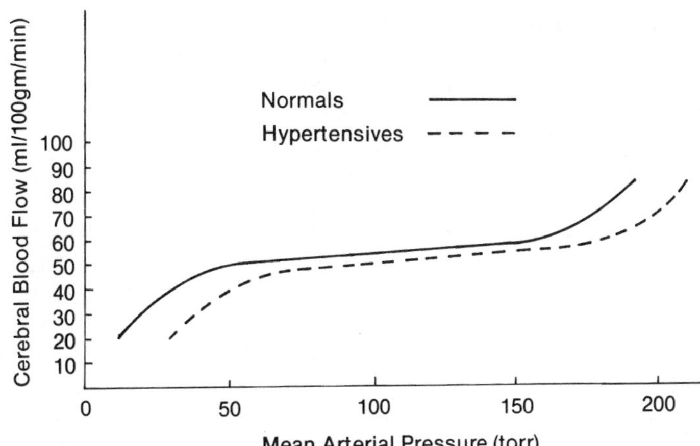


**Figure 47-1.** Cerebral blood flow in people with normal blood pressure and with chronic hypertension.

with age, even in the absence of clinical atherosclerotic disease, with flow reduction proportionally greatest in the middle cerebral artery distribution. In patients with risk factors for stroke, flow diminution is more prominent, falling roughly 25 per cent below that of normal young controls.[26] Since mean arterial pressure rises with age and resistance is equal to pressure divided by flow, age is associated with a dramatic rise in cerebrovascular resistance. The autoregulatory curve of flow versus pressure shifts to the right, raising the critical pressure below which resistance is minimized and flow falls (see Figure 47-1). Thus, episodes of hypotension, even if of a mild degree, are extremely dangerous in the elderly, particularly in the presence of stroke risk factors.

Hypotension may occur during any phase of the perioperative course. The elderly are more susceptible to postural hypotension than are younger adults, as autonomic nervous system compensatory mechanisms lose efficiency with increasing age. Preoperative medications that interfere with blood pressure control, such as narcotics, barbiturates, butyrophenones, phenothiazines, diuretics, and antidepressants, must be used with extreme caution prior to induction of anesthesia. Positional shifts of the preoperative patient from bed to stretcher to operating table must be performed slowly and gently to allow sufficient time for circulatory compensation. Dehydration from surgical disease, diuretic therapy, or lack of oral fluid intake predisposes to hypotension from all causes and must be corrected before the induction of anesthesia. Continuous IV administration of a salt-containing crystalloid solution during the evening and night prior to surgery at a rate approximately equal to 1200 ml per $m^2$ per 24 hours is an excellent way to avoid dehydration in the elderly surgical patient.

The anesthesiologist frequently encounters hypotension immediately after induction of anesthesia, as the anesthetic drugs simultaneously depress cardiac output and reflex vasoconstriction. The hypotension so induced is exaggerated in the presence of hyovolemia. Thus, preoperative maintenance of adequate circulatory volume and proportionate reduction of induction doses of anesthetic are crucial maneuvers in the elderly.

In the postoperative period, hypotension must be rapidly diagnosed and effectively treated. Frequently, it is difficult to distinguish between hypotensive states characterized by low preload, such as hypovolemia, and high preload, such as cardiac failure. In these cases, diagnosis is greatly facilitated by insertion of a thermocouple-tipped pulmonary artery catheter, with which cardiac output and left ventricular filling pressure can be measured. It must be emphasized that in the elderly, the time during which temporizing measures, such as fluid or pressor infusions, can be maintained in the face of hypotension from an undiagnosed cause may be limited. Since end-organ damage occurs swiftly, it is wise to resort to invasive monitoring for diagnosis early, if the nature of the hemodynamic situation is at all in doubt. However, if the underlying pathologic condition is irreversible, such as uncontrollable hemorrhage, disseminated sepsis, or massive myocardial infarction, invasive measures are unwarranted and contribute to needless patient suffering and expense.

## *Perioperative Renal Failure*

The occurrence of acute renal failure following surgery is a double disaster. It both places the patient in a 50 to 70 per cent mortality group and enormously complicates the treatment of the original surgical illness and the recovery.[27] The two commonest causes of perioperative renal failure are renal hypoperfusion and direct drug nephrotoxicity. The aged kidney is particularly liable to both (see Chapter 31). As in perioperative myocardial infarction and stroke, the margin for error in management of the elderly kidney is small, and prophylactic efforts may reap rich dividends. As noted elsewhere (see Chapter 31), after the fourth decade of life, perfusion and glomerular filtration rate (GFR) fall 10 per cent per decade, reaching roughly half the normal level of GFR during the eighth decade.[28] The serum creatinine level remains normal in the face of drastic decreases in GFR, rendering it a grossly deficient measure of renal reserve. Thus, determination of creatinine clearance by way of a 24-hour urine collection is a valuable aid before major surgery in the elderly and provides a quantitative measure that can be followed throughout convalescence.

Decreased renal blood flow is most marked in the cortical area, a tendency which is increased during positive pressure ventilation.[29] Since the cortical long-looped nephrons are responsible for production of the medullary osmotic gradient which enables production of a concentrated urine (and hence water conservation), elderly patients have impaired ability to conserve water and thus easily become dehydrated and hypovolemic. Hypovolemia, in turn, provokes a generalized vasoconstrictive response, which further impairs renal perfusion. Surgical blood loss, surgical evaporative water loss, respiratory water loss, and urinary loss must therefore be replaced promptly if renal function is to be optimized.

The primary monitor of the adequacy of renal perfusion is the urinary production rate. Although there is evidence of excess mortality from nosocomial urinary tract infection among the catheterized elderly,[30] we strongly believe that bladder catheterization is indicated for all elderly patients undergoing surgical procedures that entail the possibility of major blood loss or protracted duration. Criteria for Foley catheterization should be less stringent if renal function is subnormal, and, in all cases, scrupulous attention must be paid to catheter sterility and to any evidence of possible infection. If urinary output falls below 0.5 ml per kg per minute, volume loading with saline or lactated Ringer's solution should be carried out. If this fails to produce the desired result or if there is doubt about the patient's volume status, central venous or pulmonary artery catheterization should be performed without delay to guide further therapy. If central venous and pulmonary artery pressures are low, further volume is then given. If they are normal or high, low-dose dopamine and cardiotonic agents are given to improve renal perfusion and cardiac output. Diuresis induced by mannitol or furosemide may convert impending oliguric renal failure into nonoliguric renal failure, which lowers the mortality to 26 per cent.[31] Simultaneous determination of urine and serum osmolarity using the method of Miller and associates (Table 47–4) provides an excellent noninvasive diagnostic guide in distinguishing prerenal azotemia from established acute tubular necrosis, provided that laboratory facilities can rapidly make these measurements.[32] In the event of declining urine output, a urine osmolarity greater than 500 mOsm per kg and a urine : plasma osmolarity ratio greater than 1.8 are diagnostic of prerenal failure, and this determination should be followed by volume loading.

As noted in Chapter 31, the kidneys of elderly patients are more susceptible than those of young patients to nephrotoxic drugs. The commonest causes of nephrotoxic renal failure are aminoglycoside antibiotics and angiographic contrast agents. The latter are also potent osmotic diuretics and therefore promote hypovolemia and further favor renal damage. Diabetics are especially susceptible to radiocontrast nephropathy. Vigorous hydration is mandatory after angiographic studies in the elderly, by the IV route if necessary. It is often wise to wait several days after the x-ray study to perform elective surgery, to allow more time for rehydration and for excretion of the contrast agent, whose toxic potential is often underestimated. Subjection of an elderly patient with borderline hydration to the major circulatory demands of anesthesia, surgery, and recovery is an invitation to disaster. Time spent in rectifying the circulatory status prior to anesthesia is never wasted.

## REGIONAL ANESTHESIA

Despite the common belief to the contrary, there is no evidence that spinal or epidural anesthesia is inherently safer or less likely to lead to pulmonary complications than general anesthesia. Major regional anesthesia may be poorly tolerated in the elderly, and it produces rapid and profound circulatory changes that may be less controllable than those resulting from general anesthesia. Pulmonary complications are more dependent on the surgical site than on the

**Table 47–4.** URINARY INDICES IN OLIGURIC RENAL FAILURE*

| | Prerenal | ATN† |
|---|---|---|
| VOsm (mOsm/kg $H_2O$) | >500 | <350 |
| Urine sodium (mEq/L) | < 20 | > 40 |
| Urine/plasma urea nitrogen | > 8 | < 3 |
| Urine/plasma creatine | > 40 | < 20 |

* Data from Miller TR et al.: Urinary diagnostic indices in acute renal failure—a prospective study. Ann Intern Med 89:47, 1978.
† ATN = acute tubular necrosis.

anesthetic. Nevertheless, regional anesthesia offers certain advantages in specific situations. For example, preservation of consciousness during anesthesia may allow the patient to be aware of the development of myocardial ischemia as angina is provoked. The anesthesiologist thus gains a valuable monitor to guide intraoperative management. If the patient is allowed to remain awake, certain surgical complications, such as perforation of the bladder during cystoscopy and water intoxication from bladder irrigant absorption during transurethral prostate resection, can be diagnosed intraoperatively because of the pain and mental changes they provoke. When regional anesthesia is used, the small but finite risks of hypoxia from airway obstruction and serious anesthetic ventilatory depression are avoided, so long as the block is of sufficiently high quality to obviate the use of excessive doses of sedative and analgesics. Furthermore, preservation of consciousness decreases the risk of intraoperative pulmonary aspiration, as laryngeal reflexes are preserved.

Safe use of regional anesthesia in the elderly requires thorough knowledge of its effects. Spinal and epidural anesthesia may lower blood pressure and cardiac output rapidly in four ways. First, blockade of spinal somatic nerves is accompanied by simultaneous paralysis of efferent nerves, causing profound vasodilation in the anesthetized areas. Second, sympathetic blockade and motor paralysis cause peripheral venous pooling and reduce venous return to the heart. Both of these effects occur in direct proportion to the extent of the area anesthetized and are partly compensated for by reflex vasoconstriction of uninvolved areas. Third, if regional anesthesia extends cephalad as far as the mid-thoracic dermatomes, the cardiac sympathetic nerves will be blocked, potentially causing severe bradycardia. Fourth, local anesthetics themselves are potent myocardial depressants to which the elderly are especially sensitive. Although the dose administered during spinal anesthesia is quite small, it may be substantial during epidural anesthesia. A final disadvantage of regional anesthesia is that it forces one to forego the opportunity for bronchial hygiene afforded by general endotracheal anesthesia; bronchial hygiene may confer substantial benefit if pulmonary secretions are a problem. Moreover, if the sensory block afforded by the regional technique is of poor quality, the anesthesiologist may be forced to administer dangerously high doses of IV sedatives and narcotics to calm the agitated patient. The respiratory depression so induced may leave the anesthesiologist with an unplanned general anesthetic, but without the advantage of airway control which orthodox general anesthesia affords. Performance of regional anesthesia is absolutely contraindicated in those elderly patients whose mental orientation is confused or who do not understand the need for surgery. Dangerous agitation may result intraoperatively as the demented patient misinterprets the frightening situation in which he finds himself.

In general, the physiologic hazards of regional anesthesia are dose-related, being roughly proportional to the number of dermatomes that are anesthetized. Blockade of more spinal segments not only increases the overall effects of sympathetic denervation but also decreases the number of available uninvolved segments that can compensate for the initial physiologic perturbation. Hemodynamically, low spinal anesthesia (suitable for lower extremity and pelvic procedures) is therefore a completely different entity than high spinal anesthesia (capable of producing anesthesia up to the clavicles). Owing to the generally decreased compensatory abilities of the elderly vital organs, use of high spinal anesthesia should be approached with extreme trepidation because this method often produces more physiologic derangement and risk than well-controlled general anesthesia. Successful use of regional anesthesia depends on the proper selection of patient and procedure. In well-motivated elderly patients undergoing peripheral or pelvic procedures, regional anesthesia can be an excellent choice.

## CONCLUSION

As human beings age beyond the fourth decade, the maximal functional ability of all major organs declines at a predictable and measurable rate. Since these organs have large reserve capacities that are generally not necessary for daily function, people may survive to very advanced ages before this normal decay of function becomes incompatible with life, so long as major physiologic perturbations are avoided. Inevitably illness supervenes, and increased demands are made on the diminished reserves of the elderly heart, kidneys, lungs, and liver. Probability of survival is then proportional to reserve capacity. When surgery is required, the geriatric patient is faced with the stress of both the illness and the contemplated anesthetic and procedure, and the chances of survival are correspondingly decreased. In a sense, aging can be characterized by an ever-decreasing ability to restore homeostasis in the face of physiologic insult.

When the elderly patient comes to surgery, his or her physicians must perform the crucial tasks of estimating physiologic reserves, minimizing the impact of the procedure, and providing *temporary* organ system supports if reserves fail, in the hope that, in time, recovery will occur. This approach to care has achieved considerable success over the decades, as evidenced by the trend of geriatric surgical outcome to depend more on the underlying surgical disease and less on the associated conditions of the major organs.

As availability of organ reserves diminishes, measurement of function becomes more critical, and the need for quantitative data more important. Much valuable and accurate information can be gathered at low cost—a careful history regarding cardiopulmonary symptoms and exercise tolerance, clinical evaluation of risk factors of stroke and myocardial infarction, pulmonary function tests, and creatinine clearance studies are economically cheap but medically invaluable indices of vital organ reserve, which supplement the physical examination, chest x-ray, and electrocardiogram. The physician must exercise patience when obtaining this information from the elderly individual.

Monitoring of urinary output, right- and left-sided intravascular pressures, cardiac output, and arterial blood gases during surgery and recovery provides real-time quantitative measurement of organ function of high accuracy. The techniques involved are safe and effective and are most useful when physiologic function is most marginal. Thus, they have great utility in the care of the elderly. In fact, modern intensive care monitoring and support techniques are so accurate and powerful that they can often sustain life despite multiple organ failures, which may have meanwhile become irreversible. The fascination with technology may make this irreversibility easy to overlook. However, the use of such technology becomes medically and economically counterproductive as the long-term prognosis becomes less favorable. Perioperative care of the elderly requires us to be both physiologists and physicians in the broadest sense.

## References

1. Fries JF: Aging, natural death, and the compression of morbidity. N Engl J Med 303:130, 1980.
2. Anglem TJ, Bradford ML: Major surgery in the aged. N Engl J Med 249:1005, 1953.
3. Wilder RJ, Fishbein RH: Operative experience with patients over 80 years of age. Surg Gynecol Obstet 113:205, 1961.
4. Marshall WH, Fahey PJ: Operative complications and mortality in patients over 80 years of age. Arch Surg 88:896, 1964.
5. Palmberg S, Hirsjarvi E: Mortality in geriatric surgery. Gerontology 25:13, 1979.
6. Djokovic JL, Hedley-Whyte J: Prediction of outcome of surgery and anesthesia in patients over 80. JAMA 242:2301, 1979.
7. Kakkar VV, Corrigan TP, Fossard DP: Prevention of fatal postoperative pulmonary embolism by low doses of heparin. Lancet 2:45, 1975.
8. Blake R, Lynn J: Emergency abdominal surgery in the aged. Br J Surg 63:956, 1976.
9. Pontoppidan H, Beecher HK: Progressive loss of protective reflexes in the airway with the advance of age. JAMA 174:2209, 1960.
10. Evans MA et al: Gastric emptying rate in the elderly: Implications for drug therapy. J Am Geriatr Soc 29:201, 1981.
11. Maliniak K, Vakil AH: Pre-anesthetic cimetidine and gastric pH. Anesth Analg 58:309, 1979.
12. duMoulin GC et al: Aspiration of gastric bacteria in antacid-treated patient: A frequent cause of postoperative colonisation of the airway. Lancet 1:242, 1982.
13. John R, Thomas J: Chemical compositions of elastins isolated from aortas and pulmonary tissues of humans of different ages. Biochem J 127:261, 1972.
14. Brody AW et al: The residual volume-predicted values as a function of age. Am Rev Respir Dis 109:98, 1974.
15. Niewoehner DE, Kleinerman J: Morphologic basis of pulmonary resistance in the human lung and effects of aging. J Appl Physiol 36:412, 1974.
16. Pontoppidan H, Geffin B, Lowenstein E: Acute respiratory failure in the adult. N Engl J Med 287:799, 1972.
17. Kitamura H, Sawa T, Ikesona E: Postoperative hypoxemia: The contribution of age to the maldistribution of ventilation. Anesthesiology 35:238, 1972.
18. Goldman L et al: Cardiac risk factors and complications in non-cardiac surgery. Medicine 57:357, 1978.
19. Tarhan S et al: Myocardial infarction after general anesthesia. JAMA 220:1451, 1972.
20. Lakatta EG: Alterations in the cardiovascular system that occur in advanced age. Fed Proc 38:163, 1979.
21. Camm AJ et al: The rhythm of the heart in active elderly subjects. Am Heart J 99:598, 1980.
22. Port A et al: Effect of age on the response of the left ventricular ejection fraction to exercise. N Engl J Med 303:1133, 1980.
23. Crawford ES et al: Operative risk in patients with previous coronary artery bypass. Ann Thorac Surg 26:215, 1978.
24. Leonberg SC, Elliot FA: Prevention of recurrent stroke. Stroke 12:731, 1981.
25. Arnold KG: Cerebral blood flow in geriatrics—a review. Age Aging 10:5, 1981.
26. Naritomi H et al: Effects of advancing age on regional cerebral blood flow. Arch Neurol 36:410, 1979.
27. Hedley-Whyte J et al.: Applied Physiology of Respira-

tory Care. Boston, Little, Brown and Co., 1976, pp. 241.
28. Epstein J: Effects of aging on the kidney. Fed Proc 28:173, 1979.
29. Priebe HJ, Heimann JC, Hedley-Whyte J: Mechanisms of renal dysfunction during positive end-expiratory pressure ventilation. J Appl Physiol 50:643, 1981.
30. Platt R et al: Mortality associated with nosocomial urinary tract infection. N Engl J Med 307:637, 1982.
31. Anderson RJ et al.: Nonoliguric acute renal failure. N Engl J Med 296:1134, 1977.
32. Miller TR et al.: Urinary diagnostic indices in acute renal failure—a prospective study. Ann Intern Med 89:47, 1978.

## Chapter 48

# Patient Information in Geriatrics

*Shirley B. Hesslein*
*Jacqueline Levitt*

Part of the care that physicians and other health care practitioners give their patients is information about the illness in question, the course of disease, the "why's and how's" of management, and matters pertaining to health maintenance and disease prevention. This material is particularly important for elderly patients for several reasons, including the presence of multiple disease, forgetfulness or confusion on the part of the patient, and an obvious concern of the patient and family members to do all they can to help the patient maintain independence and happiness.

Although primary care physicians are limited in the amount of time they can spend with patients in answering specific questions, a large variety of informational materials for patient and family education are available from institutions and foundations. The following list includes specific publications that are currently available, often at no charge. Although individual publications may become outdated or unavailable, the organizations and their addresses change less frequently. Therefore, the listing of the source agencies should provide the physician with helpful information concerning sources of these or other materials.

The care provider should not overlook the library as an important source of patient information. The hospital medical library may be a resource, if the hospital is one that considers patient information part of its responsibility. The nearby academic medical library may have some appropriate materials if its collection development policy includes patient and/or consumer health information. The local public library may also have a policy of serving the health information needs of the community.

It is important, however, that the care provider check out the policies of these resources rather than send the patient to find out. It is quite possible that a community that has a good public library and fine teaching hospital with a good library (or even a town with a medical center with a great library) may have no collection of consumer health information or no policy of helping the patient to the materials that are potentially available.

To obtain information concerning this field, the following resources are recommended:

### The Consumer Health Information Sourcebook

Alan M. Rees and Jodith Janes, New York, Bowker, 1984, 2nd ed.

### Consumer Information Catalogue, (Quarterly)

The Consumer Information Center was established in 1970 as a "clearinghouse" for consumer information offered by almost 30 government agencies. A catalogue is published four times a year listing the materials available, many of which are free and can be ordered in quantities of up to 20 copies each.

Consumer Information Center, Dept. A, Pueblo, CO 81009.

### Consumer Health Information Service

A microfilm collection of booklets and pamphlets, collected by A.M. Rees. A print catalogue of the collection is available.

Microfilm Corporation of America, A New York Times Company, 1620 Hawkins Avenue, P.O. Box 10, Sanford, NC 27330.

## MATERIALS OF GENERAL INTEREST

### *Health Care and Disease Prevention*

Information relating to the prevention of disease, disability, premature death, and undesirable and unnecessary health problems can be obtained from the following:

Center for Health Promotion and Education, Centers for Disease Control, 1600 Clifton Road, N.E., Atlanta, GA 30333; telephone: (404) 329–3492–3698.

#### HEALTH FINDER

This is an occasional publication, which lists the federal health clearinghouses and information centers.

National Health Information Clearinghouse, P.O. Box 1133, Washington, DC 20013–1133; telephone: (800) 336–4797; Virginia only: (703) 522–2590.

#### THINKING ABOUT A NURSING HOME?

This descriptive pamphlet explains the different levels of care, such as skilled nursing and intermediate care. It reviews financial coverage of institutional care and provides specific guidelines for choosing a long term care facility.

American Health Care Association, 1200 15th Street, N.W., Washington, DC 20005.

#### DAILY HEALTH NEWS AND FEATURE STORIES

These are pre-recorded messages prepared by the American Medical Association.

American Medical Radio News, telephone: (800) 621–8094.

#### A GUIDE TO MEDICAL SELF-CARE AND SELF-HELP GROUPS FOR THE ELDERLY (NIH PUBL. NO. 80–1687)

A general information pamphlet listing a wide variety of sources of free pamphlets on health and disease as well as suggested readings on consumerism in health issues. Of particular interest is a list of the central offices of self-help groups, such as Make Today Count (for the terminally ill), SAGE (Senior Activization and Growth Explorations), and publications of the United Ostomy Association and Alzheimer's Disease and Related Disorders Association.

National Institute on Aging, National Institutes of Health, Building 31, Room 5C-36, 9000 Rockville Pike, Bethesda, MD 20205.

#### AGE PAGE

A series of one-page large print fact sheets on health issues for the older adult. Includes articles on accidents, crime, eyes, cancer, food, staying healthy after age 65, and many other topics.

National Institute on Aging, National Institutes of Health, Building 31, Room 5C-36, 9000 Rockville Pike, Bethesda, MD 20205.

### *Financial Aspects*

#### A BRIEF EXPLANATION OF MEDICARE (SSA PUBL. NO. 05–10043)

A concise, easy-to-understand explanation of this health insurance plan, including explicit mention of expenses that are covered and not covered.

Consumer Information Center, Department A, Pueblo, CO 81009.

#### INFORMATION ON MEDICARE AND HEALTH INSURANCE FOR OLDER PEOPLE

American Association of Retired Persons, 1909 K Street, N.W., Washington, DC 20049.

### *Disease Prevention*

#### STAYING HEALTHY AS YOU GET OLDER

American Society of Internal Medicine, 1101 Vermont Avenue, N.W., Suite 500, Washington, DC 20005.

#### MEDICARE: WHAT IT WILL AND WILL NOT PAY FOR

American Society of Internal Medicine, 1101 Vermont Avenue, N.W., Suite 500, Washington, DC 20005.

## *Nutrition*

Consumer inquiries about medications, nutrition, and food may be addressed to the following organization, which in turn refers questions on medications to the appropriate office.

Food and Drug Administration (FDA), Office of Consumer Affairs, Public Inquiries, 5600 Fishers Lane (HFE-88), Rockville, MD 20857; telephone: (301) 443-3170.

### Some Facts and Myths of Vitamins (Publ. No. 552-J)

This pamphlet reviews specific vitamins, including their functions and dietary sources, and clarifies some commonly held misconceptions.

Consumer Information Center, Department A, Pueblo, CO 81009.

## *Drugs*

### Substance Abuse among the Elderly

Addiction Research Foundation, 33 Russell Street, Toronto, Ontario, Canada, M5S 2S1.

### Taking Care: A Medication Guide for Older People: What Senior Citizens Should Do about Drugs and Alcohol

Do It Now Foundation, Box 5115, Phoenix, AZ 85010.

### The What If Book: Some Important Questions about Medicines You are Taking

Hoffman-La Roche, Inc., Nutley, NJ 07110.

### The What If Book: On Using Medication Correctly

Hoffman-La Roche, Inc., Nutley, NJ 07110.

### Medicines and You (1981) (NIH Publ. No. 81-2140)

National Institutes of Health, 9000 Rockville Pike, Bethesda, MD 20205.

### On Making It through the Night (Publ. No. 584-J)

This pamphlet discusses the causes of insomnia and how medication can interrupt the physiology of natural sleep. It gives suggestions for therapy without using drugs.

Consumer Information Center, Department A, Pueblo, CO 81009.

### Hemorrhoid Treatments Reviewed (Publ. No. 583-J)

A panel of experts review over-the-counter drugs available for treating hemorrhoids.

Consumer Information Center, Department A, Pueblo, CO 81009.

## *Exercise, Fitness and Rehabilitation*

Informational materials on exercise and sports and physical fitness for various groups, including the elderly, are available from

President's Council on Physical Fitness and Sports, 450 Fifth Street, N.W., Suite 7103, Washington, DC 20001; telephone: (202) 272-3430.

### Pocket Guide to Federal Help for the Disabled Person

This pamphlet describes the various services available to handicapped individuals and how to obtain them. It includes information on public transportation, medical and financial benefits, and even deductible items for income tax preparation.

Office for Handicapped Individuals, Room 338D, Hubert H. Humphrey Building, 200 Independence Ave., S.W., Washington, DC 20201.

### The Capability Collection: Ways and Means

This catalogue, with more than a thousand entries, centers on maximizing opportunities for persons with disabilities. Symbols indicate handicaps to be assisted. e.g., vision, range of motion, cardiovascular.

Ways and Means, 28001 Citrin Drive, Romulus, MI 48174.

Additional publications and audiovisual materials on rehabilitation, relevant to all disability groups, are available from:

National Rehabilitation Information Center, 4407 Eighth Street, N.E., Washington DC 20017-2277; telephone: (202) 635-5822.

# DISEASES AND CONDITIONS

## *Alzheimer's Disease*

### SENILE DEMENTIA (ALZHEIMER'S DISEASE) (1980)

National Institute of Mental Health, 5600 Fishers Lane, Rockville, MD 20857.

### THE DEMENTIAS: HOPE THROUGH RESEARCH

National Institute of Neurological and Communicative Disorders and Stroke, Building 31, Room 8A-06, 9000 Rockville Pike, Bethesda, MD 20205.

### PROGRESS REPORT ON SENILE DEMENTIA OF THE ALZHEIMER'S TYPE

National Institute on Aging, Building 31, Room 5C-36, 9000 Rockville Pike, Bethesda, MD 20205.

### "HOTLINE" ON ALZHEIMER'S DISEASE

At these toll-free numbers, information is available about publications and referrals to local chapters and support groups.

Alzheimer's Disease and Related Disorders Association, telephone: (800) 621-0379; Illinois only: (800) 572-6037.

## *Arthritis and Musculoskeletal Disease*

### ARTHRITIS INFORMATION CLEARING HOUSE

Materials are available concerning arthritis and related muscular skeletal diseases, and information is provided for individuals and organizations involved in public, professional, and patient education.

Arthritis Information Clearing House, P.O. Box 9782, Arlington, VA 22209; telephone: (703) 558-8250.

### LIVING WITH ARTHRITIS . . . AND WHERE TO TURN FOR HELP

A general discussion of arthritis, including medications, exercises and surgical treatment. Particularly useful is a list of agencies that can provide help to the disabled patient.

Arthritis Foundation, 3400 Peachtree Road, N.E., Suite 1101, Atlanta, GA 30326.

### SO YOU HAVE . . . OSTEOARTHRITIS

This publication explains in simple terms what osteoarthritis is and includes a discussion of drugs, physical therapy, exercise, and the role of rest in therapy.

Arthritis Foundation, 3400 Peachtree Road, N.E., Suite 1101, Atlanta, GA 30326.

### SO YOU HAVE . . . RHEUMATOID ARTHRITIS

Similar approach as in the publication on osteoarthritis.

Arthritis Foundation, 3400 Peachtree Road, N.E., Suite 1101, Atlanta, GA 30326.

### AIDS FOR ARTHRITIS—SELF-HELP PRODUCTS

A catalogue of home aids and applicances designed for the handicapped person. Items range from special shoe horns and zipper pulls to vegetable peeling wands and palm-operated can openers.

Aids for Arthritis, Inc., 3 Little Knoll Court, Medford, NJ 08055.

### ABOUT GOUT: A FORM OF ARTHRITIS

Arthritis Foundation, 3400 Peachtree Road, N.E., Suite 1101, Atlanta, GA 30326, or its local office.

### ARTHRITIS MEDICATION BRIEFS

Arthritis Foundation, 3400 Peachtree Road, N.E., Suite 1101, Atlanta, GA 30326, or its local office.

### ARTHRITIS QUACKERY: A $485,000,000 RACKET

Arthritis Foundation, 3400 Peachtree Road, N.E., Suite 1101, Atlanta, GA 30326, or its local office.

### ARTHRITIS: THE BASIC FACTS

Arthritis Foundation, 3400 Peachtree Road, N.E., Suite 1101, Atlanta, GA 30326, or its local office.

### GOLD TREATMENT IN RHEUMATOID ARTHRITIS: INFORMATION FOR PATIENTS (1977)

Arthritis Foundation, 3400 Peachtree Road, N.E., Suite 1101, Atlanta, GA 30326, or its local office.

**The Truth about Arthritis in Women**

Arthritis Foundation, 3400 Peachtree Road, N.E., Suite 1101, Atlanta, GA 30326, or its local office.

**The Truth about Aspirin for Arthritis**

Arthritis Foundation, 3400 Peachtree Road, N.E., Suite 1101, Atlanta, GA 30326, or its local office.

**The Truth about Diet and Arthritis**

Arthritis Foundation, 3400 Peachtree Road, N.E., Suite 1101, Atlanta, GA 30326, or its local office.

**The Mistreatment of Arthritis/The Proper Treatment of Arthritis**

Consumers Union, Mt. Vernon, NY 10550.

**Doctor, Do I Have Arthritis?**

Eli Lilly & Co., 307 E. McCarty Street, Indianapolis, IN 46286.

**Hocus-Pocus As Applied to Arthritis (1981) (HHS Publ. No. [FDA] 810-1080)**

Food and Drug Administration, 5600 Fishers Lane, Room 15B-32, Rockville, MD 20857.

**Care of the Back**

This well-illustrated pamphlet provides detailed instructions, appropriate for patient education, in a systematic series of back exercises based on the "Williams exercises." Separate editions are available for men and women. This pamphlet is directed toward relatively healthy persons in middle age; therefore, the exercise program should be scaled down to some extent for elderly persons, especially those with significant musculoskeletal disease.

William K. Ishmael and Howard B. Shorbe, J.B. Lippincott, Philadelphia, 2d ed., 1969.

## *Blindness*

**Talking Books**

For "Hotline" guides to libraries that utilize the Talking Book Service for persons who are unable to read or use standard printed materials, contact:

National Library Service for the Blind and Physically Handicapped, Library of Congress, Washington, DC 20542; telephone: (800) 424-8567; in the District of Columbia only: (202) 287-5100.

**Seeing Well As You Grow Older**

A general review of presbyopia, cataracts, floaters, glaucoma, and macular degeneration.

American Academy of Ophthalmology, 1833 Fillmore Street, P.O. Box 7424, San Francisco, CA 94120-7424

**Cataract—Clouding the Lens of Sight**

American Academy of Ophthalmology, 1833 Fillmore Street, P.O. Box 7424, San Francisco, CA 94120-7424.

**Glaucoma—It Can Take Your Sight Away**

American Academy of Ophthalmology, 1833 Fillmore Street, P.O. Box 7424, San Francisco, CA 94120-7424.

**Macular Degeneration—Major Causes of Central Vision Loss**

American Academy of Ophthalmology, 1833 Fillmore Street, P.O. Box 7424, San Francisco, CA 94120-7424.

**About Aging and Blindness**

American Foundation for the Blind, 15 W. 16th Street, New York, NY 10011.

**Keeping an Eye on Glaucoma**

Food and Drug Administration, 5600 Fishers Lane, Room 5B-32, Rockville, MD 20857.

**Glaucoma**

Lederle Pharmaceuticals, Pearl River, NY 10965.

**Saving Your Sight from Glaucoma**

Merck, Sharp & Dohme, West Point, PA 19486.

**As We Grow Older**

National Association for the Visually Handicapped, 305 East 24th Street, New York, NY 10010.

**Cataract: NEI Focus on Research (1979)**

National Eye Institute, Building 31, Room 6A-32, 9000 Rockville Pike, Bethesda, MD 20205.

**Glaucoma**

National Eye Institute, Building 31, Room 6A-32, 9000 Rockville Pike, Bethesda, MD 20205.

**Macular Degeneration (The Search for Health)**

Also available in Spanish.

National Eye Institute, Building 31, Room 6A-32, 9000 Rockville Pike, Bethesda, MD 20205.

**Senile Macular Degeneration**

National Eye Institute, Building 31, Room 6A-32, 9000 Rockville Pike, Bethesda, MD 20205.

## *Cancer*

The Office of Cancer Communications answers requests for cancer information from patients and the general public. It sponsors a toll-free telephone number to supply cancer information to everyone. The staff members do not diagnose cancer or recommend treatments for individual cases. Spanish-speaking staff members are available to callers from the following areas: California (area codes: 231, 714, 619, and 805), Florida, northern New Jersey, New York City, and Texas.

Office of Cancer Communications, National Cancer Institute, Cancer Information Service, 9000 Rockville Pike, Bethesda, MD 20205; telephone: (800) 4-CANCER; (301) 496-5583; District of Columbia area: (202) 636-5700; New York City and Long Island: (212) 794-7982; Oahu, Hawaii, and neighboring islands: (800) 524-1234.

## *Deafness and Speech*

**Sounds or Silence?**

A discussion of the types and causes of hearing loss, including several case histories illustrating various treatments. Common difficulties encountered with hearing aids with suggestions on how to overcome them are also presented.

Better Hearing Institute, 1430 K Street, N.W., Suite 600, Washington, DC 20005.

**Tuning in on Hearing Aids (No. 582-J)**

This publication details types of hearing aids, where and how to seek help, and where to go with problems with products.

Consumer Information Center, Department A, Pueblo, CO 81009.

**Communication Disorders and Aging**

American Speech-Language-Hearing Association, 10801 Rockville Pike, Rockville, MD 20852.

## *Dental Problems*

**Dentures: What You Don't Know Can Hurt You**

American Dental Association, 211 East Chicago Avenue, Chicago, IL 60611.

**Have Missing Teeth Replaced**

American Dental Association, 211 East Chicago Avenue, Chicago, IL 60611.

**Your New Dentures**

American Dental Association, 211 East Chicago Avenue, Chicago, IL 60611.

## *Cardiovascular-Pulmonary-Renal Diseases*

**An Older Person's Guide to Cardiovascular Health**

American Heart Association, National Center, 7320 Greenville Avenue, Dallas, TX 75231.

### Feelin' Fine: Living with High Blood Pressure As We Grow Older

Merck, Sharp & Dohme, West Point, PA 19486.

### Happiness Is . . . a Healthy Heart (Parts I and II)

National Institutes of Health, 9000 Rockville Pike, Bethesda, MD 20205.

### High Blood Pressure

Information is given on the detection, diagnosis, and management of high blood pressure to consumers and health professionals.

High Blood Pressure Information Center, 120/80 National Institutes of Health, Bethesda, MD 20205; telephone: (301) 496–1809.

### Heart Attacks

A thorough, basic booklet describing atherosclerosis, its symptoms, and aftermath of myocardial infarction, including a very good discussion of risk factors. It should appeal particularly to those interested in detailed information.

National Heart, Lung and Blood Institute, Office of Information, Bethesda, MD 20205.

### High Blood Pressure

A very well written booklet on the causes and effects of hypertension, including general drug categories used in treatment.

National Heart, Lung and Blood Institute, Office of Information, Bethesda, MD 20205.

### High Blood Pressure and What You Can Do about It

An easy-to-read, informative pamphlet that describes the measurement of blood pressure and dispels commonly held myths about hypertension. A current list of drugs with their possible side effects is presented.

High Blood Pressure Information Center, 120/80 National Institute of Health, Bethesda, MD 20205.

### Calling a Halt to Salt

This 14 page pamphlet lists the sodium content and calories for a wide variety of foods and unsuspected sources of sodium in commonly used food items.

Giant Food, Inc., P.O. Box 1804, Washington, DC 20013.

### Healthy Aging

Metropolitan Life Insurance Company, One Madison Avenue, New York, NY 10010.

### "Pulse"

This quarterly periodical provides information of interest to heart patients. In addition, this organization answers questions on heart disease and pacemakers.

Association of Heart Patients, P.O. Box 54305, Atlanta, GA 30308; telephone: (800) 241–6993; Georgia only: (404) 523–0826.

### Help Yourself to Better Breathing

This pamphlet gives simple answers to common questions asked by patients with lung disease. Exercises to improve breathing and information on medications commonly used are included.

The American Lung Association, 1740 Broadway, New York, NY 10019.

### "Hotline" on Kidney Disease

The American Kidney Fund provides information on direct financial aid available to pay treatment costs and on organ donations and kidney-related diseases.

American Kidney Fund, 7315 Wisconsin Avenue, Bethesda, MD 20814; telephone: (800) 638–8299; Maryland only: (800) 492–8361.

### "Hotline" on Lung Diseases

Answers to questions about asthma, emphysema, chronic bronchitis, and other respiratory and immune system disorders are provided by:

National Asthma Center, National Jewish Hospital, 3800 East Colfax Avenue, Denver, CO 80206; telephone: (800) 222–LUNG.

## *Diabetes*

### Diabetes and Aging (Bibliography)

National Diabetes Information Clearinghouse, Box NDIC, Bethesda, MD 20205.

**DIET AND NUTRITION FOR PEOPLE WITH DIABETES (BIBLIOGRAPHY)**

National Diabetes Information Clearinghouse, Box NDIC, Bethesda, MD 20205.

**THE DIABETES DICTIONARY**

National Diabetes Information Clearinghouse, Box NDIC, Bethesda, MD 20205.

**FACT SHEET: DIABETES AND CARDIOVASCULAR DISEASE (NO. 77-1212)**

A brief explanation of diabetes and the diabetic's risk of cardiovascular disease, with recommendations on how to decrease that risk.

National Heart, Lung and Blood Institute, Office of Information, Bethesda, MD 20205.

**HOW TO COPE WITH DIABETES**

Discussion of the two primary types of diabetes, their causes, symptoms, diagnosis, and treatment.

National Institute of Arthritis, Metabolism, and Digestive Disease, Information Office, Bethesda, MD 20205.

**FACT SHEET: FOOT CARE FOR THE DIABETIC PATIENT**

A single-page sheet describing in detail the elements of proper foot care, including how to bathe feet, choose shoes, and cut toenails. Essential information for all diabetics.

National Institute of Arthritis, Metabolism, and Digestive Disease, Information Office, Bethesda, MD 20205.

**THE DIABETIC NEUROPATHIES**

This pamphlet discusses the symptoms, course and treatment of the various types of diabetic neuropathy: distal symmetric polyneuropathy, autonomic neuropathy, proximal motor neuropathy, and cranial mononeuropathy. Presented in a manner that is reassuring to patients with this problem.

National Institute of Neurological and Communicative Disorders and Stroke, Building 31, Room 8A16, Bethesda, MD 20205.

**DIABETES AND YOUR EYES (NO. 81-2171)**

An explanation of diabetic retinopathy and how the risk of visual loss can be reduced by treatments such as photocoagulation and vitrectomy. Helpful illustrations and glossary of terms.

Public Health Service, National Institutes of Health, Bethesda, MD 20205.

## *Digestive Diseases*

Information on digestive diseases for health professionals and consumers is available from:

National Digestive Diseases Education and Information Clearinghouse, 1555 Wilson Boulevard, Rosslyn, VA 22209; telephone: (703) 496–9707.

## *Hypothermia*

**A WINTER HAZARD FOR THE OLD: ACCIDENTAL HYPOTHERMIA (NO. 590-J)**

A brief discussion of the signs and symptoms of this condition as well as the common risk factors, including certain medications. Suggestions are given for simple treatment measures before the victim arrives at the hospital.

Consumer Information Center, Department A, Pueblo, CO 81009.

## *Huntington's Disease*

**CARING FOR THE HUNTINGTON'S DISEASE PATIENT AT HOME**

Committee to Combat Huntington's Disease, 250 West 57th Street, New York, NY 10107.

**WHAT IS HUNTINGTON'S (CHOREA) DISEASE?**

Committee to Combat Huntington's Disease, 250 West 57th Street, New York, NY 10107.

**HUNTINGTON'S DISEASE**

National Huntington's Disease Association, 128A East 74th Street, New York, NY 10021.

### A Neurologist Speaks with Huntington's Disease Families

National Huntington's Disease Association, 128A East 74th Street, New York, NY 10021.

### Huntington's Disease: Hope through Research

National Institute of Neurological and Communicative Disorders and Stroke, Building 31, Room 8A-06, 9000 Rockville Pike, Bethesda, MD 20205.

## *Parkinson's Disease*

### Aids, Equipment, and Suggestions to Help the Patient with Parkinson's Disease in the Activities of Daily Living

This pamphlet lists adaptive equipment and useful aids that can keep patients independent in such tasks as cooking, bathing, grooming, dressing, and eating. It includes a list of suppliers of equipment.

The American Parkinson Disease Association, 116 John Street, New York, NY 10038; toll-free number: (800) 223-ADPA or (212) 732-9550.

### A Manual for Patients with Parkinson's Disease: A Guide for Patients and Their Families (1985)

A general information source that includes causes, common problems, and treatment of Parkinson's disease. There is a useful glossary of terms, and referral center locations are given.

The American Parkinson Disease Association, 116 John Street, New York, NY 10038; toll-free number: (800) 223-ADPA or (212) 732-9550.

### Speech Problems and Swallowing Problems in Parkinson's Disease (1985)

Specific exercises are described in detail on such topics as how to improve eating skills, control saliva build-up, increase voice loudness, and improve clarity of articulation. Nonverbal communication methods are also described. Particularly suitable for the self-motivated patient.

The American Parkinson Disease Association, 116 John Street, New York, NY 10038; toll-free number: (800) 223-ADPA or (212) 732-9550.

### Home Exercises for Patients with Parkinson's Disease

This pamphlet provides a well-illustrated program for strengthening muscles and improving postural stability. It gives specific steps in such motions as getting in and out of a chair and improving gait.

The American Parkinson Disease Association, 116 John Street, New York, NY 10038; toll-free number: (800) 223-ADPA or (212) 732-9550.

### The Parkinson Handbook

A handbook for the patient, including information on the disease and its treatment, exercises, psychological factors, speech impairment, and other functional activities.

National Parkinson Foundation, 1501 N.W. 9th Avenue, Miami, FL 33136.

### The Parkinson Patient—What You and Your Family Should Know

A pamphlet with hints for solving common problems and some exercises.

National Parkinson Foundation, 1501 N.W. 9th Avenue, Miami FL 33136.

### One Step at a Time

An exercise manual, including suggestions for daily living.

United Parkinson Foundation, 220 South State Street, Chicago, IL 60604.

### The Parkinson Patient at Home

A pamphlet for the patient who is not responding well to levodopa therapy. Suggestions for patients with more severe symptoms.

Parkinson's Disease Foundation, William Black Medical Research Building, Columbia University Medical Center, 650 W. 168th Street, New York, NY 10032.

### Exercises for the Parkinson Patient with Hints for Daily Living

Illustrated exercise manual, with suggestions for solving daily problems.

Parkinson's Disease Foundation, William Black Medical Research Building, Columbia University Medical Center, 650 W. 168th Street, New York, NY 10032.

### Parkinson's Disease: Hope through Research (NIH Publ. No. 83-139)

A pamphlet on recommended therapies and direction of current research.

National Institutes of Health, 9000 Rockville Pike, Bethesda, MD 20205.

# *Index*

Note: Numbers in *italics* refer to figures; numbers followed by t refer to tables.